AMA
AMERICAN MEDICAL ASSOCIATION

2019

HCPCS Level II
Professional 2019

2019 HCPCS LEVEL II, PROFESSIONAL EDITION ISBN: 978-1-62202-779-8

Notices

Knowledge and best practice in this field are constantly changing. As new research and experience broaden our understanding, changes in research methods, professional practices, or medical treatment may become necessary.

Practitioners and researchers must always rely on their own experience and knowledge in evaluating and using any information, methods, compounds, or experiments described herein. In using such information or methods they should be mindful of their own safety and the safety of others, including parties for whom they have a professional responsibility.

With respect to any drug or pharmaceutical products identified, readers are advised to check the most current information provided (i) on procedures featured or (ii) by the manufacturer of each product to be administered, to verify the recommended dose or formula, the method and duration of administration, and contraindications. It is the responsibility of practitioners, relying on their own experience and knowledge of their patients, to make diagnoses, to determine dosages and the best treatment for each individual patient, and to take all appropriate safety precautions.

To the fullest extent of the law, neither the Publisher nor the authors, contributors, or editors, assume any liability for any injury and/or damage to persons or property as a matter of products liability, negligence or otherwise, or from any use or operation of any methods, products, instructions, or ideas contained in the material herein.

International Standard Book Number: 978-1-62202-779-8

Our Commitment to Accuracy
The AMA is committed to producing accurate and reliable materials. To report corrections, please call the AMA Unified Service Center at (800) 621-8335. AMA publication and product updates, errata, and addenda can be found at amaproductupdates.org.

To purchase additional copies, contact the American Medical Association at 800-621-8335 or visit the AMA store at amastore.com. Refer to item number **OP231519**.

Content Strategist: Brandi Graham
Senior Content Development Manager: Luke Held
Content Development Specialist: Anna Miller
Publishing Services Manager: Julie Eddy
Project Manager: Abigail Bradberry
Designer: Maggie Reid

Printed in Canada

Last digit is the print number: 9 8 7 6 5 4 3 2 1

DEVELOPMENT OF THIS EDITION

Lead Technical Collaborator

Jackie Grass Koesterman, CPC
Coding and Reimbursement Specialist
Grand Forks, North Dakota

Technical Collaborators

Nancy Maguire, ACS, CRT, PCS, FCS, HCS-D, APC, AFC
Physician Consultant for Auditing and Education
Palm Bay, Florida

Patricia Cordy Henricksen, MS, CHCA, CPC-I, CPC, CCP-P, ACS-PM
AAPC/AHIMA Approved ICD-10-CM Trainer
Auditing, Coding, and Education Specialist
Soterion Medical Services/Merrick Management
Lexington, Kentucky

CONTENTS

Updates will be posted on codingupdates.com when available.

Check codingupdates.com for Practitioner and Facility Medically Unlikely Edits (MUEs) and Column 1 and Column 2 Edits.

Check the Centers for Medicare and Medicaid Services (www.cms.gov/Manuals/IOM/list.asp) website and codingupdates.com for full and select IOMs.

Notice: 2019 DMEPOS updates were unavailable at the time of printing. Check codingupdates.com for updates and DMEPOS Modifiers in January.

INTRODUCTION

2019 HCPCS quarterly updates available on the companion website at: www.codingupdates.com

The Centers for Medicare and Medicaid Services (CMS) (formerly Health Care Financing Administration [HCFA]) Healthcare Common Procedure Coding System (HCPCS) is a collection of codes and descriptors that represent procedures, supplies, products, and services that may be provided to Medicare beneficiaries and to individuals enrolled in private health insurance programs. The codes are divided as follows:

Level I: Codes and descriptors copyrighted by the American Medical Association's (AMA's) Current Procedural Terminology, ed. 4 (CPT-4). These are five-position numeric codes representing physician and nonphysician services.

Level II: Includes codes and descriptors copyrighted by the American Dental Association's current dental terminology, seventh edition (CDT-7/8). These are five-position alpha-numeric codes comprising the D series. All other Level II codes and descriptors are approved and maintained jointly by the alpha-numeric editorial panel (consisting of CMS, the Health Insurance Association of America, and the Blue Cross and Blue Shield Association). These are five-position alpha-numeric codes representing primarily items and nonphysician services that are not represented in the Level I codes.

Level III: The CMS eliminated Level III local codes. See Program Memorandum AB-02-113.

Headings are provided as a means of grouping similar or closely related items. The placement of a code under a heading does not indicate additional means of classification, nor does it relate to any health insurance coverage categories.

HCPCS also contains modifiers, which are two-position codes and descriptors used to indicate that a service or procedure that has been performed has been altered by some specific circumstance but not changed in its definition or code. Modifiers are grouped by the levels. Level I modifiers and descriptors are copyrighted by the AMA. Level II modifiers are HCPCS modifiers. Modifiers in the D series are copyrighted by the ADA.

HCPCS is designed to promote uniform reporting and statistical data collection of medical procedures, supplies, products, and services.

HCPCS Disclaimer

Inclusion or exclusion of a procedure, supply, product, or service does not imply any health insurance coverage or reimbursement policy.

HCPCS makes as much use as possible of generic descriptions, but the inclusion of brand names to describe devices or drugs is intended only for indexing purposes; it is not meant to convey endorsement of any particular product or drug.

Updating HCPCS

The primary updates are made annually. Quarterly updates are also issued by CMS.

GUIDE TO USING THE 2019 HCPCS LEVEL II CODES

Medical coding has long been a part of the health care profession. Through the years medical coding systems have become more complex and extensive. Today, medical coding is an intricate and immense process that is present in every health care setting. The increased use of electronic submissions for health care services only increases the need for coders who understand the coding process.

2019 HCPCS Level II was developed to help meet the needs of today's coder.

All material adheres to the latest government versions available at the time of printing.

Annotated

Throughout this text, revisions and additions are indicated by the following symbols:

- ▶ **New:** Additions to the previous edition are indicated by the color triangle.
- ↩ **Revised:** Revisions within the line or code from the previous edition are indicated by the color arrow.
- ✔ **Reinstated** indicates a code that was previously deleted and has now been reactivated.
- ✖ ~~deleted~~ words have been removed from this year's edition.

HCPCS Symbols

- ◎ **Special coverage instructions** apply to these codes. Usually these special coverage instructions are included in the Internet Only Manuals (IOM). References to the IOM locations are given in the form of Medicare Pub. 100 reference numbers listed below the code. IOM select references are located at codingupdates.com.
- ⃠ **Not covered or valid by Medicare** is indicated by the "No" symbol. Usually the reason for the exclusion is included in the Internet Only Manuals (IOM) select references at codingupdates.com.
- * **Carrier discretion** is an indication that you must contact the individual third-party payers to find out the coverage available for codes identified by this symbol.
- *Other* Drugs approved for Medicare Part B and other FDA-approved drugs are listed as Other.
- A2-Z3 **ASC Payment Indicators** identify the 2018 final payment for the code. A list of Payment Indicators is listed in the front material of this text.
- A-Y **OPPS Status Indicators** identify the 2018 final status assigned to the code. A list of Status Indicators is listed in the front material of this text.
- Ⓑ Bill Part B MAC.
- Ⓑ Bill DME MAC.
- Coding Clinic Indicates the American Hospital Association *Coding Clinic®* for HCPCS references by year, quarter, and page number.
- ♿ DMEPOS identifies durable medical equipment, prosthetics, orthotics, and supplies that may be eligible for payment from CMS.
- ♀ Indicates a code for female only.
- ♂ Indicates a code for male only.
- A Indicates a code with an indication of age.
- MIPS Indicates a code included in the MIPS Quality Measure Specifications.
- Qp Indicates there is a maximum allowable number of units of service, per day, per patient for physician/provider services (*see* codingupdates.com for Practitioner Medically Unlikely Edits).
- Qh Indicates there is a maximum allowable number of units of service, per day, per patient in the outpatient hospital setting (*see* codingupdates.com for Hospital Medically Unlikely Edits).

Red, green, and blue typeface terms within the Table of Drugs and tabular section are terms added by the publisher and do not appear in the official code set. Information supplementing the official HCPCS Index produced by CMS is *italicized*.

SYMBOLS AND CONVENTIONS

HCPCS Symbols

Special coverage instructions apply to these codes. Usually these instructions are included in the Internet Only Manuals (IOM). References to the IOM locations are given in the form of Medicare Pub. 100 reference numbers listed below the code. IOM select references are located at codingupdates.com.

→ ◌ **L3540** Miscellaneous shoe additions, sole, full
IOM: 100-2, 15, 290

The Internet Only Manuals (IOM) give instructions regarding use of the code. IOM select references are located at codingupdates.com.

Not covered or valid by Medicare is indicated by the "No" symbol. Usually the reason for the exclusion is included in the IOM references located at codingupdates.com.

→ ⃠ **A65331** Gradient compression stocking, thigh length, 18–30 mm Hg, each
IOM: 100-02, 15, 130; 100-03, 4, 280.1

Carrier discretion is an indication that you must contact the individual third-party payers for the coverage for these codes.

→ * **A6154** Wound pouch, each

A9541 Technetium Tc-99m sulfur colloid, diagnostic, per study dose, up to 20 millicuries **N1** ← ASC Payment Indicators **A2-Z3** identify the Final OPPS payment for the code.

A0180 Non-emergency transportation: ancillary: lodging-recipient **E** ← ASC Status Indicators **A-Y** identify the Final OPPS status assigned to the code.

A4650 Implantable radiation dosimeter; each Ⓑ ← Bill Part B MAC.

A4606 Oxygen probe for use with oximeter device; replacement Ⓓ ← Bill DME MAC.

Coding Clinic indicates the American Hospital Association *Coding Clinic®* for HCPCS references by year, quarter, and page number.

→ **A4543** Imagining, e.g., gadoteridol injection
Coding Clinic: 2001, Q3, P13-14

Codes shown are for illustration purposes only and may not be current codes.

DMEPOS symbol identifies durable medical equipment, prosthetics, orthotics, and supplies that may be eligible for payment from CMS. → **E2210** Wheelchair accessory, bearings, any type, replacement only, each ♿

✻ **A4233** Replacement battery, alkaline (other than J cell), for use with medically necessary home blood glucose monitor owned by patient, each ♿ ← On DMEPOS Fee Schedule.

If "incident to" physician service, do not bill; otherwise bill DME MAC

◌ **B9000** Enteral nutrition infusion pump - without alarm Qp Y

Pump will be denied as not medically necessary if medical necessity of pump is not documented

IOM: 100-02, 15, 120; 100-03, 3, 180.2; 100-04, 20, 100.2.2

PEN: On Fee Schedule ← On the Parenteral and Enteral Nutrition Items or Services (PEN) with modifier(s) from current PEN Fee Schedule.

A4261 Cervical cap for contraceptive use ♀ ← Indicates for female only.

A4267 Contraceptive supply, condom, male, each ♂ ← Indicates for male only.

Indicates a **reinstated** code. → ✔ **D2970** Temporary crown (fractured tooth)

Indicates **new** information or a new code. → ▶ **A4614** Peak expiratory flow rate meter, hand-held

Indicates a **revision** within the line or code. → ↩ **J0270** Injection alprostadil, per 1.25 mcg

---

Codes shown are for illustration purposes only and may not be current codes.

The strike-through indicates **deleted** information.

~~J1015 Injection, adenosine, 90 mg (not to be used to report any adenosine, phosphate compounds, instead use A9270)~~ ✖

The "✖" appears in the right margin to indicate deleted information.

Drugs approved for Medicare Part B and other FDA-approved drugs are listed as **Other**. This list may not be all inclusive.

✻ **J0135** Injection, adalimumab, 20 mg
Other: Adalimumab

Italic typeface indicates publisher-added index items.

Ambulation device, E0100–E0159
AMI, documentation, *G8006–G8011*
Amikacin Sulfate, J0278

D0145 Oral evaluation for a patient under three years of age counseling with primary care giver A

Indicates code with age indication.

Indicates the code is included in the MIPS Quality Measure Specifications.

MIPS **G0101** Cervical or vaginal cancer screening pelvic and clinical breast examination

G0104 Colorectal cancer screening; flexible sigmoidoscopy Qp

Indicates there is a maximum allowable number of units of service, per day, per patient for the **physician/provider** (*see* codingupdates.com, Medically Unlikely Edits).

G0104 Colorectal cancer screening; flexible sigmoidoscopy Qh

Indicates there is a maximum allowable number of units of service, per day, per patient for the **hospital outpatient** (*see* codingupdates.com, Medically Unlikely Edits).

Codes shown are for illustration purposes only and may not be current codes.

A2-Z3 ASC Payment Indicators

Final ASC Payment Indicators for CY 2019	
Payment Indicator	**Payment Indicator Definition**
A2	Surgical procedure on ASC list in CY 2007; payment based on OPPS relative payment weight.
B5	Alternative code may be available; no payment made
D5	Deleted/discontinued code; no payment made.
F4	Corneal tissue acquisition, hepatitis B vaccine; paid at reasonable cost.
G2	Non office-based surgical procedure added in CY 2008 or later; payment based on OPPS relative payment weight.
H2	Brachytherapy source paid separately when provided integral to a surgical procedure on ASC list; payment OPPS rate.
J7	OPPS pass-through device paid separately when provided integral to a surgical procedure on ASC list; payment contractor-priced.
J8	Device-intensive procedure; paid at adjusted rate.
K2	Drugs and biologicals paid separately when provided integral to a surgical procedure on ASC list; payment based on OPPS rate.
K7	Unclassified drugs and biologicals; payment contractor-priced.
L1	Influenza vaccine; pneumococcal vaccine. Packaged item/service; no separate payment made.
L6	New Technology Intraocular Lens (NTIOL); special payment.
N1	Packaged service/item; no separate payment made.
P2	Office-based surgical procedure added to ASC list in CY 2008 or later with MPFS nonfacility PE RVUs; payment based on OPPS relative payment weight.
P3	Office-based surgical procedure added to ASC list in CY 2008 or later with MPFS nonfacility PE RVUs; payment based on MPFS nonfacility PE RVUs.
R2	Office-based surgical procedure added to ASC list in CY 2008 or later without MPFS nonfacility PE RVUs; payment based on OPPS relative payment weight.
Z2	Radiology or diagnostic service paid separately when provided integral to a surgical procedure on ASC list; payment based on OPPS relative payment weight.
Z3	Radiology or diagnostic service paid separately when provided integral to a surgical procedure on ASC list; payment based on MPFS nonfacility PE RVUs.

CMS-1678-FC, Final Changes to the ASC Payment System and CY 2019 Payment Rates, http://www.cms.gov/Medicare/Medicare-Fee-for-Service-Payment/ASCPayment/ASC-Regulations-and-Notices.

A-Y OPPS Status Indicators

Final OPPS Payment Status Indicators for CY 2019

Indicator	Item/Code/Service	OPPS Payment Status
A	Services furnished to a hospital outpatient that are paid under a fee schedule or payment system other than OPPS,* for example:	Not paid under OPPS. Paid by MACs under a fee schedule or payment system other than OPPS. Services are subject to deductible or coinsurance unless indicated otherwise.
	• Ambulance Services	
	• Separately Payable Clinical Diagnostic Laboratory Services	Not subject to deductible or coinsurance.
	• Separately Payable Non-Implantable Prosthetics and Orthotics	
	• Physical, Occupational, and Speech Therapy	
	• Diagnostic Mammography	
	• Screening Mammography	Not subject to deductible or coinsurance.
B	Codes that are not recognized by OPPS when submitted on an outpatient hospital Part B bill type (12x and 13x)	Not paid under OPPS. • May be paid by MACs when submitted on a different bill type, for example, 75x (CORF), but not paid under OPPS. • An alternate code that is recognized by OPPS when submitted on an outpatient hospital Part B bill type (12x and 13x) may be available.
C	Inpatient Procedures	Not paid under OPPS. Admit patient. Bill as inpatient.
D	Discontinued Codes	Not paid under OPPS or any other Medicare payment system.
E1	Items, Codes and Services: • Not covered by any Medicare outpatient benefit category • Statutorily excluded by Medicare • Not reasonable and necessary	Not paid by Medicare when submitted on outpatient claims (any outpatient bill type).
E2	Items, Codes and Services: for which pricing information and claims data are not available	Not paid by Medicare when submitted on outpatient claims (any outpatient bill type).
F	Corneal Tissue Acquisition; Certain CRNA Services and Hepatitis B Vaccines	Not paid under OPPS. Paid at reasonable cost.
G	Pass-Through Drugs and Biologicals	Paid under OPPS; separate APC payment.
H	Pass-Through Device Categories	Separate cost-based pass-through payment; not subject to copayment.
J1	Hospital Part B services paid through a comprehensive APC	Paid under OPPS; all covered Part B services on the claim are packaged with the primary "J1" service for the claim, except services with OPPS status indicator of "F", "G", "H", "L" and "U"; ambulance services; diagnostic and screening mammography; all preventive services; and certain Part B inpatient services.
J2	Hospital Part B Services That May Be Paid Through a Comprehensive APC	Paid under OPPS; Addendum B displays APC assignments when services are separately payable. (1) Comprehensive APC payment based on OPPS comprehensive-specific payment criteria. Payment for all covered Part B services on the claim is packaged into a single payment for specific combinations of services, except services with OPPS status indicator of "F", "G", "H", "L" and "U"; ambulance services; diagnostic and screening mammography; all preventive services; and certain Part B inpatient services. (2) Packaged APC payment if billed on the same claim as a HCPCS code assigned status indicator "J1." (3) In other circumstances, payment is made through a separate APC payment or packaged into payment for other services.

A-Y OPPS Status Indicators—cont'd

Final OPPS Payment Status Indicators for CY 2019		
Indicator	**Item/Code/Service**	**OPPS Payment Status**
K	Nonpass-Through Drugs and Nonimplantable Biologicals, including Therapeutic Radiopharmaceuticals	Paid under OPPS: separate APC payment.
L	Influenza Vaccine; Pneumococcal Pneumonia Vaccine	Not paid under OPPS. Paid at reasonable cost; not subject to deductible or coinsurance.
M	Items and Services Not Billable to the MAC	Not paid under OPPS.
N	Items and Services Packaged into APC Rates	Paid under OPPS; payment is packaged into payment for other services. Therefore, there is no separate APC payment.
P	Partial Hospitalization	Paid under OPPS; per diem APC pay ment.
Q1	STV-Packaged Codes	Paid under OPPS; Addendum B displays APC assignments when services are separately payable. (1) Packaged APC payment if billed on the same claim as a HCPCS code assigned status indicator "S," "T," or "V." (2) Composite APC payment if billed with specific combinations of services based on OPPS composite-specific payment criteria. Payment is packaged into a single payment for specific combinations of services. (3) In other circumstances, payment is made through a separate APC payment.
Q2	T-Packaged Codes	Paid under OPPS; Addendum B displays APC assignments when services are separately payable. (1) Packaged APC payment if billed on the same claim as a HCPCS code assigned status indicator "T." (2) In other circumstances, payment is made through a separate APC payment.
Q3	Codes That May Be Paid Through a Composite APC	Paid under OPPS; Addendum B displays APC assignments when services are separately payable. Addendum M displays composite APC assignments when codes are paid through a composite APC. (1) Composite APC payment based on OPPS composite-specific payment criteria. Payment is packaged into a single payment for specific combinations of service. (2) In other circumstances, payment is made through a separate APC payment or packaged into payment for other services.
Q4	Conditionally packaged laboratory tests	Paid under OPPS or CLFS. (1) Packaged APC payment if billed on the same claim as a HCPCS code assigned published status indicator "J1," "J2," "S," "T," "V," "Q1," "Q2," or "Q3." (2) In other circumstances, laboratory tests should have an SI=A and payment is made under the CLFS.
R	Blood and Blood Products	Paid under OPPS; separate APC payment.
S	Procedure or Service, Not Discounted when Multiple	Paid under OPPS; separate APC payment.
T	Procedure or Service, Multiple Procedure Reduction Applies	Paid under OPPS; separate APC payment.
U	Brachytherapy Sources	Paid under OPPS; separate APC payment.
V	Clinic or Emergency Department Visit	Paid under OPPS; separate APC payment.
Y	Non-Implantable Durable Medical Equipment	Not paid under OPPS. All institutional providers other than home health agencies bill to a DME MAC.

*** Note — Payments "under a fee schedule or payment system other than OPPS" may be contractor priced.**

CMS-1678-FC, Final Changes to the ASC Payment System and CY 2019 Payment Rates, http://www.cms.gov/Medicare/Medicare-Fee-for-Service-Payment/HospitalOutpatientPPS/Hospital-Outpatient-Regulations-and-Notices.html.

2019 HCPCS UPDATES

2019 HCPCS New/Revised/Deleted Codes and Modifiers

HCPCS quarterly updates are posted on the companion website (www.codingupdates.com) when available.

NEW CODES/MODIFIERS

CO	G0071	G9984	M1000	M1038	Q4186
CQ	G0076	G9985	M1001	M1039	Q4187
ER	G0077	G9986	M1002	M1040	Q4188
G0	G0078	G9987	M1003	M1041	Q4189
QA	G0079	J0185	M1004	M1042	Q4190
QB	G0080	J0517	M1005	M1043	Q4191
QQ	G0081	J0567	M1006	M1044	Q4192
QR	G0082	J0584	M1007	M1045	Q4193
VM	G0083	J0599	M1008	M1046	Q4194
A4563	G0084	J0841	M1009	M1047	Q4195
A5514	G0085	J1301	M1010	M1048	Q4196
A6460	G0086	J1454	M1011	M1049	Q4197
A6461	G0087	J1628	M1012	M1050	Q4198
A9513	G2000	J1746	M1013	M1051	Q4200
A9589	G2010	J2062	M1014	M1052	Q4201
B4105	G2011	J2797	M1015	M1053	Q4202
C1823	G2012	J3245	M1016	M1054	Q4203
C8937	G9873	J3304	M1017	M1055	Q4204
C9034	G9874	J3316	M1018	M1056	Q5103
C9035	G9875	J3397	M1019	M1057	Q5104
C9036	G9876	J3398	M1020	M1058	Q5105
C9037	G9877	J3591	M1021	M1059	Q5106
C9038	G9878	J7170	M1022	M1060	Q5107
C9039	G9879	J7177	M1023	M1061	Q5108
C9407	G9880	J7203	M1024	M1062	Q5109
C9408	G9881	J7318	M1025	M1063	Q5110
C9462	G9882	J7329	M1026	M1064	Q9991
C9749	G9883	J9044	M1027	M1065	Q9992
C9751	G9884	J9057	M1028	M1066	T4545
C9752	G9885	J9153	M1029	M1067	V5171
C9753	G9890	J9173	M1030	M1068	V5172
C9754	G9891	J9229	M1031	M1069	V5181
C9755	G9978	J9311	M1032	M1070	V5211
E0447	G9979	J9312	M1033	M1071	V5212
E0467	G9980	L8608	M1034	Q2042	V5213
G0068	G9981	L8698	M1035	Q4183	V5214
G0069	G9982	L8701	M1036	Q4184	V5215
G0070	G9983	L8702	M1037	Q4185	V5221

REVISED CODES/MODIFIERS

Long Description Change
QE
QF
QG
A9273
C1889
E0218
E0483
G0499
G8647
G8648
G8649
G8650
G8651
G8652
G8653
G8654
G8655
G8656
G8657
G8658
G8659
G8660
G8661
G8662
G8663
G8664
G8665
G8666
G8667
G8668
G8669
G8670
G8671
G8672
G8673
G8674
G8709
G8749
G8806
G8880
G9428
G9429
G9431
G9454
G9457
G9509
G9511
G9530
G9531
G9532
G9537
G9573
G9574
G9594
G9596
G9612
G9614
G9625
G9627
G9628
G9630
G9631
G9633
G9649
G9651
G9683
G9685
G9727
G9729
G9731
G9733
G9735
G9737
G9739
G9755
G9764
G9765
G9772
G9773
G9803
G9804
J0834
J7178
J8655
J9041
K0037
Q2041
Q4133
Q4137
Q5101
V5190
V5200
V5230
V5240

Coverage Change
A5512

Coverage and Long Description Change
A5513

DELETED CODES/MODIFIERS

ZA
ZB
ZC
C8904
C8907
C9014
C9015
C9016
C9024
C9028
C9029
C9030
C9031
C9032
C9033
C9275
C9463
C9464
C9465
C9466
C9467
C9468
C9469
C9492
C9493
C9497
C9741
C9744
C9748
C9750
G9534
G9535
G9536
G9538
G9686
J0833
J9310
K0903
Q2040
Q4131
Q4172
Q5102
Q9993
Q9994
Q9995
V5170
V5180
V5210
V5220

NEW, REVISED, AND DELETED DENTAL CODES

New
D0412
D1516
D1517
D1526
D1527
D5282
D5283
D5876
D9130
D9613
D9944
D9945
D9946
D9961
D9990

Revised
D5211
D5212
D5630
D9219

Deleted
D1515
D1525
D5281
D9940

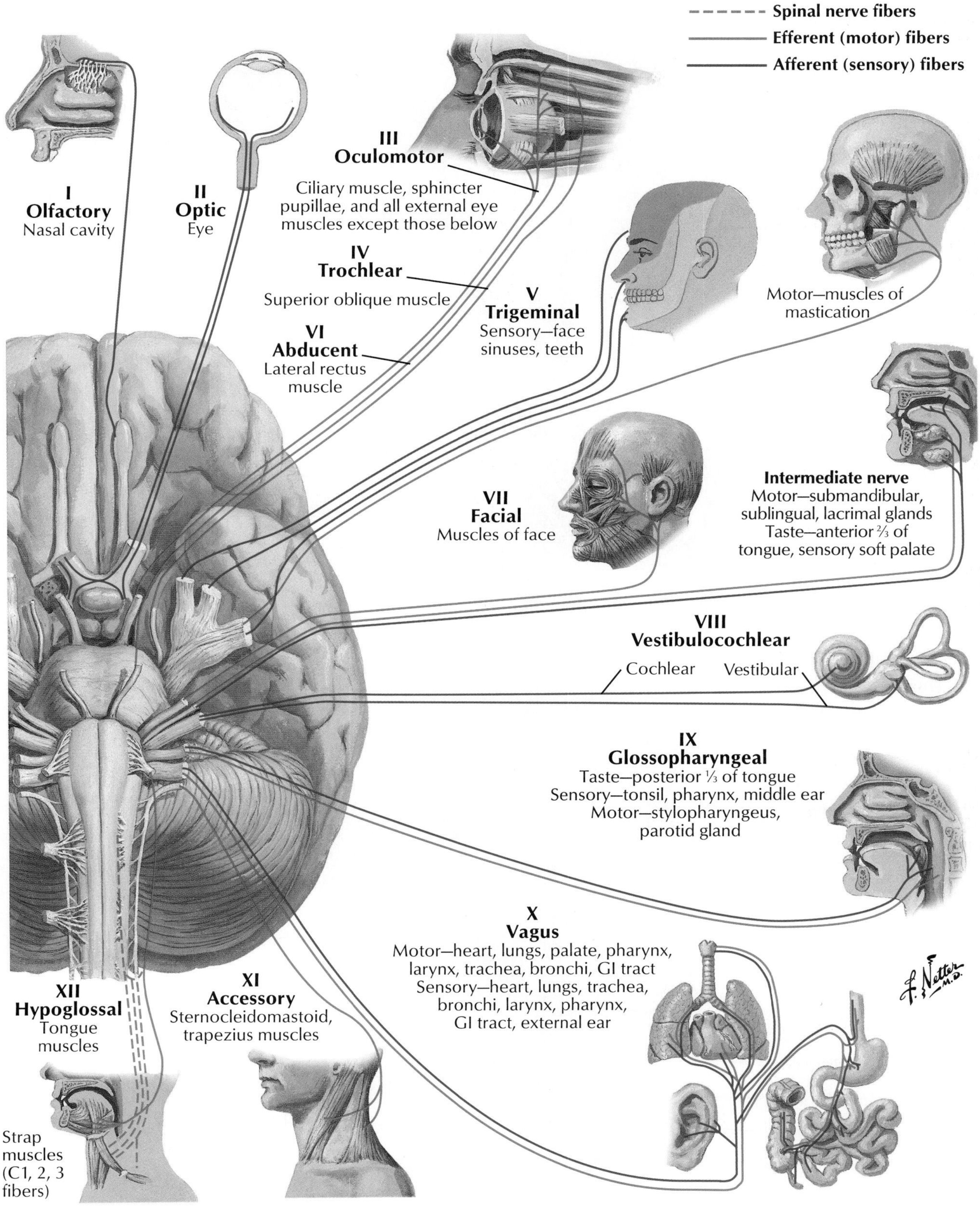

Spinal nerve fibers
Efferent (motor) fibers
Afferent (sensory) fibers
I
Olfactory
Nasal cavity
II
Optic
Eye
III
Oculomotor
Ciliary muscle, sphincter pupillae, and all external eye muscles except those below
IV
Trochlear
Superior oblique muscle
VI
Abducent
Lateral rectus muscle
V
Trigeminal
Sensory—face sinuses, teeth
Motor—muscles of mastication
VII
Facial
Muscles of face
Intermediate nerve
Motor—submandibular, sublingual, lacrimal glands
Taste—anterior ⅔ of tongue, sensory soft palate
VIII
Vestibulocochlear
Cochlear
Vestibular
IX
Glossopharyngeal
Taste—posterior ⅓ of tongue
Sensory—tonsil, pharynx, middle ear
Motor—stylopharyngeus, parotid gland
X
Vagus
Motor—heart, lungs, palate, pharynx, larynx, trachea, bronchi, GI tract
Sensory—heart, lungs, trachea, bronchi, larynx, pharynx, GI tract, external ear
XI
Accessory
Sternocleidomastoid, trapezius muscles
XII
Hypoglossal
Tongue muscles
Strap muscles (C1, 2, 3 fibers)
F. Netter M.D.

Plate 118 Cranial Nerves (Motor and Sensory Distribution): Schema. (Netter: Atlas of Human Anatomy, 4 ed, 2006, Saunders.)

NETTER'S ANATOMY ILLUSTRATIONS

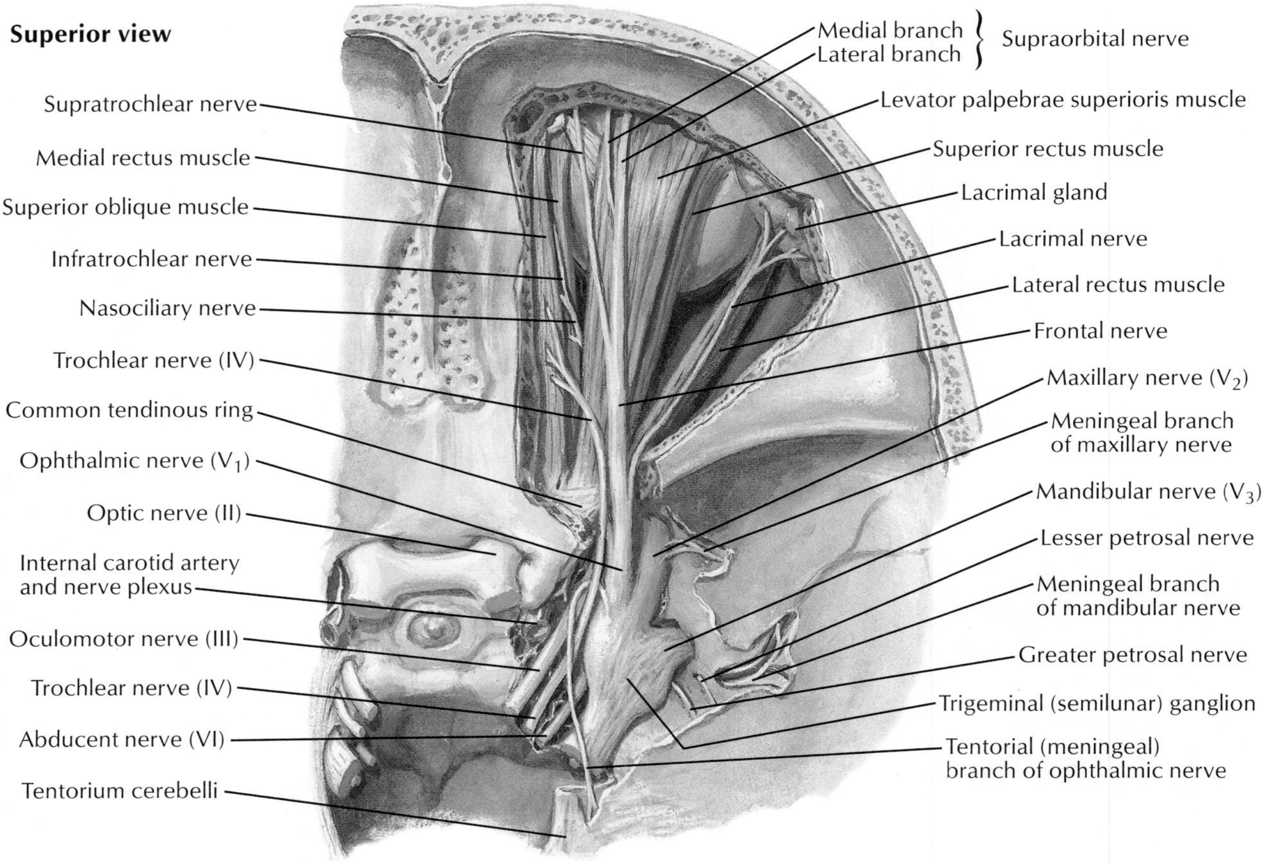
Superior view
Medial branch
Lateral branch
Supraorbital nerve
Supratrochlear nerve
Medial rectus muscle
Superior oblique muscle
Infratrochlear nerve
Nasociliary nerve
Trochlear nerve (IV)
Common tendinous ring
Ophthalmic nerve (V_1)
Optic nerve (II)
Internal carotid artery and nerve plexus
Oculomotor nerve (III)
Trochlear nerve (IV)
Abducent nerve (VI)
Tentorium cerebelli
Levator palpebrae superioris muscle
Superior rectus muscle
Lacrimal gland
Lacrimal nerve
Lateral rectus muscle
Frontal nerve
Maxillary nerve (V_2)
Meningeal branch of maxillary nerve
Mandibular nerve (V_3)
Lesser petrosal nerve
Meningeal branch of mandibular nerve
Greater petrosal nerve
Trigeminal (semilunar) ganglion
Tentorial (meningeal) branch of ophthalmic nerve

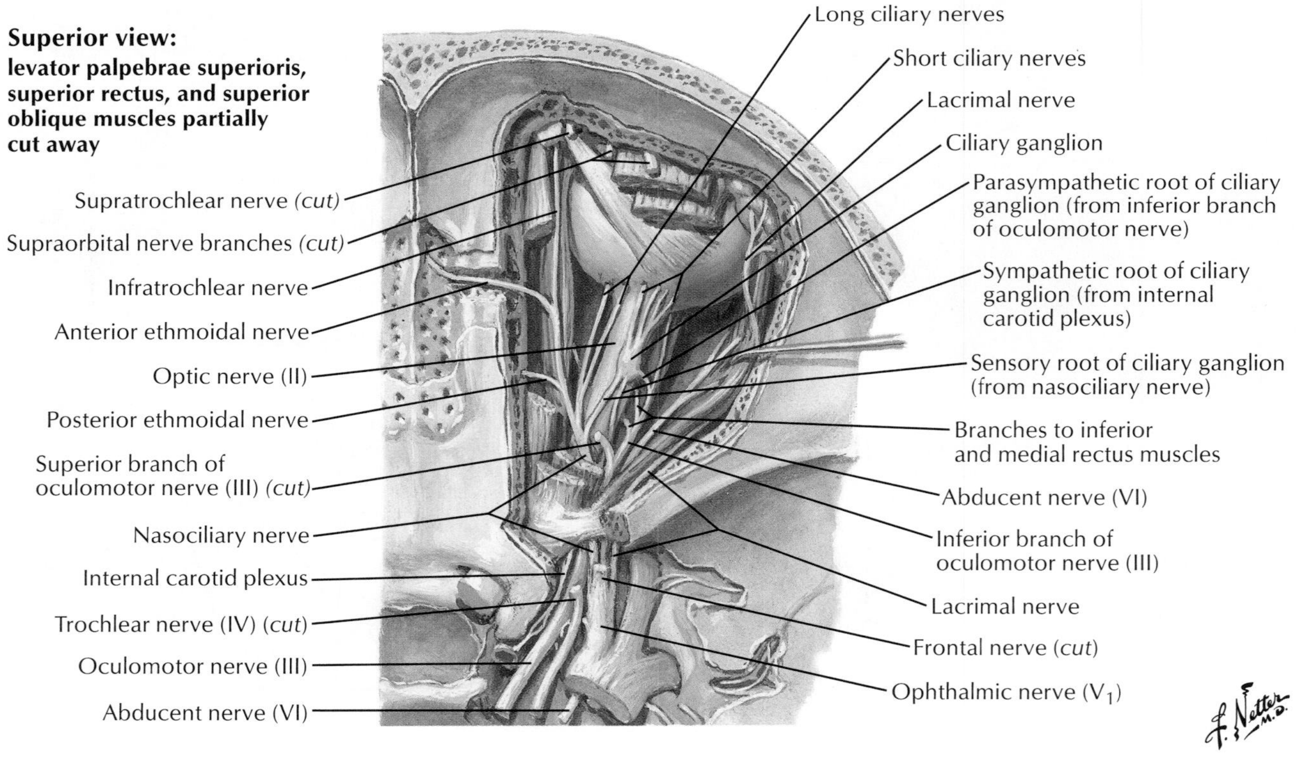
Superior view:
levator palpebrae superioris, superior rectus, and superior oblique muscles partially cut away
Supratrochlear nerve (cut)
Supraorbital nerve branches (cut)
Infratrochlear nerve
Anterior ethmoidal nerve
Optic nerve (II)
Posterior ethmoidal nerve
Superior branch of oculomotor nerve (III) (cut)
Nasociliary nerve
Internal carotid plexus
Trochlear nerve (IV) (cut)
Oculomotor nerve (III)
Abducent nerve (VI)
Long ciliary nerves
Short ciliary nerves
Lacrimal nerve
Ciliary ganglion
Parasympathetic root of ciliary ganglion (from inferior branch of oculomotor nerve)
Sympathetic root of ciliary ganglion (from internal carotid plexus)
Sensory root of ciliary ganglion (from nasociliary nerve)
Branches to inferior and medial rectus muscles
Abducent nerve (VI)
Inferior branch of oculomotor nerve (III)
Lacrimal nerve
Frontal nerve (cut)
Ophthalmic nerve (V_1)
F. Netter M.D.

Plate 86 Nerves of Orbit. (Netter: Atlas of Human Anatomy, 4 ed, 2006, Saunders.)

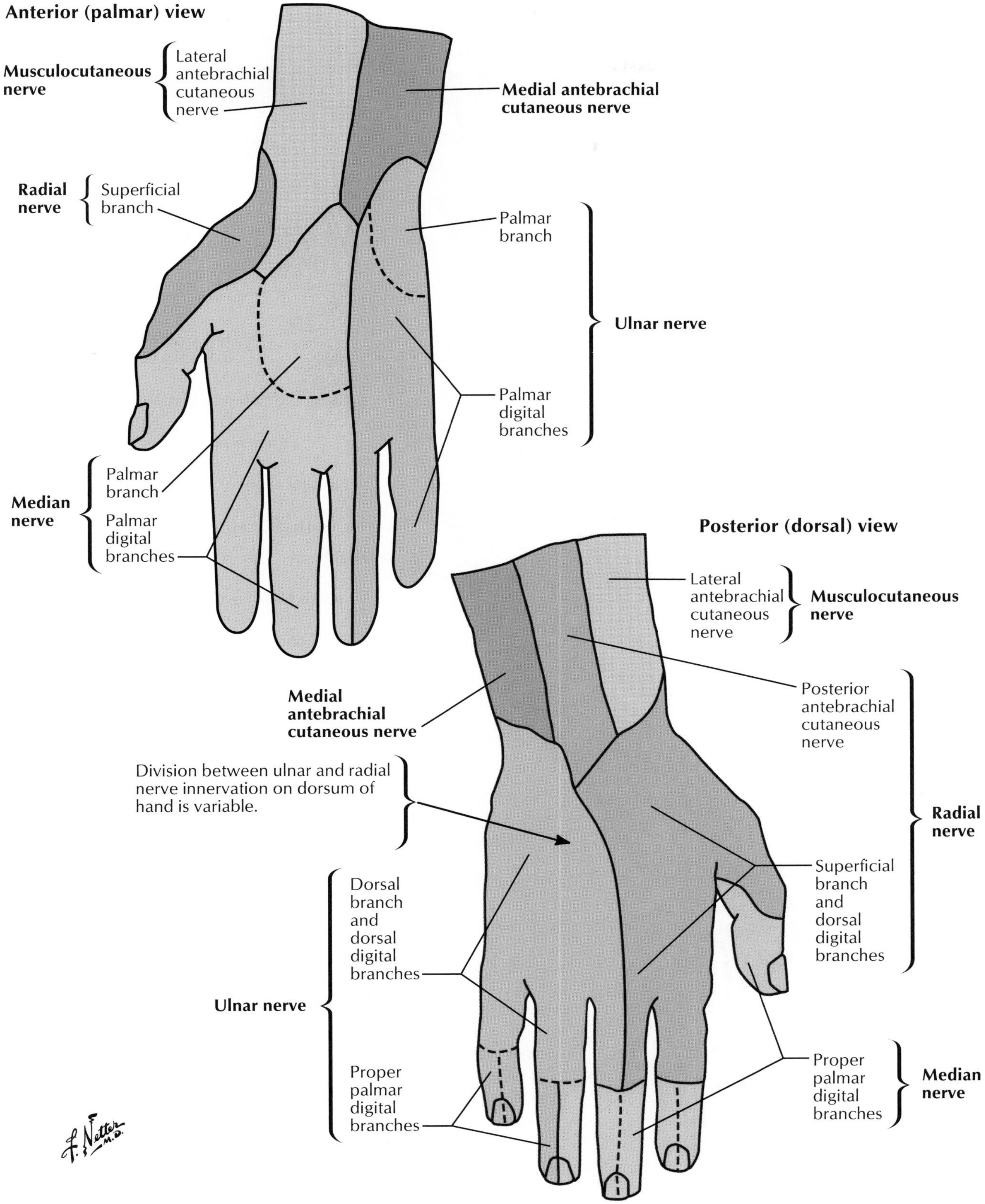

Anterior (palmar) view
Musculocutaneous nerve
Lateral antebrachial cutaneous nerve
Medial antebrachial cutaneous nerve
Radial nerve
Superficial branch
Palmar branch
Ulnar nerve
Palmar digital branches
Median nerve
Palmar branch
Palmar digital branches
Posterior (dorsal) view
Lateral antebrachial cutaneous nerve
Musculocutaneous nerve
Medial antebrachial cutaneous nerve
Posterior antebrachial cutaneous nerve
Division between ulnar and radial nerve innervation on dorsum of hand is variable.
Radial nerve
Superficial branch and dorsal digital branches
Dorsal branch and dorsal digital branches
Ulnar nerve
Proper palmar digital branches
Proper palmar digital branches
Median nerve
F. Netter M.D.

Plate 472 Cutaneous Innervation of Wrist and Hand. (Netter: Atlas of Human Anatomy, 4 ed, 2006, Saunders.)

Anterior view

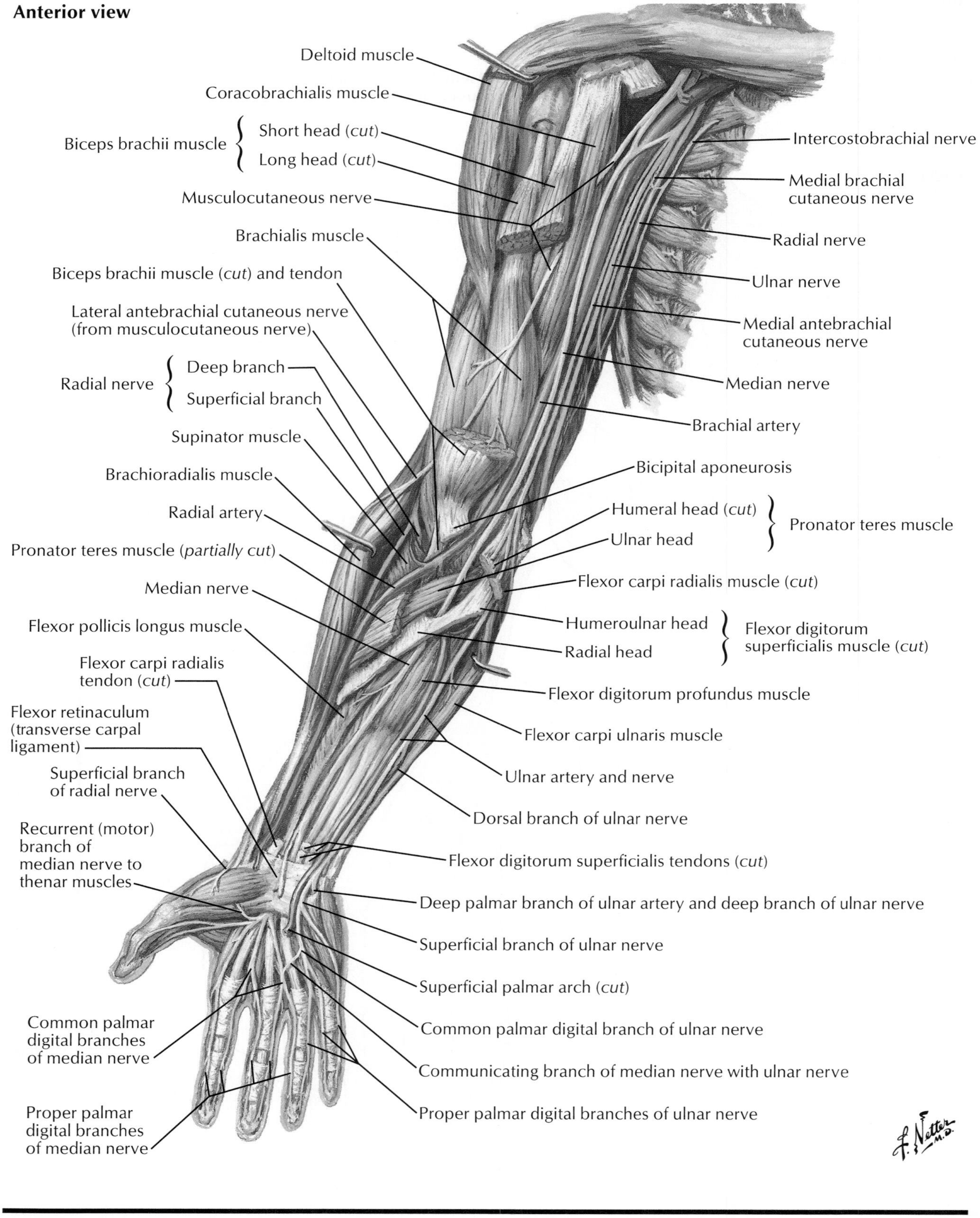

Deltoid muscle
Coracobrachialis muscle
Biceps brachii muscle
Short head (*cut*)
Long head (*cut*)
Musculocutaneous nerve
Brachialis muscle
Biceps brachii muscle (*cut*) and tendon
Lateral antebrachial cutaneous nerve (from musculocutaneous nerve)
Radial nerve
Deep branch
Superficial branch
Supinator muscle
Brachioradialis muscle
Radial artery
Pronator teres muscle (*partially cut*)
Median nerve
Flexor pollicis longus muscle
Flexor carpi radialis tendon (*cut*)
Flexor retinaculum (transverse carpal ligament)
Superficial branch of radial nerve
Recurrent (motor) branch of median nerve to thenar muscles
Common palmar digital branches of median nerve
Proper palmar digital branches of median nerve
Intercostobrachial nerve
Medial brachial cutaneous nerve
Radial nerve
Ulnar nerve
Medial antebrachial cutaneous nerve
Median nerve
Brachial artery
Bicipital aponeurosis
Humeral head (*cut*)
Ulnar head
Pronator teres muscle
Flexor carpi radialis muscle (*cut*)
Humeroulnar head
Radial head
Flexor digitorum superficialis muscle (*cut*)
Flexor digitorum profundus muscle
Flexor carpi ulnaris muscle
Ulnar artery and nerve
Dorsal branch of ulnar nerve
Flexor digitorum superficialis tendons (*cut*)
Deep palmar branch of ulnar artery and deep branch of ulnar nerve
Superficial branch of ulnar nerve
Superficial palmar arch (*cut*)
Common palmar digital branch of ulnar nerve
Communicating branch of median nerve with ulnar nerve
Proper palmar digital branches of ulnar nerve
F. Netter M.D.

Plate 473 Arteries and Nerves of Upper Limb. (Netter: Atlas of Human Anatomy, 4 ed, 2006, Saunders.)

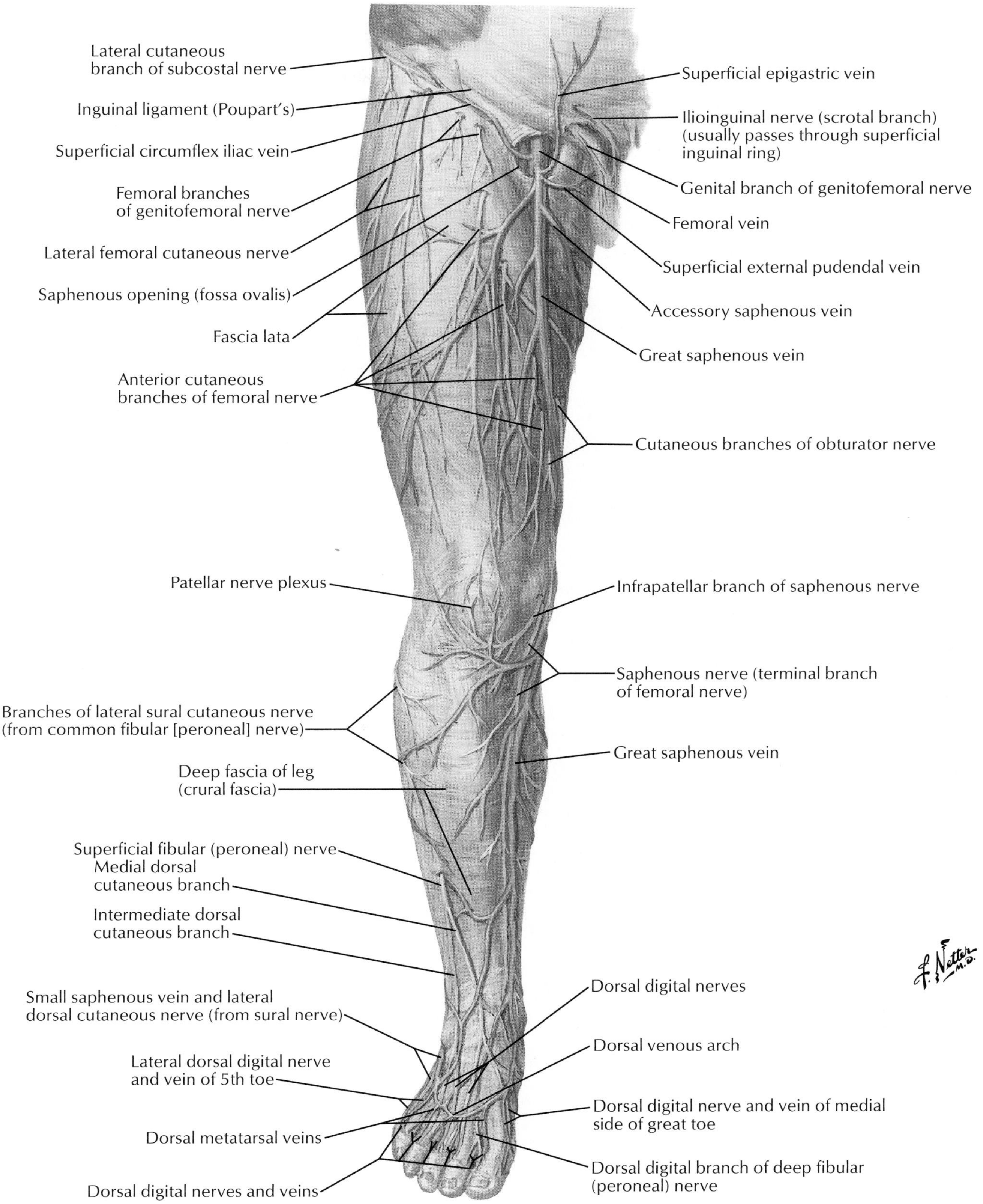
Lateral cutaneous
branch of subcostal nerve
Inguinal ligament (Poupart's)
Superficial circumflex iliac vein
Femoral branches
of genitofemoral nerve
Lateral femoral cutaneous nerve
Saphenous opening (fossa ovalis)
Fascia lata
Anterior cutaneous
branches of femoral nerve
Superficial epigastric vein
Ilioinguinal nerve (scrotal branch)
(usually passes through superficial
inguinal ring)
Genital branch of genitofemoral nerve
Femoral vein
Superficial external pudendal vein
Accessory saphenous vein
Great saphenous vein
Cutaneous branches of obturator nerve
Patellar nerve plexus
Infrapatellar branch of saphenous nerve
Saphenous nerve (terminal branch
of femoral nerve)
Branches of lateral sural cutaneous nerve
(from common fibular [peroneal] nerve)
Great saphenous vein
Deep fascia of leg
(crural fascia)
Superficial fibular (peroneal) nerve
Medial dorsal
cutaneous branch
Intermediate dorsal
cutaneous branch
Dorsal digital nerves
Small saphenous vein and lateral
dorsal cutaneous nerve (from sural nerve)
Dorsal venous arch
Lateral dorsal digital nerve
and vein of 5th toe
Dorsal digital nerve and vein of medial
side of great toe
Dorsal metatarsal veins
Dorsal digital branch of deep fibular
(peroneal) nerve
Dorsal digital nerves and veins
F. Netter M.D.

NETTER'S ANATOMY ILLUSTRATIONS

Plate 544 Superficial Nerves and Veins of Lower Limb: Anterior View. (Netter: Atlas of Human Anatomy, 4 ed, 2006, Saunders.)

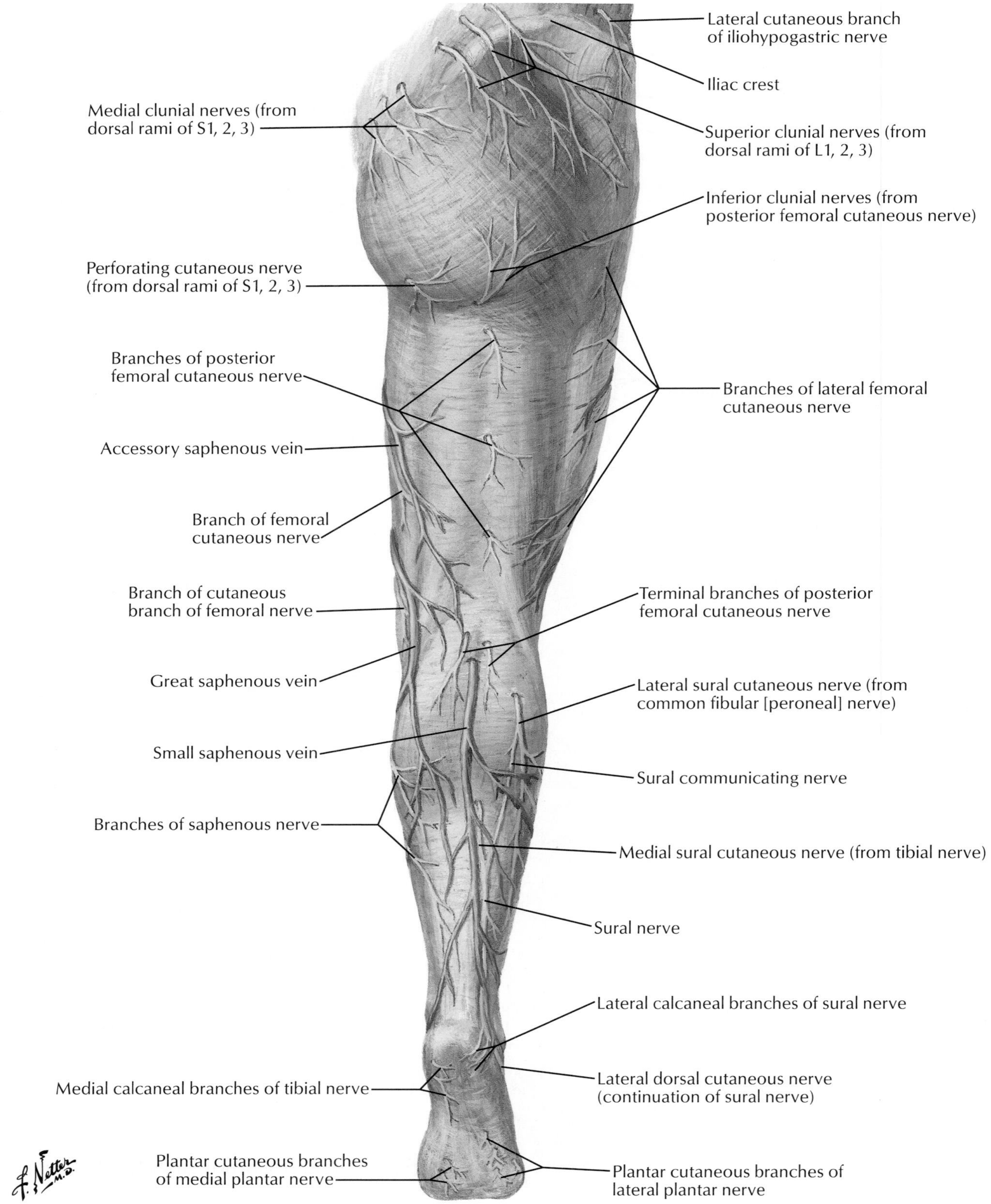

Lateral cutaneous branch of iliohypogastric nerve
Iliac crest
Medial clunial nerves (from dorsal rami of S1, 2, 3)
Superior clunial nerves (from dorsal rami of L1, 2, 3)
Inferior clunial nerves (from posterior femoral cutaneous nerve)
Perforating cutaneous nerve (from dorsal rami of S1, 2, 3)
Branches of posterior femoral cutaneous nerve
Branches of lateral femoral cutaneous nerve
Accessory saphenous vein
Branch of femoral cutaneous nerve
Branch of cutaneous branch of femoral nerve
Terminal branches of posterior femoral cutaneous nerve
Great saphenous vein
Lateral sural cutaneous nerve (from common fibular [peroneal] nerve)
Small saphenous vein
Sural communicating nerve
Branches of saphenous nerve
Medial sural cutaneous nerve (from tibial nerve)
Sural nerve
Lateral calcaneal branches of sural nerve
Medial calcaneal branches of tibial nerve
Lateral dorsal cutaneous nerve (continuation of sural nerve)
Plantar cutaneous branches of medial plantar nerve
Plantar cutaneous branches of lateral plantar nerve
F. Netter M.D.

Plate 545 Superficial Nerves and Veins of Lower Limb: Posterior View. (Netter: Atlas of Human Anatomy, 4 ed, 2006, Saunders.)

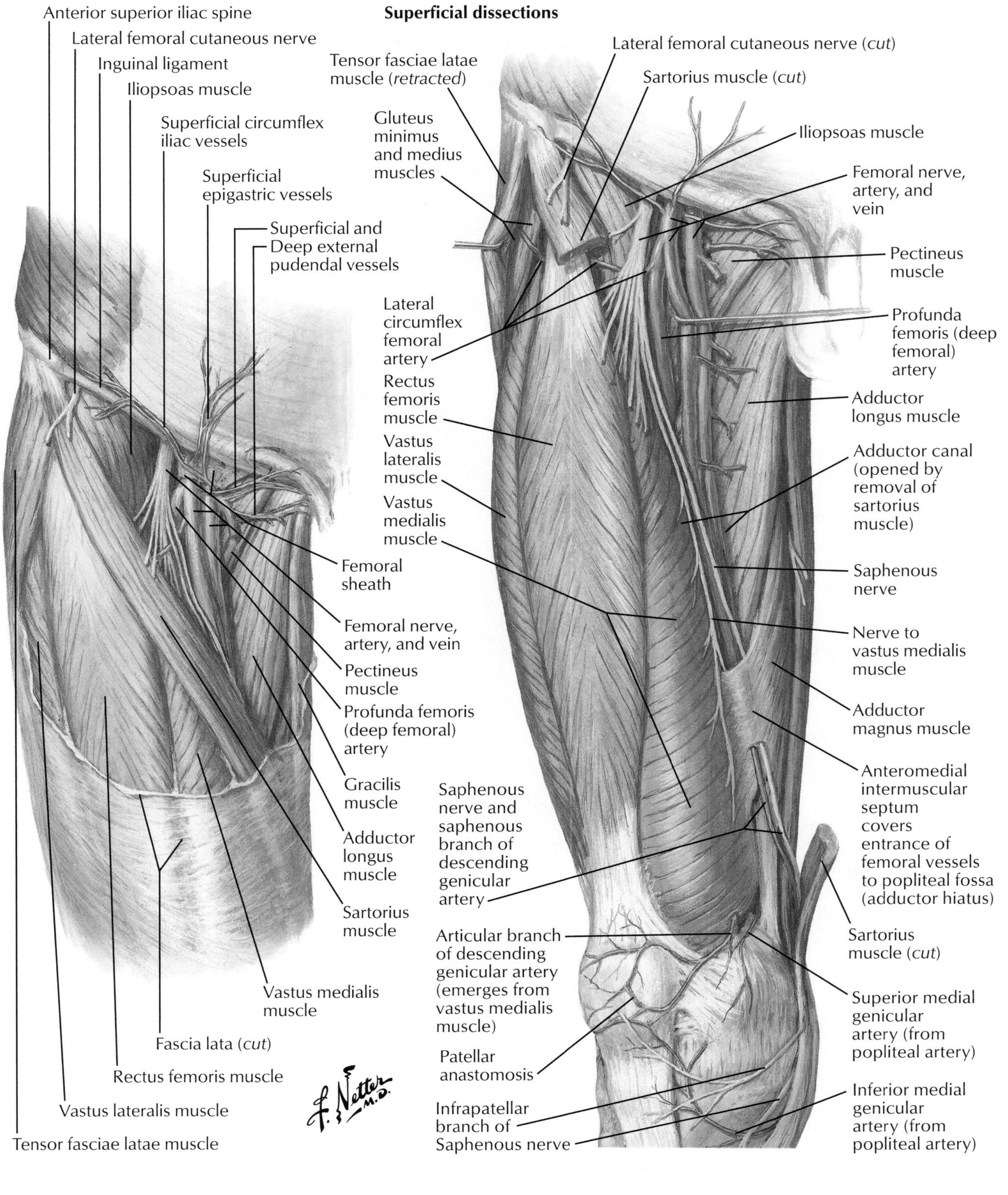
Superficial dissections
Anterior superior iliac spine
Lateral femoral cutaneous nerve
Inguinal ligament
Iliopsoas muscle
Superficial circumflex iliac vessels
Superficial epigastric vessels
Superficial and Deep external pudendal vessels
Femoral sheath
Femoral nerve, artery, and vein
Pectineus muscle
Profunda femoris (deep femoral) artery
Gracilis muscle
Adductor longus muscle
Sartorius muscle
Vastus medialis muscle
Fascia lata (cut)
Rectus femoris muscle
Vastus lateralis muscle
Tensor fasciae latae muscle
Tensor fasciae latae muscle (retracted)
Gluteus minimus and medius muscles
Lateral circumflex femoral artery
Rectus femoris muscle
Vastus lateralis muscle
Vastus medialis muscle
Saphenous nerve and saphenous branch of descending genicular artery
Articular branch of descending genicular artery (emerges from vastus medialis muscle)
Patellar anastomosis
Infrapatellar branch of Saphenous nerve
Lateral femoral cutaneous nerve (cut)
Sartorius muscle (cut)
Iliopsoas muscle
Femoral nerve, artery, and vein
Pectineus muscle
Profunda femoris (deep femoral) artery
Adductor longus muscle
Adductor canal (opened by removal of sartorius muscle)
Saphenous nerve
Nerve to vastus medialis muscle
Adductor magnus muscle
Anteromedial intermuscular septum covers entrance of femoral vessels to popliteal fossa (adductor hiatus)
Sartorius muscle (cut)
Superior medial genicular artery (from popliteal artery)
Inferior medial genicular artery (from popliteal artery)
F. Netter M.D.

Plate 500 Arteries and Nerves of Thigh: Anterior View. (Netter: Atlas of Human Anatomy, 4 ed, 2006, Saunders.)

Deep dissection

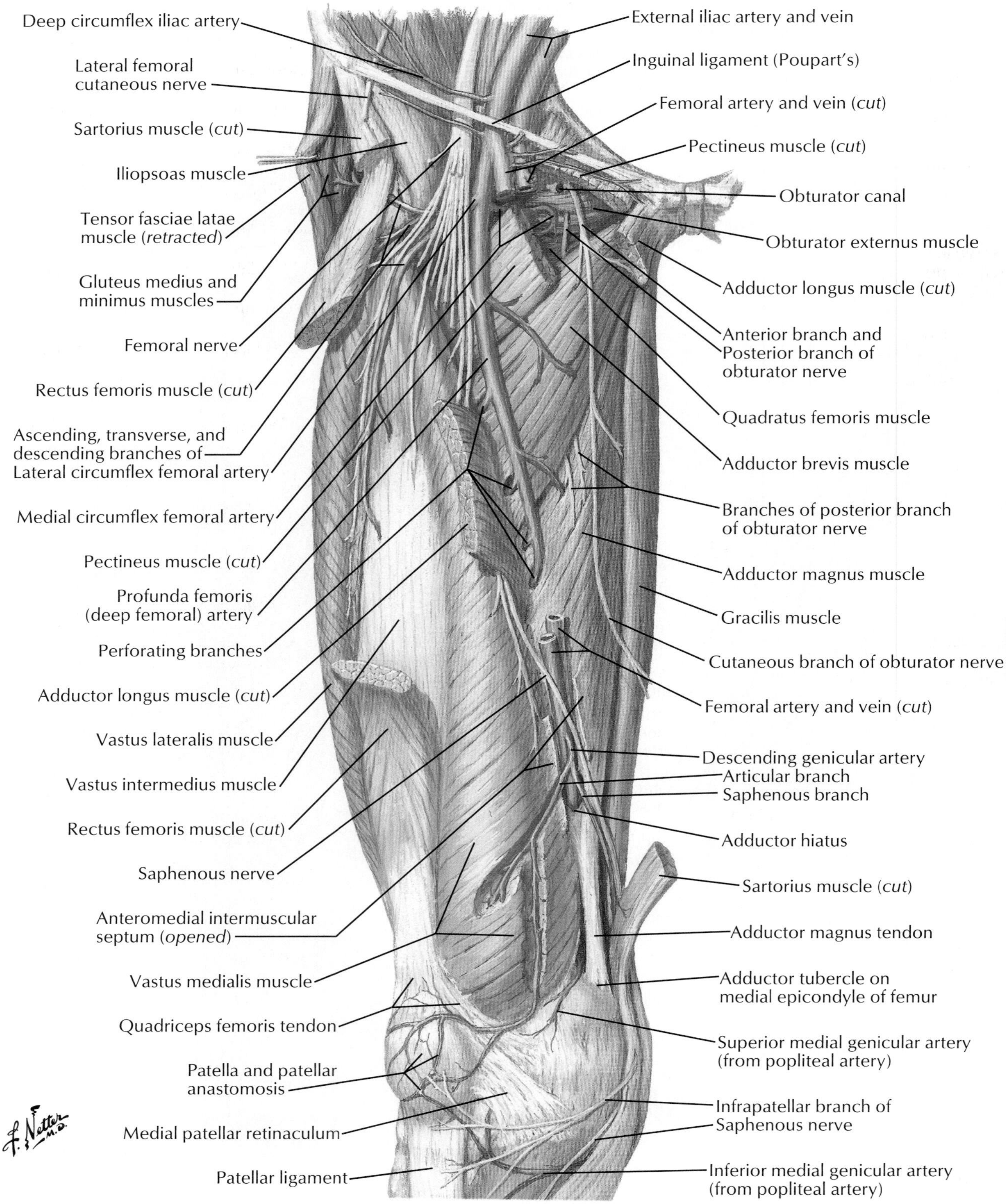
Deep circumflex iliac artery
Lateral femoral cutaneous nerve
Sartorius muscle (cut)
Iliopsoas muscle
Tensor fasciae latae muscle (retracted)
Gluteus medius and minimus muscles
Femoral nerve
Rectus femoris muscle (cut)
Ascending, transverse, and descending branches of Lateral circumflex femoral artery
Medial circumflex femoral artery
Pectineus muscle (cut)
Profunda femoris (deep femoral) artery
Perforating branches
Adductor longus muscle (cut)
Vastus lateralis muscle
Vastus intermedius muscle
Rectus femoris muscle (cut)
Saphenous nerve
Anteromedial intermuscular septum (opened)
Vastus medialis muscle
Quadriceps femoris tendon
Patella and patellar anastomosis
Medial patellar retinaculum
Patellar ligament
External iliac artery and vein
Inguinal ligament (Poupart's)
Femoral artery and vein (cut)
Pectineus muscle (cut)
Obturator canal
Obturator externus muscle
Adductor longus muscle (cut)
Anterior branch and Posterior branch of obturator nerve
Quadratus femoris muscle
Adductor brevis muscle
Branches of posterior branch of obturator nerve
Adductor magnus muscle
Gracilis muscle
Cutaneous branch of obturator nerve
Femoral artery and vein (cut)
Descending genicular artery
Articular branch
Saphenous branch
Adductor hiatus
Sartorius muscle (cut)
Adductor magnus tendon
Adductor tubercle on medial epicondyle of femur
Superior medial genicular artery (from popliteal artery)
Infrapatellar branch of Saphenous nerve
Inferior medial genicular artery (from popliteal artery)
F. Netter M.D.

Plate 501 Arteries and Nerves of Thigh: Anterior View. (Netter: Atlas of Human Anatomy, 4 ed, 2006, Saunders.)

Deep dissection

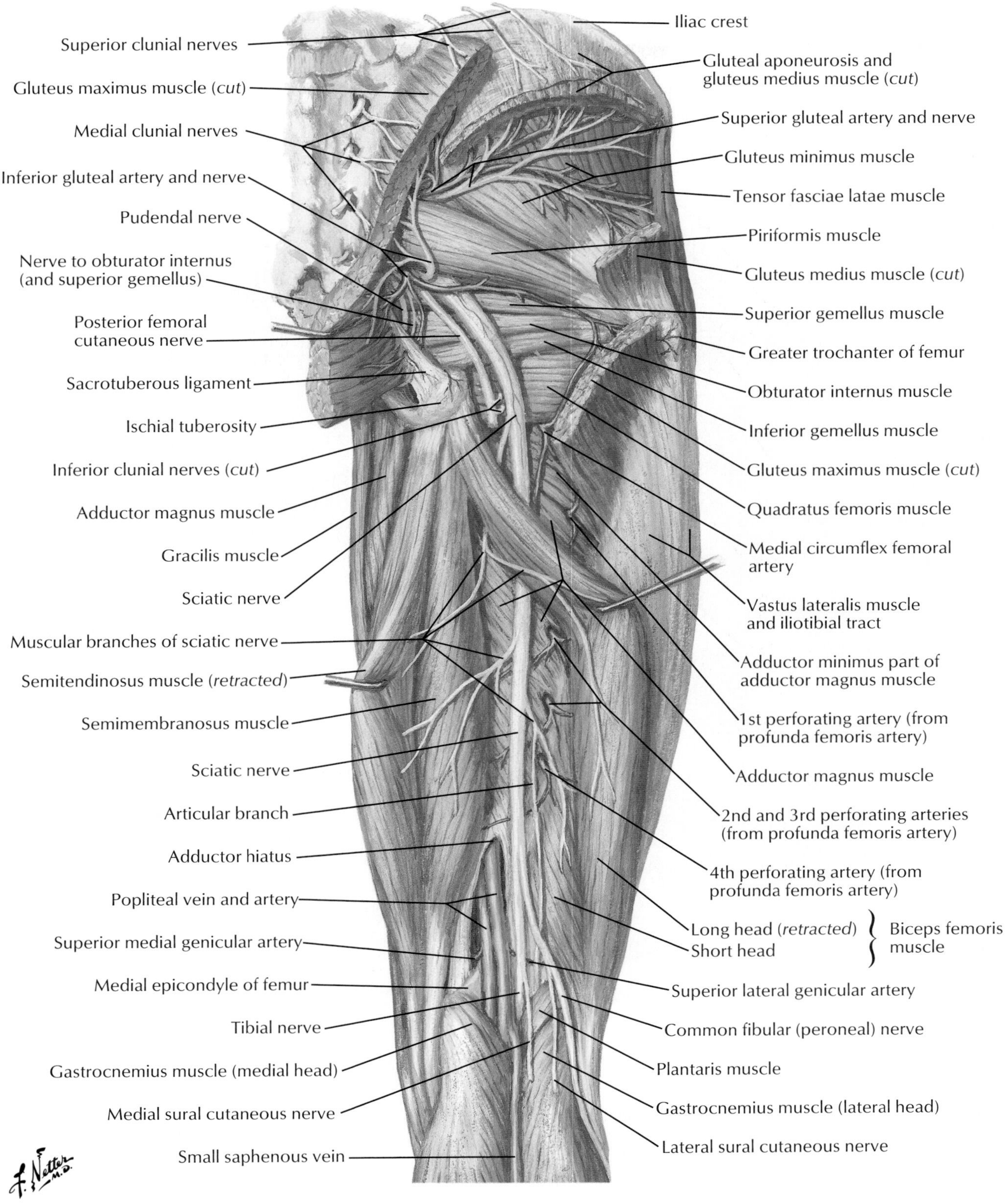

Superior clunial nerves
Gluteus maximus muscle (*cut*)
Medial clunial nerves
Inferior gluteal artery and nerve
Pudendal nerve
Nerve to obturator internus (and superior gemellus)
Posterior femoral cutaneous nerve
Sacrotuberous ligament
Ischial tuberosity
Inferior clunial nerves (*cut*)
Adductor magnus muscle
Gracilis muscle
Sciatic nerve
Muscular branches of sciatic nerve
Semitendinosus muscle (*retracted*)
Semimembranosus muscle
Sciatic nerve
Articular branch
Adductor hiatus
Popliteal vein and artery
Superior medial genicular artery
Medial epicondyle of femur
Tibial nerve
Gastrocnemius muscle (medial head)
Medial sural cutaneous nerve
Small saphenous vein
Iliac crest
Gluteal aponeurosis and gluteus medius muscle (*cut*)
Superior gluteal artery and nerve
Gluteus minimus muscle
Tensor fasciae latae muscle
Piriformis muscle
Gluteus medius muscle (*cut*)
Superior gemellus muscle
Greater trochanter of femur
Obturator internus muscle
Inferior gemellus muscle
Gluteus maximus muscle (*cut*)
Quadratus femoris muscle
Medial circumflex femoral artery
Vastus lateralis muscle and iliotibial tract
Adductor minimus part of adductor magnus muscle
1st perforating artery (from profunda femoris artery)
Adductor magnus muscle
2nd and 3rd perforating arteries (from profunda femoris artery)
4th perforating artery (from profunda femoris artery)
Long head (*retracted*)
Short head
Biceps femoris muscle
Superior lateral genicular artery
Common fibular (peroneal) nerve
Plantaris muscle
Gastrocnemius muscle (lateral head)
Lateral sural cutaneous nerve
F. Netter M.D.

Plate 502 Arteries and Nerves of Thigh: Posterior View. (Netter: Atlas of Human Anatomy, 4 ed, 2006, Saunders.)

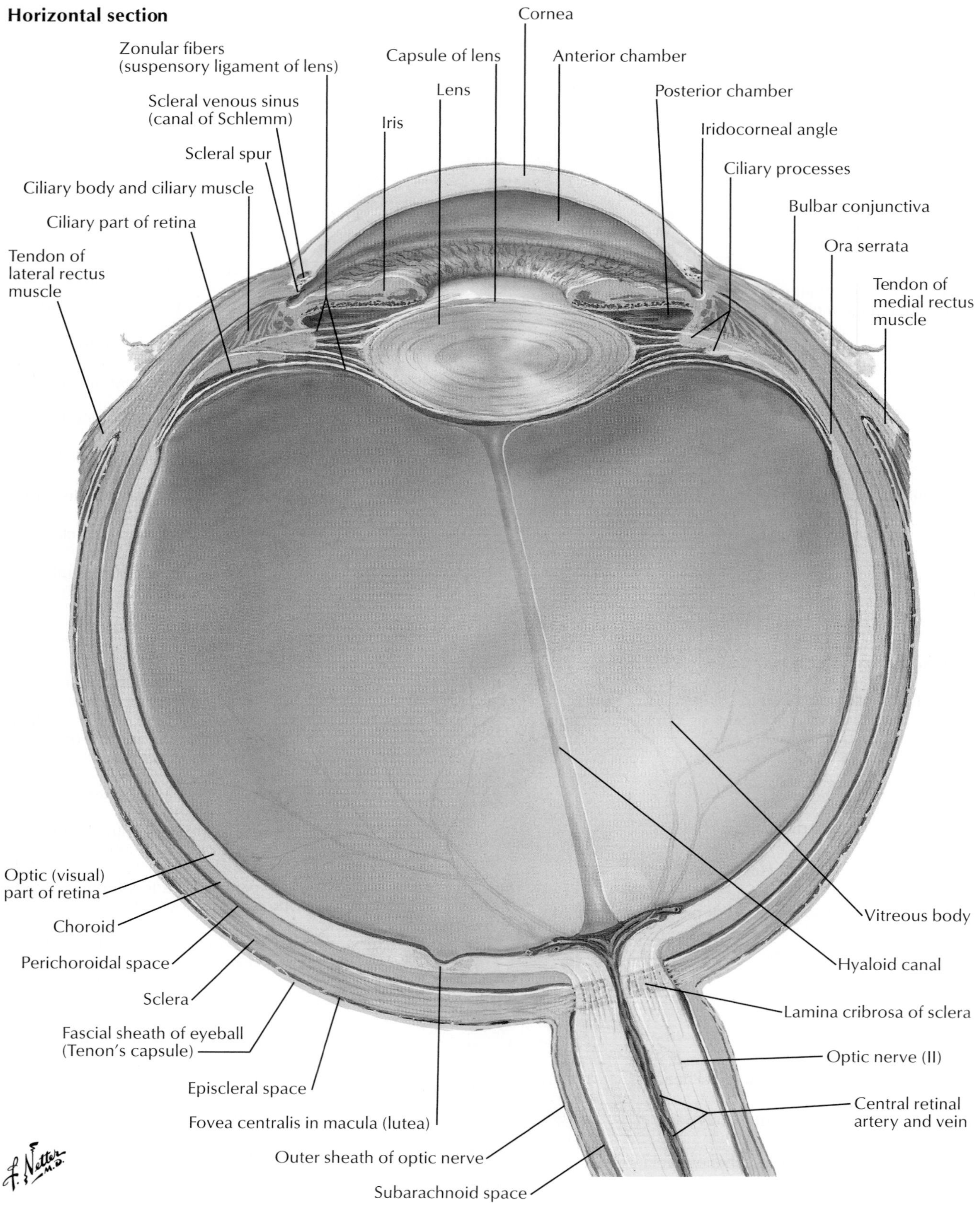
Horizontal section
Cornea
Zonular fibers
(suspensory ligament of lens)
Capsule of lens
Anterior chamber
Lens
Scleral venous sinus
(canal of Schlemm)
Posterior chamber
Iris
Iridocorneal angle
Scleral spur
Ciliary processes
Ciliary body and ciliary muscle
Bulbar conjunctiva
Ciliary part of retina
Ora serrata
Tendon of
lateral rectus
muscle
Tendon of
medial rectus
muscle
Optic (visual)
part of retina
Vitreous body
Choroid
Perichoroidal space
Hyaloid canal
Sclera
Lamina cribrosa of sclera
Fascial sheath of eyeball
(Tenon's capsule)
Optic nerve (II)
Episcleral space
Central retinal
artery and vein
Fovea centralis in macula (lutea)
Outer sheath of optic nerve
Subarachnoid space

Plate 87 Eyeball. (Netter: Atlas of Human Anatomy, 4 ed, 2006, Saunders.)

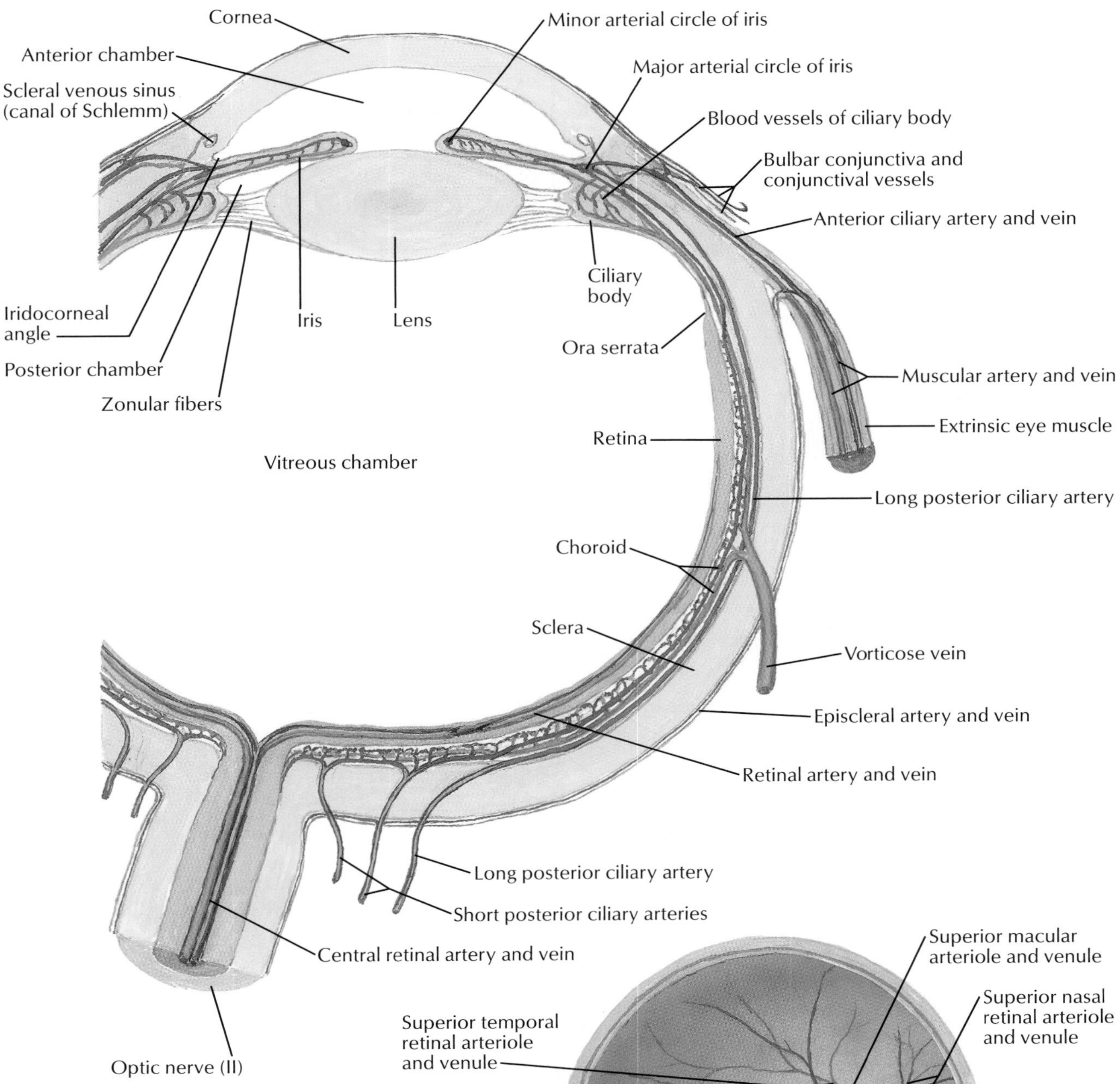
Cornea
Anterior chamber
Scleral venous sinus
(canal of Schlemm)
Minor arterial circle of iris
Major arterial circle of iris
Blood vessels of ciliary body
Bulbar conjunctiva and
conjunctival vessels
Anterior ciliary artery and vein
Ciliary
body
Iridocorneal
angle
Iris
Lens
Posterior chamber
Zonular fibers
Ora serrata
Muscular artery and vein
Extrinsic eye muscle
Retina
Vitreous chamber
Long posterior ciliary artery
Choroid
Sclera
Vorticose vein
Episcleral artery and vein
Retinal artery and vein
Long posterior ciliary artery
Short posterior ciliary arteries
Central retinal artery and vein
Optic nerve (II)

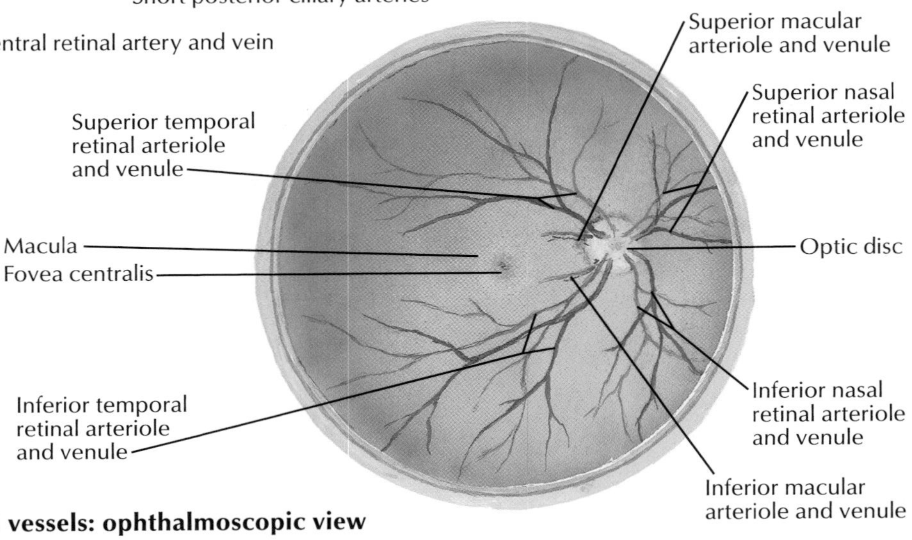
Superior macular
arteriole and venule
Superior nasal
retinal arteriole
and venule
Superior temporal
retinal arteriole
and venule
Macula
Fovea centralis
Optic disc
Inferior nasal
retinal arteriole
and venule
Inferior temporal
retinal arteriole
and venule
Inferior macular
arteriole and venule

Right retinal vessels: ophthalmoscopic view

Plate 90 Intrinsic Arteries and Veins of Eye. (Netter: Atlas of Human Anatomy, 4 ed, 2006, Saunders.)

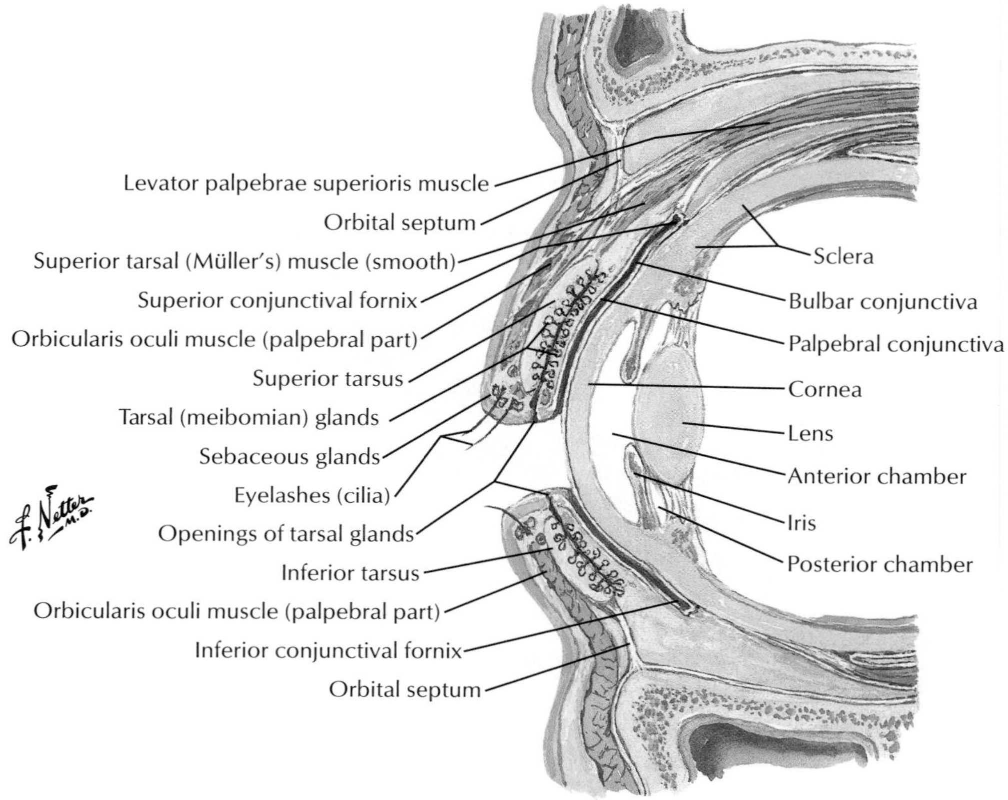

Levator palpebrae superioris muscle
Orbital septum
Superior tarsal (Müller's) muscle (smooth)
Superior conjunctival fornix
Orbicularis oculi muscle (palpebral part)
Superior tarsus
Tarsal (meibomian) glands
Sebaceous glands
Eyelashes (cilia)
Openings of tarsal glands
Inferior tarsus
Orbicularis oculi muscle (palpebral part)
Inferior conjunctival fornix
Orbital septum
Sclera
Bulbar conjunctiva
Palpebral conjunctiva
Cornea
Lens
Anterior chamber
Iris
Posterior chamber

Plate 81, Middle Eyelid. (Netter: Atlas of Human Anatomy, 4 ed, 2006, Saunders.)

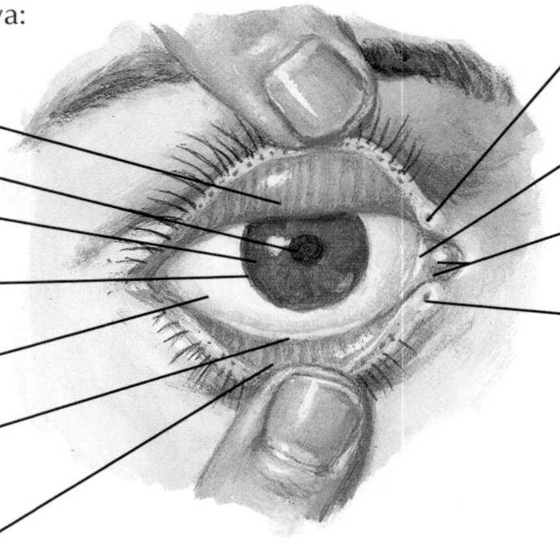

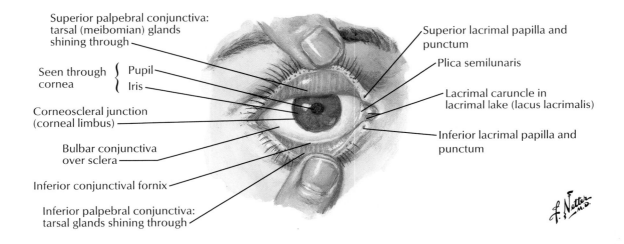

Superior palpebral conjunctiva: tarsal (meibomian) glands shining through
Seen through cornea
Pupil
Iris
Corneoscleral junction (corneal limbus)
Bulbar conjunctiva over sclera
Inferior conjunctival fornix
Inferior palpebral conjunctiva: tarsal glands shining through
Superior lacrimal papilla and punctum
Plica semilunaris
Lacrimal caruncle in lacrimal lake (lacus lacrimalis)
Inferior lacrimal papilla and punctum

Plate 81, Upper Eyelid. (Netter: Atlas of Human Anatomy, 4 ed, 2006, Saunders.)

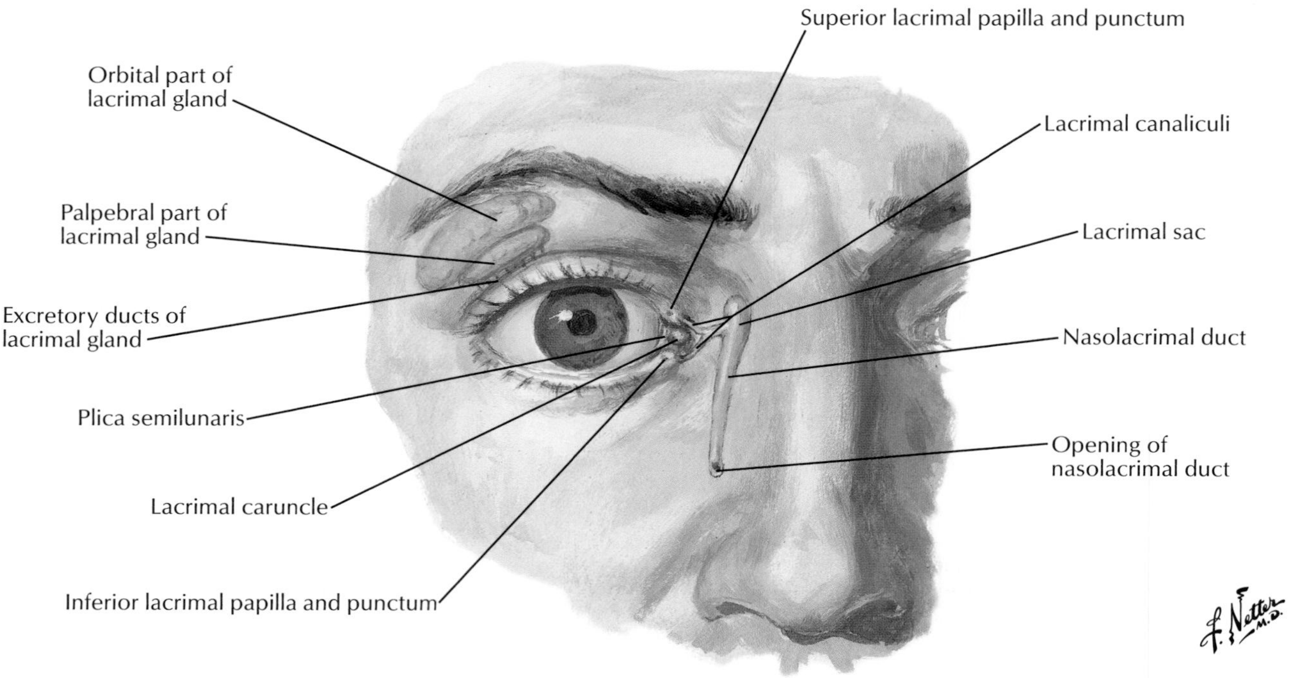
Superior lacrimal papilla and punctum
Orbital part of lacrimal gland
Lacrimal canaliculi
Palpebral part of lacrimal gland
Lacrimal sac
Excretory ducts of lacrimal gland
Nasolacrimal duct
Plica semilunaris
Opening of nasolacrimal duct
Lacrimal caruncle
Inferior lacrimal papilla and punctum

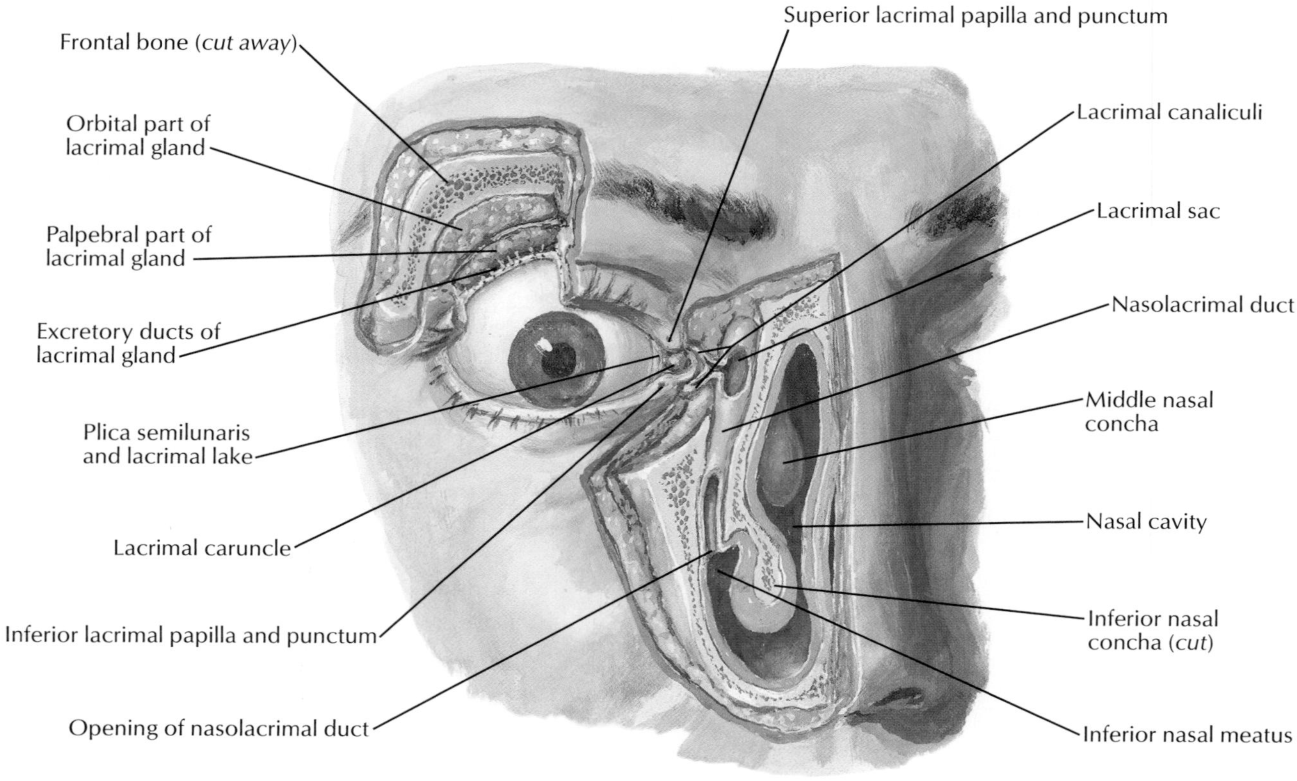
Superior lacrimal papilla and punctum
Frontal bone (*cut away*)
Lacrimal canaliculi
Orbital part of lacrimal gland
Lacrimal sac
Palpebral part of lacrimal gland
Nasolacrimal duct
Excretory ducts of lacrimal gland
Middle nasal concha
Plica semilunaris and lacrimal lake
Nasal cavity
Lacrimal caruncle
Inferior nasal concha (*cut*)
Inferior lacrimal papilla and punctum
Opening of nasolacrimal duct
Inferior nasal meatus

Plate 82 Lacrimal Apparatus. (Netter: Atlas of Human Anatomy, 4 ed, 2006, Saunders.)

Frontal section

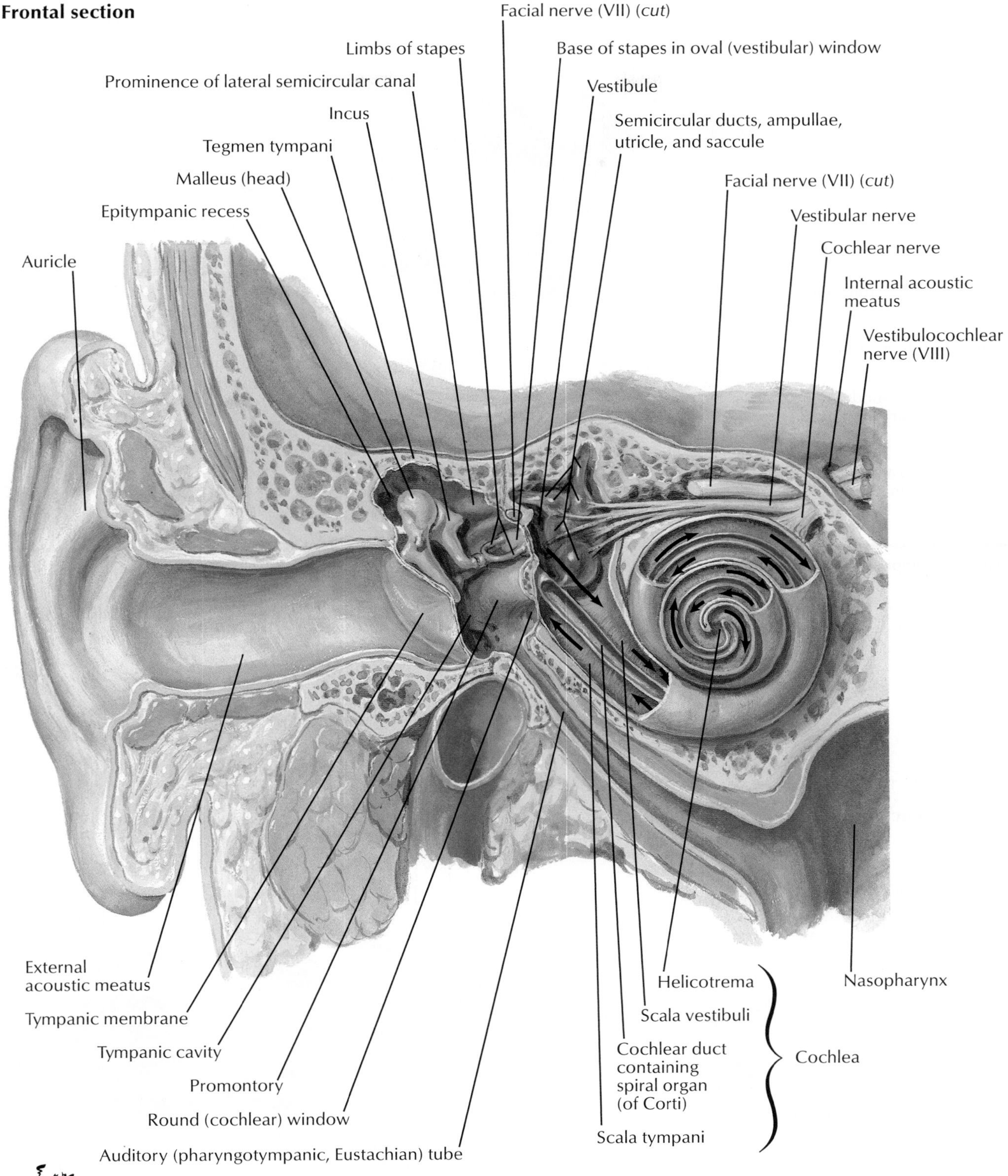
Facial nerve (VII) (*cut*)
Limbs of stapes
Base of stapes in oval (vestibular) window
Prominence of lateral semicircular canal
Vestibule
Incus
Semicircular ducts, ampullae, utricle, and saccule
Tegmen tympani
Malleus (head)
Facial nerve (VII) (*cut*)
Epitympanic recess
Vestibular nerve
Auricle
Cochlear nerve
Internal acoustic meatus
Vestibulocochlear nerve (VIII)
External acoustic meatus
Tympanic membrane
Tympanic cavity
Promontory
Round (cochlear) window
Auditory (pharyngotympanic, Eustachian) tube
Helicotrema
Scala vestibuli
Cochlear duct containing spiral organ (of Corti)
Scala tympani
Cochlea
Nasopharynx
F. Netter M.D.

Note: Arrows indicate course of sound waves.

Plate 92 Pathway of Sound Reception. (Netter: Atlas of Human Anatomy, 4 ed, 2006, Saunders.)

Medial wall of tympanic cavity: lateral view

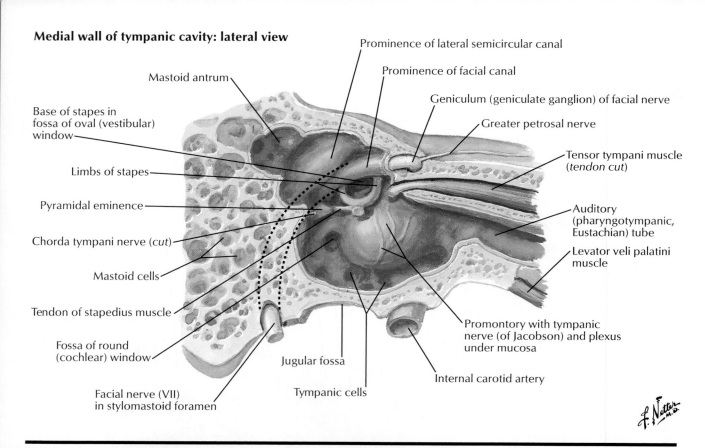

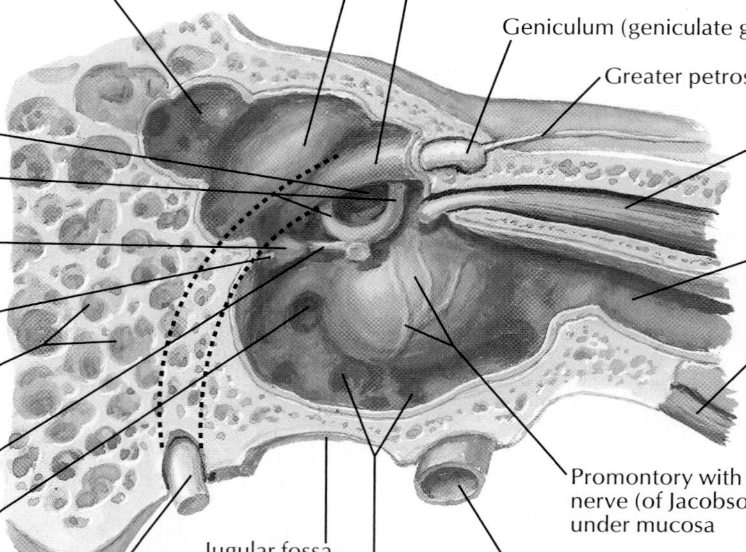
Prominence of lateral semicircular canal
Prominence of facial canal
Mastoid antrum
Geniculum (geniculate ganglion) of facial nerve
Base of stapes in fossa of oval (vestibular) window
Greater petrosal nerve
Tensor tympani muscle (*tendon cut*)
Limbs of stapes
Pyramidal eminence
Auditory (pharyngotympanic, Eustachian) tube
Chorda tympani nerve (*cut*)
Levator veli palatini muscle
Mastoid cells
Tendon of stapedius muscle
Promontory with tympanic nerve (of Jacobson) and plexus under mucosa
Fossa of round (cochlear) window
Jugular fossa
Internal carotid artery
Facial nerve (VII) in stylomastoid foramen
Tympanic cells
F. Netter M.D.

Plate 94 Tympanic Cavity. (Netter: Atlas of Human Anatomy, 4 ed, 2006, Saunders.)

Otoscopic view of right tympanic membrane

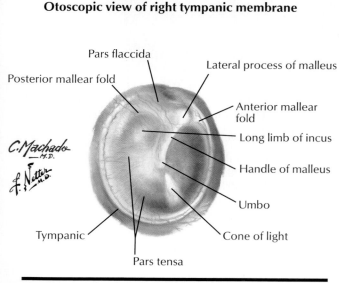

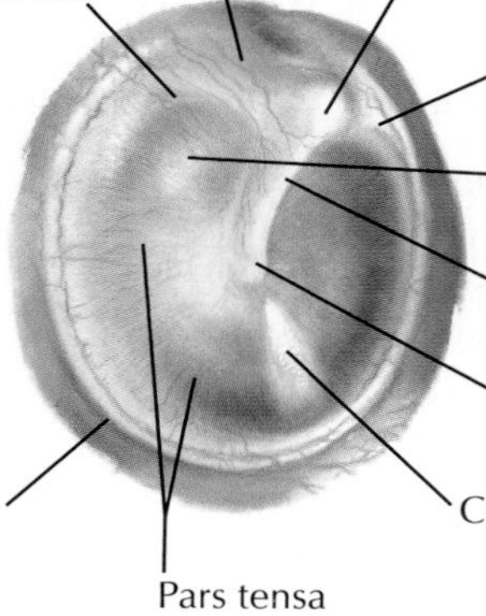
Pars flaccida
Lateral process of malleus
Posterior mallear fold
Anterior mallear fold
Long limb of incus
C. Machado M.D.
Handle of malleus
F. Netter M.D.
Umbo
Tympanic
Cone of light
Pars tensa

Plate 93 Tympanic Cavity. (Netter: Atlas of Human Anatomy, 4 ed, 2006, Saunders.)

Dissected right bony labyrinth (otic capsule): membranous labyrinth removed

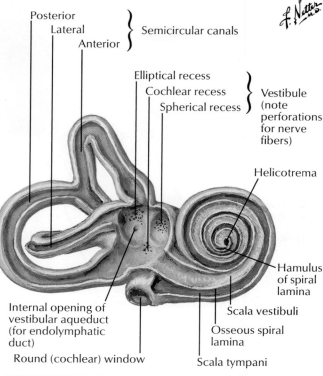

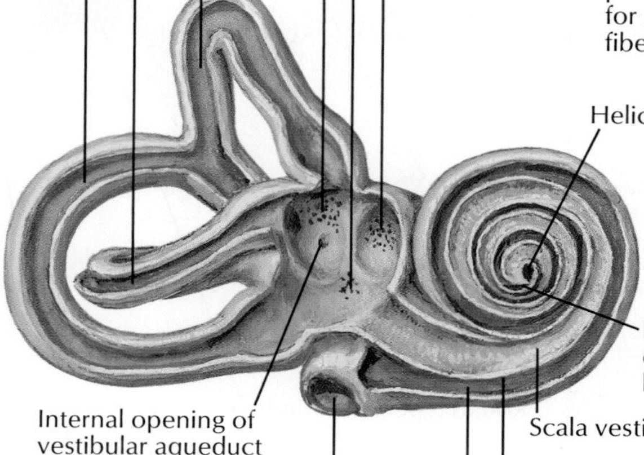
F. Netter M.D.
Posterior
Lateral
Anterior
Semicircular canals
Elliptical recess
Cochlear recess
Spherical recess
Vestibule (note perforations for nerve fibers)
Helicotrema
Hamulus of spiral lamina
Scala vestibuli
Internal opening of vestibular aqueduct (for endolymphatic duct)
Osseous spiral lamina
Round (cochlear) window
Scala tympani

Plate 95 Bony Membranous Labyrinth. (Netter: Atlas of Human Anatomy, 4 ed, 2006, Saunders.)

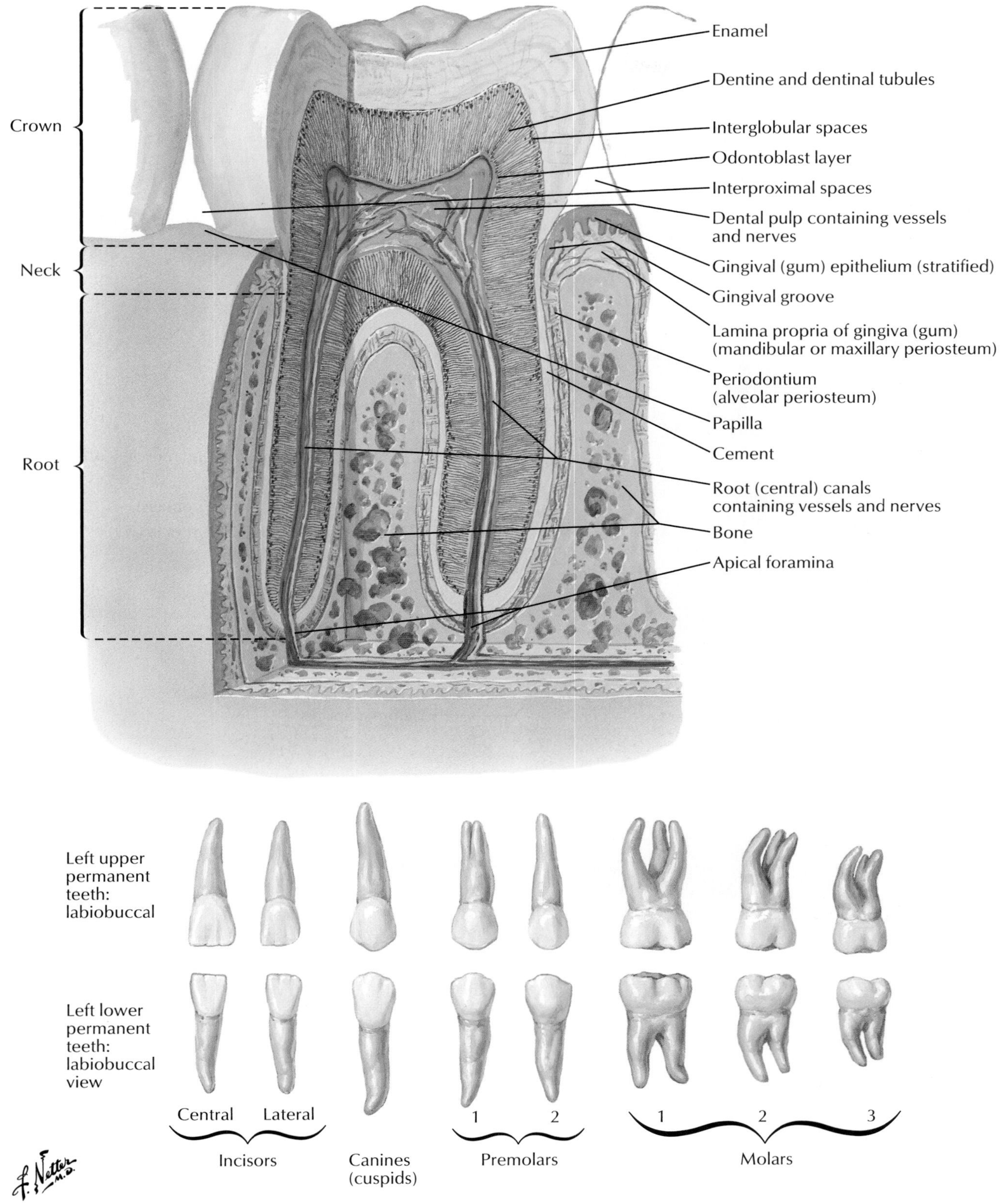
Crown
Neck
Root
Enamel
Dentine and dentinal tubules
Interglobular spaces
Odontoblast layer
Interproximal spaces
Dental pulp containing vessels and nerves
Gingival (gum) epithelium (stratified)
Gingival groove
Lamina propria of gingiva (gum) (mandibular or maxillary periosteum)
Periodontium (alveolar periosteum)
Papilla
Cement
Root (central) canals containing vessels and nerves
Bone
Apical foramina
Left upper permanent teeth: labiobuccal
Left lower permanent teeth: labiobuccal view
Central
Lateral
Incisors
Canines (cuspids)
1
2
Premolars
1
2
3
Molars

Plate 57 Teeth. (Netter: Atlas of Human Anatomy, 4 ed, 2006, Saunders.)

Tongue

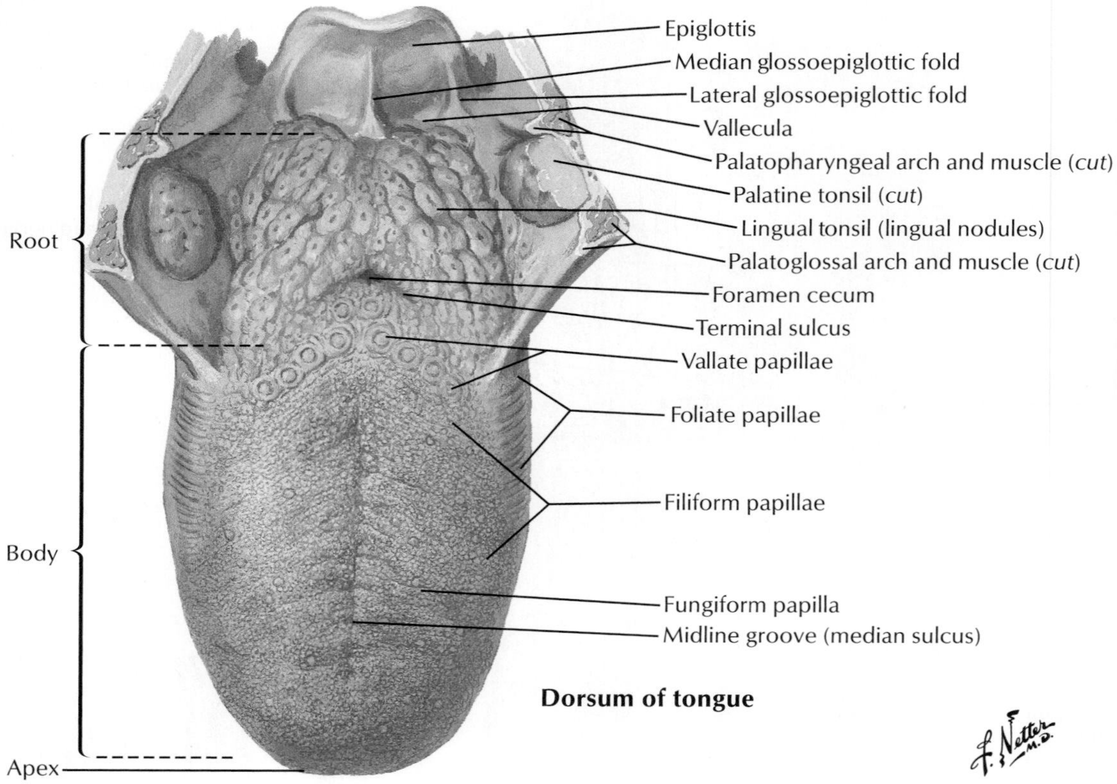
Epiglottis
Median glossoepiglottic fold
Lateral glossoepiglottic fold
Vallecula
Palatopharyngeal arch and muscle (*cut*)
Palatine tonsil (*cut*)
Lingual tonsil (lingual nodules)
Palatoglossal arch and muscle (*cut*)
Foramen cecum
Terminal sulcus
Vallate papillae
Foliate papillae
Filiform papillae
Fungiform papilla
Midline groove (median sulcus)
Root
Body
Apex
Dorsum of tongue

Plate 58 Tongue. (Netter: Atlas of Human Anatomy, 4 ed, 2006, Saunders.)

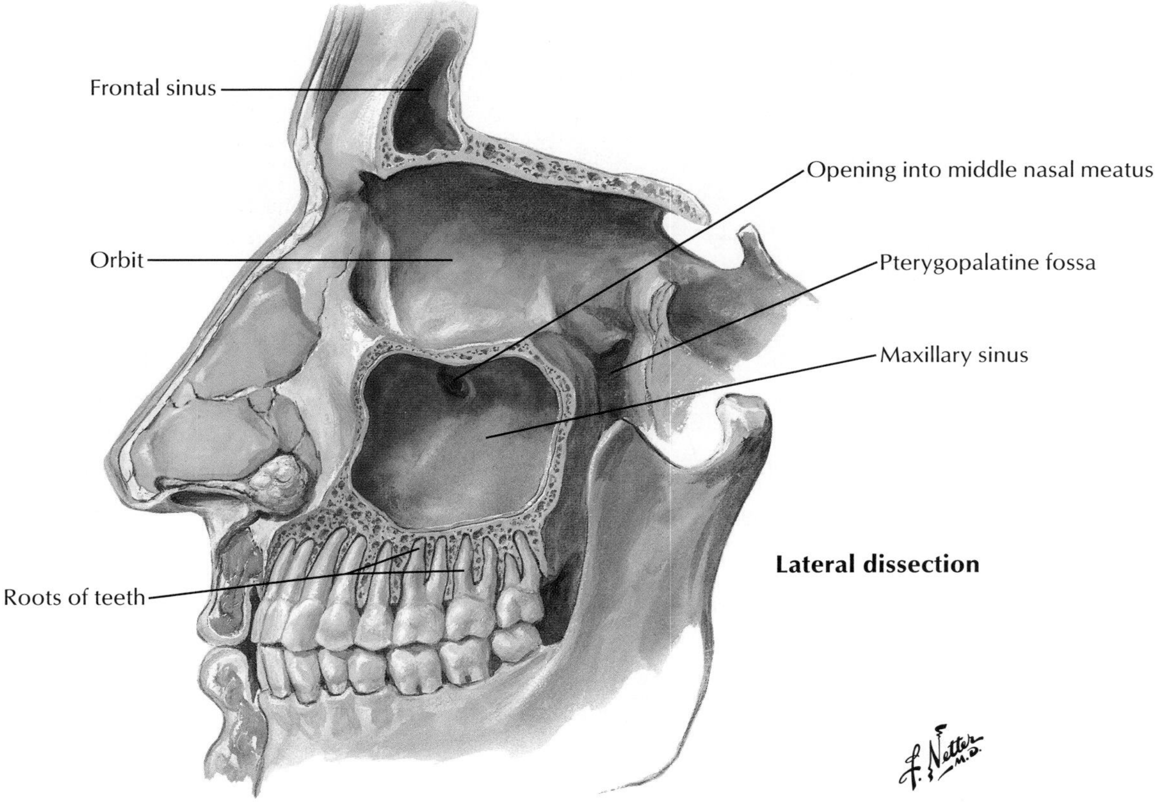
Frontal sinus
Opening into middle nasal meatus
Orbit
Pterygopalatine fossa
Maxillary sinus
Lateral dissection
Roots of teeth

Plate 49 Paranasal Sinuses. (Netter: Atlas of Human Anatomy, 4 ed, 2006, Saunders.)

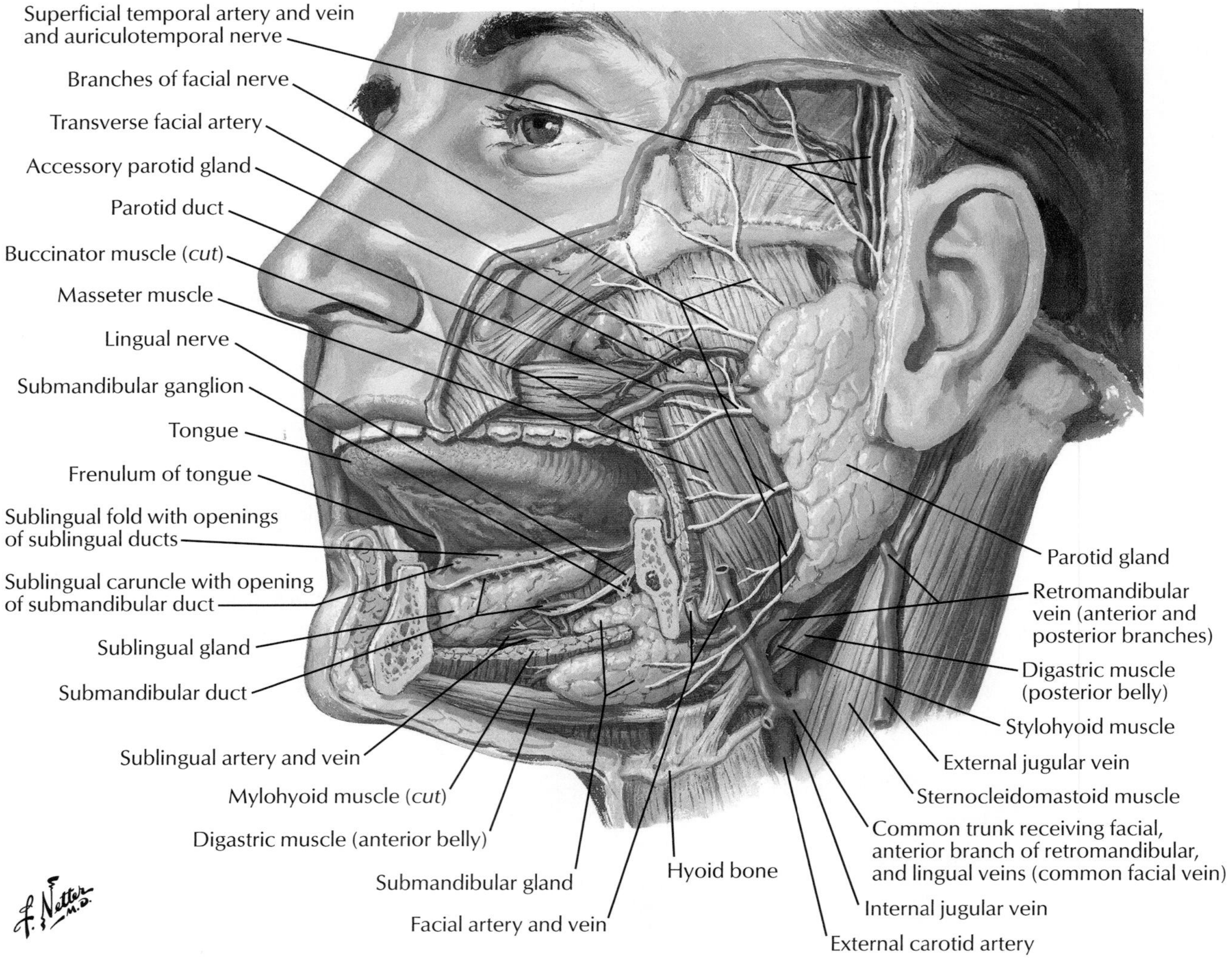
Superficial temporal artery and vein and auriculotemporal nerve
Branches of facial nerve
Transverse facial artery
Accessory parotid gland
Parotid duct
Buccinator muscle (*cut*)
Masseter muscle
Lingual nerve
Submandibular ganglion
Tongue
Frenulum of tongue
Sublingual fold with openings of sublingual ducts
Sublingual caruncle with opening of submandibular duct
Sublingual gland
Submandibular duct
Sublingual artery and vein
Mylohyoid muscle (*cut*)
Digastric muscle (anterior belly)
Submandibular gland
Facial artery and vein
Hyoid bone
External carotid artery
Internal jugular vein
Common trunk receiving facial, anterior branch of retromandibular, and lingual veins (common facial vein)
Sternocleidomastoid muscle
External jugular vein
Stylohyoid muscle
Digastric muscle (posterior belly)
Retromandibular vein (anterior and posterior branches)
Parotid gland
F. Netter M.D.

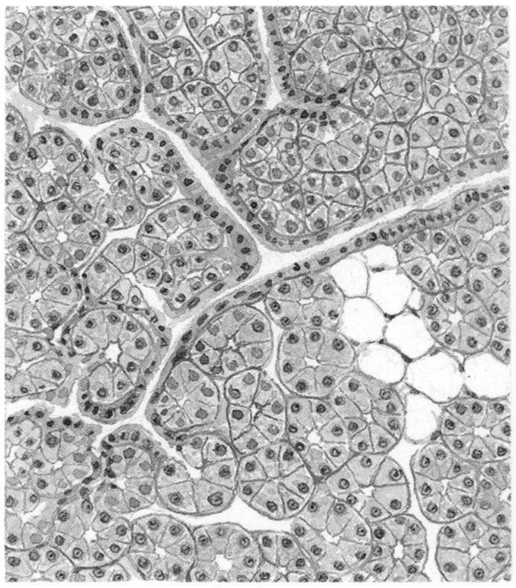
Parotid gland: totally serous

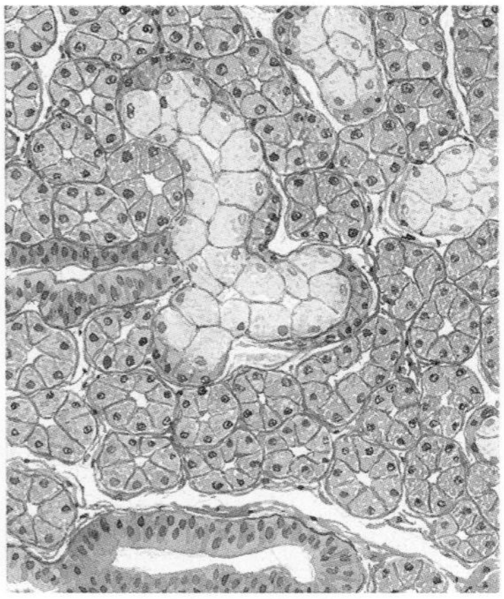
Submandibular gland: mostly serous, partially mucous

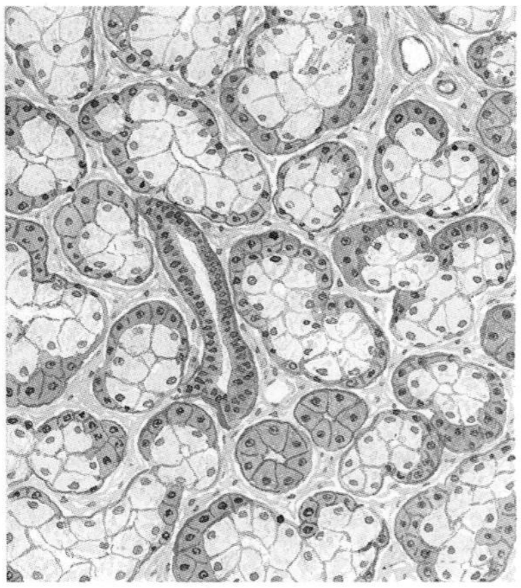
Sublingual gland: almost completely mucous

Plate 61 Salivary Glands. (Netter: Atlas of Human Anatomy, 4 ed, 2006, Saunders.)

Right coronary artery: left anterior oblique view

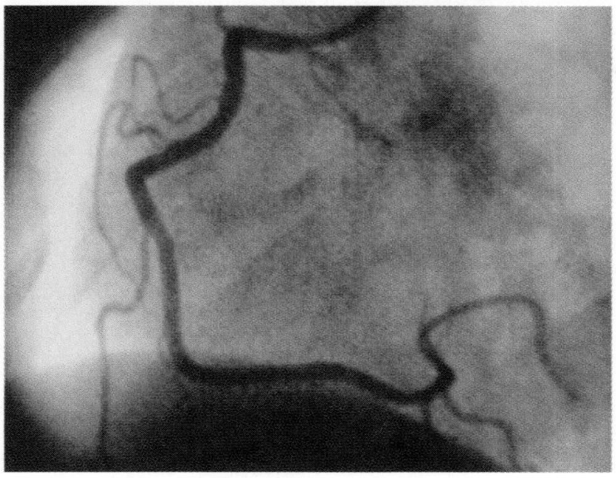

Arteriogram

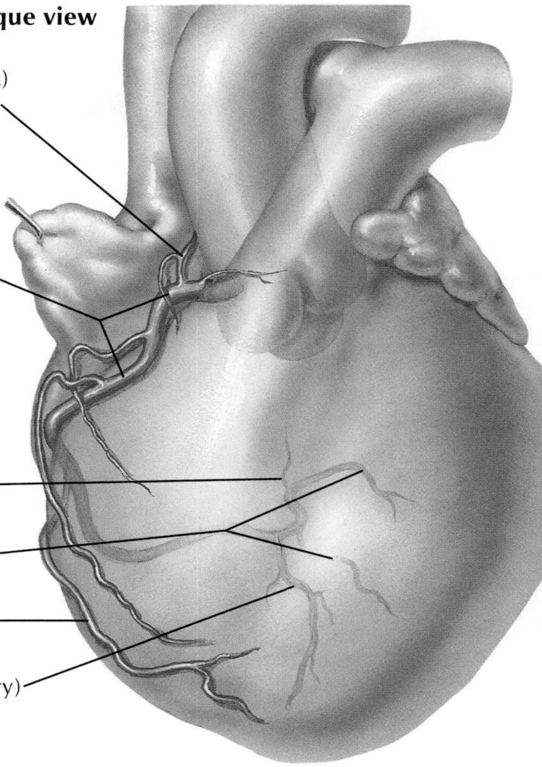
Sinuatrial (SA) nodal branch
Right coronary artery
Atrioventricular (AV) nodal branch
Branches to back of left ventricle
Right marginal branch
Posterior interventricular branch (posterior descending artery)

Right coronary artery: right anterior oblique view

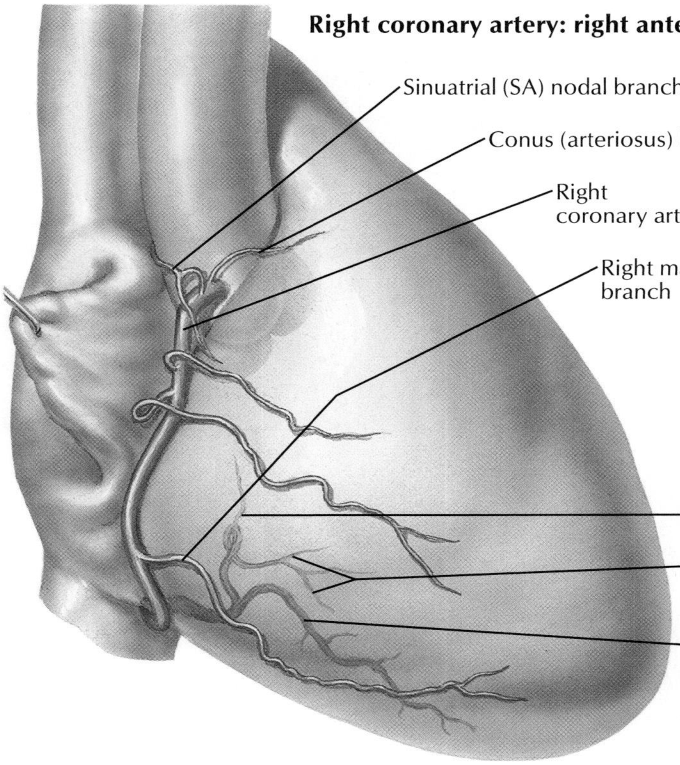
Sinuatrial (SA) nodal branch
Conus (arteriosus) branch
Right coronary artery
Right marginal branch
Atrioventricular (AV) nodal branch
Right posterolateral branches (to back of left ventricle)
Posterior interventricular branch (posterior descending artery)

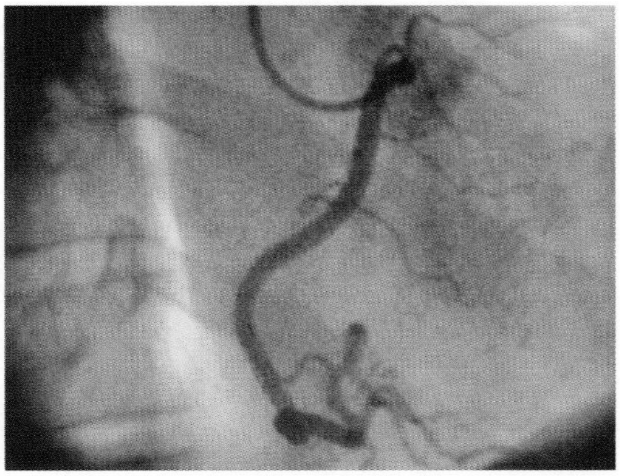

Arteriogram

Plate 218 Coronary Arteries: Arteriographic Views. (Netter: Atlas of Human Anatomy, 4 ed, 2006, Saunders.)

Left coronary artery: left anterior oblique view

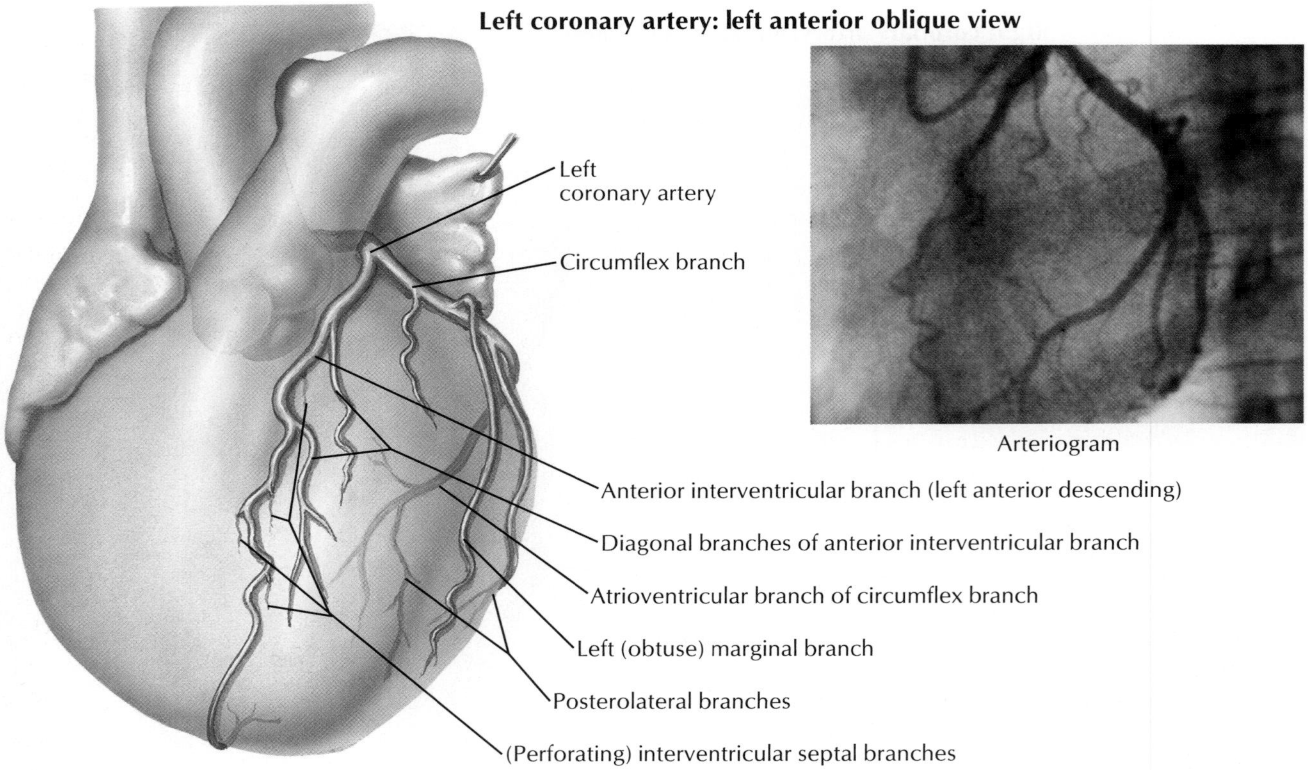
Left
coronary artery
Circumflex branch
Arteriogram
Anterior interventricular branch (left anterior descending)
Diagonal branches of anterior interventricular branch
Atrioventricular branch of circumflex branch
Left (obtuse) marginal branch
Posterolateral branches
(Perforating) interventricular septal branches

Left coronary artery: right anterior oblique view

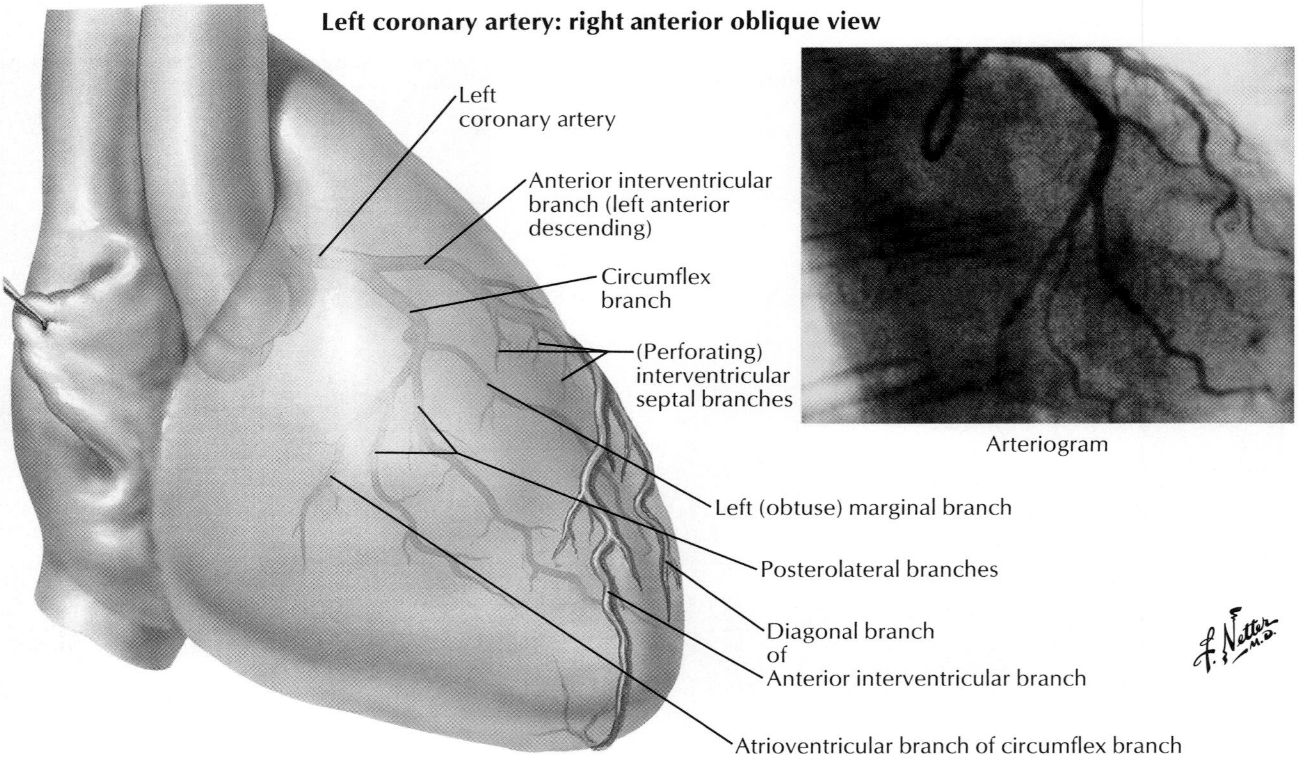
Left
coronary artery
Anterior interventricular
branch (left anterior
descending)
Circumflex
branch
(Perforating)
interventricular
septal branches
Arteriogram
Left (obtuse) marginal branch
Posterolateral branches
Diagonal branch
of
Anterior interventricular branch
Atrioventricular branch of circumflex branch

Plate 219 Coronary Arteries: Arteriographic Views. (Netter: Atlas of Human Anatomy, 4 ed, 2006, Saunders.)

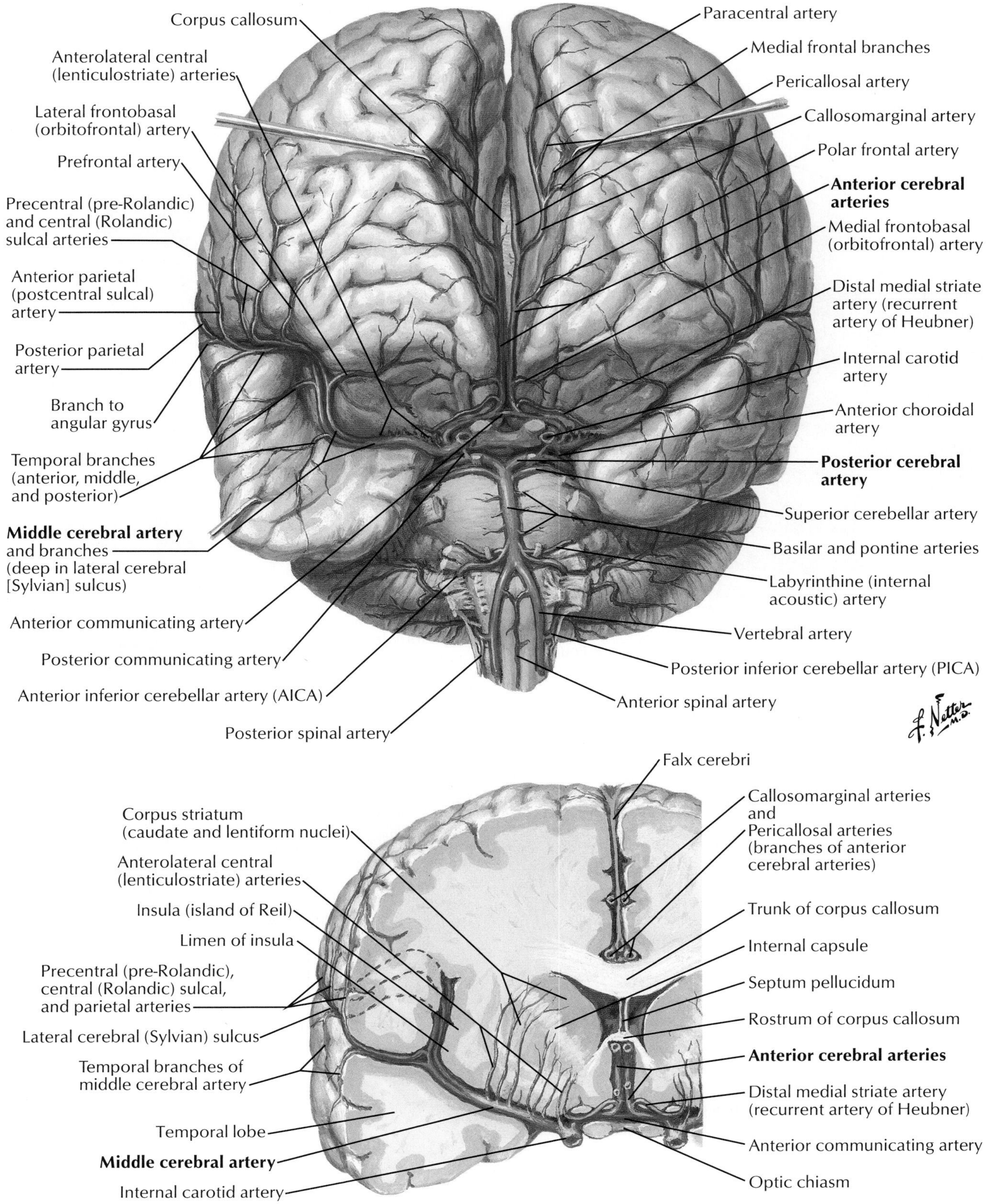
Corpus callosum
Anterolateral central (lenticulostriate) arteries
Lateral frontobasal (orbitofrontal) artery
Prefrontal artery
Precentral (pre-Rolandic) and central (Rolandic) sulcal arteries
Anterior parietal (postcentral sulcal) artery
Posterior parietal artery
Branch to angular gyrus
Temporal branches (anterior, middle, and posterior)
Middle cerebral artery and branches (deep in lateral cerebral [Sylvian] sulcus)
Anterior communicating artery
Posterior communicating artery
Anterior inferior cerebellar artery (AICA)
Posterior spinal artery
Paracentral artery
Medial frontal branches
Pericallosal artery
Callosomarginal artery
Polar frontal artery
Anterior cerebral arteries
Medial frontobasal (orbitofrontal) artery
Distal medial striate artery (recurrent artery of Heubner)
Internal carotid artery
Anterior choroidal artery
Posterior cerebral artery
Superior cerebellar artery
Basilar and pontine arteries
Labyrinthine (internal acoustic) artery
Vertebral artery
Posterior inferior cerebellar artery (PICA)
Anterior spinal artery
F. Netter M.D.
Falx cerebri
Corpus striatum (caudate and lentiform nuclei)
Anterolateral central (lenticulostriate) arteries
Insula (island of Reil)
Limen of insula
Precentral (pre-Rolandic), central (Rolandic) sulcal, and parietal arteries
Lateral cerebral (Sylvian) sulcus
Temporal branches of middle cerebral artery
Temporal lobe
Middle cerebral artery
Internal carotid artery
Callosomarginal arteries and Pericallosal arteries (branches of anterior cerebral arteries)
Trunk of corpus callosum
Internal capsule
Septum pellucidum
Rostrum of corpus callosum
Anterior cerebral arteries
Distal medial striate artery (recurrent artery of Heubner)
Anterior communicating artery
Optic chiasm

Plate 141 Arteries of Brain: Frontal View and Section. (Netter: Atlas of Human Anatomy, 4 ed, 2006, Saunders.)

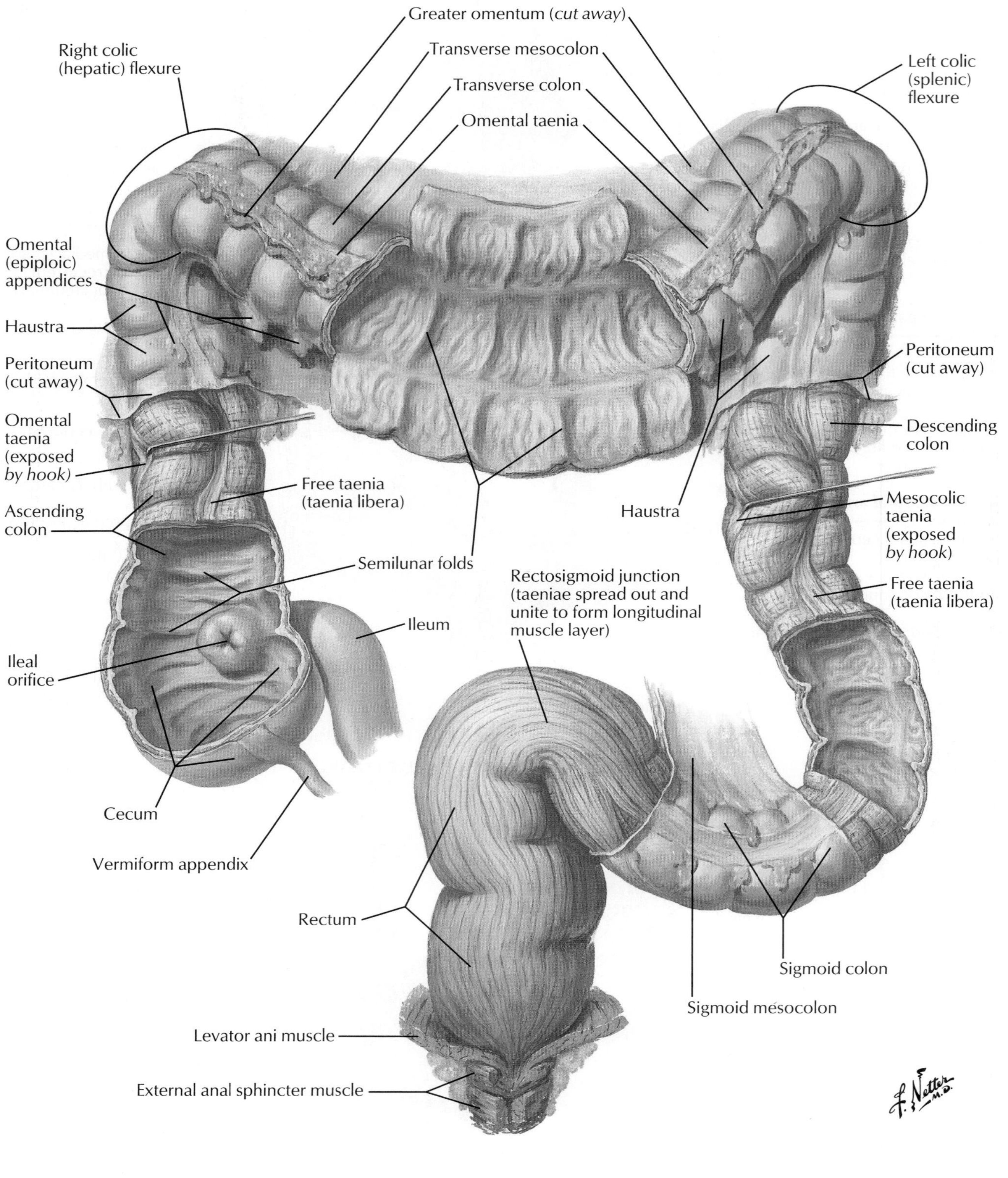
Greater omentum (*cut away*)
Transverse mesocolon
Transverse colon
Omental taenia
Right colic (hepatic) flexure
Left colic (splenic) flexure
Omental (epiploic) appendices
Haustra
Peritoneum (cut away)
Omental taenia (exposed *by hook)*
Ascending colon
Free taenia (taenia libera)
Semilunar folds
Haustra
Peritoneum (cut away)
Descending colon
Mesocolic taenia (exposed *by hook*)
Free taenia (taenia libera)
Rectosigmoid junction (taeniae spread out and unite to form longitudinal muscle layer)
Ileum
Ileal orifice
Cecum
Vermiform appendix
Rectum
Sigmoid colon
Sigmoid mesocolon
Levator ani muscle
External anal sphincter muscle

Plate 284 Mucosa and Musculature of Large Intestine. (Netter: Atlas of Human Anatomy, 4 ed, 2006, Saunders.)

Transverse Section: T3–4 Intervertebral Disc, Manubrium

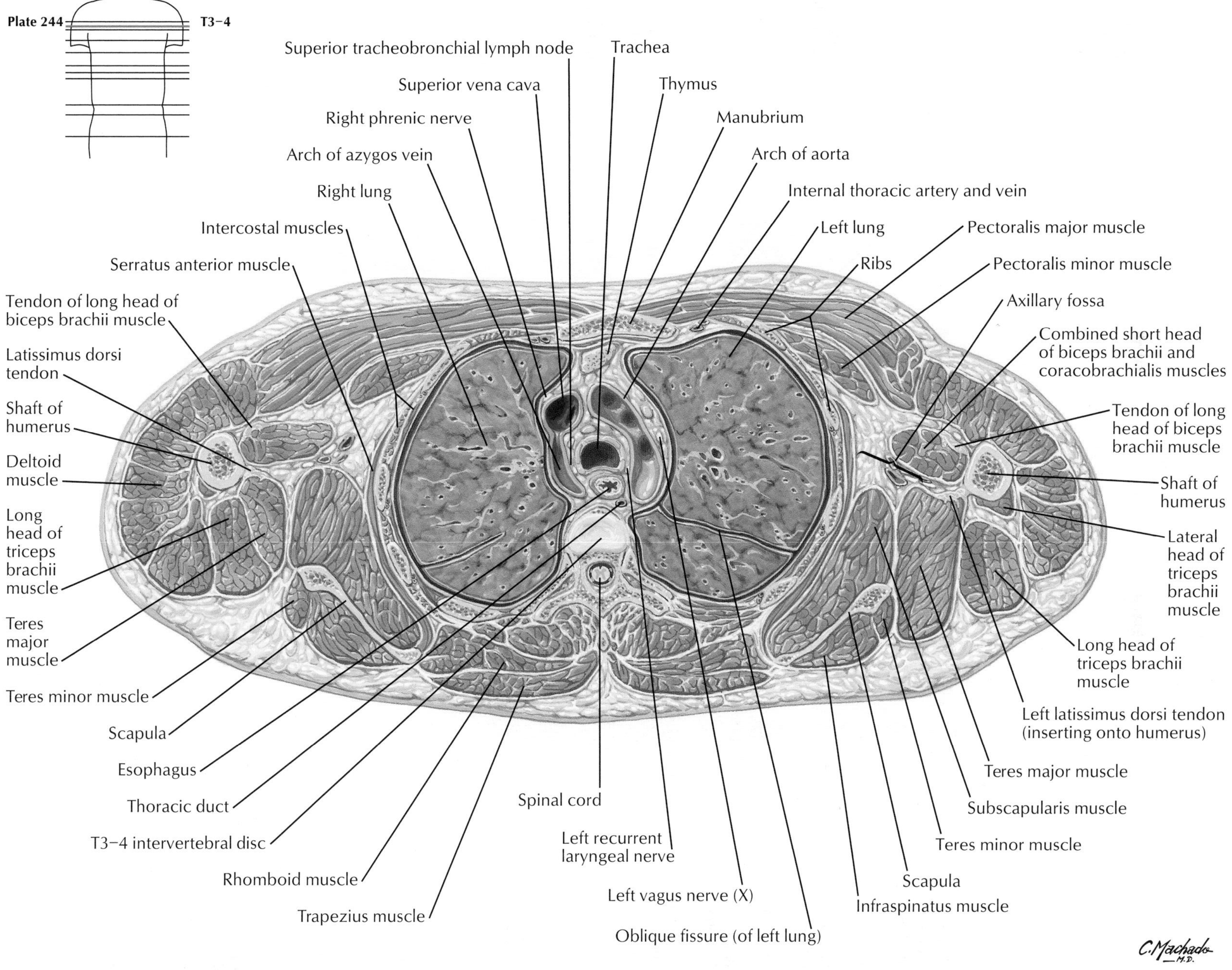

Plate 244
T3–4
Superior tracheobronchial lymph node
Superior vena cava
Right phrenic nerve
Arch of azygos vein
Right lung
Intercostal muscles
Serratus anterior muscle
Tendon of long head of biceps brachii muscle
Latissimus dorsi tendon
Shaft of humerus
Deltoid muscle
Long head of triceps brachii muscle
Teres major muscle
Teres minor muscle
Scapula
Esophagus
Thoracic duct
T3–4 intervertebral disc
Rhomboid muscle
Trapezius muscle
Trachea
Thymus
Manubrium
Arch of aorta
Internal thoracic artery and vein
Left lung
Ribs
Pectoralis major muscle
Pectoralis minor muscle
Axillary fossa
Combined short head of biceps brachii and coracobrachialis muscles
Tendon of long head of biceps brachii muscle
Shaft of humerus
Lateral head of triceps brachii muscle
Long head of triceps brachii muscle
Left latissimus dorsi tendon (inserting onto humerus)
Teres major muscle
Subscapularis muscle
Teres minor muscle
Scapula
Infraspinatus muscle
Spinal cord
Left recurrent laryngeal nerve
Left vagus nerve (X)
Oblique fissure (of left lung)
C. Machado M.D.

Plate 244 Cross Section of Thorax at T3-4 Disc Level. (Netter: Atlas of Human Anatomy, 4 ed, 2006, Saunders.)

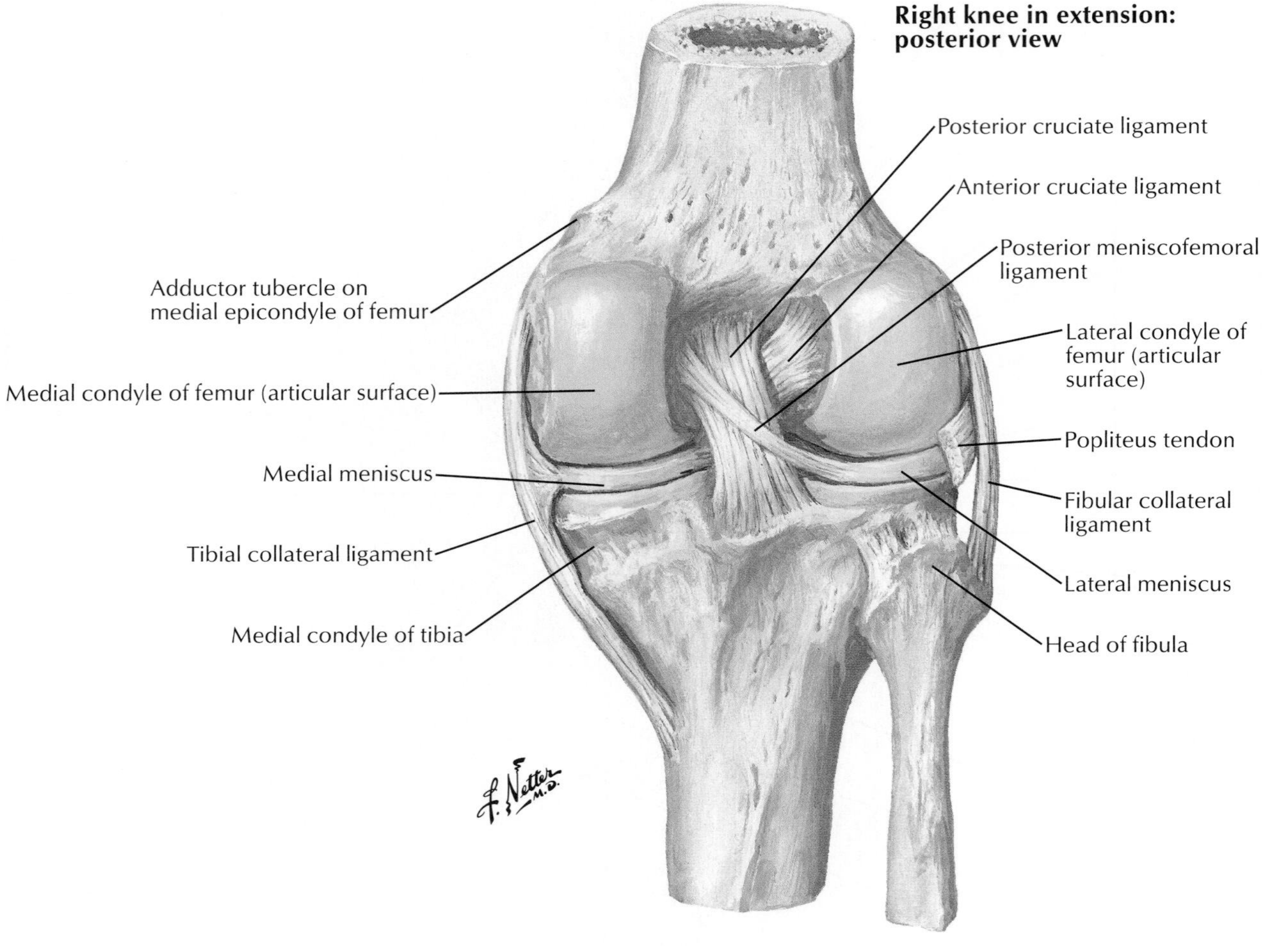
Right knee in extension: posterior view
Posterior cruciate ligament
Anterior cruciate ligament
Posterior meniscofemoral ligament
Adductor tubercle on medial epicondyle of femur
Lateral condyle of femur (articular surface)
Medial condyle of femur (articular surface)
Popliteus tendon
Medial meniscus
Fibular collateral ligament
Tibial collateral ligament
Lateral meniscus
Medial condyle of tibia
Head of fibula

Plate 509 Knee: Cruciate and Collateral Ligaments. (Netter: Atlas of Human Anatomy, 4 ed, 2006, Saunders.)

INDEX

A

◀ New ↩ Revised ✔ Reinstated ~~deleted~~ Deleted

◀ New ↩ Revised ✔ Reinstated ~~deleted~~ Deleted

◀ New ⮌ Revised ✔ Reinstated ~~deleted~~ Deleted

B

◀ New ⤾ Revised ✔ Reinstated ~~deleted~~ Deleted

◀ New ↩ Revised ✔ Reinstated ~~deleted~~ Deleted

◀ New ⮌ Revised ✔ Reinstated ~~deleted~~ Deleted

B

C

◀ New ⟲ Revised ✔ Reinstated ~~deleted~~ Deleted

D

◀ New ⮌ Revised ✔ Reinstated ~~deleted~~ Deleted

◀ New ↩ Revised ✔ Reinstated ~~deleted~~ Deleted

D

E

◀ New ↩ Revised ✔ Reinstated ~~deleted~~ Deleted

F

G

H

◀ New ↻ Revised ✔ Reinstated ~~deleted~~ Deleted

◀ New ⤾ Revised ✔ Reinstated ~~deleted~~ Deleted

I

◀ New ⤺ Revised ✔ Reinstated ~~deleted~~ Deleted

◀ New ↩ Revised ✔ Reinstated ~~deleted~~ Deleted

◀ New ↩ Revised ✔ Reinstated ~~deleted~~ Deleted

◀ New ⤾ Revised ✔ Reinstated ~~deleted~~ Deleted

M

◀ New ⮌ Revised ✔ Reinstated ~~deleted~~ Deleted

N

O

◀ New ↩ Revised ✔ Reinstated ~~deleted~~ Deleted

P

◀ New ⤺ Revised ✔ Reinstated ~~deleted~~ Deleted

Q

R

◀ New ⟲ Revised ✔ Reinstated ~~deleted~~ Deleted

S

◀ New ↩ Revised ✔ Reinstated ~~deleted~~ Deleted

◀ New ⤾ Revised ✔ Reinstated ~~deleted~~ Deleted

T

◀ New ⮌ Revised ✔ Reinstated ~~deleted~~ Deleted

◀ New ↩ Revised ✔ Reinstated ~~deleted~~ Deleted

U

V

W

◀ New ↩ Revised ✔ Reinstated ~~deleted~~ Deleted

W

X

Y

Z

◀ New ⤾ Revised ✔ Reinstated ~~deleted~~ Deleted

2019

TABLE OF DRUGS

IA	Intra-arterial administration
IU	International unit
IV	Intravenous administration
IM	Intramuscular administration
IT	Intrathecal
SC	Subcutaneous administration
INH	Administration by inhaled solution
VAR	Various routes of administration
OTH	Other routes of administration
ORAL	Administered orally

Intravenous administration includes all methods, such as gravity infusion, injections, and timed pushes. The "VAR" posting denotes various routes of administration and is used for drugs that are commonly administered into joints, cavities, tissues, or topical applications, in addition to other parenteral administrations. Listings posted with "OTH" indicate other administration methods, such as suppositories or catheter injections.

Blue typeface terms are added by publisher.

DRUG NAME	DOSAGE	METHOD OF ADMINISTRATION	HCPCS CODE
A			
Abatacept	10 mg	IV	**J0129**
Abbokinase	5,000 IU vial	IV	J3364
	250,000 IU vial	IV	J3365
Abbokinase, Open Cath	5,000 IU vial	IV	J3364
Abciximab	10 mg	IV	**J0130**
Abelcet	10 mg	IV	J0287-J0289
Abilify Maintena	1 mg		J0401
ABLC	50 mg	IV	J0285
AbobotulinumtoxintypeA	5 units	IM	**J0586**
Abraxane	1 mg		J9264
Accuneb	1 mg		J7613
Acetadote	100 mg		J0132
Acetaminophen	10 mg	IV	**J0131**
Acetazolamide sodium	up to 500 mg	IM, IV	**J1120**
Acetylcysteine			
injection	100 mg	IV	**J0132**
unit dose form	per gram	INH	**J7604, J7608**
Achromycin	up to 250 mg	IM, IV	J0120
Actemra	1 mg		J3262
ACTH	up to 40 units	IV, IM, SC	J0800
Acthar	up to 40 units	IV, IM, SC	J0800
Acthib			J3490
Acthrel	1 mcg		J0795
Actimmune	3 million units	SC	J9216
Activase	1 mg	IV	J2997

◀ New ⤾ Revised ✔ Reinstated ~~deleted~~ Deleted

DRUG NAME	DOSAGE	METHOD OF ADMINISTRATION	HCPCS CODE
Acyclovir	5 mg		J0133
			J8499
Adagen	25 IU		J2504
Adalimumab	20 mg	SC	J0135
Adcetris	1 mg	IV	J9042
Adenocard	1 mg	IV	J0153
Adenoscan	1 mg	IV	J0153
Adenosine	1 mg	IV	J0153
Ado-trastuzumab Emtansine	1 mg	IV	J9354
Adrenalin Chloride	up to 1 ml ampule	SC, IM	J0171
Adrenalin, epinephrine	0.1 mg	SC, IM	J0171
Adriamycin, PFS, RDF	10 mg	IV	J9000
Adrucil	500 mg	IV	J9190
Advate	per IU		J7192
Aflibercept	1 mg	OTH	J0178
Agalsidase beta	1 mg	IV	J0180
Aggrastat	0.25 mg	IM, IV	J3246
A-hydrocort	up to 50 mg	IV, IM, SC	J1710
	up to 100 mg		J1720
Akineton	per 5 mg	IM, IV	J0190
Akynzeo	300 mg and 0.5 mg		J8655
Alatrofloxacin mesylate, injection	100 mg	IV	J0200
Albumin			P9041, P9045, P9046, P9047
Albuterol	0.5 mg	INH	J7620
concentrated form	1 mg	INH	J7610, J7611
unit dose form	1 mg	INH	J7609, J7613
Aldesleukin	per single use vial	IM, IV	J9015
Aldomet	up to 250 mg	IV	J0210
Aldurazyme	0.1 mg		J1931
Alefacept	0.5 mg	IM, IV	J0215
Alemtuzumab	1 mg		J0202
Alferon N	250,000 IU	IM	J9215
Alglucerase	per 10 units	IV	J0205
Alglucosidase alfa	10 mg	IV	J0220, J0221
Alimta	10 mg		J9305
Alkaban-AQ	1 mg	IV	J9360
Alkeran	2 mg	ORAL	J8600
	50 mg	IV	J9245
AlloDerm	per square centimeter		Q4116

◀ New ↩ Revised ✔ Reinstated ~~deleted~~ Deleted

DRUG NAME	DOSAGE	METHOD OF ADMINISTRATION	HCPCS CODE
AlloSkin	per square centimeter		Q4115
Aloxi	25 mcg		J2469
Alpha 1-proteinase inhibitor, human	10 mg	IV	**J0256, J0257**
Alphanate			**J7186**
AlphaNine SD	per IU		J7193
Alprolix	per IU		J7201
Alprostadil			
injection	1.25 mcg	OTH	**J0270**
urethral suppository	each	OTH	**J0275**
Alteplase recombinant	1 mg	IV	**J2997**
Alupent	per 10 mg	INH	**J7667, J7668**
noncompounded, unit dose	10 mg	INH	J7669
unit does	10 mg	INH	J7670
AmBisome	10 mg	IV	J0289
Amcort	per 5 mg	IM	J3302
A-methaPred	up to 40 mg	IM, IV	J2920
	up to 125 mg	IM, IV	J2930
Amgen	1 mcg	SC	J9212
Amifostine	500 mg	IV	**J0207**
Amikacin sulfate	100 mg	IM, IV	**J0278**
Aminocaproic Acid			J3490
Aminolevalinic acid HCl	unit dose (354 mg)	OTH	**J7308**
Aminolevulinic acid Hcl 10% Gel	10 mg	OTH	**J7345**
Aminolevulinate	1 g	OTH	**J7309**
Aminophylline/Aminophyllin	up to 250 mg	IV	**J0280**
Amiodarone HCl	30 mg	IV	**J0282**
Amitriptyline HCl	up to 20 mg	IM	**J1320**
Amobarbital	up to 125 mg	IM, IV	**J0300**
Amphadase	1 ml.		J3470
Amphocin	50 mg	IV	J0285
Amphotericin B	50 mg	IV	**J0285**
Amphotericin B, lipid complex	10 mg	IV	**J0287-J0289**
Ampicillin			
sodium	up to 500 mg	IM, IV	**J0290**
sodium/sulbactam sodium	per 1.5 g	IM, IV	**J0295**
Amygdalin			J3570
Amytal	up to 125 mg	IM, IV	J0300
Anabolin LA 100	up to 50 mg	IM	J2320
Anadulafungin	1 mg	IV	**J0348**
Anascorp	up to 120 mg	IV	J0716

◀ New ↩ Revised ✔ Reinstated ~~deleted~~ Deleted

DRUG NAME	DOSAGE	METHOD OF ADMINISTRATION	HCPCS CODE
Anastrozole	1 mg		J8999
Ancef	500 mg	IV, IM	J0690
Andrest 90-4	1 mg	IM	J3121
Andro-Cyp	1 mg		J1071
Andro-Cyp 200	1 mg		J1071
Andro L.A. 200	1 mg	IM	J3121
Andro-Estro 90-4	1 mg	IM	J3121
Andro/Fem	1 mg		J1071
Androgyn L.A.	1 mg	IM	J3121
Androlone-50	up to 50 mg		J2320
Androlone-D 100	up to 50 mg	IM	J2320
Andronaq-50	up to 50 mg	IM	J3140
Andronaq-LA	1 mg		J1071
Andronate-100	1 mg		J1071
Andronate-200	1 mg		J1071
Andropository 100	1 mg	IM	J3121
Andryl 200	1 mg	IM	J3121
Anectine	up to 20 mg	IM, IV	J0330
Anergan 25	up to 50 mg	IM, IV	J2550
	12.5 mg	ORAL	Q0169
Anergan 50	up to 50 mg	IM, IV	J2550
	12.5 mg	ORAL	Q0169
Angiomax	1 mg		J0583
Anidulafungin	1 mg	IV	J0348
Anistreplase	30 units	IV	J0350
Antiflex	up to 60 mg	IM, IV	J2360
Anti-Inhibitor	per IU	IV	J7198
Antispas	up to 20 mg	IM	J0500
Antithrombin III (human)	per IU	IV	J7197
Antithrombin recombinant	50 IU	IV	J7196
Anzemet	10 mg	IV	J1260
	50 mg	ORAL	S0174
	100 mg	ORAL	Q0180
Apidra Solostar	per 50 units		J1817
A.P.L.	per 1,000 USP units	IM	J0725
Apligraf	per square centimeter		Q4101
Apomorphine Hydrochloride	1 mg	SC	J0364
Aprepitant	1 mg	IV	J0185 ◀
Aprepitant	5 mg	ORAL	J8501
Apresoline	up to 20 mg	IV, IM	J0360

◀ New ↩ Revised ✔ Reinstated ~~deleted~~ Deleted

DRUG NAME	DOSAGE	METHOD OF ADMINISTRATION	HCPCS CODE
Aprotinin	10,000 kiu		J0365
AquaMEPHYTON	per 1 mg	IM, SC, IV	J3430
Aralast	10 mg	IV	J0256
Aralen	up to 250 mg	IM	J0390
Aramine	per 10 mg	IV, IM, SC	J0380
Aranesp			
ESRD use	1 mcg		J0882
Non-ESRD use	1 mcg		J0881
Arbutamine	1 mg	IV	J0395
Arcalyst	1 mg		J2793
Aredia	per 30 mg	IV	J2430
Arfonad, *see* Trimethaphan camsylate			
Arformoterol tartrate	15 mcg	INH	J7605
Argatroban			
(for ESRD use)	1 mg	IV	J0884
(for non-ESRD use)	1 mg	IV	J0883
Aridol	25% in 50 ml	IV	J2150
	5 mg	INH	J7665
Arimidex			J8999
Aripiprazole	0.25 mg	IM	J0400
Aripiprazole, extended release	1 mg	IV	J0401
Aripiprazole lauroxil	1 mg	IV	J1942
Aristada	3.9 ml		J1942
Aristocort Forte	per 5 mg	IM	J3302
Aristocort Intralesional	per 5 mg	IM	J3302
Aristospan Intra-Articular	per 5 mg	VAR	J3303
Aristospan Intralesional	per 5 mg	VAR	J3303
Arixtra	per 0.5 m		J1652
Aromasin			J8999
Arranon	50 mg		J9261
Arrestin	up to 200 mg	IM	J3250
	250 mg	ORAL	Q0173
Arsenic trioxide	1 mg	IV	J9017
Arzerra	10 mg		J9302
Asparaginase	1,000 units	IV, IM	J9019
	10,000 units	IV, IM	J9020
Astagraf XL	0.1 mg		J7508
Astramorph PF	up to 10 mg	IM, IV, SC	J2270
Atezolizumab	10 mg	IV	J9022
Atgam	250 mg	IV	J7504

◀ New ↩ Revised ✔ Reinstated ~~deleted~~ Deleted

DRUG NAME	DOSAGE	METHOD OF ADMINISTRATION	HCPCS CODE
Ativan	2 mg	IM, IV	J2060
Atropine			
concentrated form	per mg	INH	J7635
unit dose form	per mg	INH	J7636
sulfate	0.01 mg	IV, IM, SC	J0461, J7636
Atrovent	per mg	INH	J7644, J7645
ATryn	50 IU	IV	J7196
Aurothioglucose	up to 50 mg	IM	J2910
Autologous cultured chondrocytes implant		OTH	J7330
Autoplex T	per IU	IV	J7198, J7199
AUVI-Q	0.15 mg		J0171
Avastin	10 mg		J9035
Avelox	100 mg		J2280
Avelumab	10 mg	IV	J9023
Avonex	30 mcg	IM	J1826
	1 mcg	IM	Q3027
	1 mcg	SC	Q3028
Azacitidine	1 mg	SC	J9025
Azasan	50 mg		J7500
Azathioprine	50 mg	ORAL	J7500
Azathioprine, parenteral	100 mg	IV	J7501
Azithromycin, dihydrate	1 gram	ORAL	Q0144
Azithromycin, injection	500 mg	IV	J0456
B			
Baciim			J3490
Bacitracin			J3490
Baclofen	10 mg	IT	J0475
Baclofen for intrathecal trial	50 mcg	OTH	J0476
Bactocill	up to 250 mg	IM, IV	J2700
BAL in oil	per 100 mg	IM	J0470
Banflex	up to 60 mg	IV, IM	J2360
Basiliximab	20 mg	IV	J0480
BCG (Bacillus Calmette and Guerin), live	per vial	IV	J9031
Bebulin	per IU		J7194
Beclomethasone inhalation solution, unit dose form	per mg	INH	J7622
Belatacept	1 mg	IV	J0485
Beleodaq	10 mg		J9032
Belimumab	10 mg	IV	J0490
Belinostat	10 mg	IV	J9032
Bena-D 10	up to 50 mg	IV, IM	J1200

◀ New ↩ Revised ✔ Reinstated ~~deleted~~ Deleted

DRUG NAME	DOSAGE	METHOD OF ADMINISTRATION	HCPCS CODE
Bena-D 50	up to 50 mg	IV, IM	J1200
Benadryl	up to 50 mg	IV, IM	J1200
Benahist 10	up to 50 mg	IV, IM	J1200
Benahist 50	up to 50 mg	IV, IM	J1200
Ben-Allergin-50	up to 50 mg	IV, IM	J1200
	50 mg	ORAL	Q0163
Bendamustine HCl			
Bendeka	1 mg	IV	J9034
Treanda	1 mg	IV	J9033
Benefix	per IU	IV	J7195
Benlysta	10 mg		J0490
Benoject-10	up to 50 mg	IV, IM	J1200
Benoject-50	up to 50 mg	IV, IM	J1200
Benralizumab	1 mg	IV	J0517 ◀
Bentyl	up to 20 mg	IM	J0500
Benzocaine			J3490
Benztropine mesylate	per 1 mg	IM, IV	J0515
Berinert	10 units		J0597
Berubigen	up to 1,000 mcg	IM, SC	J3420
Beta amyloid	per study dose	OTH	A9599
Betalin 12	up to 1,000 mcg	IM, SC	J3420
Betameth	per 3 mg	IM, IV	J0702
Betamethasone Acetate			J3490
Betamethasone Acetate & Betamethasone Sodium Phosphate	per 3 mg	IM	J0702
Betamethasone inhalation solution, unit dose form	per mg	INH	J7624
Betaseron	0.25 mg	SC	J1830
Bethanechol chloride	up to 5 mg	SC	J0520
Bethkis	300 mg		J7682
Bevacizumab	10 mg	IV	J9035
Bevacizumab-awwb	10 mg	IV	Q5107 ◀
Bezlotoxumab	10 mg	IV	J0565
Bicillin C-R	100,000 units		J0558
Bicillin C-R 900/300	100,000 units	IM	J0558, J0561
Bicillin L-A	100,000 units	IM	J0561
BiCNU	100 mg	IV	J9050
Biperiden lactate	per 5 mg	IM, IV	J0190
Bitolterol mesylate			
concentrated form	per mg	INH	J7628
unit dose form	per mg	INH	J7629
Bivalirudin	1 mg	IV	J0583

◀ New ⤾ Revised ✔ Reinstated ~~deleted~~ Deleted

DRUG NAME	DOSAGE	METHOD OF ADMINISTRATION	HCPCS CODE
Blenoxane	15 units	IM, IV, SC	J9040
Bleomycin sulfate	15 units	IM, IV, SC	**J9040**
Blinatumomab	1 microgram	IV	**J9039**
Blincyto	1 mcg		J9039
Boniva	1 mg		J1740
Bortezomib	0.1 mg	IV	**J9041**
Bortezomib, not otherwise specified	0.1 mg		**J9044** ◀
Botox	1 unit		J0585
Bravelle	75 IU		J3355
Brentuximab Vedotin	1 mg	IV	**J9042**
Brethine			
concentrated form	per 1 mg	INH	J7680
unit dose	per 1 mg	INH	J7681
	up to 1 mg	SC, IV	J3105
Bricanyl Subcutaneous	up to 1 mg	SC, IV	J3105
Brompheniramine maleate	per 10 mg	IM, SC, IV	**J0945**
Bronkephrine, *see* Ethylnorepinephrine HCl			
Bronkosol			
concentrated form	per mg	INH	J7647, J7648
unit dose form	per mg	INH	J7649, J7650
Brovana			J7605
Budesonide inhalation solution			
concentrated form	0.25 mg	INH	**J7633, J7634**
unit dose form	0.5 mg	INH	**J7626, J7627**
Bumetanide			J3490
Bupivacaine			J3490
Buprenex	0.3 mg		J0592
Buprenorphine Hydrochloride	0.1 mg	IM	**J0592**
Buprenorphine/Naloxone	1 mg	ORAL	**J0571**
	< = 3 mg	ORAL	**J0572**
	> 3 mg but < = 6 mg	ORAL	**J0573**
	> 6 mg but < = 10 mg	ORAL	**J0574**
	> 10 mg	ORAL	**J0575**
Buprenorphine extended release	< = 100 mg	ORAL	**Q9991** ◀
	> 100 mg	ORAL	**Q9992** ◀
Burosumab-twza	1 mg	IV	**J05894** ◀
Busulfan	1 mg	IV	**J0594**
	2 mg	ORAL	**J8510**
Butorphanol tartrate	1 mg		**J0595**

◀ **New** ↩ **Revised** ✔ **Reinstated** ~~deleted~~ **Deleted**

DRUG NAME	DOSAGE	METHOD OF ADMINISTRATION	HCPCS CODE
C			
C1 Esterase Inhibitor	10 units	IV	J0596-J0599 ↩
Cabazitaxel	1 mg	IV	J9043
Cabergoline	0.25 mg	ORAL	J8515
Cafcit	5 mg	IV	J0706
Caffeine citrate	5 mg	IV	J0706
Caine-1	10 mg	IV	J2001
Caine-2	10 mg	IV	J2001
Calcijex	0.1 mcg	IM	J0636
Calcimar	up to 400 units	SC, IM	J0630
Calcitonin-salmon	up to 400 units	SC, IM	J0630
Calcitriol	0.1 mcg	IM	J0636
Calcitrol			J8499
Calcium Disodium Versenate	up to 1,000 mg	IV, SC, IM	J0600
Calcium gluconate	per 10 ml	IV	J0610
Calcium glycerophosphate and calcium lactate	per 10 ml	IM, SC	J0620
Caldolor	100 mg	IV	J1741
Calphosan	per 10 ml	IM, SC	J0620
Camptosar	20 mg	IV	J9206
Canakinumab	1 mg	SC	J0638
Cancidas	5 mg		J0637
Capecitabine	150 mg	ORAL	J8520
	500 mg	ORAL	J8521
Capsaicin patch	per sq cm	OTH	J7336
Carbidopa 5 mg/levodopa 20 mg enteral suspension		IV	J7340
Carbocaine	per 10 ml	VAR	J0670
Carbocaine with Neo-Cobefrin	per 10 ml	VAR	J0670
Carboplatin	50 mg	IV	J9045
Carfilzomib	1 mg	IV	J9047
Carimune	500 mg		J1566
Carmustine	100 mg	IV	J9050
Carnitor	per 1 g	IV	J1955
Carticel			J7330
Caspofungin acetate	5 mg	IV	J0637
Cathflo Activase	1 mg		J2997
Caverject	per 1.25 mcg		J0270
Cayston	500 mg		S0073
Cefadyl	up to 1 g	IV, IM	J0710
Cefazolin sodium	500 mg	IV, IM	J0690
Cefepime hydrochloride	500 mg	IV	J0692

◀ New ↩ Revised ✔ Reinstated ~~deleted~~ Deleted

DRUG NAME	DOSAGE	METHOD OF ADMINISTRATION	HCPCS CODE
Cefizox	per 500 mg	IM, IV	J0715
Cefotaxime sodium	per 1 g	IV, IM	J0698
Cefotetan			J3490
Cefoxitin sodium	1 g	IV, IM	J0694
Ceftaroline fosamil	1 mg		J0712
Ceftazidime	per 500 mg	IM, IV	J0713
Ceftazidime and avibactam	0.5 g/0.125 g	IV	J0714
Ceftizoxime sodium	per 500 mg	IV, IM	J0715
Ceftolozane 50 mg and Tazobactam 25 mg		IV	J0695
Ceftriaxone sodium	per 250 mg	IV, IM	J0696
Cefuroxime sodium, sterile	per 750 mg	IM, IV	J0697
Celestone Soluspan	per 3 mg	IM	J0702
CellCept	250 mg	ORAL	J7517
Cel-U-Jec	per 4 mg	IM, IV	Q0511
Cenacort A-40	1 mg		J3300
	per 10 mg	IM	J3301
Cenacort Forte	per 5 mg	IM	J3302
Centruroides Immune F(ab)	up to 120 mg	IV	J0716
Cephalothin sodium	up to 1 g	IM, IV	J1890
Cephapirin sodium	up to 1 g	IV, IM	J0710
Ceprotin	10 IU		J2724
Ceredase	per 10 units	IV	J0205
Cerezyme	10 units		J1786
Cerliponase alfa	1 mg	IV	J0567 ◀
Certolizumab pegol	1 mg	SC	J0717
Cerubidine	10 mg	IV	J9150
Cetuximab	10 mg	IV	J9055
Chealamide	per 150 mg	IV	J3520
Chirhostim	1 mcg	IV	J2850
Chloramphenicol Sodium Succinate	up to 1 g	IV	J0720
Chlordiazepoxide HCl	up to 100 mg	IM, IV	J1990
Chloromycetin Sodium Succinate	up to 1 g	IV	J0720
Chloroprocaine HCl	per 30 ml	VAR	J2400
Chloroquine HCl	up to 250 mg	IM	J0390
Chlorothiazide sodium	per 500 mg	IV	J1205
Chlorpromazine	5 mg	ORAL	Q0161
Chlorpromazine HCl	up to 50 mg	IM, IV	J3230
Cholografin Meglumine	per ml		Q9961
Chorex-5	per 1,000 USP units	IM	J0725
Chorex-10	per 1,000 USP units	IM	J0725

◀ New ⤺ Revised ✔ Reinstated ~~deleted~~ Deleted

DRUG NAME	DOSAGE	METHOD OF ADMINISTRATION	HCPCS CODE
Chorignon	per 1,000 USP units	IM	J0725
Chorionic Gonadotropin	per 1,000 USP units	IM	**J0725**
Choron 10	per 1,000 USP units	IM	J0725
Cidofovir	375 mg	IV	**J0740**
Cilastatin sodium, imipenem	per 250 mg	IV, IM	**J0743**
Cimzia	1 mg	SC	J0717
Cinacalcet		ORAL	**J0604**
Cinryze	10 units		J0598
Cipro IV	200 mg	IV	J0706
Ciprofloxacin	200 mg	IV	**J0706**
octic suspension	6 mg	OTH	**J7342**
			J3490
Cisplatin, powder or solution	per 10 mg	IV	**J9060**
Cladribine	per mg	IV	**J9065**
Claforan	per 1 gm	IM, IV	J0698
Cleocin Phosphate			J3490
Clindamycin			J3490
Clofarabine	1 mg	IV	**J9027**
Clolar	1 mg		J9027
Clonidine Hydrochloride	1 mg	Epidural	**J0735**
Cobex	up to 1,000 mcg	IM, SC	J3420
Codeine phosphate	per 30 mg	IM, IV, SC	**J0745**
Codimal-A	per 10 mg	IM, SC, IV	J0945
Cogentin	per 1 mg	IM, IV	J0515
Colistimethate sodium	up to 150 mg	IM, IV	**J0770**
Collagenase, Clostridium Histolyticum	0.01 mg	OTH	**J0775**
Coly-Mycin M	up to 150 mg	IM, IV	J0770
Compa-Z	up to 10 mg	IM, IV	J0780
Copanlisib	1 mg	IV	**J9057** ◀
Compazine	up to 10 mg	IM, IV	J0780
	5 mg	ORAL	Q0164
			J8498
Compounded drug, not otherwise classified			**J7999**
Compro			J8498
Conray	per ml		Q9961
Conray 30	per ml		Q9958
Conray 43	per ml		Q9960
Copaxone	20 mg		J1595
Cophene-B	per 10 mg	IM, SC, IV	J0945
Copper contraceptive, intrauterine		OTH	**J7300**

◀ New ⤾ Revised ✔ Reinstated ~~deleted~~ Deleted

DRUG NAME	DOSAGE	METHOD OF ADMINISTRATION	HCPCS CODE
Cordarone	30 mg	IV	J0282
Corgonject-5	per 1,000 USP units	IM	J0725
Corifact	1 IU		J7180
Corticorelin ovine triflutate	1 mcg		J0795
Corticotropin	up to 40 units	IV, IM, SC	J0800
Cortisone Acetate Micronized			J3490
Cortrosyn	per 0.25 mg	IM, IV	J0835
Corvert	1 mg		J1742
Cosmegen	0.5 mg	IV	J9120
Cosyntropin	per 0.25 mg	IM, IV	J0833, J0834
Cotranzine	up to 10 mg	IM, IV	J0780
Crofab	up to 1 gram		J0840
Cromolyn Sodium			J8499
Cromolyn sodium, unit dose form	per 10 mg	INH	J7631, J7632
Crotalidae immune f(ab')2 (equine)	120 mg	IV	J0841 ◀
Crotalidae Polyvalent Immune Fab	up to 1 gram	IV	J0840
~~Crysticillin 300 A.S.~~	~~up to 600,000 units~~	~~IM, IV~~	~~J2510~~ ✖
Crysticillin 600 A.S.	up to 600,000 units	IM, IV	J2510
Cubicin	1 mg		J0878
Cuvitru			J7799
Cyclophosphamide	100 mg	IV	J9070
oral	25 mg	ORAL	J8530
Cyclosporine	25 mg	ORAL	J7515
	100 mg	ORAL	J7502
parenteral	250 mg	IV	J7516
Cymetra	1 cc		Q4112
Cyramza	5 mg		J9308
Cysto-Cornray II	per ml		Q9958
Cystografin	per ml		Q9958
Cytarabine	100 mg	SC, IV	J9100
Cytarabine liposome	10 mg	IT	J9098
CytoGam	per vial		J0850
Cytomegalovirus immune globulin intravenous (human)	per vial	IV	J0850
Cytosar-U	100 mg	SC, IV	J9100
Cytovene	500 mg	IV	J1570
Cytoxan	100 mg	IV	J8530, J9070
D			
D-5-W, infusion	1000 cc	IV	J7070
Dacarbazine	100 mg	IV	J9130
Daclizumab	25 mg	IV	J7513

◀ New ↩ Revised ✔ Reinstated ~~deleted~~ Deleted

DRUG NAME	DOSAGE	METHOD OF ADMINISTRATION	HCPCS CODE
Dacogen	1 mg		J0894
Dactinomycin	0.5 mg	IV	J9120
Dalalone	1 mg	IM, IV, OTH	J1100
Dalalone L.A.	1 mg	IM	J1094
Dalbavancin	5 mg	IV	J0875
Dalteparin sodium	per 2500 IU	SC	J1645
Daptomycin	1 mg	IV	J0878
Daratumumab	10 mg	IV	J9145
Darbepoetin Alfa	1 mcg	IV, SC	J0881, J0882
Darzalex	10 mg		J9145
Daunorubicin citrate, liposomal formulation	10 mg	IV	J9151
Daunorubicin HCl	10 mg	IV	J9150
Daunoxome	10 mg	IV	J9151
DDAVP	1 mcg	IV, SC	J2597
Decadron	1 mg	IM, IV, OTH	J1100
	0.25 mg		J8540
Decadron Phosphate	1 mg	IM, IV, OTH	J1100
Decadron-LA	1 mg	IM	J1094
Deca-Durabolin	up to 50 mg	IM	J2320
Decaject	1 mg	IM, IV, OTH	J1100
Decaject-L.A.	1 mg	IM	J1094
Decitabine	1 mg	IV	J0894
Decolone-50	up to 50 mg	IM	J2320
Decolone-100	up to 50 mg	IM	J2320
De-Comberol	1 mg		J1071
Deferoxamine mesylate	500 mg	IM, SC, IV	J0895
Definity	per ml		J3490, Q9957
Degarelix	1 mg	SC	J9155
Dehist	per 10 mg	IM, SC, IV	J0945
Deladumone	1 mg	IM	J3121
Deladumone OB	1 mg	IM	J3121
Delatest	1 mg	IM	J3121
Delatestadiol	1 mg	IM	J3121
Delatestryl	1 mg	IM	J3121
Delestrogen	up to 10 mg	IM	J1380
Delta-Cortef	5 mg	ORAL	J7510
Demadex	10 mg/ml	IV	J3265
Demerol HCl	per 100 mg	IM, IV, SC	J2175
Denileukin diftitox	300 mcg	IV	J9160
Denosumab	1 mg	SC	J0897
DepAndro 100	1 mg		J1071

◀ New ↩ Revised ✓ Reinstated ~~deleted~~ Deleted

DRUG NAME	DOSAGE	METHOD OF ADMINISTRATION	HCPCS CODE
DepAndro 200	1 mg		J1071
DepAndrogyn	1 mg		J1071
DepGynogen	up to 5 mg	IM	J1000
DepMedalone 40	20 mg	IM	J1020
	40 mg	IM	J1030
	80 mg	IM	J1040
DepMedalone 80	20 mg	IM	J1020
	40 mg	IM	J1030
	80 mg	IM	J1040
DepoCyt	10 mg		J9098
Depo-estradiol cypionate	up to 5 mg	IM	J1000
Depogen	up to 5 mg	IM	J1000
Depoject	20 mg	IM	J1020
	40 mg	IM	J1030
	80 mg	IM	J1040
Depo-Medrol	20 mg	IM	J1020
	40 mg	IM	J1030
	80 mg	IM	J1040
Depopred-40	20 mg	IM	J1020
	40 mg	IM	J1030
	80 mg	IM	J1040
Depopred-80	20 mg	IM	J1020
	40 mg	IM	J1030
	80 mg	IM	J1040
Depo-Provera Contraceptive	1 mg		J1050
Depotest	1 mg		J1071
Depo-Testadiol	1 mg		J1071
Depo-Testosterone	1 mg		J1071
Depotestrogen	1 mg		J1071
Dermagraft	per square centimeter		Q4106
Desferal Mesylate	500 mg	IM, SC, IV	J0895
Desmopressin acetate	1 mcg	IV, SC	J2597
Dexacen-4	1 mg	IM, IV, OTH	J1100
Dexacen LA-8	1 mg	IM	J1094
Dexamethasone			
concentrated form	per mg	INH	J7637
intravitreal implant	0.1 mg	OTH	J7312
unit form	per mg	INH	J7638
oral	0.25 mg	ORAL	J8540
acetate	1 mg	IM	J1094
sodium phosphate	1 mg	IM, IV, OTH	J1100

◀ New ↩ Revised ✔ Reinstated ~~deleted~~ Deleted

DRUG NAME	DOSAGE	METHOD OF ADMINISTRATION	HCPCS CODE
Dexasone	1 mg	IM, IV, OTH	J1100
Dexasone L.A.	1 mg	IM	J1094
Dexferrum	50 mg		J1750
Dexone	0.25 mg	ORAL	J8540
	1 mg	IM, IV, OTH	J1100
Dexone LA	1 mg	IM	J1094
Dexpak	0.25 mg	ORAL	J8540
Dexrazoxane hydrochloride	250 mg	IV	**J1190**
Dextran 40	500 ml	IV	**J7100**
Dextran 75	500 ml	IV	**J7110**
Dextrose 5%/normal saline solution	500 ml = 1 unit	IV	**J7042**
Dextrose/water (5%)	500 ml = 1 unit	IV	**J7060**
D.H.E. 45	per 1 mg		J1110
Diamox	up to 500 mg	IM, IV	J1120
Diazepam	up to 5 mg	IM, IV	**J3360**
Diazoxide	up to 300 mg	IV	**J1730**
Dibent	up to 20 mg	IM	J0500
Diclofenac sodium	37.5	IV	**J1130**
Dicyclomine HCl	up to 20 mg	IM	**J0500**
Didronel	per 300 mg	IV	J1436
Diethylstilbestrol diphosphate	250 mg	IV	**J9165**
Diflucan	200 mg	IV	J1450
DigiFab	per vial		J1162
Digoxin	up to 0.5 mg	IM, IV	**J1160**
Digoxin immune fab (ovine)	per vial		**J1162**
Dihydrex	up to 50 mg	IV, IM	J1200
	50 mg	ORAL	Q0163
Dihydroergotamine mesylate	per 1 mg	IM, IV	**J1110**
Dilantin	per 50 mg	IM, IV	J1165
Dilaudid	up to 4 mg	SC, IM, IV	J1170
	250 mg	OTH	S0092
Dilocaine	10 mg	IV	J2001
Dilomine	up to 20 mg	IM	J0500
Dilor	up to 500 mg	IM	J1180
Dimenhydrinate	up to 50 mg	IM, IV	**J1240**
Dimercaprol	per 100 mg	IM	**J0470**
Dimethyl sulfoxide	50%, 50 ml	OTH	J1212
Dinate	up to 50 mg	IM, IV	J1240
Dioval	up to 10 mg	IM	J1380
Dioval 40	up to 10 mg	IM	J1380

◀ New ↩ Revised ✔ Reinstated ~~deleted~~ Deleted

DRUG NAME	DOSAGE	METHOD OF ADMINISTRATION	HCPCS CODE
Dioval XX	up to 10 mg	IM	J1380
Diphenacen-50	up to 50 mg	IV, IM	J1200
	50 mg	ORAL	Q0163
Diphenhydramine HCl			
injection	up to 50 mg	IV, IM	J1200
oral	50 mg	ORAL	Q0163
Diprivan	10 mg		J2704
			J3490
Dipyridamole	per 10 mg	IV	J1245
Disotate	per 150 mg	IV	J3520
Di-Spaz	up to 20 mg	IM	J0500
Ditate-DS	1 mg	IM	J3121
Diuril Sodium	per 500 mg	IV	J1205
D-Med 80	20 mg	IM	J1020
	40 mg	IM	J1030
	80 mg	IM	J1040
DMSO, Dimethyl sulfoxide 50%	50 ml	OTH	J1212
Dobutamine HCl	per 250 mg	IV	J1250
Dobutrex	per 250 mg	IV	J1250
Docefrez	1 mg		J9171
Docetaxel	20 mg	IV	J9170
Dolasetron mesylate			
injection	10 mg	IV	J1260
tablets	100 mg	ORAL	Q0180
Dolophine HCl	up to 10 mg	IM, SC	J1230
Dommanate	up to 50 mg	IM, IV	J1240
Donbax	10 mg		J1267
Dopamine	40 mg		J1265
Dopamine HCl	40 mg		J1265
Doribax	10 mg		J1267
Doripenem	10 mg	IV	J1267
Dornase alpha, unit dose form	per mg	INH	J7639
Dotarem	0.1 ml		A9575
Doxercalciferol	1 mcg	IV	J1270
Doxil	10 mg	IV	J9000, Q2050
Doxorubicin HCL	10 mg	IV	J9000
Doxy	100 mg		J3490
Dramamine	up to 50 mg	IM, IV	J1240
Dramanate	up to 50 mg	IM, IV	J1240
Dramilin	up to 50 mg	IM, IV	J1240

◀ New ↩ Revised ✔ Reinstated ~~deleted~~ Deleted

DRUG NAME	DOSAGE	METHOD OF ADMINISTRATION	HCPCS CODE	
Dramocen	up to 50 mg	IM, IV	J1240	
Dramoject	up to 50 mg	IM, IV	J1240	
Dronabinol	2.5 mg	ORAL	**Q0167**	
Droperidol	up to 5 mg	IM, IV	**J1790**	
Droperidol and fentanyl citrate	up to 2 ml ampule	IM, IV	**J1810**	
Droxia		ORAL	J8999	
Drug administered through a metered dose inhaler		INH	**J3535**	
DTIC-Dome	100 mg	IV	J9130	
Dua-Gen L.A.	1 mg	IM	J3121	
DuoNeb	up to 2.5 mg		J7620	
Duopa	20 ml		J7340	
Duoval P.A.	1 mg	IM	J3121	
Durabolin	up to 50 mg	IM	J2320	
Duracillin A.S.	up to 600,000 units	IM, IV	J2510	
Duraclon	1 mg	Epidural	J0735	
Dura-Estrin	up to 5 mg	IM	J1000	
Duragen-10	up to 10 mg	IM	J1380	
Duragen-20	up to 10 mg	IM	J1380	
Duragen-40	up to 10 mg	IM	J1380	
Duralone-40	20 mg	IM	J1020	
	40 mg	IM	J1030	
	80 mg	IM	J1040	
Duralone-80	20 mg	IM	J1020	
	40 mg	IM	J1030	
	80 mg	IM	J1040	
Duralutin, *see* Hydroxyprogesterone Caproate				
Duramorph	up to 10 mg	IM, IV, SC	J2270, J2274	
Duratest-100	1 mg		J1071	
Duratest-200	1 mg		J1071	
Duratestrin	1 mg		J1071	
Durathate-200	1 mg	IM	J3121	
Durvalumab	10 mg	IV	**J9173**	◀
Dymenate	up to 50 mg	IM, IV	J1240	
Dyphylline	up to 500 mg	IM	**J1180**	
Dysport	5 units		J0586	
Dalvance	5 mg		J0875	
E				
Ecallantide	1 mg	SC	**J1290**	
Eculizumab	10 mg	IV	**J1300**	
Edaravone	1 mg	IV	**J1301**	◀

◀ **New** ⮌ **Revised** ✔ **Reinstated** ~~deleted~~ **Deleted**

DRUG NAME	DOSAGE	METHOD OF ADMINISTRATION	HCPCS CODE
Edetate calcium disodium	up to 1,000 mg	IV, SC, IM	**J0600**
Edetate disodium	per 150 mg	IV	**J3520**
Elaprase	1 mg		J1743
Elavil	up to 20 mg	IM	J1320
Elelyso	10 units		J3060
Eligard	7.5 mg		J9217
Elitek	0.5 mg		J2783
Ellence	2 mg		J9178
Elliotts B solution	1 ml	OTH	**J9175**
Eloctate	per IU		J7205
Elosulfase alfa	1 mg	IV	**J1322**
Elotuzumab	1 mg	IV	**J9176**
Eloxatin	0.5 mg		J9263
Elspar	10,000 units	IV, IM	J9020
Emend			J1453, J8501
Emete-Con, *see* Benzquinamide			
Eminase	30 units	IV	J0350
Empliciti	1 mg		J9176
Enbrel	25 mg	IM, IV	J1438
Endrate ethylenediamine-tetra-acetic acid	per 150 mg	IV	J3520
Enfuvirtide	1 mg	SC	**J1324**
Engerix-B			J3490
Enovil	up to 20 mg	IM	J1320
Enoxaparin sodium	10 mg	SC	**J1650**
Entyvio			J3380
Eovist	1 ml		A9581
Epinephrine			J7799
Epinephrine, adrenalin	0.1 mg	SC, IM	**J0171**
Epirubicin hydrochloride	2 mg		**J9178**
Epoetin alfa	100 units	IV, SC	**Q4081**
Epoetin alfa, non-ESRD use	1000 units	IV	**J0885**
Epoetin alfa, ESRD use	100 mg	IV, SC	**Q5105** ◀
Epoetin alfa, non-ESRD use	1000 units	IV	**Q5106** ◀
Epoetin beta, ESRD use	1 mcg	IV	**J0887**
Epoetin beta, non-ESRD use	1 mcg	IV	**J0888**
Epogen	1,000 units		J0885
			Q4081
Epoprostenol	0.5 mg	IV	**J1325**
Eptifibatide, injection	5 mg	IM, IV	**J1327**
Eraxis	1 mg	IV	J0348

◀ **New** ⮐ **Revised** ✔ **Reinstated** ~~deleted~~ **Deleted**

DRUG NAME	DOSAGE	METHOD OF ADMINISTRATION	HCPCS CODE
Erbitux	10 mg		J9055
Ergonovine maleate	up to 0.2 mg	IM, IV	J1330
Eribulin mesylate	0.1 mg	IV	J9179
Erivedge	150 mg		J8999
Ertapenem sodium	500 mg	IM, IV	J1335
Erwinase	1,000 units	IV, IM	J9019
	10,000 units	IV, IM	J9020
Erythromycin lactobionate	500 mg	IV	J1364
Estra-D	up to 5 mg	IM	J1000
Estradiol			
L.A.	up to 10 mg	IM	J1380
L.A. 20	up to 10 mg	IM	J1380
L.A. 40	up to 10 mg	IM	J1380
Estradiol Cypionate	up to 5 mg	IM	J1000
Estradiol valerate	up to 10 mg	IM	J1380
Estra-L 20	up to 10 mg	IM	J1380
Estra-L 40	up to 10 mg	IM	J1380
Estra-Testrin	1 mg	IM	J3121
Estro-Cyp	up to 5 mg	IM	J1000
Estrogen, conjugated	per 25 mg	IV, IM	J1410
Estroject L.A.	up to 5 mg	IM	J1000
Estrone	per 1 mg	IM	J1435
Estrone 5	per 1 mg	IM	J1435
Estrone Aqueous	per 1 mg	IM	J1435
Estronol	per 1 mg	IM	J1435
Estronol-L.A.	up to 5 mg	IM	J1000
Etanercept, injection	25 mg	IM, IV	J1438
Etelcalcetide	0.1 mg	IV	Q4078 ↩
Eteplirsen	10 mg	IV	J1428
Ethamolin	100 mg		J1430
Ethanolamine	100 mg		J1430, J3490
Ethyol	500 mg	IV	J0207
Etidronate disodium	per 300 mg	IV	J1436
Etonogestrel implant			J7307
Etopophos	10 mg	IV	J9181
Etoposide	10 mg	IV	J9181
oral	50 mg	ORAL	J8560
Euflexxa	per dose	OTH	J7323
Everolimus	0.25 mg	ORAL	J7527
Everone	1 mg	IM	J3121

◀ New ↩ Revised ✔ Reinstated ~~deleted~~ Deleted

DRUG NAME	DOSAGE	METHOD OF ADMINISTRATION	HCPCS CODE
Evomela	50 mg		J9245
Eylea	1 mg	OTH	J0178
F			
Fabrazyme	1 mg	IV	J0180
Factor IX			
anti-hemophilic factor, purified, non-recombinant	per IU	IV	**J7193**
anti-hemophilic factor, recombinant	per IU	IV	**J7195, J7200-J7202**
complex	per IU	IV	**J7194**
Factor VIIa (coagulation factor, recombinant)	1 mcg	IV	**J7189**
Factor VIII (anti-hemophilic factor)			
human	per IU	IV	**J7190**
porcine	per IU	IV	**J7191**
recombinant	per IU	IV	**J7182, J7185, J7192, J7188**
Factor VIII (anti-hemophilic factor recombinant)			
(Afstyla)	per IU	IV	**J7210**
(Kovaltry)	per IU	IV	**J7211**
Factor VIII Fc fusion (recombinant)	per IU	IV	**J7205, J7207, J7209**
Factor X (human)	per IU	IV	**J7175**
Factor XIII A-subunit (recombinant)	per IU	IV	**J7181**
Factors, other hemophilia clotting	per IU	IV	**J7196**
Factrel	per 100 mcg	SC, IV	J1620
Famotidine			J3490
Faslodex	25 mg		J9395
Feiba NF			J7198
Feiba VH Immuno	per IU	IV	J7196
Fentanyl citrate	0.1 mg	IM, IV	**J3010**
Feraheme	1 mg		Q0138, Q0139
Ferric carboxymaltose	1 mg	IV	**J1439**
Ferric pyrophosphate citrate solution	0.1 mg of iron	IV	**J1443**
Ferrlecit	12.5 mg		J2916
Ferumoxytol	1 mg		**Q0138, Q0139**
Filgrastim-aafi	1 mcg	IV	**Q5110** ◀
Filgrastim			
(G-CSF)	1 mcg	SC, IV	**J1442, Q5101**
(TBO)	1 mcg	IV	**J1447**
Firazyr	1 mg	SC	J1744
Firmagon	1 mg		J9155
Flebogamma	500 mg	IV	**J1572**
	1 cc		J1460

◀ **New** ↩ **Revised** ✔ **Reinstated** ~~deleted~~ **Deleted**

DRUG NAME	DOSAGE	METHOD OF ADMINISTRATION	HCPCS CODE
Flexoject	up to 60 mg	IV, IM	J2360
Flexon	up to 60 mg	IV, IM	J2360
Flolan	0.5 mg	IV	J1325
Flo-Pred	5 mg		J7510
Florbetaben f18, diagnostic	per study dose	IV	Q9983
Floxuridine	500 mg	IV	J9200
Fluconazole	200 mg	IV	J1450
Fludara	1 mg	ORAL	J8562
	50 mg	IV	J9185
Fludarabine phosphate	1 mg	ORAL	J8562
	50 mg	IV	J9185
Flunisolide inhalation solution, unit dose form	per mg	INH	J7641
Fluocinolone		OTH	J7311, J7313
Fluorouracil	500 mg	IV	J9190
Fluphenazine decanoate	up to 25 mg		J2680
Flutamide			J8999
Flutemetamol f18, diagnostic	per study dose	IV	Q9982
Folex	5 mg	IA, IM, IT, IV	J9250
	50 mg	IA, IM, IT, IV	J9260
Folex PFS	5 mg	IA, IM, IT, IV	J9250
	50 mg	IA, IM, IT, IV	J9260
Follutein	per 1,000 USP units	IM	J0725
Folotyn	1 mg		J9307
Fomepizole	15 mg		J1451
Fomivirsen sodium	1.65 mg	Intraocular	J1452
Fondaparinux sodium	0.5 mg	SC	J1652
Formoterol	12 mcg	INH	J7640
Formoterol fumarate	20 mcg	INH	J7606
Fortaz	per 500 mg	IM, IV	J0713
Fosaprepitant	1 mg	IV	J1453
Foscarnet sodium	per 1,000 mg	IV	J1455
Foscavir	per 1,000 mg	IV	J1455
Fosnetupitant 235 mg and palonosetron 0.25 mg		IV	J1454 ◀
Fosphenytoin	50 mg	IV	Q2009
Fragmin	per 2,500 IU		J1645
FUDR	500 mg	IV	J9200
Fulvestrant	25 mg	IM	J9395
Fungizone intravenous	50 mg	IV	J0285
Furomide M.D.	up to 20 mg	IM, IV	J1940
Furosemide	up to 20 mg	IM, IV	J1940

◀ **New** ⤺ **Revised** ✔ **Reinstated** ~~deleted~~ **Deleted**

DRUG NAME	DOSAGE	METHOD OF ADMINISTRATION	HCPCS CODE
G			
Gablofen	10 mg		J0475
	50 mcg		J0476
Gadavist	0.1 ml		A9585
Gadoxetate disodium	1 ml	IV	**A9581**
Gallium nitrate	1 mg	IV	**J1457**
Galsulfase	1 mg	IV	**J1458**
Gamastan	1 cc	IM	J1460
	over 10 cc	IM	J1560
Gamma globulin	1 cc	IM	**J1460**
	over 10 cc	IM	**J1560**
Gammagard Liquid	500 mg	IV	**J1569**
Gammagard S/D			J1566
GammaGraft	per square centimeter		Q4111
Gammaplex	500 mg	IV	**J1557**
Gammar	1 cc	IM	J1460
	over 10 cc	IM	J1560
Gammar-IV, *see* Immune globin intravenous (human)			
Gamulin RH			
immune globulin, human	100 IU		J2791
	1 dose package, 300 mcg	IM	J2790
immune globulin, human, solvent detergent	100 IU	IV	J2792
Gamunex	500 mg	IV	**J1561**
Ganciclovir, implant	4.5 mg	OTH	**J7310**
Ganciclovir sodium	500 mg	IV	**J1570**
Ganirelix			J3490
Garamycin, gentamicin	up to 80 mg	IM, IV	**J1580**
Gastrografin	per ml		Q9963
Gatifloxacin	10 mg	IV	**J1590**
Gazyva	10 mg		J9301
Gefitinib	250 mg	ORAL	**J8565**
Gel-One	per dose	OTH	**J7326**
Gemcitabine HCl	200 mg	IV	**J9201**
Gemsar	200 mg	IV	J9201
Gemtuzumab ozogamicin	5 mg	IV	**J9300** ↩
Gengraf	100 mg		J7502
	25 mg	ORAL	J7515
Genotropin	1 mg		J2941
Gentamicin Sulfate	up to 80 mg	IM, IV	J1580, J7699

◀ New ↩ Revised ✔ Reinstated ~~deleted~~ Deleted

DRUG NAME	DOSAGE	METHOD OF ADMINISTRATION	HCPCS CODE
Gentran	500 ml	IV	J7100
Gentran 75	500 ml	IV	J7110
Geodon	10 mg		J3486
Gesterol 50	per 50 mg		J2675
Glassia	10 mg	IV	J0257
Glatiramer Acetate	20 mg	SC	J1595
Gleevec (Film-Coated)	400 mg		J8999
GlucaGen	per 1 mg		J1610
Glucagon HCl	per 1 mg	SC, IM, IV	J1610
Glukor	per 1,000 USP units	IM	J0725
Glycopyrrolate			
concentrated form	per 1 mg	INH	J7642
unit dose form	per 1 mg	INH	J7643
Gold sodium thiomalate	up to 50 mg	IM	J1600
Golimumab	1 mg	IV	J1602
Gonadorelin HCl	per 100 mcg	SC, IV	J1620
Gonal-F			J3490
Gonic	per 1,000 USP units	IM	J0725
Goserelin acetate implant	per 3.6 mg	SC	J9202
Graftjacket	per square centimeter		Q4107
Graftjacket Xpress	1 cc		Q4113
Granisetron HCl			
extended release	0.1 mg	IV	J1627
injection	100 mcg	IV	J1626
oral	1 mg	ORAL	Q0166
Guselkumab	1 mg	IV	J1628 ◀
Gynogen L.A. A10	up to 10 mg	IM	J1380
Gynogen L.A. A20	up to 10 mg	IM	J1380
Gynogen L.A. A40	up to 10 mg	IM	J1380
H			
Halaven	0.1 mg		J9179
Haldol	up to 5 mg	IM, IV	J1630
Haloperidol	up to 5 mg	IM, IV	J1630
Haloperidol decanoate	per 50 mg	IM	J1631
Haloperidol Lactate	up to 5 mg		J1630
Hectoral	1 mcg	IV	J1270
Helixate FS	per IU		J7192
Hemin	1 mg		J1640
Hemofil M	per IU	IV	J7190
Hemophilia clotting factors (e.g., anti-inhibitors)	per IU	IV	J7198
NOC	per IU	IV	J7199

◀ New ⤺ Revised ✔ Reinstated ~~deleted~~ Deleted

DRUG NAME	DOSAGE	METHOD OF ADMINISTRATION	HCPCS CODE	
Hepagam B	0.5 ml	IM	**J1571**	
	0.5 ml	IV	**J1573**	
Heparin sodium	1,000 units	IV, SC	**J1644**	
Heparin sodium (heparin lock flush)	10 units	IV	**J1642**	
Heparin Sodium (Procine)	per 1,000 units		J1644	
Hep-Lock	10 units	IV	J1642	
Hep-Lock U/P	10 units	IV	J1642	
Herceptin	10 mg	IV	J9355	
Hexabrix 320	per ml		Q9967	
Hexadrol Phosphate	1 mg	IM, IV, OTH	J1100	
Hexaminolevulinate hydrochloride	100 mg	IV	**A9589**	◀
Histaject	per 10 mg	IM, SC, IV	J0945	
Histerone 50	up to 50 mg	IM	J3140	
Histerone 100	up to 50 mg	IM	J3140	
Histrelin				
acetate	10 mcg		**J1675**	
implant	50 mg	OTH	**J9225,** J9226	
Hizentra, *see* Immune globulin				
Humalog	per 5 units		J1815	
	per 50 units		J1817	
Human fibrinogen concentrate	100 mg	IV	**J7178**	
Human fibrinogen concentrate (fibryga)	1 mg	IV	**J7177**	◀
Humate-P	per IU		J7187	
Humatrope	1 mg		J2941	
Humira	20 mg		J0135	
Humulin	per 5 units		J1815	
	per 50 units		J1817	
Hyalgan, Spurtaz or VISCO-3		IA	**J7321**	
Hyaluronan or derivative	per dose	IV	**J7327**	
Durolane	1 mg	IA	**J7318**	◀
Gel-Syn	0.1 mg	IA	**J7328**	
Gelsyn-3	0.1 mg	IV	**J7328**	
Gen Visc 850	1 mg	IA	**J7320**	
Hymovis	1 mg	IA	**J7322**	
Trivisc	1 mg	IV	**J7329**	◀
Hyaluronic Acid			J3490	
Hyaluronidase	up to 150 units	SC, IV	**J3470**	
Hyaluronidase				
ovine	up to 999 units	VAR	**J3471**	
ovine	per 1000 units	VAR	**J3472**	
recombinant	1 usp	SC	**J3473**	

◀ **New** ↩ **Revised** ✔ **Reinstated** ~~deleted~~ **Deleted**

DRUG NAME	DOSAGE	METHOD OF ADMINISTRATION	HCPCS CODE
Hyate:C	per IU	IV	J7191
Hybolin Decanoate	up to 50 mg	IM	J2320
Hybolin Improved, *see* Nandrolone phenpropionate			
Hycamtin	0.25 mg	ORAL	J8705
	4 mg	IV	J9351
Hydralazine HCl	up to 20 mg	IV, IM	**J0360**
Hydrate	up to 50 mg	IM, IV	J1240
Hydrea			J8999
Hydrocortisone acetate	up to 25 mg	IV, IM, SC	**J1700**
Hydrocortisone sodium phosphate	up to 50 mg	IV, IM, SC	**J1710**
Hydrocortisone succinate sodium	up to 100 mg	IV, IM, SC	**J1720**
Hydrocortone Acetate	up to 25 mg	IV, IM, SC	J1700
Hydrocortone Phosphate	up to 50 mg	IM, IV, SC	J1710
Hydromorphone HCl	up to 4 mg	SC, IM, IV	**J1170**
Hydroxyprogesterone Caproate	1 mg	IM	**J1725**
(Makena)	10 mg	IV	**J1726**
NOS	10 mg	IV	**J1729**
Hydroxyurea			J8999
Hydroxyzine HCl	up to 25 mg	IM	**J3410**
Hydroxyzine Pamoate	25 mg	ORAL	**Q0177**
Hylan G-F 20		OTH	**J7322**
Hylenex	1 USP unit		J3473
Hyoscyamine sulfate	up to 0.25 mg	SC, IM, IV	**J1980**
Hyperrho S/D	300 mcg		J2790
	100 IU		J2792
Hyperstat IV	up to 300 mg	IV	J1730
Hyper-Tet	up to 250 units	IM	J1670
HypRho-D	300 mcg	IM	J2790
			J2791
	50 mcg		J2788
Hyrexin-50	up to 50 mg	IV, IM	J1200
Hyzine-50	up to 25 mg	IM	J3410
I			
Ibalizumab-uiyk	10 mg	IV	**J1746** ◀
Ibandronate sodium	1 mg	IV	**J1740**
Ibuprofen	100 mg	IV	**J1741**
Ibutilide fumarate	1 mg	IV	**J1742**
Icatibant	1 mg	SC	**J1744**
Idamycin	5 mg	IV	J9211
Idarubicin HCl	5 mg	IV	**J9211**
Idursulfase	1 mg	IV	**J1743**

◀ New   ↩ Revised   ✔ Reinstated   ~~deleted~~ Deleted

DRUG NAME	DOSAGE	METHOD OF ADMINISTRATION	HCPCS CODE
Ifex	1 g	IV	J9208
Ifosfamide	1 g	IV	J9208
Ilaris	1 mg		J0638
Iloprost	20 mcg	INH	Q4074
Ilotycin, *see* Erythromycin gluceptate			
Iluvien	0.01 mg		J7313
Imferon	50 mg		J1750
Imiglucerase	10 units	IV	J1786
Imitrex	6 mg	SC	J3030
Imlygic	per 1 million plaque forming units		J9325, J9999
Immune globulin			
Bivigam	500 mg	IV	J1556
Cuvitru	100 mg	IV	J1555
Flebogamma	500 mg	IV	J1572
Gammagard Liquid	500 mg	IV	J1569
Gammaplex	500 mg	IV	J1557
Gamunex	500 mg	IV	J1561
HepaGam B	0.5 ml	IM	J1571
	0.5 ml	IV	J1573
Hizentra	100 mg	SC	J1559
Hyaluronidase, (HYQVIA)	100 mg	IV	J1575
NOS	500 mg	IV	J1566, J1599
Octagam	500 mg	IV	J1568
Privigen	500 mg	IV	J1459
Rhophylac	100 IU	IM	J2791
Subcutaneous	100 mg	SC	J1562
Immunosuppressive drug, not otherwise classified			J7599
Imuran	50 mg	ORAL	J7500
	100 mg	IV	J7501
Inapsine	up to 5 mg	IM, IV	J1790
Incobotulinumtoxin type A	1 unit	IM	J0588
Increlex	1 mg		J2170
Inderal	up to 1 mg	IV	J1800
Infed	50 mg		J1750
Infergen	1 mcg	SC	J9212
Inflectra			Q5102
Infliximab			◀
dyyb	10 mg	IM, IV	Q5103 ◀
abda	10 mg	IM, IV	Q5104 ◀
qbtx	10 mg	IM, IV	Q5109 ◀

◀ **New** ↩ **Revised** ✔ **Reinstated** ~~deleted~~ **Deleted**

DRUG NAME	DOSAGE	METHOD OF ADMINISTRATION	HCPCS CODE	
~~Infliximab, injection~~	~~10 mg~~	~~IM, IV~~	~~J1745, Q5102~~	✖
Infumorph	10 mg		J2274	
Injectafer	1 mg		J1439	
Injection factor ix, glycopegylated	1 iu	IV	**J7203**	◀
Injection sulfur hexafluoride lipid microspheres	per ml	IV	**Q9950**	
Innohep	1,000 iu	SC	J1655	
Innovar	up to 2 ml ampule	IM, IV	J1810	
Inotuzumab orogamicin	0.1 mg	IV	**J9229**	◀
Insulin	5 units	SC	**J1815**	
Insulin-Humalog	per 50 units		J1817	
Insulin lispro	50 units	SC	**J1817**	
Intal	per 10 mg	INH	J7631, J7632	
Integra				
Bilayer Matrix Wound Dressing (BMWD)	per square centimeter		Q4104	
Dermal Regeneration Template (DRT)	per square centimeter		Q4105	
Flowable Wound Matrix	1 cc		Q4114	
Matrix	per square centimeter		Q4108	
Integrilin	5 mg	IM, IV	J1327	
Interferon alfa-2a, recombinant	3 million units	SC, IM	**J9213**	
Interferon alfa-2b, recombinant	1 million units	SC, IM	**J9214**	
Interferon alfa-n3 (human leukocyte derived)	250,000 IU	IM	**J9215**	
Interferon alphacon-1, recombinant	1 mcg	SC	**J9212**	
Interferon beta-1a	30 mcg	IM	**J1826**	
	1 mcg	IM	**Q3027**	
	1 mcg	SC	**Q3028**	
Interferon beta-1b	0.25 mg	SC	**J1830**	
Interferon gamma-1b	3 million units	SC	**J9216**	
Intrauterine copper contraceptive		OTH	J7300	
Intron-A	1 million units		J9214	
Invanz	500 mg		J1335	
Invega Sustenna	1 mg		J2426	
Ipilimumab	1 mg	IV	**J9228**	
Ipratropium bromide, unit dose form	per mg	INH	J3535, J7620, **J7644, J7645**	
Iressa	250 mg		J8565	
Irinotecan	20 mg	IV	**J9206, J9205**	
Iron dextran	50 mg	IV, IM	**J1750**	
Iron sucrose	1 mg	IV	**J1756**	
Irrigation solution for Tx of bladder calculi	per 50 ml	OTH	**Q2004**	
Isavuconazonium	1 mg	IV	**J1833**	
Isocaine HCl	per 10 ml	VAR	J0670	

◀ **New** ↩ **Revised** ✔ **Reinstated** ~~deleted~~ **Deleted**

DRUG NAME	DOSAGE	METHOD OF ADMINISTRATION	HCPCS CODE
Isoetharine HCl			
concentrated form	per mg	INH	**J7647, J7648**
unit dose form	per mg	INH	**J7649, J7650**
Isoproterenol HCl			
concentrated form	per mg	INH	**J7657, J7658**
unit dose form	per mg	INH	**J7659, J7660**
Isovue	per ml		Q9966, Q9967
Istodax	1 mg		J9315
Isuprel			
concentrated form	per mg	INH	J7657, J7658
unit dose form	per mg	INH	J7659, J7660
Itraconazole	50 mg	IV	**J1835**
Ixabepilone	1 mg	IV	**J9207**
Ixempra	1 mg		J9207
J			
Jenamicin	up to 80 mg	IM, IV	J1580
Jetrea	0.125 mg		J7316
Jevtana	1 mg		J9043
K			
Kabikinase	per 250,000 IU	IV	J2995
Kadcyla	1 mg		J9354
Kalbitor	1 mg		J1290
Kaleinate	per 10 ml	IV	J0610
Kanamycin sulfate	up to 75 mg	IM, IV	**J1850**
	up to 500 mg	IM, IV	**J1840**
Kantrex	up to 75 mg	IM, IV	J1850
	up to 500 mg	IM, IV	J1840
Keflin	up to 1 g	IM, IV	J1890
Kefurox	per 750 mg		J0697
Kefzol	500 mg	IV, IM	J0690
Kenaject-40	1 mg		J3300
	per 10 mg	IM	J3301
Kenalog-10	1 mg		J3300
	per 10 mg	IM	J3301
Kenalog-40	1 mg		J3300
	per 10 mg	IM	J3301
Kepivance	50 mcg		J2425
Keppra	10 mg		J1953
Keroxx	1 cc	IV	**Q4202** ◀
Kestrone 5	per 1 mg	IM	J1435

◀ New ↩ Revised ✔ Reinstated ~~deleted~~ Deleted

DRUG NAME	DOSAGE	METHOD OF ADMINISTRATION	HCPCS CODE
Ketorolac tromethamine	per 15 mg	IM, IV	J1885
Key-Pred 25	up to 1 ml	IM	J2650
Key-Pred 50	up to 1 ml	IM	J2650
Key-Pred-SP, *see* Prednisolone sodium phosphate			
Keytruda	1 mg		J9271
K-Flex	up to 60 mg	IV, IM	J2360
Kinevac	5 mcg	IV	J2805
Kitabis PAK	per 300 mg		J7682
Klebcil	up to 75 mg	IM, IV	J1850
	up to 500 mg	IM, IV	J1840
Koate-HP (anti-hemophilic factor)			
human	per IU	IV	J7190
porcine	per IU	IV	J7191
recombinant	per IU	IV	J7192
Kogenate			
human	per IU	IV	J7190
porcine	per IU	IV	J7191
recombinant	per IU	IV	J7192
Konakion	per 1 mg	IM, SC, IV	J3430
Konyne-80	per IU	IV	J7194
Krystexxa	1 mg		J2507
Kyleena	19.5 mg	OTH	J7296 ⮐
Kyprolis	1 mg		J9047
Kytril	1 mg	ORAL	Q0166
	1 mg	IV	S0091
	100 mcg	IV	J1626
L			
L.A.E. 20	up to 10 mg	IM	J1380
Laetrile, Amygdalin, vitamin B-17			J3570
Lanoxin	up to 0.5 mg	IM, IV	J1160
Lanreotide	1 mg	SC	J1930
Lantus	per 5 units		J1815
Largon, *see* Propiomazine HCl			
Laronidase	0.1 mg	IV	J1931
Lasix	up to 20 mg	IM, IV	J1940
L-Caine	10 mg	IV	J2001
Lemtrada	1 mg		J0202
Lepirudin	50 mg		J1945
Leucovorin calcium	per 50 mg	IM, IV	J0640
Leukeran			J8999

◀ New ⮐ Revised ✔ Reinstated ~~deleted~~ Deleted

DRUG NAME	DOSAGE	METHOD OF ADMINISTRATION	HCPCS CODE
Leukine	50mcg	IV	J2820
Leuprolide acetate	per 1 mg	IM	**J9218**
Leuprolide acetate (for depot suspension)	per 3.75 mg	IM	**J1950**
	7.5 mg	IM	**J9217**
Leuprolide acetate implant	65 mg	OTH	**J9219**
Leustatin	per mg	IV	J9065
Levalbuterol HCl			
concentrated form	0.5 mg	INH	**J7607, J7612**
unit dose form	0.5 mg	INH	**J7614, J7615**
Levaquin I.U.	250 mg	IV	J1956
Levetiracetam	10 mg	IV	**J1953**
Levocarnitine	per 1 gm	IV	**J1955**
Levo-Dromoran	up to 2 mg	SC, IV	J1960
Levofloxacin	250 mg	IV	**J1956**
Levoleucovorin calcium	0.5 mg	IV	**J0641**
Levonorgestrel implant		OTH	**J7306**
Levonorgestrel-releasing intrauterine contraceptive system	52 mg	OTH	**J7297, J7298**
Kyleena	19.5 mg	OTH	**J7296**
Levorphanol tartrate	up to 2 mg	SC, IV	**J1960**
Levsin	up to 0.25 mg	SC, IM, IV	J1980
Levulan Kerastick	unit dose (354 mg)	OTH	J7308
Lexiscan	0.1 mg		J2785
Librium	up to 100 mg	IM, IV	J1990
Lidocaine HCl	10 mg	IV	**J2001**
Lidoject-1	10 mg	IV	J2001
Lidoject-2	10 mg	IV	J2001
Liletta	52 mg	OTH	J7297
Lincocin	up to 300 mg	IV	J2010
Lincomycin HCl	up to 300 mg	IV	**J2010**
Linezolid	200 mg	IV	**J2020**
Lioresal	10 mg	IT	J0475
			J0476
Liposomal			◀
Cytarabine	2.27 mg	IV	**J9153** ◀
Daunorubicin	1 mg	IV	**J9153** ◀
Liquaemin Sodium	1,000 units	IV, SC	J1644
LMD (10%)	500 ml	IV	J7100
Locort	1.5 mg		J8540
Lorazepam	2 mg	IM, IV	**J2060**
Lovenox	10 mg	SC	J1650

◀ **New** ⤾ **Revised** ✓ **Reinstated** ~~deleted~~ **Deleted**

DRUG NAME	DOSAGE	METHOD OF ADMINISTRATION	HCPCS CODE
Loxapine	1 mg	OTH	J2062 ◀
Lucentis	0.1 mg		J2778
Lufyllin	up to 500 mg	IM	J1180
Lumason	per ml		Q9950
Luminal Sodium	up to 120 mg	IM, IV	J2560
Lumizyme	10 mg		J0221
Lupon Depot	7.5 mg		J9217
	3.75 mg		J1950
Lupron	per 1 mg	IM	J9218
	per 3.75 mg	IM	J1950
	7.5 mg	IM	J9217
Lyophilized, *see* Cyclophosphamide, lyophilized			
M			
Macugen	0.3 mg		J2503
Magnesium sulfate	500 mg		J3475
Magnevist	per ml		A9579
Makena	1 mg		J1725
Mannitol	25% in 50 ml	IV	J2150
	5 mg	INH	J7665
Marcaine			J3490
Marinol	2.5 mg	ORAL	Q0167
Marmine	up to 50 mg	IM, IV	J1240
Matulane	50 mg		J8999
Maxipime	500 mg	IV	J0692
MD-76R	per ml		Q9963
MD Gastroview	per ml		Q9963
Mecasermin	1 mg	SC	J2170
Mechlorethamine HCl (nitrogen mustard), HN2	10 mg	IV	J9230
Medralone 40	20 mg	IM	J1020
	40 mg	IM	J1030
	80 mg	IM	J1040
Medralone 80	20 mg	IM	J1020
	40 mg	IM	J1030
	80 mg	IM	J1040
Medrol	per 4 mg	ORAL	J7509
Medroxyprogesterone acetate	1 mg	IM	J1050
Mefoxin	1 g	IV, IM	J0694
Megestrol Acetate			J8999
Melphalan HCl	50 mg	IV	J9245
Melphalan, oral	2 mg	ORAL	J8600

◀ **New** ↩ **Revised** ✓ **Reinstated** ~~deleted~~ **Deleted**

DRUG NAME	DOSAGE	METHOD OF ADMINISTRATION	HCPCS CODE
Menoject LA	1 mg		J1071
Mepergan injection	up to 50 mg	IM, IV	J2180
Meperidine and promethazine HCl	up to 50 mg	IM, IV	**J2180**
Meperidine HCl	per 100 mg	IM, IV, SC	**J2175**
Mepivacaine HCl	per 10 ml	VAR	**J0670**
Mepolizumab	1 mg	IV	**J2182**
Mercaptopurine			J8999
Meropenem	100 mg	IV	**J2185**
Merrem	100 mg		J2185
Mesna	200 mg	IV	**J9209**
Mesnex	200 mg	IV	J9209
Metaprel			
concentrated form	per 10 mg	INH	J7667, J7668
unit dose form	per 10 mg	INH	J7669, J7670
Metaproterenol sulfate			
concentrated form	per 10 mg	INH	**J7667, J7668**
unit dose form	per 10 mg	INH	**J7669, J7670**
Metaraminol bitartrate	per 10 mg	IV, IM, SC	**J0380**
Metastron	per millicurie		A9600
Methacholine chloride	1 mg	INH	**J7674**
Methadone HCl	up to 10 mg	IM, SC	**J1230**
Methergine	up to 0.2 mg		J2210
Methocarbamol	up to 10 ml	IV, IM	**J2800**
Methotrexate LPF	5mg	IV, IM, IT, IA	J9250
	50 mg	IV, IM, IT, IA	J9260
Methotrexate, oral	2.5 mg	ORAL	**J8610**
Methotrexate sodium	5 mg	IV, IM, IT, IA	**J9250**
	50 mg	IV, IM, IT, IA	**J9260**
Methyldopate HCl	up to 250 mg	IV	**J0210**
Methylergonovine maleate	up to 0.2 mg		J2210
Methylnaltrexone	0.1 mg	SC	**J2212**
Methylprednisolone acetate	20 mg	IM	**J1020**
	40 mg	IM	**J1030**
	80 mg	IM	**J1040**
Methylprednisolone, oral	per 4 mg	ORAL	**J7509**
Methylprednisolone sodium succinate	up to 40 mg	IM, IV	**J2920**
	up to 125 mg	IM, IV	**J2930**
Metoclopramide HCl	up to 10 mg	IV	**J2765**
Metrodin	75 IU		J3355
Metronidazole			J3490

◀ **New** ↩ **Revised** ✔ **Reinstated** ~~deleted~~ **Deleted**

DRUG NAME	DOSAGE	METHOD OF ADMINISTRATION	HCPCS CODE
Metvixia	1 g	OTH	J7309
Miacalcin	up to 400 units	SC, IM	J0630
Micafungin sodium	1 mg		J2248
MicRhoGAM	50 mcg		J2788
Midazolam HCl	per 1 mg	IM, IV	J2250
Milrinone lactate	5 mg	IV	J2260
Minocine	1 mg		J2265
Minocycline Hydrochloride	1 mg	IV	J2265
Mircera	1 mcg		J0887, J0888
Mirena	52 mg	OTH	J7297, J7298
Mithracin	2,500 mcg	IV	J9270
Mitomycin	0.2 mg	Ophthalmic	J7315
	5 mg	IV	J9280
Mitosol	0.2 mg	Ophthalmic	J7315
	5 mg	IV	J9280
Mitoxantrone HCl	per 5 mg	IV	J9293
Monocid, *see* Cefonicic sodium			
Monoclate-P			
human	per IU	IV	J7190
porcine	per IU	IV	J7191
Monoclonal antibodies, parenteral	5 mg	IV	J7505
Mononine	per IU	IV	J7193
Monovisc			J7327
Morphine sulfate	up to 10 mg	IM, IV, SC	J2270
preservative-free	10 mg	SC, IM, IV	J2274
Moxifloxacin	100 mg	IV	J2280
Mozobil	1 mg		J2562
M-Prednisol-40	20 mg	IM	J1020
	40 mg	IM	J1030
	80 mg	IM	J1040
M-Prednisol-80	20 mg	IM	J1020
	40 mg	IM	J1030
	80 mg	IM	J1040
Mucomyst			
unit dose form	per gram	INH	J7604, J7608
Mucosol			
injection	100 mg	IV	J0132
unit dose	per gram	INH	J7604, J7608
MultiHance	per ml		A9577
MultiHance Multipack	per ml		A9578

◀ New ⤾ Revised ✔ Reinstated ~~deleted~~ Deleted

DRUG NAME	DOSAGE	METHOD OF ADMINISTRATION	HCPCS CODE
Muromonab-CD3	5 mg	IV	**J7505**
Muse		OTH	J0275
	1.25 mcg	OTH	J0270
Mustargen	10 mg	IV	J9230
Mutamycin			
	0.2 mg	Ophthalmic	**J7315**
	5 mg	IV	**J9280**
Mycamine	1 mg		J2248
Mycophenolate Mofetil	250 mg	ORAL	**J7517**
Mycophenolic acid	180 mg	ORAL	**J7518**
Myfortic	180 mg		J7518
Myleran	1 mg		J0594
	2 mg	ORAL	J8510
Mylotarg	5mg	IV	J9300
Myobloc	per 100 units	IM	J0587
Myochrysine	up to 50 mg	IM	J1600
Myolin	up to 60 mg	IV, IM	J2360
N			
Nabilone	1 mg	ORAL	**J8650**
Nafcillin			J3490
Naglazyme	1 mg		J1458
Nalbuphine HCl	per 10 mg	IM, IV, SC	**J2300**
Naloxone HCl	per 1 mg	IM, IV, SC	**J2310,** J3490
Naltrexone			J3490
Naltrexone, depot form	1 mg	IM	**J2315**
Nandrobolic L.A.	up to 50 mg	IM	J2320
Nandrolone decanoate	up to 50 mg	IM	**J2320**
Narcan	1 mg	IM, IV, SC	J2310
Naropin	1 mg		J2795
Nasahist B	per 10mg	IM, SC, IV	J0945
Nasal vaccine inhalation		INH	**J3530**
Natalizumab	1 mg	IV	**J2323**
Natrecor	0.1 mg		J2325
Navane, *see* Thiothixene			
Navelbine	per 10 mg	IV	J9390
ND Stat	per 10 mg	IM, SC, IV	J0945
Nebcin	up to 80 mg	IM, IV	J3260
NebuPent	per 300 mg	INH	J2545, J7676
Necitumumab	1 mg	IV	**J9295**
Nelarabine	50 mg	IV	**J9261**

◀ **New** ↩ **Revised** ✔ **Reinstated** ~~deleted~~ **Deleted**

DRUG NAME	DOSAGE	METHOD OF ADMINISTRATION	HCPCS CODE
Nembutal Sodium Solution	per 50 mg	IM, IV, OTH	J2515
Neocyten	up to 60 mg	IV, IM	J2360
Neo-Durabolic	up to 50 mg	IM	J2320
Neoquess	up to 20 mg	IM	J0500
Neoral	100 mg		J7502
	25 mg		J7515
Neosar	100 mg	IV	J9070
Neostigmine methylsulfate	up to 0.5 mg	IM, IV, SC	J2710
Neo-Synephrine	up to 1 ml	SC, IM, IV	J2370
Nervocaine 1%	10 mg	IV	J2001
Nervocaine 2%	10 mg	IV	J2001
Nesacaine	per 30 ml	VAR	J2400
Nesacaine-MPF	per 30 ml	VAR	J2400
Nesiritide	0.1 mg	IV	J2325
Netupitant 300 mg and palonosetron 0.5 mg		ORAL	J8655
Neulasta	6 mg		J2505
Neumega	5 mg	SC	J2355
Neupogen			
(G-CSF)	1 mcg	SC, IV	J1442
Neutrexin	per 25 mg	IV	J3305
Nipent	per 10 mg	IV	J9268
Nivolumab	1 mg	IV	J9299
Nolvadex			J8999
Nordryl	up to 50mg	IV, IM	J1200
	50mg	ORAL	Q0163
Norflex	up to 60 mg	IV, IM	J2360
Norzine	up to 10 mg	IM	J3280
Not otherwise classified drugs			J3490
other than inhalation solution administered through DME			J7799
inhalation solution administered through DME			J7699
anti-neoplastic			J9999
chemotherapeutic		ORAL	J8999
immunosuppressive			J7599
nonchemotherapeutic		ORAL	J8499
Novantrone	per 5 mg	IV	J9293
Novarel	per 1,000 USP Units		J0725
Novolin	per 5 units		J1815
	per 50 units		J1817
Novolog	per 5 units		J1815
	per 50 units		J1817

◀ New   ⤾ Revised   ✔ Reinstated   ~~deleted~~ Deleted

DRUG NAME	DOSAGE	METHOD OF ADMINISTRATION	HCPCS CODE
Novo Seven	1 mcg	IV	J7189
Novoeight			J7182
NPH	5 units	SC	J1815
Nplate	100 units		J0587
	10 mcg		J2796
Nubain	per 10 mg	IM, IV, SC	J2300
Nulecit	12.5 mg		J2916
Nulicaine	10 mg	IV	J2001
Nulojix	1 mg	IV	J0485
Numorphan	up to 1 mg	IV, SC, IM	J2410
Numorphan H.P.	up to 1 mg	IV, SC, IM	J2410
Nusinersen	0.1 mg	IV	J2326
Nutropin	1 mg		J2941
O			
Oasis Burn Matrix	per square centimeter		Q4103
Oasis Wound Matrix	per square centimeter		Q4102
Obinutuzumab	10 mg		J9301
Ocriplasmin	0.125 mg	IV	J7316
Ocrelizumab	1 mg	IV	J2350
Octagam	500 mg	IV	J1568
Octreotide Acetate, injection	1 mg	IM	J2353
	25 mcg	IV, SQ	J2354
Oculinum	per unit	IM	J0585
Ofatumumab	10 mg	IV	J9302
Ofev			J8499
Ofirmev	10 mg	IV	J0131
O-Flex	up to 60 mg	IV, IM	J2360
Oforta	10 mg		J8562
Olanzapine	1 mg	IM	J2358
Olaratumab	10 mg	IV	J9285
Omacetaxine Mepesuccinate	0.01 mg	IV	J9262
Omalizumab	5 mg	SC	J2357
Omnipaque	per ml		Q9965, Q9966, Q9967
Omnipen-N	up to 500 mg	IM, IV	J0290
	per 1.5 gm	IM, IV	J0295
Omniscan	per ml		A9579
Omnitrope	1 mg		J2941
Omontys	0.1 mg	IV, SC	J0890
OnabotulinumtoxinA	1 unit	IM	J0585

◀ New ↩ Revised ✔ Reinstated ~~deleted~~ Deleted

DRUG NAME	DOSAGE	METHOD OF ADMINISTRATION	HCPCS CODE
Oncaspar	per single dose vial	IM, IV	J9266
Oncovin	1 mg	IV	J9370
Ondansetron HCl	1 mg	IV	J2405
	1 mg	ORAL	Q0162
Onivyde	1 mg		J9205
Opana	up to 1 mg		J2410
Opdivo	1 mg		J9299
Oprelvekin	5 mg	SC	J2355
Optimark	per ml		A9579
Optiray	per ml		Q9966, Q9967
Optison	per ml		Q9956
Oraminic II	per10mg	IM, SC, IV	J0945
Orapred	per 5 mg	ORAL	J7510
Orbactiv	10 mg		J2407
Orencia	10 mg		J0129
Oritavancin	10 mg	IV	J2407
Ormazine	up to 50 mg	IM, IV	J3230
Orphenadrine citrate	up to 60 mg	IV, IM	J2360
Orphenate	up to 60 mg	IV, IM	J2360
Orthovisc		OTH	J7324
Or-Tyl	up to 20 mg	IM	J0500
Osmitrol			J7799
Ovidrel			J3490
Oxacillin sodium	up to 250 mg	IM, IV	J2700
Oxaliplatin	0.5 mg	IV	J9263
Oxilan	per ml		Q9967
Oxymorphone HCl	up to 1 mg	IV, SC, IM	J2410
Oxytetracycline HCl	up to 50 mg	IM	J2460
Oxytocin	up to 10 units	IV, IM	J2590
Ozurdex	0.1 mg		J7312
P			
Paclitaxel	1 mg	IV	J9267
Paclitaxel protein-bound particles	1 mg	IV	J9264
Palifermin	50 mcg	IV	J2425
Paliperidone Palmitate	1 mg	IM	J2426
Palonosetron HCl	25 mcg	IV	J2469
Netupitant 300 mg and palonosetron 0.5 mg		ORAL	J8655
Pamidronate disodium	per 30 mg	IV	J2430
Panhematin	1 mg		J1640
Panitumumab	10 mg	IV	J9303

◀ New ⤾ Revised ✔ Reinstated ~~deleted~~ Deleted

DRUG NAME	DOSAGE	METHOD OF ADMINISTRATION	HCPCS CODE	
Papaverine HCl	up to 60 mg	IV, IM	J2440	
Paragard T 380 A		OTH	J7300	
Paraplatin	50 mg	IV	J9045	
Paricalcitol, injection	1 mcg	IV, IM	J2501	
Pasireotide, long acting	1 mg	IV	J2502	
Pathogen(s) test for platelets		OTH	P9100	
Peforomist	20 mcg		J7606	
Pegademase bovine	25 IU		J2504	
Pegaptinib	0.3 mg	OTH	J2503	
Pegaspargase	per single dose vial	IM, IV	J9266	
Pegasys			J3490	
Pegfilgrastim	0.5 mg	SC	J2505	↩
Pegfilgrastim-jmdb	0.5 mg	SC	Q5108	◀
Peginesatide	0.1 mg	IV, SC	J0890	
Peg-Intron			J3490	
Pegloticase	1 mg	IV	J2507	
Pembrolizumab	1 mg	IV	J9271	
Pemetrexed	10 mg	IV	J9305	
Penicillin G Benzathine	100,000 units	IM	J0561	
Penicillin G Benzathine and Penicillin G Procaine	100,000 units	IM	J0558	
Penicillin G potassium	up to 600,000 units	IM, IV	J2540	
Penicillin G procaine, aqueous	up to 600,000 units	IM, IV	J2510	
Penicillin G Sodium			J3490	
Pentam	per 300 mg		J7676	
Pentamidine isethionate	per 300 mg	INH, IM	J2545, J7676	
Pentastarch, 10%	100 ml		J2513	
Pentazocine HCl	30 mg	IM, SC, IV	J3070	
Pentobarbital sodium	per 50 mg	IM, IV, OTH	J2515	
Pentostatin	per 10 mg	IV	J9268	
Peramivir	1 mg	IV	J2547	
Perjeta	1 mg		J9306	
Permapen	up to 600,000	IM	J0561	
Perphenazine				
Injection	up to 5 mg	IM, IV	J3310	
tablets	4 mg	ORAL	Q0175	
Persantine IV	per 10 mg	IV	J1245	
Pertuzumab	1 mg	IV	J9306	
Pet Imaging				
Fluciclovine F-18, diagnostic	1 millcurie	IV	A9588	
Gallium Ga-68, dotatate, diagnostic	0.1 millicurie	IV	A9587	

◀ New ↩ Revised ✔ Reinstated ~~deleted~~ Deleted

DRUG NAME	DOSAGE	METHOD OF ADMINISTRATION	HCPCS CODE
Pfizerpen	up to 600,000 units	IM, IV	J2540
Pfizerpen A.S.	up to 600,000 units	IM, IV	J2510
Phenadoz			J8498
Phenazine 25	up to 50 mg	IM, IV	J2550
	12.5 mg	ORAL	Q0169
Phenazine 50	up to 50 mg	IM, IV	J2550
	12.5 mg	ORAL	Q0169
Phenergan	12.5 mg	ORAL	Q0169
	up to 50 mg	IM, IV	J2550
			J8498
Phenobarbital sodium	up to 120 mg	IM, IV	J2560
Phentolamine mesylate	up to 5 mg	IM, IV	J2760
Phenylephrine HCl	up to 1 ml	SC, IM, IV	J2370, J7799
Phenytoin sodium	per 50 mg	IM, IV	J1165
Photofrin	75 mg	IV	J9600
Phytonadione (Vitamin K)	per 1 mg	IM, SC, IV	J3430
Piperacillin/Tazobactam Sodium, injection	1.125 g	IV	J2543
Pitocin	up to 10 units	IV, IM	J2590
Plantinol AQ	10 mg	IV	J9060
Plasma			
cryoprecipitate reduced	each unit	IV	P9044
pooled multiple donor, frozen	each unit	IV	P9023, P9070
(single donor), pathogen reduced, frozen	each unit	IV	P9071
Plas+SD	each unit	IV	P9023
Platelets, pheresis, pathogen reduced	each unit	IV	P9073
Pathogen(s) test for platelets		OTH	P9100
Platinol	10 mg	IV, IM	J9060
Plerixafor	1 mg	SC	J2562
Plicamycin	2,500 mcg	IV	J9270
Polocaine	per 10 ml	VAR	J0670
Polycillin-N	up to 500 mg	IM, IV	J0290
	per 1.5 gm	IM, IV	J0295
Polygam	500 mg		J1566
Porfimer Sodium	75 mg	IV	J9600
Portrazza	1 mg		J9295
Positron emission tomography radiopharmaceutical, diagnostic			
for non-tumor identification, NOC		IV	A9598
for tumor identification, NOC		IV	A9597
Potassium chloride	per 2 mEq	IV	J3480
Potassium Chloride	up to 1,000 cc		J7120

◀ New ↩ Revised ✓ Reinstated ~~deleted~~ Deleted

DRUG NAME	DOSAGE	METHOD OF ADMINISTRATION	HCPCS CODE
Pralatrexate	1 mg	IV	J9307
Pralidoxime chloride	up to 1 g	IV, IM, SC	J2730
Predalone-50	up to 1 ml	IM	J2650
Predcor-25	up to 1 ml	IM	J2650
Predcor-50	up to 1 ml	IM	J2650
Predicort-50	up to 1 ml	IM	J2650
Prednisolone acetate	up to 1 ml	IM	J2650
Prednisolone, oral	5 mg	ORAL	J7510
Prednisone, immediate release or delayed release	1 mg	ORAL	J7512
Predoject-50	up to 1 ml	IM	J2650
Pregnyl	per 1,000 USP units	IM	J0725
Premarin Intravenous	per 25 mg	IV, IM	J1410
Prescription, chemotherapeutic, not otherwise specified		ORAL	J8999
Prescription, nonchemotherapeutic, not otherwise specified		ORAL	J8499
Prialt	1 mcg		J2278
Primacor	5 mg	IV	J2260
Primatrix	per square centimeter		Q4110
Primaxin	per 250 mg	IV, IM	J0743
Priscoline HCl	up to 25 mg	IV	J2670
Privigen	500 mg	IV	J1459
Probuphine System Kit			J0570
Procainamide HCl	up to 1 g	IM, IV	J2690
Prochlorperazine	up to 10 mg	IM, IV	J0780
			J8498
Prochlorperazine maleate	5 mg	ORAL	Q0164
	5 mg		S0183
Procrit			J0885
			Q4081
Pro-Depo, *see* Hydroxyprogesterone Caproate			
Profasi HP	per 1,000 USP units	IM	J0725
Profilnine Heat-Treated			
non-recombinant	per IU	IV	J7193
recombinant	per IU	IU	J7195, J7200-J7202
complex	per IU	IV	J7194
Profonol	10 mg/ml		J3490
Progestaject	per 50 mg		J2675
Progesterone	per 50 mg	IM	J2675
Prograf			
oral	1 mg	ORAL	J7507
parenteral	5mg		J7525

◀ New ⤺ Revised ✔ Reinstated ~~deleted~~ Deleted

DRUG NAME	DOSAGE	METHOD OF ADMINISTRATION	HCPCS CODE
Prohance Multipack	per ml		A9576
Prokine	50 mcg	IV	J2820
Prolastin	10 mg	IV	J0256
Proleukin	per single use vial	IM, IV	J9015
Prolia	1 mg		J0897
Prolixin Decanoate	up to 25 mg	IM, SC	J2680
Promazine HCl	up to 25 mg	IM	J2950
Promethazine			J8498
Promethazine HCl			
injection	up to 50 mg	IM, IV	J2550
oral	12.5 mg	ORAL	Q0169
Promethegan			J8498
Pronestyl	up to 1 g	IM, IV	J2690
Proplex SX-T			
non-recombinant	per IU	IV	J7193
recombinant	per IU		J7195, J7200-J7202
complex	per IU	IV	J7194
Proplex T			
non-recombinant	per IU	IV	J7193
recombinant	per IU		J7195, J7200-J7202
complex	per IU	IV	J7194
Propofol	10 mg	IV	J2704
Propranolol HCl	up to 1 mg	IV	J1800
Prorex-25			
	up to 50 mg	IM, IV	J2550
	12.5 mg	ORAL	Q0169
Prorex-50	up to 50 mg	IM, IV	J2550
	12.5 mg	ORAL	Q0169
Prostaglandin E1	per 1.25 mcg		J0270
Prostaphlin	up to 1 g	IM, IV	J2690
Prostigmin	up to 0.5 mg	IM, IV, SC	J2710
Prostin VR Pediatric	0.5 mg		J0270
Protamine sulfate	per 10 mg	IV	J2720
Protein C Concentrate	10 IU	IV	J2724
Prothazine	up to 50 mg	IM, IV	J2550
	12.5 mg	ORAL	Q0169
Protirelin	per 250 mcg	IV	J2725
Protonix			J3490
Protopam Chloride	up to 1 g	IV, IM, SC	J2730
Provenge			Q2043

◀ New ↩ Revised ✔ Reinstated ~~deleted~~ Deleted

DRUG NAME	DOSAGE	METHOD OF ADMINISTRATION	HCPCS CODE
Proventil			
concentrated form	1 mg	INH	J7610, J7611
unit dose form	1 mg	INH	J7609, J7613
Provocholine	per 1 mg		J7674
Prozine-50	up to 25 mg	IM	J2950
Pulmicort Respules			
concentrated form	0.25 mg	INH	J7633, J7634
unit does	0.5 mg	INH	J7626, J7627
Pulmozyme	per mg		J7639
Pyridoxine HCl	100 mg		**J3415**
Q			
Quelicin	up to 20 mg	IV, IM	J0330
Quinupristin/dalfopristin	500 mg (150/350)	IV	**J2770**
Qutenza	per square cm		J7336
R			
Ramucirumab	5 mg	IV	**J9308**
Ranibizumab	0.1 mg	OTH	**J2778**
Ranitidine HCl, injection	25 mg	IV, IM	**J2780**
Rapamune	1 mg	ORAL	J7520
Rasburicase	0.5 mg	IV	**J2783**
Rebif	11 mcg		Q3026
Reclast	1 mg		J3489
Recombinate			
human	per IU	IV	J7190
porcine	per IU	IV	J7191
recombinant	per IU	IV	J7192
Recombivax			J3490
Redisol	up to 1,000 mcg	IM, SC	J3420
Regadenoson	0.1 mg	IV	**J2785**
Regitine	up to 5 mg	IM, IV	J2760
Reglan	up to 10 mg	IV	J2765
Regular	5 units	SC	J1815
Relefact TRH	per 250 mcg	IV	J2725
Relistor	0.1 mg	SC	J2212
Remicade	10 mg	IM, IV	J1745
Remodulin	1 mg		J3285
Renflexis			Q5102
ReoPro	10 mg	IV	J0130
Rep-Pred 40	20 mg	IM	J1020
	40 mg	IM	J1030
	80 mg	IM	J1040

◀ New ⤾ Revised ✔ Reinstated ~~deleted~~ Deleted

DRUG NAME	DOSAGE	METHOD OF ADMINISTRATION	HCPCS CODE
Rep-Pred 80	20 mg	IM	J1020
	40 mg	IM	J1030
	80 mg	IM	J1040
Resectisol			J7799
Reslizumab	1 mg	IV	J2786
Retavase	18.1 mg	IV	J2993
Reteplase	18.8 mg	IV	J2993
Retisert			J7311
Retrovir	10 mg	IV	J3485
Rheomacrodex	500 ml	IV	J7100
Rhesonativ	300 mcg	IM	J2790
	50 mg		J2788
Rheumatrex Dose Pack	2.5 mg	ORAL	J8610
Rho(D)			
immune globulin		IM, IV	J2791
immune globulin, human	1 dose package/ 300 mcg	IM	J2790
	50 mg	IM	J2788
immune globulin, human, solvent detergent	100	IV, IU	J2792
RhoGAM	300 mcg	IM	J2790
	50 mg		J2788
Rhophylac	100 IU	IM, IV	J2791
Riastap	100 mg		J7178
Rifadin			J3490
Rifampin			J3490
Rilonacept	1 mg	SC	J2793
RimabotulinumtoxinB	100 units	IM	J0587
Rimso-50	50 ml		J1212
Ringers lactate infusion	up to 1,000 cc	IV	J7120, J7121
Risperdal Costa	0.5 mg		J2794
Risperidone	0.5 mg	IM	J2794
Rituxan	100 mg	IV	J9310
Rituximab	100 mg	IV	J9310
Rixubis			J7200
Robaxin	up to 10 ml	IV, IM	J2800
Rocephin	per 250 mg	IV, IM	J0696
Roferon-A	3 million units	SC, IM	J9213
Rolapitant	0.5 mg	IV	J2797 ◀
Rolapitant, oral, 1 mg	1 mg	ORAL	J8670
Romidepsin	1 mg	IV	J9315
Romiplostim	10 mcg	SC	J2796

◀ New ⤼ Revised ✔ Reinstated ~~deleted~~ Deleted

DRUG NAME	DOSAGE	METHOD OF ADMINISTRATION	HCPCS CODE
Ropivacaine Hydrochloride	1 mg	OTH	J2795
Rubex	10 mg	IV	J9000
Rubramin PC	up to 1,000 mcg	IM, SC	J3420
S			
Saizen	1 mg		J2941
Saline solution	10 ml		A4216
5% dextrose	500 ml	IV	J7042
infusion	250 cc	IV	J7050
	1,000 cc	IV	J7030
sterile	500 ml = 1 unit	IV, OTH	J7040
Sandimmune	25 mg	ORAL	J7515
	100 mg	ORAL	J7502
	250 mg	OTH	J7516
Sandoglobulin, *see* Immune globin intravenous (human)			
Sandostatin, Lar Depot	25 mcg		J2354
	1 mg	IM	J2353
Sargramostim (GM-CSF)	50 mcg	IV	J2820
Sculptra	0.5 mg	IV	Q2028
Sebelelipase alfa	1 mg	IV	J2840
Selestoject	per 4 mg	IM, IV	J0702
Sermorelin acetate	1 mcg	SC	Q0515
Serostim	1 mg		J2941
Signifor LAR	20 ml		J2502
Siltuximab	10 mg	IV	J2860
Simponi Aria	1 mg		J1602
Simulect	20 mg		J0480
Sincalide	5 mcg	IV	J2805
Sinografin	per ml		Q9963
Sinusol-B	per 10 mg	IM, SC, IV	J0945
Sirolimus	1 mg	ORAL	J7520
Sivextro	1 mg		J3090
Skyla	13.5 mg	OTH	J7301
Smz-TMP			J3490
Sodium Chloride	1,000 cc		J7030
	500 ml = 1 unit		J7040
	500 ml		A4217
	250 cc		J7050
Bacteriostatic	10 ml		A4216
Sodium Chloride Concentrate			J7799
Sodium ferricgluconate in sucrose	12.5 mg		J2916

◀ New ↩ Revised ✔ Reinstated ~~deleted~~ Deleted

DRUG NAME	DOSAGE	METHOD OF ADMINISTRATION	HCPCS CODE
Sodium Hyaluronate			J3490
Euflexxa			**J7323**
Hyalgan~~, Spurtaz, Visco-3~~			**J7321**
Orthovisc			**J7324**
Solganal	up to 50 mg	IM	J2910
Soliris	10 mg		J1300
Solu-Cortef	up to 50 mg	IV, IM, SC	J1710
	100 mg		J1720
Solu-Medrol	up to 40 mg	IM, IV	J2920
	up to 125 mg	IM, IV	J2930
Solurex	1 mg	IM, IV, OTH	J1100
Solurex LA	1 mg	IM	J1094
Somatrem	1 mg	SC	**J2940**
Somatropin	1 mg	SC	**J2941**
Somatulin Depot	1 mg		J1930
Sparine	up to 25 mg	IM	J2950
Spasmoject	up to 20 mg	IM	J0500
Spectinomycin HCl	up to 2 g	IM	**J3320**
Sporanox	50 mg	IV	J1835
Staphcillin, *see* Methicillin sodium			
Stelara	1 mg		J3357
Stilphostrol	250 mg	IV	J9165
Streptase	250,000 IU	IV	J2995
Streptokinase	per 250,000	IU, IV	**J2995**
Streptomycin	up to 1 g	IM	**J3000**
Streptomycin Sulfate	up to 1 g	IM	J3000
Streptozocin	1 gm	IV	**J9320**
Strontium-89 chloride	per millicurie		**A9600**
Sublimaze	0.1 mg	IM, IV	J3010
Succinylcholine chloride	up to 20 mg	IV, IM	**J0330**
Sufentanil Citrate			J3490
Sumarel Dosepro	6 mg		J3030
Sumatriptan succinate	6 mg	SC	**J3030**
Supartz		OTH	**J7321**
Supprelin LA	50 mg		J9226
Surostrin	up to 20 mg	IV, IM	**J0330**
Sus-Phrine	up to 1 ml ampule	SC, IM	J0171
Synercid	500 mg (150/350)	IV	J2770
Synkavite	per 1 mg	IM, SC, IV	J3430
Synribo	0.01 mg		J9262

◀ **New** ↩ **Revised** ✔ **Reinstated** ~~deleted~~ **Deleted**

DRUG NAME	DOSAGE	METHOD OF ADMINISTRATION	HCPCS CODE
Syntocinon	up to 10 units	IV, IM	J2590
Synvisc and Synvisc-One	1 mg	OTH	J7325
Syrex	10 ml		A4216
Sytobex	1,000 mcg	IM, SC	J3420
T			
Tacrolimus			
(Envarsus XR)	0.25 mg	ORAL	J7503
oral, extended release	0.1 mg	ORAL	J7508
oral, immediate release	1 mg	ORAL	J7507
parenteral	5 mg	IV	J7525
Taliglucerase Alfa	10 units	IV	J3060
Talimogene laherparepvec	per 1 million plaque forming units	IV	J9325
Talwin	30 mg	IM, SC, IV	J3070
Tamoxifen Citrate			J8999
Taractan, *see* Chlorprothixene			
Taxol	1 mg	IV	J9267
Taxotere	20mg	IV	J9171
Tazicef	per 500 mg		J0713
Tazidime, *see* Ceftazidime Technetium TC Sestambi	per dose		A9500
			J0713
Tedizolid phosphate	1 mg	IV	J3090
TEEV	1 mg	IM	J3121
Teflaro	1 mg		J0712
Telavancin	10 mg	IV	J3095
Temodar	5 mg	ORAL	J8700, J9328
Temozolomide	1 mg	IV	J9328
	5 mg	ORAL	J8700
Temsirolimus	1 mg	IV	J9330
Tenecteplase	1 mg	IV	J3101
Teniposide	50 mg		Q2017
Tepadina	15 mg		J9340
Tequin	10 mg	IV	J1590
Terbutaline sulfate	up to 1 mg	SC, IV	J3105
concentrated form	per 1 mg	INH	J7680
unit dose form	per 1 mg	INH	J7681
Teriparatide	10 mcg	SC	J3110
Terramycin IM	up to 50 mg	IM	J2460
Testa-C	1 mg		J1071
Testadiate	1 mg	IM	J3121

◀ New ⤾ Revised ✔ Reinstated ~~deleted~~ Deleted

DRUG NAME	DOSAGE	METHOD OF ADMINISTRATION	HCPCS CODE
Testadiate-Depo	1 mg		J1071
Testaject-LA	1 mg		J1071
Testaqua	up to 50 mg	IM	J3140
Test-Estro Cypionates	1 mg		J1071
Test-Estro-C	1 mg		J1071
Testex	up to 100 mg	IM	J3150
Testo AQ	up to 50 mg		J3140
Testoject-50	up to 50 mg	IM	J3140
Testoject-LA	1 mg		J1071
Testone			
LA 100	1 mg	IM	J3121
LA 200	1 mg	IM	J3121
Testopel Pellets			J3490
Testosterone Aqueous	up to 50 mg	IM	J3140
Testosterone cypionate	1 mg	IM	**J1071**
Testosterone enanthate	1 mg	IM	**J3121**
Testosterone undecanoate	1 mg	IM	**J3145**
Testradiol 90/4	1 mg	IM	J3121
Testrin PA	1 mg	IM	J3121
Testro AQ	up to 50 mg		J3140
Tetanus immune globulin, human	up to 250 units	IM	**J1670**
Tetracycline	up to 250 mg	IM, IV	**J0120**
Thallous Chloride TI-201	per MCI		**A9505**
Theelin Aqueous	per 1 mg	IM	J1435
Theophylline	per 40 mg	IV	**J2810**
TheraCys	per vial	IV	J9031
Thiamine HCl	100 mg		**J3411**
Thiethylperazine maleate			
injection	up to 10 mg	IM	**J3280**
oral	10 mg	ORAL	**Q0174**
Thiotepa	15 mg	IV	**J9340**
Thorazine	up to 50 mg	IM, IV	J3230
Thrombate III	per IU		J7197
Thymoglobulin (*see also* Immune globin)			
anti-thymocyte globulin, equine	250 mg	IV	**J7504**
anti-thymocyte globulin, rabbit	25 mg	IV	**J7511**
Thypinone	per 250 mcg	IV	J2725
Thyrogen	0.9 mg	IM, SC	J3240
Thyrotropin Alfa, injection	0.9 mg	IM, SC	**J3240**
Tice BCG	per vial	IV	J9031

◀ New ↩ Revised ✔ Reinstated ~~deleted~~ Deleted

DRUG NAME	DOSAGE	METHOD OF ADMINISTRATION	HCPCS CODE
Ticon			
injection	up to 200 mg	IM	J3250
oral	250 mg	ORAL	Q0173
Tigan			
injection	up to 200 mg	IM	J3250
oral	250 mg	ORAL	Q0173
Tigecycline	1 mg	IV	**J3243**
Tiject-20			
injection	up to 200 mg	IM	J3250
oral	250 mg	ORAL	Q0173
Tinzaparin	1,000 IU	SC	**J1655**
Tirofiban Hydrochloride, injection	0.25 mg	IM, IV	**J3246**
TNKase	1 mg	IV	J3101
Tobi	300 mg	INH	J7682, J7685
Tobramycin, inhalation solution	300 mg	INH	**J7682, J7685**
Tobramycin sulfate	up to 80 mg	IM, IV	**J3260**
Tocilizumab	1 mg	IV	**J3262**
Tofranil, *see* Imipramine HCl			
Tolazoline HCl	up to 25 mg	IV	**J2670**
Toposar	10 mg		J9181
Topotecan	0.25 mg	ORAL	**J8705**
	0.1 mg	IV	**J9351**
Toradol	per 15 mg	IM, IV	J1885
Torecan			
injection	up to 10 mg	IM	J3280
oral	10 mg	ORAL	Q0174
Torisel	1 mg		**J9330**
Tornalate			
concentrated form	per mg	INH	J7628
unit dose	per mg	INH	J7629
Torsemide	10 mg/ml	IV	**J3265**
Totacillin-N	up to 500 mg	IM, IV	J0290
	per 1.5 gm	IM, IV	J0295
Trabectedin	0.1 mg	IV	**J9352**
Trastuzumab	10 mg	IV	**J9355**
Treanda	1 mg	IV	J3490, J9033
Trelstar	3.75 mg		J3315
Treprostinil	1 mg		**J3285,** J7686
Trexall	2.5 mg	ORAL	J8610

◀ New ↩ Revised ✔ Reinstated ~~deleted~~ Deleted

DRUG NAME	DOSAGE	METHOD OF ADMINISTRATION	HCPCS CODE	
Triam-A	1 mg		J3300	
	per 10 mg	IM	J3301	
Triamcinolone				
concentrated form	per 1 mg	INH	**J7683**	
unit dose	per 1 mg	INH	**J7684**	
Triamcinolone acetonide	1 mg		**J3300**	
	per 10 mg	IM	**J3301**	
Triamcinolone acetonide XR	1 mg	IM	**J3304**	◀
Triamcinolone diacetate	per 5 mg	IM	**J3302**	
Triamcinolone hexacetonide	per 5 mg	VAR	**J3303**	
Triesence	1 mg		J3300	
	per 10 mg	IM	J3301	
Triethylene thio-Phosphoramide/T	15 mg		J9340	
Triflupromazine HCl	up to 20 mg	IM, IV	**J3400**	
Tri-Kort	1 mg		J3300	
	per 10 mg	IM	J3301	
Trilafon	4 mg	ORAL	Q0175	
	up to 5 mg	IM, IV	J3310	
Trilog	1 mg		J3300	
	per 10 mg	IM	J3301	
Trilone	per 5 mg		J3302	
Trimethobenzamide HCl				
injection	up to 200 mg	IM	**J3250**	
oral	250 mg	ORAL	**Q0173**	
Trimetrexate glucuronate	per 25 mg	IV	**J3305**	
Triptorelin Pamoate	3.75 mg	SC	**J3315**	
Triptorelin XR	3.75 mg	SC	**J3316**	◀
Trisenox	1 mg	IV	J9017	
Trobicin	up to 2 g	IM	J3320	
Trovan	100 mg	IV	J0200	
Tysabri	1 mg		J2323	
Tyvaso	1.74 mg		J7686	
U				
Ultravist 240	per ml		Q9966	
Ultravist 300	per ml		Q9967	
Ultravist 370	per ml		Q9967	
Ultrazine-10	up to 10 mg	IM, IV	J0780	
Unasyn	per 1.5 gm	IM, IV	J0295	
Unclassified drugs (*see also* Not elsewhere classified)			**J3490**	
Unclassified drugs or biological used for ESRD on dialysis		IV	**J3591**	◀

◀ **New** ⤾ **Revised** ✔ **Reinstated** ~~deleted~~ **Deleted**

DRUG NAME	DOSAGE	METHOD OF ADMINISTRATION	HCPCS CODE
Unspecified oral antiemetic			Q0181
Urea	up to 40 g	IV	J3350
Ureaphil	up to 40 g	IV	J3350
Urecholine	up to 5 mg	SC	J0520
Urofollitropin	75 IU		J3355
Urokinase	5,000 IU vial	IV	J3364
	250,000 IU vial	IV	J3365
Ustekinumab	1 mg	SC	J3357
	1 mg	IV	J3358
V			
Valcyte			J3490
Valergen 10	10 mg	IM	J1380
Valergen 20	10 mg	IM	J1380
Valergen 40	up to 10 mg	IM	J1380
Valertest No. 1	1 mg	IM	J3121
Valertest No. 2	1 mg	IM	J3121
Valganciclovir HCL			J8499
Valium	up to 5 mg	IM, IV	J3360
Valrubicin, intravesical	200 mg	OTH	J9357
Valstar	200 mg	OTH	J9357
Vancocin	500 mg	IV, IM	J3370
Vancoled	500 mg	IV, IM	J3370
Vancomycin HCl	500 mg	IV, IM	J3370
Vantas	50 mg		J9226, J9225
Varubi	90 mg		J8670
Vasceze	per 10 mg		J1642
Vasoxyl, *see* Methoxamine HCl			
Vectibix	10 mg		J9303
Vedolizumab	1 mg	IV	J3380
Velaglucerase alfa	100 units	IV	J3385
Velban	1 mg	IV	J9360
Velcade	0.1 mg		J9041
Veletri	0.5 mg		J1325
Velsar	1 mg	IV	J9360
Venofer	1 mg	IV	J1756
Ventavis	20 mcg		Q4074
Ventolin	0.5 mg	INH	J7620
concentrated form	1 mg	INH	J7610, J7611
unit dose form	1 mg	INH	J7609, J7613
VePesid	50 mg	ORAL	J8560

◀ New ↩ Revised ✔ Reinstated ~~deleted~~ Deleted

DRUG NAME	DOSAGE	METHOD OF ADMINISTRATION	HCPCS CODE	
Veritas Collagen Matrix			J3490	
Versed	per 1 mg	IM, IV	J2250	
Verteporfin	0.1 mg	IV	J3396	
Vesprin	up to 20 mg	IM, IV	J3400	
Vestronidase alfa-vjbk	1 mg	IV	J3397	◀
VFEND IV	10 mg	IV	J3465	
V-Gan 25	up to 50 mg	IM, IV	J2550	
	12.5 mg	ORAL	Q0169	
V-Gan 50	up to 50 mg	IM, IV	J2550	
	12.5 mg	ORAL	Q0169	
Viadur	65 mg	OTH	J9219	
Vibativ	10 mg		J3095	
Vinblastine sulfate	1 mg	IV	J9360	
Vincasar PFS	1 mg	IV	J9370	
Vincristine sulfate	1 mg	IV	J9370	
Vincristine sulfate Liposome	1 mg	IV	J9371	
Vinorelbine tartrate	per 10 mg	IV	J9390	
Vispaque	per ml		Q9966, Q9967	
Vistaject-25	up to 25 mg	IM	J3410	
Vistaril	up to 25 mg	IM	J3410	
	25mg	ORAL	Q0177	
Vistide	375 mg	IV	J0740	
Visudyne	0.1 mg	IV	J3396	
Vitamin B-12 cyanocobalamin	up to 1,000 mcg	IM, SC	J3420	
Vitamin K, phytonadione, menadione, menadiol sodium diphosphate	per 1 mg	IM, SC, IV	J3430	
Vitrase	per 1 USP unit		J3471	
Vivaglobin	100 mg		J1562	
Vivitrol	1 mg		J2315	
Von Willebrand Factor Complex, human	per IU VWF:RCo	IV	J7187	
Wilate	per IU VWF	IV	J7183	
Vonvendi	per IU VWF	IV	J7179	
Voretigene neparvovec-rzyl	1 billion vector genomes	IV	J3398	◀
Voriconazole	10 mg	IV	J3465	
Vpriv	100 units		J3385	
W				
Wehamine	up to 50 mg	IM, IV	J1240	
Wehdryl	up to 50 mg	IM, IV	J1200	
	50 mg	ORAL	Q0163	
Wellcovorin	per 50 mg	IM, IV	J0640	

◀ New   ⤻ Revised   ✔ Reinstated   ~~deleted~~ Deleted

DRUG NAME	DOSAGE	METHOD OF ADMINISTRATION	HCPCS CODE
Wilate	per IU	IV	J7183
Win Rho SD	100 IU	IV	J2792
Wyamine Sulfate, *see* Mephentermine sulfate			
Wycillin	up to 600,000 units	IM, IV	J2510
Wydase	up to 150 units	SC, IV	J3470
X			
Xeloda	150 mg	ORAL	J8520
	500 mg	ORAL	J8521
Xeomin	1 unit		J0588
Xgera	1 mg		J0987
Xgeva	1 mg		J0897
Xiaflex	0.01 mg		J0775
Xolair	5 mg		J2357
Xopenex	0.5 mg	INH	J7620
concentrated form	1 mg	INH	J7610, J7611, J7612
unit dose form	1 mg	INH	J7609, J7613, J7614
Xylocaine HCl	10 mg	IV	J2001
Xyntha	per IU	IV	J7185, J7192, J7182, J7188
Y			
Yervoy *see* Ipilimumab			
Yondelis	0.1 mg		J9352, J9999
Z			
Zaltrap	1 mg		J9400
Zanosar	1 g	IV	J9320
Zantac	25 mg	IV, IM	J2780
Zarxio	1 mcg		Q5101
Zemaira	10 mg	IV	J0256
Zemplar	1 mcg	IM, IV	J2501
Zenapax	25 mg	IV	J7513
Zerbaxa	1 gm		J0695
Zetran	up to 5 mg	IM, IV	J3360
Ziconotide	1 mcg	OTH	J2278
Zidovudine	10 mg	IV	J3485
Zinacef	per 750 mg	IM, IV	J0697
Zinecard	per 250 mg		J1190
Ziprasidone Mesylate	10 mg	IM	J3486
Zithromax	1 gm	ORAL	Q0144
Injection	500 mg	IV	J0456

◀ New ⤺ Revised ✔ Reinstated ~~deleted~~ Deleted

DRUG NAME	DOSAGE	METHOD OF ADMINISTRATION	HCPCS CODE
Ziv-Aflibercept	1 mg	IV	J9400
Zmax	1 g		Q0144
Zofran	1 mg	IV	J2405
	1 mg	ORAL	Q0162
Zoladex	per 3.6 mg	SC	J9202
Zoledronic Acid	1 mg	IV	J3489
Zolicef	500 mg	IV, IM	J0690
Zometra	1 mg		J3489
Zorbtive	1 mg		J2941
Zortress	0.25 mg	ORAL	J7527
Zosyn	1.125 g	IV	J2543
Zovirax	5 mg		J8499
Zyprexa Relprevv	1 mg		J2358
Zyvox	200 mg	IV	J2020

◀ New ⤾ Revised ✔ Reinstated ~~deleted~~ Deleted

LEVEL II NATIONAL CODES

2019 HCPCS quarterly updates available on the companion website at: http://www.codingupdates.com

DISCLAIMER

Every effort has been made to make this text complete and accurate, but no guarantee, warranty, or representation is made for its accuracy or completeness. This text is based on the Centers for Medicare and Medicaid Services Healthcare Common Procedure Coding System (HCPCS).

Do not report HCPCS modifiers with PQRI CPT Category II codes, rather use Category II modifiers (i.e., 1P, 2P, 3P, or 8P) or the claim may be returned or denied.

LEVEL II NATIONAL MODIFIERS

* ✻ **A1** Dressing for one wound
* ✻ **A2** Dressing for two wounds
* ✻ **A3** Dressing for three wounds
* ✻ **A4** Dressing for four wounds
* ✻ **A5** Dressing for five wounds
* ✻ **A6** Dressing for six wounds
* ✻ **A7** Dressing for seven wounds
* ✻ **A8** Dressing for eight wounds
* ✻ **A9** Dressing for nine or more wounds
* ◌ **AA** Anesthesia services performed personally by anesthesiologist
  IOM: 100-04, 12, 90.4
* ◌ **AD** Medical supervision by a physician: more than four concurrent anesthesia procedures
  IOM: 100-04, 12, 90.4
* ✻ **AE** Registered dietician
* ✻ **AF** Specialty physician
* ✻ **AG** Primary physician
* ◌ **AH** Clinical psychologist
  IOM: 100-04, 12, 170
* ✻ **AI** Principal physician of record
* ◌ **AJ** Clinical social worker
  IOM: 100-04, 12, 170; 100-04, 12, 150
* ✻ **AK** Nonparticipating physician
* ◌ **AM** Physician, team member service
  Not assigned for Medicare
  Cross Reference QM
* ✻ **AO** Alternate payment method declined by provider of service
* ✻ **AP** Determination of refractive state was not performed in the course of diagnostic ophthalmological examination
* ✻ **AQ** Physician providing a service in an unlisted health professional shortage area (HPSA)
* ✻ **AR** Physician provider services in a physician scarcity area
* ✻ **AS** Physician assistant, nurse practitioner, or clinical nurse specialist services for assistant at surgery
* ✻ **AT** Acute treatment (this modifier should be used when reporting service 98940, 98941, 98942)
* ✻ **AU** Item furnished in conjunction with a urological, ostomy, or tracheostomy supply
* ✻ **AV** Item furnished in conjunction with a prosthetic device, prosthetic or orthotic
* ✻ **AW** Item furnished in conjunction with a surgical dressing
* ✻ **AX** Item furnished in conjunction with dialysis services
* ✻ **AY** Item or service furnished to an ESRD patient that is not for the treatment of ESRD
* ⃠ **AZ** Physician providing a service in a dental health professional shortage area for the purpose of an electronic health record incentive payment
* ✻ **BA** Item furnished in conjunction with parenteral enteral nutrition (PEN) services
* ✻ **BL** Special acquisition of blood and blood products
* ✻ **BO** Orally administered nutrition, not by feeding tube
* ✻ **BP** The beneficiary has been informed of the purchase and rental options and has elected to purchase the item
* ✻ **BR** The beneficiary has been informed of the purchase and rental options and has elected to rent the item
* ✻ **BU** The beneficiary has been informed of the purchase and rental options and after 30 days has not informed the supplier of his/her decision
* ✻ **CA** Procedure payable only in the inpatient setting when performed emergently on an outpatient who expires prior to admission
* ✻ **CB** Service ordered by a renal dialysis facility (RDF) physician as part of the ESRD beneficiary's dialysis benefit, is not part of the composite rate, and is separately reimbursable
* ✻ **CC** Procedure code change (Use CC when the procedure code submitted was changed either for administrative reasons or because an incorrect code was filed)
* ◌ **CD** AMCC test has been ordered by an ESRD facility or MCP physician that is part of the composite rate and is not separately billable

▶ New ⤺ Revised ✔ Reinstated ~~deleted~~ Deleted ⃠ Not covered or valid by Medicare
◌ Special coverage instructions ✻ Carrier discretion Ⓑ Bill Part B MAC Ⓔ Bill DME MAC

CE AMCC test has been ordered by an ESRD facility or MCP physician that is a composite rate test but is beyond the normal frequency covered under the rate and is separately reimbursable based on medical necessity

CF AMCC test has been ordered by an ESRD facility or MCP physician that is not part of the composite rate and is separately billable

* **CG** Policy criteria applied

CH 0 percent impaired, limited or restricted

CI At least 1 percent but less than 20 percent impaired, limited or restricted

CJ At least 20 percent but less than 40 percent impaired, limited or restricted

CK At least 40 percent but less than 60 percent impaired, limited or restricted

CL At least 60 percent but less than 80 percent impaired, limited or restricted

CM At least 80 percent but less than 100 percent impaired, limited or restricted

CN 100 percent impaired, limited or restricted

▶* **CO** Outpatient occupational therapy services furnished in whole or in part by an occupational therapy assistant

* **CR** Catastrophe/Disaster related

* **CS** Item or service related, in whole or in part, to an illness, injury, or condition that was caused by or exacerbated by the effects, direct or indirect, of the 2010 oil spill in the Gulf of Mexico, including but not limited to subsequent clean-up activities

* **CT** Computed tomography services furnished using equipment that does not meet each of the attributes of the national electrical manufacturers association (NEMA) XR-29-2013 standard

Coding Clinic: 2017, Q1, P6

▶* **CQ** Outpatient physical therapy services furnished in whole or in part by a physical therapist assistant

* **DA** Oral health assessment by a licensed health professional other than a dentist

* **E1** Upper left, eyelid

Coding Clinic: 2016, Q3, P3

* **E2** Lower left, eyelid

Coding Clinic: 2016, Q3, P3

* **E3** Upper right, eyelid

Coding Clinic: 2011, Q3, P6

* **E4** Lower right, eyelid

EA Erythropoetic stimulating agent (ESA) administered to treat anemia due to anti-cancer chemotherapy

CMS requires claims for non-ESRD ESAs (J0881 and J0885) to include one of three modifiers: EA, EB, EC.

EB Erythropoetic stimulating agent (ESA) administered to treat anemia due to anti-cancer radiotherapy

CMS requires claims for non-ESRD ESAs (J0881 and J0885) to include one of three modifiers: EA, EB, EC.

EC Erythropoetic stimulating agent (ESA) administered to treat anemia not due to anti-cancer radiotherapy or anti-cancer chemotherapy

CMS requires claims for non-ESRD ESAs (J0881 and J0885) to include one of three modifiers: EA, EB, EC.

ED Hematocrit level has exceeded 39% (or hemoglobin level has exceeded 13.0 g/dl) for 3 or more consecutive billing cycles immediately prior to and including the current cycle

EE Hematocrit level has not exceeded 39% (or hemoglobin level has not exceeded 13.0 g/dl) for 3 or more consecutive billing cycles immediately prior to and including the current cycle

EJ Subsequent claims for a defined course of therapy, e.g., EPO, sodium hyaluronate, infliximab

EM Emergency reserve supply (for ESRD benefit only)

* **EP** Service provided as part of Medicaid early periodic screening diagnosis and treatment (EPSDT) program

▶* **ER** Items and services furnished by a provider-based, off-campus emergency department

* **ET** Emergency services

* **EX** Expatriate beneficiary

* **EY** No physician or other licensed health care provider order for this item or service

Items billed before a signed and dated order has been received by the supplier must be submitted with an EY modifier added to each related HCPCS code.

* **F1** Left hand, second digit

* **F2** Left hand, third digit

MIPS | Qp Quantity Physician | Qh Quantity Hospital | ♀ Female only
♂ Male only | A Age | DMEPOS | A2-Z3 ASC Payment Indicator | A-Y ASC Status Indicator | Coding Clinic

✻ **F3** Left hand, fourth digit

✻ **F4** Left hand, fifth digit

✻ **F5** Right hand, thumb

✻ **F6** Right hand, second digit

✻ **F7** Right hand, third digit

✻ **F8** Right hand, fourth digit

✻ **F9** Right hand, fifth digit

✻ **FA** Left hand, thumb

⃠ **FB** Item provided without cost to provider, supplier or practitioner, or full credit received for replaced device (examples, but not limited to, covered under warranty, replaced due to defect, free samples)

◎ **FC** Partial credit received for replaced device

✻ **FP** Service provided as part of family planning program

✻ **FX** X-ray taken using film

Coding Clinic: 2017, Q1, P6

✻ **FY** X-ray taken using computed radiography technology/cassette-based imaging

▶ ✻ **G0** Telehealth services for diagnosis, evaluation, or treatment, of symptoms of an acute stroke

✻ **G1** Most recent URR reading of less than 60

IOM: 100-04, 8, 50.9

✻ **G2** Most recent URR reading of 60 to 64.9

IOM: 100-04, 8, 50.9

✻ **G3** Most recent URR reading of 65 to 69.9

IOM: 100-04, 8, 50.9

✻ **G4** Most recent URR reading of 70 to 74.9

IOM: 100-04, 8, 50.9

✻ **G5** Most recent URR reading of 75 or greater

IOM: 100-04, 8, 50.9

✻ **G6** ESRD patient for whom less than six dialysis sessions have been provided in a month

IOM: 100-04, 8, 50.9

◎ **G7** Pregnancy resulted from rape or incest or pregnancy certified by physician as life threatening

IOM: 100-02, 15, 20.1; 100-03, 3, 170.3

✻ **G8** Monitored anesthesia care (MAC) for deep complex, complicated, or markedly invasive surgical procedure

✻ **G9** Monitored anesthesia care for patient who has history of severe cardiopulmonary condition

✻ **GA** Waiver of liability statement issued as required by payer policy, individual case

An item/service is expected to be denied as not reasonable and necessary and an ABN is on file. Modifier GA can be used on either a specific or a miscellaneous HCPCS code. Modifiers GA and GY should never be reported together on the same line for the same HCPCS code.

✻ **GB** Claim being resubmitted for payment because it is no longer covered under a global payment demonstration

◎ **GC** This service has been performed in part by a resident under the direction of a teaching physician

IOM: 100-04, 12, 90.4, 100

✻ **GD** Units of service exceeds medically unlikely edit value and represents reasonable and necessary services

◎ **GE** This service has been performed by a resident without the presence of a teaching physician under the primary care exception

✻ **GF** Non-physician (e.g., nurse practitioner (NP), certified registered nurse anesthetist (CRNA), certified registered nurse (CRN), clinical nurse specialist (CNS), physician assistant (PA)) services in a critical access hospital

✻ **GG** Performance and payment of a screening mammogram and diagnostic mammogram on the same patient, same day

✻ **GH** Diagnostic mammogram converted from screening mammogram on same day

✻ **GJ** "Opt out" physician or practitioner emergency or urgent service

✻ **GK** Reasonable and necessary item/service associated with a GA or GZ modifier

An upgrade is defined as an item that goes beyond what is medically necessary under Medicare's coverage requirements. An item can be considered an upgrade even if the physician has signed an order for it. When suppliers know that an item will not be paid in full because it does not meet the coverage criteria stated in the LCD, the supplier can still obtain partial payment at the time of initial determination if the claim is billed using one of the upgrade modifiers (GK or GL). (https://www.cms.gov/manuals/downloads/clm104c01.pdf)

▶ New ↻ Revised ✔ Reinstated ~~deleted~~ Deleted ⃠ Not covered or valid by Medicare
◎ Special coverage instructions ✻ Carrier discretion Ⓑ Bill Part B MAC Ⓑ Bill DME MAC

* **GL** Medically unnecessary upgrade provided instead of non-upgraded item, no charge, no Advance Beneficiary Notice (ABN)
* **GM** Multiple patients on one ambulance trip
* **GN** Services delivered under an outpatient speech language pathology plan of care
* **GO** Services delivered under an outpatient occupational therapy plan of care
* **GP** Services delivered under an outpatient physical therapy plan of care
* **GQ** Via asynchronous telecommunications system
* **GR** This service was performed in whole or in part by a resident in a department of Veterans Affairs medical center or clinic, supervised in accordance with VA policy
* **GS** Dosage of erythropoietin-stimulating agent has been reduced and maintained in response to hematocrit or hemoglobin level
* **GT** Via interactive audio and video telecommunication systems
* **GU** Waiver of liability statement issued as required by payer policy, routine notice
* **GV** Attending physician not employed or paid under arrangement by the patient's hospice provider
* **GW** Service not related to the hospice patient's terminal condition
* **GX** Notice of liability issued, voluntary under payer policy

  GX modifier must be submitted with non-covered charges only. This modifier differentiates from the required uses in conjunction with ABN. (https://www.cms.gov/manuals/downloads/clm104c01.pdf)
* **GY** Item or service statutorily excluded, does not meet the definition of any Medicare benefit or, for non-Medicare insurers, is not a contract benefit

  Examples of "statutorily excluded" include: Infusion drug not administered using a durable infusion pump, a wheelchair that is for use for mobility outside the home or hearing aids. GA and GY should never be coded together on the same line for the same HCPCS code. (https://www.cms.gov/manuals/downloads/clm104c01.pdf)
* **GZ** Item or service expected to be denied as not reasonable or necessary

  Used when an ABN is not on file and can be used on either a specific or a miscellaneous HCPCS code. It would never be correct to place any combination of GY, GZ or GA modifiers on the same claim line and will result in rejected or denied claim for invalid coding. (https://www.cms.gov/manuals/downloads/clm104c01.pdf)
* **H9** Court-ordered
* **HA** Child/adolescent program
* **HB** Adult program, nongeriatric
* **HC** Adult program, geriatric
* **HD** Pregnant/parenting women's program
* **HE** Mental health program
* **HF** Substance abuse program
* **HG** Opioid addiction treatment program
* **HH** Integrated mental health/substance abuse program
* **HI** Integrated mental health and intellectual disability/developmental disabilities program
* **HJ** Employee assistance program
* **HK** Specialized mental health programs for high-risk populations
* **HL** Intern
* **HM** Less than bachelor degree level
* **HN** Bachelors degree level
* **HO** Masters degree level
* **HP** Doctoral level
* **HQ** Group setting
* **HR** Family/couple with client present
* **HS** Family/couple without client present
* **HT** Multi-disciplinary team
* **HU** Funded by child welfare agency
* **HV** Funded by state addictions agency
* **HW** Funded by state mental health agency
* **HX** Funded by county/local agency
* **HY** Funded by juvenile justice agency
* **HZ** Funded by criminal justice agency
* **J1** Competitive acquisition program no-pay submission for a prescription number
* **J2** Competitive acquisition program, restocking of emergency drugs after emergency administration

MIPS | Qp Quantity Physician | Qh Quantity Hospital | ♀ Female only
♂ Male only | A Age | DMEPOS | A2-Z3 ASC Payment Indicator | A-Y ASC Status Indicator | Coding Clinic

✻ **J3** Competitive acquisition program (CAP), drug not available through CAP as written, reimbursed under average sales price methodology

✻ **J4** DMEPOS item subject to DMEPOS competitive bidding program that is furnished by a hospital upon discharge

✻ **JA** Administered intravenously

This modifier is informational only (not a payment modifier) and may be submitted with all injection codes. According to Medicare, reporting this modifier is voluntary. (CMS Pub. 100-04, chapter 8, section 60.2.3.1 and Pub. 100-04, chapter 17, section 80.11)

✻ **JB** Administered subcutaneously

✻ **JC** Skin substitute used as a graft

✻ **JD** Skin substitute not used as a graft

✻ **JE** Administered via dialysate

✻ **JG** Drug or biological acquired with 340B drug pricing program discount

✻ **JW** Drug amount discarded/not administered to any patient

Use JW to identify unused drugs or biologicals from single use vial/package that are appropriately discarded. Bill on separate line for payment of discarded drug/biological.

IOM: 100-4, 17, 40

Coding Clinic: 2016, Q4, P4-7; 2010, Q3, P10

✻ **K0** Lower extremity prosthesis functional Level 0 - does not have the ability or potential to ambulate or transfer safely with or without assistance and a prosthesis does not enhance their quality of life or mobility.

✻ **K1** Lower extremity prosthesis functional Level 1 - has the ability or potential to use a prosthesis for transfers or ambulation on level surfaces at fixed cadence. Typical of the limited and unlimited household ambulator.

✻ **K2** Lower extremity prosthesis functional Level 2 - has the ability or potential for ambulation with the ability to traverse low level environmental barriers such as curbs, stairs or uneven surfaces. Typical of the limited community ambulator.

✻ **K3** Lower extremity prosthesis functional Level 3 - has the ability or potential for ambulation with variable cadence. Typical of the community ambulator who has the ability to traverse most environmental barriers and may have vocational, therapeutic, or exercise activity that demands prosthetic utilization beyond simple locomotion.

✻ **K4** Lower extremity prosthesis functional Level 4 - has the ability or potential for prosthetic ambulation that exceeds the basic ambulation skills, exhibiting high impact, stress, or energy levels, typical of the prosthetic demands of the child, active adult, or athlete.

✻ **KA** Add on option/accessory for wheelchair

✻ **KB** Beneficiary requested upgrade for ABN, more than 4 modifiers identified on claim

✻ **KC** Replacement of special power wheelchair interface

✻ **KD** Drug or biological infused through DME

✻ **KE** Bid under round one of the DMEPOS competitive bidding program for use with non-competitive bid base equipment

✻ **KF** Item designated by FDA as Class III device

✻ **KG** DMEPOS item subject to DMEPOS competitive bidding program number 1

✻ **KH** DMEPOS item, initial claim, purchase or first month rental

✻ **KI** DMEPOS item, second or third month rental

✻ **KJ** DMEPOS item, parenteral enteral nutrition (PEN) pump or capped rental, months four to fifteen

✻ **KK** DMEPOS item subject to DMEPOS competitive bidding program number 2

✻ **KL** DMEPOS item delivered via mail

✻ **KM** Replacement of facial prosthesis including new impression/moulage

✻ **KN** Replacement of facial prosthesis using previous master model

✻ **KO** Single drug unit dose formulation

✻ **KP** First drug of a multiple drug unit dose formulation

✻ **KQ** Second or subsequent drug of a multiple drug unit dose formulation

✻ **KR** Rental item, billing for partial month

KS Glucose monitor supply for diabetic beneficiary not treated with insulin

✻ **KT** Beneficiary resides in a competitive bidding area and travels outside that competitive bidding area and receives a competitive bid item

✻ **KU** DMEPOS item subject to DMEPOS competitive bidding program number 3

✻ **KV** DMEPOS item subject to DMEPOS competitive bidding program that is furnished as part of a professional service

✻ **KW** DMEPOS item subject to DMEPOS competitive bidding program number 4

✻ **KX** Requirements specified in the medical policy have been met

Used for physical, occupational, or speech-language therapy to request an exception to therapy payment caps and indicate the services are reasonable and necessary and that there is documentation of medical necessity in the patient's medical record. (Pub 100-04 Attachment - Business Requirements Centers for Medicare and Medicaid Services, Transmittal 2457, April 27, 2012)

Medicare requires modifier KX for implanted permanent cardiac pacemakers, single chamber or duel chamber, for one of the following CPT codes: 33206, 33207, 33208.

✻ **KY** DMEPOS item subject to DMEPOS competitive bidding program number 5

✻ **KZ** New coverage not implemented by managed care

✻ **LC** Left circumflex coronary artery

✻ **LD** Left anterior descending coronary artery

✻ **LL** Lease/rental (use the LL modifier when DME equipment rental is to be applied against the purchase price)

✻ **LM** Left main coronary artery

✻ **LR** Laboratory round trip

LS FDA-monitored intraocular lens implant

✻ **LT** Left side (used to identify procedures performed on the left side of the body)

Modifiers LT and RT identify procedures which can be performed on paired organs. Used for procedures performed on one side only. Should also be used when the procedures are similar but not identical and are performed on paired body parts.

Coding Clinic: 2016, Q3, P5

✻ **M2** Medicare secondary payer (MSP)

✻ **MS** Six month maintenance and servicing fee for reasonable and necessary parts and labor which are not covered under any manufacturer or supplier warranty

✻ **NB** Nebulizer system, any type, FDA-cleared for use with specific drug

✻ **NR** New when rented (use the NR modifier when DME which was new at the time of rental is subsequently purchased)

✻ **NU** New equipment

✻ **P1** A normal healthy patient

✻ **P2** A patient with mild systemic disease

✻ **P3** A patient with severe systemic disease

✻ **P4** A patient with severe systemic disease that is a constant threat to life

✻ **P5** A moribund patient who is not expected to survive without the operation

✻ **P6** A declared brain-dead patient whose organs are being removed for donor purposes

⊘ **PA** Surgical or other invasive procedure on wrong body part

⊘ **PB** Surgical or other invasive procedure on wrong patient

⊘ **PC** Wrong surgery or other invasive procedure on patient

✻ **PD** Diagnostic or related non diagnostic item or service provided in a wholly owned or operated entity to a patient who is admitted as an inpatient within 3 days

✻ **PI** Positron emission tomography (PET) or PET/computed tomography (CT) to inform the initial treatment strategy of tumors that are biopsy proven or strongly suspected of being cancerous based on other diagnostic testing

✻ **PL** Progressive addition lenses

✻ **PM** Post mortem

✻ **PN** Non-excepted service provided at an off-campus, outpatient, provider-based department of a hospital

✻ **PO** Expected services provided at off-campus, outpatient, provider-based department of a hospital

✻ **PS** Positron emission tomography (PET) or PET/computed tomography (CT) to inform the subsequent treatment strategy of cancerous tumors when the beneficiary's treating physician determines that the PET study is needed to inform subsequent anti-tumor strategy

*	**PT**	Colorectal cancer screening test; converted to diagnostic text or other procedure Assign this modifier with the appropriate CPT procedure code for colonoscopy, flexible sigmoidoscopy, or barium enema when the service is initiated as a colorectal cancer screening service but then becomes a diagnostic service. (MLN Matters article MM7012 (PDF, 75 KB) Reference Medicare Transmittal 3232 April 3, 2015. Coding Clinic: 2011, Q1, P10
◎	**Q0**	Investigational clinical service provided in a clinical research study that is in an approved clinical research study
◎	**Q1**	Routine clinical service provided in a clinical research study that is in an approved clinical research study
*	**Q2**	Demonstration procedure/service
*	**Q3**	Live kidney donor surgery and related services
*	**Q4**	Service for ordering/referring physician qualifies as a service exemption
◎	**Q5**	Service furnished under a reciprocal billing arrangement by a substitute physician or by a substitute physical therapist furnishing outpatient physical therapy services in a health professional shortage area, a medically underserved area, or a rural area *IOM: 100-04, 1, 30.2.10*
◎	**Q6**	Service furnished under a fee-for-time compensation arrangement by a substitute physician or by a substitute physical therapist furnishing outpatient physical therapy services in a health professional shortage area, a medically underserved area, or a rural area *IOM: 100-04, 1, 30.2.11*
*	**Q7**	One Class A finding
*	**Q8**	Two Class B findings
*	**Q9**	One Class B and two Class C findings
▶ *	**QA**	Prescribed amounts of stationary oxygen for daytime use while at rest and nighttime use differ and the average of the two amounts is less than 1 liter per minute (lpm)
▶ *	**QB**	Prescribed amounts of stationary oxygen for daytime use while at rest and nighttime use differ and the average of the two amounts exceeds 4 liters per minute (lpm) and portable oxygen is prescribed
*	**QC**	Single channel monitoring
*	**QD**	Recording and storage in solid state memory by a digital recorder
⮌ *	**QE**	Prescribed amount of stationary oxygen while at rest is less than 1 liter per minute (LPM)
⮌ *	**QF**	Prescribed amount of stationary oxygen while at rest exceeds 4 liters per minute (LPM) and portable oxygen is prescribed
⮌ *	**QG**	Prescribed amount of stationary oxygen while at rest is greater than 4 liters per minute (LPM)
*	**QH**	Oxygen conserving device is being used with an oxygen delivery system
◎	**QJ**	Services/items provided to a prisoner or patient in state or local custody, however, the state or local government, as applicable, meets the requirements in 42 CFR 411.4 (B)
◎	**QK**	Medical direction of two, three, or four concurrent anesthesia procedures involving qualified individuals *IOM: 100-04, 12, 50K, 90*
*	**QL**	Patient pronounced dead after ambulance called
*	**QM**	Ambulance service provided under arrangement by a provider of services
*	**QN**	Ambulance service furnished directly by a provider of services
◎	**QP**	Documentation is on file showing that the laboratory test(s) was ordered individually or ordered as a CPT-recognized panel other than automated profile codes 80002-80019, G0058, G0059, and G0060.
*	**QQ**	Ordering professional consulted a qualified clinical decision support mechanism for this service and the related data was provided to the furnishing professional
▶ *	**QR**	Prescribed amounts of stationary oxygen for daytime use while at rest and nighttime use differ and the average of the two amounts is greater than 4 liters per minute (lpm)
◎	**QS**	Monitored anesthesia care service *IOM: 100-04, 12, 30.6, 501*
*	**QT**	Recording and storage on tape by an analog tape recorder
*	**QW**	CLIA-waived test
*	**QX**	CRNA service: with medical direction by a physician

▶ New ⮌ Revised ✔ Reinstated ~~deleted~~ Deleted ⊘ Not covered or valid by Medicare
◎ Special coverage instructions * Carrier discretion Ⓑ Bill Part B MAC Ⓑ Bill DME MAC

QY Medical direction of one certified registered nurse anesthetist (CRNA) by an anesthesiologist

IOM: 100-04, 12, 50K, 90

QZ CRNA service: without medical direction by a physician

RA Replacement of a DME, orthotic or prosthetic item

Contractors will deny claims for replacement parts when furnished in conjunction with the repair of a capped rental item and billed with modifier RB, including claims for parts submitted using code E1399, that are billed during the capped rental period (i.e., the last day of the 13th month of continuous use or before). Repair includes all maintenance, servicing, and repair of capped rental DME because it is included in the allowed rental payment amounts. (Pub 100-20 One-Time Notification Centers for Medicare & Medicaid Services, Transmittal: 901, May 13, 2011)

RB Replacement of a part of a DME, orthotic or prosthetic item furnished as part of a repair

RC Right coronary artery

RD Drug provided to beneficiary, but not administered "incident-to"

RE Furnished in full compliance with FDA-mandated risk evaluation and mitigation strategy (REMS)

RI Ramus intermedius coronary artery

RR Rental (use the 'RR' modifier when DME is to be rented)

RT Right side (used to identify procedures performed on the right side of the body)

Modifiers LT and RT identify procedures which can be performed on paired organs. Used for procedures performed on one side only. Should also be used when the procedures are similar but not identical and are performed on paired body parts.

Coding Clinic: 2016, Q3, P5

SA Nurse practitioner rendering service in collaboration with a physician

SB Nurse midwife

SC Medically necessary service or supply

SD Services provided by registered nurse with specialized, highly technical home infusion training

SE State and/or federally funded programs/services

SF Second opinion ordered by a professional review organization (PRO) per Section 9401, P.L. 99-272 (100% reimbursement – no Medicare deductible or coinsurance)

SG Ambulatory surgical center (ASC) facility service

Only valid for surgical codes. After 1/1/08 not required for ASC facility charges.

SH Second concurrently administered infusion therapy

SJ Third or more concurrently administered infusion therapy

SK Member of high risk population (use only with codes for immunization)

SL State supplied vaccine

SM Second surgical opinion

SN Third surgical opinion

SQ Item ordered by home health

SS Home infusion services provided in the infusion suite of the IV therapy provider

ST Related to trauma or injury

SU Procedure performed in physician's office (to denote use of facility and equipment)

SV Pharmaceuticals delivered to patient's home but not utilized

SW Services provided by a certified diabetic educator

SY Persons who are in close contact with member of high-risk population (use only with codes for immunization)

T1 Left foot, second digit

T2 Left foot, third digit

T3 Left foot, fourth digit

T4 Left foot, fifth digit

T5 Right foot, great toe

T6 Right foot, second digit

T7 Right foot, third digit

T8 Right foot, fourth digit

T9 Right foot, fifth digit

TA Left foot, great toe

TB Drug or biological acquired with 340B drug pricing program discount, reported for informational purposes

MIPS | Qp Quantity Physician | Qh Quantity Hospital | ♀ Female only
♂ Male only | A Age | DMEPOS | A2-Z3 ASC Payment Indicator | A-Y ASC Status Indicator | Coding Clinic

✻	**TC**	Technical component; under certain circumstances, a charge may be made for the technical component alone; under those circumstances the technical component charge is identified by adding modifier TC to the usual procedure number; technical component charges are institutional charges and not billed separately by physicians; however, portable x-ray suppliers only bill for technical component and should utilize modifier TC; the charge data from portable x-ray suppliers will then be used to build customary and prevailing profiles.
⃠	**TD**	RN
⃠	**TE**	LPN/LVN
⃠	**TF**	Intermediate level of care
⃠	**TG**	Complex/high tech level of care
⃠	**TH**	Obstetrical treatment/services, prenatal or postpartum
⃠	**TJ**	Program group, child and/or adolescent
⃠	**TK**	Extra patient or passenger, non-ambulance
⃠	**TL**	Early intervention/individualized family service plan (IFSP)
⃠	**TM**	Individualized education program (IEP)
⃠	**TN**	Rural/outside providers' customary service area
⃠	**TP**	Medical transport, unloaded vehicle
⃠	**TQ**	Basic life support transport by a volunteer ambulance provider
⃠	**TR**	School-based individual education program (IEP) services provided outside the public school district responsible for the student
✻	**TS**	Follow-up service
⃠	**TT**	Individualized service provided to more than one patient in same setting
⃠	**TU**	Special payment rate, overtime
⃠	**TV**	Special payment rates, holidays/ weekends
⃠	**TW**	Back-up equipment
⃠	**U1**	Medicaid Level of Care 1, as defined by each State
⃠	**U2**	Medicaid Level of Care 2, as defined by each State
⃠	**U3**	Medicaid Level of Care 3, as defined by each State
⃠	**U4**	Medicaid Level of Care 4, as defined by each State
⃠	**U5**	Medicaid Level of Care 5, as defined by each State
⃠	**U6**	Medicaid Level of Care 6, as defined by each State
⃠	**U7**	Medicaid Level of Care 7, as defined by each State
⃠	**U8**	Medicaid Level of Care 8, as defined by each State
⃠	**U9**	Medicaid Level of Care 9, as defined by each State
⃠	**UA**	Medicaid Level of Care 10, as defined by each State
⃠	**UB**	Medicaid Level of Care 11, as defined by each State
⃠	**UC**	Medicaid Level of Care 12, as defined by each State
⃠	**UD**	Medicaid Level of Care 13, as defined by each State
✻	**UE**	Used durable medical equipment
⃠	**UF**	Services provided in the morning
⃠	**UG**	Services provided in the afternoon
⃠	**UH**	Services provided in the evening
✻	**UJ**	Services provided at night
⃠	**UK**	Services provided on behalf of the client to someone other than the client (collateral relationship)
✻	**UN**	Two patients served
✻	**UP**	Three patients served
✻	**UQ**	Four patients served
✻	**UR**	Five patients served
✻	**US**	Six or more patients served
✻	**V1**	Demonstration Modifier 1
✻	**V2**	Demonstration Modifier 2
✻	**V3**	Demonstration Modifier 3
✻	**V5**	Vascular catheter (alone or with any other vascular access)
✻	**V6**	Arteriovenous graft (or other vascular access not including a vascular catheter)
✻	**V7**	Arteriovenous fistula only (in use with two needles)
✻	**VM**	Medicare diabetes prevention program (MDPP) virtual make-up session
✻	**VP**	Aphakic patient

✻ **X1** Continuous/broad services: for reporting services by clinicians, who provide the principal care for a patient, with no planned endpoint of the relationship; services in this category represent comprehensive care, dealing with the entire scope of patient problems, either directly or in a care coordination role; reporting clinician service examples include, but are not limited to: primary care, and clinicians providing comprehensive care to patients in addition to specialty care

✻ **X2** Continuous/focused services: for reporting services by clinicians whose expertise is needed for the ongoing management of a chronic disease or a condition that needs to be managed and followed with no planned endpoint to the relationship; reporting clinician service examples include but are not limited to: a rheumatologist taking care of the patient's rheumatoid arthritis longitudinally but not providing general primary care services

✻ **X3** Episodic/broad services: for reporting services by clinicians who have broad responsibility for the comprehensive needs of the patient that is limited to a defined period and circumstance such as a hospitalization; reporting clinician service examples include but are not limited to the hospitalist's services rendered providing comprehensive and general care to a patient while admitted to the hospital

✻ **X4** Episodic/focused services: for reporting services by clinicians who provide focused care on particular types of treatment limited to a defined period and circumstance; the patient has a problem, acute or chronic, that will be treated with surgery, radiation, or some other type of generally time-limited intervention; reporting clinician service examples include but are not limited to, the orthopedic surgeon performing a knee replacement and seeing the patient through the postoperative period

✻ **X5** Diagnostic services requested by another clinician: for reporting services by a clinician who furnishes care to the patient only as requested by another clinician or subsequent and related services requested by another clinician; this modifier is reported for patient relationships that may not be adequately captured by the above alternative categories; reporting clinician service examples include but are not limited to, the radiologist's interpretation of an imaging study requested by another clinician

✻ **XE** Separate encounter, a service that is distinct because it occurred during a separate encounter

✻ **XP** Separate practitioner, a service that is distinct because it was performed by a different practitioner

✻ **XS** Separate structure, a service that is distinct because it was performed on a separate organ/structure

✻ **XU** Unusual non-overlapping service, the use of a service that is distinct because it does not overlap usual components of the main service

~~ZA~~ ~~Novartis/Sandoz~~ ✖

~~ZB~~ ~~Pfizer/Hospira~~ ✖

~~ZC~~ ~~Merck/Samsung Bioepis~~ ✖

Ambulance Modifiers

Modifiers that are used on claims for ambulance services are created by combining two alpha characters. Each alpha character, with the exception of X, represents an origin (source) code or a destination code. The pair of alpha codes creates one modifier. The first position alpha-code = origin; the second position alpha-code = destination. On form CMS-1491, used to report ambulance services, Item 12 should contain the origin code and Item 13 should contain the destination code. Origin and destination codes and their descriptions are as follows:

D	Diagnostic or therapeutic site other than P or H when these are used as origin codes
E	Residential, domiciliary, custodial facility (other than an 1819 facility)
G	Hospital-based ESRD facility
H	Hospital
I	Site of transfer (e.g., airport or helicopter pad) between modes of ambulance transport
J	Freestanding ESRD facility
N	Skilled nursing facility
P	Physician's office
R	Residence
S	Scene of accident or acute event
X	Intermediate stop at physician's office on way to hospital (destination code only)

TRANSPORT SERVICES INCLUDING AMBULANCE (A0000-A0999)

⃠ **A0021** Ambulance service, outside state per mile, transport (Medicaid only) Ⓑ Qp Qh E1

Cross Reference A0030

⃠ **A0080** Non-emergency transportation, per mile - vehicle provided by volunteer (individual or organization), with no vested interest Ⓑ Qp Qh E1

⃠ **A0090** Non-emergency transportation, per mile - vehicle provided by individual (family member, self, neighbor) with vested interest Ⓑ Qp Qh E1

⃠ **A0100** Non-emergency transportation; taxi Ⓑ Qp Qh E1

⃠ **A0110** Non-emergency transportation and bus, intra- or interstate carrier Ⓑ Qp Qh E1

⃠ **A0120** Non-emergency transportation: mini-bus, mountain area transports, or other transportation systems Ⓑ Qp Qh E1

⃠ **A0130** Non-emergency transportation: wheelchair van Ⓑ Qp Qh E1

⃠ **A0140** Non-emergency transportation and air travel (private or commercial), intra- or interstate Ⓑ Qp Qh E1

⃠ **A0160** Non-emergency transportation: per mile - caseworker or social worker Ⓑ Qp Qh E1

⃠ **A0170** Transportation: ancillary: parking fees, tolls, other Ⓑ Qp Qh E1

⃠ **A0180** Non-emergency transportation: ancillary: lodging - recipient Ⓑ Qp Qh E1

⃠ **A0190** Non-emergency transportation: ancillary: meals - recipient Ⓑ Qp Qh E1

⃠ **A0200** Non-emergency transportation: ancillary: lodging - escort Ⓑ Qp Qh E1

⃠ **A0210** Non-emergency transportation: ancillary: meals - escort Ⓑ Qp Qh E1

⃠ **A0225** Ambulance service, neonatal transport, base rate, emergency transport, one way Ⓑ Qp Qh E1

⃠ **A0380** BLS mileage (per mile) Ⓑ Qp Qh E1

Cross Reference A0425

⃠ **A0382** BLS routine disposable supplies Ⓑ Qp Qh E1

⃠ **A0384** BLS specialized service disposable supplies; defibrillation (used by ALS ambulances and BLS ambulances in jurisdictions where defibrillation is permitted in BLS ambulances) Ⓑ Qp Qh E1

⃠ **A0390** ALS mileage (per mile) Ⓑ Qp Qh E1

Cross Reference A0425

⃠ **A0392** ALS specialized service disposable supplies; defibrillation (to be used only in jurisdictions where defibrillation cannot be performed in BLS ambulances) Ⓑ Qp Qh E1

⃠ **A0394** ALS specialized service disposable supplies; IV drug therapy Ⓑ Qp Qh E1

⃠ **A0396** ALS specialized service disposable supplies; esophageal intubation Ⓑ Qp Qh E1

⃠ **A0398** ALS routine disposable supplies Ⓑ Qp Qh E1

⃠ **A0420** Ambulance waiting time (ALS or BLS), one half (½) hour increments Ⓑ Qp Qh E1

Waiting Time Table

UNITS	TIME	UNITS	TIME
1	½ to 1 hr.	6	3 to 3½ hrs.
2	1 to 1½ hrs.	7	3½ to 4 hrs.
3	1½ to 2 hrs.	8	4 to 4½ hrs.
4	2 to 2½ hrs.	9	4½ to 5 hrs.
5	2½ to 3 hrs.	10	5 to 5½ hrs.

⃠ **A0422** Ambulance (ALS or BLS) oxygen and oxygen supplies, life sustaining situation Ⓑ Qp Qh E1

⃠ **A0424** Extra ambulance attendant, ground (ALS or BLS) or air (fixed or rotary winged); (requires medical review) Ⓑ Qp Qh E1

* **A0425** Ground mileage, per statute mile Ⓑ Qp Qh A

* **A0426** Ambulance service, advanced life support, non-emergency transport, Level 1 (ALS 1) Ⓑ Qp Qh A

* **A0427** Ambulance service, advanced life support, emergency transport, Level 1 (ALS 1-Emergency) Ⓑ Qp Qh A

* **A0428** Ambulance service, basic life support, non-emergency transport (BLS) Ⓑ Qp Qh A

* **A0429** Ambulance service, basic life support, emergency transport (BLS-Emergency) Ⓑ Qp Qh A

MIPS | Qp Quantity Physician | Qh Quantity Hospital | ♀ Female only
♂ Male only | A Age | DMEPOS | A2-Z3 ASC Payment Indicator | A-Y ASC Status Indicator | Coding Clinic

* **A0430** Ambulance service, conventional air services, transport, one way (fixed wing) Ⓑ Qp Qh A

* **A0431** Ambulance service, conventional air services, transport, one way (rotary wing) Ⓑ Qp Qh A

* **A0432** Paramedic intercept (PI), rural area, transport furnished by a volunteer ambulance company, which is prohibited by state law from billing third party payers Ⓑ Qp Qh A

* **A0433** Advanced life support, Level 2 (ALS2) Ⓑ Qp Qh A

* **A0434** Specialty care transport (SCT) Ⓑ Qp Qh A

* **A0435** Fixed wing air mileage, per statute mile Ⓑ Qp Qh A

* **A0436** Rotary wing air mileage, per statute mile Ⓑ Qp Qh A

⊘ **A0888** Noncovered ambulance mileage, per mile (e.g., for miles traveled beyond closest appropriate facility) Ⓑ Qp Qh E1

MCM: 2125

⊘ **A0998** Ambulance response and treatment, no transport Ⓑ Qp Qh E1

IOM: 100-02, 10, 20

◌ **A0999** Unlisted ambulance service Ⓑ A

IOM: 100-02, 10, 20

MEDICAL AND SURGICAL SUPPLIES (A4000-A8004)

Injection and Infusion

* **A4206** Syringe with needle, sterile 1 cc or less, each Ⓑ Ⓔ N

* **A4207** Syringe with needle, sterile 2 cc, each Ⓑ Ⓔ N

* **A4208** Syringe with needle, sterile 3 cc, each Ⓑ Ⓔ N

* **A4209** Syringe with needle, sterile 5 cc or greater, each Ⓑ Ⓔ N

⊘ **A4210** Needle-free injection device, each Ⓔ Qp Qh E1

IOM: 100-03, 4, 280.1

◌ **A4211** Supplies for self-administered injections Ⓑ Ⓔ Qp Qh N

IOM: 100-02, 15, 50

* **A4212** Non-coring needle or stylet with or without catheter Ⓑ Qp Qh N

* **A4213** Syringe, sterile, 20 cc or greater, each Ⓑ Ⓔ N

* **A4215** Needle, sterile, any size, each Ⓑ Ⓔ N

◌ **A4216** Sterile water, saline and/or dextrose diluent/flush, 10 ml Ⓑ Ⓔ ♿ N

Other: Sodium Chloride, Bacteriostatic, Syrex

IOM: 100-02, 15, 50

◌ **A4217** Sterile water/saline, 500 ml Ⓑ Ⓔ ♿ N

Other: Sodium Chloride

IOM: 100-02, 15, 50

◌ **A4218** Sterile saline or water, metered dose dispenser, 10 ml Ⓑ Ⓔ N

Other: Sodium Chloride

◌ **A4220** Refill kit for implantable infusion pump Ⓑ Qp Qh N

Do not report with 95990 or 95991 since Medicare payment for these codes includes the refill kit.

IOM: 100-03, 4, 280.1

* **A4221** Supplies for maintenance of non-insulin drug infusion catheter, per week (list drugs separately) Ⓔ Qp Qh ♿ N

Includes dressings for catheter site and flush solutions not directly related to drug infusion.

* **A4222** Infusion supplies for external drug infusion pump, per cassette or bag (list drug separately) Ⓔ Qp Qh ♿ N

Includes cassette or bag, diluting solutions, tubing and/or administration supplies, port cap changes, compounding charges, and preparation charges.

* **A4223** Infusion supplies not used with external infusion pump, per cassette or bag (list drugs separately) Ⓔ N

IOM: 100-03, 4, 280.1

* **A4224** Supplies for maintenance of insulin infusion catheter, per week Ⓔ Qp Qh ♿ N

◌ **A4225** Supplies for external insulin infusion pump, syringe type cartridge, sterile, each Ⓔ Qp Qh ♿ N

IOM: 100-03, 1, 50.3

◌ **A4230** Infusion set for external insulin pump, non-needle cannula type Ⓔ N

Requires prior authorization and copy of invoice.

IOM: 100-03, 4, 280.1

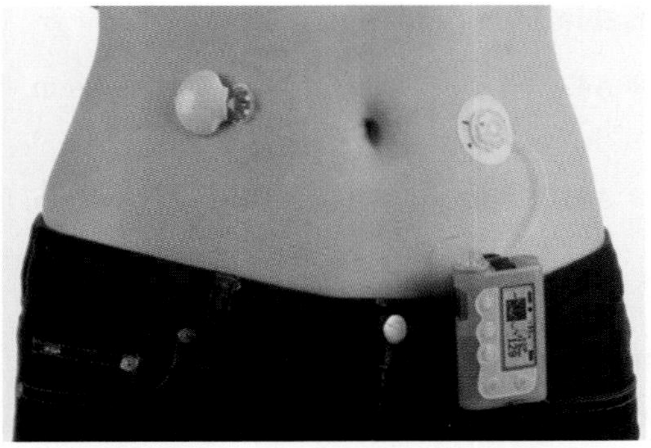

Figure 1 Insulin pump.

A4231 Infusion set for external insulin pump, needle type N

Requires prior authorization and copy of invoice.

IOM: 100-03, 4, 280.1

A4232 Syringe with needle for external insulin pump, sterile, 3 cc Qp Qh E1

Reports insulin reservoir for use with external insulin infusion pump (E0784); may be glass or plastic; includes needle for drawing up insulin. Does not include insulin for use in reservoir.

IOM: 100-03, 4, 280.1

Replacement Batteries

* A4233 Replacement battery, alkaline (other than J cell), for use with medically necessary home blood glucose monitor owned by patient, each Qh E1

* A4234 Replacement battery, alkaline, J cell, for use with medically necessary home blood glucose monitor owned by patient, each Qh E1

* A4235 Replacement battery, lithium, for use with medically necessary home blood glucose monitor owned by patient, each Qp Qh E1

* A4236 Replacement battery, silver oxide, for use with medically necessary home blood glucose monitor owned by patient, each Qh E1

Miscellaneous Supplies

* A4244 Alcohol or peroxide, per pint N

* A4245 Alcohol wipes, per box N

* A4246 Betadine or pHisoHex solution, per pint N

* A4247 Betadine or iodine swabs/wipes, per box N

* A4248 Chlorhexidine containing antiseptic, 1 ml N

A4250 Urine test or reagent strips or tablets (100 tablets or strips) Qp Qh E1

IOM: 100-02, 15, 110

A4252 Blood ketone test or reagent strip, each Qp Qh E1

Medicare Statute 1861(n)

A4253 Blood glucose test or reagent strips for home blood glucose monitor, per 50 strips Qp Qh N

Test strips (1 unit = 50 strips); non-insulin treated (every 3 months) 100 test strips (1×/day testing), 100 lancets (1×/day testing); modifier KS

IOM: 100-03, 1, 40.2

A4255 Platforms for home blood glucose monitor, 50 per box Qp Qh N

IOM: 100-03, 1, 40.2

A4256 Normal, low and high calibrator solution/chips Qp Qh N

IOM: 100-03, 1, 40.2

* A4257 Replacement lens shield cartridge for use with laser skin piercing device, each Qp Qh E1

A4258 Spring-powered device for lancet, each Qp Qh N

IOM: 100-03, 1, 40.2

A4259 Lancets, per box of 100 Qp Qh N

IOM: 100-03, 1, 40.2

A4261 Cervical cap for contraceptive use Qp Qh ♀ E1

Medicare Statute 1862A1

A4262 Temporary, absorbable lacrimal duct implant, each Qp Qh N

IOM: 100-04, 12, 20.3, 30.4

A4263 Permanent, long term, non-dissolvable lacrimal duct implant, each Qp Qh N

Bundled with insertion if performed in physician office.

IOM: 100-04, 12, 30.4

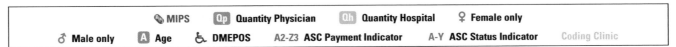

MIPS | Qp Quantity Physician | Qh Quantity Hospital | ♀ Female only
♂ Male only | A Age | DMEPOS | A2-Z3 ASC Payment Indicator | A-Y ASC Status Indicator | Coding Clinic

⃠ **A4264** Permanent implantable contraceptive intratubal occlusion device(s) and delivery system Ⓑ Qp Qh ♀ E1

Reports the Essure device.

A4265 Paraffin, per pound Ⓑ Ⓓ Qp Qh ♿ N

IOM: 100-03, 4, 280.1

⃠ **A4266** Diaphragm for contraceptive use Ⓑ Qp Qh ♀ E1

⃠ **A4267** Contraceptive supply, condom, male, each Ⓑ Qp Qh ♂ E1

⃠ **A4268** Contraceptive supply, condom, female, each Ⓑ Qp Qh ♀ E1

⃠ **A4269** Contraceptive supply, spermicide (e.g., foam, gel), each Ⓑ Qp Qh E1

✻ **A4270** Disposable endoscope sheath, each Ⓑ Qp Qh N

✻ **A4280** Adhesive skin support attachment for use with external breast prosthesis, each Ⓓ Qh ♀ ♿ N

✻ **A4281** Tubing for breast pump, replacement Ⓓ ♀ E1

✻ **A4282** Adapter for breast pump, replacement Ⓓ ♀ E1

✻ **A4283** Cap for breast pump bottle, replacement Ⓓ ♀ E1

✻ **A4284** Breast shield and splash protector for use with breast pump, replacement Ⓓ ♀ E1

✻ **A4285** Polycarbonate bottle for use with breast pump, replacement Ⓓ ♀ E1

✻ **A4286** Locking ring for breast pump, replacement Ⓓ ♀ E1

✻ **A4290** Sacral nerve stimulation test lead, each Ⓑ N

Service not separately priced by Part B (e.g., services not covered, bundled, used by Part A only)

Implantable Catheters

A4300 Implantable access catheter, (e.g., venous, arterial, epidural subarachnoid, or peritoneal, etc.) external access Ⓑ Qp Qh N

IOM: 100-02, 15, 120

✻ **A4301** Implantable access total; catheter, port/reservoir (e.g., venous, arterial, epidural, subarachnoid, peritoneal, etc.) Ⓑ Qp Qh N

Disposable Drug Delivery System

✻ **A4305** Disposable drug delivery system, flow rate of 50 ml or greater per hour Ⓑ Ⓓ Qp Qh N

✻ **A4306** Disposable drug delivery system, flow rate of less than 50 ml per hour Ⓑ Ⓓ Qp Qh N

Incontinence Appliances and Care Supplies

A4310 Insertion tray without drainage bag and without catheter (accessories only) Ⓑ Ⓓ Qp Qh ♿ N

IOM: 100-02, 15, 120

A4311 Insertion tray without drainage bag with indwelling catheter, Foley type, two-way latex with coating (Teflon, silicone, silicone elastomer, or hydrophilic, etc.) Ⓑ Ⓓ Qp Qh ♿ N

IOM: 100-02, 15, 120

A4312 Insertion tray without drainage bag with indwelling catheter, Foley type, two-way, all silicone Ⓑ Ⓓ Qp Qh ♿ N

Must meet criteria for indwelling catheter and medical record must justify need for:

- Recurrent encrustation
- Inability to pass a straight catheter
- Sensitivity to latex

Must be medically necessary.

IOM: 100-02, 15, 120

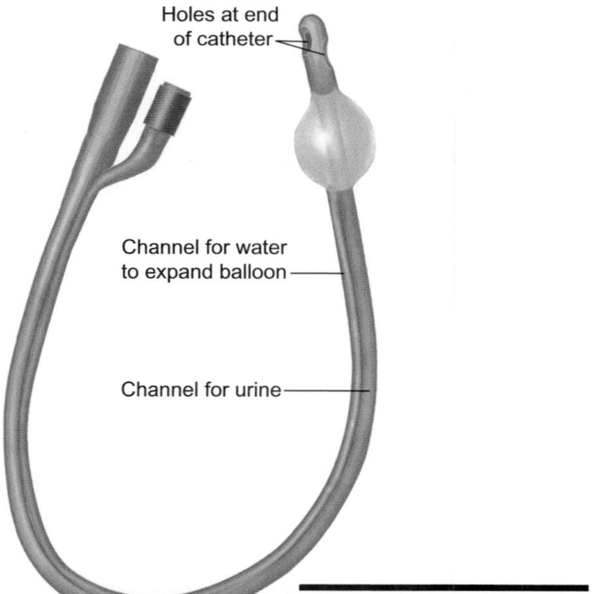
Holes at end of catheter
Channel for water to expand balloon
Channel for urine

Figure 2 Foley catheter.

▶ New ↻ Revised ✔ Reinstated ~~deleted~~ Deleted ⃠ Not covered or valid by Medicare
Special coverage instructions ✻ Carrier discretion Ⓑ Bill Part B MAC Ⓓ Bill DME MAC

A4313 Insertion tray without drainage bag with indwelling catheter, Foley type, three-way, for continuous irrigation Qp Qh N

Must meet criteria for indwelling catheter and medical record must justify need for:

- Recurrent encrustation
- Inability to pass a straight catheter
- Sensitivity to latex

Must be medically necessary.

IOM: 100-02, 15, 120

A4314 Insertion tray with drainage bag with indwelling catheter, Foley type, two-way latex with coating (Teflon, silicone, silicone elastomer or hydrophilic, etc.) Qp Qh N

IOM: 100-02, 15, 120

A4315 Insertion tray with drainage bag with indwelling catheter, Foley type, two-way, all silicone Qp Qh N

IOM: 100-02, 15, 120

A4316 Insertion tray with drainage bag with indwelling catheter, Foley type, three-way, for continuous irrigation Qp Qh N

IOM: 100-02, 15, 120

A4320 Irrigation tray with bulb or piston syringe, any purpose Qp Qh N

IOM: 100-02, 15, 120

A4321 Therapeutic agent for urinary catheter irrigation N

IOM: 100-02, 15, 120

A4322 Irrigation syringe, bulb, or piston, each Qp Qh N

IOM: 100-02, 15, 120

A4326 Male external catheter with integral collection chamber, any type, each Qp Qh ♂ N

IOM: 100-02, 15, 120

A4327 Female external urinary collection device; meatal cup, each Qp Qh ♀ N

IOM: 100-02, 15, 120

A4328 Female external urinary collection device; pouch, each Qp Qh ♀ N

IOM: 100-02, 15, 120

A4330 Perianal fecal collection pouch with adhesive, each Qp Qh N

IOM: 100-02, 15, 120

A4331 Extension drainage tubing, any type, any length, with connector/adaptor, for use with urinary leg bag or urostomy pouch, each Qh N

IOM: 100-02, 15, 120

A4332 Lubricant, individual sterile packet, each Qp Qh N

IOM: 100-02, 15, 120

A4333 Urinary catheter anchoring device, adhesive skin attachment, each N

IOM: 100-02, 15, 120

A4334 Urinary catheter anchoring device, leg strap, each N

IOM: 100-02, 15, 120

A4335 Incontinence supply; miscellaneous Qp Qh N

IOM: 100-02, 15, 120

A4336 Incontinence supply, urethral insert, any type, each N

IOM: 100-02, 15, 120

A4337 Incontinence supply, rectal insert, any type, each Qp Qh N

IOM: 100-02, 15, 120

A4338 Indwelling catheter; Foley type, two-way latex with coating (Teflon, silicone, silicone elastomer, or hydrophilic, etc.), each Qp Qh N

IOM: 100-02, 15, 120

A4340 Indwelling catheter; specialty type (e.g., coude, mushroom, wing, etc.), each Qp Qh N

Must meet criteria for indwelling catheter and medical record must justify need for:

- Recurrent encrustation
- Inability to pass a straight catheter
- Sensitivity to latex

Must be medically necessary.

IOM: 100-02, 15, 120

A4344 Indwelling catheter, Foley type, two-way, all silicone, each Qp Qh N

Must meet criteria for indwelling catheter and medical record must justify need for:

- Recurrent encrustation
- Inability to pass a straight catheter
- Sensitivity to latex

Must be medically necessary.

IOM: 100-02, 15, 120

MIPS | Qp Quantity Physician | Qh Quantity Hospital | ♀ Female only
♂ Male only | A Age | DMEPOS | A2-Z3 ASC Payment Indicator | A-Y ASC Status Indicator | Coding Clinic

A4346 Indwelling catheter; Foley type, three way for continuous irrigation, each N

IOM: 100-02, 15, 120

A4349 Male external catheter, with or without adhesive, disposable, each N

IOM: 100-02, 15, 120

A4351 Intermittent urinary catheter; straight tip, with or without coating (Teflon, silicone, silicone elastomer, or hydrophilic, etc.), each N

IOM: 100-02, 15, 120

A4352 Intermittent urinary catheter; coude (curved) tip, with or without coating (Teflon, silicone, silicone elastomeric, or hydrophilic, etc.), each N

IOM: 100-02, 15, 120

A4353 Intermittent urinary catheter, with insertion supplies N

IOM: 100-02, 15, 120

A4354 Insertion tray with drainage bag but without catheter N

IOM: 100-02, 15, 120

A4355 Irrigation tubing set for continuous bladder irrigation through a three-way indwelling Foley catheter, each N

IOM: 100-02, 15, 120

External Urinary Supplies

A4356 External urethral clamp or compression device (not to be used for catheter clamp), each N

IOM: 100-02, 15, 120

A4357 Bedside drainage bag, day or night, with or without anti-reflux device, with or without tube, each N

IOM: 100-02, 15, 120

A4358 Urinary drainage bag, leg or abdomen, vinyl, with or without tube, with straps, each N

IOM: 100-02, 15, 120

A4360 Disposable external urethral clamp or compression device, with pad and/or pouch, each N

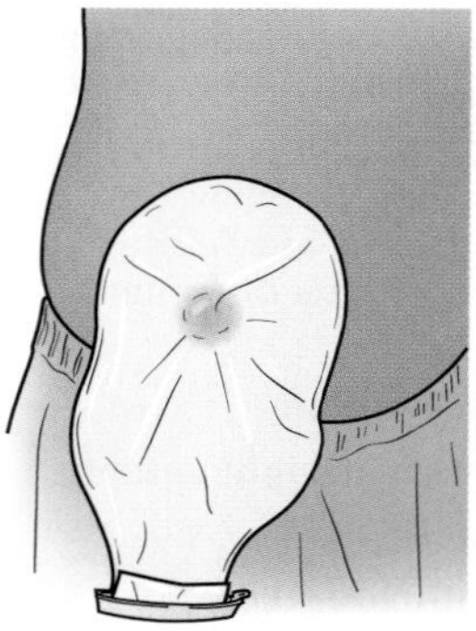

Figure 3 Ostomy pouch.

Ostomy Supplies

A4361 Ostomy faceplate, each N

IOM: 100-02, 15, 120

A4362 Skin barrier; solid, 4 × 4 or equivalent; each N

IOM: 100-02, 15, 120

A4363 Ostomy clamp, any type, replacement only, each E1

A4364 Adhesive, liquid or equal, any type, per oz N

Fee schedule category: Ostomy, tracheostomy, and urologicals items.

IOM: 100-02, 15, 120

* **A4366** Ostomy vent, any type, each N

A4367 Ostomy belt, each N

IOM: 100-02, 15, 120

* **A4368** Ostomy filter, any type, each N

A4369 Ostomy skin barrier, liquid (spray, brush, etc.), per oz N

IOM: 100-02, 15, 120

A4371 Ostomy skin barrier, powder, per oz N

IOM: 100-02, 15, 120

A4372 Ostomy skin barrier, solid 4 × 4 or equivalent, standard wear, with built-in convexity, each N

IOM: 100-02, 15, 120

A4373 Ostomy skin barrier, with flange (solid, flexible, or accordion), with built-in convexity, any size, each N

IOM: 100-02, 15, 120

▶ New ↩ Revised ✔ Reinstated ~~deleted~~ Deleted ⊘ Not covered or valid by Medicare
Special coverage instructions * Carrier discretion Bill Part B MAC Bill DME MAC

A4375 Ostomy pouch, drainable, with faceplate attached, plastic, each Qp Qh N
IOM: 100-02, 15, 120

A4376 Ostomy pouch, drainable, with faceplate attached, rubber, each Qp Qh N
IOM: 100-02, 15, 120

A4377 Ostomy pouch, drainable, for use on faceplate, plastic, each Qp Qh N
IOM: 100-02, 15, 120

A4378 Ostomy pouch, drainable, for use on faceplate, rubber, each Qp Qh N
IOM: 100-02, 15, 120

A4379 Ostomy pouch, urinary, with faceplate attached, plastic, each Qp Qh N
IOM: 100-02, 15, 120

A4380 Ostomy pouch, urinary, with faceplate attached, rubber, each Qp Qh N
IOM: 100-02, 15, 120

A4381 Ostomy pouch, urinary, for use on faceplate, plastic, each Qp Qh N
IOM: 100-02, 15, 120

A4382 Ostomy pouch, urinary, for use on faceplate, heavy plastic, each Qp Qh N
IOM: 100-02, 15, 120

A4383 Ostomy pouch, urinary, for use on faceplate, rubber, each Qp Qh N
IOM: 100-02, 15, 120

A4384 Ostomy faceplate equivalent, silicone ring, each Qp Qh N
IOM: 100-02, 15, 120

A4385 Ostomy skin barrier, solid 4 × 4 or equivalent, extended wear, without built-in convexity, each Qp Qh N
IOM: 100-02, 15, 120

A4387 Ostomy pouch closed, with barrier attached, with built-in convexity (1 piece), each Qh N
IOM: 100-02, 15, 120

A4388 Ostomy pouch, drainable, with extended wear barrier attached (1 piece), each Qh N
IOM: 100-02, 15, 120

A4389 Ostomy pouch, drainable, with barrier attached, with built-in convexity (1 piece), each Qp Qh N
IOM: 100-02, 15, 120

A4390 Ostomy pouch, drainable, with extended wear barrier attached, with built-in convexity (1 piece), each Qh N
IOM: 100-02, 15, 120

A4391 Ostomy pouch, urinary, with extended wear barrier attached (1 piece), each Qh N
IOM: 100-02, 15, 120

A4392 Ostomy pouch, urinary, with standard wear barrier attached, with built-in convexity (1 piece), each Qp Qh N
IOM: 100-02, 15, 120

A4393 Ostomy pouch, urinary, with extended wear barrier attached, with built-in convexity (1 piece), each Qh N
IOM: 100-02, 15, 120

A4394 Ostomy deodorant, with or without lubricant, for use in ostomy pouch, per fluid ounce N
IOM: 100-02, 15, 20

A4395 Ostomy deodorant for use in ostomy pouch, solid, per tablet N
IOM: 100-02, 15, 20

A4396 Ostomy belt with peristomal hernia support Qh N
IOM: 100-02, 15, 120

A4397 Irrigation supply; sleeve, each Qp Qh N
IOM: 100-02, 15, 120

A4398 Ostomy irrigation supply; bag, each Qp Qh N
IOM: 100-02, 15, 120

A4399 Ostomy irrigation supply; cone/catheter, with or without brush Qp Qh N
IOM: 100-02, 15, 120

A4400 Ostomy irrigation set Qp Qh N
IOM: 100-02, 15, 120

A4402 Lubricant, per ounce Qp Qh N
IOM: 100-02, 15, 120

A4404 Ostomy ring, each Qp Qh N
IOM: 100-02, 15, 120

A4405 Ostomy skin barrier, non-pectin based, paste, per ounce N
IOM: 100-02, 15, 120

MIPS | Qp Quantity Physician | Qh Quantity Hospital | ♀ Female only
♂ Male only | A Age | DMEPOS | A2-Z3 ASC Payment Indicator | A-Y ASC Status Indicator | Coding Clinic

○ **A4406** Ostomy skin barrier, pectin-based, paste, per ounce (B) (D) N

IOM: 100-02, 15, 120

○ **A4407** Ostomy skin barrier, with flange (solid, flexible, or accordion), extended wear, with built-in convexity, 4 × 4 inches or smaller, each (B) (D) Qp Qh N

IOM: 100-02, 15, 120

○ **A4408** Ostomy skin barrier, with flange (solid, flexible, or accordion), extended wear, with built-in convexity, larger than 4 × 4 inches, each (B) (D) Qh N

IOM: 100-02, 15, 120

○ **A4409** Ostomy skin barrier, with flange (solid, flexible, or accordion), extended wear, without built-in convexity, 4 × 4 inches or smaller, each (B) (D) Qh N

IOM: 100-02, 15, 120

○ **A4410** Ostomy skin barrier, with flange (solid, flexible, or accordion), extended wear, without built-in convexity, larger than 4 × 4 inches, each (B) (D) Qp Qh N

IOM: 100-02, 15, 120

○ **A4411** Ostomy skin barrier, solid 4 × 4 or equivalent, extended wear, with built-in convexity, each (B) (D) Qh N

○ **A4412** Ostomy pouch, drainable, high output, for use on a barrier with flange (2 piece system), without filter, each (B) (D) Qh N

IOM: 100-02, 15, 120

○ **A4413** Ostomy pouch, drainable, high output, for use on a barrier with flange (2 piece system), with filter, each (B) (D) Qp Qh N

IOM: 100-02, 15, 120

○ **A4414** Ostomy skin barrier, with flange (solid, flexible, or accordion), without built-in convexity, 4 × 4 inches or smaller, each (B) (D) Qh N

IOM: 100-02, 15, 120

○ **A4415** Ostomy skin barrier, with flange (solid, flexible, or accordion), without built-in convexity, larger than 4 × 4 inches, each (B) (D) Qh N

IOM: 100-02, 15, 120

* **A4416** Ostomy pouch, closed, with barrier attached, with filter (1 piece), each (B) (D) Qp Qh N

* **A4417** Ostomy pouch, closed, with barrier attached, with built-in convexity, with filter (1 piece), each (B) (D) Qh N

* **A4418** Ostomy pouch, closed; without barrier attached, with filter (1 piece), each (B) (D) Qh N

* **A4419** Ostomy pouch, closed; for use on barrier with non-locking flange, with filter (2 piece), each (B) (D) Qp Qh N

* **A4420** Ostomy pouch, closed; for use on barrier with locking flange (2 piece), each (B) (D) Qh N

* **A4421** Ostomy supply; miscellaneous (B) (D) N

○ **A4422** Ostomy absorbent material (sheet/pad/crystal packet) for use in ostomy pouch to thicken liquid stomal output, each (B) (D) N

IOM: 100-02, 15, 120

* **A4423** Ostomy pouch, closed; for use on barrier with locking flange, with filter (2 piece), each (B) (D) Qp Qh N

* **A4424** Ostomy pouch, drainable, with barrier attached, with filter (1 piece), each (B) (D) Qh N

* **A4425** Ostomy pouch, drainable; for use on barrier with non-locking flange, with filter (2 piece system), each (B) (D) Qh N

* **A4426** Ostomy pouch, drainable; for use on barrier with locking flange (2 piece system), each (B) (D) Qp Qh N

* **A4427** Ostomy pouch, drainable; for use on barrier with locking flange, with filter (2 piece system), each (B) (D) Qh N

* **A4428** Ostomy pouch, urinary, with extended wear barrier attached, with faucet-type tap with valve (1 piece), each (B) (D) Qh N

* **A4429** Ostomy pouch, urinary, with barrier attached, with built-in convexity, with faucet-type tap with valve (1 piece), each (B) (D) Qp Qh N

* **A4430** Ostomy pouch, urinary, with extended wear barrier attached, with built-in convexity, with faucet-type tap with valve (1 piece), each (B) (D) Qh N

* **A4431** Ostomy pouch, urinary; with barrier attached, with faucet-type tap with valve (1 piece), each (B) (D) Qh N

* **A4432** Ostomy pouch, urinary; for use on barrier with non-locking flange, with faucet-type tap with valve (2 piece), each (B) (D) Qp Qh N

* **A4433** Ostomy pouch, urinary; for use on barrier with locking flange (2 piece), each (B) (D) Qh N

* **A4434** Ostomy pouch, urinary; for use on barrier with locking flange, with faucet-type tap with valve (2 piece), each Qh N
* **A4435** Ostomy pouch, drainable, high output, with extended wear barrier (one-piece system), with or without filter, each Qp Qh N

Miscellaneous Supplies

A4450 Tape, non-waterproof, per 18 square inches N

If used with surgical dressings, billed with AW modifier (in addition to appropriate A1-A9 modifier).

IOM: 100-02, 15, 120

A4452 Tape, waterproof, per 18 square inches N

If used with surgical dressings, billed with AW modifier (in addition to appropriate A1-A9 modifier).

IOM: 100-02, 15, 120

A4455 Adhesive remover or solvent (for tape, cement or other adhesive), per ounce Qp Qh N

IOM: 100-02, 15, 120

A4456 Adhesive remover, wipes, any type, each N

May be reimbursed for male or female clients to home health DME providers and DME medical suppliers in the home setting.

IOM: 100-02, 15, 120

* **A4458** Enema bag with tubing, reusable N
* **A4459** Manual pump-operated enema system, includes balloon, catheter and all accessories, reusable, any type Qp Qh N
* **A4461** Surgical dressing holder, non-reusable, each Qp Qh N
* **A4463** Surgical dressing holder, reusable, each Qh N
* **A4465** Non-elastic binder for extremity Qp Qh N

A4467 Belt, strap, sleeve, garment, or covering, any type Qp Qh E1

A4470 Gravlee jet washer Qp Qh N

Symptoms suggestive of endometrial disease must be present for this disposable diagnostic tool to be covered.

IOM: 100-02, 16, 90; 100-03, 4, 230.5

A4480 VABRA aspirator Qp Qh N

Symptoms suggestive of endometrial disease must be present for this disposable diagnostic tool to be covered.

IOM: 100-02, 16, 90; 100-03, 4, 230.6

A4481 Tracheostoma filter, any type, any size, each Qh N

IOM: 100-02, 15, 120

A4483 Moisture exchanger, disposable, for use with invasive mechanical ventilation N

IOM: 100-02, 15, 120

A4490 Surgical stockings above knee length, each Qp Qh E1

IOM: 100-02, 15, 100; 100-02, 15, 110; 100-03, 4, 280.1

A4495 Surgical stockings thigh length, each Qp Qh E1

IOM: 100-02, 15, 100; 100-02, 15, 110; 100-03, 4, 280.1

A4500 Surgical stockings below knee length, each Qp Qh E1

IOM: 100-02, 15, 100; 100-02, 15, 110; 100-03, 4, 280.1

A4510 Surgical stockings full length, each Qp Qh E1

IOM: 100-02, 15, 100; 100-02, 15, 110; 100-03, 4, 280.1

A4520 Incontinence garment, any type (e.g., brief, diaper), each Qp Qh E1

IOM: 100-03, 4, 280.1

A4550 Surgical trays Qp Qh B

No longer payable by Medicare; included in practice expense for procedures. Some private payers may pay, most private payers follow Medicare guidelines.

IOM: 100-04, 12, 20.3, 30.4

A4553 Non-disposable underpads, all sizes Qp Qh E1

IOM: 100-03, 4, 280.1

A4554 Disposable underpads, all sizes Qp Qh E1

IOM: 100-03, 4, 280.1

A4555 Electrode/transducer for use with electrical stimulation device used for cancer treatment, replacement only Qp Qh E1

* **A4556** Electrodes (e.g., apnea monitor), per pair Qp Qh N

MIPS | Qp Quantity Physician | Qh Quantity Hospital | ♀ Female only
♂ Male only | A Age | DMEPOS | A2-Z3 ASC Payment Indicator | A-Y ASC Status Indicator | Coding Clinic

MEDICAL AND SURGICAL SUPPLIES A4434 – A4556

* **A4557** Lead wires (e.g., apnea monitor), per pair Qp Qh — N
* **A4558** Conductive gel or paste, for use with electrical device (e.g., TENS, NMES), per oz Qp Qh — N
* **A4559** Coupling gel or paste, for use with ultrasound device, per oz — N
* **A4561** Pessary, rubber, any type Qp Qh ♀ — N
* **A4562** Pessary, non-rubber, any type Qp Qh ♀ — N
* ▶ **A4563** Rectal control system for vaginal insertion, for long term use, includes pump and all supplies and accessories, any type each — N
* **A4565** Slings Qp Qh — N
* ⃠ **A4566** Shoulder sling or vest design, abduction restrainer, with or without swathe control, prefabricated, includes fitting and adjustment Qp Qh — E1
* ⃠ **A4570** Splint Qp Qh — E1

  IOM: 100-02, 6, 10; 100-02, 15, 100; 100-04, 4, 240
* **A4575** Topical hyperbaric oxygen chamber, disposable Qp Qh — A
* ⃠ **A4580** Cast supplies (e.g., plaster) Qp Qh — E1

  IOM: 100-02, 6, 10; 100-02, 15, 100; 100-04, 4, 240
* ⃠ **A4590** Special casting material (e.g., fiberglass) Qp Qh — E1

  IOM: 100-02, 6, 10; 100-02, 15, 100; 100-04, 4, 240
* **A4595** Electrical stimulator supplies, 2 lead, per month (e.g., TENS, NMES) Qp Qh — N

  IOM: 100-03, 2, 160.13
* **A4600** Sleeve for intermittent limb compression device, replacement only, each — E1

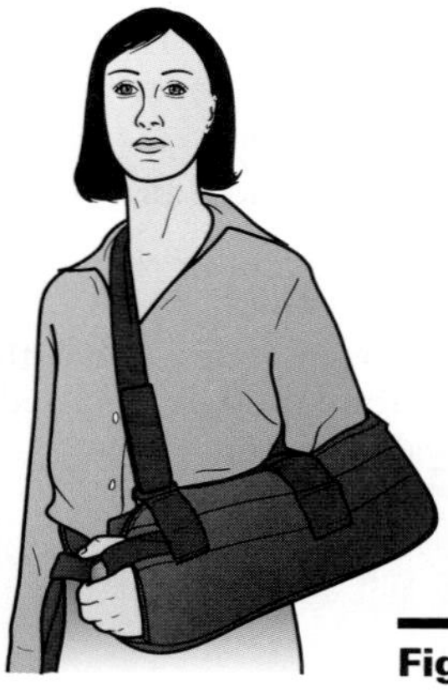

Figure 4 Arm sling.

* **A4601** Lithium ion battery, rechargeable, for non-prosthetic use, replacement — E1
* **A4602** Replacement battery for external infusion pump owned by patient, lithium, 1.5 volt, each Qp Qh — N
* **A4604** Tubing with integrated heating element for use with positive airway pressure device Qh — N
* **A4605** Tracheal suction catheter, closed system, each Qh — N
* **A4606** Oxygen probe for use with oximeter device, replacement Qp Qh — N
* **A4608** Transtracheal oxygen catheter, each — N

Supplies for Respiratory and Oxygen Equipment

* ⃠ **A4611** Battery, heavy duty; replacement for patient owned ventilator Qp Qh — E1

  Medicare Statute 1834(a)(3)(a)
* ⃠ **A4612** Battery cables; replacement for patient-owned ventilator Qh — E1

  Medicare Statute 1834(a)(3)(a)
* ⃠ **A4613** Battery charger; replacement for patient-owned ventilator Qh — E1

  Medicare Statute 1834(a)(3)(a)
* **A4614** Peak expiratory flow rate meter, hand held Qp Qh — N
* **A4615** Cannula, nasal — N

  IOM: 100-03, 2, 160.6; 100-04, 20, 100.2
* **A4616** Tubing (oxygen), per foot — N

  IOM: 100-03, 2, 160.6; 100-04, 20, 100.2

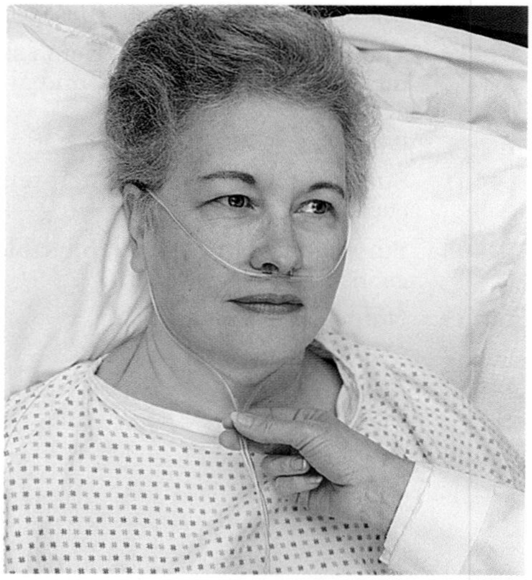

Figure 5 Nasal cannula.

▶ New ↩ Revised ✔ Reinstated ~~deleted~~ Deleted ⃠ Not covered or valid by Medicare
Special coverage instructions * Carrier discretion Bill Part B MAC Bill DME MAC

A4617 Mouth piece N

IOM: 100-03, 2, 160.6; 100-04, 20, 100.2

A4618 Breathing circuits Qp Qh N

IOM: 100-03, 2, 160.6; 100-04, 20, 100.2

A4619 Face tent N

IOM: 100-03, 2, 160.6; 100-04, 20, 100.2

A4620 Variable concentration mask N

IOM: 100-03, 2, 160.6; 100-04, 20, 100.2

A4623 Tracheostomy, inner cannula Qh N

IOM: 100-02, 15, 120; 100-03, 1, 20.9

* **A4624** Tracheal suction catheter, any type, other than closed system, each Qh N

Sterile suction catheters are medically necessary only for tracheostomy suctioning. Limitations include three suction catheters per day when covered for medically necessary tracheostomy suctioning. Assign DX V44.0 or V55.0 on the claim form. (CMS Manual System, Pub. 100-3, NCD manual, Chapter 1, Section 280-1)

A4625 Tracheostomy care kit for new tracheostomy Qp Qh N

Dressings used with tracheostomies are included in the allowance for the code. This starter kit is covered after a surgical tracheostomy. (https://www . noridianmedicare.com/dme/coverage/docs/lcds/current_lcds/tracheostomy_care_supplies.htm)

IOM: 100-02, 15, 120

A4626 Tracheostomy cleaning brush, each N

IOM: 100-02, 15, 120

A4627 Spacer, bag, or reservoir, with or without mask, for use with metered dose inhaler Qp Qh E1

IOM: 100-02, 15, 110

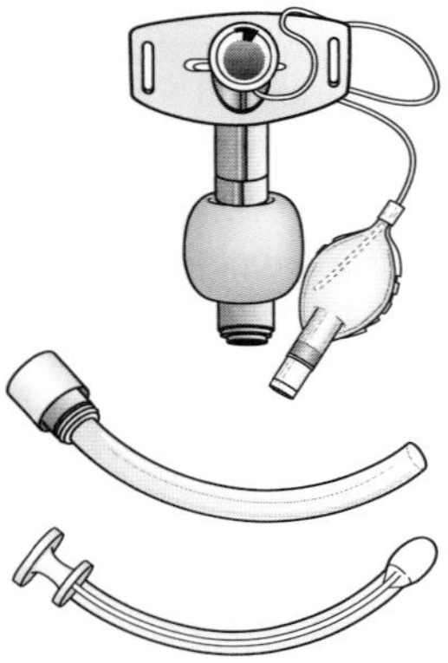

Figure 6 Tracheostomy cannula.

* **A4628** Oropharyngeal suction catheter, each Qh N

No more than three catheters per week are covered for medically necessary oropharyngeal suctioning because the catheters can be reused if cleansed and disinfected. (MS Manual System, Pub. 100-3, NCD manual, Chapter 1, Section 280-1)

A4629 Tracheostomy care kit for established tracheostomy Qh N

IOM: 100-02, 15, 120

Replacement Parts

A4630 Replacement batteries, medically necessary, transcutaneous electrical stimulator, owned by patient E1

IOM: 100-03, 3, 160.7

* **A4633** Replacement bulb/lamp for ultraviolet light therapy system, each Qp Qh E1

* **A4634** Replacement bulb for therapeutic light box, tabletop model N

A4635 Underarm pad, crutch, replacement, each Qp Qh E1

IOM: 100-03, 4, 280.1

A4636 Replacement, handgrip, cane, crutch, or walker, each Qh E1

IOM: 100-03, 4, 280.1

A4637 Replacement, tip, cane, crutch, walker, each Qh E1

IOM: 100-03, 4, 280.1

* **A4638** Replacement battery for patient-owned ear pulse generator, each Qp Qh E1

* **A4639** Replacement pad for infrared heating pad system, each E1

A4640 Replacement pad for use with medically necessary alternating pressure pad owned by patient Qp Qh E1

IOM: 100-03, 4, 280.1; 100-08, 5, 5.2.3

Supplies for Radiological Procedures

* **A4641** Radiopharmaceutical, diagnostic, not otherwise classified N

Is not an applicable tracer for PET scans

* **A4642** Indium In-111 satumomab pendetide, diagnostic, per study dose, up to 6 millicuries Qp Qh N

MIPS | Qp Quantity Physician | Qh Quantity Hospital | ♀ Female only
♂ Male only | A Age | DMEPOS | A2-Z3 ASC Payment Indicator | A-Y ASC Status Indicator | Coding Clinic

Miscellaneous Supplies

* **A4648** Tissue marker, implantable, any type, each Ⓟ Qp Qh N

Coding Clinic: 2018, Q2, P4,5; 2013, Q3, P9

* **A4649** Surgical supply miscellaneous Ⓟ Ⓔ Qp N

* **A4650** Implantable radiation dosimeter, each Ⓟ Qp Qh N

A4651 Calibrated microcapillary tube, each Ⓔ N

IOM: 100-04, 3, 40.3

A4652 Microcapillary tube sealant Ⓔ N

IOM: 100-04, 3, 40.3

Supplies for Dialysis

* **A4653** Peritoneal dialysis catheter anchoring device, belt, each Ⓔ Qp Qh N

A4657 Syringe, with or without needle, each Ⓔ Qp Qh N

IOM: 100-04, 8, 90.3.2

A4660 Sphygmomanometer/blood pressure apparatus with cuff and stethoscope Ⓔ Qp Qh N

IOM: 100-04, 8, 90.3.2

A4663 Blood pressure cuff only Ⓔ Qp Qh N

IOM: 100-04, 8, 90.3.2

⊘ **A4670** Automatic blood pressure monitor Ⓔ Qp Qh E1

IOM: 100-04, 8, 90.3.2

A4671 Disposable cycler set used with cycler dialysis machine, each Ⓔ Qp Qh B

IOM: 100-04, 8, 90.3.2

A4672 Drainage extension line, sterile, for dialysis, each Ⓔ Qp Qh B

IOM: 100-04, 8, 90.3.2

A4673 Extension line with easy lock connectors, used with dialysis Ⓔ Qp Qh B

IOM: 100-04, 8, 90.3.2

A4674 Chemicals/antiseptics solution used to clean/sterilize dialysis equipment, per 8 oz Ⓔ Qp Qh B

IOM: 100-04, 8, 90.3.2

A4680 Activated carbon filters for hemodialysis, each Ⓔ Qp Qh N

IOM: 100-04, 8, 90.3.2

A4690 Dialyzers (artificial kidneys), all types, all sizes, for hemodialysis, each Ⓔ Qp Qh N

IOM: 100-04, 8, 90.3.2

A4706 Bicarbonate concentrate, solution, for hemodialysis, per gallon Ⓔ Qp Qh N

IOM: 100-04, 8, 90.3.2

A4707 Bicarbonate concentrate, powder, for hemodialysis, per packet Ⓔ Qp Qh N

IOM: 100-04, 8, 90.3.2

A4708 Acetate concentrate solution, for hemodialysis, per gallon Ⓔ Qp Qh N

IOM: 100-04, 8, 90.3.2

A4709 Acid concentrate, solution, for hemodialysis, per gallon Ⓔ Qp Qh N

IOM: 100-04, 8, 90.3.2

A4714 Treated water (deionized, distilled, or reverse osmosis) for peritoneal dialysis, per gallon Ⓔ Qp Qh N

IOM: 100-03, 4, 230.7; 100-04, 3, 40.3

A4719 "Y set" tubing for peritoneal dialysis Ⓔ Qp Qh N

IOM: 100-04, 8, 90.3.2

A4720 Dialysate solution, any concentration of dextrose, fluid volume greater than 249 cc, but less than or equal to 999 cc, for peritoneal dialysis Ⓔ Qp Qh N

Do not use AX modifier.

IOM: 100-04, 8, 90.3.2

A4721 Dialysate solution, any concentration of dextrose, fluid volume greater than 999 cc but less than or equal to 1999 cc, for peritoneal dialysis Ⓔ Qp Qh N

IOM: 100-04, 8, 90.3.2

A4722 Dialysate solution, any concentration of dextrose, fluid volume greater than 1999 cc but less than or equal to 2999 cc, for peritoneal dialysis Ⓔ Qp Qh N

IOM: 100-04, 8, 90.3.2

A4723 Dialysate solution, any concentration of dextrose, fluid volume greater than 2999 cc but less than or equal to 3999 cc, for peritoneal dialysis Ⓔ Qp Qh N

IOM: 100-04, 8, 90.3.2

A4724 Dialysate solution, any concentration of dextrose, fluid volume greater than 3999 cc but less than or equal to 4999 cc for peritoneal dialysis Ⓔ Qp Qh N

IOM: 100-04, 8, 90.3.2

A4725 Dialysate solution, any concentration of dextrose, fluid volume greater than 4999 cc but less than or equal to 5999 cc, for peritoneal dialysis Qp Qh N
IOM: 100-04, 8, 90.3.2

A4726 Dialysate solution, any concentration of dextrose, fluid volume greater than 5999 cc, for peritoneal dialysis Qp Qh N
IOM: 100-04, 8, 90.3.2

* A4728 Dialysate solution, non-dextrose containing, 500 ml Qp Qh B

A4730 Fistula cannulation set for hemodialysis, each Qp Qh N
IOM: 100-04, 8, 90.3.2

A4736 Topical anesthetic, for dialysis, per gram Qp Qh N
IOM: 100-04, 8, 90.3.2

A4737 Injectable anesthetic, for dialysis, per 10 ml Qp Qh N
IOM: 100-04, 8, 90.3.2

A4740 Shunt accessory, for hemodialysis, any type, each Qp Qh N
IOM: 100-04, 8, 90.3.2

A4750 Blood tubing, arterial or venous, for hemodialysis, each Qp Qh N
IOM: 100-04, 8, 90.3.2

A4755 Blood tubing, arterial and venous combined, for hemodialysis, each Qp Qh N
IOM: 100-04, 8, 90.3.2

A4760 Dialysate solution test kit, for peritoneal dialysis, any type, each Qp Qh N
IOM: 100-04, 8, 90.3.2

A4765 Dialysate concentrate, powder, additive for peritoneal dialysis, per packet Qp Qh N
IOM: 100-04, 8, 90.3.2

A4766 Dialysate concentrate, solution, additive for peritoneal dialysis, per 10 ml Qp Qh N
IOM: 100-04, 8, 90.3.2

A4770 Blood collection tube, vacuum, for dialysis, per 50 Qp Qh N
IOM: 100-04, 8, 90.3.2

A4771 Serum clotting time tube, for dialysis, per 50 Qp Qh N
IOM: 100-04, 8, 90.3.2

A4772 Blood glucose test strips, for dialysis, per 50 Qp Qh N
IOM: 100-04, 8, 90.3.2

A4773 Occult blood test strips, for dialysis, per 50 Qp Qh N
IOM: 100-04, 8, 90.3.2

A4774 Ammonia test strips, for dialysis, per 50 Qp Qh N
IOM: 100-04, 8, 90.3.2

A4802 Protamine sulfate, for hemodialysis, per 50 mg Qp Qh N
IOM: 100-04, 8, 90.3.2

A4860 Disposable catheter tips for peritoneal dialysis, per 10 Qp Qh N
IOM: 100-04, 8, 90.3.2

A4870 Plumbing and/or electrical work for home hemodialysis equipment Qp Qh N
IOM: 100-04, 8, 90.3.2

A4890 Contracts, repair and maintenance, for hemodialysis equipment Qp Qh N
IOM: 100-02, 15, 110.2

A4911 Drain bag/bottle, for dialysis, each Qp Qh N

A4913 Miscellaneous dialysis supplies, not otherwise specified Qp Qh N
Items not related to dialysis must not be billed with the miscellaneous codes A4913 or E1699.

A4918 Venous pressure clamp, for hemodialysis, each Qp Qh N

A4927 Gloves, non-sterile, per 100 Qp Qh N

A4928 Surgical mask, per 20 Qp Qh N

A4929 Tourniquet for dialysis, each Qp Qh N

A4930 Gloves, sterile, per pair Qp Qh N

* A4931 Oral thermometer, reusable, any type, each Qp Qh N

* A4932 Rectal thermometer, reusable, any type, each Qp Qh N

Additional Ostomy Supplies

A5051 Ostomy pouch, closed; with barrier attached (1 piece), each Qp Qh N
IOM: 100-02, 15, 120

A5052 Ostomy pouch, closed; without barrier attached (1 piece), each Qp Qh N
IOM: 100-02, 15, 120

MIPS | Qp Quantity Physician | Qh Quantity Hospital | ♀ Female only
♂ Male only | A Age | DMEPOS | A2-Z3 ASC Payment Indicator | A-Y ASC Status Indicator | Coding Clinic

A5053 Ostomy pouch, closed; for use on faceplate, each Qp Qh N
IOM: 100-02, 15, 120

A5054 Ostomy pouch, closed; for use on barrier with flange (2 piece), each Qp N
IOM: 100-02, 15, 120

A5055 Stoma cap Qp Qh N
IOM: 100-02, 15, 120

A5056 Ostomy pouch, drainable, with extended wear barrier attached, with filter (1 piece), each Qp Qh N
IOM: 100-02, 15, 120

A5057 Ostomy pouch, drainable, with extended wear barrier attached, with built in convexity, with filter (1 piece), each Qp Qh N
IOM: 100-02, 15, 120

* **A5061** Ostomy pouch, drainable; with barrier attached (1 piece), each Qp Qh N
IOM: 100-02, 15, 120

A5062 Ostomy pouch, drainable; without barrier attached (1 piece), each Qp Qh N
IOM: 100-02, 15, 120

A5063 Ostomy pouch, drainable; for use on barrier with flange (2 piece system), each Qp Qh N
IOM: 100-02, 15, 120

A5071 Ostomy pouch, urinary; with barrier attached (1 piece), each Qp Qh N
IOM: 100-02, 15, 120

A5072 Ostomy pouch, urinary; without barrier attached (1 piece), each Qp Qh N
IOM: 100-02, 15, 120

A5073 Ostomy pouch, urinary; for use on barrier with flange (2 piece), each Qp Qh N
IOM: 100-02, 15, 120

A5081 Stoma plug or seal, any type Qp Qh N
IOM: 100-02, 15, 120

A5082 Continent device; catheter for continent stoma Qp Qh N
IOM: 100-02, 15, 120

* **A5083** Continent device, stoma absorptive cover for continent stoma Qh N

A5093 Ostomy accessory; convex insert Qp Qh N
IOM: 100-02, 15, 120

Additional Incontinence and Ostomy Supplies

A5102 Bedside drainage bottle with or without tubing, rigid or expandable, each Qp Qh N
IOM: 100-02, 15, 120

A5105 Urinary suspensory, with leg bag, with or without tube, each Qp Qh N
IOM: 100-02, 15, 120

A5112 Urinary drainage bag, leg bag, leg or abdomen, latex, with or without tube, with straps, each Qp Qh N
IOM: 100-02, 15, 120

A5113 Leg strap; latex, replacement only, per set Qp Qh E1
IOM: 100-02, 15, 120

A5114 Leg strap; foam or fabric, replacement only, per set Qp Qh E1
IOM: 100-02, 15, 120

A5120 Skin barrier, wipes or swabs, each Qp Qh N
IOM: 100-02, 15, 120

A5121 Skin barrier; solid, 6 × 6 or equivalent, each Qp Qh N
IOM: 100-02, 15, 120

A5122 Skin barrier; solid, 8 × 8 or equivalent, each Qp Qh N
IOM: 100-02, 15, 120

A5126 Adhesive or non-adhesive; disk or foam pad Qp Qh N
IOM: 100-02, 15, 120

A5131 Appliance cleaner, incontinence and ostomy appliances, per 16 oz Qp Qh N
IOM: 100-02, 15, 120

A5200 Percutaneous catheter/tube anchoring device, adhesive skin attachment Qh N
IOM: 100-02, 15, 120

▶ New ↩ Revised ✔ Reinstated ~~deleted~~ Deleted ⊘ Not covered or valid by Medicare
Special coverage instructions * Carrier discretion Bill Part B MAC Bill DME MAC

Diabetic Shoes, Fitting, and Modifications

A5500 For diabetics only, fitting (including follow-up), custom preparation and supply of off-the-shelf depth-inlay shoe manufactured to accommodate multi-density insert(s), per shoe Qp Qh Y

IOM: 100-02, 15, 140

A5501 For diabetics only, fitting (including follow-up), custom preparation and supply of shoe molded from cast(s) of patient's foot (custom-molded shoe), per shoe Qp Qh Y

The diabetic patient must have at least one of the following conditions: peripheral neuropathy with evidence of callus formation, pre-ulcerative calluses, previous ulceration, foot deformity, previous amputation or poor circulation.

IOM: 100-02, 15, 140

A5503 For diabetics only, modification (including fitting) of off-the-shelf depth-inlay shoe or custom-molded shoe with roller or rigid rocker bottom, per shoe Qp Qh Y

IOM: 100-02, 15, 140

A5504 For diabetics only, modification (including fitting) of off-the-shelf depth-inlay shoe or custom-molded shoe with wedge(s), per shoe Qp Qh Y

IOM: 100-02, 15, 140

A5505 For diabetics only, modification (including fitting) of off-the-shelf depth-inlay shoe or custom-molded shoe with metatarsal bar, per shoe Qp Qh Y

IOM: 100-02, 15, 140

A5506 For diabetics only, modification (including fitting) of off-the-shelf depth-inlay shoe or custom-molded shoe with off-set heel(s), per shoe Qp Qh Y

IOM: 100-02, 15, 140

A5507 For diabetics only, not otherwise specified modification (including fitting) of off-the-shelf depth-inlay shoe or custom-molded shoe, per shoe Qp Qh Y

Only used for not otherwise specified therapeutic modifications to shoe or for repairs to a diabetic shoe(s)

IOM: 100-02, 15, 140

A5508 For diabetics only, deluxe feature of off-the-shelf depth-inlay shoe or custom-molded shoe, per shoe Qp Qh Y

IOM: 100-02, 15, 40

A5510 For diabetics only, direct formed, compression molded to patient's foot without external heat source, multiple-density insert(s) prefabricated, per shoe Qp Qh N

IOM: 100-02, 15, 140

* **A5512** For diabetics only, multiple density insert, direct formed, molded to foot after external heat source of 230 degrees Fahrenheit or higher, total contact with patient's foot, including arch, base layer minimum of 1/4 inch material of shore a 35 durometer or 3/16 inch material of shore a 40 durometer (or higher), prefabricated, each Qp Qh Y

* **A5513** For diabetics only, multiple density insert, custom molded from model of patient's foot, total contact with patient's foot, including arch, base layer minimum of 3/16 inch material of shore a 35 durometer (or higher), includes arch filler and other shaping material, custom fabricated, each Qp Qh Y

▶ **A5514** For diabetics only, multiple density insert, made by direct carving with cam technology from a rectified CAD model created from a digitized scan of the patient, total contact with patient's foot, including arch, base layer minimum of 3/16 inch material of shore a 35 durometer (or higher), includes arch filler and other shaping material, custom fabricated, each Y

Dressings

A6000 Non-contact wound warming wound cover for use with the non-contact wound warming device and warming card Qp Qh E1

IOM: 100-02, 16, 20

A6010 Collagen based wound filler, dry form, sterile, per gram of collagen N

IOM: 100-02, 15, 100

A6011 Collagen based wound filler, gel/paste, per gram of collagen N

IOM: 100-02, 15, 100

A6021 Collagen dressing, sterile, size 16 sq. in. or less, each N

IOM: 100-02, 15, 100

A6022 Collagen dressing, sterile, size more than 16 sq. in. but less than or equal to 48 sq. in., each Qp N

IOM: 100-02, 15, 100

MIPS | Qp Quantity Physician | Qh Quantity Hospital | ♀ Female only
♂ Male only | A Age | DMEPOS | A2-Z3 ASC Payment Indicator | A-Y ASC Status Indicator | Coding Clinic

A6023 Collagen dressing, sterile, size more than 48 sq. in., each N

IOM: 100-02, 15, 100

A6024 Collagen dressing wound filler, sterile, per 6 inches N

IOM: 100-02, 15, 100

* **A6025** Gel sheet for dermal or epidermal application (e.g., silicone, hydrogel, other), each N

If used for the treatment of keloids or other scars, a silicone gel sheet will not meet the definition of the surgical dressing benefit and will be denied as noncovered.

A6154 Wound pouch, each Qp Qh N

Waterproof collection device with drainable port that adheres to skin around wound. Usual dressing change is up to 3 times per week.

IOM: 100-02, 15, 100

A6196 Alginate or other fiber gelling dressing, wound cover, sterile, pad size 16 sq. in. or less, each dressing Qp N

IOM: 100-02, 15, 100

A6197 Alginate or other fiber gelling dressing, wound cover, sterile, pad size more than 16 sq. in., but less than or equal to 48 sq. in., each dressing Qp N

IOM: 100-02, 15, 100

A6198 Alginate or other fiber gelling dressing, wound cover, sterile, pad size more than 48 sq. in., each dressing Qp N

IOM: 100-02, 15, 100

A6199 Alginate or other fiber gelling dressing, wound filler, sterile, per 6 inches Qp N

IOM: 100-02, 15, 100

A6203 Composite dressing, sterile, pad size 16 sq. in. or less, with any size adhesive border, each dressing Qp N

Usual composite dressing change is up to 3 times per week, one wound cover per dressing change.

IOM: 100-02, 15, 100

A6204 Composite dressing, sterile, pad size more than 16 sq. in. but less than or equal to 48 sq. in., with any size adhesive border, each dressing Qp N

Usual composite dressing change is up to 3 times per week, one wound cover per dressing change.

IOM: 100-02, 15, 100

A6205 Composite dressing, sterile, pad size more than 48 sq. in., with any size adhesive border, each dressing Qp Qh N

Usual composite dressing change is up to 3 times per week, one wound cover per dressing change.

IOM: 100-02, 15, 100

A6206 Contact layer, sterile, 16 sq. in. or less, each dressing Qp N

Contact layers are porous to allow wound fluid to pass through for absorption by separate overlying dressing and are not intended to be changed with each dressing change. Usual dressing change is up to once per week.

IOM: 100-02, 15, 100

A6207 Contact layer, sterile, more than 16 sq. in. but less than or equal to 48 sq. in., each dressing Qp N

Contact layer dressings are used to line the entire wound; they are not intended to be changed with each dressing change. Usual dressing change is up to once per week.

IOM: 100-02, 15, 100

A6208 Contact layer, sterile, more than 48 sq. in., each dressing Qp N

Contact layer dressings are used to line the entire wound; they are not intended to be changed with each dressing change. Usual dressing change is up to once per week.

IOM: 100-02, 15, 100

A6209 Foam dressing, wound cover, sterile, pad size 16 sq. in. or less, without adhesive border, each dressing Qp N

Made of open cell, medical grade expanded polymer; with nonadherent property over wound site.

IOM: 100-02, 15, 100

▶ New ↩ Revised ✔ Reinstated ~~deleted~~ Deleted ⊘ Not covered or valid by Medicare
Special coverage instructions * Carrier discretion Ⓑ Bill Part B MAC Ⓑ Bill DME MAC

A6210 Foam dressing, wound cover, sterile, pad size more than 16 sq. in. but less than or equal to 48 sq. in., without adhesive border, each dressing Qp N

Foam dressings are covered items when used on full thickness wounds (e.g., stage III or IV ulcers) with moderate to heavy exudates. Usual dressing change for a foam wound cover when used as primary dressing is up to 3 times per week. When foam wound cover is used as a secondary dressing for wounds with very heavy exudates, dressing change may be up to 3 times per week. Usual dressing change for foam wound fillers is up to once per day (A6209-A6215).

IOM: 100-02, 15, 100

A6211 Foam dressing, wound cover, sterile, pad size more than 48 sq. in., without adhesive border, each dressing Qp N

IOM: 100-02, 15, 100

A6212 Foam dressing, wound cover, sterile, pad size 16 sq. in. or less, with any size adhesive border, each dressing Qp N

IOM: 100-02, 15, 100

A6213 Foam dressing, wound cover, sterile, pad size more than 16 sq. in. but less than or equal to 48 sq. in., with any size adhesive border, each dressing Qp N

IOM: 100-02, 15, 100

A6214 Foam dressing, wound cover, sterile, pad size more than 48 sq. in., with any size adhesive border, each dressing Qp N

IOM: 100-02, 15, 100

A6215 Foam dressing, wound filler, sterile, per gram Qp N

IOM: 100-02, 15, 100

A6216 Gauze, non-impregnated, non-sterile, pad size 16 sq. in. or less, without adhesive border, each dressing Qp N

IOM: 100-02, 15, 100

A6217 Gauze, non-impregnated, non-sterile, pad size more than 16 sq. in. but less than or equal to 48 sq. in., without adhesive border, each dressing Qp N

IOM: 100-02, 15, 100

A6218 Gauze, non-impregnated, non-sterile, pad size more than 48 sq. in., without adhesive border, each dressing Qp N

IOM: 100-02, 15, 100

A6219 Gauze, non-impregnated, sterile, pad size 16 sq. in. or less, with any size adhesive border, each dressing Qp N

IOM: 100-02, 15, 100

A6220 Gauze, non-impregnated, sterile, pad size more than 16 sq. in. but less than or equal to 48 sq. in., with any size adhesive border, each dressing Qp N

IOM: 100-02, 15, 100

A6221 Gauze, non-impregnated, sterile, pad size more than 48 sq. in., with any size adhesive border, each dressing N

IOM: 100-02, 15, 100

A6222 Gauze, impregnated with other than water, normal saline, or hydrogel, sterile, pad size 16 sq. in. or less, without adhesive border, each dressing Qp N

Substances may have been incorporated into dressing material (i.e., iodinated agents, petrolatum, zinc paste, crystalline sodium chloride, chlorhexadine gluconate [CHG], bismuth tribromophenate [BTP], water, aqueous saline, hydrogel, or agents).

IOM: 100-02, 15, 100

A6223 Gauze, impregnated with other than water, normal saline, or hydrogel, sterile, pad size more than 16 sq. in. but less than or equal to 48 sq. in., without adhesive border, each dressing Qp N

IOM: 100-02, 15, 100

A6224 Gauze, impregnated with other than water, normal saline, or hydrogel, sterile, pad size more than 48 sq. in., without adhesive border, each dressing Qp N

IOM: 100-02, 15, 100

A6228 Gauze, impregnated, water or normal saline, sterile, pad size 16 sq. in. or less, without adhesive border, each dressing Qp Qh N

IOM: 100-02, 15, 100

MIPS | Qp Quantity Physician | Qh Quantity Hospital | ♀ Female only
♂ Male only | A Age | DMEPOS | A2-Z3 ASC Payment Indicator | A-Y ASC Status Indicator | Coding Clinic

A6229 Gauze, impregnated, water or normal saline, sterile, pad size more than 16 sq. in. but less than or equal to 48 sq. in., without adhesive border, each dressing Qp N

IOM: 100-02, 15, 100

A6230 Gauze, impregnated, water or normal saline, sterile, pad size more than 48 sq. in., without adhesive border, each dressing Qp Qh N

IOM: 100-02, 15, 100

A6231 Gauze, impregnated, hydrogel, for direct wound contact, sterile, pad size 16 sq. in. or less, each dressing Qp N

IOM: 100-02, 15, 100

A6232 Gauze, impregnated, hydrogel, for direct wound contact, sterile, pad size greater than 16 sq. in., but less than or equal to 48 sq. in., each dressing N

IOM: 100-02, 15, 100

A6233 Gauze, impregnated, hydrogel, for direct wound contact, sterile, pad size more than 48 sq. in., each dressing N

IOM: 100-02, 15, 100

A6234 Hydrocolloid dressing, wound cover, sterile, pad size 16 sq. in. or less, without adhesive border, each dressing Qp N

This type of dressing is usually used on wounds with light to moderate exudate with an average of three dressing changes per week.

IOM: 100-02, 15, 100

A6235 Hydrocolloid dressing, wound cover, sterile, pad size more than 16 sq. in. but less than or equal to 48 sq. in., without adhesive border, each dressing Qp N

IOM: 100-02, 15, 100

A6236 Hydrocolloid dressing, wound cover, sterile, pad size more than 48 sq. in., without adhesive border, each dressing Qp Qh N

IOM: 100-02, 15, 100

A6237 Hydrocolloid dressing, wound cover, sterile, pad size 16 sq. in. or less, with any size adhesive border, each dressing Qp N

IOM: 100-02, 15, 100

A6238 Hydrocolloid dressing, wound cover, sterile, pad size more than 16 sq. in. but less than or equal to 48 sq. in., with any size adhesive border, each dressing Qp Qh N

IOM: 100-02, 15, 100

A6239 Hydrocolloid dressing, wound cover, sterile, pad size more than 48 sq. in., with any size adhesive border, each dressing Qp Qh N

IOM: 100-02, 15, 100

A6240 Hydrocolloid dressing, wound filler, paste, sterile, per ounce Qp Qh N

IOM: 100-02, 15, 100

A6241 Hydrocolloid dressing, wound filler, dry form, sterile, per gram Qp Qh N

IOM: 100-02, 15, 100

A6242 Hydrogel dressing, wound cover, sterile, pad size 16 sq. in. or less, without adhesive border, each dressing Qp N

Considered medically necessary when used on full thickness wounds with minimal or no exudate (e.g., stage III or IV ulcers).

Usually up to one dressing change per day is considered medically necessary, but if well documented and medically necessary, the payer may allow more frequent dressing changes.

IOM: 100-02, 15, 100

A6243 Hydrogel dressing, wound cover, sterile, pad size more than 16 sq. in. but less than or equal to 48 sq. in., without adhesive border, each dressing Qp N

IOM: 100-02, 15, 100

A6244 Hydrogel dressing, wound cover, sterile, pad size more than 48 sq. in., without adhesive border, each dressing Qp Qh N

IOM: 100-02, 15, 100

A6245 Hydrogel dressing, wound cover, sterile, pad size 16 sq. in. or less, with any size adhesive border, each dressing Qp N

Coverage of a non-elastic gradient compression wrap is limited to one per 6 months per leg.

IOM: 100-02, 15, 100

A6246 Hydrogel dressing, wound cover, sterile, pad size more than 16 sq. in. but less than or equal to 48 sq. in., with any size adhesive border, each dressing Qp Qh N

IOM: 100-02, 15, 100

A6247 Hydrogel dressing, wound cover, sterile, pad size more than 48 sq. in., with any size adhesive border, each dressing Qp Qh N

IOM: 100-02, 15, 100

A6248 Hydrogel dressing, wound filler, gel, per fluid ounce Qp N

IOM: 100-02, 15, 100

A6250 Skin sealants, protectants, moisturizers, ointments, any type, any size Qp Qh N

IOM: 100-02, 15, 100

A6251 Specialty absorptive dressing, wound cover, sterile, pad size 16 sq. in. or less, without adhesive border, each dressing Qp N

IOM: 100-02, 15, 100

A6252 Specialty absorptive dressing, wound cover, sterile, pad size more than 16 sq. in. but less than or equal to 48 sq. in., without adhesive border, each dressing Qp N

IOM: 100-02, 15, 100

A6253 Specialty absorptive dressing, wound cover, sterile, pad size more than 48 sq. in., without adhesive border, each dressing Qp N

IOM: 100-02, 15, 100

A6254 Specialty absorptive dressing, wound cover, sterile, pad size 16 sq. in. or less, with any size adhesive border, each dressing Qp N

IOM: 100-02, 15, 100

A6255 Specialty absorptive dressing, wound cover, sterile, pad size more than 16 sq. in. but less than or equal to 48 sq. in., with any size adhesive border, each dressing Qp N

IOM: 100-02, 15, 100

A6256 Specialty absorptive dressing, wound cover, sterile, pad size more than 48 sq. in., with any size adhesive border, each dressing Qp Qh N

Considered medically necessary when used for moderately or highly exudative wounds (e.g., stage III or IV ulcers).

IOM: 100-02, 15, 100

A6257 Transparent film, sterile, 16 sq. in. or less, each dressing Qp N

Considered medically necessary when used on open partial thickness wounds with minimal exudate or closed wounds.

IOM: 100-02, 15, 100

A6258 Transparent film, sterile, more than 16 sq. in. but less than or equal to 48 sq. in., each dressing Qp N

IOM: 100-02, 15, 100

A6259 Transparent film, sterile, more than 48 sq. in., each dressing Qp Qh N

IOM: 100-02, 15, 100

A6260 Wound cleansers, any type, any size Qp N

IOM: 100-02, 15, 100

A6261 Wound filler, gel/paste, per fluid ounce, not otherwise specified Qp Qh N

Units of service for wound fillers are 1 gram, 1 fluid ounce, 6 inch length, or 1 yard depending on product.

IOM: 100-02, 15, 100

A6262 Wound filler, dry form, per gram, not otherwise specified Qp Qh N

Dry forms (e.g., powder, granules, beads) are used to eliminate dead space in an open wound.

IOM: 100-02, 15, 100

A6266 Gauze, impregnated, other than water, normal saline, or zinc paste, sterile, any width, per linear yard Qp N

IOM: 100-02, 15, 100

A6402 Gauze, non-impregnated, sterile, pad size 16 sq. in. or less, without adhesive border, each dressing Qp N

IOM: 100-02, 15, 100

A6403 Gauze, non-impregnated, sterile, pad size more than 16 sq. in., less than or equal to 48 sq. in., without adhesive border, each dressing Qp N

IOM: 100-02, 15, 100

A6404 Gauze, non-impregnated, sterile, pad size more than 48 sq. in., without adhesive border, each dressing Qp Qh N

IOM: 100-02, 15, 100

* **A6407** Packing strips, non-impregnated, sterile, up to 2 inches in width, per linear yard N

IOM: 100-02, 15, 100

A6410 Eye pad, sterile, each Qp Qh N

IOM: 100-02, 15, 100

MIPS | Qp Quantity Physician | Qh Quantity Hospital | ♀ Female only
♂ Male only | A Age | DMEPOS | A2-Z3 ASC Payment Indicator | A-Y ASC Status Indicator | Coding Clinic

A6411 Eye pad, non-sterile, each N

IOM: 100-02, 15, 100

* **A6412** Eye patch, occlusive, each N

Bandages

A6413 Adhesive bandage, first-aid type, any size, each Qp Qh E1

First aid type bandage is a wound cover with a pad size of less than 4 sq. in. Does not meet the definition of the surgical dressing benefit and will be denied as non-covered.

Medicare Statute 1861(s)(5)

* **A6441** Padding bandage, non-elastic, non-woven/non-knitted, width greater than or equal to three inches and less than five inches, per yard N

* **A6442** Conforming bandage, non-elastic, knitted/woven, non-sterile, width less than three inches, per yard N

Non-elastic, moderate or high compression that is typically sustained for one week

* **A6443** Conforming bandage, non-elastic, knitted/woven, non-sterile, width greater than or equal to three inches and less than five inches, per yard N

* **A6444** Conforming bandage, non-elastic, knitted/woven, non-sterile, width greater than or equal to five inches, per yard N

* **A6445** Conforming bandage, non-elastic, knitted/woven, sterile, width less than three inches, per yard N

* **A6446** Conforming bandage, non-elastic, knitted/woven, sterile, width greater than or equal to three inches and less than five inches, per yard N

* **A6447** Conforming bandage, non-elastic, knitted/woven, sterile, width greater than or equal to five inches, per yard N

* **A6448** Light compression bandage, elastic, knitted/woven, width less than three inches, per yard N

Used to hold wound cover dressings in place over a wound. Example is an ACE type elastic bandage.

* **A6449** Light compression bandage, elastic, knitted/woven, width greater than or equal to three inches and less than five inches, per yard N

* **A6450** Light compression bandage, elastic, knitted/woven, width greater than or equal to five inches, per yard N

* **A6451** Moderate compression bandage, elastic, knitted/woven, load resistance of 1.25 to 1.34 foot pounds at 50% maximum stretch, width greater than or equal to three inches and less than five inches, per yard N

Elastic bandages that produce moderate compression that is typically sustained for one week

Medicare considers coverage if part of a multi-layer compression bandage system for the treatment of a venous stasis ulcer. Do not assign for strains or sprains.

* **A6452** High compression bandage, elastic, knitted/woven, load resistance greater than or equal to 1.35 foot pounds at 50% maximum stretch, width greater than or equal to three inches and less than five inches, per yard N

Elastic bandages that produce high compression that is typically sustained for one week

* **A6453** Self-adherent bandage, elastic, non-knitted/non-woven, width less than three inches, per yard N

* **A6454** Self-adherent bandage, elastic, non-knitted/non-woven, width greater than or equal to three inches and less than five inches, per yard N

* **A6455** Self-adherent bandage, elastic, non-knitted/non-woven, width greater than or equal to five inches, per yard N

* **A6456** Zinc paste impregnated bandage, non-elastic, knitted/woven, width greater than or equal to three inches and less than five inches, per yard N

* **A6457** Tubular dressing with or without elastic, any width, per linear yard N

▶ * **A6460** Synthetic resorbable wound dressing, sterile, pad size 16 sq. in. or less, without adhesive border, each dressing N

▶ * **A6461** Synthetic resorbable wound dressing, sterile, pad size more than 16 sq. in. but less than or equal to 48 sq. in., without adhesive border, each dressing N

▶ New ↩ Revised ✔ Reinstated ~~deleted~~ Deleted ⃠ Not covered or valid by Medicare
Special coverage instructions * Carrier discretion Bill Part B MAC Bill DME MAC

Compression Garments

A6501 Compression burn garment, bodysuit (head to foot), custom fabricated Qp Qh N

Garments used to reduce hypertrophic scarring and joint contractures following burn injury

IOM: 100-02, 15, 100

A6502 Compression burn garment, chin strap, custom fabricated Qp Qh N

IOM: 100-02, 15, 100

A6503 Compression burn garment, facial hood, custom fabricated Qp Qh N

IOM: 100-02, 15, 100

A6504 Compression burn garment, glove to wrist, custom fabricated Qp Qh N

IOM: 100-02, 15, 100

A6505 Compression burn garment, glove to elbow, custom fabricated Qp Qh N

IOM: 100-02, 15, 100

A6506 Compression burn garment, glove to axilla, custom fabricated Qp Qh N

IOM: 100-02, 15, 100

A6507 Compression burn garment, foot to knee length, custom fabricated Qp Qh N

IOM: 100-02, 15, 100

A6508 Compression burn garment, foot to thigh length, custom fabricated Qp Qh N

IOM: 100-02, 15, 100

A6509 Compression burn garment, upper trunk to waist including arm openings (vest), custom fabricated Qp Qh N

IOM: 100-02, 15, 100

A6510 Compression burn garment, trunk, including arms down to leg openings (leotard), custom fabricated Qp Qh N

IOM: 100-02, 15, 100

A6511 Compression burn garment, lower trunk including leg openings (panty), custom fabricated Qp Qh N

IOM: 100-02, 15, 100

A6512 Compression burn garment, not otherwise classified N

IOM: 100-02, 15, 100

* **A6513** Compression burn mask, face and/or neck, plastic or equal, custom fabricated Qp Qh B

A6530 Gradient compression stocking, below knee, 18-30 mmHg, each Qp Qh E1

IOM: 100-03, 4, 280.1

A6531 Gradient compression stocking, below knee, 30-40 mmHg, each Qp Qh N

Covered when used in treatment of open venous stasis ulcer. Modifiers A1-A9 are not assigned. Must be billed with AW, RT, or LT.

IOM: 100-02, 15, 100

A6532 Gradient compression stocking, below knee, 40-50 mmHg, each Qp Qh N

Covered when used in treatment of open venous stasis ulcer. Modifiers A1-A9 are not assigned. Must be billed with AW, RT, or LT.

IOM: 100-02, 15, 100

A6533 Gradient compression stocking, thigh length, 18-30 mmHg, each Qp Qh E1

IOM: 100-02, 15, 130; 100-03, 4, 280.1

A6534 Gradient compression stocking, thigh length, 30-40 mmHg, each Qp Qh E1

IOM: 100-02, 15, 130; 100-03, 4, 280.1

A6535 Gradient compression stocking, thigh length, 40-50 mmHg, each Qp Qh E1

IOM: 100-02, 15, 130; 100-03, 4, 280.1

A6536 Gradient compression stocking, full length/chap style, 18-30 mmHg, each Qp Qh E1

IOM: 100-02, 15, 130; 100-03, 4, 280.1

A6537 Gradient compression stocking, full length/chap style, 30-40 mmHg, each Qp Qh E1

IOM: 100-02, 15, 130; 100-03, 4, 280.1

A6538 Gradient compression stocking, full length/chap style, 40-50 mmHg, each Qp Qh E1

IOM: 100-02, 15, 130; 100-03, 4, 280.1

A6539 Gradient compression stocking, waist length, 18-30 mmHg, each Qp Qh E1

IOM: 100-02, 15, 130; 100-03, 4, 280.1

A6540 Gradient compression stocking, waist length, 30-40 mmHg, each Qp Qh E1

IOM: 100-02, 15, 130; 100-03, 4, 280.1

⊘ **A6541** Gradient compression stocking, waist length, 40-50 mmHg, each Ⓑ Qp Qh — E1

IOM: 100-02, 15, 130; 100-03, 4, 280.1

⊘ **A6544** Gradient compression stocking, garter belt Ⓑ Qp Qh — E1

IOM: 100-02, 15, 130; 100-03, 4, 280.1

A6545 Gradient compression wrap, non-elastic, below knee, 30-50 mm hg, each Ⓑ Qp Qh ♿ — N

Modifiers RT and/or LT must be appended. When assigned for bilateral items (left/right) on the same date of service, bill both items on the same claim line using RT/LT modifiers and 2 units of service.

IOM: 10-02, 15, 100

⊘ **A6549** Gradient compression stocking/sleeve, not otherwise specified Ⓑ Qp Qh — E1

IOM: 100-02, 15, 130; 100-03, 4, 280.1

Wound Care

* **A6550** Wound care set, for negative pressure wound therapy electrical pump, includes all supplies and accessories Ⓑ Qh ♿ — N

Respiratory Supplies

* **A7000** Canister, disposable, used with suction pump, each Ⓑ Qp Qh ♿ — Y
* **A7001** Canister, non-disposable, used with suction pump, each Ⓑ Qh ♿ — Y
* **A7002** Tubing, used with suction pump, each Ⓑ Qh ♿ — Y
* **A7003** Administration set, with small volume nonfiltered pneumatic nebulizer, disposable Ⓑ Qp Qh ♿ — Y
* **A7004** Small volume nonfiltered pneumatic nebulizer, disposable Ⓑ Qh ♿ — Y
* **A7005** Administration set, with small volume nonfiltered pneumatic nebulizer, non-disposable Ⓑ Qp Qh ♿ — Y
* **A7006** Administration set, with small volume filtered pneumatic nebulizer Ⓑ Qp Qh ♿ — Y
* **A7007** Large volume nebulizer, disposable, unfilled, used with aerosol compressor Ⓑ Qh ♿ — Y
* **A7008** Large volume nebulizer, disposable, prefilled, used with aerosol compressor Ⓑ ♿ — Y
* **A7009** Reservoir bottle, nondisposable, used with large volume ultrasonic nebulizer Ⓑ ♿ — Y
* **A7010** Corrugated tubing, disposable, used with large volume nebulizer, 100 feet Ⓑ Qh ♿ — Y
* **A7012** Water collection device, used with large volume nebulizer Ⓑ Qh ♿ — Y
* **A7013** Filter, disposable, used with aerosol compressor or ultrasonic generator Ⓑ Qp Qh ♿ — Y
* **A7014** Filter, non-disposable, used with aerosol compressor or ultrasonic generator Ⓑ Qp Qh ♿ — Y
* **A7015** Aerosol mask, used with DME nebulizer Ⓑ Qh ♿ — Y
* **A7016** Dome and mouthpiece, used with small volume ultrasonic nebulizer Ⓑ Qp Qh ♿ — Y

A7017 Nebulizer, durable, glass or autoclavable plastic, bottle type, not used with oxygen Ⓑ Qp Qh ♿ — Y

IOM: 100-03, 4, 280.1

* **A7018** Water, distilled, used with large volume nebulizer, 1000 ml Ⓑ Qh ♿ — Y
* **A7020** Interface for cough stimulating device, includes all components, replacement only Ⓑ Qp Qh ♿ — Y
* **A7025** High frequency chest wall oscillation system vest, replacement for use with patient owned equipment, each Ⓑ Qp Qh ♿ — N
* **A7026** High frequency chest wall oscillation system hose, replacement for use with patient owned equipment, each Ⓑ Qp Qh ♿ — Y
* **A7027** Combination oral/nasal mask, used with continuous positive airway pressure device, each Ⓑ Qp Qh ♿ — Y
* **A7028** Oral cushion for combination oral/nasal mask, replacement only, each Ⓑ Qp Qh ♿ — Y
* **A7029** Nasal pillows for combination oral/nasal mask, replacement only, pair Ⓑ Qp Qh ♿ — Y
* **A7030** Full face mask used with positive airway pressure device, each Ⓑ Qh ♿ — Y
* **A7031** Face mask interface, replacement for full face mask, each Ⓑ Qh ♿ — Y
* **A7032** Cushion for use on nasal mask interface, replacement only, each Ⓑ Qp Qh ♿ — Y

▶ New ⤺ Revised ✓ Reinstated ~~deleted~~ Deleted ⊘ Not covered or valid by Medicare
Special coverage instructions * Carrier discretion Ⓑ Bill Part B MAC Ⓑ Bill DME MAC

* A7033 Pillow for use on nasal cannula type interface, replacement only, pair Qh Y
* A7034 Nasal interface (mask or cannula type) used with positive airway pressure device, with or without head strap Qh Y
* A7035 Headgear used with positive airway pressure device Qp Qh Y
* A7036 Chinstrap used with positive airway pressure device Qp Qh Y
* A7037 Tubing used with positive airway pressure device Qp Qh Y
* A7038 Filter, disposable, used with positive airway pressure device Qh Y
* A7039 Filter, non disposable, used with positive airway pressure device Qp Qh Y
* A7040 One way chest drain valve Qp Qh N
* A7041 Water seal drainage container and tubing for use with implanted chest tube Qp Qh N
* A7044 Oral interface used with positive airway pressure device, each Qp Qh Y
* A7045 Exhalation port with or without swivel used with accessories for positive airway devices, replacement only Qh Y
  IOM: 100-03, 4, 230.17
* A7046 Water chamber for humidifier, used with positive airway pressure device, replacement, each Qh Y
  IOM: 100-03, 4, 230.17
* A7047 Oral interface used with respiratory suction pump, each Qp Qh N
* A7048 Vacuum drainage collection unit and tubing kit, including all supplies needed for collection unit change, for use with implanted catheter, each Qp Qh N

Tracheostomy Supplies

* A7501 Tracheostoma valve, including diaphragm, each Qp Qh N
  IOM: 100-02, 15, 120
* A7502 Replacement diaphragm/faceplate for tracheostoma valve, each Qh N
  IOM: 100-02, 15, 120
* A7503 Filter holder or filter cap, reusable, for use in a tracheostoma heat and moisture exchange system, each Qh N
  IOM: 100-02, 15, 120
* A7504 Filter for use in a tracheostoma heat and moisture exchange system, each Qp Qh N
  IOM: 100-02, 15, 120
* A7505 Housing, reusable without adhesive, for use in a heat and moisture exchange system and/or with a tracheostoma valve, each Qh N
  IOM: 100-02, 15, 120
* A7506 Adhesive disc for use in a heat and moisture exchange system and/or with tracheostoma valve, any type, each Qh N
  IOM: 100-02, 15, 120
* A7507 Filter holder and integrated filter without adhesive, for use in a tracheostoma heat and moisture exchange system, each Qp Qh N
  IOM: 100-02, 15, 120
* A7508 Housing and integrated adhesive, for use in a tracheostoma heat and moisture exchange system and/or with a tracheostoma valve, each Qh N
  IOM: 100-02, 15, 120
* A7509 Filter holder and integrated filter housing, and adhesive, for use as a tracheostoma heat and moisture exchange system, each Qh N
  IOM: 100-02, 15, 120
* A7520 Tracheostomy/laryngectomy tube, non-cuffed, polyvinylchloride (PVC), silicone or equal, each Qp Qh N
* A7521 Tracheostomy/laryngectomy tube, cuffed, polyvinylchloride (PVC), silicone or equal, each Qh N
* A7522 Tracheostomy/laryngectomy tube, stainless steel or equal (sterilizable and reusable), each Qh N
* A7523 Tracheostomy shower protector, each N
* A7524 Tracheostoma stent/stud/button, each Qp Qh N
* A7525 Tracheostomy mask, each Qh N
* A7526 Tracheostomy tube collar/holder, each Qh N
* A7527 Tracheostomy/laryngectomy tube plug/stop, each Qp Qh N

MIPS | Qp Quantity Physician | Qh Quantity Hospital | ♀ Female only
♂ Male only | A Age | DMEPOS | A2-Z3 ASC Payment Indicator | A-Y ASC Status Indicator | Coding Clinic

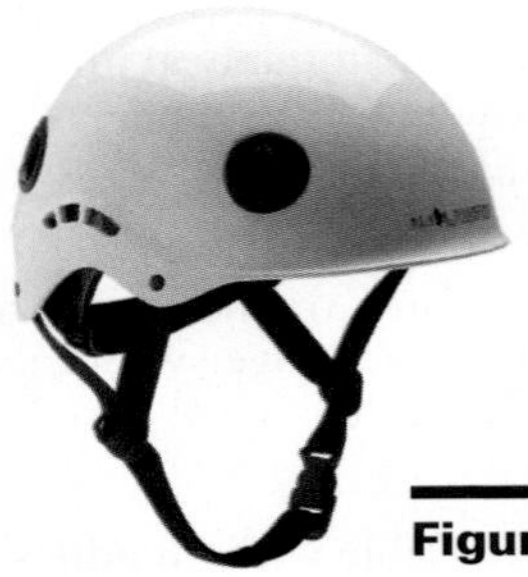

Figure 7 Helmet.

Helmets

*	**A8000**	Helmet, protective, soft, prefabricated, includes all components and accessories	Y
*	**A8001**	Helmet, protective, hard, prefabricated, includes all components and accessories	Y
*	**A8002**	Helmet, protective, soft, custom fabricated, includes all components and accessories	Y
*	**A8003**	Helmet, protective, hard, custom fabricated, includes all components and accessories	Y
*	**A8004**	Soft interface for helmet, replacement only	Y

ADMINISTRATIVE, MISCELLANEOUS, AND INVESTIGATIONAL (A9000-A9999)

Note: The following codes do not imply that codes in other sections are necessarily covered.

Miscellaneous Supplies

◌	**A9150**	Non-prescription drugs *IOM: 100-02, 15, 50*	B
⃠	**A9152**	Single vitamin/mineral/trace element, oral, per dose, not otherwise specified Qp Qh	E1
⃠	**A9153**	Multiple vitamins, with or without minerals and trace elements, oral, per dose, not otherwise specified Qp Qh	E1
*	**A9155**	Artificial saliva, 30 ml Qp Qh	B
⃠	**A9180**	Pediculosis (lice infestation) treatment, topical, for administration by patient/caretaker Qp Qh	E1
⃠	**A9270**	Non-covered item or service Qp Qh *IOM: 100-02, 16, 20*	E1
⃠	**A9272**	Wound suction, disposable, includes dressing, all accessories and components, any type, each Qp Qh *Medicare Statute 1861(n)*	E1
⮌ ⃠	**A9273**	Cold or hot water bottle, ice cap or collar, heat and/or cold wrap, any type Qp Qh	E1
⃠	**A9274**	External ambulatory insulin delivery system, disposable, each, includes all supplies and accessories Qp Qh *Medicare Statute 1861(n)*	E1
⃠	**A9275**	Home glucose disposable monitor, includes test strips Qp Qh	E1
⃠	**A9276**	Sensor; invasive (e.g., subcutaneous), disposable, for use with interstitial continuous glucose monitoring system, one unit = 1 day supply Qp Qh *Medicare Statute 1861(n)*	E1
⃠	**A9277**	Transmitter; external, for use with interstitial continuous glucose monitoring system Qp Qh *Medicare Statute 1861(n)*	E1
⃠	**A9278**	Receiver (monitor); external, for use with interstitial continuous glucose monitoring system Qp Qh *Medicare Statute 1861(n)*	E1
⃠	**A9279**	Monitoring feature/device, stand-alone or integrated, any type, includes all accessories, components and electronics, not otherwise classified Qp Qh *Medicare Statute 1861(n)*	E1
⃠	**A9280**	Alert or alarm device, not otherwise classified Qp Qh *Medicare Statute 1861*	E1
⃠	**A9281**	Reaching/grabbing device, any type, any length, each Qp Qh *Medicare Statute 1862 SSA*	E1
⃠	**A9282**	Wig, any type, each Qp Qh *Medicare Statute 1862 SSA*	E1
⃠	**A9283**	Foot pressure off loading/supportive device, any type, each Qp Qh *Medicare Statute 1862A(i)13*	E1
◌	**A9284**	Spirometer, non-electronic, includes all accessories Qp Qh	N
*	**A9285**	Inversion/eversion correction device Qp Qh	A
⃠	**A9286**	Hygienic item or device, disposable or non-disposable, any type, each Qp Qh *Medicare Statute 1834*	E1

▶ New ⮌ Revised ✔ Reinstated ~~deleted~~ Deleted ⃠ Not covered or valid by Medicare
◌ Special coverage instructions * Carrier discretion Ⓑ Bill Part B MAC Ⓓ Bill DME MAC

⦸ **A9300** Exercise equipment Qp Qh E1
IOM: 100-02, 15, 110.1; 100-03, 4, 280.1

Supplies for Radiology Procedures (Radiopharmaceuticals)

* **A9500** Technetium Tc-99m sestamibi, diagnostic, per study dose Qp Qh N1 N
Should be filed on same claim as procedure code reporting radiopharmaceutical. Verify with payer definition of a "study."
Coding Clinic: 2006, Q2, P5

* **A9501** Technetium Tc-99m teboroxime, diagnostic, per study dose Qp Qh N1 N

* **A9502** Technetium Tc-99m tetrofosmin, diagnostic, per study dose Qp Qh N1 N
Coding Clinic: 2006, Q2, P5

* **A9503** Technetium Tc-99m medronate, diagnostic, per study dose, up to 30 millicuries Qp Qh N1 N

* **A9504** Technetium Tc-99m apcitide, diagnostic, per study dose, up to 20 millicuries Qp Qh N1 N

* **A9505** Thallium Tl-201 thallous chloride, diagnostic, per millicurie Qp Qh N1 N

* **A9507** Indium In-111 capromab pendetide, diagnostic, per study dose, up to 10 millicuries Qp Qh N1 N

* **A9508** Iodine I-131 iobenguane sulfate, diagnostic, per 0.5 millicurie Qp Qh N1 N

* **A9509** Iodine I-123 sodium iodide, diagnostic, per millicurie Qp Qh N1 N

* **A9510** Technetium Tc-99m disofenin, diagnostic, per study dose, up to 15 millicuries Qp Qh N1 N

* **A9512** Technetium Tc-99m pertechnetate, diagnostic, per millicurie Qp Qh N1 N

▶ **A9513** Lutetium lu 177, dotatate, therapeutic, 1 millicurie G

* **A9515** Choline C-11, diagnostic, per study dose up to 20 millicuries Qp Qh K2 G

* **A9516** Iodine I-123 sodium iodide, diagnostic, per 100 microcuries, up to 999 microcuries Qp Qh N1 N

* **A9517** Iodine I-131 sodium iodide capsule(s), therapeutic, per millicurie Qp Qh K

* **A9520** Technetium Tc-99m tilmanocept, diagnostic, up to 0.5 millicuries Qp Qh N1 N

* **A9521** Technetium Tc-99m exametazime, diagnostic, per study dose, up to 25 millicuries Qp Qh N1 N

* **A9524** Iodine I-131 iodinated serum albumin, diagnostic, per 5 microcuries Qp Qh N1 N

* **A9526** Nitrogen N-13 ammonia, diagnostic, per study dose, up to 40 millicuries Qp Qh N1 N

* **A9527** Iodine I-125, sodium iodide solution, therapeutic, per millicurie Qp Qh H2 U

* **A9528** Iodine I-131 sodium iodide capsule(s), diagnostic, per millicurie Qp Qh N1 N

* **A9529** Iodine I-131 sodium iodide solution, diagnostic, per millicurie Qp Qh N1 N

* **A9530** Iodine I-131 sodium iodide solution, therapeutic, per millicurie Qp Qh K

* **A9531** Iodine I-131 sodium iodide, diagnostic, per microcurie (up to 100 microcuries) Qp Qh N1 N

* **A9532** Iodine I-125 serum albumin, diagnostic, per 5 microcuries Qp Qh N1 N

* **A9536** Technetium Tc-99m depreotide, diagnostic, per study dose, up to 35 millicuries Qp Qh N1 N

* **A9537** Technetium Tc-99m mebrofenin, diagnostic, per study dose, up to 15 millicuries Qp Qh N1 N

* **A9538** Technetium Tc-99m pyrophosphate, diagnostic, per study dose, up to 25 millicuries Qp Qh N1 N

* **A9539** Technetium Tc-99m pentetate, diagnostic, per study dose, up to 25 millicuries Qp Qh N1 N

* **A9540** Technetium Tc-99m macroaggregated albumin, diagnostic, per study dose, up to 10 millicuries Qp Qh N1 N

* **A9541** Technetium Tc-99m sulfur colloid, diagnostic, per study dose, up to 20 millicuries Qp Qh N1 N

* **A9542** Indium In-111 ibritumomab tiuxetan, diagnostic, per study dose, up to 5 millicuries Qp Qh N1 N
Specifically for diagnostic use.

* **A9543** Yttrium Y-90 ibritumomab tiuxetan, therapeutic, per treatment dose, up to 40 millicuries Qp Qh K
Specifically for therapeutic use.

✻ **A9546** Cobalt Co-57/58, cyanocobalamin, diagnostic, per study dose, up to 1 microcurie Ⓑ Qp Qh N1 N

✻ **A9547** Indium In-111 oxyquinoline, diagnostic, per 0.5 millicurie Ⓑ Qp Qh N1 N

✻ **A9548** Indium In-111 pentetate, diagnostic, per 0.5 millicurie Ⓑ Qp Qh N1 N

✻ **A9550** Technetium Tc-99m sodium gluceptate, diagnostic, per study dose, up to 25 millicuries Ⓑ Qp Qh N1 N

✻ **A9551** Technetium Tc-99m succimer, diagnostic, per study dose, up to 10 millicuries Ⓑ Qp Qh N1 N

✻ **A9552** Fluorodeoxyglucose F-18 FDG, diagnostic, per study dose, up to 45 millicuries Ⓑ Qp Qh N1 N

Coding Clinic: 2008, Q3, P7

✻ **A9553** Chromium Cr-51 sodium chromate, diagnostic, per study dose, up to 250 microcuries Ⓑ Qp Qh N1 N

✻ **A9554** Iodine I-125 sodium Iothalamate, diagnostic, per study dose, up to 10 microcuries Ⓑ Qp Qh N1 N

✻ **A9555** Rubidium Rb-82, diagnostic, per study dose, up to 60 millicuries Ⓑ Qp Qh N1 N

✻ **A9556** Gallium Ga-67 citrate, diagnostic, per millicurie Ⓑ Qp Qh N1 N

✻ **A9557** Technetium Tc-99m bicisate, diagnostic, per study dose, up to 25 millicuries Ⓑ Qp Qh N1 N

✻ **A9558** Xenon Xe-133 gas, diagnostic, per 10 millicuries Ⓑ Qp Qh N1 N

✻ **A9559** Cobalt Co-57 cyanocobalamin, oral, diagnostic, per study dose, up to 1 microcurie Ⓑ Qp Qh N1 N

✻ **A9560** Technetium Tc-99m labeled red blood cells, diagnostic, per study dose, up to 30 millicuries Ⓑ Qp Qh N1 N

Coding Clinic: 2008, Q3, P7

✻ **A9561** Technetium Tc-99m oxidronate, diagnostic, per study dose, up to 30 millicuries Ⓑ Qp Qh N1 N

✻ **A9562** Technetium Tc-99m mertiatide, diagnostic, per study dose, up to 15 millicuries Ⓑ Qp Qh N1 N

✻ **A9563** Sodium phosphate P-32, therapeutic, per millicurie Ⓑ Qp Qh K

✻ **A9564** Chromic phosphate P-32 suspension, therapeutic, per millicurie Ⓑ Qp Qh E1

✻ **A9566** Technetium Tc-99m fanolesomab, diagnostic, per study dose, up to 25 millicuries Ⓑ Qp Qh N1 N

✻ **A9567** Technetium Tc-99m pentetate, diagnostic, aerosol, per study dose, up to 75 millicuries Ⓑ Qp Qh N1 N

✻ **A9568** Technetium TC-99m arcitumomab, diagnostic, per study dose, up to 45 millicuries Ⓑ Qp Qh N1 N

✻ **A9569** Technetium Tc-99m exametazime labeled autologous white blood cells, diagnostic, per study dose Ⓑ Qp Qh N1 N

✻ **A9570** Indium In-111 labeled autologous white blood cells, diagnostic, per study dose Ⓑ Qp Qh N1 N

✻ **A9571** Indium In-111 labeled autologous platelets, diagnostic, per study dose Ⓑ Qp Qh N1 N

✻ **A9572** Indium In-111 pentetreotide, diagnostic, per study dose, up to 6 millicuries Ⓑ Qp Qh N1 N

✻ **A9575** Injection, gadoterate meglumine, 0.1 ml Ⓑ Qp Qh N1 N

Other: Dotarem

✻ **A9576** Injection, gadoteridol, (ProHance Multipack), per ml Ⓑ Qp Qh N1 N

✻ **A9577** Injection, gadobenate dimeglumine (MultiHance), per ml Ⓑ Qp Qh N1 N

✻ **A9578** Injection, gadobenate dimeglumine (MultiHance Multipack), per ml Ⓑ Qp Qh N1 N

✻ **A9579** Injection, gadolinium-based magnetic resonance contrast agent, not otherwise specified (NOS), per ml Ⓑ Qp Qh N1 N

Other: Magnevist, Omniscan, Optimark, Prohance

✻ **A9580** Sodium fluoride F-18, diagnostic, per study dose, up to 30 millicuries Ⓑ Qp Qh N1 N

✻ **A9581** Injection, gadoxetate disodium, 1 ml Ⓑ Qp Qh N1 N

Local Medicare contractors may require the use of modifier JW to identify unused product from single-dose vials that are appropriately discarded.

Other: Eovist

✻ **A9582** Iodine I-123 iobenguane, diagnostic, per study dose, up to 15 millicuries Ⓑ Qp Qh N1 N

Molecular imaging agent that assists in the identification of rare neuroendocrine tumors.

▶ New ⟲ Revised ✔ Reinstated ~~deleted~~ Deleted ⊘ Not covered or valid by Medicare
Special coverage instructions ✻ Carrier discretion Ⓑ Bill Part B MAC Ⓓ Bill DME MAC

* **A9583** Injection, gadofosveset trisodium, 1 ml Qp Qh N1 N
* **A9584** Iodine 1-123 ioflupane, diagnostic, per study dose, up to 5 millicuries Qp Qh N1 N

  Coding Clinic: 2012, Q1, P9
* **A9585** Injection, gadobutrol, 0.1 ml Qp Qh N1 N

  Other: Gadavist

  Coding Clinic: 2012, Q1, P8
* **A9586** Florbetapir F18, diagnostic, per study dose, up to 10 millicuries Qp Qh N1 N
* **A9587** Gallium Ga-68, dotatate, diagnostic, 0.1 millicurie Qp Qh K2 G

  Coding Clinic: 2017, Q1, P9
* ▶ **A9589** Instillation, hexaminolevulinate hydrochloride, 100 mg N1 N
* **A9588** Fluciclovine F-18, diagnostic, 1 millicurie Qp Qh K2 G

  Coding Clinic: 2017, Q1, P9
* **A9597** Positron emission tomography radiopharmaceutical, diagnostic, for tumor identification, not otherwise classified N1 N

  Coding Clinic: 2017, Q1, P8-9
* **A9598** Positron emission tomography radiopharmaceutical, diagnostic, for non-tumor identification, not otherwise classified N1 N

  Coding Clinic: 2017, Q1, P8-9
* **A9600** Strontium Sr-89 chloride, therapeutic, per millicurie Qp Qh K
* **A9604** Samarium SM-153 lexidronam, therapeutic, per treatment dose, up to 150 millicuries Qp Qh K
* **A9606** Radium Ra-223 dichloride, therapeutic, per microcurie Qp Qh K
* **A9698** Non-radioactive contrast imaging material, not otherwise classified, per study N1 N

  IOM: 100-04, 12, 70; 100-04, 13, 20

  Coding Clinic: 2017, Q1, P8
* **A9699** Radiopharmaceutical, therapeutic, not otherwise classified N
* **A9700** Supply of injectable contrast material for use in echocardiography, per study Qp Qh N1 N

  IOM: 100-04, 12, 30.4

  Coding Clinic: 2017, Q1, P8

Miscellaneous Service Component

* **A9900** Miscellaneous DME supply, accessory, and/or service component of another HCPCS code Y

  On DMEPOS fee schedule as a payable replacement for miscellaneous implanted or non-implanted items.
* **A9901** DME delivery, set up, and/or dispensing service component of another HCPCS code A
* **A9999** Miscellaneous DME supply or accessory, not otherwise specified Y

  On DMEPOS fee schedule as a payable replacement for miscellaneous implanted or non-implanted items.

ENTERAL AND PARENTERAL THERAPY (B4000-B9999)

Enteral Feeding Supplies

B4034 Enteral feeding supply kit; syringe fed, per day, includes but not limited to feeding/flushing syringe, administration set tubing, dressings, tape Qh Y

Dressings used with gastrostomy tubes for enteral nutrition (covered under the prosthetic device benefit) are included in the payment.

IOM: 100-02, 15, 120; 100-03, 3, 180.2; 100-04, 20, 100.2.2

PEN: On Fee Schedule

B4035 Enteral feeding supply kit; pump fed, per day, includes but not limited to feeding/flushing syringe, administration set tubing, dressings, tape Qh Y

IOM: 100-02, 15, 120; 100-03, 3, 180.2; 100-04, 20, 100.2.2

PEN: On Fee Schedule

B4036 Enteral feeding supply kit; gravity fed, per day, includes but not limited to feeding/flushing syringe, administration set tubing, dressings, tape Qh Y

IOM: 100-02, 15, 120; 100-03, 3, 180.2; 100-04, 20, 100.2.2

PEN: On Fee Schedule

B4081 Nasogastric tubing with stylet Qp Qh Y

More than 3 nasogastric tubes (B4081-B4083), or 1 gastrostomy/jejunostomy tube (B4087-B4088) every three months is rarely medically necessary.

IOM: 100-02, 15, 120; 100-03, 3, 180.2; 100-04, 20, 100.2.2

PEN: On Fee Schedule

B4082 Nasogastric tubing without stylet Qp Qh Y

IOM: 100-02, 15, 120; 100-03, 3, 180.2; 100-04, 20, 100.2.2

PEN: On Fee Schedule

B4083 Stomach tube - Levine type Qp Qh Y

IOM: 100-02, 15, 120; 100-03, 3, 180.2; 100-04, 20, 100.2.2

PEN: On Fee Schedule

* **B4087** Gastrostomy/jejunostomy tube, standard, any material, any type, each Qp Qh A

PEN: On Fee Schedule

* **B4088** Gastrostomy/jejunostomy tube, low-profile, any material, any type, each Qp Qh A

PEN: On Fee Schedule

Enteral Formulas and Additives

⃠ **B4100** Food thickener, administered orally, per ounce E1

B4102 Enteral formula, for adults, used to replace fluids and electrolytes (e.g., clear liquids), 500 ml = 1 unit A Y

IOM: 100-03, 3, 180.2

B4103 Enteral formula, for pediatrics, used to replace fluids and electrolytes (e.g., clear liquids), 500 ml = 1 unit A Y

IOM: 100-03, 3, 180.2

B4104 Additive for enteral formula (e.g., fiber) E1

IOM: 100-03, 3, 180.2

▶ **B4105** In-line cartridge containing digestive enzyme(s) for enteral feeding, each Y

Cross Reference Q9994

B4149 Enteral formula, manufactured blenderized natural foods with intact nutrients, includes proteins, fats, carbohydrates, vitamins and minerals, may include fiber, administered through an enteral feeding tube, 100 calories = 1 unit Qp Qh Y

Produced to meet unique nutrient needs for specific disease conditions; medical record must document specific condition and need for special nutrient.

IOM: 100-02, 15, 120; 100-03, 3, 180.2; 100-04, 20, 100.2.2

PEN: On Fee Schedule

B4150 Enteral formulae, nutritionally complete with intact nutrients, includes proteins, fats, carbohydrates, vitamins, and minerals, may include fiber, administered through an enteral feeding tube, 100 calories = 1 unit Qh Y

IOM: 100-02, 15, 120; 100-03, 3, 180.2; 100-04, 20, 100.2.2

PEN: On Fee Schedule

▶ New ↩ Revised ✔ Reinstated ~~deleted~~ Deleted ⃠ Not covered or valid by Medicare
Special coverage instructions * Carrier discretion Bill Part B MAC Bill DME MAC

B4152 Enteral formula, nutritionally complete, calorically dense (equal to or greater than 1.5 kcal/ml) with intact nutrients, includes proteins, fats, carbohydrates, vitamins and minerals, may include fiber, administered through an enteral feeding tube, 100 calories = 1 unit Ⓑ Qh Y

IOM: 100-02, 15, 120; 100-03, 3, 180.2; 100-04, 20, 100.2.2

PEN: On Fee Schedule

B4153 Enteral formula, nutritionally complete, hydrolyzed proteins (amino acids and peptide chain), includes fats, carbohydrates, vitamins and minerals, may include fiber, administered through an enteral feeding tube, 100 calories = 1 unit Ⓑ Qp Qh Y

If 2 enteral nutrition products described by same HCPCS code and provided at same time billed on single claim line with units of service reflecting total calories of both nutrients

IOM: 100-02, 15, 120; 100-03, 3, 180.2; 100-04, 20, 100.2.2

PEN: On Fee Schedule

B4154 Enteral formula, nutritionally complete, for special metabolic needs, excludes inherited disease of metabolism, includes altered composition of proteins, fats, carbohydrates, vitamins and/or minerals, may include fiber, administered through an enteral feeding tube, 100 calories = 1 unit Ⓑ Qh Y

IOM: 100-02, 15, 120; 100-03, 3, 180.2; 100-04, 20, 100.2.2

PEN: On Fee Schedule

B4155 Enteral formula, nutritionally incomplete/modular nutrients, includes specific nutrients, carbohydrates (e.g., glucose polymers), proteins/amino acids (e.g., glutamine, arginine), fat (e.g., medium chain triglycerides) or combination, administered through an enteral feeding tube, 100 calories = 1 unit Ⓑ Qh Y

IOM: 100-02, 15, 120; 100-03, 3, 180.2; 100-04, 20, 100.2.2

PEN: On Fee Schedule

B4157 Enteral formula, nutritionally complete, for special metabolic needs for inherited disease of metabolism, includes proteins, fats, carbohydrates, vitamins and minerals, may include fiber, administered through an enteral feeding tube, 100 calories = 1 unit Ⓑ Qp Qh Y

IOM: 100-03, 3, 180.2

B4158 Enteral formula, for pediatrics, nutritionally complete with intact nutrients, includes proteins, fats, carbohydrates, vitamins and minerals, may include fiber and/or iron, administered through an enteral feeding tube, 100 calories = 1 unit Ⓑ Qh A Y

IOM: 100-03, 3, 180.2

B4159 Enteral formula, for pediatrics, nutritionally complete soy based with intact nutrients, includes proteins, fats, carbohydrates, vitamins and minerals, may include fiber and/or iron, administered through an enteral feeding tube, 100 calories = 1 unit Ⓑ Qh A Y

IOM: 100-03, 3, 180.2

B4160 Enteral formula, for pediatrics, nutritionally complete calorically dense (equal to or greater than 0.7 kcal/ml) with intact nutrients, includes proteins, fats, carbohydrates, vitamins and minerals, may include fiber, administered through an enteral feeding tube, 100 calories = 1 unit Ⓑ Qp Qh A Y

IOM: 100-03, 3, 180.2

B4161 Enteral formula, for pediatrics, hydrolyzed/amino acids and peptide chain proteins, includes fats, carbohydrates, vitamins and minerals, may include fiber, administered through an enteral feeding tube, 100 calories = 1 unit Ⓑ Qh A Y

IOM: 100-03, 3, 180.2

B4162 Enteral formula, for pediatrics, special metabolic needs for inherited disease of metabolism, includes proteins, fats, carbohydrates, vitamins and minerals, may include fiber, administered through an enteral feeding tube, 100 calories = 1 unit Ⓑ Qh A Y

IOM: 100-03, 3, 180.2

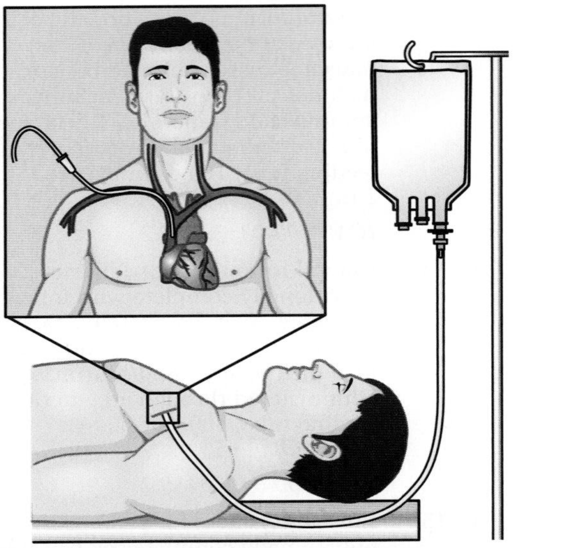

Figure 8 Total Parenteral Nutrition (TPN) involves percutaneous placement of central venous catheter into vena cava or right atrium.

Parenteral Nutritional Solutions and Supplies

B4164 Parenteral nutrition solution: carbohydrates (dextrose), 50% or less (500 ml = 1 unit) - home mix Ⓑ Qp Qh Y

IOM: 100-02, 15, 120; 100-03, 3, 180.2; 100-04, 20, 100.2.2

PEN: On Fee Schedule

B4168 Parenteral nutrition solution; amino acid, 3.5%, (500 ml = 1 unit) - home mix Ⓑ Qp Qh Y

IOM: 100-02, 15, 120; 100-03, 3, 180.2; 100-04, 20, 100.2.2

PEN: On Fee Schedule

B4172 Parenteral nutrition solution; amino acid, 5.5% through 7%, (500 ml = 1 unit) - home mix Ⓑ Qp Qh Y

IOM: 100-02, 15, 120; 100-03, 3, 180.2; 100-04, 20, 100.2.2

B4176 Parenteral nutrition solution; amino acid, 7% through 8.5%, (500 ml = 1 unit) - home mix Ⓑ Qp Qh Y

IOM: 100-02, 15, 120; 100-03, 3, 180.2; 100-04, 20, 100.2.2

PEN: On Fee Schedule

B4178 Parenteral nutrition solution: amino acid, greater than 8.5% (500 ml = 1 unit) - home mix Ⓑ Qp Qh Y

IOM: 100-02, 15, 120; 100-03, 3, 180.2; 100-04, 20, 100.2.2

PEN: On Fee Schedule

B4180 Parenteral nutrition solution; carbohydrates (dextrose), greater than 50% (500 ml = 1 unit) - home mix Ⓑ Qp Qh Y

IOM: 100-02, 15, 120; 100-03, 3, 180.2; 100-04, 20, 100.2.2

PEN: On Fee Schedule

B4185 Parenteral nutrition solution, per 10 grams lipids Ⓑ B

PEN: On Fee Schedule

B4189 Parenteral nutrition solution; compounded amino acid and carbohydrates with electrolytes, trace elements, and vitamins, including preparation, any strength, 10 to 51 grams of protein - premix Ⓑ Qp Qh Y

IOM: 100-02, 15, 120; 100-03, 3, 180.2; 100-04, 20, 100.2.2

PEN: On Fee Schedule

B4193 Parenteral nutrition solution; compounded amino acid and carbohydrates with electrolytes, trace elements, and vitamins, including preparation, any strength, 52 to 73 grams of protein - premix Ⓑ Qh Y

IOM: 100-02, 15, 120; 100-03, 3, 180.2; 100-04, 20, 100.2.2

PEN: On Fee Schedule

B4197 Parenteral nutrition solution; compounded amino acid and carbohydrates with electrolytes, trace elements and vitamins, including preparation, any strength, 74 to 100 grams of protein - premix Ⓑ Qh Y

IOM: 100-02, 15, 120; 100-03, 3, 180.2; 100-04, 20, 100.2.2

PEN: On Fee Schedule

B4199 Parenteral nutrition solution; compounded amino acid and carbohydrates with electrolytes, trace elements and vitamins, including preparation, any strength, over 100 grams of protein - premix Ⓑ Qp Qh Y

IOM: 100-02, 15, 120; 100-03, 3, 180.2; 100-04, 20, 100.2.2

PEN: On Fee Schedule

▶ New ⤺ Revised ✔ Reinstated ~~deleted~~ Deleted ⊘ Not covered or valid by Medicare
Special coverage instructions ✻ Carrier discretion Ⓑ Bill Part B MAC Ⓑ Bill DME MAC

B4216 Parenteral nutrition; additives (vitamins, trace elements, heparin, electrolytes) home mix per day Ⓑ Qh Y

IOM: 100-02, 15, 120; 100-03, 3, 180.2; 100-04, 20, 100.2.2

PEN: On Fee Schedule

B4220 Parenteral nutrition supply kit; premix, per day Ⓑ Qh Y

IOM: 100-02, 15, 120; 100-03, 3, 180.2; 100-04, 20, 100.2.2

PEN: On Fee Schedule

B4222 Parenteral nutrition supply kit; home mix, per day Ⓑ Qh Y

IOM: 100-02, 15, 120; 100-03, 3, 180.2; 100-04, 20, 100.2.2

PEN: On Fee Schedule

B4224 Parenteral nutrition administration kit, per day Ⓑ Qh Y

Dressings used with parenteral nutrition (covered under the prosthetic device benefit) are included in the payment. (www.cms.gov/medicare-coverage-database/)

IOM: 100-02, 15, 120; 100-03, 3, 180.2; 100-04, 20, 100.2.2

PEN: On Fee Schedule

B5000 Parenteral nutrition solution compounded amino acid and carbohydrates with electrolytes, trace elements, and vitamins, including preparation, any strength, renal - Aminosyn-RF, NephrAmine, RenAmine - premix Ⓑ Qp Qh Y

IOM: 100-02, 15, 120; 100-03, 3, 180.2; 100-04, 20, 100.2.2

PEN: On Fee Schedule

B5100 Parenteral nutrition solution compounded amino acid and carbohydrates with electrolytes, trace elements, and vitamins, including preparation, any strength, hepatic, HepatAmine - premix Ⓑ Qp Qh Y

IOM: 100-02, 15, 120; 100-03, 3, 180.2; 100-04, 20, 100.2.2

PEN: On Fee Schedule

B5200 Parenteral nutrition solution compounded amino acid and carbohydrates with electrolytes, trace elements, and vitamins, including preparation, any strength, stress-branch chain amino acids-FreAmine-HBC - premix Ⓑ Qp Qh Y

IOM: 100-02, 15, 120; 100-03, 3, 180.2; 100-04, 20, 100.2.2

Enteral and Parenteral Pumps

B9002 Enteral nutrition infusion pump, any type Ⓑ Qh Y

IOM: 100-02, 15, 120; 100-03, 3, 180.2; 100-04, 20, 100.2.2

PEN: On Fee Schedule

B9004 Parenteral nutrition infusion pump, portable Ⓑ Qh Y

IOM: 100-02, 15, 120; 100-03, 3, 180.2; 100-04, 20, 100.2.2

PEN: On Fee Schedule

B9006 Parenteral nutrition infusion pump, stationary Ⓑ Qh Y

IOM: 100-02, 15, 120; 100-03, 3, 180.2; 100-04, 20, 100.2.2

PEN: On Fee Schedule

B9998 NOC for enteral supplies Ⓑ Y

IOM: 100-02, 15, 120; 100-03, 3, 180.2; 100-04, 20, 100.2.2

B9999 NOC for parenteral supplies Ⓑ Y

Determine if an alternative HCPCS Level II or a CPT code better describes the service being reported. This code should be reported only if a more specific code is unavailable.

IOM: 100-02, 15, 120; 100-03, 3, 180.2; 100-04, 20, 100.2.2

CMS HOSPITAL OUTPATIENT PAYMENT SYSTEM (C1000-C9999)

NOTE: C-codes are used on Medicare Ambulatory Surgical Center (ASC) and Hospital Outpatient Prospective Payment System (OPPS) claims, but may also be recognized on claims from other providers or by other payment systems. As of 10/01/2006, the following non-OPPS providers have been able to bill Medicare using the C-codes, or an appropriate CPT code on Types of Bill (TOBs) 12X, 13X, or 85X:

- Critical Access Hospitals (CAHs);
- Indian Health Service Hospitals (IHS);
- Hospitals located in American Samoa, Guam, Saipan or the Virgin Islands; and
- Maryland waiver hospitals.

The billing of C-codes by Method I and Method II Critical Access Hospitals (CAHs) is limited to the billing for facility (technical) services. The C-codes shall not be billed by Method II CAHs for professional services with revenue codes (RCs) 96X, 97X, or 98X.

C codes are updated quarterly by the Centers for Medicare and Medicaid Services (CMS).

Devices and Supplies

C1713 Anchor/Screw for opposing bone-to-bone or soft tissue-to-bone (implantable) Qh N1 N

Medicare Statute 1833(t)

Coding Clinic: 2018, Q2, P5; Q1, P4; 2016, Q3, P16; 2015, Q3, P2; 2010, Q2, P3

C1714 Catheter, transluminal atherectomy, directional Qh N1 N

Medicare Statute 1833(t)

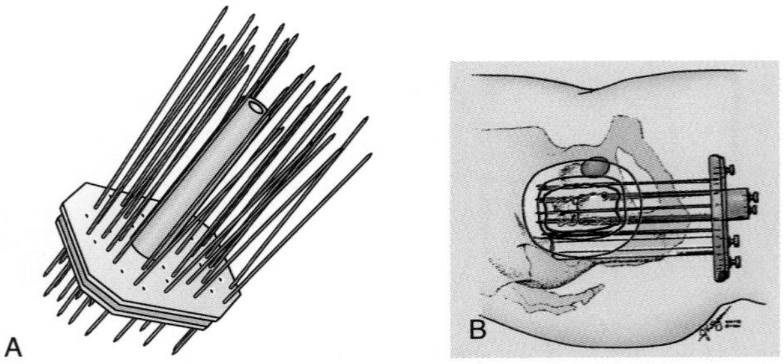
A
B

Figure 9 (A) Brachytherapy device, (B) Brachytherapy device inserted.

C1715 Brachytherapy needle Qh N1 N

Medicare Statute 1833(t)

Brachytherapy Sources

C1716 Brachytherapy source, non-stranded, gold-198, per source Qp Qh H2 U

Medicare Statute 1833(t)

C1717 Brachytherapy source, non-stranded, high dose rate iridium 192, per source Qp Qh H2 U

Medicare Statute 1833(t)

C1719 Brachytherapy source, non-stranded, non-high dose rate iridium-192, per source Qp Qh H2 U

Medicare Statute 1833(t)

Cardioverter-Defibrilators

C1721 Cardioverter-defibrillator, dual chamber (implantable) Qp Qh N1 N

Related CPT codes: 33224, 33240, 33249.

Medicare Statute 1833(t)

C1722 Cardioverter-defibrillator, single chamber (implantable) Qp Qh N1 N

Related CPT codes: 33240, 33249.

Medicare Statute 1833(t)

Coding Clinic: 2017, Q2, P5; 2006, Q2, P9

Catheters

C1724 Catheter, transluminal atherectomy, rotational Qh N1 N

Medicare Statute 1833(t)

Coding Clinic: 2016, Q3, P9

C1725 Catheter, transluminal angioplasty, non-laser (may include guidance, infusion/perfusion capability) Qh N1 N

Medicare Statute 1833(t)

Coding Clinic: 2016, Q3, P16, P19

C1726 Catheter, balloon dilatation, non-vascular Qh N1 N

Medicare Statute 1833(t)

Coding Clinic: 2016, Q3, P16, P19

C1727 Catheter, balloon tissue dissector, non-vascular (insertable) Qh N1 N

Medicare Statute 1833(t)

Coding Clinic: 2016, Q3, P16

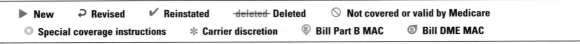

C1728 Catheter, brachytherapy seed administration Qh N1 N
Medicare Statute 1833(t)

C1729 Catheter, drainage Qh N1 N
Medicare Statute 1833(t)
Coding Clinic: 2016, Q3, P17

C1730 Catheter, electrophysiology, diagnostic, other than 3D mapping (19 or fewer electrodes) Qp Qh N1 N
Medicare Statute 1833(t)
Coding Clinic: 2016, Q3, P17

C1731 Catheter, electrophysiology, diagnostic, other than 3D mapping (20 or more electrodes) Qp Qh N1 N
Medicare Statute 1833(t)
Coding Clinic: 2016, Q3, P17

C1732 Catheter, electrophysiology, diagnostic/ablation, 3D or vector mapping Qp Qh N1 N
Medicare Statute 1833(t)
Coding Clinic: 2016, Q3, P15, P17, P19

C1733 Catheter, electrophysiology, diagnostic/ablation, other than 3D or vector mapping, other than cool-tip Qp Qh N1 N
Medicare Statute 1833(t)
Coding Clinic: 2016, Q3, P17

C1749 Endoscope, retrograde imaging/illumination colonoscope device (implantable) Qp Qh N1 N
Medicare Statute 1833(t)

C1750 Catheter, hemodialysis/peritoneal, long-term Qh N1 N
Medicare Statute 1833(t)
Coding Clinic: 2015, Q4, P6

C1751 Catheter, infusion, inserted peripherally, centrally, or midline (other than hemodialysis) Qh N1 N
Medicare Statute 1833(t)

C1752 Catheter, hemodialysis/peritoneal, short-term Qh N1 N
Medicare Statute 1833(t)

C1753 Catheter, intravascular ultrasound Qh N1 N
Medicare Statute 1833(t)

C1754 Catheter, intradiscal Qh N1 N
Medicare Statute 1833(t)

C1755 Catheter, instraspinal Qh N1 N
Medicare Statute 1833(t)

C1756 Catheter, pacing, transesophageal Qh N1 N
Medicare Statute 1833(t)

C1757 Catheter, thrombectomy/embolectomy Qh N1 N
Medicare Statute 1833(t)

C1758 Catheter, ureteral Qh N1 N
Medicare Statute 1833(t)

C1759 Catheter, intracardiac echocardiography Qh N1 N
Medicare Statute 1833(t)

Devices

C1760 Closure device, vascular (implantable/insertable) Qh N1 N
Medicare Statute 1833(t)
Coding Clinic: 2016, Q3, P19

C1762 Connective tissue, human (includes fascia lata) Qh N1 N
Medicare Statute 1833(t)
Coding Clinic: 2016, Q3, P9, P16, P19; 2015, Q3, P2; 2003, Q3, P12

C1763 Connective tissue, non-human (includes synthetic) Qh N1 N
Medicare Statute 1833(t)
Coding Clinic: 2016, Q3, P9, P17, P19; 2010, Q4, P3; Q2, P3; 2003, Q3, P12

C1764 Event recorder, cardiac (implantable) Qp Qh N1 N
Medicare Statute 1833(t)
Coding Clinic: 2015, Q2, P8

C1765 Adhesion barrier Qh N1 N
Medicare Statute 1833(t)
Coding Clinic: 2016, Q3, P16

C1766 Introducer/sheath, guiding, intracardiac electrophysiological, steerable, other than peel-away Qh N1 N
Medicare Statute 1833(t)

C1767 Generator, neurostimulator (implantable), nonrechargeable Qp Qh N1 N
Related CPT codes: 61885, 61886, 63685, 64590.
Medicare Statute 1833(t)
Coding Clinic: 2007, Q1, P8

C1768 Graft, vascular Qh N1 N
Medicare Statute 1833(t)

◎ **C1769** Guide wire Qh N1 N
Medicare Statute 1833(t)
Coding Clinic: 2016, Q3, P3; 2007, Q2, P7-8

◎ **C1770** Imaging coil, magnetic reasonance (insertable) Qh N1 N
Medicare Statute 1833(t)

◎ **C1771** Repair device, urinary, incontinence, with sling graft Qp Qh N1 N
Medicare Statute 1833(t)
Coding Clinic: 2016, Q3, P19; 2008, Q3, P7

◎ **C1772** Infusion pump, programmable (implantable) Qp Qh N1 N
Medicare Statute 1833(t)

◎ **C1773** Retrieval device, insertable (used to retrieve fractured medical devices) Qh N1 N
Medicare Statute 1833(t)
Coding Clinic: 2016, Q3, P19

◎ **C1776** Joint device (implantable) Qp Qh N1 N
Medicare Statute 1833(t)
Coding Clinic: 2018, Q3, P6; 2016, Q3, P3, P18; 2010, Q3, P6; 2008, Q4, P10

◎ **C1777** Lead, cardioverter-defibrillator, endocardial single coil (implantable) Qh N1 N
Related CPT codes: 33216, 33217, 33249.
Medicare Statute 1833(t)
Coding Clinic: 2017, Q2, P5; 2006, Q2, P9

◎ **C1778** Lead, neurostimulator (implantable) Qp Qh N1 N
Related CPT codes: 43647, 63650, 63655, 63663, 63664, 64553, 64555, 64560, 64561, 64565, 64573, 64575, 64577, 64580, 64581.
Medicare Statute 1833(t)
Coding Clinic: 2007, Q1, P8

◎ **C1779** Lead, pacemaker, trasvenous VDD single pass Qh N1 N
Related CPT codes: 33206, 33207, 33208, 33210, 33211, 33214, 33216, 33217, 33249.
Medicare Statute 1833(t)
Coding Clinic: 2016, Q3, P19

◎ **C1780** Lens, intraocular (new technology) Qh N1 N
Medicare Statute 1833(t)
Coding Clinic: 2016, Q3, P18

◎ **C1781** Mesh (implantable) Qh N1 N
Medicare Statute 1833(t)
Coding Clinic: 2016, Q3, P18-19; 2012, Q2, P3; 2010, Q2, P2-3

◎ **C1782** Morcellator Qp Qh N1 N
Medicare Statute 1833(t)
Coding Clinic: 2016, Q3, P18

◎ **C1783** Ocular implant, aqueous drainage assist device Qh N1 N
Medicare Statute 1833(t)
Coding Clinic: 2017, Q1, P5

◎ **C1784** Ocular device, intraoperative, detached retina Qh N1 N
Medicare Statute 1833(t)
Coding Clinic: 2016, Q3, P18

◎ **C1785** Pacemaker, dual chamber, rate-responsive (implantable) Qp Qh N1 N
Related CPT codes: 33206, 33207, 33208, 33213, 33214, 33224.
Medicare Statute 1833(t)

◎ **C1786** Pacemaker, single chamber, rate-responsive (implantable) Qp Qh N1 N
Related CPT codes: 33206, 33207, 33212.
Medicare Statute 1833(t)

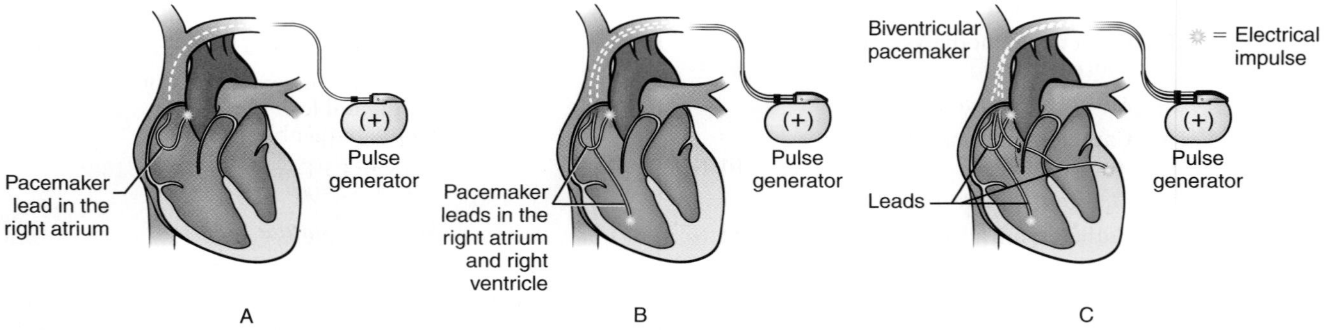
Pacemaker lead in the right atrium
(+)
Pulse generator
A
Pacemaker leads in the right atrium and right ventricle
(+)
Pulse generator
B
Biventricular pacemaker
= Electrical impulse
Leads
(+)
Pulse generator
C

Figure 10 (A) Single pacemaker, (B) Dual pacemaker, (C) Biventricular pacemaker.

▶ New ⤴ Revised ✔ Reinstated ~~deleted~~ Deleted ⊘ Not covered or valid by Medicare
◎ Special coverage instructions ✻ Carrier discretion Ⓑ Bill Part B MAC Ⓓ Bill DME MAC

C1787 Patient programmer, neurostimulator Qh N1 N
Medicare Statute 1833(t)
Coding Clinic: 2016, Q3, P19

C1788 Port, indwelling (implantable) Qh N1 N
Medicare Statute 1833(t)

C1789 Prosthesis, breast (implantable) Qh N1 N
Medicare Statute 1833(t)

C1813 Prosthesis, penile, inflatable Qp Qh ♂ N1 N
Medicare Statute 1833(t)

C1814 Retinal tamponade device, silicone oil Qh N1 N
Medicare Statute 1833(t)
Coding Clinic: 2016, Q3, P19; 2006, Q2, P9

C1815 Prosthesis, urinary sphincter (implantable) Qp Qh N1 N
Medicare Statute 1833(t)

C1816 Receiver and/or transmitter, neurostimulator (implantable) Qh N1 N
Medicare Statute 1833(t)

C1817 Septal defect implant system, intracardiac Qp Qh N1 N
Medicare Statute 1833(t)
Coding Clinic: 2016, Q3, P19

C1818 Integrated keratoprosthesic Qh N1 N
Medicare Statute 1833(t)
Coding Clinic: 2016, Q3, P18

C1819 Surgical tissue localization and excision device (implantable) Qh N1 N
Medicare Statute 1833(t)

C1820 Generator, neurostimulator (implantable), with rechargeable battery and charging system Qp Qh N1 N
Related CPT codes: 61885, 61886, 63685, 64590.
Medicare Statute 1833(t)
Coding Clinic: 2016, Q2, P7

C1821 Interspinous process distraction device (implantable) Qh N1 N
Medicare Statute 1833(t)

C1822 Generator, neurostimulator (implantable), high frequency, with rechargeable battery and charging system Qp Qh N1 N
Medicare Statute 1833(T)
Coding Clinic: 2016, Q2, P7

▶ C1823 Generator, neurostimulator (implantable), non-rechargeable, with transvenous sensing and stimulation leads H
Medicare Statute 1833(t)

C1830 Powered bone marrow biopsy needle Qp Qh N1 N
Medicare Statute 1833(t)

C1840 Lens, intraocular (telescopic) Qp Qh N1 N
Medicare Statute 1833(t)
Coding Clinic: 2012, Q3, P10

C1841 Retinal prosthesis, includes all internal and external components Qp Qh J7 N
Medicare Statute 1833(t)

C1842 Retinal prosthesis, includes all internal and external components; add-on to C1841 Qp Qh J7 E1
Medicare Statute 1833(t)
Coding Clinic: 2017, Q1, P6

C1874 Stent, coated/covered, with delivery system Qh N1 N
Medicare Statute 1833(t)
Coding Clinic: 2016, Q3, P16-17, P19

C1875 Stent, coated/covered, without delivery system Qh N1 N
Medicare Statute 1833(t)
Coding Clinic: 2016, Q3, P16-17

C1876 Stent, non-coated/non-covered, with delivery system Qh N1 N
Medicare Statute 1833(t)
Coding Clinic: 2016, Q3, P19

C1877 Stent, non-coated/non-covered, without delivery system Qh N1 N
Medicare Statute 1833(t)

C1878 Material for vocal cord medialization, synthetic (implantable) Qh N1 N
Medicare Statute 1833(t)
Coding Clinic: 2016, Q3, P18

C1880 Vena cava filter Qh N1 N
Medicare Statute 1833(t)

C1881 Dialysis access system (implantable) Qh N1 N
Medicare Statute 1833(t)

C1882 Cardioverter-defibrillator, other than single or dual chamber (implantable) Qp Qh N1 N
Related CPT codes: 33224, 33240, 33249.
Medicare Statute 1833(t)
Coding Clinic: 2016, Q3, P16; 2012, Q2, P9; 2006, Q2, P9

C1883 Adapter/Extension, pacing lead or neurostimulator lead (implantable) Qh N1 N
Medicare Statute 1833(t)
Coding Clinic: 2016, Q3, P15, P17; 2007, Q1, P8

C1884 Embolization protective system Qh N1 N
Medicare Statute 1833(t)
Coding Clinic: 2016, Q3, P17

C1885 Catheter, transluminal angioplasty, laser Qh N1 N
Medicare Statute 1833(t)
Coding Clinic: 2016, Q3, p16, Q1, P5

C1886 Catheter, extravascular tissue ablation, any modality (insertable) Qp Qh N1 N
Medicare Statute 1833(t)

C1887 Catheter, guiding (may include infusion/perfusion capability) Qh N1 N
Medicare Statute 1833(t)
Coding Clinic: 2016, Q3, P17

C1888 Catheter, ablation, non-cardiac, endovascular (implantable) Qh N1 N
Medicare Statute 1833(t)
Coding Clinic: 2016, Q3, P16

C1889 Implantable/insertable device, not otherwise classified N1 N
Medicare Statute 1833(T)

C1891 Infusion pump, non-programmable, permanent (implantable) Qp Qh N1 N
Medicare Statute 1833(t)

C1892 Introducer/sheath, guiding, intracardiac electrophysiological, fixed-curve, peel-away Qh N1 N
Medicare Statute 1833(t)
Coding Clinic: 2016, Q3, P19

C1893 Introducer/sheath, guiding, intracardiac electrophysiological, fixed-curve, other than peel-away Qh N1 N
Medicare Statute 1833(t)

C1894 Introducer/sheath, other than guiding, other than intracardiac electrophysiological, non-laser Qh N1 N
Medicare Statute 1833(t)

C1895 Lead, cardioverter-defibrillator, endocardial dual coil (implantable) Qh N1 N
Related CPT codes: 33216, 33217, 33249.
Medicare Statute 1833(t)
Coding Clinic: 2006, Q2, P9

C1896 Lead, cardioverter-defibrillator, other than endocardial single or dual coil (implantable) Qh N1 N
Related CPT codes: 33216, 33217, 33249.
Medicare Statute 1833(t)

C1897 Lead, neurostimulator test kit (implantable) Qh N1 N
Related CPT codes: 43647, 63650, 63655, 63663, 63664, 64553, 64555, 64560, 64561, 64565, 64575, 64577, 64580, 64581.
Medicare Statute 1833(t)
Coding Clinic: 2007, Q1, P8

C1898 Lead, pacemaker, other than transvenous VDD single pass Qh N1 N
Related CPT codes: 33206, 33207, 33208, 33210, 33211, 33214, 33216, 33217, 33249.
Medicare Statute 1833(t)
Coding Clinic: 2002, Q3, P8

C1899 Lead, pacemaker/cardioverter-defibrillator combination (implantable) Qh N1 N
Related CPT codes: 33216, 33217, 33249.
Medicare Statute 1833(t)

C1900 Lead, left ventricular coronary venous system Qp Qh N1 N
Related CPT codes: 33224, 33225.
Medicare Statute 1833(t)
Coding Clinic: 2016, Q3, P18

C2613 Lung biopsy plug with delivery system Qp Qh N1 N
Medicare Statute 1833(t)
Coding Clinic: 2015, Q2, P11

C2614 Probe, percutaneous lumbar discectomy Qh N1 N
Medicare Statute 1833(t)

C2615 Sealant, pulmonary, liquid Qh N1 N
Medicare Statute 1833(t)
Coding Clinic: 2016, Q3, P18

Brachytherapy Source

C2616 Brachytherapy source, non-stranded, yttrium-90, per source Qp Qh H2 U
Medicare Statute 1833(t)

Cardiovascular and Genitourinary Devices

C2617 Stent, non-coronary, temporary, without delivery system Qh N1 N
Medicare Statute 1833(t)
Coding Clinic: 2018, Q1, P4; 2016, Q3, P3, P19

C2618 Probe/needle, cryoablation Qh N1 N
Medicare Statute 1833(t)

C2619 Pacemaker, dual chamber, non rate-responsive (implantable) Qp Qh N1 N
Related CPT codes: 33206, 33207, 33208, 33213, 33214, 33224.
Medicare Statute 1833(t)

C2620 Pacemaker, single chamber, non rate-responsive (implantable) Qp Qh N1 N
Related CPT codes: 33206, 33207, 33212, 33224.
Medicare Statute 1833(t)

C2621 Pacemaker, other than single or dual chamber (implantable) Qp Qh N1 N
Related CPT codes: 33206, 33207, 33208, 33212, 33213, 33214, 33224.
Medicare Statute 1833(t)
Coding Clinic: 2016, Q3, P18; 2002, Q3, P8

C2622 Prosthesis, penile, non-inflatable Qp Qh ♂ N1 N
Medicare Statute 1833(t)

C2623 Catheter, transluminal angioplasty, drug-coated, non-laser Qp Qh N1 N
Medicare Statute 1833(t)

C2624 Implantable wireless pulmonary artery pressure sensor with delivery catheter, including all system components Qp Qh N1 N
Medicare Statute 1833(t)
Coding Clinic: 2015, Q3, P2

C2625 Stent, non-coronary, temporary, with delivery system Qh N1 N
Medicare Statute 1833(t)
Coding Clinic: 2016, Q3, P19; 2015, Q2, P9

C2626 Infusion pump, non-programmable, temporary (implantable) Qp Qh N1 N
Medicare Statute 1833(t)
Coding Clinic: 2016, Q3, P18

C2627 Catheter, suprapubic/cystoscopic Qh N1 N
Medicare Statute 1833(t)

C2628 Catheter, occlusion Qh N1 N
Medicare Statute 1833(t)

C2629 Introducer/Sheath, other than guiding, other than intracardiac electrophysiological, laser Qh N1 N
Medicare Statute 1833(t)

C2630 Catheter, electrophysiology, diagnostic/ablation, other than 3D or vector mapping, cool-tip Qp Qh N1 N
Medicare Statute 1833(t)
Coding Clinic: 2016, Q3, P17

C2631 Repair device, urinary, incontinence, without sling graft Qp Qh N1 N
Medicare Statute 1833(t)

Brachytherapy Sources

C2634 Brachytherapy source, non-stranded, high activity, iodine-125, greater than 1.01 mci (NIST), per source Qp Qh H2 U
Medicare Statute 1833(t)

C2635 Brachytherapy source, non-stranded, high activity, palladium-103, greater than 2.2 mci (NIST), per source Qp Qh H2 U
Medicare Statute 1833(t)

C2636 Brachytherapy linear source, non-stranded, palladium-103, per 1 mm Qp Qh H2 U

C2637 Brachytherapy source, non-stranded, Ytterbium-169, per source Qp Qh B
Medicare Statute 1833(t)

C2638 Brachytherapy source, stranded, iodine-125, per source Qp Qh H2 U
Medicare Statute 1833(t)(2)

C2639 Brachytherapy source, non-stranded, iodine-125, per source Qp Qh H2 U
Medicare Statute 1833(t)(2)

C2640 Brachytherapy source, stranded, palladium-103, per source Qp Qh H2 U
Medicare Statute 1833(t)(2)

C2641 Brachytherapy source, non-stranded, palladium-103, per source Qp Qh H2 U
Medicare Statute 1833(t)(2)

C2642 Brachytherapy source, stranded, cesium-131, per source Qp Qh H2 U
Medicare Statute 1833(t)(2)

C2643 Brachytherapy source, non-stranded, cesium-131, per source Qp Qh H2 U
Medicare Statute 1833(t)(2)

C2644 Brachytherapy source, Cesium-131 chloride solution, per millicurie Qp Qh H2 U
Medicare Statute 1833(t)

C2645 Brachytherapy planar source, palladium-103, per square millimeter Qp Qh H2 U

Medicare Statute 1833(T)

C2698 Brachytherapy source, stranded, not otherwise specified, per source H2 U

Medicare Statute 1833(t)(2)

C2699 Brachytherapy source, non-stranded, not otherwise specified, per source H2 U

Medicare Statute 1833(t)(2)

Skin Substitute Graft Application

C5271 Application of low cost skin substitute graft to trunk, arms, legs, total wound surface area up to 100 sq cm; first 25 sq cm or less wound surface area Qp Qh T

Medicare Statute 1833(t)

C5272 Application of low cost skin substitute graft to trunk, arms, legs, total wound surface area up to 100 sq cm; each additional 25 sq cm wound surface area, or part thereof (list separately in addition to code for primary procedure) Qp Qh N

Medicare Statute 1833(t)

C5273 Application of low cost skin substitute graft to trunk, arms, legs, total wound surface area greater than or equal to 100 sq cm; first 100 sq cm wound surface area, or 1% of body area of infants and children Qp Qh A T

Medicare Statute 1833(t)

C5274 Application of low cost skin substitute graft to trunk, arms, legs, total wound surface area greater than or equal to 100 sq cm; each additional 100 sq cm wound surface area, or part thereof, or each additional 1% of body area of infants and children, or part thereof (list separately in addition to code for primary procedure) Qp Qh A N

Medicare Statute 1833(t)

C5275 Application of low cost skin substitute graft to face, scalp, eyelids, mouth, neck, ears, orbits, genitalia, hands, feet, and/or multiple digits, total wound surface area up to 100 sq cm; first 25 sq cm or less wound surface area Qp Qh T

Medicare Statute 1833(t)

C5276 Application of low cost skin substitute graft to face, scalp, eyelids, mouth, neck, ears, orbits, genitalia, hands, feet, and/or multiple digits, total wound surface area up to 100 sq cm; each additional 25 sq cm wound surface area, or part thereof (list separately in addition to code for primary procedure) Qp Qh N

Medicare Statute 1833(t)

C5277 Application of low cost skin substitute graft to face, scalp, eyelids, mouth, neck, ears, orbits, genitalia, hands, feet, and/or multiple digits, total wound surface area greater than or equal to 100 sq cm; first 100 sq cm wound surface area, or 1% of body area of infants and children Qp Qh A T

Medicare Statute 1833(t)

C5278 Application of low cost skin substitute graft to face, scalp, eyelids, mouth, neck, ears, orbits, genitalia, hands, feet, and/or multiple digits, total wound surface area greater than or equal to 100 sq cm; each additional 100 sq cm wound surface area, or part thereof, or each additional 1% of body area of infants and children, or part thereof (list separately in addition to code for primary procedure) Qp Qh A N

Medicare Statute 1833(t)

Magnetic Resonance Angiography: Trunk and Lower Extremities

C8900 Magnetic resonance angiography with contrast, abdomen Qp Qh Z2 Q3

Medicare Statute 1833(t)(2)

C8901 Magnetic resonance angiography without contrast, abdomen Qp Qh Z2 Q3

Medicare Statute 1833(t)(2)

C8902 Magnetic resonance angiography without contrast followed by with contrast, abdomen Qp Qh Z2 Q3

Medicare Statute 1833(t)(2)

C8903 Magnetic resonance imaging with contrast, breast; unilateral Qp Qh Z2 Q3

Medicare Statute 1833(t)(2)

~~C8904 Magnetic resonance imaging without contrast, breast; unilateral~~ ✖

C8905 Magnetic resonance imaging without contrast followed by with contrast, breast; unilateral Qp Qh Z2 Q3

Medicare Statute 1833(t)(2)

▶ New ↩ Revised ✔ Reinstated ~~deleted~~ Deleted ⊘ Not covered or valid by Medicare
Special coverage instructions ✱ Carrier discretion Bill Part B MAC Bill DME MAC

C8906 Magnetic resonance imaging with contrast, breast; bilateral Qp Qh Z2 Q3

Medicare Statute 1833(t)(2)

~~C8907 Magnetic resonance imaging without contrast, breast; bilateral~~ ✖

C8908 Magnetic resonance imaging without contrast followed by with contrast, breast; bilateral Qp Qh Z2 Q3

Medicare Statute 1833(t)(2)

C8909 Magnetic resonance angiography with contrast, chest (excluding myocardium) Qp Qh Z2 Q3

Medicare Statute 1833(t)(2)

C8910 Magnetic resonance angiography without contrast, chest (excluding myocardium) Qp Qh Z2 Q3

Medicare Statute 1833(t)(2)

C8911 Magnetic resonance angiography without contrast followed by with contrast, chest (excluding myocardium) Qp Qh Z2 Q3

Medicare Statute 1833(t)(2)

C8912 Magnetic resonance angiography with contrast, lower extremity Qp Qh Z2 Q3

Medicare Statute 1833(t)(2)

C8913 Magnetic resonance angiography without contrast, lower extremity Qp Qh Z2 Q3

Medicare Statute 1833(t)(2)

C8914 Magnetic resonance angiography without contrast followed by with contrast, lower extremity Qp Qh Z2 Q3

Medicare Statute 1833(t)(2)

C8918 Magnetic resonance angiography with contrast, pelvis Qp Qh Z2 Q3

Medicare Statute 1833(t)(2)

C8919 Magnetic resonance angiography without contrast, pelvis Qp Qh Z2 Q3

Medicare Statute 1833(t)(2)

C8920 Magnetic resonance angiography without contrast followed by with contrast, pelvis Qp Qh Z2 Q3

Medicare Statute 1833(t)(2)

Transthoracic and Transesophageal Echocardiography

C8921 Transthoracic echocardiography with contrast, or without contrast followed by with contrast, for congenital cardiac anomalies; complete Qp Qh S

Medicare Statute 1833(t)(2)

Coding Clinic: 2012, Q3, P8

C8922 Transthoracic echocardiography with contrast, or without contrast followed by with contrast, for congenital cardiac anomalies; follow-up or limited study Qp Qh S

Medicare Statute 1833(t)(2)

Coding Clinic: 2012, Q3, P8

C8923 Transthoracic echocardiography with contrast, or without contrast followed by with contrast, real-time with image documentation (2D), includes M-mode recording, when performed, complete, without spectral or color Doppler echocardiography Qp Qh S

Medicare Statute 1833(t)(2)

Coding Clinic: 2012, Q3, P8

C8924 Transthoracic echocardiography with contrast, or without contrast followed by with contrast, real-time with image documentation (2D), includes M-mode recording, when performed, follow-up or limited study Qp Qh S

Medicare Statute 1833(t)(2)

Coding Clinic: 2012, Q3, P8

C8925 Transesophageal echocardiography (TEE) with contrast, or without contrast followed by with contrast, real time with image documentation (2D) (with or without M-mode recording); including probe placement, image acquisition, interpretation and report Qp Qh S

Medicare Statute 1833(t)(2)

Coding Clinic: 2012, Q3, P8

C8926 Transesophageal echocardiography (TEE) with contrast, or without contrast followed by with contrast, for congenital cardiac anomalies; including probe placement, image acquisition, interpretation and report Qp Qh S

Medicare Statute 1833(t)(2)

Coding Clinic: 2012, Q3, P8

C8927 Transesophageal echocardiography (TEE) with contrast, or without contrast followed by with contrast, for monitoring purposes, including probe placement, real time 2-dimensional image acquisition and interpretation leading to ongoing (continuous) assessment of (dynamically changing) cardiac pumping function and to therapeutic measures on an immediate time basis Qp Qh S

Medicare Statute 1833(t)(2)

Coding Clinic: 2012, Q3, P8

C8928 Transthoracic echocardiography with contrast, or without contrast followed by with contrast, real-time with image documentation (2D), includes M-mode recording, when performed, during rest and cardiovascular stress test using treadmill, bicycle exercise and/or pharmacologically induced stress, with interpretation and report Qp Qh S
Medicare Statute 1833(t)(2)
Coding Clinic: 2012, Q3, P8

C8929 Transthoracic echocardiography with contrast, or without contrast followed by with contrast, real-time with image documentation (2D), includes M-mode recording, when performed, complete, with spectral Doppler echocardiography, and with color flow Doppler echocardiography Qp Qh S
Medicare Statute 1833(t)(2)
Coding Clinic: 2012, Q3, P8

C8930 Transthoracic echocardiography, with contrast, or without contrast followed by with contrast, real-time with image documentation (2D), includes M-mode recording, when performed, during rest and cardiovascular stress test using treadmill, bicycle exercise and/or pharmacologically induced stress, with interpretation and report; including performance of continuous electrocardiographic monitoring, with physician supervision Qp Qh S
Medicare Statute 1833(t)(2)
Coding Clinic: 2012, Q3, P8

Magnetic Resonance Angiography: Spine and Upper Extremities

C8931 Magnetic resonance angiography with contrast, spinal canal and contents Qp Qh Z2 Q3
Medicare Statute 1833(t)

C8932 Magnetic resonance angiography without contrast, spinal canal and contents Qp Qh Z2 Q3
Medicare Statute 1833(t)

C8933 Magnetic resonance angiography without contrast followed by with contrast, spinal canal and contents Qp Qh Z2 Q3
Medicare Statute 1833(t)

C8934 Magnetic resonance angiography with contrast, upper extremity Qh Z2 Q3
Medicare Statute 1833(t)

C8935 Magnetic resonance angiography without contrast, upper extremity Qh Z2 Q3
Medicare Statute 1833(t)

C8936 Magnetic resonance angiography without contrast followed by with contrast, upper extremity Qh Z2 Q3
Medicare Statute 1833(t)

▶ **C8937** Computer-aided detection, including computer algorithm analysis of breast MRI image data for lesion detection/ characterization, pharmacokinetic analysis, with further physician review for interpretation (list separately in addition to code for primary procedure) N
Medicare Statute 1833(t)

Drugs and Biologicals

C8957 Intravenous infusion for therapy/ diagnosis; initiation of prolonged infusion (more than 8 hours), requiring use of portable or implantable pump Qp Qh S
Medicare Statute 1833(t)
Coding Clinic: 2008, Q3, P8

~~C9014 Injection, cerliponase alfa, 1 mg~~ ✖

~~C9015 Injection, C-1 esterase inhibitor (human), haegarda, 10 units~~ ✖

~~C9016 Injection, triptorelin extended release, 3.75 mg~~ ✖

~~C9024 Injection, liposomal, 1 mg daunorubicin and 2.27 mg cytarabine~~ ✖

~~C9028 Injection, inotuzumab ozogamicin, 0.1 mg~~ ✖

~~C9029 Injection, guselkumab, 1 mg~~ ✖

▶ **C9034** Injection, dexamethasone 9%, intraocular, 1 mcg G
Medicare Statute 1833(t)

▶ **C9035** Injection, aripiprazole lauroxil (aristada initio), 1 mg G
Medicare Statute 1833(t)

▶ **C9036** Injection, patisiran, 0.1 mg G
Medicare Statute 1833(t)

▶ **C9037** Injection, risperidone (perseris), 0.5 mg G
Medicare Statute 1833(t)

▶ **C9038** Injection, mogamulizumab-kpkc, 1 mg G
Medicare Statute 1833(t)

▶ **C9039** Injection, plazomicin, 5 mg G
Medicare Statute 1833(t)

C9113 Injection, pantoprazole sodium, per vial Qp Qh N1 N
Medicare Statute 1833(t)

C9132 Prothrombin complex concentrate (human), Kcentra, per i.u. of Factor IX activity Qp Qh K2 K
Medicare Statute 1833(t)

C9248 Injection, clevidipine butyrate, 1 mg Qp Qh N1 N
Medicare Statute 1833(t)

C9250 Human plasma fibrin sealant, vapor-heated, solvent-detergent (ARTISS), 2 ml Qp Qh K2 K
Example of diagnosis codes to be reported with C9250: T20.00-T25.799.
Medicare Statute 621MMA

C9254 Injection, lacosamide, 1 mg Qp Qh N1 N
Medicare Statute 621MMA

C9257 injection, bevacizumab, 0.25 mg Qp Qh K2 K
Medicare Statute 1833(t)

~~C9275 Injection, hexaminolevulinate hydrochloride, 100 mg, per study dose~~ ✖

C9285 Lidocaine 70 mg/tetracaine 70 mg, per patch Qp Qh N1 N
Medicare Statute 1833(t)
Coding Clinic: 2011, Q3, P9

C9290 Injection, bupivacine liposome, 1 mg Qp Qh N1 N
Medicare Statute 1833(t)

C9293 Injection, glucarpidase, 10 units Qp Qh K2 K
Medicare Statute 1833(t)

C9352 Microporous collagen implantable tube (NeuraGen Nerve Guide), per centimeter length Qp Qh N1 N
Medicare Statute 621MMA

C9353 Microporous collagen implantable slit tube (NeuraWrap Nerve Protector), per centimeter length Qp Qh N1 N
Medicare Statute 621MMA

C9354 Acellular pericardial tissue matrix of non-human origin (Veritas), per square centimeter Qp Qh N1 N
Medicare Statute 621MMA

C9355 Collagen nerve cuff (NeuroMatrix), per 0.5 centimeter length Qp Qh N1 N
Medicare Statute 621MMA

C9356 Tendon, porous matrix of cross-linked collagen and glycosaminoglycan matrix (TenoGlide Tendon Protector Sheet), per square centimeter Qp Qh N1 N
Medicare Statute 621MMA

C9358 Dermal substitute, native, non-denatured collagen, fetal bovine origin (SurgiMend Collagen Matrix), per 0.5 square centimeters Qp Qh N1 N
Medicare Statute 621MMA
Coding Clinic: 2013, Q3, P9; 2012, Q2, P7

C9359 Porous purified collagen matrix bone void filler (Integra Mozaik Osteoconductive Scaffold Putty, Integra OS Osteoconductive Scaffold Putty), per 0.5 cc Qp Qh N1 N
Medicare Statute 1833(t)
Coding Clinic: 2015, Q3, P2

C9360 Dermal substitute, native, non-denatured collagen, neonatal bovine origin (SurgiMend Collagen Matrix), per 0.5 square centimeters Qp Qh N1 N
Medicare Statute 621MMA
Coding Clinic: 2012, Q2, P7

C9361 Collagen matrix nerve wrap (NeuroMend Collagen Nerve Wrap), per 0.5 centimeter length Qp Qh N1 N
Medicare Statute 621MMA

C9362 Porous purified collagen matrix bone void filler (Integra Mozaik Osteoconductive Scaffold Strip), per 0.5 cc Qp Qh N1 N
Medicare Statute 621MMA
Coding Clinic: 2010, Q2, P8

C9363 Skin substitute, Integra Meshed Bilayer Wound Matrix, per square centimeter Qp Qh N1 N
Medicare Statute 621MMA
Coding Clinic: 2012, Q2, P7; 2010, Q2, P8

C9364 Porcine implant, Permacol, per square centimeter Qp Qh N1 N
Medicare Statute 621MMA

C9399 Unclassified drugs or biologicals K7 A
Medicare Statute 621MMA
Coding Clinic: 2017, Q1, P1-3, P8; 2016, Q4, P10; 2014, Q2, P8; 2013, Q2, P3; 2010, Q3, P8

▶ **C9407** Iodine i-131 iobenguane, diagnostic, 1 millicurie G
Medicare Statute 1833(t)

▶ **C9408** Iodine i-131 iobenguane, therapeutic, 1 millicurie G
Medicare Statute 1833(t)

C9447 Injection, phenylephrine and ketorolac, 4 ml vial Qp Qh N1 N
Medicare Statute 1833(t)

C9460 Injection, cangrelor, 1 mg Qp Qh K2 G
Medicare Statute 1833(t)

▶ ◎ **C9462** Injection, delafloxacin, 1 mg K2 G
Medicare Statute 1833(t)

◎ **C9482** Injection, sotalol hydrochloride, 1 mg Qp Qh K2 G
Medicare Statute 1833(t)
Coding Clinic: 2016, Q4, P9

◎ **C9488** Injection, conivaptan hydrochloride, 1 mg K2 G
Medicare Statute 1833(t)

~~C9492 Injection, durvalumab, 10 mg~~ ✖

~~C9493 Injection, edaravone, 1 mg~~ ✖

~~C9497 Loxapine, inhalation powder, 10 mg~~ ✖

Percutaneous Transcatheter and Transluminal Coronary Procedures

◎ **C9600** Percutaneous transcatheter placement of drug eluting intracoronary stent(s), with coronary angioplasty when performed; a single major coronary artery or branch Qp Qh J1
Medicare Statute 1833(t)

◎ **C9601** Percutaneous transcatheter placement of drug-eluting intracoronary stent(s), with coronary angioplasty when performed; each additional branch of a major coronary artery (list separately in addition to code for primary procedure) Qp Qh N
Medicare Statute 1833(t)

◎ **C9602** Percutaneous transluminal coronary atherectomy, with drug eluting intracoronary stent, with coronary angioplasty when performed; a single major coronary artery or branch Qp Qh J1
Medicare Statute 1833(t)

◎ **C9603** Percutaneous transluminal coronary atherectomy, with drug-eluting intracoronary stent, with coronary angioplasty when performed; each additional branch of a major coronary artery (list separately in addition to code for primary procedure) Qp Qh N
Medicare Statute 1833(t)

◎ **C9604** Percutaneous transluminal revascularization of or through coronary artery bypass graft (internal mammary, free arterial, venous), any combination of drug-eluting intracoronary stent, atherectomy and angioplasty, including distal protection when performed; a single vessel Qp Qh J1

◎ **C9605** Percutaneous transluminal revascularization of or through coronary artery bypass graft (internal mammary, free arterial, venous), any combination of drug-eluting intracoronary stent, atherectomy and angioplasty, including distal protection when performed; each additional branch subtended by the bypass graft (list separately in addition to code for primary procedure) Qp Qh N
Medicare Statute 1833(t)

◎ **C9606** Percutaneous transluminal revascularization of acute total/subtotal occlusion during acute myocardial infarction, coronary artery or coronary artery bypass graft, any combination of drug-eluting intracoronary stent, atherectomy and angioplasty, including aspiration thrombectomy when performed, single vessel Qp Qh J1
Medicare Statute 1833(t)

◎ **C9607** Percutaneous transluminal revascularization of chronic total occlusion, coronary artery, coronary artery branch, or coronary artery bypass graft, any combination of drug-eluting intracoronary stent, atherectomy and angioplasty; single vessel Qp Qh J1
Medicare Statute 1833(t)

◎ **C9608** Percutaneous transluminal revascularization of chronic total occlusion, coronary artery, coronary artery branch, or coronary artery bypass graft, any combination of drug-eluting intracoronary stent, atherectomy and angioplasty; each additional coronary artery, coronary artery branch, or bypass graft (list separately in addition to code for primary procedure) Qp Qh N
Medicare Statute 1833(t)

Therapeutic Services and Supplies

◎ **C9725** Placement of endorectal intracavitary applicator for high intensity brachytherapy Qp Qh T
Medicare Statute 1833(t)

◎ **C9726** Placement and removal (if performed) of applicator into breast for intraoperative radiation therapy, add-on to primary breast procedure Qh N
Medicare Statute 1833(t)

◎ **C9727** Insertion of implants into the soft palate; minimum of three implants Qp Qh T
Medicare Statute 1833(t)

▶ New ⮌ Revised ✔ Reinstated ~~deleted~~ Deleted ⊘ Not covered or valid by Medicare
◎ Special coverage instructions ✻ Carrier discretion Ⓑ Bill Part B MAC Ⓓ Bill DME MAC

C9728 Placement of interstitial device(s) for radiation therapy/surgery guidance (e.g., fiducial markers, dosimeter), for other than the following sites (any approach): abdomen, pelvis, prostate, retroperitoneum, thorax, single or multiple Qp Qh S

Medicare Statute 1833(t)

Coding Clinic: 2018, Q2, P4

C9733 Non-ophthalmic fluorescent vascular angiography Qp Qh Q2

Medicare Statute 1833(t)

Coding Clinic: 2012, Q1, P7

C9734 Focused ultrasound ablation/therapeutic intervention, other than uterine leiomyomata, with magnetic resonance (MR) guidance Qp Qh J1

Medicare Statute 1833(t)

C9738 Adjunctive blue light cystoscopy with fluorescent imaging agent (list separately in addition to code for primary procedure) N1 N

Medicare Statute 1833(t)

C9739 Cystourethroscopy, with insertion of transprostatic implant; 1 to 3 implants Qp Qh J1

Medicare Statute 1833(t)

Coding Clinic: 2014, Q2, P6

C9740 Cystourethroscopy, with insertion of transprostatic implant; 4 or more implants Qp Qh J1

Medicare Statute 1833(t)

Coding Clinic: 2014, Q2, P6

~~C9741 Right heart catheterization with implantation of wireless pressure sensor in the pulmonary artery, including any type of measurement, angiography, imaging supervision, interpretation, and report~~ ✖

~~C9744 Ultrasound, abdominal, with contrast~~ ✖

C9745 Nasal endoscopy, surgical; balloon dilation of eustachian tube J1

Medicare Statute 1833(t)

C9746 Transperineal implantation of permanent adjustable balloon continence device, with cystourethroscopy, when performed and/or fluoroscopy, when performed J1

Medicare Statute 1833(t)

C9747 Ablation of prostate, transrectal, high intensity focused ultrasound (HIFU), including imaging guidance J1

Medicare Statute 1833(t)

~~C9748 Transurethral destruction of prostate tissue; by radiofrequency water vapor (steam) thermal therapy~~ ✖

▶ **C9749** Repair of nasal vestibular lateral wall stenosis with implant(s) J1

Medicare Statute 1833(t)

▶ **C9751** Bronchoscopy, rigid or flexible, transbronchial ablation of lesion(s) by microwave energy, including fluoroscopic guidance, when performed, with computed tomography acquisition(s) and 3-D rendering, computer-assisted, image-guided navigation, and endobronchial ultrasound (EBUS) guided transtracheal and/or transbronchial sampling (e.g., aspiration[s]/biopsy[ies]) and all mediastinal and/or hilar lymph node stations or structures and therapeutic intervention(s) T

Medicare Statute 1833(t)

▶ **C9752** Destruction of intraosseous basivertebral nerve, first two vertebral bodies, including imaging guidance (e.g., fluoroscopy), lumbar/sacrum J1

Medicare Statute 1833(t)

▶ **C9753** Destruction of intraosseous basivertebral nerve, each additional vertebral body, including imaging guidance (e.g., fluoroscopy), lumbar/sacrum (list separately in addition to code for primary procedure) N

Medicare Statute 1833(t)

▶ **C9754** Creation of arteriovenous fistula, percutaneous; direct, any site, including all imaging and radiologic supervision and interpretation, when performed and secondary procedures to redirect blood flow (e.g., transluminal balloon angioplasty, coil embolization, when performed) J1

Medicare Statute 1833(t)

▶ **C9755** Creation of arteriovenous fistula, percutaneous using magnetic-guided arterial and venous catheters and radiofrequency energy, including flow-directing procedures (e.g., vascular coil embolization with radiologic supervision and interpretation, when performed) and fistulogram(s), angiography, venography, and/or ultrasound, with radiologic supervision and interpretation, when performed J1

Medicare Statute 1833(t)

C9898 Radiolabeled product provided during a hospital inpatient stay Qh N

C9899 Implanted prosthetic device, payable only for inpatients who do not have inpatient coverage A

Medicare Statute 1833(t)

DENTAL PROCEDURES (D0000-D9999)

Diagnostic (D0120-D0999)

Clinical Oral Evaluations

D0120 Periodic oral evaluation - established patient Ⓑ E1

An evaluation performed on a patient of record to determine any changes in the patient's dental and medical health status since a previous comprehensive or periodic evaluation. This includes an oral cancer evaluation and periodontal screening where indicated, and may require interpretation of information acquired through additional diagnostic procedures. Report additional diagnostic procedures separately.

D0140 Limited oral evaluation - problem focused Ⓑ E1

An evaluation limited to a specific oral health problem or complaint. This may require interpretation of information acquired through additional diagnostic procedures. Report additional diagnostic procedures separately. Definitive procedures may be required on the same date as the evaluation. Typically, patients receiving this type of evaluation present with a specific problem and/or dental emergencies, trauma, acute infections, etc.

D0145 Oral evaluation for a patient under three years of age and counseling with primary caregiver Ⓑ A E1

Diagnostic services performed for a child under the age of three, preferably within the first six months of the eruption of the first primary tooth, including recording the oral and physical health history, evaluation of caries susceptibility, development of an appropriate preventive oral health regimen and communication with and counseling of the child's parent, legal guardian and/or primary caregiver.

D0150 Comprehensive oral evaluation - new or established patient Ⓑ S

Used by a general dentist and/or a specialist when evaluating a patient comprehensively. This applies to new patients; established patients who have had a significant change in health conditions or other unusual circumstances, by report, or established patients who have been absent from active treatment for three or more years. It is a thorough evaluation and recording of the extraoral and intraoral hard and soft tissues. It may require interpretation of information acquired through additional diagnostic procedures. Additional diagnostic procedures should be reported separately. This includes an evaluation for oral cancer where indicated, the evaluation and recording of the patient's dental and medical history and a general health assessment. It may include the evaluation and recording of dental caries, missing or unerupted teeth, restorations, existing prostheses, occlusal relationships, periodontal conditions (including periodontal screening and/or charting), hard and soft tissue anomalies, etc.

D0160 Detailed and extensive oral evaluation - problem focused, by report Ⓑ E1

A detailed and extensive problem focused evaluation entails extensive diagnostic and cognitive modalities based on the findings of a comprehensive oral evaluation. Integration of more extensive diagnostic modalities to develop a treatment plan for a specific problem is required. The condition requiring this type of evaluation should be described and documented. Examples of conditions requiring this type of evaluation may include dentofacial anomalies, complicated perio-prosthetic conditions, complex temporomandibular dysfunction, facial pain of unknown origin, conditions requiring multi-disciplinary consultation, etc.

D0170 Re-evaluation - limited, problem focused (established patient; not post-operative visit) Ⓑ E1

Assessing the status of a previously existing condition. For example: - a traumatic injury where no treatment was rendered but patient needs follow-up monitoring; - evaluation for undiagnosed continuing pain; - soft tissue lesion requiring follow-up evaluation.

D0171 Re-evaluation - post-operative office visit Ⓑ E1

D0180 Comprehensive periodontal evaluation - new or established patient Ⓑ E1

This procedure is indicated for patients showing signs or symptoms of periodontal disease and for patients with risk factors such as smoking or diabetes. It includes evaluation of periodontal conditions, probing and charting, evaluation and recording of the patient's dental and medical history and general health assessment. It may include the evaluation and recording of dental caries, missing or unerupted teeth, restorations, occlusal relationships and oral cancer evaluation.

Pre-Diagnostic Services

D0190 Screening of a patient Ⓑ E1

A screening, including state or federally mandated screenings, to determine an individual's need to be seen by a dentist for diagnosis.

D0191 Assessment of a patient Ⓑ E1

A limited clinical inspection that is performed to identify possible signs of oral or systemic disease, malformation, or injury, and the potential need for referral for diagnosis and treatment.

Diagnostic Imaging

D0210 Intraoral - complete series of radiographic image Ⓑ E1

A radiographic survey of the whole mouth, usually consisting of 14-22 periapical and posterior bitewing images intended to display the crowns and roots of all teeth, periapical areas and alveolar bone.

Cross Reference 70320

D0220 Intraoral - periapical first radiographic image Ⓑ E1

Cross Reference 70300

D0230 Intraoral - periapical each additional radiographic image Ⓑ E1

Cross Reference 70310

D0240 Intraoral - occlusal radiographic image Ⓑ S

D0250 Extra-oral — 2D projection radiographic image created using a stationary radiation source, detector Ⓑ S

These images include, but are not limited to: Lateral Skull; Posterior-Anterior Skull; Submentovertex; Waters; Reverse Tomes; Oblique Mandibular Body; Lateral Ramus.

D0251 Extra-oral posterior dental radiographic image Ⓑ Q1

Image limited to exposure of complete posterior teeth in both dental arches. This is a unique image that is not derived from another image.

D0270 Bitewing - single radiographic image Ⓑ S

D0272 Bitewings - two radiographic images Ⓑ S

D0273 Bitewings - three radiographic images Ⓑ E1

D0274 Bitewings - four radiographic images Ⓑ S

D0277 Vertical bitewings - 7 to 8 radiographic images Ⓑ S

This does not constitute a full mouth intraoral radiographic series.

D0310 Sialography Ⓑ E1

Cross Reference 70390

D0320 Temporomandibular joint arthrogram, including injection Ⓑ E1

Cross Reference 70332

D0321 Other temporomandibular joint radiographic image, by report Ⓑ E1

Cross Reference 76499

D0322 Tomographic survey Ⓑ E1

D0330 Panoramic radiographic image Ⓑ E1

Cross Reference 70320

D0340 2D cephalometric radiographic image - acquisition, measurement and analysis Ⓑ E1

Image of the head made using a cephalostat to standardize anatomic positioning, and with reproducible x-ray beam geometry.

Cross Reference 70350

D0350 2D oral/facial photographic image obtained intra-orally or extra-orally Ⓑ E1

D0351 3D photographic image Ⓑ E1

This procedure is for dental or maxillofacial diagnostic purposes. Not applicable for a CAD-CAM procedure.

D0364 Cone beam CT capture and interpretation with limited field of view - less than one whole jaw Ⓑ E1

D0365 Cone beam CT capture and interpretation with field of view of one full dental arch - mandible Ⓑ E1

D0366 Cone beam CT capture and interpretation with field of view of one full dental arch - maxilla, with or without cranium Ⓑ E1

D0367 Cone beam CT capture and interpretation with field of view of both jaws, with or without cranium Ⓑ E1

D0368 Cone beam CT capture and interpretation for TMJ series including two or more exposures Ⓑ E1

D0369 Maxillofacial MRI capture and interpretation Ⓑ E1

D0370 Maxillofacial ultrasound capture and interpretation Ⓑ E1

D0371 Sialoendoscopy capture and interpretation Ⓑ E1

D0380 Cone beam CT image capture with limited field of view - less than one whole jaw Ⓑ E1

D0381 Cone beam CT image capture with field of view of one full dental arch - mandible Ⓑ E1

D0382 Cone beam CT image capture with field of view of one full dental arch - maxilla, with or without cranium Ⓑ E1

D0383 Cone beam CT image capture with field of view of both jaws, with or without cranium Ⓑ E1

D0384 Cone beam CT image capture for TMJ series including two or more exposures Ⓑ E1

D0385 Maxillofacial MRI image capture Ⓑ E1

D0386 Maxillofacial ultrasound image capture Ⓑ E1

D0391 Interpretation of diagnostic image by a practitioner not associated with capture of the image, including report Ⓑ E1

D0393 Treatment simulation using 3D image volume Ⓑ E1

The use of 3D image volumes for simulation of treatment including, but not limited to, dental implant placement, orthognathic surgery and orthodontic tooth movement.

D0394 Digital subtraction of two or more images or image volumes of the same modality Ⓑ E1

To demonstrate changes that have occurred over time.

D0395 Fusion of two or more 3D image volumes of one or more modalities Ⓑ E1

Tests and Examinations

D0411 HbA1c in-office point of service testing Ⓑ E1

▶ **D0412** Blood gucose level test - in-office using a glucose meter Ⓑ E1

D0414 Laboratory processing of microbial specimen to include culture and sensitivity studies, preparation and transmission of written report Ⓑ E1

D0415 Collection of microorganisms for culture and sensitivity Ⓑ E1

Cross Reference D0410

D0416 Viral culture Ⓑ B

A diagnostic test to identify viral organisms, most often herpes virus.

D0417 Collection and preparation of saliva sample for laboratory diagnostic testing Ⓑ E1

D0418 Analysis of saliva sample Ⓑ E1

Chemical or biological analysis of saliva sample for diagnostic purposes.

D0422 Collection and preparation of genetic sample material for laboratory analysis and report Ⓑ E1

D0423 Genetic test for susceptibility to diseases - specimen analysis Ⓑ E1

Certified laboratory analysis to detect specific genetic variations associated with increased susceptibility for diseases.

D0425 Caries susceptibility tests E1

Not to be used for carious dentin staining.

D0431 Adjunctive pre-diagnostic test that aids in detection of mucosal abnormalities including premalignant and malignant lesions, not to include cytology or biopsy procedures B

D0460 Pulp vitality tests S

Includes multiple teeth and contra lateral comparison(s), as indicated.

D0470 Diagnostic casts E1

Also known as diagnostic models or study models.

Oral Pathology Laboratory (Use Codes D0472 – D0502)

D0472 Accession of tissue, gross examination, preparation and transmission of written report B

To be used in reporting architecturally intact tissue obtained by invasive means.

D0473 Accession of tissue, gross and microscopic examination, preparation and transmission of written report B

To be used in reporting architecturally intact tissue obtained by invasive means.

D0474 Accession of tissue, gross and microscopic examination, including assessment of surgical margins for presence of disease, preparation and transmission of written report B

To be used in reporting architecturally intact tissue obtained by invasive means.

D0475 Decalcification procedure B

Procedure in which hard tissue is processed in order to allow sectioning and subsequent microscopic examination.

D0476 Special stains for microorganisms B

Procedure in which additional stains are applied to biopsy or surgical specimen in order to identify microorganisms.

D0477 Special stains, not for microorganisms B

Procedure in which additional stains are applied to a biopsy or surgical specimen in order to identify such things as melanin, mucin, iron, glycogen, etc.

D0478 Immunohistochemical stains B

A procedure in which specific antibody based reagents are applied to tissue samples in order to facilitate diagnosis.

D0479 Tissue in-situ hybridization, including interpretation B

A procedure which allows for the identification of nucleic acids, DNA and RNA, in the tissue sample in order to aid in the diagnosis of microorganisms and tumors.

D0480 Accession of exfoliative cytologic smears, microscopic examination, preparation and transmission of written report B

To be used in reporting disaggregated, non-transepithelial cell cytology sample via mild scraping of the oral mucosa.

D0481 Electron microscopy B

D0482 Direct immunofluorescence B

A technique used to identify immunoreactants which are localized to the patient's skin or mucous membranes.

D0483 Indirect immunofluorescence B

A technique used to identify circulating immunoreactants.

D0484 Consultation on slides prepared elsewhere B

A service provided in which microscopic slides of a biopsy specimen prepared at another laboratory are evaluated to aid in the diagnosis of a difficult case or to offer a consultative opinion at the patient's request. The findings are delivered by written report.

D0485 Consultation, including preparation of slides from biopsy material supplied by referring source B

A service that requires the consulting pathologist to prepare the slides as well as render a written report. The slides are evaluated to aid in the diagnosis of a difficult case or to offer a consultative opinion at the patient's request.

D0486 Laboratory accession of transepithelial cytologic sample, microscopic examination, preparation and transmission of written report E1

Analysis, and written report of findings, of cytologic sample of disaggregated transepithelial cells.

D0502 Other oral pathology procedures, by report B

Tests and Examinations

D0600 Non-ionizing diagnostic procedure capable of quantifying, monitoring, and recording changes in structure of enamel, dentin, and cementum Ⓑ S

D0601 Caries risk assessment and documentation, with a finding of low risk Ⓑ E1

Using recognized assessment tools.

D0602 Caries risk assessment and documentation, with a finding of moderate risk Ⓑ E1

Using recognized assessment tools.

D0603 Caries risk assessment and documentation, with a finding of high risk Ⓑ E1

Using recognized assessment tools.

None

D0999 Unspecified diagnostic procedure, by report Ⓑ B

Used for procedure that is not adequately described by a code. Describe procedure.

Preventative (D1110-D1999)

Dental Prophylaxis

D1110 Prophylaxis - adult Ⓑ A E1

Removal of plaque, calculus and stains from the tooth structures in the permanent and transitional dentition. It is intended to control local irritational factors.

D1120 Prophylaxis - child Ⓑ A E1

Removal of plaque, calculus and stains from the tooth structures in the primary and transitional dentition. It is intended to control local irritational factors.

Topical Fluoride Treatment (Office Procedure)

D1206 Topical application of fluoride varnish Ⓑ E1

D1208 Topical application of fluoride — excluding varnish Ⓑ E1

Other Preventative Services

D1310 Nutritional counseling for the control of dental disease Ⓑ E1

Counseling on food selection and dietary habits as a part of treatment and control of periodontal disease and caries.

D1320 Tobacco counseling for the control and prevention of oral disease Ⓑ E1

Tobacco prevention and cessation services reduce patient risks of developing tobacco-related oral diseases and conditions and improves prognosis for certain dental therapies.

D1330 Oral hygiene instruction Ⓑ E1

This may include instructions for home care. Examples include tooth brushing technique, flossing, use of special oral hygiene aids.

D1351 Sealant - per tooth Ⓑ E1

Mechanically and/or chemically prepared enamel surface sealed to prevent decay.

D1352 Preventive resin restoration in a moderate to high caries risk patient — permanent tooth Ⓑ E1

Conservative restoration of an active cavitated lesion in a pit or fissure that does not extend into dentin; includes placement of a sealant in any radiating non-carious fissures or pits.

D1353 Sealant repair — per tooth Ⓑ E1

D1354 Interim caries arresting medicament application — per tooth Ⓑ E1

Conservative treatment of an active, non-symptomatic carious lesion by topical application of a caries arresting or inhibiting medicament and without mechanical removal of sound tooth structure.

Space Maintenance (Passive Appliances)

D1510 Space maintainer - fixed - unilateral Ⓑ S

Excludes a distal shoe space maintainer.

▶ **D1516** Space Maintainer - fixed - bilateral, maxillary Ⓑ S

▶ **D1517** Space Maintainer - fixed - bilateral, mandibular Ⓑ S

D1520 Space maintainer - removable - unilateral Ⓑ S

▶ New ⮌ Revised ✔ Reinstated ~~deleted~~ Deleted ⃠ Not covered or valid by Medicare
Special coverage instructions ✻ Carrier discretion Ⓑ Bill Part B MAC Ⓑ Bill DME MAC

▶ **D1526** Space maintainer - removable - bilateral, maxillary Ⓑ S

▶ **D1527** Space maintainer - removable - bilateral, mandibular Ⓑ S

D1550 Re-cement or re-bond space maintainer Ⓑ S

D1555 Removal of fixed space maintainer Ⓑ E1

Procedure performed by dentist or practice that did not originally place the appliance.

Space Maintainers

D1575 Distal shoe space maintainer - fixed - unilateral Ⓑ S

Fabrication and delivery of fixed appliance extending subgingivally and distally to guide the eruption of the first permanent molar. Does not include ongoing follow-up or adjustments, or replacement appliances, once the tooth has erupted.

None

D1999 Unspecified preventive procedure, by report Ⓑ E1

Used for procedure that is not adequately described by another CDT Code. Describe procedure.

Restorative (D2140-D2999)

Amalgam Restorations (Including Polishing)

D2140 Amalgam - one surface, primary or permanent Ⓑ E1

D2150 Amalgam - two surfaces, primary or permanent Ⓑ E1

D2160 Amalgam - three surfaces, primary or permanent Ⓑ E1

D2161 Amalgam - four or more surfaces, primary or permanent Ⓑ E1

Resin-Based Composite Restorations – Direct

D2330 Resin-based composite - one surface, anterior Ⓑ E1

D2331 Resin-based composite - two surfaces, anterior Ⓑ E1

D2332 Resin-based composite - three surfaces, anterior Ⓑ E1

D2335 Resin-based composite - four or more surfaces or involving incisal angle (anterior) Ⓑ E1

Incisal angle to be defined as one of the angles formed by the junction of the incisal and the mesial or distal surface of an anterior tooth.

D2390 Resin-based composite crown, anterior Ⓑ E1

Full resin-based composite coverage of tooth.

D2391 Resin-based composite - one surface, posterior Ⓑ E1

Used to restore a carious lesion into the dentin or a deeply eroded area into the dentin. Not a preventive procedure.

D2392 Resin-based composite - two surfaces, posterior Ⓑ E1

D2393 Resin-based composite - three surfaces, posterior Ⓑ E1

D2394 Resin-based composite - four or more surfaces, posterior Ⓑ E1

Gold Foil Restorations

D2410 Gold foil - one surface Ⓑ E1

D2420 Gold foil - two surfaces Ⓑ E1

D2430 Gold foil - three surfaces Ⓑ E1

Inlay/Onlay Restorations

D2510 Inlay - metallic - one surface Ⓑ E1

D2520 Inlay - metallic - two surfaces Ⓑ E1

D2530 Inlay - metallic - three or more surfaces Ⓑ E1

D2542 Onlay - metallic - two surfaces Ⓑ E1

D2543 Onlay - metallic - three surfaces Ⓑ E1

D2544 Onlay - metallic - four or more surfaces Ⓑ E1

D2610 Inlay - porcelain/ceramic - one surface Ⓑ E1

D2620 Inlay - porcelain/ceramic - two surfaces Ⓑ E1

D2630 Inlay - porcelain/ceramic - three or more surfaces Ⓑ E1

D2642 Onlay - porcelain/ceramic - two surfaces Ⓑ E1

D2643 Onlay - porcelain/ceramic - three surfaces Ⓑ E1

D2644 Onlay - porcelain/ceramic - four or more surfaces Ⓑ E1

D2650 Inlay - resin-based composite - one surface Ⓑ E1

D2651 Inlay - resin-based composite - two surfaces Ⓑ E1

D2652 Inlay - resin-based composite - three or more surfaces Ⓑ E1

D2662 Onlay - resin-based composite - two surfaces Ⓑ E1

D2663 Onlay - resin-based composite - three surfaces Ⓑ E1

D2664 Onlay - resin-based composite - four or more surfaces Ⓑ E1

Crowns – Single Restoration Only

D2710 Crown - resin-based composite (indirect) Ⓑ E1

D2712 Crown - 3/4 resin-based composite (indirect) Ⓑ E1

This procedure does not include facial veneers.

D2720 Crown - resin with high noble metal Ⓑ E1

D2721 Crown - resin with predominantly base metal Ⓑ E1

D2722 Crown - resin with noble metal Ⓑ E1

D2740 Crown - porcelain/ceramic Ⓑ E1

D2750 Crown - porcelain fused to high noble metal Ⓑ E1

D2751 Crown - porcelain fused to predominantly base metal Ⓑ E1

D2752 Crown - porcelain fused to noble metal Ⓑ E1

D2780 Crown - 3/4 cast high noble metal Ⓑ E1

D2781 Crown - 3/4 cast predominantly base metal Ⓑ E1

D2782 Crown - 3/4 cast noble metal Ⓑ E1

D2783 Crown - 3/4 porcelain/ceramic Ⓑ E1

This procedure does not include facial veneers.

D2790 Crown - full cast high noble metal Ⓑ E1

D2791 Crown - full cast predominantly base metal Ⓑ E1

D2792 Crown - full cast noble metal Ⓑ E1

D2794 Crown - titanium Ⓑ E1

D2799 Provisional crown - further treatment or completion of diagnosis necessary prior to final impression Ⓑ E1

Not to be used as a temporary crown for a routine prosthetic restoration.

Other Restorative Services

D2910 Re-cement or re-bond inlay, onlay, veneer or partial coverage restoration Ⓑ E1

D2915 Re-cement or re-bond indirectly fabricated cast or prefabricated post and core Ⓑ E1

D2920 Re-cement or re-bond crown Ⓑ E1

D2921 Reattachment of tooth fragment, incisal edge or cusp Ⓑ E1

D2929 Prefabricated porcelain/ceramic crown - primary tooth Ⓑ E1

D2930 Prefabricated stainless steel crown - primary tooth Ⓑ E1

D2931 Prefabricated stainless steel crown - permanent tooth Ⓑ E1

D2932 Prefabricated resin crown Ⓑ E1

D2933 Prefabricated stainless steel crown with resin window Ⓑ E1

Open-face stainless steel crown with aesthetic resin facing or veneer.

D2934 Prefabricated esthetic coated stainless steel crown - primary tooth Ⓑ E1

Stainless steel primary crown with exterior esthetic coating.

D2940 Protective restoration Ⓑ E1

Direct placement of a restorative material to protect tooth and/or tissue form. This procedure may be used to relieve pain, promote healing, or prevent further deterioration. Not to be used for endodontic access closure, or as a base or liner under a restoration.

D2941 Interim therapeutic restoration - primary dentition Ⓑ E1

Placement of an adhesive restorative material following caries debridement by hand or other method for the management of early childhood caries. Not considered a definitive restoration.

D2949 Restorative foundation for an indirect restoration Ⓑ E1

Placement of restorative material to yield a more ideal form, including elimination of undercuts.

D2950 Core build-up, including any pins when required Ⓑ E1

Refers to building up of coronal structure when there is insufficient retention for a separate extracoronal restorative procedure. A core buildup is not a filler to eliminate any undercut, box form, or concave irregularity in a preparation.

▶ **New** ↻ **Revised** ✔ **Reinstated** ~~deleted~~ **Deleted** ⊘ **Not covered or valid by Medicare**
⊙ **Special coverage instructions** ✳ **Carrier discretion** Ⓑ **Bill Part B MAC** Ⓑ **Bill DME MAC**

D2951 Pin retention - per tooth, in addition to restoration Ⓑ E1

D2952 Post and core in addition to crown, indirectly fabricated Ⓑ E1

Post and core are custom fabricated as a single unit.

D2953 Each additional indirectly fabricated post - same tooth Ⓑ E1

To be used with D2952.

D2954 Prefabricated post and core in addition to crown Ⓑ E1

Core is built around a prefabricated post. This procedure includes the core material.

D2955 Post removal Ⓑ E1

D2957 Each additional prefabricated post - same tooth Ⓑ E1

To be used with D2954.

D2960 Labial veneer (laminate) - chairside Ⓑ E1

Refers to labial/facial direct resin bonded veneers.

D2961 Labial veneer (resin laminate) - laboratory Ⓑ E1

Refers to labial/facial indirect resin bonded veneers.

D2962 Labial veneer (porcelain laminate) - laboratory Ⓑ E1

Refers also to facial veneers that extend interproximally and/or cover the incisal edge. Porcelain/ceramic veneers presently include all ceramic and porcelain veneers.

D2971 Additional procedures to construct new crown under existing partial denture framework Ⓑ E1

To be reported in addition to a crown code.

D2975 Coping Ⓑ E1

A thin covering of the coronal portion of a tooth, usually devoid of anatomic contour, that can be used as a definitive restoration.

D2980 Crown repair, necessitated by restorative material failure Ⓑ E1

D2981 Inlay repair necessitated by restorative material failure Ⓑ E1

D2982 Onlay repair necessitated by restorative material failure Ⓑ E1

D2983 Veneer repair necessitated by restorative material failure Ⓑ E1

D2990 Resin infiltration of incipient smooth surface lesions Ⓑ E1

Placement of an infiltrating resin restoration for strengthening, stabilizing and/or limiting the progression of the lesion.

None

D2999 Unspecified restorative procedure, by report Ⓑ S

Use for procedure that is not adequately described by a code. Describe procedure.

Endodontics (D3110-D3999)

Pulp Capping

D3110 Pulp cap - direct (excluding final restoration) Ⓑ E1

Procedure in which the exposed pulp is covered with a dressing or cement that protects the pulp and promotes healing and repair.

D3120 Pulp cap - indirect (excluding final restoration) Ⓑ E1

Procedure in which the nearly exposed pulp is covered with a protective dressing to protect the pulp from additional injury and to promote healing and repair via formation of secondary dentin. This code is not to be used for bases and liners when all caries has been removed.

Pulpotomy

D3220 Therapeutic pulpotomy (excluding final restoration) removal of pulp coronal to the dentinocemental junction and application of medicament Ⓑ E1

Pulpotomy is the surgical removal of a portion of the pulp with the aim of maintaining the vitality of the remaining portion by means of an adequate dressing.

– To be performed on primary or permanent teeth.

– This is not to be construed as the first stage of root canal therapy.

– Not to be used for apexogenesis.

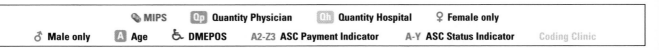

D3221 Pulpal debridement, primary and permanent teeth Ⓑ E1

Pulpal debridement for the relief of acute pain prior to conventional root canal therapy. This procedure is not to be used when endodontic treatment is completed on the same day.

D3222 Partial pulpotomy for apexogenesis - permanent tooth with incomplete root development Ⓑ E1

Removal of a portion of the pulp and application of a medicament with the aim of maintaining the vitality of the remaining portion to encourage continued physiological development and formation of the root. This procedure is not to be construed as the first stage of root canal therapy.

Endodontic Therapy on Primary Teeth

D3230 Pulpal therapy (resorbable filling) - anterior, primary tooth (excluding final restoration) Ⓑ E1

Primary incisors and cuspids.

D3240 Pulpal therapy (resorbable filling) - posterior, primary tooth (excluding final restoration) Ⓑ E1

Primary first and second molars.

Endodontic Therapy (Including Treatment Plan, Clinical Procedures and Follow-Up Care)

D3310 Endodontic therapy, anterior tooth (excluding final restoration) Ⓑ E1

D3320 Endodontic therapy, premolar tooth (excluding final restoration) Ⓑ E1

D3330 Endodontic therapy, molar (excluding final restoration) Ⓑ E1

D3331 Treatment of root canal obstruction; non-surgical access Ⓑ E1

In lieu of surgery, the formation of a pathway to achieve an apical seal without surgical intervention because of a non-negotiable root canal blocked by foreign bodies, including but not limited to separated instruments, broken posts or calcification of 50% or more of the length of the tooth root.

D3332 Incomplete endodontic therapy; inoperable, unrestorable or fractured tooth Ⓑ E1

Considerable time is necessary to determine diagnosis and/or provide initial treatment before the fracture makes the tooth unretainable.

D3333 Internal root repair of perforation defects Ⓑ E1

Non-surgical seal of perforation caused by resorption and/or decay but not iatrogenic by provider filing claim.

Endodontic Retreatment

D3346 Retreatment of previous root canal therapy - anterior Ⓑ E1

D3347 Retreatment of previous root canal therapy - premolar Ⓑ E1

D3348 Retreatment of previous root canal therapy - molar Ⓑ E1

Apexification/Recalcification

D3351 Apexification/recalcification - initial visit (apical closure/calcific repair of perforations, root resorption, etc.) Ⓑ E1

Includes opening tooth, preparation of canal spaces, first placement of medication and necessary radiographs. (This procedure may include first phase of complete root canal therapy.)

D3352 Apexification/recalcification - interim medication replacement (apical closure/calcific repair of perforations, root resorption, pulp space disinfection, etc.) Ⓑ E1

For visits in which the intra-canal medication is replaced with new medication. Includes any necessary radiographs.

D3353 Apexification/recalcification - final visit (includes completed root canal therapy - apical closure/calcific repair of perforations, root resorption, etc.) Ⓑ E1

Includes removal of intra-canal medication and procedures necessary to place final root canal filling material including necessary radiographs. (This procedure includes last phase of complete root canal therapy.)

Pulpal Regeneration

D3355 Pulpal regeneration - initial visit Ⓑ E1

Includes opening tooth, preparation of canal spaces, placement of medication.

D3356 Pulpal regeneration - interim medication replacement Ⓑ E1

D3357 Pulpal regeneration - completion of treatment Ⓑ E1

Does not include final restoration.

Apicoectomy/Periradicular Services

D3410 Apicoectomy - anterior Ⓑ E1

For surgery on root of anterior tooth. Does not include placement of retrograde filling material.

D3421 Apicoectomy - premolar (first root) Ⓑ E1

For surgery on one root of a premolar. Does not include placement of retrograde filling material. If more than one root is treated, see D3426.

D3425 Apicoectomy - molar (first root) Ⓑ E1

For surgery on one root of a molar tooth. Does not include placement of retrograde filling material. If more than one root is treated, see D3426.

D3426 Apicoectomy (each additional root) Ⓑ E1

Typically used for premolar and molar surgeries when more than one root is treated during the same procedure. This does not include retrograde filling material placement.

D3427 Periradicular surgery without apicoectomy Ⓑ E1

D3428 Bone graft in conjunction with periradicular surgery - per tooth, single site Ⓑ E1

Includes non-autogenous graft material.

D3429 Bone graft in conjunction with periradicular surgery - each additional contiguous tooth in the same surgical site Ⓑ E1

Includes non-autogenous graft material.

D3430 Retrograde filling - per root Ⓑ E1

For placement of retrograde filling material during periradicular surgery procedures. If more than one filling is placed in one root - report as D3999 and describe.

D3431 Bologic materials to aid in soft and osseous tissue regeneration in conjunction with periradicular surgery Ⓑ E1

D3432 Guided tissue regeneration, resorbable barrier, per site, in conjunction with periradicular surgery Ⓑ E1

D3450 Root amputation - per root Ⓑ E1

Root resection of a multi-rooted tooth while leaving the crown. If the crown is sectioned, see D3920.

D3460 Endodontic endosseous implant Ⓑ S

Placement of implant material, which extends from a pulpal space into the bone beyond the end of the root.

D3470 Intentional replantation (including necessary splinting) Ⓑ E1

For the intentional removal, inspection and treatment of the root and replacement of a tooth into its own socket. This does not include necessary retrograde filling material placement.

Other Endodontic Procedures

D3910 Surgical procedure for isolation of tooth with rubber dam Ⓑ E1

D3920 Hemisection (including any root removal), not including root canal therapy Ⓑ E1

Includes separation of a multi-rooted tooth into separate sections containing the root and the overlying portion of the crown. It may also include the removal of one or more of those sections.

D3950 Canal preparation and fitting of preformed dowel or post Ⓑ E1

Should not be reported in conjunction with D2952, D2953, D2954 or D2957 by the same practitioner.

None

D3999 Unspecified endodontic procedure, by report Ⓑ S

Used for procedure that is not adequately described by a code. Describe procedure.

Periodontics (D4210-D4999)

Surgical Services (Including Usual Postoperative Care)

D4210 Gingivectomy or gingivoplasty - four or more contiguous teeth or tooth bounded spaces per quadrant Ⓑ E1

It is performed to eliminate suprabony pockets or to restore normal architecture when gingival enlargements or asymmetrical or unaesthetic topography is evident with normal bony configuration.

Cross Reference 41820

D4211 Gingivectomy or gingivoplasty - one to three contiguous teeth or tooth bounded spaces per quadrant Ⓑ E1

It is performed to eliminate suprabony pockets or to restore normal architecture when gingival enlargements or asymmetrical or unaesthetic topography is evident with normal bony configuration.

D4212 Gingivectomy or gingivoplasty to allow access for restorative procedure, per tooth Ⓑ E1

D4230 Anatomical crown exposure - four or more contiguous teeth or bounded tooth spaces per quadrant Ⓑ E1

This procedure is utilized in an otherwise periodontally healthy area to remove enlarged gingival tissue and supporting bone (ostectomy) to provide an anatomically correct gingival relationship.

D4231 Anatomical crown exposure - one to three teeth or bounded tooth spaces per quadrant Ⓑ E1

This procedure is utilized in an otherwise periodontally healthy area to remove enlarged gingival tissue and supporting bone (ostectomy) to provide an anatomically correct gingival relationship.

D4240 Gingival flap procedure, including root planing - four or more contiguous teeth or tooth bounded spaces per quadrant Ⓑ E1

A soft tissue flap is reflected or resected to allow debridement of the root surface and the removal of granulation tissue. Osseous recontouring is not accomplished in conjunction with this procedure. May include open flap curettage, reverse bevel flap surgery, modified Kirkland flap procedure, and modified Widman surgery. This procedure is performed in the presence of moderate to deep probing depths, loss of attachment, need to maintain esthetics, need for increased access to the root surface and alveolar bone, or to determine the presence of a cracked tooth, fractured root, or external root resorption. Other procedures may be required concurrent to D4240 and should be reported separately using their own unique codes.

D4241 Gingival flap procedure, including root planing - one to three contiguous teeth or tooth bounded spaces per quadrant Ⓑ E1

A soft tissue flap is reflected or resected to allow debridement of the root surface and the removal of granulation tissue. Osseous recontouring is not accomplished in conjunction with this procedure. May include open flap curettage, reverse bevel flap surgery, modified Kirkland flap procedure, and modified Widman surgery. This procedure is performed in the presence of moderate to deep probing depths, loss of attachment, need to maintain esthetics, need for increased access to the root surface and alveolar bone, or to determine the presence of a cracked tooth, fractured root, or external root resorption. Other procedures may be required concurrent to D4241 and should be reported separately using their own unique codes.

D4245 Apically positioned flap Ⓑ E1

Procedure is used to preserve keratinized gingiva in conjunction with osseous resection and second stage implant procedure. Procedure may also be used to preserve keratinized/ attached gingiva during surgical exposure of labially impacted teeth, and may be used during treatment of peri-implantitis.

D4249 Clinical crown lengthening - hard tissue Ⓑ E1

This procedure is employed to allow a restorative procedure on a tooth with little or no tooth structure exposed to the oral cavity. Crown lengthening requires reflection of a full thickness flap and removal of bone, altering the crown to root ratio. It is performed in a healthy periodontal environment, as opposed to osseous surgery, which is performed in the presence of periodontal disease.

D4260 Osseous surgery (including elevation of a full thickness flap and closure) - four or more contiguous teeth or tooth bounded spaces per quadrant Ⓑ S

This procedure modifies the bony support of the teeth by reshaping the alveolar process to achieve a more physiologic form during the surgical procedure. This must include the removal of supporting bone (ostectomy) and/or non-supporting bone (osteoplasty). Other procedures may be required concurrent to D4260 and should be reported using their own unique codes.

D4261 Osseous surgery (including elevation of a full thickness flap and closure) - one to three contiguous teeth or tooth bounded spaces per quadrant Ⓑ E1

This procedure modifies the bony support of the teeth by reshaping the alveolar process to achieve a more physiologic form during the surgical procedure. This must include the removal of supporting bone (ostectomy) and/or non-supporting bone (osteoplasty). Other procedures may be required concurrent to D4261 and should be reported using their own unique codes.

D4263 Bone replacement graft - retained natural tooth - first site in quadrant Ⓑ S

This procedure involves the use of grafts to stimulate periodontal regeneration when the disease process has led to a deformity of the bone. This procedure does not include flap entry and closure, wound debridement, osseous contouring, or the placement of biologic materials to aid in osseous tissue regeneration or barrier membranes. Other separate procedures delivered concurrently are documented with their own codes. Not to be reported for an edentulous space or an extraction site.

D4264 Bone replacement graft - retained natural tooth - each additional site in quadrant Ⓑ S

This procedure involves the use of grafts to stimulate periodontal regeneration when the disease process has led to a deformity of the bone. This procedure does not include flap entry and closure, wound debridement, osseous contouring, or the placement of biologic materials to aid in osseous tissue regeneration or barrier membranes. This procedure is performed concurrently with one or more bone replacement grafts to document the number of sites involved. Not to be reported for an edentulous space or an extraction site.

D4265 Biologic materials to aid in soft and osseous tissue regeneration Ⓑ E1

Biologic materials may be used alone or with other regenerative substrates such as bone and barrier membranes, depending upon their formulation and the presentation of the periodontal defect. This procedure does not include surgical entry and closure, wound debridement, osseous contouring, or the placement of graft materials and/or barrier membranes. Other separate procedures may be required concurrent to D4265 and should be reported using their own unique codes.

D4266 Guided tissue regeneration - resorbable barrier, per site Ⓑ E1

This procedure does not include flap entry and closure, or, when indicated, wound debridement, osseous contouring, bone replacement grafts, and placement of biologic materials to aid in osseous regeneration. This procedure can be used for periodontal and peri-implant defects.

D4267 Guided tissue regeneration - nonresorbable barrier, per site, (includes membrane removal) Ⓑ E1

This procedure does not include flap entry and closure, or, when indicated, wound debridement, osseous contouring, bone replacement grafts, and placement of biologic materials to aid in osseous regeneration. This procedure can be used for periodontal and peri-implant defects.

D4268 Surgical revision procedure, per tooth Ⓑ S

This procedure is to refine the results of a previously provided surgical procedure. This may require a surgical procedure to modify the irregular contours of hard or soft tissue. A mucoperiosteal flap may be elevated to allow access to reshape alveolar bone. The flaps are replaced or repositioned and sutured.

D4270 Pedicle soft tissue graft procedure Ⓑ S

A pedicle flap of gingiva can be raised from an edentulous ridge, adjacent teeth, or from the existing gingiva on the tooth and moved laterally or coronally to replace alveolar mucosa as marginal tissue. The procedure can be used to cover an exposed root or to eliminate a gingival defect if the root is not too prominent in the arch.

D4273 Autogenous connective tissue graft procedure (including donor and recipient surgical sites) first tooth, implant, or edentulous tooth position in graft Ⓑ S

There are two surgical sites. The recipient site utilizes a split thickness incision, retaining the overlapping flap of gingiva and/or mucosa. The connective tissue is dissected from a separate donor site leaving an epithelialized flap for closure.

D4274 Mesial/distal wedge procedure, single tooth (when not performed in conjuction with surgical procedures in the same anatomical area) Ⓑ E1

This procedure is performed in an edentulous area adjacent to a tooth, allowing removal of a tissue wedge to gain access for debridement, permit close flap adaptation, and reduce pocket depths.

D4275 Non-autogenous connective tissue graft (including recipient site and donor material) first tooth, implant, or edentulous tooth position in graft Ⓑ E1

There is only a recipient surgical site utilizing split thickness incision, retaining the overlaying flap of gingiva and/or mucosa. A donor surgical site is not present.

D4276 Combined connective tissue and double pedicle graft, per tooth Ⓑ E1

Advanced gingival recession often cannot be corrected with a single procedure. Combined tissue grafting procedures are needed to achieve the desired outcome.

D4277 Free soft tissue graft procedure (including recipient and donor surgical sites) first tooth, implant or edentulous tooth position in graft Ⓑ E1

D4278 Free soft tissue graft procedure (including recipient and donor surgical sites) each additional contiguous tooth, implant or edentulous tooth position in same graft site Ⓑ E1

Used in conjunction with D4277.

D4283 Autogenous connective tissue graft procedure (including donor and recipient surgical sites) - each additional contiguous tooth, implant or edentulous tooth position in same graft site Ⓑ E1

Used in conjunction with D4273.

D4285 Non-autogenous connective tissue graft procedure (including recipient surgical site and donor material) - each additional contiguous tooth, implant or edentulous tooth position in same graft site Ⓑ E1

Used in conjunction with D4275.

Non-Surgical Periodontal Services

D4320 Provisional splinting - intracoronal Ⓑ E1

This is an interim stabilization of mobile teeth. A variety of methods and appliances may be employed for this purpose. Identify the teeth involved.

D4321 Provisional splinting - extracoronal Ⓑ E1

This is an interim stabilization of mobile teeth. A variety of methods and appliances may be employed for this purpose. Identify the teeth involved.

D4341 Periodontal scaling and root planing - four or more teeth per quadrant Ⓑ E1

This procedure involves instrumentation of the crown and root surfaces of the teeth to remove plaque and calculus from these surfaces. It is indicated for patients with periodontal disease and is therapeutic, not prophylactic, in nature. Root planing is the definitive procedure designed for the removal of cementum and dentin that is rough, and/or permeated by calculus or contaminated with toxins or microorganisms. Some soft tissue removal occurs. This procedure may be used as a definitive treatment in some stages of periodontal disease and/or as a part of pre-surgical procedures in others.

D4342 Periodontal scaling and root planing - one to three teeth, per quadrant Ⓑ E1

This procedure involves instrumentation of the crown and root surfaces of the teeth to remove plaque and calculus from these surfaces. It is indicated for patients with periodontal disease and is therapeutic, not prophylactic, in nature. Root planing is the definitive procedure designed for the removal of cementum and dentin that is rough, and/or permeated by calculus or contaminated with toxins or microorganisms. Some soft tissue removal occurs. This procedure may be used as a definitive treatment in some stages of periodontal disease and/or as a part of pre-surgical procedures in others.

D4346 Scaling in presence of generalized moderate or severe gingival inflammation - full mouth, after oral evaluation Ⓑ E1

The removal of plaque, calculus and stains from supra- and sub-gingival tooth surfaces when there is generalized moderate or severe gingival inflammation in the absence of periodontitis. It is indicated for patients who have swollen, inflamed gingiva, generalized suprabony pockets, and moderate to severe bleeding on probing. Should not be reported in conjunction with prophylaxis, scaling and root planing, or debridement procedures.

D4355 Full mouth debridement to enable a comprehensive oral evaluation and diagnosis on a subsequent visit Ⓑ S

Full mouth debridement involves the preliminary removal of plaque and calculus that interferes with the ability of the dentist to perform a comprehensive oral evaluation. Not to be completed on the same day as D0150, D0160, or D0180.

D4381 Localized delivery of antimicrobial agents via a controlled release vehicle into diseased crevicular tissue, per tooth Ⓑ S

FDA approved subgingival delivery devices containing antimicrobial medication(s) are inserted into periodontal pockets to suppress the pathogenic microbiota. These devices slowly release the pharmacological agents so they can remain at the intended site of action in a therapeutic concentration for a sufficient length of time.

Other Periodontal Services

D4910 Periodontal maintenance Ⓑ E1

This procedure is instituted following periodontal therapy and continues at varying intervals, determined by the clinical evaluation of the dentist, for the life of the dentition or any implant replacements. It includes removal of the bacterial plaque and calculus from supragingival and subgingival regions, site specific scaling and root planing where indicated, and polishing the teeth. If new or recurring periodontal disease appears, additional diagnostic and treatment procedures must be considered.

D4920 Unscheduled dressing change (by someone other than treating dentist or their staff) Ⓑ E1

D4921 Gingival irrigation - per quadrant Ⓑ E1

Irrigation of gingival pockets with medicinal agent. Not to be used to report use of mouth rinses or non-invasive chemical debridement.

None

D4999 Unspecified periodontal procedure, by report Ⓑ E1

Use for procedure that is not adequately described by a code. Describe procedure.

Prosthodontics (removable)

Complete Dentures (Including Routine Post-Delivery Care)

D5110 Complete denture - maxillary Ⓑ E1

D5120 Complete denture - mandibular Ⓑ E1

D5130 Immediate denture - maxillary Ⓑ E1

Includes limited follow-up care only; does not include required future rebasing/relining procedure(s).

D5140 Immediate denture - mandibular Ⓑ E1

Includes limited follow-up care only; does not include required future rebasing/relining procedure(s).

Partial Dentures (Including Routine Post-Delivery Care)

↩ **D5211** Maxillary partial denture-resin base (including retentive/clasping materials, rests and teeth) Ⓑ E1

Includes acrylic resin base denture with resin or wrought wire clasps.

↩ **D5212** Mandibular partial denture-resin base (including, retentive/clasping materials, rests and teeth) Ⓑ E1

Includes acrylic resin base denture with resin or wrought wire clasps.

D5213 Maxillary partial denture - cast metal framework with resin denture bases (including any conventional clasps, rests and teeth) Ⓑ E1

D5214 Mandibular partial denture - cast metal framework with resin denture bases (including any conventional clasps, rests and teeth) Ⓑ E1

D5221 Immediate maxillary partial denture - resin base (including any conventional clasps, rests and teeth) Ⓑ E1

Includes limited follow-up care only; does not include future rebasing/ relining procedure(s).

D5222 Immediate mandibular partial denture - resin base (including any conventional clasps, rests and teeth) Ⓑ E1

Includes limited follow-up care only; does not include future rebasing/ relining procedure(s).

D5223 Immediate maxillary partial denture - cast metal framework with resin denture bases (including any conventional clasps, rests and teeth) Ⓑ E1

Includes limited follow-up care only; does not include future rebasing/ relining procedure(s).

D5224 Immediate mandibular partial denture - cast metal framework with resin denture bases (including any conventional clasps, rests and teeth) Ⓑ E1

Includes limited follow-up care only; does not include future rebasing/ relining procedure(s).

D5225 Maxillary partial denture - flexible base (including any clasps, rests and teeth) Ⓑ E1

D5226 Mandibular partial denture - flexible base (including any clasps, rests and teeth) Ⓑ E1

▶ **D5282** Removable unilateral partial denture - one piece cast metal (including clasps and teeth), maxillary Ⓑ E1

▶ **D5283** Removable unilateral partial denture - one piece cast metal (including clasps and teeth), mandibular Ⓑ E1

Adjustment to Dentures

D5410 Adjust complete denture - maxillary Ⓑ E1

D5411 Adjust complete denture - mandibular Ⓑ E1

D5421 Adjust partial denture - maxillary Ⓑ E1

D5422 Adjust partial denture - mandibular Ⓑ E1

Repairs to Complete Dentures

D5511 Repair broken complete denture base, mandibular Ⓑ E1

D5512 Repair broken complete denture base, maxillary Ⓑ E1

D5520 Replace missing or broken teeth-complete denture (each tooth) Ⓑ E1

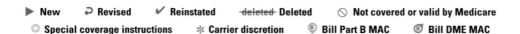

Repairs to Partial Dentures

D5611 Repair resin partial denture base, mandibular E1

D5612 Repair resin partial denture base, maxillary E1

D5621 Repair cast partial framework, mandibular E1

D5622 Repair cast partial framework, maxillary E1

D5630 Repair or replace broken, retentive clasping materials - per tooth E1

D5640 Replace broken teeth - per tooth E1

D5650 Add tooth to existing partial denture E1

D5660 Add clasp to existing partial denture - per tooth E1

D5670 Replace all teeth and acrylic on cast metal framework (maxillary) E1

D5671 Replace all teeth and acrylic on cast metal framework (mandibular) E1

Denture Rebase Procedures

D5710 Rebase complete maxillary denture E1

D5711 Rebase complete mandibular denture E1

D5720 Rebase maxillary partial denture E1

D5721 Rebase mandibular partial denture E1

Denture Reline Procedures

D5730 Reline complete maxillary denture (chairside) E1

D5731 Reline lower complete mandibular denture (chairside) E1

D5740 Reline maxillary partial denture (chairside) E1

D5741 Reline mandibular partial denture (chairside) E1

D5750 Reline complete maxillary denture (laboratory) E1

D5751 Reline complete mandibular denture (laboratory) E1

D5760 Reline maxillary partial denture (laboratory) E1

D5761 Reline mandibular partial denture (laboratory) E1

Interim Prosthesis

D5810 Interim complete denture (maxillary) E1

D5811 Interim complete denture (mandibular) E1

D5820 Interim partial denture (maxillary) E1

Includes any necessary clasps and rests.

D5821 Interim partial denture (mandibular) E1

Includes any necessary clasps and rests.

Other Removable Prosthetic Services

D5850 Tissue conditioning, maxillary E1

Treatment reline using materials designed to heal unhealthy ridges prior to more definitive final restoration.

D5851 Tissue conditioning, mandibular E1

Treatment reline using materials designed to heal unhealthy ridges prior to more definitive final restoration.

D5862 Precision attachment, by report E1

Each set of male and female components should be reported as one precision attachment. Describe the type of attachment used.

D5863 Overdenture - complete maxillary E1

D5864 Overdenture - partial maxillary E1

D5865 Overdenture - complete mandibular E1

D5866 Overdenture - partial mandibular E1

D5867 Replacement of replaceable part of semi-precision or precision attachment (male or female component) E1

D5875 Modification of removable prosthesis following implant surgery E1

Attachment assemblies are reported using separate codes.

▶ **D5876** Add metal substructure to acrylic full denture (per arch) E1

None

D5899 Unspecified removable prosthodontic procedure, by report E1

Use for a procedure that is not adequately described by a code. Describe procedure.

Maxillofacial Prosthetics

D5911 Facial moulage (sectional) Ⓑ S

A sectional facial moulage impression is a procedure used to record the soft tissue contours of a portion of the face. Occasionally several separate sectional impressions are made, then reassembled to provide a full facial contour cast. The impression is utilized to create a partial facial moulage and generally is not reusable.

D5912 Facial moulage (complete) Ⓑ S

Synonymous terminology: facial impression, face mask impression. A complete facial moulage impression is a procedure used to record the soft tissue contours of the whole face. The impression is utilized to create a facial moulage and generally is not reusable.

D5913 Nasal prosthesis Ⓑ E1

Synonymous terminology: artificial nose. A removable prosthesis attached to the skin, which artificially restores part or all of the nose. Fabrication of a nasal prosthesis requires creation of an original mold. Additional prostheses usually can be made from the same mold, and assuming no further tissue changes occur, the same mold can be utilized for extended periods of time. When a new prosthesis is made from the existing mold, this procedure is termed a nasal prosthesis replacement.

Cross Reference 21087

D5914 Auricular prosthesis Ⓑ E1

Synonymous terminology: artificial ear, ear prosthesis. A removable prosthesis, which artificially restores part or all of the natural ear. Usually, replacement prostheses can be made from the original mold if tissue bed changes have not occurred. Creation of an auricular prosthesis requires fabrication of a mold, from which additional prostheses usually can be made, as needed later (auricular prosthesis, replacement).

Cross Reference 21086

D5915 Orbital prosthesis Ⓑ E1

A prosthesis, which artificially restores the eye, eyelids, and adjacent hard and soft tissue, lost as a result of trauma or surgery. Fabrication of an orbital prosthesis requires creation of an original mold. Additional prostheses usually can be made from the same mold, and assuming no further tissue changes occur, the same mold can be utilized for extended periods of time. When a new prosthesis is made from the existing mold, this procedure is termed an orbital prosthesis replacement.

Cross Reference L8611

D5916 Ocular prosthesis Ⓑ E1

Synonymous terminology: artificial eye, glass eye. A prosthesis, which artificially replaces an eye missing as a result of trauma, surgery or congenital absence. The prosthesis does not replace missing eyelids or adjacent skin, mucosa or muscle. Ocular prostheses require semiannual or annual cleaning and polishing. Also, occasional revisions to re-adapt the prosthesis to the tissue bed may be necessary. Glass eyes are rarely made and cannot be re-adapted.

Cross Reference V2623, V2629

D5919 Facial prosthesis Ⓑ E1

Synonymous terminology: prosthetic dressing. A removable prosthesis, which artificially replaces a portion of the face, lost due to surgery, trauma or congenital absence. Flexion of natural tissues may preclude adaptation and movement of the prosthesis to match the adjacent skin. Salivary leakage, when communicating with the oral cavity, adversely affects retention.

Cross Reference 21088

D5922 Nasal septal prosthesis Ⓑ E1

Synonymous terminology: septal plug, septal button. Removable prosthesis to occlude (obturate) a hole within the nasal septal wall. Adverse chemical degradation in this moist environment may require frequent replacement. Silicone prostheses are occasionally subject to fungal invasion.

Cross Reference 30220

D5923 Ocular prosthesis, interim E1

Synonymous terminology: eye shell, shell, ocular conformer, conformer. A temporary replacement generally made of clear acrylic resin for an eye lost due to surgery or trauma. No attempt is made to re-establish esthetics. Fabrication of an interim ocular prosthesis generally implies subsequent fabrication of an aesthetic ocular prosthesis.

Cross Reference 92330

D5924 Cranial prosthesis E1

Synonymous terminology: skull plate, cranioplasty prosthesis, cranial implant. A biocompatible, permanently implanted replacement of a portion of the skull bones; an artificial replacement for a portion of the skull bone.

Cross Reference 62143

D5925 Facial augmentation implant prosthesis E1

Synonymous terminology: facial implant. An implantable biocompatible material generally onlayed upon an existing bony area beneath the skin tissue to fill in or collectively raise portions of the overlaying facial skin tissues to create acceptable contours. Although some forms of pre-made surgical implants are commercially available, the facial augmentation is usually custom made for surgical implantation for each individual patient due to the irregular or extensive nature of the facial deficit.

Cross Reference 21208

D5926 Nasal prosthesis, replacement E1

Synonymous terminology: replacement nose. An artificial nose produced from a previously made mold. A replacement prosthesis does not require fabrication of a new mold. Generally, several prostheses can be made from the same mold assuming no changes occur in the tissue bed due to surgery or age related topographical variations.

Cross Reference 21087

D5927 Auricular prosthesis, replacement E1

Synonymous terminology: replacement ear. An artificial ear produced from a previously made mold. A replacement prosthesis does not require fabrication of a new mold. Generally, several prostheses can be made from the same mold assuming no changes occur in the tissue bed due to surgery or age related topographical variations.

Cross Reference 21086

D5928 Orbital prosthesis, replacement E1

A replacement for a previously made orbital prosthesis. A replacement prosthesis does not require fabrication of a new mold. Generally, several prostheses can be made from the same mold assuming no changes occur in the tissue bed due to surgery or age related topographical variations.

Cross Reference 67550

D5929 Facial prosthesis, replacement E1

A replacement facial prosthesis made from the original mold. A replacement prosthesis does not require fabrication of a new mold. Generally, several prostheses can be made from the same mold assuming no changes occur in the tissue bed due to further surgery or age related topographical variations.

Cross Reference 21088

D5931 Obturator prosthesis, surgical E1

Synonymous terminology: obturator, surgical stayplate, immediate temporary obturator. A temporary prosthesis inserted during or immediately following surgical or traumatic loss of a portion or all of one or both maxillary bones and contiguous alveolar structures (e.g., gingival tissue, teeth). Frequent revisions of surgical obturators are necessary during the ensuing healing phase (approximately six months). Some dentists prefer to replace many or all teeth removed by the surgical procedure in the surgical obturator, while others do not replace any teeth. Further surgical revisions may require fabrication of another surgical obturator (e.g., an initially planned small defect may be revised and greatly enlarged after the final pathology report indicates margins are not free of tumor).

Cross Reference 21079

D5932 Obturator prosthesis, definitive Ⓑ E1

Synonymous terminology: obturator. A prosthesis, which artificially replaces part or all of the maxilla and associated teeth, lost due to surgery, trauma or congenital defects. A definitive obturator is made when it is deemed that further tissue changes or recurrence of tumor are unlikely and a more permanent prosthetic rehabilitation can be achieved; it is intended for long-term use.

Cross Reference 21080

D5933 Obturator prosthesis, modification Ⓑ E1

Synonymous terminology: adjustment, denture adjustment, temporary or office reline. Revision or alteration of an existing obturator (surgical, interim, or definitive); possible modifications include relief of the denture base due to tissue compression, augmentation of the seal or peripheral areas to affect adequate sealing or separation between the nasal and oral cavities.

Cross Reference 21080

D5934 Mandibular resection prosthesis with guide flange Ⓑ E1

Synonymous terminology: resection device, resection appliance. A prosthesis which guides the remaining portion of the mandible, left after a partial resection, into a more normal relationship with the maxilla. This allows for some tooth-to-tooth or an improved tooth contact. It may also artificially replace missing teeth and thereby increase masticatory efficiency.

Cross Reference 21081

D5935 Mandibular resection prosthesis without guide flange Ⓑ E1

A prosthesis which helps guide the partially resected mandible to a more normal relation with the maxilla allowing for increased tooth contact. It does not have a flange or ramp, however, to assist in directional closure. It may replace missing teeth and thereby increase masticatory efficiency. Dentists who treat mandibulectomy patients may prefer to replace some, all or none of the teeth in the defect area. Frequently, the defect's margins preclude even partial replacement. Use of a guide (a mandibular resection prosthesis with a guide flange) may not be possible due to anatomical limitations or poor patient tolerance. Ramps, extended occlusal arrangements and irregular occlusal positioning relative to the denture foundation frequently preclude stability of the prostheses, and thus some prostheses are poorly tolerated under such adverse circumstances.

Cross Reference 21081

D5936 Obturator/prosthesis, interim Ⓑ E1

Synonymous terminology: immediate postoperative obturator. A prosthesis which is made following completion of the initial healing after a surgical resection of a portion or all of one or both the maxillae; frequently many or all teeth in the defect area are replaced by this prosthesis. This prosthesis replaces the surgical obturator, which is usually inserted at, or immediately following the resection.

Generally, an interim obturator is made to facilitate closure of the resultant defect after initial healing has been completed. Unlike the surgical obturator, which usually is made prior to surgery and frequently revised in the operating room during surgery, the interim obturator is made when the defect margins are clearly defined and further surgical revisions are not planned. It is a provisional prosthesis, which may replace some or all lost teeth, and other lost bone and soft tissue structures. Also, it frequently must be revised (termed an obturator prosthesis modification) during subsequent dental procedures (e.g., restorations, gingival surgery) as well as to compensate for further tissue shrinkage before a definitive obturator prosthesis is made.

Cross Reference 21079

D5937 Trismus appliance (not for tm treatment) ® E1

Synonymous terminology: occlusal device for mandibular trismus, dynamic bite opener. A prosthesis, which assists the patient in increasing their oral aperture width in order to eat as well as maintain oral hygiene. Several versions and designs are possible, all intending to ease the severe lack of oral opening experienced by many patients immediately following extensive intraoral surgical procedures.

D5951 Feeding aid ® E1

Synonymous terminology: feeding prosthesis. A prosthesis, which maintains the right and left maxillary segments of an infant cleft palate patient in their proper orientation until surgery is performed to repair the cleft. It closes the oral-nasal cavity defect, thus enhancing sucking and swallowing. Used on an interim basis, this prosthesis achieves separation of the oral and nasal cavities in infants born with wide clefts necessitating delayed closure. It is eliminated if surgical closure can be affected or, alternatively, with eruption of the deciduous dentition a pediatric speech aid may be made to facilitate closure of the defect.

D5952 Speech aid prosthesis, pediatric ® A E1

Synonymous terminology: nasopharyngeal obturator, speech appliance, obturator, cleft palate appliance, prosthetic speech aid, speech bulb. A temporary or interim prosthesis used to close a defect in the hard and/or soft palate. It may replace tissue lost due to developmental or surgical alterations. It is necessary for the production of intelligible speech. Normal lateral growth of the palatal bones necessitates occasional replacement of this prosthesis. Intermittent revisions of the obturator section can assist in maintenance of palatalpharyngeal closure (termed a speech aid prosthesis modification). Frequently, such prostheses are not fabricated before the deciduous dentition is fully erupted since clasp retention is often essential.

Cross Reference 21084

D5953 Speech aid prosthesis, adult ® A E1

Synonymous terminology: prosthetic speech appliance, speech aid, speech bulb. A definitive prosthesis, which can improve speech in adult cleft palate patients either by obturating (sealing off) a palatal cleft or fistula, or occasionally by assisting an incompetent soft palate. Both mechanisms are necessary to achieve velopharyngeal competency. Generally, this prosthesis is fabricated when no further growth is anticipated and the objective is to achieve long-term use. Hence, more precise materials and techniques are utilized. Occasionally such procedures are accomplished in conjunction with precision attachments in crown work undertaken on some or all maxillary teeth to achieve improved aesthetics.

Cross Reference 21084

D5954 Palatal augmentation prosthesis ® E1

Synonymous terminology: superimposed prosthesis, maxillary glossectomy prosthesis, maxillary speech prosthesis, palatal drop prosthesis. A removable prosthesis which alters the hard and/or soft palate's topographical form adjacent to the tongue.

Cross Reference 21082

D5955 Palatal lift prosthesis, definitive ® E1

A prosthesis which elevates the soft palate superiorly and aids in restoration of soft palate functions which may be lost due to an acquired, congenital or developmental defect. A definitive palatal lift is usually made for patients whose experience with an interim palatal lift has been successful, especially if surgical alterations are deemed unwarranted.

Cross Reference 21083

D5958 Palatal lift prosthesis, interim Ⓑ E1

Synonymous terminology: diagnostic palatal lift. A prosthesis which elevates and assists in restoring soft palate function which may be lost due to clefting, surgery, trauma or unknown paralysis. It is intended for interim use to determine its usefulness in achieving palatalpharyngeal competency or enhance swallowing reflexes. This prosthesis is intended for interim use as a diagnostic aid to assess the level of possible improvement in speech intelligibility. Some clinicians believe use of a palatal lift on an interim basis may stimulate an otherwise flaccid soft palate to increase functional activity, subsequently lessening its need.

Cross Reference 21083

D5959 Palatal lift prosthesis, modification Ⓑ E1

Synonymous terminology: revision of lift, adjustment. Alterations in the adaptation, contour, form or function of an existing palatal lift necessitated due to tissue impingement, lack of function, poor clasp adaptation or the like.

Cross Reference 21083

D5960 Speech aid prosthesis, modification Ⓑ E1

Synonymous terminology: adjustment, repair, revision. Any revision of a pediatric or adult speech aid not necessitating its replacement. Frequently, revisions of the obturating section of any speech aid is required to facilitate enhanced speech intelligibility. Such revisions or repairs do not require complete remaking of the prosthesis, thus extending its longevity.

Cross Reference 21084

D5982 Surgical stent Ⓑ E1

Synonymous terminology: periodontal stent, skin graft stent, columellar stent. Stents are utilized to apply pressure to soft tissues to facilitate healing and prevent cicatrization or collapse. A surgical stent may be required in surgical and post-surgical revisions to achieve close approximation of tissues. Usually such materials as temporary or interim soft denture liners, gutta percha, or dental modeling impression compound may be used.

Cross Reference 21085

D5983 Radiation carrier Ⓑ S

Synonymous terminology: radiotherapy prosthesis, carrier prosthesis, radiation applicator, radium carrier, intracavity carrier, intracavity applicator. A device used to administer radiation to confined areas by means of capsules, beads or needles of radiation emitting materials such as radium or cesium. Its function is to hold the radiation source securely in the same location during the entire period of treatment. Radiation oncologists occasionally request these devices to achieve close approximation and controlled application of radiation to a tumor deemed amiable to eradication.

D5984 Radiation shield Ⓑ S

Synonymous terminology: radiation stent, tongue protector, lead shield. An intraoral prosthesis designed to shield adjacent tissues from radiation during orthovoltage treatment of malignant lesions of the head and neck region.

D5985 Radiation cone locator Ⓑ S

Synonymous terminology: docking device, cone locator. A prosthesis utilized to direct and reduplicate the path of radiation to an oral tumor during a split course of irradiation.

D5986 Fluoride gel carrier Ⓑ E1

Synonymous terminology: fluoride applicator. A prosthesis, which covers the teeth in either dental arch and is used to apply topical fluoride in close proximity to tooth enamel and dentin for several minutes daily.

D5987 Commissure splint Ⓑ S

Synonymous terminology: lip splint. A device placed between the lips, which assists in achieving increased opening between the lips. Use of such devices enhances opening where surgical, chemical or electrical alterations of the lips has resulted in severe restriction or contractures.

D5988 Surgical splint E1

Synonymous terminology: Gunning splint, modified Gunning splint, labiolingual splint, fenestrated splint, Kingsley splint, cast metal splint. Splints are designed to utilize existing teeth and/or alveolar processes as points of anchorage to assist in stabilization and immobilization of broken bones during healing. They are used to re-establish, as much as possible, normal occlusal relationships during the process of immobilization. Frequently, existing prostheses (e.g., a patient's complete dentures) can be modified to serve as surgical splints. Frequently, surgical splints have arch bars added to facilitate intermaxillary fixation. Rubber elastics may be used to assist in this process. Circummandibular eyelet hooks can be utilized for enhanced stabilization with wiring to adjacent bone.

D5991 Vesicobullous disease medicament carrier E1

A custom fabricated carrier that covers the teeth and alveolar mucosa, or alveolar mucosa alone, and is used to deliver prescription medicaments for treatment of immunologically mediated vesiculobullous disease.

D5992 Adjust maxillofacial prosthetic appliance, by report E1

D5993 Maintenance and cleaning of a maxillofacial prosthesis (extra or intra-oral) other than required adjustments, by report E1

D5994 Periodontal medicament carrier with peripheral seal - laboratory processed E1

A custom fabricated, laboratory processed carrier that covers the teeth and alveolar mucosa. Used as a vehicle to deliver prescribed medicaments for sustained contact with the gingiva, alveolar mucosa, and into the periodontal sulcus or pocket.

D5999 Unspecified maxillofacial prosthesis, by report E1

Used for procedure that is not adequately described by a code. Describe procedure.

Implant Services (D6010-D6199)

D6010-D6199: FPD = fixed partial denture

Surgical Services

D6010 Surgical placement of implant body: endosteal implant E1

Cross Reference 21248

D6011 Second stage implant surgery E1

Surgical access to an implant body for placement of a healing cap or to enable placement of an abutment.

D6012 Surgical placement of interim implant body for transitional prosthesis: endosteal implant E1

Includes removal during later therapy to accommodate the definitive restoration, which may include placement of other implants.

D6013 Surgical placement of mini implant E1

D6040 Surgical placement: eposteal implant E1

An eposteal (subperiosteal) framework of a biocompatible material designed and fabricated to fit on the surface of the bone of the mandible or maxilla with permucosal extensions which provide support and attachment of a prosthesis. This may be a complete arch or unilateral appliance. Eposteal implants rest upon the bone and under the periosteum.

Cross Reference 21245

D6050 Surgical placement: transosteal implant E1

A transosteal (transosseous) biocompatible device with threaded posts penetrating both the superior and inferior cortical bone plates of the mandibular symphysis and exiting through the permucosa providing support and attachment for a dental prosthesis. Transosteal implants are placed completely through the bone and into the oral cavity from extraoral or intraoral.

Cross Reference 21244

Implant Supported Prosthetics

D6051 Interim abutment - includes placement and removal Ⓑ E1

Includes placement and removal. A healing cap is not an interim abutment.

D6052 Semi-precision attachment abutment Ⓑ E1

Includes placement of keeper assembly.

D6055 Connecting bar — implant supported or abutment supported Ⓑ E1

Utilized to stabilize and anchor a prosthesis.

D6056 Prefabricated abutment - includes modification and placement Ⓑ E1

Modification of a prefabricated abutment may be necessary.

D6057 Custom fabricated abutment - includes placement Ⓑ E1

Created by a laboratory process, specific for an individual application.

D6058 Abutment supported porcelain/ceramic crown Ⓑ E1

A single crown restoration that is retained, supported and stabilized by an abutment on an implant.

D6059 Abutment supported porcelain fused to metal crown (high noble metal) Ⓑ E1

A single metal-ceramic crown restoration that is retained, supported and stabilized by an abutment on an implant.

D6060 Abutment supported porcelain fused to metal crown (predominantly base metal) Ⓑ E1

A single metal-ceramic crown restoration that is retained, supported and stabilized by an abutment on an implant.

D6061 Abutment supported porcelain fused to metal crown (noble metal) Ⓑ E1

A single metal-ceramic crown restoration that is retained, supported and stabilized by an abutment on an implant.

D6062 Abutment supported cast metal crown (high noble metal) Ⓑ E1

A single cast metal crown restoration that is retained, supported and stabilized by an abutment on an implant.

D6063 Abutment supported cast metal crown (predominantly base metal) Ⓑ E1

A single cast metal crown restoration that is retained, supported and stabilized by an abutment on an implant.

D6064 Abutment supported cast metal crown (noble metal) Ⓑ E1

A single cast metal crown restoration that is retained, supported and stabilized by an abutment on an implant.

D6065 Implant supported porcelain/ceramic crown Ⓑ E1

A single crown restoration that is retained, supported and stabilized by an implant.

D6066 Implant supported porcelain fused to metal crown (titanium, titanium alloy, high noble metal) Ⓑ E1

A single metal-ceramic crown restoration that is retained, supported and stabilized by an implant.

D6067 Implant supported metal crown (titanium, titanium alloy, high noble metal) Ⓑ E1

A single cast metal or milled crown restoration that is retained, supported and stabilized by an implant.

D6068 Abutment supported retainer for porcelain/ceramic FPD Ⓑ E1

A ceramic retainer for a fixed partial denture that gains retention, support and stability from an abutment on an implant.

D6069 Abutment supported retainer for porcelain fused to metal FPD (high noble metal) Ⓑ E1

A metal-ceramic retainer for a fixed partial denture that gains retention, support and stability from an abutment on an implant.

D6070 Abutment supported retainer for porcelain fused to metal FPD (predominantly base metal) Ⓑ E1

A metal-ceramic retainer for a fixed partial denture that gains retention, support and stability from an abutment on an implant.

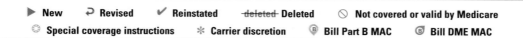

D6071 Abutment supported retainer for porcelain fused to metal FPD (noble metal) Ⓑ E1

A metal-ceramic retainer for a fixed partial denture that gains retention, support and stability from an abutment on an implant.

D6072 Abutment supported retainer for cast metal FPD (high noble metal) Ⓑ E1

A cast metal retainer for a fixed partial denture that gains retention, support and stability from an abutment on an implant.

D6073 Abutment supported retainer for cast metal FPD (predominantly base metal) Ⓑ E1

A cast metal retainer for a fixed partial denture that gains retention, support and stability from an abutment on an implant.

D6074 Abutment supported retainer for cast metal FPD (noble metal) Ⓑ E1

A cast metal retainer for a fixed partial denture that gains retention, support and stability from an abutment on an implant.

D6075 Implant supported retainer for ceramic FPD Ⓑ E1

A ceramic retainer for a fixed partial denture that gains retention, support and stability from an implant.

D6076 Implant supported retainer for porcelain fused to metal FPD (titanium, titanium alloy, or high noble metal) Ⓑ E1

A metal-ceramic retainer for a fixed partial denture that gains retention, support and stability from an implant.

D6077 Implant supported retainer for cast metal FPD (titanium, titanium alloy, or high noble metal) Ⓑ E1

A cast metal retainer for a fixed partial denture that gains retention, support and stability from an implant.

Other Implant Services

D6080 Implant maintenance procedures when prostheses are removed and reinserted, including cleansing of prostheses and abutments Ⓑ E1

This procedure includes active debriding of the implant(s) and examination of all aspects of the implant system(s), including the occlusion and stability of the superstructure. The patient is also instructed in thorough daily cleansing of the implant(s). This is not a per implant code, and is indicated for implant supported fixed prostheses.

D6081 Scaling and debridement in the presence of inflammation or mucositis of a single implant, including cleaning of the implant surfaces, without flap entry and closure Ⓑ E1

This procedure is not performed in conjunction with D1110, D4910, or D4346.

D6085 Provisional implant crown Ⓑ E1

Used when a period of healing is necessary prior to fabrication and placement of permanent prosthetic.

D6090 Repair implant supported prosthesis by report Ⓑ E1

This procedure involves the repair or replacement of any part of the implant supported prosthesis.

Cross Reference 21299

D6091 Replacement of semi-precision or precision attachment (male or female component) of implant/abutment supported prosthesis, per attachment Ⓑ E1

This procedure applies to the replaceable male or female component of the attachment.

D6092 Re-cement or re-bond implant/ abutment supported crown Ⓑ E1

D6093 Re-cement or re-bond implant/ abutment supported fixed partial denture Ⓑ E1

D6094 Abutment supported crown - (titanium) Ⓑ E1

A single crown restoration that is retained, supported and stabilized by an abutment on an implant. May be cast or milled.

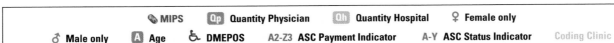

D6095 Repair implant abutment, by report Ⓑ E1

This procedure involves the repair or replacement of any part of the implant abutment.

Cross Reference 21299

D6096 Remove broken implant retaining screw Ⓑ E1

Surgical Services

D6100 Implant removal, by report Ⓑ E1

This procedure involves the surgical removal of an implant. Describe procedure.

Cross Reference 21299

D6101 Debridement of a peri-implant defect or defects surrounding a single implant, and surface cleaning of exposed implant surfaces, including flap entry and closure Ⓑ E1

D6102 Debridement and osseous contouring of a peri-implant defect or defects surrounding a single implant and includes surface cleaning of the exposed implant surfaces and flap entry and closure Ⓑ E1

D6103 Bone graft for repair of peri-implant defect - does not include flap entry and closure Ⓑ E1

Placement of a barrier membrane or biologic materials to aid in osseous regeneration, are reported separately.

D6104 Bone graft at time of implant placement Ⓑ E1

Placement of a barrier membrane, or biologic materials to aid in osseous regeneration are reported separately.

Implant Supported Prosthetics

D6110 Implant /abutment supported removable denture for edentulous arch - maxillary Ⓑ E1

D6111 Implant /abutment supported removable denture for edentulous arch - mandibular Ⓑ E1

D6112 Implant/abutment supported removable denture for partially edentulous arch - maxillary Ⓑ E1

D6113 Implant/abutment supported removable denture for partially edentulous arch - mandibular Ⓑ E1

D6114 Implant/abutment supported fixed denture for edentulous arch - maxillary Ⓑ E1

D6115 Implant/abutment supported fixed denture for edentulous arch - mandibular Ⓑ E1

D6116 Implant/abutment supported fixed denture for partially edentulous arch - maxillary Ⓑ E1

D6117 Implant/abutment supported fixed denture for partially edentulous arch - mandibular Ⓑ E1

D6118 Implant/abutment supported interim fixed denture for edentulous arch mandibular Ⓑ E1

Used when a period of healing is necessary prior to fabrication and placement of a permanent prosthetic.

D6119 Implant/abutment supported interim fixed denture for edentulous arch maxillary Ⓑ E1

Used when a period of healing is necessary prior to fabrication and placement of a permanent prosthetic.

D6190 Radiographic/surgical implant index, by report Ⓑ E1

An appliance, designed to relate osteotomy or fixture position to existing anatomic structures, to be utilized during radiographic exposure for treatment planning and/or during osteotomy creation for fixture installation.

D6194 Abutment supported retainer crown for FPD (titanium) Ⓑ E1

A retainer for a fixed partial denture that gains retention, support and stability from an abutment on an implant. May be cast or milled.

None

D6199 Unspecified implant procedure, by report Ⓑ E1

Use for procedure that is not adequately described by a code. Describe procedure.

Cross Reference 21299

▶ New ⤾ Revised ✔ Reinstated ~~deleted~~ Deleted ⃠ Not covered or valid by Medicare
Special coverage instructions ✻ Carrier discretion Ⓑ Bill Part B MAC Ⓓ Bill DME MAC

Prosthodontics, fixed (D6205-D6999)

Fixed Partial Denture Pontics

D6205 Pontic - indirect resin based composite Ⓑ E1

Not to be used as a temporary or provisional prosthesis.

D6210 Pontic - cast high noble metal Ⓑ E1

D6211 Pontic - cast predominantly base metal Ⓑ E1

D6212 Pontic - cast noble metal Ⓑ E1

D6214 Pontic - titanium Ⓑ E1

D6240 Pontic - porcelain fused to high noble metal Ⓑ E1

D6241 Pontic - porcelain fused to predominantly base metal Ⓑ E1

D6242 Pontic - porcelain fused to noble metal Ⓑ E1

IOM: 100-02, 15, 150

D6245 Pontic - porcelain/ceramic Ⓑ E1

D6250 Pontic - resin with high noble metal Ⓑ E1

D6251 Pontic - resin with predominantly base metal Ⓑ E1

D6252 Pontic - resin with noble metal Ⓑ E1

D6253 Provisional pontic - further treatment or completion of diagnosis necessary prior to final impression Ⓑ E1

Not to be used as a temporary pontic for routine prosthetic fixed partial dentures.

Fixed Partial Denture Retainers – Inlays/Onlays

D6545 Retainer - cast metal for resin bonded fixed prosthesis Ⓑ E1

D6548 Retainer - porcelain/ceramic for resin bonded fixed prosthesis Ⓑ E1

D6549 Retainer - for resin bonded fixed prosthesis Ⓑ E1

D6600 Retainer inlay - porcelain/ceramic, two surfaces Ⓑ E1

D6601 Retainer inlay - porcelain/ceramic, three or more surfaces Ⓑ E1

D6602 Retainer inlay - cast high noble metal, two surfaces Ⓑ E1

D6603 Retainer inlay - cast high noble metal, three or more surfaces Ⓑ E1

D6604 Retainer inlay - cast predominantly base metal, two surfaces Ⓑ E1

D6605 Retainer inlay - cast predominantly base metal, three or more surfaces Ⓑ E1

D6606 Retainer inlay - cast noble metal, two surfaces Ⓑ E1

D6607 Retainer inlay - cast noble metal, three or more surfaces Ⓑ E1

D6608 Retainer onlay - porcelain/ceramic, two surfaces Ⓑ E1

D6609 Retainer onlay - porcelain/ceramic, three or more surfaces Ⓑ E1

D6610 Retainer onlay - cast high noble metal, two surfaces Ⓑ E1

D6611 Retainer onlay - cast high noble metal, three or more surfaces Ⓑ E1

D6612 Retainer onlay - cast predominantly base metal, two surfaces Ⓑ E1

D6613 Retainer onlay - cast predominantly base metal, three or more surfaces Ⓑ E1

D6614 Retainer onlay - cast noble metal, two surfaces Ⓑ E1

D6615 Retainer onlay - cast noble metal, three or more surfaces Ⓑ E1

D6624 Retainer inlay - titanium Ⓑ E1

D6634 Retainer onlay - titanium Ⓑ E1

Fixed Partial Denture Retainers – Crowns

D6710 Retainer crown - indirect resin based composite Ⓑ E1

Not to be used as a temporary or provisional prosthesis.

D6720 Retainer crown - resin with high noble metal Ⓑ E1

D6721 Retainer crown - resin with predominantly base metal Ⓑ E1

D6722 Retainer crown - resin with noble metal Ⓑ E1

D6740 Retainer crown - porcelain/ceramic Ⓑ E1

D6750 Retainer crown - porcelain fused to high noble metal Ⓑ E1

D6751 Retainer crown - porcelain fused to predominantly base metal Ⓑ E1

D6752 Retainer crown - porcelain fused to noble metal Ⓑ E1

D6780 Retainer crown - 3/4 cast high noble metal Ⓑ E1

D6781 Retainer crown - 3/4 cast predominantly based metal Ⓑ E1

D6782 Retainer crown - 3/4 cast noble metal Ⓑ E1

D6783 Retainer crown - 3/4 porcelain/ceramic Ⓑ E1

D6790 Retainer crown - full cast high noble metal Ⓑ E1

D6791 Retainer crown - full cast predominantly base metal Ⓑ E1

D6792 Retainer crown - full cast noble metal Ⓑ E1

D6793 Provisional retainer crown - further treatment or completion of diagnosis necessary prior to final impression Ⓑ E1

Not to be used as a temporary retainer crown for routine prosthetic fixed partial dentures.

D6794 Retainer crown - titanium Ⓑ E1

Other Fixed Partial Denture Services

D6920 Connector bar Ⓑ S

A device attached to fixed partial denture retainer or coping which serves to stabilize and anchor a removable overdenture prosthesis.

D6930 Re-cement or re-bond fixed partial denture Ⓑ E1

D6940 Stress breaker Ⓑ E1

A non-rigid connector.

D6950 Precision attachment Ⓑ E1

A male and female pair constitutes one precision attachment, and is separate from the prosthesis.

D6980 Bridge repair necessitated by restorative material failure Ⓑ E1

D6985 Pediatric partial denture, fixed Ⓑ A E1

This prosthesis is used primarily for aesthetic purposes.

None

D6999 Unspecified fixed prosthodontic procedure, by report Ⓑ E1

Used for procedure that is not adequately described by a code. Describe procedure.

Oral and Maxillofacial Surgery (D7111-D7999)

Extractions (Includes Local Anesthesia, Suturing, If Needed, and Routine Postoperative Care)

D7111 Extraction, coronal remnants - primary tooth Ⓑ S

Removal of soft tissue-retained coronal remnants.

D7140 Extraction, erupted tooth or exposed root (elevation and/or forceps removal) Ⓑ S

Includes removal of tooth structure, minor smoothing of socket bone, and closure, as necessary.

D7210 Extraction, erupted tooth requiring removal of bone and/or sectioning of tooth, and including elevation of mucoperiosteal flap if indicated Ⓑ S

Includes related cutting of gingiva and bone, removal of tooth structure, minor smoothing of socket bone and closure.

D7220 Removal of impacted tooth - soft tissue Ⓑ S

Occlusal surface of tooth covered by soft tissue; requires mucoperiosteal flap elevation.

D7230 Removal of impacted tooth - partially bony Ⓑ S

Part of crown covered by bone; requires mucoperiosteal flap elevation and bone removal.

D7240 Removal of impacted tooth - completely bony Ⓑ S

Most or all of crown covered by bone; requires mucoperiosteal flap elevation and bone removal.

D7241 Removal of impacted tooth - completely bony, with unusual surgical complications Ⓑ S

Most or all of crown covered by bone; unusually difficult or complicated due to factors such as nerve dissection required, separate closure of maxillary sinus required or aberrant tooth position.

D7250 Removal of residual tooth roots (cutting procedure) Ⓑ S

Includes cutting of soft tissue and bone, removal of tooth structure, and closure.

D7251 Coronectomy — intentional partial tooth removal Ⓑ E1

Intentional partial tooth removal is performed when a neurovascular complication is likely if the entire impacted tooth is removed.

Other Surgical Procedures

D7260 Oral antral fistula closure Ⓑ S

Excision of fistulous tract between maxillary sinus and oral cavity and closure by advancement flap.

D7261 Primary closure of a sinus perforation Ⓑ S

Subsequent to surgical removal of tooth, exposure of sinus requiring repair, or immediate closure of oroantral or oralnasal communication in absence of fistulous tract.

D7270 Tooth reimplantation and/or stabilization of accidentally evulsed or displaced tooth Ⓑ E1

Includes splinting and/or stabilization.

D7272 Tooth transplantation (includes reimplantation from one site to another and splinting and/or stabilization) Ⓑ E1

D7280 Exposure of an unerupted tooth Ⓑ E1

An incision is made and the tissue is reflected and bone removed as necessary to expose the crown of an impacted tooth not intended to be extracted.

D7282 Mobilization of erupted or malpositioned tooth to aid eruption Ⓑ E1

To move/luxate teeth to eliminate ankylosis; not in conjunction with an extraction.

D7283 Placement of device to facilitate eruption of impacted tooth Ⓑ B

Placement of an orthodontic bracket, band or other device on an unerupted tooth, after its exposure, to aid in its eruption. Report the surgical exposure separately using D7280.

D7285 Incisional biopsy of oral tissue - hard (bone, tooth) Ⓑ E1

For partial removal of specimen only. This procedure involves biopsy of osseous lesions and is not used for apicoectomy/periradicular surgery. This procedure does not entail an excision.

Cross Reference 20220, 20225, 20240, 20245

D7286 Incisional biopsy of oral tissue - soft Ⓑ E1

For partial removal of an architecturally intact specimen only. This procedure is not used at the same time as codes for apicoectomy/periradicular curettage. This procedure does not entail an excision.

Cross Reference 40808

D7287 Exfoliative cytological sample collection Ⓑ E1

For collection of non-transepithelial cytology sample via mild scraping of the oral mucosa.

D7288 Brush biopsy - transepithelial sample collection Ⓑ B

For collection of oral disaggregated transepithelial cells via rotational brushing of the oral mucosa.

D7290 Surgical repositioning of teeth Ⓑ E1

Grafting procedure(s) is/are additional.

D7291 Transseptal fiberotomy/supra crestal fiberotomy, by report Ⓑ S

The supraosseous connective tissue attachment is surgically severed around the involved teeth. Where there are adjacent teeth, the transseptal fiberotomy of a single tooth will involve a minimum of three teeth. Since the incisions are within the gingival sulcus and tissue and the root surface is not instrumented, this procedure heals by the reunion of connective tissue with the root surface on which viable periodontal tissue is present (reattachment).

D7292 Placement of temporary anchorage device [screw retained plate] requiring flap; includes device removal Ⓑ E1

D7293 Placement of temporary anchorage device requiring flap; includes device removal Ⓑ E1

D7294 Placement of temporary anchorage device without flap; includes device removal Ⓑ E1

D7295 Harvest of bone for use in autogenous grafting procedure Ⓑ E1

Reported in addition to those autogenous graft placement procedures that do not include harvesting of bone.

D7296 Corticotomy one to three teeth or tooth spaces, per quadrant Ⓑ E1

This procedure involves creating multiple cuts, perforations, or removal of cortical, alveolar or basal bone of the jaw for the purpose of facilitating orthodontic repositioning of the dentition. This procedure includes flap entry and closure. Graft material and membrane, if used, should be reported separately.

D7297 Corticotomy four or more teeth or tooth spaces, per quadrant Ⓑ E1

This procedure involves creating multiple cuts, perforations, or removal of cortical, alveolar or basal bone of the jaw for the purpose of facilitating orthodontic repositioning of the dentition. This procedure includes flap entry and closure. Graft material and membrane, if used, should be reported separately.

Alveoloplasty – Preparation of Ridge

D7310 Alveoloplasty in conjunction with extractions - four or more teeth or tooth spaces, per quadrant Ⓑ E1

The alveoloplasty is distinct (separate procedure) from extractions. Usually in preparation for a prosthesis or other treatments such as radiation therapy and transplant surgery.

Cross Reference 41874

D7311 Alveoloplasty in conjunction with extractions - one to three teeth or tooth spaces, per quadrant Ⓑ E1

The alveoloplasty is distinct (separate procedure) from extractions. Usually in preparation for a prosthesis or other treatments such as radiation therapy and transplant surgery.

D7320 Alveoloplasty not in conjunction with extractions - four or more teeth or tooth spaces, per quadrant Ⓑ E1

No extractions performed in an edentulous area. See D7310 if teeth are being extracted concurrently with the alveoloplasty. Usually in preparation for a prosthesis or other treatments such as radiation therapy and transplant surgery.

Cross Reference 41870

D7321 Alveoloplasty not in conjunction with extractions - one to three teeth or tooth spaces, per quadrant Ⓑ B

No extractions performed in an edentulous area. See D7311 if teeth are being extracted concurrently with the alveoloplasty. Usually in preparation for a prosthesis or other treatments such as radiation therapy and transplant surgery.

Vestibuloplasty

D7340 Vestibuloplasty - ridge extension (second epithelialization) Ⓑ E1

Cross Reference 40840, 40842, 40843, 40844

D7350 Vestibuloplasty - ridge extension (including soft tissue grafts, muscle reattachments, revision of soft tissue attachment, and management of hypertrophied and hyperplastic tissue) Ⓑ E1

Cross Reference 40845

Excision of Soft Tissue Lesions

D7410 Excision of benign lesion up to 1.25 cm Ⓑ E1

D7411 Excision of benign lesion greater than 1.25 cm Ⓑ E1

D7412 Excision of benign lesion, complicated Ⓑ E1

Requires extensive undermining with advancement or rotational flap closure.

D7413 Excision of malignant lesion up to 1.25 cm Ⓑ E1

D7414 Excision of malignant lesion greater than 1.25 cm Ⓑ E1

D7415 Excision of malignant lesion, complicated Ⓑ E1

Requires extensive undermining with advancement or rotational flap closure.

Excision of Intra-Osseous Lesions

D7440 Excision of malignant tumor - lesion diameter up to 1.25 cm Ⓑ E1

D7441 Excision of malignant tumor - lesion diameter greater than 1.25 cm Ⓑ E1

D7450 Removal of benign odontogenic cyst or tumor - lesion diameter up to 1.25 cm Ⓑ E1

D7451 Removal of benign odontogenic cyst or tumor - lesion diameter greater than 1.25 cm Ⓑ E1

D7460 Removal of benign nonodontogenic cyst or tumor - lesion diameter up to 1.25 cm Ⓑ E1

D7461 Removal of benign nonodontogenic cyst or tumor - lesion diameter greater than 1.25 cm Ⓑ E1

Excision of Soft Tissue Lesions

D7465 Destruction of lesion(s) by physical or chemical methods, by report Ⓑ E1

Examples include using cryo, laser or electro surgery.

Cross Reference 41850

Excision of Bone Tissue

D7471 Removal of lateral exostosis (maxilla or mandible) Ⓑ E1

Cross Reference 21031, 21032

D7472 Removal of torus palatinus Ⓑ E1

D7473 Removal of torus mandibularis Ⓑ E1

D7485 Reduction of osseous tuberosity Ⓑ E1

D7490 Radical resection of maxilla or mandible Ⓑ E1

Partial resection of maxilla or mandible; removal of lesion and defect with margin of normal appearing bone. Reconstruction and bone grafts should be reported separately.

Cross Reference 21095

Surgical Incision

D7510 Incision and drainage of abscess - intraoral soft tissue Ⓑ E1

Involves incision through mucosa, including periodontal origins.

Cross Reference 41800

D7511 Incision and drainage of abscess - intraoral soft tissue - complicated (includes drainage of multiple fascial spaces) Ⓑ B

Incision is made intraorally and dissection is extended into adjacent fascial space(s) to provide adequate drainage of abscess/cellulitis.

D7520 Incision and drainage of abscess - extraoral soft tissue Ⓑ E1

Involves incision through skin.

Cross Reference 41800

D7521 Incision and drainage of abscess - extraoral soft tissue - complicated (includes drainage of multiple fascial spaces) Ⓑ B

Incision is made extraorally and dissection is extended into adjacent fascial space(s) to provide adequate drainage of abscess/cellulitis.

D7530 Removal of foreign body from mucosa, skin, or subcutaneous alveolar tissue Ⓑ E1

Cross Reference 41805, 41828

D7540 Removal of reaction-producing foreign bodies, musculoskeletal system Ⓑ E1

May include, but is not limited to, removal of splinters, pieces of wire, etc., from muscle and/or bone.

Cross Reference 20520, 41800, 41806

D7550 Partial ostectomy/sequestrectomy for removal of non-vital bone Ⓑ E1

Removal of loose or sloughed-off dead bone caused by infection or reduced blood supply.

Cross Reference 20999

D7560 Maxillary sinusotomy for removal of tooth fragment or foreign body Ⓑ E1

Cross Reference 31020

Treatment of Closed Fractures

D7610 Maxilla - open reduction (teeth immobilized, if present) Ⓑ E1

Teeth may be wired, banded or splinted together to prevent movement. Incision required for interosseous fixation.

D7620 Maxilla - closed reduction (teeth immobilized if present) Ⓑ E1

No incision required to reduce fracture. See D7610 if interosseous fixation is applied.

D7630 Mandible - open reduction (teeth immobilized, if present) Ⓑ E1

Teeth may be wired, banded or splinted together to prevent movement. Incision required to reduce fracture.

D7640 Mandible - closed reduction (teeth immobilized if present) Ⓑ E1

No incision required to reduce fracture. See D7630 if interosseous fixation is applied.

D7650 Malar and/or zygomatic arch - open reduction Ⓑ E1

D7660 Malar and/or zygomatic arch - closed reduction Ⓑ E1

D7670 Alveolus - closed reduction, may include stabilization of teeth Ⓑ E1

Teeth may be wired, banded or splinted together to prevent movement.

D7671 Alveolus - open reduction, may include stabilization of teeth Ⓑ E1

Teeth may be wired, banded or splinted together to prevent movement.

D7680 Facial bones - complicated reduction with fixation and multiple surgical approaches Ⓑ E1

Facial bones include upper and lower jaw, cheek, and bones around eyes, nose, and ears.

Treatment of Open Fractures

D7710 Maxilla - open reduction Ⓑ E1

Incision required to reduce fracture.

Cross Reference 21346

D7720 Maxilla - closed reduction Ⓑ E1

Cross Reference 21345

D7730 Mandible - open reduction Ⓑ E1

Incision required to reduce fracture.

Cross Reference 21461, 21462

D7740 Mandible - closed reduction Ⓑ E1

Cross Reference 21455

D7750 Malar and/or zygomatic arch - open reduction Ⓑ E1

Incision required to reduce fracture.

Cross Reference 21360, 21365

D7760 Malar and/or zygomatic arch - closed reduction Ⓑ E1

Cross Reference 21355

D7770 Alveolus - open reduction stabilization of teeth Ⓑ E1

Fractured bone(s) are exposed to mouth or outside the face. Incision required to reduce fracture.

Cross Reference 21422

D7771 Alveolus, closed reduction stabilization of teeth Ⓑ E1

Fractured bone(s) are exposed to mouth or outside the face.

D7780 Facial bones - complicated reduction with fixation and multiple approaches Ⓑ E1

Incision required to reduce fracture. Facial bones include upper and lower jaw, cheek, and bones around eyes, nose, and ears.

Cross Reference 21433, 21435

Reduction of Dislocation and Management of Other Temporomandibular Joint Dysfunction

D7810 Open reduction of dislocation Ⓑ E1

Access to TMJ via surgical opening.

Cross Reference 21490

D7820 Closed reduction of dislocation Ⓑ E1

Joint manipulated into place; no surgical exposure.

Cross Reference 21480

D7830 Manipulation under anesthesia Ⓑ E1

Usually done under general anesthesia or intravenous sedation.

Cross Reference 00190

D7840 Condylectomy Ⓑ E1

Removal of all or portion of the mandibular condyle (separate procedure).

Cross Reference 21050

D7850 Surgical discectomy, with/without implant Ⓑ E1

Excision of the intra-articular disc of a joint.

Cross Reference 21060

D7852 Disc repair Ⓑ E1

Repositioning and/or sculpting of disc; repair of perforated posterior attachment.

Cross Reference 21299

D7854 Synovectomy Ⓑ E1

Excision of a portion or all of the synovial membrane of a joint.

Cross Reference 21299

D7856 Myotomy Ⓑ E1

Cutting of muscle for therapeutic purposes (separate procedure).

Cross Reference 21299

D7858 Joint reconstruction Ⓑ E1

Reconstruction of osseous components including or excluding soft tissues of the joint with autogenous, homologous, or alloplastic materials.

Cross Reference 21242, 21243

D7860 Arthrotomy Ⓑ E1

Cutting into joint (separate procedure).

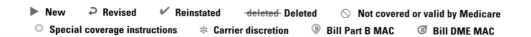

D7865 Arthroplasty Ⓑ E1

Reduction of osseous components of the joint to create a pseudoarthrosis or eliminate an irregular remodeling pattern (osteophytes).

Cross Reference 21240

D7870 Arthrocentesis Ⓑ E1

Withdrawal of fluid from a joint space by aspiration.

Cross Reference 21060

D7871 Non-arthroscopic lysis and lavage Ⓑ E1

Inflow and outflow catheters are placed into the joint space. The joint is lavaged and manipulated as indicated in an effort to release minor adhesions and synovial vacuum phenomenon as well as to remove inflammation products from the joint space.

D7872 Arthroscopy - diagnosis, with or without biopsy Ⓑ E1

Cross Reference 29800

D7873 Arthroscopy: lavage and lysis of adhesions Ⓑ E1

Removal of adhesions using the arthroscope and lavage of the joint cavities.

Cross Reference 29804

D7874 Arthroscopy: disc repositioning and stabilization Ⓑ E1

Repositioning and stabilization of disc using arthroscopic techniques.

Cross Reference 29804

D7875 Arthroscopy: synovectomy Ⓑ E1

Removal of inflamed and hyperplastic synovium (partial/complete) via an arthroscopic technique.

Cross Reference 29804

D7876 Arthroscopy: discectomy Ⓑ E1

Removal of disc and remodeled posterior attachment via the arthroscope.

Cross Reference 29804

D7877 Arthroscopy: debridement Ⓑ E1

Removal of pathologic hard and/or soft tissue using the arthroscope.

Cross Reference 29804

D7880 Occlusal orthotic device, by report Ⓑ E1

Presently includes splints provided for treatment of temporomandibular joint dysfunction.

Cross Reference 21499

D7881 Occlusal orthotic device adjustment Ⓑ E1

D7899 Unspecified TMD therapy, by report Ⓑ E1

Used for procedure that is not adequately described by a code. Describe procedure.

Cross Reference 21499

Repair of Traumatic Wounds

D7910 Suture of recent small wounds up to 5 cm Ⓑ E1

Cross Reference 12011, 12013

Complicated Suturing (Reconstruction Requiring Delicate Handling of Tissue and Wide Undermining for Meticulous Closure)

D7911 Complicated suture - up to 5 cm Ⓑ E1

Cross Reference 12051, 12052

D7912 Complicated suture - greater than 5 cm Ⓑ E1

Cross Reference 13132

Other Repair Procedures

D7920 Skin graft (identify defect covered, location, and type of graft) Ⓑ E1

D7921 Collection and application of autologous blood concentrate product Ⓑ E1

D7940 Osteoplasty - for orthognathic deformities Ⓑ S

Reconstruction of jaws for correction of congenital, developmental or acquired traumatic or surgical deformity.

D7941 Osteotomy - mandibular rami Ⓑ E1

Cross Reference 21193, 21195, 21196

D7943 Osteotomy - mandibular rami with bone graft; includes obtaining the graft Ⓑ E1

Cross Reference 21194

D7944 Osteotomy - segmented or subapical Ⓑ E1

Report by range of tooth numbers within segment.

Cross Reference 21198, 21206

DURABLE MEDICAL EQUIPMENT (E0100-E8002)

Canes

E0100 Cane, includes canes of all materials, adjustable or fixed, with tip Ⓑ Qp Qh ♿ Y

IOM: 100-02, 15, 110.1; 100-03, 4, 280.1; 100-03, 4, 280.2

E0105 Cane, quad or three prong, includes canes of all materials, adjustable or fixed, with tips Ⓑ Qp Qh ♿ Y

IOM: 100-02, 15, 110.1; 100-03, 4, 280.1; 100-03, 4, 280.2

Coding Clinic: 2016, Q3, P3

Crutches

E0110 Crutches, forearm, includes crutches of various materials, adjustable or fixed, pair, complete with tips and handgrips Ⓑ Qp Qh ♿ Y

Crutches are covered when prescribed for a patient who is normally ambulatory but suffers from a condition that impairs ambulation. Provides minimal to moderate weight support while ambulating.

IOM: 100-02, 15, 110.1; 100-03, 4, 280.1

E0111 Crutch forearm, includes crutches of various materials, adjustable or fixed, each, with tips and handgrips Ⓑ Qp Qh ♿ Y

IOM: 100-02, 15, 110.1; 100-03, 4, 280.1

E0112 Crutches, underarm, wood, adjustable or fixed, pair, with pads, tips, and handgrips Ⓑ Qp Qh ♿ Y

IOM: 100-02, 15, 110.1; 100-03, 4, 280.1

E0113 Crutch underarm, wood, adjustable or fixed, each, with pad, tip, and handgrip Ⓑ Qp Qh ♿ Y

IOM: 100-02, 15, 110.1; 100-03, 4, 280.1

E0114 Crutches, underarm, other than wood, adjustable or fixed, pair, with pads, tips and handgrips Ⓑ Qp Qh ♿ Y

IOM: 100-02, 15, 110.1; 100-03, 4, 280.1

E0116 Crutch, underarm, other than wood, adjustable or fixed, with pad, tip, handgrip, with or without shock absorber, each Ⓑ Qp Qh ♿ Y

IOM: 100-02, 15, 110.1; 100-03, 4, 280.1

E0117 Crutch, underarm, articulating, spring assisted, each Ⓑ Qp Qh ♿ Y

IOM: 100-02, 15, 110.1

* **E0118** Crutch substitute, lower leg platform, with or without wheels, each Ⓑ Qp Qh E1

Walkers

E0130 Walker, rigid (pickup), adjustable or fixed height Ⓑ Qp Qh ♿ Y

Standard walker criteria for payment: Individual has a mobility limitation that significantly impairs ability to participate in mobility-related activities of daily living that cannot be adequately or safely addressed by a cane. The patient is able to use the walker safely; the functional mobility deficit can be resolved with use of a standard walker.

IOM: 100-02, 15, 110.1; 100-03, 4, 280.1

E0135 Walker, folding (pickup), adjustable or fixed height Ⓑ Qp Qh ♿ Y

IOM: 100-02, 15, 110.1; 100-03, 4, 280.1

E0140 Walker, with trunk support, adjustable or fixed height, any type Ⓑ Qp Qh ♿ Y

IOM: 100-02, 15, 110.1; 100-03, 4, 280.1

E0141 Walker, rigid, wheeled, adjustable or fixed height Ⓑ Qp Qh ♿ Y

IOM: 100-02, 15, 110.1; 100-03, 4, 280.1

E0143 Walker, folding, wheeled, adjustable or fixed height Ⓑ Qp Qh ♿ Y

IOM: 100-02, 15, 110.1; 100-03, 4, 280.1

E0144 Walker, enclosed, four sided framed, rigid or folding, wheeled, with posterior seat Ⓑ Qp Qh ♿ Y

IOM: 100-02, 15, 110.1; 100-03, 4, 280.1

E0147 Walker, heavy duty, multiple braking system, variable wheel resistance Ⓑ Qp Qh ♿ Y

Heavy-duty walker is labeled as capable of supporting more than 300 pounds

IOM: 100-02, 15, 110.1; 100-03, 4, 280.1

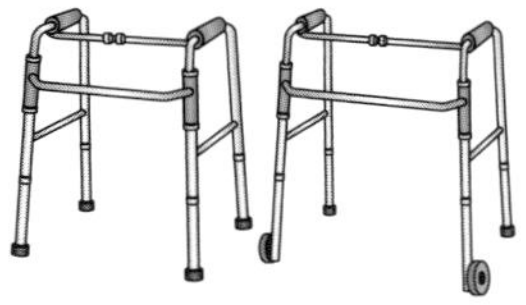

Figure 11 Walkers.

✻ **E0148** Walker, heavy duty, without wheels, rigid or folding, any type, each Ⓑ Qp Qh ♿ Y

Heavy-duty walker is labeled as capable of supporting more than 300 pounds

✻ **E0149** Walker, heavy duty, wheeled, rigid or folding, any type Ⓑ Qp Qh ♿ Y

Heavy-duty walker is labeled as capable of supporting more than 300 pounds

✻ **E0153** Platform attachment, forearm crutch, each Ⓑ Qp Qh ♿ Y

✻ **E0154** Platform attachment, walker, each Ⓑ Qp Qh ♿ Y

✻ **E0155** Wheel attachment, rigid pick-up walker, per pair Ⓑ Qp Qh ♿ Y

Attachments

✻ **E0156** Seat attachment, walker Ⓑ Qp Qh ♿ Y

✻ **E0157** Crutch attachment, walker, each Ⓑ Qp Qh ♿ Y

✻ **E0158** Leg extensions for walker, per set of four (4) Ⓑ Qp Qh ♿ Y

Leg extensions are considered medically necessary DME for patients 6 feet tall or more.

✻ **E0159** Brake attachment for wheeled walker, replacement, each Ⓑ Qp Qh ♿ Y

Sitz Bath/Equipment

E0160 Sitz type bath or equipment, portable, used with or without commode Ⓑ Qp Qh ♿ Y

IOM: 100-03, 4, 280.1

E0161 Sitz type bath or equipment, portable, used with or without commode, with faucet attachment/s Ⓑ Qp Qh ♿ Y

IOM: 100-03, 4, 280.1

E0162 Sitz bath chair Ⓑ Qp Qh ♿ Y

IOM: 100-03, 4, 280.1

Commodes

E0163 Commode chair, mobile or stationary, with fixed arms Ⓑ Qp Qh ♿ Y

IOM: 100-02, 15, 110.1; 100-03, 4, 280.1

E0165 Commode chair, mobile or stationary, with detachable arms Ⓑ Qp Qh ♿ Y

IOM: 100-02, 15, 110.1; 100-03, 4, 280.1

E0167 Pail or pan for use with commode chair, replacement only Ⓑ Qp Qh ♿ Y

IOM: 100-03, 4, 280.1

✻ **E0168** Commode chair, extra wide and/or heavy duty, stationary or mobile, with or without arms, any type, each Ⓑ Qp Qh ♿ Y

Extra-wide or heavy duty commode chair is labeled as capable of supporting more than 300 pounds

✻ **E0170** Commode chair with integrated seat lift mechanism, electric, any type Ⓑ Qp Qh ♿ Y

✻ **E0171** Commode chair with integrated seat lift mechanism, non-electric, any type Ⓑ Qp Qh ♿ Y

⊘ **E0172** Seat lift mechanism placed over or on top of toilet, any type Ⓑ Qp Qh E1

Medicare Statute 1861 SSA

✻ **E0175** Foot rest, for use with commode chair, each Ⓑ Qp Qh ♿ Y

Decubitus Care Equipment

E0181 Powered pressure reducing mattress overlay/pad, alternating, with pump, includes heavy duty Ⓑ Qp Qh ♿ Y

Requires the provider to determine medical necessity compliance. To demonstrate the requirements in the medical policy were met, attach KX.

IOM: 100-03, 4, 280.1; 100-08, 5, 5.2.3

E0182 Pump for alternating pressure pad, for replacement only Ⓑ Qp Qh ♿ Y

IOM: 100-03, 4, 280.1; 100-08, 5, 5.2.3

E0184 Dry pressure mattress Ⓑ Qp Qh ♿ Y

IOM: 100-03, 4, 280.1; 100-08, 5, 5.2.3

E0185 Gel or gel-like pressure pad for mattress, standard mattress length and width Ⓑ Qp Qh ♿ Y

IOM: 100-03, 4, 280.1; 100-08, 5, 5.2.3

E0186 Air pressure mattress Ⓑ Qp Qh ♿ Y

IOM: 100-03, 4, 280.1

E0187 Water pressure mattress Ⓑ Qp Qh ♿ Y

IOM: 100-03, 4, 280.1

E0188 Synthetic sheepskin pad Ⓑ Qp Qh ♿ Y

IOM: 100-03, 4, 280.1; 100-08, 5, 5.2.3

E0189 Lambswool sheepskin pad, any size Ⓑ Qp Qh ♿ Y

IOM: 100-03, 4, 280.1; 100-08, 5, 5.2.3

E0190 Positioning cushion/pillow/wedge, any shape or size, includes all components and accessories E1
IOM: 100-02, 15, 110.1

* **E0191** Heel or elbow protector, each Y

* **E0193** Powered air flotation bed (low air loss therapy) Y

E0194 Air fluidized bed Y
IOM: 100-03, 4, 280.1

E0196 Gel pressure mattress Y
IOM: 100-03, 4, 280.1

E0197 Air pressure pad for mattress, standard mattress length and width Y
IOM: 100-03, 4, 280.1

E0198 Water pressure pad for mattress, standard mattress length and width Y
IOM: 100-03, 4, 280.1

E0199 Dry pressure pad for mattress, standard mattress length and width Y
IOM: 100-03, 4, 280.1

Heat/Cold Application

E0200 Heat lamp, without stand (table model), includes bulb, or infrared element Y
Covered when medical review determines patient's medical condition is one for which application of heat by heat lamp is therapeutically effective
IOM: 100-02, 15, 110.1; 100-03, 4, 280.1

* **E0202** Phototherapy (bilirubin) light with photometer Y

⃠ **E0203** Therapeutic lightbox, minimum 10,000 lux, table top model E1
IOM: 100-03, 4, 280.1

E0205 Heat lamp, with stand, includes bulb, or infrared element Y
IOM: 100-02, 15, 110.1; 100-03, 4, 280.1

E0210 Electric heat pad, standard Y
Flexible device containing electric resistive elements producing heat; has fabric cover to prevent burns; with or without timing devices for automatic shut-off
IOM: 100-03, 4, 280.1

E0215 Electric heat pad, moist Y
Flexible device containing electric resistive elements producing heat. Must have component that will absorb and retain liquid (water).
IOM: 100-03, 4, 280.1

E0217 Water circulating heat pad with pump Y
Consists of flexible pad containing series of channels through which water is circulated by means of electrical pumping mechanism and heated in external reservoir
IOM: 100-03, 4, 280.1

E0218 Fluid circulating cold pad with pump, any type Y
IOM: 100-03, 4, 280.1

* **E0221** Infrared heating pad system Y

E0225 Hydrocollator unit, includes pads Y
IOM: 100-02, 15, 230; 100-03, 4, 280.1

⃠ **E0231** Non-contact wound warming device (temperature control unit, AC adapter and power cord) for use with warming card and wound cover E1
IOM: 100-02, 16, 20

⃠ **E0232** Warming card for use with the non-contact wound warming device and non-contact wound warming wound cover E1
IOM: 100-02, 16, 20

E0235 Paraffin bath unit, portable, (see medical supply code A4265 for paraffin) Y
Ordered by physician and patient's condition expected to be relieved by long-term use of modality
IOM: 100-02, 15, 230; 100-03, 4, 280.1

E0236 Pump for water circulating pad Y
IOM: 100-03, 4, 280.1

E0239 Hydrocollator unit, portable Y
IOM: 100-02, 15, 230; 100-03, 4, 280.1

Bath and Toilet Aids

⃠ **E0240** Bath/shower chair, with or without wheels, any size E1
IOM: 100-03, 4, 280.1

▶ New ↩ Revised ✔ Reinstated ~~deleted~~ Deleted ⃠ Not covered or valid by Medicare
Special coverage instructions * Carrier discretion Bill Part B MAC Bill DME MAC

⃠ **E0241** Bath tub wall rail, each ⓑ Qp Qh E1
IOM: 100-02, 15, 110.1; 100-03, 4, 280.1

⃠ **E0242** Bath tub rail, floor base ⓑ Qp Qh E1
IOM: 100-02, 15, 110.1; 100-03, 4, 280.1

⃠ **E0243** Toilet rail, each ⓑ Qp Qh E1
IOM: 100-02, 15, 110.1; 100-03, 4, 280.1

⃠ **E0244** Raised toilet seat ⓑ Qp Qh E1
IOM: 100-03, 4, 280.1

⃠ **E0245** Tub stool or bench ⓑ Qp Qh E1
IOM: 100-03, 4, 280.1

* **E0246** Transfer tub rail attachment ⓑ Qp Qh E1

E0247 Transfer bench for tub or toilet with or without commode opening ⓑ Qp Qh E1
IOM: 100-03, 4, 280.1

E0248 Transfer bench, heavy duty, for tub or toilet with or without commode opening ⓑ Qp Qh E1
Heavy duty transfer bench is labeled as capable of supporting more than 300 pounds
IOM: 100-03, 4, 280.1

Pad for Heating Unit

E0249 Pad for water circulating heat unit, for replacement only ⓑ Qp Qh ♿ Y
Describes durable replacement pad used with water circulating heat pump system
IOM: 100-03, 4, 280.1

Hospital Beds and Accessories

E0250 Hospital bed, fixed height, with any type side rails, with mattress ⓑ Qp Qh ♿ Y
IOM: 100-02, 15, 110.1; 100-03, 4, 280.7

E0251 Hospital bed, fixed height, with any type side rails, without mattress ⓑ Qp Qh ♿ Y
IOM: 100-02, 15, 110.1; 100-03, 4, 280.7

E0255 Hospital bed, variable height, hi-lo, with any type side rails, with mattress ⓑ Qp Qh ♿ Y
IOM: 100-02, 15, 110.1; 100-03, 4, 280.7

E0256 Hospital bed, variable height, hi-lo, with any type side rails, without mattress ⓑ Qp Qh ♿ Y
IOM: 100-02, 15, 110.1; 100-03, 4, 280.7

E0260 Hospital bed, semi-electric (head and foot adjustment), with any type side rails, with mattress ⓑ Qp Qh ♿ Y
IOM: 100-02, 15, 110.1; 100-03, 4, 280.7

E0261 Hospital bed, semi-electric (head and foot adjustment), with any type side rails, without mattress ⓑ Qp Qh ♿ Y
IOM: 100-02, 15, 110.1; 100-03, 4, 280.7

E0265 Hospital bed, total electric (head, foot and height adjustments), with any type side rails, with mattress ⓑ Qp Qh ♿ Y
IOM: 100-02, 15, 110.1; 100-03, 4, 280.7

E0266 Hospital bed, total electric (head, foot and height adjustments), with any type side rails, without mattress ⓑ Qp Qh ♿ Y
IOM: 100-02, 15, 110.1; 100-03, 4, 280.7

⃠ **E0270** Hospital bed, institutional type includes: oscillating, circulating and Stryker frame, with mattress ⓑ Qp Qh E1
IOM: 100-03, 4, 280.1

E0271 Mattress, innerspring ⓑ Qp Qh ♿ Y
IOM: 100-03, 4, 280.1; 100-03, 4, 280.7

E0272 Mattress, foam rubber ⓑ Qp Qh ♿ Y
IOM: 100-03, 4, 280.1; 100-03, 4, 280.7

⃠ **E0273** Bed board ⓑ Qp Qh E1
IOM: 100-03, 4, 280.1

⃠ **E0274** Over-bed table ⓑ Qp Qh E1
IOM: 100-03, 4, 280.1

E0275 Bed pan, standard, metal or plastic ⓑ Qp Qh ♿ Y
IOM: 100-03, 4, 280.1

E0276 Bed pan, fracture, metal or plastic ⓑ Qp Qh ♿ Y
IOM: 100-03, 4, 280.1

E0277 Powered pressure-reducing air mattress ⓑ Qp Qh ♿ Y
IOM: 100-03, 4, 280.1

* **E0280** Bed cradle, any type ⓑ Qp Qh ♿ Y

E0290 Hospital bed, fixed height, without side rails, with mattress ⓑ Qp Qh ♿ Y
IOM: 100-02, 15, 110.1; 100-03, 4, 280.7

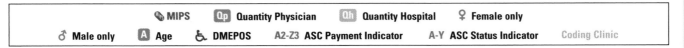

E0291 Hospital bed, fixed height, without side rails, without mattress Qp Qh Y
IOM: 100-02, 15, 110.1; 100-03, 4, 280.7

E0292 Hospital bed, variable height, hi-lo, without side rails, with mattress Qp Qh Y
IOM: 100-02, 15, 110.1; 100-03, 4, 280.7

E0293 Hospital bed, variable height, hi-lo, without side rails, without mattress Qp Qh Y
IOM: 100-02, 15, 110.1; 100-03, 4, 280.7

E0294 Hospital bed, semi-electric (head and foot adjustment), without side rails, with mattress Qp Qh Y
IOM: 100-02, 15, 110.1; 100-03, 4, 280.7

E0295 Hospital bed, semi-electric (head and foot adjustment), without side rails, without mattress Qp Qh Y
IOM: 100-02, 15, 110.1; 100-03, 4, 280.7

E0296 Hospital bed, total electric (head, foot and height adjustments), without side rails, with mattress Qp Qh Y
IOM: 100-02, 15, 110.1; 100-03, 4, 280.7

E0297 Hospital bed, total electric (head, foot and height adjustments), without side rails, without mattress Qp Qh Y
IOM: 100-02, 15, 110.1; 100-03, 4, 280.7

* **E0300** Pediatric crib, hospital grade, fully enclosed, with or without top enclosure Qp Qh A Y

E0301 Hospital bed, heavy duty, extra wide, with weight capacity greater than 350 pounds, but less than or equal to 600 pounds, with any type side rails, without mattress Qp Qh Y
IOM: 100-03, 4, 280.7

E0302 Hospital bed, extra heavy duty, extra wide, with weight capacity greater than 600 pounds, with any type side rails, without mattress Qp Qh Y
IOM: 100-03, 4, 280.7

E0303 Hospital bed, heavy duty, extra wide, with weight capacity greater than 350 pounds, but less than or equal to 600 pounds, with any type side rails, with mattress Qp Qh Y
IOM: 100-03, 4, 280.7

E0304 Hospital bed, extra heavy duty, extra wide, with weight capacity greater than 600 pounds, with any type side rails, with mattress Qp Qh Y
IOM: 100-03, 4, 280.7

E0305 Bed side rails, half length Qp Qh Y
IOM: 100-03, 4, 280.7

E0310 Bed side rails, full length Qp Qh Y
IOM: 100-03, 4, 280.7

⃠ **E0315** Bed accessory: board, table, or support device, any type Qp Qh E1
IOM: 100-03, 4, 280.1

* **E0316** Safety enclosure frame/canopy for use with hospital bed, any type Qp Qh Y

E0325 Urinal; male, jug-type, any material Qp Qh ♂ Y
IOM: 100-03, 4, 280.1

E0326 Urinal; female, jug-type, any material Qp Qh ♀ Y
IOM: 100-03, 4, 280.1

* **E0328** Hospital bed, pediatric, manual, 360 degree side enclosures, top of headboard, footboard and side rails up to 24 inches above the spring, includes mattress Qp Qh A Y

* **E0329** Hospital bed, pediatric, electric or semi-electric, 360 degree side enclosures, top of headboard, footboard and side rails up to 24 inches above the spring, includes mattress Qp Qh A Y

* **E0350** Control unit for electronic bowel irrigation/evacuation system Qp Qh E1

Pulsed Irrigation Enhanced Evacuation (PIEE) is pulsed irrigation of severely impacted fecal material and may be necessary for patients who have not responded to traditional bowel program.

* **E0352** Disposable pack (water reservoir bag, speculum, valving mechanism and collection bag/box) for use with the electronic bowel irrigation/evacuation system Qp Qh E1

Therapy kit includes 1 B-Valve circuit, 2 containment bags, 1 lubricating jelly, 1 bed pad, 1 tray liner-waste disposable bag, and 2 hose clamps

* **E0370** Air pressure elevator for heel Qp Qh E1

▶ New ↻ Revised ✔ Reinstated ~~deleted~~ Deleted ⃠ Not covered or valid by Medicare
Special coverage instructions * Carrier discretion Bill Part B MAC Bill DME MAC

* **E0371** Non powered advanced pressure reducing overlay for mattress, standard mattress length and width Ⓑ Qp Qh ♿ Y

  Patient has at least one large Stage III or Stage IV pressure sore (greater than 2 × 2 cm.) on trunk, with only two turning surfaces on which to lie

* **E0372** Powered air overlay for mattress, standard mattress length and width Ⓑ Qp Qh ♿ Y

* **E0373** Non powered advanced pressure reducing mattress Ⓑ Qp Qh ♿ Y

Oxygen and Related Respiratory Equipment

E0424 Stationary compressed gaseous oxygen system, rental; includes container, contents, regulator, flowmeter, humidifier, nebulizer, cannula or mask, and tubing Ⓑ Qp Qh ♿ Y

IOM: 100-03, 4, 280.1; 100-04, 20, 30.6

E0425 Stationary compressed gas system, purchase; includes regulator, flowmeter, humidifier, nebulizer, cannula or mask, and tubing Ⓑ Qp Qh E1

IOM: 100-03, 4, 280.1; 100-04, 20, 30.6

E0430 Portable gaseous oxygen system, purchase; includes regulator, flowmeter, humidifier, cannula or mask, and tubing Ⓑ Qp Qh E1

IOM: 100-03, 4, 280.1; 100-04, 20, 30.6

E0431 Portable gaseous oxygen system, rental; includes portable container, regulator, flowmeter, humidifier, cannula or mask, and tubing Ⓑ Qp Qh ♿ Y

IOM: 100-03, 4, 280.1; 100-04, 20, 30.6

* **E0433** Portable liquid oxygen system, rental; home liquefier used to fill portable liquid oxygen containers, includes portable containers, regulator, flowmeter, humidifier, cannula or mask and tubing, with or without supply reservoir and contents gauge Ⓑ Qh ♿ Y

E0434 Portable liquid oxygen system, rental; includes portable container, supply reservoir, humidifier, flowmeter, refill adaptor, contents gauge, cannula or mask, and tubing Ⓑ Qp Qh ♿ Y

Fee schedule payments for stationary oxygen system rentals are all-inclusive and represent monthly allowance for beneficiary. Non-Medicare payers may rent device to beneficiaries, or arrange for purchase of device.

IOM: 100-03, 4, 280.1; 100-04, 20, 30.6

E0435 Portable liquid oxygen system, purchase; includes portable container, supply reservoir, flowmeter, humidifier, contents gauge, cannula or mask, tubing and refill adaptor Ⓑ Qp Qh E1

IOM: 100-03, 4, 280.1; 100-04, 20, 30.6

E0439 Stationary liquid oxygen system, rental; includes container, contents, regulator, flowmeter, humidifier, nebulizer, cannula or mask, and tubing Ⓑ Qp Qh ♿ Y

This allowance includes payment for equipment, contents, and accessories furnished during rental month

IOM: 100-03, 4, 280.1; 100-04, 20, 30.6

E0440 Stationary liquid oxygen system, purchase; includes use of reservoir, contents indicator, regulator, flowmeter, humidifier, nebulizer, cannula or mask, and tubing Ⓑ Qp Qh E1

IOM: 100-03, 4, 280.1; 100-04, 20, 30.6

E0441 Stationary oxygen contents, gaseous, 1 month's supply = 1 unit Ⓑ Qp Qh ♿ Y

IOM: 100-03, 4, 280.1; 100-04, 20, 30.6

E0442 Stationary oxygen contents, liquid, 1 month's supply = 1 unit Ⓑ Qp Qh ♿ Y

IOM: 100-03, 4, 280.1; 100-04, 20, 30.6

E0443 Portable oxygen contents, gaseous, 1 month's supply = 1 unit Ⓑ Qp Qh ♿ Y

IOM: 100-03, 4, 280.1; 100-04, 20, 30.6

E0444 Portable oxygen contents, liquid, 1 month's supply = 1 unit Ⓑ Qp Qh ♿ Y

IOM: 100-03, 4, 280.1; 100-04, 20, 30.6

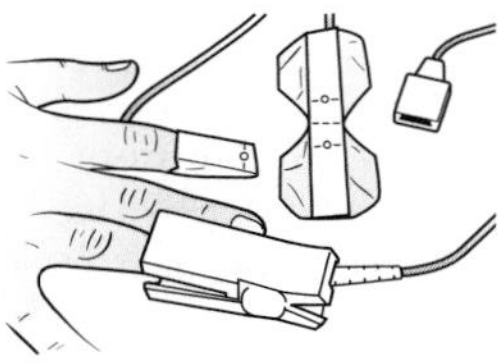

Figure 12 Oximeter device.

✻ **E0445** Oximeter device for measuring blood oxygen levels non-invasively Ⓑ Qp Qh N

✻ **E0446** Topical oxygen delivery system, not otherwise specified, includes all supplies and accessories Ⓑ Qp Qh A

▶ ◌ **E0447** Portable oxygen contents, liquid, 1 month's supply = 1 unit, prescribed amount at rest or nighttime exceeds 4 liters per minute (lpm) Y

◌ **E0455** Oxygen tent, excluding croup or pediatric tents Ⓑ Qp Qh Y

IOM: 100-03, 4, 280.1; 100-04, 20, 30.6

⃠ **E0457** Chest shell (cuirass) Ⓑ Qp Qh E1

⃠ **E0459** Chest wrap Ⓑ Qp Qh E1

✻ **E0462** Rocking bed with or without side rails Ⓑ Qp Qh ♿ Y

◌ **E0465** Home ventilator, any type, used with invasive interface (e.g., tracheostomy tube) Ⓑ Qp Qh ♿ Y

IOM: 100-03, 4, 280.1

◌ **E0466** Home ventilator, any type, used with non-invasive interface (e.g., mask, chest shell) Ⓑ Qp Qh ♿ Y

IOM: 100-03, 4, 280.1

▶ ◌ **E0467** Home ventilator, multi-function respiratory device, also performs any or all of the additional functions of oxygen concentration, drug nebulization, aspiration, and cough stimulation, includes all accessories, components and supplies for all functions Y

◌ **E0470** Respiratory assist device, bi-level pressure capability, without backup rate feature, used with noninvasive interface, e.g., nasal or facial mask (intermittent assist device with continuous positive airway pressure device) Ⓑ Qp Qh ♿ Y

IOM: 100-03, 4, 240.2

◌ **E0471** Respiratory assist device, bi-level pressure capability, with back-up rate feature, used with noninvasive interface, e.g., nasal or facial mask (intermittent assist device with continuous positive airway pressure device) Ⓑ Qp Qh ♿ Y

IOM: 100-03, 4, 240.2

◌ **E0472** Respiratory assist device, bi-level pressure capability, with backup rate feature, used with invasive interface, e.g., tracheostomy tube (intermittent assist device with continuous positive airway pressure device) Ⓑ Qp Qh ♿ Y

IOM: 100-03, 4, 240.2

◌ **E0480** Percussor, electric or pneumatic, home model Ⓑ Qp Qh ♿ Y

IOM: 100-03, 4, 240.2

⃠ **E0481** Intrapulmonary percussive ventilation system and related accessories Ⓑ Qp Qh E1

IOM: 100-03, 4, 240.2

✻ **E0482** Cough stimulating device, alternating positive and negative airway pressure Ⓑ Qp Qh ♿ Y

↩ ✻ **E0483** High frequency chest wall oscillation system, includes all accessories and supplies, each Ⓑ Qp Qh ♿ Y

✻ **E0484** Oscillatory positive expiratory pressure device, non-electric, any type, each Ⓑ Qp Qh ♿ Y

✻ **E0485** Oral device/appliance used to reduce upper airway collapsibility, adjustable or non-adjustable, prefabricated, includes fitting and adjustment Ⓑ Qp Qh ♿ Y

✻ **E0486** Oral device/appliance used to reduce upper airway collapsibility, adjustable or non-adjustable, custom fabricated, includes fitting and adjustment Ⓑ Qp Qh ♿ Y

◌ **E0487** Spirometer, electronic, includes all accessories Ⓑ Qp Qh N

IPPB Machines

◌ **E0500** IPPB machine, all types, with built-in nebulization; manual or automatic valves; internal or external power source Ⓑ Qp Qh ♿ Y

IOM: 100-03, 4, 240.2

Humidifiers/Nebulizers/Compressors for Use with Oxygen IPPB Equipment

◌ **E0550** Humidifier, durable for extensive supplemental humidification during IPPB treatments or oxygen delivery Ⓑ Qp Qh ♿ Y

IOM: 100-03, 4, 240.2

◌ **E0555** Humidifier, durable, glass or autoclavable plastic bottle type, for use with regulator or flowmeter Ⓑ Qp Qh Y

IOM: 100-03, 4, 280.1; 100-04, 20, 30.6

◌ **E0560** Humidifier, durable for supplemental humidification during IPPB treatment or oxygen delivery Ⓑ Qp Qh ♿ Y

IOM: 100-03, 4, 280.1

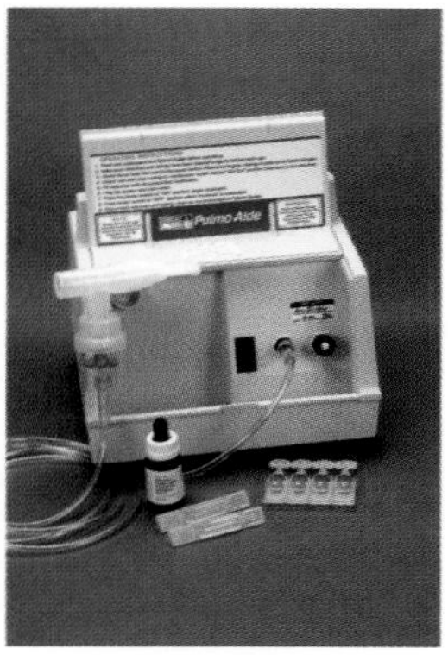

Figure 13 Nebulizer

* **E0561** Humidifier, non-heated, used with positive airway pressure device Ⓑ Qp Qh ♿ Y
* **E0562** Humidifier, heated, used with positive airway pressure device Ⓑ Qp Qh ♿ Y
* **E0565** Compressor, air power source for equipment which is not self-contained or cylinder driven Ⓑ Qp Qh ♿ Y
* **E0570** Nebulizer, with compressor Ⓑ Qp Qh ♿ Y
  IOM: 100-03, 4, 240.2; 100-03, 4, 280.1
* **E0572** Aerosol compressor, adjustable pressure, light duty for intermittent use Ⓑ Qp Qh ♿ Y
* **E0574** Ultrasonic/electronic aerosol generator with small volume nebulizer Ⓑ Qp Qh ♿ Y
* **E0575** Nebulizer, ultrasonic, large volume Ⓑ Qp Qh ♿ Y
  IOM: 100-03, 4, 240.2
* **E0580** Nebulizer, durable, glass or autoclavable plastic, bottle type, for use with regulator or flowmeter Ⓑ Qp Qh ♿ Y
  IOM: 100-03, 4, 240.2; 100-03, 4, 280.1
* **E0585** Nebulizer, with compressor and heater Ⓑ Qp Qh ♿ Y
  IOM: 100-03, 4, 240.2; 100-03, 4, 280.1

Suction Pump/CPAP

* **E0600** Respiratory suction pump, home model, portable or stationary, electric Ⓑ Qp Qh ♿ Y
  IOM: 100-03, 4, 240.2
* **E0601** Continuous positive airway pressure (CPAP) device Ⓑ Qp Qh ♿ Y
  IOM: 100-03, 4, 240.4

Breast Pump

* **E0602** Breast pump, manual, any type Ⓑ Qp Qh ♀ ♿ Y
  Bill either manual breast pump or breast pump kit
* **E0603** Breast pump, electric (AC and/or DC), any type Ⓑ Qp Qh ♀ N
* **E0604** Breast pump, hospital grade, electric (AC and/or DC), any type Ⓑ Qp Qh ♀ A

Other Breathing Aids

* **E0605** Vaporizer, room type Ⓑ Qp Qh ♿ Y
  IOM: 100-03, 4, 240.2
* **E0606** Postural drainage board Ⓑ Qp Qh ♿ Y
  IOM: 100-03, 4, 240.2

Monitoring Equipment

* **E0607** Home blood glucose monitor Ⓑ Qp Qh ♿ Y
  Document recipient or caregiver is competent to monitor equipment and that device is designed for home rather than clinical use
  IOM: 100-03, 4, 280.1; 100-03, 1, 40.2
* **E0610** Pacemaker monitor, self-contained, (checks battery depletion, includes audible and visible check systems) Ⓑ Qp Qh ♿ Y
  IOM: 100-03, 1, 20.8
* **E0615** Pacemaker monitor, self-contained, checks battery depletion and other pacemaker components, includes digital/visible check systems Ⓑ Qp Qh ♿ Y
  IOM: 100-03, 1, 20.8
* **E0616** Implantable cardiac event recorder with memory, activator and programmer Ⓟ Qp Qh N
  Assign when two 30-day pre-symptom external loop recordings fail to establish a definitive diagnosis.

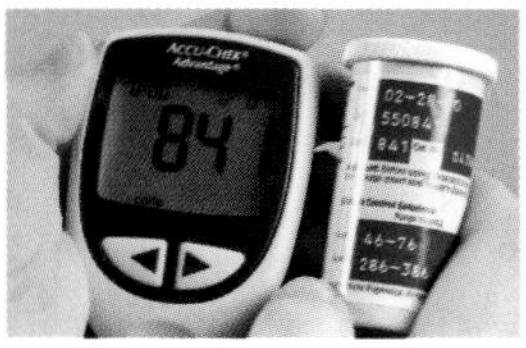

Figure 14 Glucose monitor.

* **E0617** External defibrillator with integrated electrocardiogram analysis Ⓑ Qp Qh ♿ Y
* **E0618** Apnea monitor, without recording feature Ⓑ Qp Qh ♿ Y
* **E0619** Apnea monitor, with recording feature Ⓑ Qp Qh ♿ Y
* **E0620** Skin piercing device for collection of capillary blood, laser, each Ⓑ Qp Qh ♿ Y

Patient Lifts

E0621 Sling or seat, patient lift, canvas or nylon Ⓑ Qp Qh ♿ Y

IOM: 100-03, 4, 240.2, 280.4

⊘ **E0625** Patient lift, bathroom or toilet, not otherwise classified Ⓑ Qp Qh E1

IOM: 100-03, 4, 240.2

E0627 Seat lift mechanism, electric, any type Ⓑ Qp Qh ♿ Y

IOM: 100-03, 4, 280.4; 100-04, 4, 20

E0629 Seat lift mechanism, non-electric, any type Ⓑ Qp Qh ♿ Y

IOM: 100-04, 4, 20

E0630 Patient lift, hydraulic or mechanical, includes any seat, sling, strap(s) or pad(s) Ⓑ Qp Qh ♿ Y

IOM: 100-03, 4, 240.2

E0635 Patient lift, electric, with seat or sling Ⓑ Qp Qh ♿ Y

IOM: 100-03, 4, 240.2

* **E0636** Multipositional patient support system, with integrated lift, patient accessible controls Ⓑ Qp Qh ♿ Y

⊘ **E0637** Combination sit to stand frame/table system, any size including pediatric, with seat lift feature, with or without wheels Ⓑ Qp Qh E1

IOM: 100-03, 4, 240.2

⊘ **E0638** Standing frame/table system, one position (e.g., upright, supine or prone stander), any size including pediatric, with or without wheels Ⓑ Qp Qh E1

IOM: 100-03, 4, 240.2

* **E0639** Patient lift, moveable from room to room with disassembly and reassembly, includes all components/accessories Ⓑ Qp Qh ♿ E1
* **E0640** Patient lift, fixed system, includes all components/accessories Ⓑ Qp Qh ♿ E1

⊘ **E0641** Standing frame/table system, multi-position (e.g., three-way stander), any size including pediatric, with or without wheels Ⓑ Qp Qh E1

IOM: 100-03, 4, 240.2

⊘ **E0642** Standing frame/table system, mobile (dynamic stander), any size including pediatric Ⓑ Qp Qh E1

IOM: 100-03, 4, 240.2

Pneumatic Compressor and Appliances

E0650 Pneumatic compressor, non-segmental home model Ⓑ Qp Qh ♿ Y

Lymphedema pumps are classified as segmented or nonsegmented, depending on whether distinct segments of devices can be inflated sequentially.

IOM: 100-03, 4, 280.6

E0651 Pneumatic compressor, segmental home model without calibrated gradient pressure Ⓑ Qp Qh ♿ Y

IOM: 100-03, 4, 280.6

E0652 Pneumatic compressor, segmental home model with calibrated gradient pressure Ⓑ Qp Qh ♿ Y

IOM: 100-03, 4, 280.6

E0655 Non-segmental pneumatic appliance for use with pneumatic compressor, half arm Ⓑ Qp Qh ♿ Y

IOM: 100-03, 4, 280.6

E0656 Segmental pneumatic appliance for use with pneumatic compressor, trunk Ⓑ Qp Qh ♿ Y

E0657 Segmental pneumatic appliance for use with pneumatic compressor, chest Ⓑ Qp Qh ♿ Y

E0660 Non-segmental pneumatic appliance for use with pneumatic compressor, full leg Ⓑ Qp Qh ♿ Y

IOM: 100-03, 4, 280.6

E0665 Non-segmental pneumatic appliance for use with pneumatic compressor, full arm Ⓑ Qp Qh ♿ Y

IOM: 100-03, 4, 280.6

E0666 Non-segmental pneumatic appliance for use with pneumatic compressor, half leg Ⓑ Qp Qh ♿ Y

IOM: 100-03, 4, 280.6

▶ New ↩ Revised ✔ Reinstated ~~deleted~~ Deleted ⊘ Not covered or valid by Medicare
Special coverage instructions * Carrier discretion Ⓑ Bill Part B MAC Ⓑ Bill DME MAC

E0667 Segmental pneumatic appliance for use with pneumatic compressor, full leg Qp Qh Y
IOM: 100-03, 4, 280.6

E0668 Segmental pneumatic appliance for use with pneumatic compressor, full arm Qp Qh Y
IOM: 100-03, 4, 280.6

E0669 Segmental pneumatic appliance for use with pneumatic compressor, half leg Qp Qh Y
IOM: 100-03, 4, 280.6

E0670 Segmental pneumatic appliance for use with pneumatic compressor, integrated, 2 full legs and trunk Qp Qh Y
IOM: 100-03, 4, 280.6

E0671 Segmental gradient pressure pneumatic appliance, full leg Qp Qh Y
IOM: 100-03, 4, 280.6

E0672 Segmental gradient pressure pneumatic appliance, full arm Qp Qh Y
IOM: 100-03, 4, 280.6

E0673 Segmental gradient pressure pneumatic appliance, half leg Qp Qh Y
IOM: 100-03, 4, 280.6

* E0675 Pneumatic compression device, high pressure, rapid inflation/deflation cycle, for arterial insufficiency (unilateral or bilateral system) Qp Qh Y

* E0676 Intermittent limb compression device (includes all accessories), not otherwise specified Qp Qh Y

Ultraviolet Light Therapy Systems

* E0691 Ultraviolet light therapy system, includes bulbs/lamps, timer and eye protection; treatment area 2 square feet or less Qp Qh Y

* E0692 Ultraviolet light therapy system panel, includes bulbs/lamps, timer and eye protection, 4 foot panel Qp Qh Y

* E0693 Ultraviolet light therapy system panel, includes bulbs/lamps, timer and eye protection, 6 foot panel Qp Qh Y

* E0694 Ultraviolet multidirectional light therapy system in 6 foot cabinet, includes bulbs/lamps, timer and eye protection Qp Qh Y

Safety Equipment

* E0700 Safety equipment, device or accessory, any type Qp Qh E1

E0705 Transfer device, any type, each Qp Qh B

Restraints

* E0710 Restraints, any type (body, chest, wrist or ankle) Qp Qh E1

Transcutaneous and/or Neuromuscular Electrical Nerve Stimulators (TENS)

E0720 Transcutaneous electrical nerve stimulation (TENS) device, two lead, localized stimulation Qp Qh Y
A Certificate of Medical Necessity (CMN) is not needed for a TENS rental, but is needed purchase.
IOM: 100-03, 2, 160.2; 100-03, 4, 280.1

E0730 Transcutaneous electrical nerve stimulation (TENS) device, four or more leads, for multiple nerve stimulation Qp Qh Y
IOM: 100-03, 2, 160.2; 100-03, 4, 280.1

E0731 Form fitting conductive garment for delivery of TENS or NMES (with conductive fibers separated from the patient's skin by layers of fabric) Qp Qh Y
IOM: 100-03, 2, 160.13

E0740 Non-implanted pelvic floor electrical stimulator, complete system Qp Qh Y
IOM: 100-03, 4, 230.8

* E0744 Neuromuscular stimulator for scoliosis Qp Qh Y

E0745 Neuromuscular stimulator, electronic shock unit Qp Qh Y
IOM: 100-03, 2, 160.12

E0746 Electromyography (EMG), biofeedback device Qp Qh N
IOM: 100-03, 1, 30.1

E0747 Osteogenesis stimulator, electrical, non-invasive, other than spinal applications Y

Devices are composed of two basic parts: Coils that wrap around cast and pulse generator that produces electric current

E0748 Osteogenesis stimulator, electrical, non-invasive, spinal applications Y

Device should be applied within 30 days as adjunct to spinal fusion surgery

E0749 Osteogenesis stimulator, electrical, surgically implanted N

* **E0755** Electronic salivary reflex stimulator (intra-oral/non-invasive) E1

* **E0760** Osteogenesis stimulator, low intensity ultrasound, non-invasive Y

Ultrasonic osteogenesis stimulator may not be used concurrently with other noninvasive stimulators

E0761 Non-thermal pulsed high frequency radiowaves, high peak power electromagnetic energy treatment device E1

* **E0762** Transcutaneous electrical joint stimulation device system, includes all accessories B

E0764 Functional neuromuscular stimulator, transcutaneous stimulation of sequential muscle groups of ambulation with computer control, used for walking by spinal cord injured, entire system, after completion of training program Y

IOM: 100-03, 2, 160.12

* **E0765** FDA approved nerve stimulator, with replaceable batteries, for treatment of nausea and vomiting Y

* **E0766** Electrical stimulation device used for cancer treatment, includes all accessories, any type Y

E0769 Electrical stimulation or electromagnetic wound treatment device, not otherwise classified B

IOM: 100-04, 32, 11.1

E0770 Functional electrical stimulator, transcutaneous stimulation of nerve and/or muscle groups, any type, complete system, not otherwise specified Y

Infusion Supplies

* **E0776** IV pole Y

PEN: On Fee Schedule

* **E0779** Ambulatory infusion pump, mechanical, reusable, for infusion 8 hours or greater Y

Requires prior authorization and copy of invoice

This is a capped rental infusion pump modifier. The correct monthly modifier (KH, KI, KJ) is used to indicate which month the rental is for (i.e., KH, month 1; KI, months 2 and 3; KJ, months 4 through 13).

* **E0780** Ambulatory infusion pump, mechanical, reusable, for infusion less than 8 hours Y

Requires prior authorization and copy of invoice

E0781 Ambulatory infusion pump, single or multiple channels, electric or battery operated with administrative equipment, worn by patient Y

IOM: 100-03, 1, 50.3

E0782 Infusion pump, implantable, non-programmable (includes all components, e.g., pump, cathether, connectors, etc.) N

IOM: 100-03, 1, 50.3

E0783 Infusion pump system, implantable, programmable (includes all components, e.g., pump, catheter, connectors, etc.) N

IOM: 100-03, 1, 50.3

E0784 External ambulatory infusion pump, insulin Y

IOM: 100-03, 4, 280.14

E0785 Implantable intraspinal (epidural/intrathecal) catheter used with implantable infusion pump, replacement N

IOM: 100-03, 1, 50.3

E0786 Implantable programmable infusion pump, replacement (excludes implantable intraspinal catheter) N

IOM: 100-03, 1, 50.3

E0791 Parenteral infusion pump, stationary, single or multi-channel Y

IOM: 100-02, 15, 120; 100-03, 3, 180.2; 100-04, 20, 100.2.2

▶ New ↩ Revised ✔ Reinstated ~~deleted~~ Deleted ⊘ Not covered or valid by Medicare
Special coverage instructions * Carrier discretion Bill Part B MAC Bill DME MAC

Traction Equipment and Orthopedic Devices

E0830 Ambulatory traction device, all types, each Ⓑ Qp Qh N
IOM: 100-03, 4, 280.1

E0840 Traction frame, attached to headboard, cervical traction Ⓑ Qp Qh ♿ Y
IOM: 100-03, 4, 280.1

* **E0849** Traction equipment, cervical, free-standing stand/frame, pneumatic, applying traction force to other than mandible Ⓑ Qp Qh ♿ Y

E0850 Traction stand, free standing, cervical traction Ⓑ Qp Qh ♿ Y
IOM: 100-03, 4, 280.1

* **E0855** Cervical traction equipment not requiring additional stand or frame Ⓑ Qp Qh ♿ Y

* **E0856** Cervical traction device, with inflatable air bladder(s) Ⓑ Qp Qh ♿ Y

E0860 Traction equipment, overdoor, cervical Ⓑ Qp Qh ♿ Y
IOM: 100-03, 4, 280.1

E0870 Traction frame, attached to footboard, extremity traction, (e.g., Buck's) Ⓑ Qp Qh ♿ Y
IOM: 100-03, 4, 280.1

E0880 Traction stand, free standing, extremity traction (e.g., Buck's) Ⓑ Qp Qh ♿ Y
IOM: 100-03, 4, 280.1

E0890 Traction frame, attached to footboard, pelvic traction Ⓑ Qp Qh ♿ Y
IOM: 100-03, 4, 280.1

E0900 Traction stand, free standing, pelvic traction (e.g., Buck's) Ⓑ Qp Qh ♿ Y
IOM: 100-03, 4, 280.1

E0910 Trapeze bars, A/K/A patient helper, attached to bed, with grab bar Ⓑ Qp Qh ♿ Y
IOM: 100-03, 4, 280.1

E0911 Trapeze bar, heavy duty, for patient weight capacity greater than 250 pounds, attached to bed, with grab bar Ⓑ Qp Qh ♿ Y
IOM: 100-03, 4, 280.1

E0912 Trapeze bar, heavy duty, for patient weight capacity greater than 250 pounds, free standing, complete with grab bar Ⓑ Qp Qh ♿ Y
IOM: 100-03, 4, 280.1

E0920 Fracture frame, attached to bed, includes weights Ⓑ Qp Qh ♿ Y
IOM: 100-03, 4, 280.1

E0930 Fracture frame, free standing, includes weights Ⓑ Qp Qh ♿ Y
IOM: 100-03, 4, 280.1

E0935 Continuous passive motion exercise device for use on knee only Ⓑ Qp Qh ♿ Y
To qualify for coverage, use of device must commence within two days following surgery
IOM: 100-03, 4, 280.1

⊘ **E0936** Continuous passive motion exercise device for use other than knee Ⓑ Qp Qh E1

E0940 Trapeze bar, free standing, complete with grab bar Ⓑ Qp Qh ♿ Y
IOM: 100-03, 4, 280.1

E0941 Gravity assisted traction device, any type Ⓑ Qp Qh ♿ Y
IOM: 100-03, 4, 280.1

* **E0942** Cervical head harness/halter Ⓑ Qp Qh ♿ Y

* **E0944** Pelvic belt/harness/boot Ⓑ Qp Qh ♿ Y

* **E0945** Extremity belt/harness Ⓑ Qp Qh ♿ Y

E0946 Fracture, frame, dual with cross bars, attached to bed (e.g., Balken, 4 poster) Ⓑ Qp Qh ♿ Y
IOM: 100-03, 4, 280.1

E0947 Fracture frame, attachments for complex pelvic traction Ⓑ Qp Qh ♿ Y
IOM: 100-03, 4, 280.1

E0948 Fracture frame, attachments for complex cervical traction Ⓑ Qp Qh ♿ Y
IOM: 100-03, 4, 280.1

Wheelchair Accessories

E0950 Wheelchair accessory, tray, each Ⓑ Qp Qh ♿ Y
IOM: 100-03, 4, 280.1

* **E0951** Heel loop/holder, any type, with or without ankle strap, each Ⓑ Qp Qh ♿ Y

E0952 Toe loop/holder, any type, each Ⓑ Qp Qh ♿ Y
IOM: 100-03, 4, 280.1

✻ **E0953** Wheelchair accessory, lateral thigh or knee support, any type, including fixed mounting hardware, each Y

✻ **E0954** Wheelchair accessory, foot box, any type, includes attachment and mounting hardware, each foot Y

✻ **E0955** Wheelchair accessory, headrest, cushioned, any type, including fixed mounting hardware, each Ⓑ Qp Qh ♿ Y

✻ **E0956** Wheelchair accessory, lateral trunk or hip support, any type, including fixed mounting hardware, each Ⓑ Qp Qh ♿ Y

✻ **E0957** Wheelchair accessory, medial thigh support, any type, including fixed mounting hardware, each Ⓑ Qp Qh ♿ Y

E0958 Manual wheelchair accessory, one-arm drive attachment, each Ⓑ Qp Qh ♿ Y

IOM: 100-03, 4, 280.1

✻ **E0959** Manual wheelchair accessory, adapter for amputee, each Ⓑ Qp Qh ♿ B

IOM: 100-03, 4, 280.1

✻ **E0960** Wheelchair accessory, shoulder harness/straps or chest strap, including any type mounting hardware Ⓑ Qp Qh ♿ Y

✻ **E0961** Manual wheelchair accessory, wheel lock brake extension (handle), each Ⓑ Qp Qh ♿ B

IOM: 100-03, 4, 280.1

✻ **E0966** Manual wheelchair accessory, headrest extension, each Ⓑ Qp Qh ♿ B

IOM: 100-03, 4, 280.1

E0967 Manual wheelchair accessory, hand rim with projections, any type, replacement only, each Ⓑ Qp Qh ♿ Y

IOM: 100-03, 4, 280.1

E0968 Commode seat, wheelchair Ⓑ Qp Qh ♿ Y

IOM: 100-03, 4, 280.1

E0969 Narrowing device, wheelchair Ⓑ ♿ Y

IOM: 100-03, 4, 280.1

⊘ **E0970** No. 2 footplates, except for elevating leg rest Ⓑ Qp Qh E1

IOM: 100-03, 4, 280.1

Cross Reference K0037, K0042

✻ **E0971** Manual wheelchair accessory, anti-tipping device, each Ⓑ Qp Qh ♿ B

IOM: 100-03, 4, 280.1

Cross Reference K0021

E0973 Wheelchair accessory, adjustable height, detachable armrest, complete assembly, each Ⓑ Qp Qh ♿ B

IOM: 100-03, 4, 280.1

E0974 Manual wheelchair accessory, anti-rollback device, each Ⓑ Qp Qh ♿ B

IOM: 100-03, 4, 280.1

✻ **E0978** Wheelchair accessory, positioning belt/safety belt/pelvic strap, each Ⓑ Qp Qh ♿ B

✻ **E0980** Safety vest, wheelchair Ⓑ ♿ Y

✻ **E0981** Wheelchair accessory, seat upholstery, replacement only, each Ⓑ Qp Qh ♿ Y

✻ **E0982** Wheelchair accessory, back upholstery, replacement only, each Ⓑ Qp Qh ♿ Y

✻ **E0983** Manual wheelchair accessory, power add-on to convert manual wheelchair to motorized wheelchair, joystick control Ⓑ Qp Qh ♿ Y

✻ **E0984** Manual wheelchair accessory, power add-on to convert manual wheelchair to motorized wheelchair, tiller control Ⓑ Qp Qh ♿ Y

✻ **E0985** Wheelchair accessory, seat lift mechanism Ⓑ Qp Qh ♿ Y

✻ **E0986** Manual wheelchair accessory, push-rim activated power assist system Ⓑ Qp Qh ♿ Y

✻ **E0988** Manual wheelchair accessory, lever-activated, wheel drive, pair Ⓑ Qp Qh ♿ Y

✻ **E0990** Wheelchair accessory, elevating leg rest, complete assembly, each Ⓑ Qp Qh ♿ B

IOM: 100-03, 4, 280.1

✻ **E0992** Manual wheelchair accessory, solid seat insert Ⓑ Qp Qh ♿ B

E0994 Arm rest, each Ⓑ Qp Qh ♿ Y

IOM: 100-03, 4, 280.1

✻ **E0995** Wheelchair accessory, calf rest/pad, replacement only, each Ⓑ Qp Qh ♿ B

IOM: 100-03, 4, 280.1

✻ **E1002** Wheelchair accessory, power seating system, tilt only Ⓑ Qp Qh ♿ Y

* **E1003** Wheelchair accessory, power seating system, recline only, without shear reduction Ⓑ Qp Qh ♿ Y

* **E1004** Wheelchair accessory, power seating system, recline only, with mechanical shear reduction Ⓑ Qp Qh ♿ Y

* **E1005** Wheelchair accessory, power seating system, recline only, with power shear reduction Ⓑ Qp Qh ♿ Y

* **E1006** Wheelchair accessory, power seating system, combination tilt and recline, without shear reduction Ⓑ Qp Qh ♿ Y

* **E1007** Wheelchair accessory, power seating system, combination tilt and recline, with mechanical shear reduction Ⓑ Qp Qh ♿ Y

* **E1008** Wheelchair accessory, power seating system, combination tilt and recline, with power shear reduction Ⓑ Qp Qh ♿ Y

* **E1009** Wheelchair accessory, addition to power seating system, mechanically linked leg elevation system, including pushrod and leg rest, each Ⓑ Qp Qh ♿ Y

* **E1010** Wheelchair accessory, addition to power seating system, power leg elevation system, including leg rest, pair Ⓑ Qp Qh ♿ Y

○ **E1011** Modification to pediatric size wheelchair, width adjustment package (not to be dispensed with initial chair) Ⓑ Qp Qh A ♿ Y

IOM: 100-03, 4, 280.1

* **E1012** Wheelchair accessory, addition to power seating system, center mount power elevating leg rest/platform, complete system, any type, each Qp Qh ♿ Y

○ **E1014** Reclining back, addition to pediatric size wheelchair Ⓑ Qp Qh A ♿ Y

IOM: 100-03, 4, 280.1

○ **E1015** Shock absorber for manual wheelchair, each Ⓑ Qp Qh ♿ Y

IOM: 100-03, 4, 280.1

○ **E1016** Shock absorber for power wheelchair, each Ⓑ Qp Qh ♿ Y

IOM: 100-03, 4, 280.1

○ **E1017** Heavy duty shock absorber for heavy duty or extra heavy duty manual wheelchair, each Ⓑ Qp Qh ♿ Y

IOM: 100-03, 4, 280.1

○ **E1018** Heavy duty shock absorber for heavy duty or extra heavy duty power wheelchair, each Ⓑ Qp Qh ♿ Y

IOM: 100-03, 4, 280.1

○ **E1020** Residual limb support system for wheelchair, any type Ⓑ Qp Qh ♿ Y

IOM: 100-03, 3, 280.3

* **E1028** Wheelchair accessory, manual swing-away, retractable or removable mounting hardware for joystick, other control interface or positioning accessory Ⓑ Qp Qh ♿ Y

* **E1029** Wheelchair accessory, ventilator tray, fixed Ⓑ Qp Qh ♿ Y

* **E1030** Wheelchair accessory, ventilator tray, gimbaled Ⓑ Qp Qh ♿ Y

Rollabout Chair, Transfer System, Transport Chair

○ **E1031** Rollabout chair, any and all types with casters 5" or greater Ⓑ Qp Qh ♿ Y

IOM: 100- 03, 4, 280.1

○ **E1035** Multi-positional patient transfer system, with integrated seat, operated by care giver, patient weight capacity up to and including 300 lbs Ⓑ Qp Qh ♿ Y

IOM: 100-02, 15, 110

* **E1036** Multi-positional patient transfer system, extra-wide, with integrated seat, operated by caregiver, patient weight capacity greater than 300 lbs Ⓑ Qh ♿ Y

○ **E1037** Transport chair, pediatric size Ⓑ Qp Qh A ♿ Y

IOM: 100-03, 4, 280.1

○ **E1038** Transport chair, adult size, patient weight capacity up to and including 300 pounds Ⓑ Qp Qh A ♿ Y

IOM: 100-03, 4, 280.1

* **E1039** Transport chair, adult size, heavy duty, patient weight capacity greater than 300 pounds Ⓑ Qp Qh A ♿ Y

Wheelchair: Fully Reclining

○ **E1050** Fully-reclining wheelchair, fixed full length arms, swing away detachable elevating leg rests Ⓑ Qp Qh ♿ Y

IOM: 100-03, 4, 280.1

MIPS | Qp Quantity Physician | Qh Quantity Hospital | ♀ Female only
♂ Male only | A Age | ♿ DMEPOS | A2-Z3 ASC Payment Indicator | A-Y ASC Status Indicator | Coding Clinic

E1060 Fully-reclining wheelchair, detachable arms, desk or full length, swing away detachable elevating legrests Qp Qh Y

IOM: 100-03, 4, 280.1

E1070 Fully-reclining wheelchair, detachable arms (desk or full length) swing away detachable footrests Qp Qh Y

IOM: 100-03, 4, 280.1

Wheelchair: Hemi

E1083 Hemi-wheelchair, fixed full length arms, swing away detachable elevating leg rest Qp Qh Y

IOM: 100-03, 4, 280.1

E1084 Hemi-wheelchair, detachable arms desk or full length arms, swing away detachable elevating leg rests Qp Qh Y

IOM: 100-03, 4, 280.1

E1085 Hemi-wheelchair, fixed full length arms, swing away detachable foot rests Qp Qh E1

IOM: 100-03, 4, 280.1

Cross Reference K0002

E1086 Hemi-wheelchair, detachable arms desk or full length, swing away detachable footrests Qp Qh E1

IOM: 100-03, 4, 280.1

Cross Reference K0002

Wheelchair: High-strength Lightweight

E1087 High strength lightweight wheelchair, fixed full length arms, swing away detachable elevating leg rests Qp Qh Y

IOM: 100-03, 4, 280.1

E1088 High strength lightweight wheelchair, detachable arms desk or full length, swing away detachable elevating leg rests Qp Qh Y

IOM: 100-03, 4, 280.1

E1089 High strength lightweight wheelchair, fixed length arms, swing away detachable footrest Qp Qh E1

IOM: 100-03, 4, 280.1

Cross Reference K0004

E1090 High strength lightweight wheelchair, detachable arms desk or full length, swing away detachable foot rests Qp Qh E1

IOM: 100-03, 4, 280.1

Cross Reference K0004

Wheelchair: Wide Heavy Duty

E1092 Wide heavy duty wheelchair, detachable arms (desk or full length) swing away detachable elevating leg rests Qp Qh Y

IOM: 100-03, 4, 280.1

E1093 Wide heavy duty wheelchair, detachable arms (desk or full length arms), swing away detachable foot rests Qp Qh Y

IOM: 100-03, 4, 280.1

Wheelchair: Semi-reclining

E1100 Semi-reclining wheelchair, fixed full length arms, swing away detachable elevating leg rests Qp Qh Y

IOM: 100-03, 4, 280.1

E1110 Semi-reclining wheelchair, detachable arms (desk or full length), elevating leg rest Qp Qh Y

IOM: 100-03, 4, 280.1

Wheelchair: Standard

E1130 Standard wheelchair, fixed full length arms, fixed or swing away detachable footrests Qp Qh E1

IOM: 100-03, 4, 280.1

Cross Reference K0001

E1140 Wheelchair, detachable arms, desk or full length, swing away detachable footrests Qp Qh E1

IOM: 100-03, 4, 280.1

Cross Reference K0001

E1150 Wheelchair, detachable arms, desk or full length, swing away detachable elevating legrests Qp Qh Y

IOM: 100-03, 4, 280.1

New | Revised | Reinstated | ~~deleted~~ Deleted | Not covered or valid by Medicare
Special coverage instructions | Carrier discretion | Bill Part B MAC | Bill DME MAC

E1160 Wheelchair, fixed full length arms, swing away detachable elevating legrests Ⓑ Qp Qh ♿ Y
IOM: 100-03, 4, 280.1

✻ **E1161** Manual adult size wheelchair, includes tilt in space Ⓑ Qp Qh A ♿ Y

Wheelchair: Amputee

E1170 Amputee wheelchair, fixed full length arms, swing away detachable elevating legrests Ⓑ Qp Qh ♿ Y
IOM: 100-03, 4, 280.1

E1171 Amputee wheelchair, fixed full length arms, without footrests or legrest Ⓑ Qp Qh ♿ Y
IOM: 100-03, 4, 280.1

E1172 Amputee wheelchair, detachable arms (desk or full length) without footrests or legrest Ⓑ Qp Qh ♿ Y
IOM: 100-03, 4, 280.1

E1180 Amputee wheelchair, detachable arms (desk or full length) swing away detachable footrests Ⓑ Qp Qh ♿ Y
IOM: 100-03, 4, 280.1

E1190 Amputee wheelchair, detachable arms (desk or full length), swing away detachable elevating legrests Ⓑ Qp Qh ♿ Y
IOM: 100-03, 4, 280.1

E1195 Heavy duty wheelchair, fixed full length arms, swing away detachable elevating legrests Ⓑ Qp Qh ♿ Y
IOM: 100-03, 4, 280.1

E1200 Amputee wheelchair, fixed full length arms, swing away detachable footrest Ⓑ Qp Qh ♿ Y
IOM: 100-03, 4, 280.1

Wheelchair: Other and Accessories

E1220 Wheelchair; specially sized or constructed (indicate brand name, model number, if any) and justification Ⓑ Qp Qh Y
IOM: 100-03, 4, 280.3

E1221 Wheelchair with fixed arm, footrests Ⓑ Qp Qh ♿ Y
IOM: 100-03, 4, 280.3

E1222 Wheelchair with fixed arm, elevating legrests Ⓑ Qp Qh ♿ Y
IOM: 100-03, 4, 280.3

E1223 Wheelchair with detachable arms, footrests Ⓑ Qp Qh ♿ Y
IOM: 100-03, 4, 280.3

E1224 Wheelchair with detachable arms, elevating legrests Ⓑ Qp Qh ♿ Y
IOM: 100-03, 4, 280.3

E1225 Wheelchair accessory, manual semi-reclining back, (recline greater than 15 degrees, but less than 80 degrees), each Ⓑ Qp Qh ♿ Y
IOM: 100-03, 4, 280.3

E1226 Wheelchair accessory, manual fully reclining back, (recline greater than 80 degrees), each Ⓑ Qp Qh ♿ B
IOM: 100-03, 4, 280.1

E1227 Special height arms for wheelchair Ⓑ ♿ Y
IOM: 100-03, 4, 280.3

E1228 Special back height for wheelchair Ⓑ Qp Qh ♿ Y
IOM: 100-03, 4, 280.3

Wheelchair: Pediatric

✻ **E1229** Wheelchair, pediatric size, not otherwise specified Ⓑ Qp Qh A Y

E1230 Power operated vehicle (three or four wheel non-highway), specify brand name and model number Ⓑ Qp Qh ♿ Y
Patient is unable to operate manual wheelchair; patient capable of safely operating controls for scooter; patient can transfer safely in and out of scooter
IOM: 100-08, 5, 5.2.3

E1231 Wheelchair, pediatric size, tilt-in-space, rigid, adjustable, with seating system Ⓑ Qp Qh A ♿ Y
IOM: 100-03, 4, 280.1

E1232 Wheelchair, pediatric size, tilt-in-space, folding, adjustable, with seating system Ⓑ Qp Qh A ♿ Y
IOM: 100-03, 4, 280.1

E1233 Wheelchair, pediatric size, tilt-in-space, rigid, adjustable, without seating system Ⓑ Qp Qh A ♿ Y
IOM: 100-03, 4, 280.1

⊙ **E1234** Wheelchair, pediatric size, tilt-in-space, folding, adjustable, without seating system ⑧ Qp Qh A ⎣ Y

IOM: 100-03, 4, 280.1

⊙ **E1235** Wheelchair, pediatric size, rigid, adjustable, with seating system ⑧ Qp Qh A ⎣ Y

IOM: 100-03, 4, 280.1

⊙ **E1236** Wheelchair, pediatric size, folding, adjustable, with seating system ⑧ Qp Qh A ⎣ Y

IOM: 100-03, 4, 280.1

⊙ **E1237** Wheelchair, pediatric size, rigid, adjustable, without seating system ⑧ Qp Qh A ⎣ Y

IOM: 100-03, 4, 280.1

⊙ **E1238** Wheelchair, pediatric size, folding, adjustable, without seating system ⑧ Qp Qh A ⎣ Y

IOM: 100-03, 4, 280.1

✳ **E1239** Power wheelchair, pediatric size, not otherwise specified ⑧ Qh A Y

Wheelchair: Lightweight

⊙ **E1240** Lightweight wheelchair, detachable arms, (desk or full length) swing away detachable, elevating leg rests ⑧ Qp Qh ⎣ Y

IOM: 100-03, 4, 280.1

⊘ **E1250** Lightweight wheelchair, fixed full length arms, swing away detachable footrest ⑧ Qp Qh E1

IOM: 100-03, 4, 280.1

Cross Reference K0003

⊘ **E1260** Lightweight wheelchair, detachable arms (desk or full length) swing away detachable footrest ⑧ Qp Qh E1

IOM: 100-03, 4, 280.1

Cross Reference K0003

⊙ **E1270** Lightweight wheelchair, fixed full length arms, swing away detachable elevating legrests ⑧ Qp Qh ⎣ Y

IOM: 100-03, 4, 280.1

Wheelchair: Heavy Duty

⊙ **E1280** Heavy duty wheelchair, detachable arms (desk or full length), elevating legrests ⑧ Qp Qh ⎣ Y

IOM: 100-03, 4, 280.1

⊘ **E1285** Heavy duty wheelchair, fixed full length arms, swing away detachable footrest ⑧ Qp Qh E1

IOM: 100-03, 4, 280.1

Cross Reference K0006

⊘ **E1290** Heavy duty wheelchair, detachable arms (desk or full length) swing away detachable footrest ⑧ Qp Qh E1

IOM: 100-03, 4, 280.1

Cross Reference K0006

⊙ **E1295** Heavy duty wheelchair, fixed full length arms, elevating legrest ⑧ Qp Qh ⎣ Y

IOM: 100-03, 4, 280.1

⊙ **E1296** Special wheelchair seat height from floor ⑧ ⎣ Y

IOM: 100-03, 4, 280.3

⊙ **E1297** Special wheelchair seat depth, by upholstery ⑧ ⎣ Y

IOM: 100-03, 4, 280.3

⊙ **E1298** Special wheelchair seat depth and/or width, by construction ⑧ ⎣ Y

IOM: 100-03, 4, 280.3

Whirlpool Equipment

⊘ **E1300** Whirlpool, portable (overtub type) ⑧ Qp Qh E1

IOM: 100-03, 4, 280.1

⊙ **E1310** Whirlpool, non-portable (built-in type) ⑧ Qp Qh ⎣ Y

IOM: 100-03, 4, 280.1

Additional Oxygen Related Equipment

✳ **E1352** Oxygen accessory, flow regulator capable of positive inspiratory pressure ⑧ Qp Qh Y

⊙ **E1353** Regulator ⑧ Qp Qh ⎣ Y

IOM: 100-03, 4, 240.2

✳ **E1354** Oxygen accessory, wheeled cart for portable cylinder or portable concentrator, any type, replacement only, each ⑧ Qp Qh Y

⊙ **E1355** Stand/rack ⑧ Qp Qh ⎣ Y

IOM: 100-03, 4, 240.2

✳ **E1356** Oxygen accessory, battery pack/cartridge for portable concentrator, any type, replacement only, each ⑧ Qp Qh Y

▶ **New** ⤾ **Revised** ✔ **Reinstated** ~~deleted~~ **Deleted** ⊘ **Not covered or valid by Medicare**

* **E1357** Oxygen accessory, battery charger for portable concentrator, any type, replacement only, each Ⓑ Qp Qh Y
E1358 Oxygen accessory, DC power adapter for portable concentrator, any type, replacement only, each Ⓑ Qp Qh Y
E1372 Immersion external heater for nebulizer Ⓑ Qp Qh ♿ Y
IOM: 100-03, 4, 240.2
E1390 Oxygen concentrator, single delivery port, capable of delivering 85 percent or greater oxygen concentration at the prescribed flow rate Ⓑ Qp Qh ♿ Y
IOM: 100-03, 4, 240.2
E1391 Oxygen concentrator, dual delivery port, capable of delivering 85 percent or greater oxygen concentration at the prescribed flow rate, each Ⓑ Qp Qh ♿ Y
IOM: 100-03, 4, 240.2
E1392 Portable oxygen concentrator, rental Ⓑ Qp Qh ♿ Y
IOM: 100-03, 4, 240.2
* **E1399** Durable medical equipment, miscellaneous Ⓑ Y
Example: Therapeutic exercise putty; rubber exercise tubing; anti-vibration gloves.
On DMEPOS fee schedule as a payable replacement for miscellaneous implanted or non-implanted items.
E1405 Oxygen and water vapor enriching system with heated delivery Ⓑ Qp Qh ♿ Y
IOM: 100-03, 4, 240.2
E1406 Oxygen and water vapor enriching system without heated delivery Ⓑ Qp Qh ♿ Y
IOM: 100-03, 4, 240.2

Artificial Kidney Machines and Accessories

E1500 Centrifuge, for dialysis Ⓑ Qp Qh A
E1510 Kidney, dialysate delivery syst kidney machine, pump recirculating, air removal syst. flowrate meter, power off, heater and temperature control with alarm, I.V. poles, pressure gauge, concentrate container Ⓑ Qp Qh A
E1520 Heparin infusion pump for hemodialysis Ⓑ Qp Qh A
E1530 Air bubble detector for hemodialysis, each, replacement Ⓑ Qp Qh A
E1540 Pressure alarm for hemodialysis, each, replacement Ⓑ Qp Qh A
E1550 Bath conductivity meter for hemodialysis, each Ⓑ Qp Qh A
E1560 Blood leak detector for hemodialysis, each, replacement Ⓑ Qp Qh A
E1570 Adjustable chair, for ESRD patients Ⓑ Qp Qh A
E1575 Transducer protectors/fluid barriers for hemodialysis, any size, per 10 Ⓑ Qp Qh A
E1580 Unipuncture control system for hemodialysis Ⓑ Qp Qh A
E1590 Hemodialysis machine Ⓑ Qp Qh A
E1592 Automatic intermittent peritoneal dialysis system Ⓑ Qp Qh A
E1594 Cycler dialysis machine for peritoneal dialysis Ⓑ Qp Qh A
E1600 Delivery and/or installation charges for hemodialysis equipment Ⓑ Qp Qh A
E1610 Reverse osmosis water purification system, for hemodialysis Ⓑ Qp Qh A
IOM: 100-03, 4, 230.7
E1615 Deionizer water purification system, for hemodialysis Ⓑ Qp Qh A
IOM: 100-03, 4, 230.7
E1620 Blood pump for hemodialysis replacement Ⓑ Qp Qh A
E1625 Water softening system, for hemodialysis Ⓑ Qp Qh A
IOM: 100-03, 4, 230.7
* **E1630** Reciprocating peritoneal dialysis system Ⓑ Qp Qh A
E1632 Wearable artificial kidney, each Ⓑ Qp Qh A
E1634 Peritoneal dialysis clamps, each Ⓑ Qp Qh B
IOM: 100-04, 8, 60.4.2; 100-04, 8, 90.1; 100-04, 18, 80; 100-04, 18, 90
E1635 Compact (portable) travel hemodialyzer system Ⓑ Qp Qh A
E1636 Sorbent cartridges, for hemodialysis, per 10 Ⓑ Qp Qh A
E1637 Hemostats, each Ⓑ Qp Qh A
E1639 Scale, each Ⓑ Qp Qh A
E1699 Dialysis equipment, not otherwise specified Ⓑ A

Jaw Motion Rehabilitation System

* E1700 Jaw motion rehabilitation system Ⓑ Qp Qh ♿ Y
  Must be prescribed by physician
* E1701 Replacement cushions for jaw motion rehabilitation system, pkg. of 6 Ⓑ Qp Qh ♿ Y
* E1702 Replacement measuring scales for jaw motion rehabilitation system, pkg. of 200 Ⓑ Qp Qh ♿ Y

Other Orthopedic Devices

* E1800 Dynamic adjustable elbow extension/ flexion device, includes soft interface material Ⓑ Qp Qh ♿ Y
* E1801 Static progressive stretch elbow device, extension and/or flexion, with or without range of motion adjustment, includes all components and accessories Ⓑ Qp Qh ♿ Y
* E1802 Dynamic adjustable forearm pronation/ supination device, includes soft interface material Ⓑ Qp Qh ♿ Y
* E1805 Dynamic adjustable wrist extension/ flexion device, includes soft interface material Ⓑ Qp Qh ♿ Y
* E1806 Static progressive stretch wrist device, flexion and/or extension, with or without range of motion adjustment, includes all components and accessories Ⓑ Qp Qh ♿ Y
* E1810 Dynamic adjustable knee extension/ flexion device, includes soft interface material Ⓑ Qp Qh ♿ Y
* E1811 Static progressive stretch knee device, extension and/or flexion, with or without range of motion adjustment, includes all components and accessories Ⓑ Qp Qh ♿ Y
* E1812 Dynamic knee, extension/flexion device with active resistance control Ⓑ Qp Qh ♿ Y
* E1815 Dynamic adjustable ankle extension/ flexion device, includes soft interface material Ⓑ Qp Qh ♿ Y
* E1816 Static progressive stretch ankle device, flexion and/or extension, with or without range of motion adjustment, includes all components and accessories Ⓑ Qp Qh ♿ Y
* E1818 Static progressive stretch forearm pronation/supination device with or without range of motion adjustment, includes all components and accessories Ⓑ Qp Qh ♿ Y
* E1820 Replacement soft interface material, dynamic adjustable extension/flexion device Ⓑ Qp Qh ♿ Y
* E1821 Replacement soft interface material/cuffs for bi-directional static progressive stretch device Ⓑ Qp Qh ♿ Y
* E1825 Dynamic adjustable finger extension/ flexion device, includes soft interface material Ⓑ Qp Qh ♿ Y
* E1830 Dynamic adjustable toe extension/ flexion device, includes soft interface material Ⓑ Qp Qh ♿ Y
* E1831 Static progressive stretch toe device, extension and/or flexion, with or without range of motion adjustment, includes all components and accessories Ⓑ Qp Qh ♿ Y
* E1840 Dynamic adjustable shoulder flexion/ abduction/rotation device, includes soft interface material Ⓑ Qp Qh ♿ Y
* E1841 Static progressive stretch shoulder device, with or without range of motion adjustment, includes all components and accessories Ⓑ Qp Qh ♿ Y

Miscellaneous

* E1902 Communication board, non-electronic augmentative or alternative communication device Ⓑ Qp Qh Y
* E2000 Gastric suction pump, home model, portable or stationary, electric Ⓑ Qp Qh ♿ Y
○ E2100 Blood glucose monitor with integrated voice synthesizer Ⓑ Qp Qh ♿ Y
  IOM: 100-03, 4, 230.16
○ E2101 Blood glucose monitor with integrated lancing/blood sample Ⓑ Qp Qh ♿ Y
  IOM: 100-03, 4, 230.16
* E2120 Pulse generator system for tympanic treatment of inner ear endolymphatic fluid Ⓑ Qp Qh ♿ Y

▶ New ↩ Revised ✔ Reinstated ~~deleted~~ Deleted ⊘ Not covered or valid by Medicare
○ Special coverage instructions * Carrier discretion Ⓑ Bill Part B MAC Ⓑ Bill DME MAC

Wheelchair Assessories: Manual and Power

✻ **E2201** Manual wheelchair accessory, nonstandard seat frame, width greater than or equal to 20 inches and less than 24 inches Ⓑ Qp Qh ♿ Y

✻ **E2202** Manual wheelchair accessory, nonstandard seat frame width, 24-27 inches Ⓑ Qp Qh ♿ Y

✻ **E2203** Manual wheelchair accessory, nonstandard seat frame depth, 20 to less than 22 inches Ⓑ Qp Qh ♿ Y

✻ **E2204** Manual wheelchair accessory, nonstandard seat frame depth, 22 to 25 inches Ⓑ Qp Qh ♿ Y

✻ **E2205** Manual wheelchair accessory, handrim without projections (includes ergonomic or contoured), any type, replacement only, each Ⓑ Qp Qh ♿ Y

✻ **E2206** Manual wheelchair accessory, wheel lock assembly, complete, replacement only, each Ⓑ Qp Qh ♿ Y

✻ **E2207** Wheelchair accessory, crutch and cane holder, each Ⓑ Qp Qh ♿ Y

✻ **E2208** Wheelchair accessory, cylinder tank carrier, each Ⓑ Qp Qh ♿ Y

✻ **E2209** Accessory arm trough, with or without hand support, each Ⓑ Qp Qh ♿ Y

✻ **E2210** Wheelchair accessory, bearings, any type, replacement only, each Ⓑ Qp Qh ♿ Y

✻ **E2211** Manual wheelchair accessory, pneumatic propulsion tire, any size, each Ⓑ Qp Qh ♿ Y

✻ **E2212** Manual wheelchair accessory, tube for pneumatic propulsion tire, any size, each Ⓑ Qp Qh ♿ Y

✻ **E2213** Manual wheelchair accessory, insert for pneumatic propulsion tire (removable), any type, any size, each Ⓑ Qp Qh ♿ Y

✻ **E2214** Manual wheelchair accessory, pneumatic caster tire, any size, each Ⓑ Qp Qh ♿ Y

✻ **E2215** Manual wheelchair accessory, tube for pneumatic caster tire, any size, each Ⓑ Qp Qh ♿ Y

✻ **E2216** Manual wheelchair accessory, foam filled propulsion tire, any size, each Ⓑ Qp Qh ♿ Y

✻ **E2217** Manual wheelchair accessory, foam filled caster tire, any size, each Ⓑ Qp Qh ♿ Y

✻ **E2218** Manual wheelchair accessory, foam propulsion tire, any size, each Ⓑ Qp Qh ♿ Y

✻ **E2219** Manual wheelchair accessory, foam caster tire, any size, each Ⓑ Qp Qh ♿ Y

✻ **E2220** Manual wheelchair accessory, solid (rubber/plastic) propulsion tire, any size, replacement only, each Ⓑ Qp Qh ♿ Y

✻ **E2221** Manual wheelchair accessory, solid (rubber/plastic) caster tire (removable), any size, replacement only, each Ⓑ Qp Qh ♿ Y

✻ **E2222** Manual wheelchair accessory, solid (rubber/plastic) caster tire with integrated wheel, any size, replacement only, each Ⓑ Qp Qh ♿ Y

✻ **E2224** Manual wheelchair accessory, propulsion wheel excludes tire, any size, replacement only, each Ⓑ Qp Qh ♿ Y

✻ **E2225** Manual wheelchair accessory, caster wheel excludes tire, any size, replacement only, each Ⓑ Qp Qh ♿ Y

✻ **E2226** Manual wheelchair accessory, caster fork, any size, replacement only, each Ⓑ Qp Qh ♿ Y

✻ **E2227** Manual wheelchair accessory, gear reduction drive wheel, each Ⓑ Qp Qh ♿ Y

✻ **E2228** Manual wheelchair accessory, wheel braking system and lock, complete, each Ⓑ Qp Qh ♿ Y

✻ **E2230** Manual wheelchair accessory, manual standing system Ⓑ Qp Qh Y

✻ **E2231** Manual wheelchair accessory, solid seat support base (replaces sling seat), includes any type mounting hardware Ⓑ Qp Qh ♿ Y

✻ **E2291** Back, planar, for pediatric size wheelchair including fixed attaching hardware Ⓑ Qp Qh A Y

✻ **E2292** Seat, planar, for pediatric size wheelchair including fixed attaching hardware Ⓑ Qp Qh A Y

✻ **E2293** Back, contoured, for pediatric size wheelchair including fixed attaching hardware Ⓑ Qp Qh A Y

✻ **E2294** Seat, contoured, for pediatric size wheelchair including fixed attaching hardware Ⓑ Qp Qh A Y

✻ **E2295** Manual wheelchair accessory, for pediatric size wheelchair, dynamic seating frame, allows coordinated movement of multiple positioning features Ⓑ Qp Qh A Y

✻ **E2300** Wheelchair accessory, power seat elevation system, any type Ⓑ Qp Qh Y

* **E2301** Wheelchair accessory, power standing system, any type Qp Qh Y
* **E2310** Power wheelchair accessory, electronic connection between wheelchair controller and one power seating system motor, including all related electronics, indicator feature, mechanical function selection switch, and fixed mounting hardware Qp Qh ♿ Y
* **E2311** Power wheelchair accessory, electronic connection between wheelchair controller and two or more power seating system motors, including all related electronics, indicator feature, mechanical function selection switch, and fixed mounting hardware Qp Qh ♿ Y
* **E2312** Power wheelchair accessory, hand or chin control interface, mini-proportional remote joystick, proportional, including fixed mounting hardware Qp Qh ♿ Y
* **E2313** Power wheelchair accessory, harness for upgrade to expandable controller, including all fasteners, connectors and mounting hardware, each Qp Qh ♿ Y
* **E2321** Power wheelchair accessory, hand control interface, remote joystick, nonproportional, including all related electronics, mechanical stop switch, and fixed mounting hardware Qp Qh ♿ Y
* **E2322** Power wheelchair accessory, hand control interface, multiple mechanical switches, nonproportional, including all related electronics, mechanical stop switch, and fixed mounting hardware Qp Qh ♿ Y
* **E2323** Power wheelchair accessory, specialty joystick handle for hand control interface, prefabricated Qp Qh ♿ Y
* **E2324** Power wheelchair accessory, chin cup for chin control interface Qp Qh ♿ Y
* **E2325** Power wheelchair accessory, sip and puff interface, nonproportional, including all related electronics, mechanical stop switch, and manual swingaway mounting hardware Qp Qh ♿ Y
* **E2326** Power wheelchair accessory, breath tube kit for sip and puff interface Qp Qh ♿ Y
* **E2327** Power wheelchair accessory, head control interface, mechanical, proportional, including all related electronics, mechanical direction change switch, and fixed mounting hardware Qp Qh ♿ Y
* **E2328** Power wheelchair accessory, head control or extremity control interface, electronic, proportional, including all related electronics and fixed mounting hardware Qp Qh ♿ Y
* **E2329** Power wheelchair accessory, head control interface, contact switch mechanism, nonproportional, including all related electronics, mechanical stop switch, mechanical direction change switch, head array, and fixed mounting hardware Qp Qh ♿ Y
* **E2330** Power wheelchair accessory, head control interface, proximity switch mechanism, nonproportional, including all related electronics, mechanical stop switch, mechanical direction change switch, head array, and fixed mounting hardware Qp Qh ♿ Y
* **E2331** Power wheelchair accessory, attendant control, proportional, including all related electronics and fixed mounting hardware Qp Qh Y
* **E2340** Power wheelchair accessory, nonstandard seat frame width, 20-23 inches Qp Qh ♿ Y
* **E2341** Power wheelchair accessory, nonstandard seat frame width, 24-27 inches Qp Qh ♿ Y
* **E2342** Power wheelchair accessory, nonstandard seat frame depth, 20 or 21 inches Qp Qh ♿ Y
* **E2343** Power wheelchair accessory, nonstandard seat frame depth, 22-25 inches Qp Qh ♿ Y
* **E2351** Power wheelchair accessory, electronic interface to operate speech generating device using power wheelchair control interface Qp Qh ♿ Y
* **E2358** Power wheelchair accessory, Group 34 non-sealed lead acid battery, each Qp Qh Y
* **E2359** Power wheelchair accessory, Group 34 sealed lead acid battery, each (e.g., gel cell, absorbed glassmat) Qp Qh ♿ Y
* **E2360** Power wheelchair accessory, 22 NF non-sealed lead acid battery, each ♿ Y

✻ **E2361** Power wheelchair accessory, 22NF sealed lead acid battery, each (e.g., gel cell, absorbed glassmat) Ⓑ Qp Qh ♿ Y

✻ **E2362** Power wheelchair accessory, group 24 non-sealed lead acid battery, each Ⓑ ♿ Y

✻ **E2363** Power wheelchair accessory, group 24 sealed lead acid battery, each (e.g., gel cell, absorbed glassmat) Ⓑ Qp Qh ♿ Y

✻ **E2364** Power wheelchair accessory, U-1 non-sealed lead acid battery, each Ⓑ ♿ Y

✻ **E2365** Power wheelchair accessory, U-1 sealed lead acid battery, each (e.g., gel cell, absorbed glassmat) Ⓑ Qp Qh ♿ Y

✻ **E2366** Power wheelchair accessory, battery charger, single mode, for use with only one battery type, sealed or non-sealed, each Ⓑ Qp Qh ♿ Y

✻ **E2367** Power wheelchair accessory, battery charger, dual mode, for use with either battery type, sealed or non-sealed, each Ⓑ Qp Qh ♿ Y

✻ **E2368** Power wheelchair component, drive wheel motor, replacement only Ⓑ Qp Qh ♿ Y

✻ **E2369** Power wheelchair component, drive wheel gear box, replacement only Ⓑ Qp Qh ♿ Y

✻ **E2370** Power wheelchair component, integrated drive wheel motor and gear box combination, replacement only Ⓑ Qp Qh ♿ Y

✻ **E2371** Power wheelchair accessory, group 27 sealed lead acid battery, (e.g., gel cell, absorbed glass mat), each Ⓑ Qp Qh ♿ Y

✻ **E2372** Power wheelchair accessory, group 27 non-sealed lead acid battery, each Ⓑ ♿ Y

✻ **E2373** Power wheelchair accessory, hand or chin control interface, compact remote joystick, proportional, including fixed mounting hardware Ⓑ Qp Qh ♿ Y

○ **E2374** Power wheelchair accessory, hand or chin control interface, standard remote joystick (not including controller), proportional, including all related electronics and fixed mounting hardware, replacement only Ⓑ Qp Qh ♿ Y

○ **E2375** Power wheelchair accessory, non-expandable controller, including all related electronics and mounting hardware, replacement only Ⓑ Qp Qh ♿ Y

○ **E2376** Power wheelchair accessory, expandable controller, including all related electronics and mounting hardware, replacement only Ⓑ Qp Qh ♿ Y

○ **E2377** Power wheelchair accessory, expandable controller, including all related electronics and mounting hardware, upgrade provided at initial issue Ⓑ Qp Qh ♿ Y

✻ **E2378** Power wheelchair component, actuator, replacement only Ⓑ Qp Qh ♿ Y

○ **E2381** Power wheelchair accessory, pneumatic drive wheel tire, any size, replacement only, each Ⓑ Qp Qh ♿ Y

○ **E2382** Power wheelchair accessory, tube for pneumatic drive wheel tire, any size, replacement only, each Ⓑ Qp Qh ♿ Y

○ **E2383** Power wheelchair accessory, insert for pneumatic drive wheel tire (removable), any type, any size, replacement only, each Ⓑ Qp Qh ♿ Y

○ **E2384** Power wheelchair accessory, pneumatic caster tire, any size, replacement only, each Ⓑ Qp Qh ♿ Y

○ **E2385** Power wheelchair accessory, tube for pneumatic caster tire, any size, replacement only, each Ⓑ Qp Qh ♿ Y

○ **E2386** Power wheelchair accessory, foam filled drive wheel tire, any size, replacement only, each Ⓑ Qp Qh ♿ Y

○ **E2387** Power wheelchair accessory, foam filled caster tire, any size, replacement only, each Ⓑ Qp Qh ♿ Y

○ **E2388** Power wheelchair accessory, foam drive wheel tire, any size, replacement only, each Ⓑ Qp Qh ♿ Y

○ **E2389** Power wheelchair accessory, foam caster tire, any size, replacement only, each Ⓑ Qp Qh ♿ Y

○ **E2390** Power wheelchair accessory, solid (rubber/plastic) drive wheel tire, any size, replacement only, each Ⓑ Qp Qh ♿ Y

○ **E2391** Power wheelchair accessory, solid (rubber/plastic) caster tire (removable), any size, replacement only, each Ⓑ Qp Qh ♿ Y

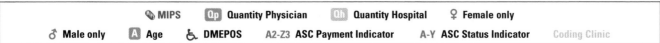

◌ **E2392** Power wheelchair accessory, solid (rubber/plastic) caster tire with integrated wheel, any size, replacement only, each Ⓔ Qp Qh ♿ Y

◌ **E2394** Power wheelchair accessory, drive wheel excludes tire, any size, replacement only, each Ⓔ Qp Qh ♿ Y

◌ **E2395** Power wheelchair accessory, caster wheel excludes tire, any size, replacement only, each Ⓔ Qp Qh ♿ Y

◌ **E2396** Power wheelchair accessory, caster fork, any size, replacement only, each Ⓔ Qp Qh ♿ Y

* **E2397** Power wheelchair accessory, lithium-based battery, each Ⓔ Qp Qh ♿ Y

Negative Pressure

* **E2402** Negative pressure wound therapy electrical pump, stationary or portable Ⓔ Qp Qh ♿ Y

Document at least every 30 calendar days the quantitative wound characteristics, including wound surface area (length, width and depth).

Medicare coverage up to a maximum of 15 dressing kits (A6550) per wound per month unless documentation states that the wound size requires more than one dressing kit for each dressing change.

Speech Device

◌ **E2500** Speech generating device, digitized speech, using pre-recorded messages, less than or equal to 8 minutes recording time Ⓔ Qp Qh ♿ Y

IOM: 100-03, 1, 50.1

◌ **E2502** Speech generating device, digitized speech, using pre-recorded messages, greater than 8 minutes but less than or equal to 20 minutes recording time Ⓔ Qp Qh ♿ Y

IOM: 100-03, 1, 50.1

◌ **E2504** Speech generating device, digitized speech, using pre-recorded messages, greater than 20 minutes but less than or equal to 40 minutes recording time Ⓔ Qp Qh ♿ Y

IOM: 100-03, 1, 50.1

◌ **E2506** Speech generating device, digitized speech, using pre-recorded messages, greater than 40 minutes recording time Ⓔ Qp Qh ♿ Y

IOM: 100-03, 1, 50.1

◌ **E2508** Speech generating device, synthesized speech, requiring message formulation by spelling and access by physical contact with the device Ⓔ Qp Qh ♿ Y

IOM: 100-03, 1, 50.1

◌ **E2510** Speech generating device, synthesized speech, permitting multiple methods of message formulation and multiple methods of device access Ⓔ Qp Qh ♿ Y

IOM: 100-03, 1, 50.1

◌ **E2511** Speech generating software program, for personal computer or personal digital assistant Ⓔ Qp Qh ♿ Y

IOM: 100-03, 1, 50.1

◌ **E2512** Accessory for speech generating device, mounting system Ⓔ Qp Qh ♿ Y

IOM: 100-03, 1, 50.1

◌ **E2599** Accessory for speech generating device, not otherwise classified Ⓔ Y

IOM: 100-03, 1, 50.1

Wheelchair: Cushion

* **E2601** General use wheelchair seat cushion, width less than 22 inches, any depth Ⓔ Qp Qh ♿ Y

* **E2602** General use wheelchair seat cushion, width 22 inches or greater, any depth Ⓔ Qp Qh ♿ Y

* **E2603** Skin protection wheelchair seat cushion, width less than 22 inches, any depth Ⓔ Qp Qh ♿ Y

* **E2604** Skin protection wheelchair seat cushion, width 22 inches or greater, any depth Ⓔ Qp Qh ♿ Y

* **E2605** Positioning wheelchair seat cushion, width less than 22 inches, any depth Ⓔ Qp Qh ♿ Y

* **E2606** Positioning wheelchair seat cushion, width 22 inches or greater, any depth Ⓔ Qp Qh ♿ Y

* **E2607** Skin protection and positioning wheelchair seat cushion, width less than 22 inches, any depth Ⓔ Qp Qh ♿ Y

* **E2608** Skin protection and positioning wheelchair seat cushion, width 22 inches or greater, any depth Ⓔ Qp Qh ♿ Y

* **E2609** Custom fabricated wheelchair seat cushion, any size Ⓔ Qp Qh Y

* **E2610** Wheelchair seat cushion, powered Ⓔ B

* **E2611** General use wheelchair back cushion, width less than 22 inches, any height, including any type mounting hardware Ⓑ Qp Qh ♿ Y

* **E2612** General use wheelchair back cushion, width 22 inches or greater, any height, including any type mounting hardware Ⓑ Qp Qh ♿ Y

* **E2613** Positioning wheelchair back cushion, posterior, width less than 22 inches, any height, including any type mounting hardware Ⓑ Qp Qh ♿ Y

* **E2614** Positioning wheelchair back cushion, posterior, width 22 inches or greater, any height, including any type mounting hardware Ⓑ Qp Qh ♿ Y

* **E2615** Positioning wheelchair back cushion, posterior-lateral, width less than 22 inches, any height, including any type mounting hardware Ⓑ Qp Qh ♿ Y

* **E2616** Positioning wheelchair back cushion, posterior-lateral, width 22 inches or greater, any height, including any type mounting hardware Ⓑ Qp Qh ♿ Y

* **E2617** Custom fabricated wheelchair back cushion, any size, including any type mounting hardware Ⓑ Qp Qh Y

* **E2619** Replacement cover for wheelchair seat cushion or back cushion, each Ⓑ Qp Qh ♿ Y

* **E2620** Positioning wheelchair back cushion, planar back with lateral supports, width less than 22 inches, any height, including any type mounting hardware Ⓑ Qp Qh ♿ Y

* **E2621** Positioning wheelchair back cushion, planar back with lateral supports, width 22 inches or greater, any height, including any type mounting hardware Ⓑ Qp Qh ♿ Y

Wheelchair: Skin Protection

* **E2622** Skin protection wheelchair seat cushion, adjustable, width less than 22 inches, any depth Ⓑ Qp Qh ♿ Y

* **E2623** Skin protection wheelchair seat cushion, adjustable, width 22 inches or greater, any depth Ⓑ Qp Qh ♿ Y

* **E2624** Skin protection and positioning wheelchair seat cushion, adjustable, width less than 22 inches, any depth Ⓑ Qp Qh ♿ Y

* **E2625** Skin protection and positioning wheelchair seat cushion, adjustable, width 22 inches or greater, any depth Ⓑ Qp Qh ♿ Y

Wheelchair: Arm Support

* **E2626** Wheelchair accessory, shoulder elbow, mobile arm support attached to wheelchair, balanced, adjustable Ⓑ Qp Qh ♿ Y

* **E2627** Wheelchair accessory, shoulder elbow, mobile arm support attached to wheelchair, balanced, adjustable rancho type Ⓑ Qp Qh ♿ Y

* **E2628** Wheelchair accessory, shoulder elbow, mobile arm support attached to wheelchair, balanced, reclining Ⓑ Qp Qh ♿ Y

* **E2629** Wheelchair accessory, shoulder elbow, mobile arm support attached to wheelchair, balanced, friction arm support (friction dampening to proximal and distal joints) Ⓑ Qp Qh ♿ Y

* **E2630** Wheelchair accessory, shoulder elbow, mobile arm support, monosuspension arm and hand support, overhead elbow forearm hand sling support, yoke type suspension support Ⓑ Qp Qh ♿ Y

* **E2631** Wheelchair accessory, addition to mobile arm support, elevating proximal arm Ⓑ Qp Qh ♿ Y

* **E2632** Wheelchair accessory, addition to mobile arm support, offset or lateral rocker arm with elastic balance control Ⓑ Qp Qh ♿ Y

* **E2633** Wheelchair accessory, addition to mobile arm support, supinator Ⓑ Qp Qh ♿ Y

Pediatric Gait Trainer

⊘ **E8000** Gait trainer, pediatric size, posterior support, includes all accessories and components Ⓑ A E1

⊘ **E8001** Gait trainer, pediatric size, upright support, includes all accessories and components Ⓑ A E1

⊘ **E8002** Gait trainer, pediatric size, anterior support, includes all accessories and components Ⓑ A E1

TEMPORARY PROCEDURES/ PROFESSIONAL SERVICES (G0000-G9999)

NOTE: Series "G", "K", and "Q" in the Level II coding are reserved for CMS assignment. "G", "K", and "Q" codes are temporary national codes for items or services requiring uniform national coding between one year's update and the next. Sometimes "temporary" codes remain for more than one update. If "G", "K", and "Q" codes are not converted to permanent codes in Level I or Level II series in the following update, they will remain active until converted in following years or until CMS notifies contractors to delete them. All active "G", "K", and "Q" codes at the time of update will be included on the update file for contractors. In addition, deleted codes are retained on the file for informational purposes, with a deleted indicator, for four years.

Vaccine Administration

✻ **G0008** Administration of influenza virus vaccine Ⓑ Qp Qh S

Coinsurance and deductible do not apply. If provided, report significant, separately identifiable E/M for medically necessary services (V04.81).

Coding Clinic: 2016, Q4, P3

✻ **G0009** Administration of pneumococcal vaccine Ⓑ Qp Qh S

Reported once in a lifetime based on risk; Medicare covers cost of vaccine and administration (V03.82)

Copayment, coinsurance, and deductible waived. (https://www.cms.gov/MLNProducts/downloads/MPS_QuickReferenceChart_1.pdf)

Coding Clinic: 2016, Q4, P3

✻ **G0010** Administration of hepatitis B vaccine Ⓑ Qp Qh S

Report for other than OPPs. Coinsurance and deductible apply; Medicare covers both cost of vaccine and administration (V05.3)

Copayment/coinsurance and deductible are waived. (https://www.cms.gov/MLNProducts/downloads/MPS_QuickReferenceChart_1.pdf)

Coding Clinic: 2016, Q4, P3

Semen Analysis

✻ **G0027** Semen analysis; presence and/or motility of sperm excluding Huhner Ⓑ Qp Qh ♂ Q4

Laboratory Certification: Hematology

Administration, Payment and Care Management Services

▶ ✻ **G0068** Professional services for the administration of anti-infective, pain management, chelation, pulmonary hypertension, and/or inotropic infusion drug(s) for each infusion drug administration calendar day in the individual's home, each 15 minutes A

▶ ✻ **G0069** Professional services for the administration of subcutaneous immunotherapy for each infusion drug administration calendar day in the individual's home, each 15 minutes A

▶ ✻ **G0070** Professional services for the administration of chemotherapy for each infusion drug administration calendar day in the individual's home, each 15 minutes A

▶ ✻ **G0071** Payment for communication technology-based services for 5 minutes or more of a virtual (non-face-to-face) communication between an rural health clinic (RHC) or federally qualified health center (FQHC) practitioner and RHC or FQHC patient, or 5 minutes or more of remote evaluation of recorded video and/or images by an RHC or FQHC practitioner, occurring in lieu of an office visit; RHC or FQHC only A

▶ ✻ **G0076** Brief (20 minutes) care management home visit for a new patient. For use only in a Medicare-approved CMMI model. (Services must be furnished within a beneficiary's home, domiciliary, rest home, assisted living and/or nursing facility.) B

▶ ✻ **G0077** Limited (30 minutes) care management home visit for a new patient. For use only in a Medicare-approved CMMI model. (Services must be furnished within a beneficiary's home, domiciliary, rest home, assisted living and/or nursing facility.) B

▶ ✻ **G0078** Moderate (45 minutes) care management home visit for a new patient. For use only in a Medicare-approved CMMI model. (Services must be furnished within a beneficiary's home, domiciliary, rest home, assisted living and/or nursing facility.) B

▶ * **G0079** Comprehensive (60 minutes) care management home visit for a new patient. For use only in a Medicare-approved CMMI model. (Services must be furnished within a beneficiary's home, domiciliary, rest home, assisted living and/or nursing facility.) B

▶ * **G0080** Extensive (75 minutes) care management home visit for a new patient. For use only in a Medicare-approved CMMI model. (Services must be furnished within a beneficiary's home, domiciliary, rest home, assisted living and/or nursing facility.) B

▶ * **G0081** Brief (20 minutes) care management home visit for an existing patient. For use only in a Medicare-approved CMMI model. (Services must be furnished within a beneficiary's home, domiciliary, rest home, assisted living and/or nursing facility.) B

▶ * **G0082** Limited (30 minutes) care management home visit for an existing patient. For use only in a Medicare-approved CMMI model. (Services must be furnished within a beneficiary's home, domiciliary, rest home, assisted living and/or nursing facility.) B

▶ * **G0083** Moderate (45 minutes) care management home visit for an existing patient. For use only in a Medicare-approved CMMI model. (Services must be furnished within a beneficiary's home, domiciliary, rest home, assisted living and/or nursing facility.) B

▶ * **G0084** Comprehensive (60 minutes) care management home visit for an existing patient. For use only in a Medicare-approved CMMI model. (Services must be furnished within a beneficiary's home, domiciliary, rest home, assisted living and/or nursing facility.) B

▶ * **G0085** Extensive (75 minutes) care management home visit for an existing patient. For use only in a Medicare-approved CMMI model. (Services must be furnished within a beneficiary's home, domiciliary, rest home, assisted living and/or nursing facility.) B

▶ * **G0086** Limited (30 minutes) care management home care plan oversight. For use only in a Medicare-approved CMMI model. (Services must be furnished within a beneficiary's home, domiciliary, rest home, assisted living and/or nursing facility.) B

▶ * **G0087** Comprehensive (60 minutes) care management home care plan oversight. For use only in a Medicare-approved CMMI model. (Services must be furnished within a beneficiary's home, domiciliary, rest home, assisted living and/or nursing facility.) B

Screening Services

MIPS **G0101** Cervical or vaginal cancer screening; pelvic and clinical breast examination Ⓑ Qp Qh S

Covered once every two years and annually if high risk for cervical/vaginal cancer, or if childbearing age patient has had an abnormal Pap smear in preceding three years. High risk diagnosis, V15.89

Coding Clinic: 2002, Q4, P8

MIPS **G0102** Prostate cancer screening; digital rectal examination Ⓑ Qp Qh N

Covered annually by Medicare (V76.44). Not separately payable with an E/M code (99201-99499).

IOM: 100-02, 6, 10; 100-04, 4, 240; 100-04, 18, 50.1

G0103 Prostate cancer screening; prostate specific antigen test (PSA) Ⓑ Qp Qh A

Covered annually by Medicare (V76.44)

IOM: 100-02, 6, 10; 100-04, 4, 240; 100-04, 18, 50

Laboratory Certification: Routine chemistry

MIPS **G0104** Colorectal cancer screening; flexible sigmoidoscopy Ⓑ Qp Qh T

Covered once every 48 months for beneficiaries age 50+

Co-insurance waived under Section 4104.

Coding Clinic: 2011, Q2, P4

MIPS **G0105** Colorectal cancer screening; colonoscopy on individual at high risk Ⓑ Qp Qh T

Screening colonoscopy covered once every 24 months for high risk for developing colorectal cancer. May use modifier 53 if appropriate (physician fee schedule).

Co-insurance waived under Section 4104.

Coding Clinic: 2018, Q2, P4; 2011, Q2, P4

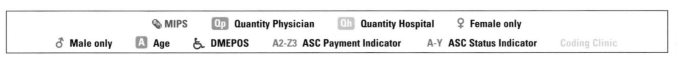

G0106 Colorectal cancer screening; alternative to G0104, screening sigmoidoscopy, barium enema Qp Qh S

Barium enema (not high risk) (alternative to G0104). Covered once every 4 years for beneficiaries age 50+. Use modifier 26 for professional component only.

Coding Clinic: 2011, Q2, P4

Diabetes Management Training Services

* **G0108** Diabetes outpatient self-management training services, individual, per 30 minutes Qp Qh A

Report for beneficiaries diagnosed with diabetes.

Effective January 2011, DSMT will be included in the list of reimbursable Medicare telehealth services.

* **G0109** Diabetes outpatient self-management training services, group session (2 or more) per 30 minutes Qp Qh A

Report for beneficiaries diagnosed with diabetes.

Effective January 2011, DSMT will be included in the list of reimbursable Medicare telehealth services.

Screening Services

* **G0117** Glaucoma screening for high risk patients furnished by an optometrist or ophthalmologist Qp Qh S

Covered once per year (full 11 months between screenings). Bundled with all other ophthalmic services provided on same day. Diagnosis code V80.1.

* **G0118** Glaucoma screening for high risk patient furnished under the direct supervision of an optometrist or ophthalmologist Qp Qh S

Covered once per year (full 11 months between screenings). Diagnosis code V80.1.

G0120 Colorectal cancer screening; alternative to G0105, screening colonoscopy, barium enema. Qp Qh S

Barium enema for patients with a high risk of developing colorectal. Covered once every 2 years. Used as an alternative to G0105. Use modifier 26 for professional component only.

G0121 Colorectal cancer screening; colonoscopy on individual not meeting criteria for high risk Qp Qh T

Screening colonoscopy for patients that are not high risk. Covered once every 10 years, but not within 48 months of a G0104. For non-Medicare patients report 45378.

Co-insurance waived under Section 4104.

Coding Clinic: 2018, Q2, P4

⊘ **G0122** Colorectal cancer screening; barium enema E1

Medicare: this service is denied as noncovered, because it fails to meet the requirements of the benefit. The beneficiary is liable for payment.

G0123 Screening cytopathology, cervical or vaginal (any reporting system), collected in preservative fluid, automated thin layer preparation, screening by cytotechnologist under physician supervision Qp Qh ♀ A

Use G0123 or G0143 or G0144 or G0145 or G0147 or G0148 or P3000 for Pap smears NOT requiring physician interpretation (technical component).

IOM: 100-03, 3, 190.2; 100-04, 18, 30

Laboratory Certification: Cytology

G0124 Screening cytopathology, cervical or vaginal (any reporting system), collected in preservative fluid, automated thin layer preparation, requiring interpretation by physician Qp Qh ♀ B

Report professional component for Pap smears requiring physician interpretation.

IOM: 100-03, 3, 190.2; 100-04, 18, 30

Laboratory Certification: Cytology

Miscellaneous Services, Diagnostic and Therapeutic

G0127 Trimming of dystrophic nails, any number Qp Qh Q1

Must be used with a modifier (Q7, Q8, or Q9) to show that the foot care service is needed because the beneficiary has a systemic disease. Limit 1 unit of service.

IOM: 100-02, 15, 290

▶ New ⤺ Revised ✓ Reinstated ~~deleted~~ Deleted ⊘ Not covered or valid by Medicare
Special coverage instructions * Carrier discretion Bill Part B MAC Bill DME MAC

G0128 Direct (face-to-face with patient) skilled nursing services of a registered nurse provided in a comprehensive outpatient rehabilitation facility, each 10 minutes beyond the first 5 minutes Qp Qh B

A separate nursing service that is clearly identifiable in the Plan of Treatment and not part of other services. Documentation must support this service. Examples include: Insertion of a urinary catheter, intramuscular injections, bowel disimpaction, nursing assessment, and education. Restricted coverage by Medicare.

Medicare Statute 1833(a)

* **G0129** Occupational therapy services requiring the skills of a qualified occupational therapist, furnished as a component of a partial hospitalization treatment program, per session (45 minutes or more) Qh P

G0130 Single energy x-ray absorptiometry (SEXA) bone density study, one or more sites; appendicular skeleton (peripheral) (e.g., radius, wrist, heel) Qp Qh Z3 S

Covered every 24 months (more frequently if medically necessary). Use modifier 26 for professional component only.

Preventive service; no deductible

IOM: 100-03, 2, 150.3; 100-04, 13, 140.1

* **G0141** Screening cytopathology smears, cervical or vaginal, performed by automated system, with manual rescreening, requiring interpretation by physician Qp Qh ♀ B

Co-insurance, copay, and deductible waived

Report professional component for Pap smears requiring physician interpretation. Refer to diagnosis of V15.89, V76.2, V76.47, or V76.49 to report appropriate risk level.

Laboratory Certification: Cytology

* **G0143** Screening cytopathology, cervical or vaginal (any reporting system), collected in preservative fluid, automated thin layer preparation, with manual screening and rescreening by cytotechnologist under physician supervision Qp Qh ♀ A

Co-insurance, copay, and deductible waived

Laboratory Certification: Cytology

* **G0144** Screening cytopathology, cervical or vaginal (any reporting system), collected in preservative fluid, automated thin layer preparation, with screening by automated system, under physician supervision Qp Qh ♀ A

Co-insurance, copay, and deductible waived

Laboratory Certification: Cytology

* **G0145** Screening cytopathology, cervical or vaginal (any reporting system), collected in preservative fluid, automated thin layer preparation, with screening by automated system and manual rescreening under physician supervision Qp Qh ♀ A

Co-insurance, copay, and deductible waived

Laboratory Certification: Cytology

* **G0147** Screening cytopathology smears, cervical or vaginal; performed by automated system under physician supervision Qp Qh ♀ A

Co-insurance, copay, and deductible waived

Laboratory Certification: Cytology

* **G0148** Screening cytopathology smears, cervical or vaginal; performed by automated system with manual rescreening Qp Qh ♀ A

Co-insurance, copay, and deductible waived

Laboratory Certification: Cytology

* **G0151** Services performed by a qualified physical therapist in the home health or hospice setting, each 15 minutes B

* **G0152** Services performed by a qualified occupational therapist in the home health or hospice setting, each 15 minutes B

* **G0153** Services performed by a qualified speech-language pathologist in the home health or hospice setting, each 15 minutes B

* **G0155** Services of clinical social worker in home health or hospice settings, each 15 minutes B

* **G0156** Services of home health/health aide in home health or hospice settings, each 15 minutes B

* **G0157** Services performed by a qualified physical therapist assistant in the home health or hospice setting, each 15 minutes B

MIPS | Qp Quantity Physician | Qh Quantity Hospital | ♀ Female only
♂ Male only | A Age | DMEPOS | A2-Z3 ASC Payment Indicator | A-Y ASC Status Indicator | Coding Clinic

* **G0158** Services performed by a qualified occupational therapist assistant in the home health or hospice setting, each 15 minutes Ⓑ B

* **G0159** Services performed by a qualified physical therapist, in the home health setting, in the establishment or delivery of a safe and effective physical therapy maintenance program, each 15 minutes Ⓑ B

* **G0160** Services performed by a qualified occupational therapist, in the home health setting, in the establishment or delivery of a safe and effective occupational therapy maintenance program, each 15 minutes Ⓑ B

* **G0161** Services performed by a qualified speech-language pathologist, in the home health setting, in the establishment or delivery of a safe and effective speech-language pathology maintenance program, each 15 minutes Ⓑ B

* **G0162** Skilled services by a registered nurse (RN) for management and evaluation of the plan of care; each 15 minutes (the patient's underlying condition or complication requires an RN to ensure that essential non-skilled care achieves its purpose in the home health or hospice setting) Ⓑ B

Transmittal No. 824 (CR7182)

G0166 External counterpulsation, per treatment session Ⓑ Qp Qh Q1

IOM: 100-03, 1, 20.20

* **G0168** Wound closure utilizing tissue adhesive(s) only Ⓑ Qp Qh B

Report for wound closure with only tissue adhesive. If a practitioner utilizes tissue adhesive in addition to staples or sutures to close a wound, HCPCS code G0168 is not separately reportable, but is included in the tissue repair.

The only closure material used for a simple repair, coverage based on payer.

Coding Clinic: 2005, Q1, P5; 2001, Q4, P12; Q3, P13

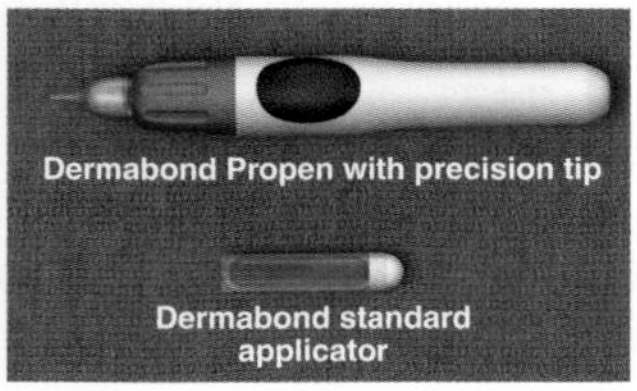
Dermabond Propen with precision tip
Dermabond standard applicator

Figure 15 Tissue adhesive.

* **G0175** Scheduled interdisciplinary team conference (minimum of three exclusive of patient care nursing staff) with patient present Ⓑ Qp Qh V

G0176 Activity therapy, such as music, dance, art or play therapies not for recreation, related to the care and treatment of patient's disabling mental health problems, per session (45 minutes or more) Ⓑ Qh P

Paid in partial hospitalization

G0177 Training and educational services related to the care and treatment of patient's disabling mental health problems per session (45 minutes or more) Ⓑ Qp Qh N

Paid in partial hospitalization

* **G0179** Physician recertification for Medicare-covered home health services under a home health plan of care (patient not present), including contacts with home health agency and review of reports of patient status required by physicians to affirm the initial implementation of the plan of care that meets patient's needs, per recertification period Ⓑ Qp Qh M

The recertification code is used after a patient has received services for at least 60 days (or one certification period) when the physician signs the certification after the initial certification period.

* **G0180** Physician certification for Medicare-covered home health services under a home health plan of care (patient not present), including contacts with home health agency and review of reports of patient status required by physicians to affirm the initial implementation of the plan of care that meets patient's needs, per certification period Ⓑ Qp Qh M

This code can be billed only when the patient has not received Medicare covered home health services for at least 60 days.

▶ New ⤺ Revised ✔ Reinstated ~~deleted~~ Deleted ⊘ Not covered or valid by Medicare
Special coverage instructions * Carrier discretion Ⓑ Bill Part B MAC Ⓑ Bill DME MAC

* **G0181** Physician supervision of a patient receiving Medicare-covered services provided by a participating home health agency (patient not present) requiring complex and multidisciplinary care modalities involving regular physician development and/or revision of care plans, review of subsequent reports of patient status, review of laboratory and other studies, communication (including telephone calls) with other health care professionals involved in the patient's care, integration of new information into the medical treatment plan and/or adjustment of medical therapy, within a calendar month, 30 minutes or more Qp Qh M

Coding Clinic: 2015, Q2, P10

* **G0182** Physician supervision of a patient under a Medicare-approved hospice (patient not present) requiring complex and multidisciplinary care modalities involving regular physician development and/or revision of care plans, review of subsequent reports of patient status, review of laboratory and other studies, communication (including telephone calls) with other health care professionals involved in the patient's care, integration of new information into the medical treatment plan and/or adjustment of medical therapy, within a calendar month, 30 minutes or more Qp Qh M

Coding Clinic: 2015, Q2, P10

* **G0186** Destruction of localized lesion of choroid (for example, choroidal neovascularization); photocoagulation, feeder vessel technique (one or more sessions) Qp Qh T

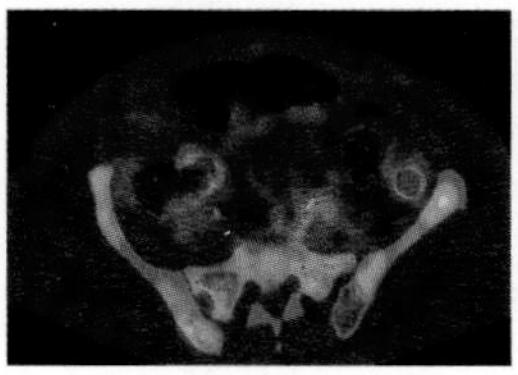

Figure 16 PET scan.

⊘ **G0219** PET imaging whole body; melanoma for non-covered indications E1

Example: Assessing regional lymph nodes in melanoma.

IOM: 100-03, 4, 220.6

Coding Clinic: 2007, Q1, P6

⊘ **G0235** PET imaging, any site, not otherwise specified Qp Qh E1

Example: Prostate cancer diagnosis and initial staging.

IOM: 100-03, 4, 220.6

Coding Clinic: 2007, Q1, P6

* **G0237** Therapeutic procedures to increase strength or endurance of respiratory muscles, face to face, one on one, each 15 minutes (includes monitoring) Qp Qh S

* **G0238** Therapeutic procedures to improve respiratory function, other than described by G0237, one on one, face to face, per 15 minutes (includes monitoring) Qp Qh S

* **G0239** Therapeutic procedures to improve respiratory function or increase strength or endurance of respiratory muscles, two or more individuals (includes monitoring) Qp Qh S

G0245 Initial physician evaluation and management of a diabetic patient with diabetic sensory neuropathy resulting in a loss of protective sensation (LOPS) which must include (1) the diagnosis of LOPS, (2) a patient history, (3) a physical examination that consist of at least the following elements: (A) visual inspection of the forefoot, hindfoot and toe web spaces, (B) evaluation of a protective sensation, (C) evaluation of foot structure and biomechanics, (D) evaluation of vascular status and skin integrity, and (E) evaluation and recommendation of footwear, and (4) patient education Qp Qh V

IOM: 100-03, 1, 70.2.1

G0246 Follow-up physician evaluation and management of a diabetic patient with diabetic sensory neuropathy resulting in a loss of protective sensation (LOPS) to include at least the following: (1) a patient history, (2) a physical examination that includes: (A) visual inspection of the forefoot, hindfoot and toe web spaces, (B) evaluation of protective sensation, (C) evaluation of foot structure and biomechanics, (D) evaluation of vascular status and skin integrity, and (E) evaluation and recommendation of footwear, and (3) patient education Qp Qh V

IOM: 100-03, 1, 70.2.1; 100-02, 15, 290

G0247 Routine foot care by a physician of a diabetic patient with diabetic sensory neuropathy resulting in a loss of protective sensation (LOPS) to include, the local care of superficial wounds (i.e., superficial to muscle and fascia) and at least the following if present: (1) local care of superficial wounds, (2) debridement of corns and calluses, and (3) trimming and debridement of nails Qp Qh Q1

IOM: 100-03, 1, 70.2.1

G0248 Demonstration, prior to initiation, of home INR monitoring for patient with either mechanical heart valve(s), chronic atrial fibrillation, or venous thromboembolism who meets Medicare coverage criteria, under the direction of a physician; includes: face-to-face demonstration of use and care of the INR monitor, obtaining at least one blood sample, provision of instructions for reporting home INR test results, and documentation of patient's ability to perform testing and report results Qp Qh V

G0249 Provision of test materials and equipment for home INR monitoring of patient with either mechanical heart valve(s), chronic atrial fibrillation, or venous thromboembolism who meets Medicare coverage criteria; includes provision of materials for use in the home and reporting of test results to physician; testing not occurring more frequently than once a week; testing materials, billing units of service include 4 tests Qp Qh V

G0250 Physician review, interpretation, and patient management of home INR testing for patient with either mechanical heart valve(s), chronic atrial fibrillation, or venous thromboembolism who meets Medicare coverage criteria; testing not occurring more frequently than once a week; billing units of service include 4 tests Qp Qh M

G0252 PET imaging, full and partial-ring PET scanners only, for initial diagnosis of breast cancer and/or surgical planning for breast cancer (e.g., initial staging of axillary lymph nodes) E1

IOM: 100-03, 4, 220.6

Coding Clinic: 2007, Q1, P6

G0255 Current perception threshold/sensory nerve conduction test (SNCT), per limb, any nerve E1

IOM: 100-03, 2, 160.23

G0257 Unscheduled or emergency dialysis treatment for an ESRD patient in a hospital outpatient department that is not certified as an ESRD facility Qp Qh S

Coding Clinic: 2003, Q1, P9

G0259 Injection procedure for sacroiliac joint; arthrography Qp Qh N

Replaces 27096 for reporting injections for Medicare beneficiaries

Used by Part A only (facility), not priced by Part B Medicare.

G0260 Injection procedure for sacroiliac joint; provision of anesthetic, steroid and/or other therapeutic agent, with or without arthrography Qp Qh T

ASCs report when a therapeutic sacroiliac joint injection is administered in ASC

* **G0268** Removal of impacted cerumen (one or both ears) by physician on same date of service as audiologic function testing Qp Qh N

Report only when a physician, not an audiologist, performs the procedure.

Use with DX 380.4 when performed by physician.

Coding Clinic: 2016, Q2, P2-3; 2003, Q1, P12

▶ New ⤾ Revised ✔ Reinstated ~~deleted~~ Deleted ⊘ Not covered or valid by Medicare
Special coverage instructions * Carrier discretion Bill Part B MAC Bill DME MAC

G0269 Placement of occlusive device into either a venous or arterial access site, post surgical or interventional procedure (e.g., angioseal plug, vascular plug) Qh N

Report for replacement of vasoseal. Hospitals may report the closure device as a supply with C1760. Bundled status on Physician Fee Schedule.

Coding Clinic: 2011, Q3, P4; 2010, Q4, P6

* **G0270** Medical nutrition therapy; reassessment and subsequent intervention(s) following second referral in same year for change in diagnosis, medical condition or treatment regimen (including additional hours needed for renal disease), individual, face to face with the patient, each 15 minutes Qp Qh A

Requires physician referral for beneficiaries with diabetes or renal disease. Services must be provided by dietitian/nutritionist. Co-insurance and deductible waived.

* **G0271** Medical nutrition therapy, reassessment and subsequent intervention(s) following second referral in same year for change in diagnosis, medical condition, or treatment regimen (including additional hours needed for renal disease), group (2 or more individuals), each 30 minutes Qp Qh A

Requires physician referral for beneficiaries with diabetes or renal disease. Services must be provided by dietitian/nutritionist. Co-insurance and deductible waived.

G0276 Blinded procedure for lumbar stenosis, percutaneous image-guided lumbar decompression (PILD) or placebo-control, performed in an approved coverage with evidence development (CED) clinical trial Qp Qh J1

G0277 Hyperbaric oxygen under pressure, full body chamber, per 30 minute interval Qp Qh S

IOM: 100-03, 1, 20.29

Coding Clinic: 2015, Q3, P7

* **G0278** Iliac and/or femoral artery angiography, non-selective, bilateral or ipsilateral to catheter insertion, performed at the same time as cardiac catheterization and/or coronary angiography, includes positioning or placement of the catheter in the distal aorta or ipsilateral femoral or iliac artery, injection of dye, production of permanent images, and radiologic supervision and interpretation (list separately in addition to primary procedure) Qp Qh N

Medicare specific code not reported for iliac injection used as a guiding shot for a closure device

Coding Clinic: 2011, Q3, P4; 2006, Q4, P7

* **G0279** Diagnostic digital breast tomosynthesis, unilateral or bilateral (list separately in addition to G0204 or G0206) A

* **G0281** Electrical stimulation, (unattended), to one or more areas, for chronic stage III and stage IV pressure ulcers, arterial ulcers, diabetic ulcers, and venous stasis ulcers not demonstrating measurable signs of healing after 30 days of conventional care, as part of a therapy plan of care Qp Qh A

Reported by encounter/areas and not by site. Therapists report G0281 and G0283 rather than 97014.

G0282 Electrical stimulation, (unattended), to one or more areas, for wound care other than described in G0281 E1

IOM: 100-03, 4, 270.1

* **G0283** Electrical stimulation (unattended), to one or more areas for indication(s) other than wound care, as part of a therapy plan of care Qp Qh A

Reported by encounter/areas and not by site. Therapists report G0281 and G0283 rather than 97014.

* **G0288** Reconstruction, computed tomographic angiography of aorta for surgical planning for vascular surgery Qp Qh N

MIPS | Qp Quantity Physician | Qh Quantity Hospital | ♀ Female only
♂ Male only | A Age | DMEPOS | A2-Z3 ASC Payment Indicator | A-Y ASC Status Indicator | Coding Clinic

✻ **G0289** Arthroscopy, knee, surgical, for removal of loose body, foreign body, debridement/shaving of articular cartilage (chondroplasty) at the time of other surgical knee arthroscopy in a different compartment of the same knee Ⓑ Qp Qh **N**

Add-on code reported with knee arthroscopy code for major procedure performed-reported once per extra compartment

"The code may be reported twice (or with a unit of two) if the physician performs these procedures in two compartments, in addition to the compartment where the main procedure was performed." (http://www.ama-assn.org/resources/doc/cpt/orthopaedics.pdf)

⚙ **G0293** Noncovered surgical procedure(s) using conscious sedation, regional, general or spinal anesthesia in a Medicare qualifying clinical trial, per day Ⓑ Qp Qh **Q1**

⚙ **G0294** Noncovered procedure(s) using either no anesthesia or local anesthesia only, in a Medicare qualifying clinical trial, per day Ⓑ Qp Qh **Q1**

⊘ **G0295** Electromagnetic therapy, to one or more areas, for wound care other than described in G0329 or for other uses Ⓑ **E1**

IOM: 100-03, 4, 270.1

✻ **G0296** Counseling visit to discuss need for lung cancer screening (LDCT) using low dose CT scan (service is for eligibility determination and shared decision making) Ⓑ Qp Qh **S**

✻ **G0297** Low dose CT scan (LDCT) for lung cancer screening Ⓑ Qp Qh **S**

✻ **G0299** Direct skilled nursing services of a registered nurse (RN) in the home health or hospice setting, each 15 minutes Ⓑ **B**

✻ **G0300** Direct skilled nursing services of a licensed practical nurse (LPN) in the home health or hospice setting, each 15 minutes Ⓑ **B**

✻ **G0302** Pre-operative pulmonary surgery services for preparation for LVRS, complete course of services, to include a minimum of 16 days of services Ⓑ Qp Qh **S**

✻ **G0303** Pre-operative pulmonary surgery services for preparation for LVRS, 10 to 15 days of services Ⓑ Qp Qh **S**

✻ **G0304** Pre-operative pulmonary surgery services for preparation for LVRS, 1 to 9 days of services Ⓑ Qp Qh **S**

✻ **G0305** Post-discharge pulmonary surgery services after LVRS, minimum of 6 days of services Ⓑ Qp Qh **S**

✻ **G0306** Complete CBC, automated (HgB, HCT, RBC, WBC, without platelet count) and automated WBC differential count Ⓑ Qp Qh **Q4**

Laboratory Certification: Hematology

✻ **G0307** Complete CBC, automated (HgB, HCT, RBC, WBC; without platelet count) Ⓑ Qp Qh **Q4**

Laboratory Certification: Hematology

⚙ **G0328** Colorectal cancer screening; fecal occult blood test, immunoassay, 1-3 simultaneous Ⓑ Qp Qh **A**

Co-insurance and deductible waived

Reported for Medicare patients 501; one FOBT per year, with either G0107 (guaiac-based) or G0328 (immunoassay-based)

Laboratory Certification: Routine chemistry, Hematology

Coding Clinic: 2012, Q2, P9

✻ **G0329** Electromagnetic therapy, to one or more areas for chronic stage III and stage IV pressure ulcers, arterial ulcers, and diabetic ulcers and venous stasis ulcers not demonstrating measurable signs of healing after 30 days of conventional care as part of a therapy plan of care Ⓑ Qp Qh **A**

⚙ **G0333** Pharmacy dispensing fee for inhalation drug(s); initial 30-day supply as a beneficiary Ⓔ Qp Qh **M**

Medicare will reimburse an initial dispensing fee to a pharmacy for initial 30-day period of inhalation drugs furnished through DME.

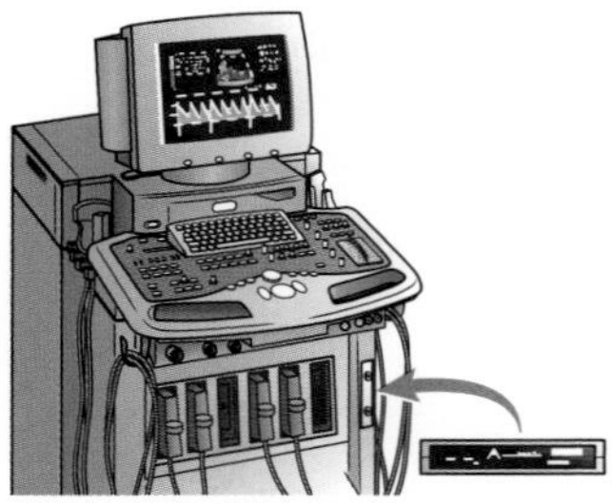
US machine
Electromagnetic device

Figure 17 Electromagnetic device.

▶ New ↻ Revised ✔ Reinstated ~~deleted~~ Deleted ⊘ Not covered or valid by Medicare
⚙ Special coverage instructions ✻ Carrier discretion Ⓑ Bill Part B MAC Ⓔ Bill DME MAC

* **G0337** Hospice evaluation and counseling services, pre-election Qp Qh B

* **G0339** Image-guided robotic linear accelerator-based stereotactic radiosurgery, complete course of therapy in one session or first session of fractionated treatment Qp Qh B

* **G0340** Image-guided robotic linear accelerator-based stereotactic radiosurgery, delivery including collimator changes and custom plugging, fractionated treatment, all lesions, per session, second through fifth sessions, maximum five sessions per course of treatment Qp Qh B

G0341 Percutaneous islet cell transplant, includes portal vein catheterization and infusion Qp Qh C

IOM: 100-03, 4, 260.3; 100-04, 32, 70

G0342 Laparoscopy for islet cell transplant, includes portal vein catheterization and infusion Qp Qh C

IOM: 100-03, 4, 260.3

G0343 Laparotomy for islet cell transplant, includes portal vein catheterization and infusion Qp Qh C

IOM: 100-03, 4, 260.3

* **G0365** Vessel mapping of vessels for hemodialysis access (services for preoperative vessel mapping prior to creation of hemodialysis access using an autogenous hemodialysis conduit, including arterial inflow and venous outflow) Qp Qh S

Includes evaluation of the relevant arterial and venous vessels. Use modifier 26 for professional component only.

G0372 Physician service required to establish and document the need for a power mobility device Qp Qh M

Providers should bill the E/M code and G0372 on the same claim.

Hospital Services: Observation and Emergency Department

G0378 Hospital observation service, per hour Qh N

Report all related services in addition to G0378. Report units of hours spent in observation (rounded to the nearest hour). Hospitals report the ED or clinic visit with a CPT code or, if applicable, G0379 (direct admit to observation) and G0378 (hospital observation services, per hour).

Coding Clinic: 2007, Q1, P10; 2006, Q3, P7-8

G0379 Direct admission of patient for hospital observation care Qp Qh J2

Report all related services in addition to G0379. Report units of hours spent in observation (rounded to the nearest hour). Hospitals report the ED or clinic visit with a CPT code or, if applicable, G0379 (direct admit to observation) and G0378 (hospital observation services, per hour).

Coding Clinic: 2007, Q1, P7

* **G0380** Level 1 hospital emergency department visit provided in a type B emergency department; (the ED must meet at least one of the following requirements: (1) it is licensed by the state in which it is located under applicable state law as an emergency room or emergency department; (2) it is held out to the public (by name, posted signs, advertising, or other means) as a place that provides care for emergency medical conditions on an urgent basis without requiring a previously scheduled appointment; or (3) during the calendar year immediately preceding the calendar year in which a determination under 42 CFR 489.24 is being made, based on a representative sample of patient visits that occurred during that calendar year, it provides at least one-third of all of its outpatient visits for the treatment of emergency medical conditions on an urgent basis without requiring a previously scheduled appointment) Qh J2

Coding Clinic: 2009, Q1, P4; 2007, Q2, P1

* **G0381** Level 2 hospital emergency department visit provided in a type B emergency department; (the ED must meet at least one of the following requirements: (1) it is licensed by the state in which it is located under applicable state law as an emergency room or emergency department; (2) it is held out to the public (by name, posted signs, advertising, or other means) as a place that provides care for emergency medical conditions on an urgent basis without requiring a previously scheduled appointment; or (3) during the calendar year immediately preceding the calendar year in which a determination under 42 CFR 489.24 is being made, based on a representative sample of patient visits that occurred during that calendar year, it provides at least one-third of all of its outpatient visits for the treatment of emergency medical conditions on an urgent basis without requiring a previously scheduled appointment) Ⓑ Qh J2

Coding Clinic: 2009, Q1, P4; 2007, Q2, P1

* **G0382** Level 3 hospital emergency department visit provided in a type B emergency department; (the ED must meet at least one of the following requirements: (1) it is licensed by the state in which it is located under applicable state law as an emergency room or emergency department; (2) it is held out to the public (by name, posted signs, advertising, or other means) as a place that provides care for emergency medical conditions on an urgent basis without requiring a previously scheduled appointment; or (3) during the calendar year immediately preceding the calendar year in which a determination under 42 CFR 489.24 is being made, based on a representative sample of patient visits that occurred during that calendar year, it provides at least one-third of all of its outpatient visits for the treatment of emergency medical conditions on an urgent basis without requiring a previously scheduled appointment) Ⓑ Qh J2

Coding Clinic: 2009, Q1, P4; 2007, Q2, P1

* **G0383** Level 4 hospital emergency department visit provided in a type B emergency department; (the ED must meet at least one of the following requirements: (1) it is licensed by the state in which it is located under applicable state law as an emergency room or emergency department; (2) it is held out to the public (by name, posted signs, advertising, or other means) as a place that provides care for emergency medical conditions on an urgent basis without requiring a previously scheduled appointment; or (3) during the calendar year immediately preceding the calendar year in which a determination under 42 CFR 489.24 is being made, based on a representative sample of patient visits that occurred during that calendar year, it provides at least one-third of all of its outpatient visits for the treatment of emergency medical conditions on an urgent basis without requiring a previously scheduled appointment) Ⓑ Qh J2

Coding Clinic: 2009, Q1, P4; 2007, Q2, P1

* **G0384** Level 5 hospital emergency department visit provided in a type B emergency department; (the ED must meet at least one of the following requirements: (1) it is licensed by the state in which it is located under applicable state law as an emergency room or emergency department; (2) it is held out to the public (by name, posted signs, advertising, or other means) as a place that provides care for emergency medical conditions on an urgent basis without requiring a previously scheduled appointment; or (3) during the calendar year immediately preceding the calendar year in which a determination under 42 CFR 489.24 is being made, based on a representative sample of patient visits that occurred during that calendar year, it provides at least one-third of all of its outpatient visits for the treatment of emergency medical conditions on an urgent basis without requiring a previously scheduled appointment) Ⓑ Qh J2

Coding Clinic: 2009, Q1, P4; 2007, Q2, P1

Trauma Response Team

G0390 Trauma response team associated with hospital critical care service Ⓑ Qh S

Coding Clinic: 2007, Q2, P5

Alcohol Substance Abuse Assessment and Intervention

* G0396 Alcohol and/or substance (other than tobacco) abuse structured assessment (e.g., audit, DAST), and brief intervention 15 to 30 minutes Qp Qh S

Bill instead of 99408 and 99409

* G0397 Alcohol and/or substance (other than tobacco) abuse structured assessment (e.g., audit, DAST), and intervention, greater than 30 minutes Qp Qh S

Bill instead of 99408 and 99409

Home Sleep Study Test

* G0398 Home sleep study test (HST) with type II portable monitor, unattended; minimum of 7 channels: EEG, EOG, EMG, ECG/heart rate, airflow, respiratory effort and oxygen saturation Qp Qh S

* G0399 Home sleep test (HST) with type III portable monitor, unattended; minimum of 4 channels: 2 respiratory movement/airflow, 1 ECG/heart rate and 1 oxygen saturation Qp Qh S

* G0400 Home sleep test (HST) with type IV portable monitor, unattended; minimum of 3 channels Qp Qh S

Initial Examination for Medicare Enrollment

* G0402 Initial preventive physical examination; face-to-face visit, services limited to new beneficiary during the first 12 months of Medicare enrollment Qp Qh V

Depending on circumstances, 99201-99215 may be assigned with modifier 25 to report an E/M service as a significant, separately identifiable service in addition to the Initial Preventive Physical Examination (IPPE), G0402.

Copayment and coinsurance waived, deductible waived.

Coding Clinic: 2009, Q4, P8

Electrocardiogram

* G0403 Electrocardiogram, routine ECG with 12 leads; performed as a screening for the initial preventive physical examination with interpretation and report Qp Qh M

Optional service may be ordered or performed at discretion of physician. Once in a life-time screening, stemming from a referral from Initial Preventive Physical Examination (IPPE). Both deductible and co-payment apply.

* G0404 Electrocardiogram, routine ECG with 12 leads; tracing only, without interpretation and report, performed as a screening for the initial preventive physical examination Qp Qh S

* G0405 Electrocardiogram, routine ECG with 12 leads; interpretation and report only, performed as a screening for the initial preventive physical examination Qp Qh B

Follow-up Telehealth Consultation

* G0406 Follow-up inpatient consultation, limited, physicians typically spend 15 minutes communicating with the patient via telehealth Qp Qh B

These telehealth modifers are required when billing for telehealth services with codes G0406-G0408 and G0425-G0427:

- GT, via interactive audio and video telecommunications system
- GQ, via asynchronous telecommunications system

* G0407 Follow-up inpatient consultation, intermediate, physicians typically spend 25 minutes communicating with the patient via telehealth Qp Qh B

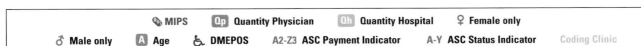

* G0408 Follow-up inpatient consultation, complex, physicians typically spend 35 minutes communicating with the patient via telehealth Qp Qh B

Psychological Services

* G0409 Social work and psychological services, directly relating to and/or furthering the patient's rehabilitation goals, each 15 minutes, face-to-face; individual (services provided by a CORF-qualified social worker or psychologist in a CORF) Ⓑ — B

* G0410 Group psychotherapy other than of a multiple-family group, in a partial hospitalization setting, approximately 45 to 50 minutes Ⓑ Qp Qh — P

  Coding Clinic: 2009, Q4, P9, 10

* G0411 Interactive group psychotherapy, in a partial hospitalization setting, approximately 45 to 50 minutes Ⓑ Qp Qh — P

  Coding Clinic: 2009, Q4, P9, 10

Fracture Treatment

* G0412 Open treatment of iliac spine(s), tuberosity avulsion, or iliac wing fracture(s), unilateral or bilateral for pelvic bone fracture patterns which do not disrupt the pelvic ring includes internal fixation, when performed Ⓑ Qp Qh — C

* G0413 Percutaneous skeletal fixation of posterior pelvic bone fracture and/or dislocation, for fracture patterns which disrupt the pelvic ring, unilateral or bilateral, (includes ilium, sacroiliac joint and/or sacrum) Ⓑ Qp Qh — J1

* G0414 Open treatment of anterior pelvic bone fracture and/or dislocation for fracture patterns which disrupt the pelvic ring, unilateral or bilateral, includes internal fixation when performed (includes pubic symphysis and/or superior/inferior rami) Ⓑ Qp Qh — C

* G0415 Open treatment of posterior pelvic bone fracture and/or dislocation, for fracture patterns which disrupt the pelvic ring, unilateral or bilateral, includes internal fixation, when performed (includes ilium, sacroiliac joint and/or sacrum) Ⓑ Qp Qh — C

Surgical Pathology: Prostate Biopsy

* G0416 Surgical pathology, gross and microscopic examinations for prostate needle biopsy, any method Ⓑ Qp Qh ♂ — Q2

  This testing requires a facility to have either a CLIA certificate of registration (certificate type code 9), a CLIA certificate of compliance (certificate type code 1), or a CLIA certificate of accreditation (certificate type code 3). A facility without a valid, current, CLIA certificate, with a current CLIA certificate of waiver (certificate type code 2) or with a current CLIA certificate for provider-performed microscopy procedures (certificate type code 4), must not be permitted to be paid for these tests. This code has a TC, 26 (physician), or gobal component.

  Laboratory Certification: Histopathology

  Coding Clinic: 2013, Q2, P6

Educational Services

* G0420 Face-to-face educational services related to the care of chronic kidney disease; individual, per session, per one hour Ⓑ Qp Qh — A

  CKD is kidney damage of 3 months or longer, regardless of the cause of kidney damage. Sessions billed in increments of one hour (if session is less than one hour, it must last at least 31 minutes to be billable. Sessions less than one hour and longer than 31 minutes is billable as one session. No more than 6 sessions of KDE services in a beneficiary's lifetime.

* G0421 Face-to-face educational services related to the care of chronic kidney disease; group, per session, per one hour Ⓑ Qp Qh — A

  Group setting: 2 to 20, report codes G0420 and G0421 with diagnosis code 585.4.

▶ New ↩ Revised ✔ Reinstated ~~deleted~~ Deleted ⊘ Not covered or valid by Medicare
Special coverage instructions * Carrier discretion Ⓑ Bill Part B MAC Ⓓ Bill DME MAC

Cardiac and Pulmonary Rehabilitation

* **G0422** Intensive cardiac rehabilitation; with or without continuous ECG monitoring with exercise, per session Qp Qh S

  Includes the same service as 93798 but at a greater frequency; may be reported with as many as six hourly sessions on a single date of service. Includes medical nutrition services to reduce cardiac disease risk factors.

* **G0423** Intensive cardiac rehabilitation; with or without continuous ECG monitoring; without exercise, per session Qp Qh S

  Includes the same service as 93797 but at a greater frequency; may be reported with as many as six hourly sessions on a single date of service. Includes medical nutrition services to reduce cardiac disease risk factors.

* **G0424** Pulmonary rehabilitation, including exercise (includes monitoring), one hour, per session, up to two sessions per day Qp Qh S

  Includes therapeutic services and all related monitoring services to inprove respiratory function. Do not report with G0237, G0238, or G0239.

Initial Telehealth Consultation

* **G0425** Telehealth consultation, emergency department or initial inpatient, typically 30 minutes communicating with the patient via telehealth Qp Qh B

  Problem Focused: Problem focused history and examination, with straightforward medical decision making complexity. Typically 30 minutes communicating with patient via telehealth.

* **G0426** Initial inpatient telehealth consultation, emergency department or initial inpatient, typically 50 minutes communicating with the patient via telehealth Qp Qh B

  Detailed: Detailed history and examination, with moderate medical decision making complexity. Typically 50 minutes communicating with patient via telehealth.

* **G0427** Initial inpatient telehealth consultation, emergency department or initial inpatient, typically 70 minutes or more communicating with the patient via telehealth Qp Qh B

  Comprehensive: Comprehensive history and examination, with high medical decision making complexity. Typically 70 minutes or more communicating with patient via telehealth.

Fillers

⊘ **G0428** Collagen meniscus implant procedure for filling meniscal defects (e.g., cmi, collagen scaffold, menaflex) E1

* **G0429** Dermal filler injection(s) for the treatment of facial lipodystrophy syndrome (LDS) (e.g., as a result of highly active antiretroviral therapy) Qp Qh T

  Designated for dermal fillers Sculptra® and Radiesse (Medicare). (https://www.cms.gov/ContractorLearningResources/downloads/JA6953.pdf)

  Coding Clinic: 2010, Q3, P8

Laboratory Screening

* **G0432** Infectious agent antibody detection by enzyme immunoassay (EIA) technique, HIV-1 and/or HIV-2, screening Qp Qh A

  Laboratory Certification: Virology, General immunology

  Coding Clinic: 2010, Q2, P10

* **G0433** Infectious agent antibody detection by enzyme-linked immunosorbent assay (ELISA) technique, HIV-1 and/or HIV-2, screening Qp Qh A

  Laboratory Certification: Virology, General immunology

  Coding Clinic: 2010, Q2, P10

* **G0435** Infectious agent antibody detection by rapid antibody test, HIV-1 and/or HIV-2, screening Qp Qh A

  Coding Clinic: 2010, Q2, P10

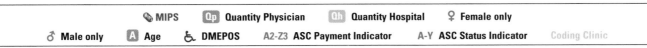

Counselling, Wellness, and Screening Services

* G0438 Annual wellness visit; includes a personalized prevention plan of service (pps), initial visit Ⓑ Qp Qh A
* G0439 Annual wellness visit, includes a personalized prevention plan of service (pps), subsequent visit Ⓑ Qp Qh A
* G0442 Annual alcohol misuse screening, 15 minutes Ⓑ Qp Qh S

Coding Clinic: 2012, Q1, P7

* G0443 Brief face-to-face behavioral counseling for alcohol misuse, 15 minutes Ⓑ Qp Qh S

Coding Clinic: 2012, Q1, P7

* G0444 Annual depression screening, 15 minutes Ⓑ Qp Qh S
* G0445 High intensity behavioral counseling to prevent sexually transmitted infection; face-to-face, individual, includes: education, skills training and guidance on how to change sexual behavior; performed semi-annually, 30 minutes Ⓑ Qp Qh S
* G0446 Annual, face-to-face intensive behavioral therapy for cardiovascular disease, individual, 15 minutes Ⓑ Qp Qh S

Coding Clinic: 2012, Q2, P8

* G0447 Face-to-face behavioral counseling for obesity, 15 minutes Ⓑ Qp Qh S

Coding Clinic: 2012, Q1, P8

* G0448 Insertion or replacement of a permanent pacing cardioverter-defibrillator system with transvenous lead(s), single or dual chamber with insertion of pacing electrode, cardiac venous system, for left ventricular pacing Ⓑ Qp Qh B
* G0451 Development testing, with interpretation and report, per standardized instrument form Ⓑ Qp Qh Q3

Miscellaneous Services

* G0452 Molecular pathology procedure; physician interpretation and report Ⓑ Qp Qh B
* G0453 Continuous intraoperative neurophysiology monitoring, from outside the operating room (remote or nearby), per patient, (attention directed exclusively to one patient) each 15 minutes (list in addition to primary procedure) Ⓑ Qp Qh N
* G0454 Physician documentation of face-to-face visit for durable medical equipment determination performed by nurse practitioner, physician assistant or clinical nurse specialist Ⓑ Qp Qh B
* G0455 Preparation with instillation of fecal microbiota by any method, including assessment of donor specimen Ⓑ Qp Qh Q1

Coding Clinic: 2013, Q3, P8

* G0458 Low dose rate (LDR) prostate brachytherapy services, composite rate Ⓑ Qp Qh B
* G0459 Inpatient telehealth pharmacologic management, including prescription, use, and review of medication with no more than minimal medical psychotherapy Ⓑ Qp Qh B
* G0460 Autologous platelet rich plasma for chronic wounds/ulcers, including phlebotomy, centrifugation, and all other preparatory procedures, administration and dressings, per treatment Ⓑ Qp Qh T
* G0463 Hospital outpatient clinic visit for assessment and management of a patient Ⓑ Qp Qh J2
* G0464 Colorectal cancer screening; stool-based DNA and fecal occult hemoglobin (e.g., KRAS, NDRG4 and BMP3) Ⓑ

Cross Reference 81528

Laboratory Certification: General immunology, Routine chemistry,Clinical cytogenetics

Federally Qualified Health Center Visits

* G0466 Federally qualified health center (FQHC) visit, new patient; a medically-necessary, face-to-face encounter (one-on-one) between a new patient and a FQHC practitioner during which time one or more FQHC services are rendered and includes a typical bundle of Medicare-covered services that would be furnished per diem to a patient receiving a FQHC visit Ⓑ Qp Qh A

▶ New ↩ Revised ✔ Reinstated ~~deleted~~ Deleted ⃠ Not covered or valid by Medicare
Special coverage instructions * Carrier discretion Ⓑ Bill Part B MAC Ⓓ Bill DME MAC

* **G0467** Federally qualified health center (FQHC) visit, established patient; a medically-necessary, face-to-face encounter (one-on-one) between an established patient and a FQHC practitioner during which time one or more FQHC services are rendered and includes a typical bundle of Medicare-covered services that would be furnished per diem to a patient receiving a FQHC visit Qp Qh A

* **G0468** Federally qualified health center (FQHC) visit, IPPE or AWV; a FQHC visit that includes an initial preventive physical examination (IPPE) or annual wellness visit (AWV) and includes a typical bundle of Medicare-covered services that would be furnished per diem to a patient receiving an IPPE or AWV Qp Qh A

* **G0469** Federally qualified health center (FQHC) visit, mental health, new patient; a medically-necessary, face-to-face mental health encounter (one-on-one) between a new patient and a FQHC practitioner during which time one or more FQHC services are rendered and includes a typical bundle of Medicare-covered services that would be furnished per diem to a patient receiving a mental health visit Qp Qh A

* **G0470** Federally qualified health center (FQHC) visit, mental health, established patient; a medically-necessary, face-to-face mental health encounter (one-on-one) between an established patient and a FQHC practitioner during which time one or more FQHC services are rendered and includes a typical bundle of Medicare-covered services that would be furnished per diem to a patient receiving a mental health visit Qp Qh A

Other Miscellaneous Services

* **G0471** Collection of venous blood by venipuncture or urine sample by catheterization from an individual in a skilled nursing facility (SNF) or by a laboratory on behalf of a home health agency (HHA) Qp Qh A

G0472 Hepatitis C antibody screening, for individual at high risk and other covered indication(s) Qp Qh A

Medicare Statute 1861SSA

Laboratory Certification: General immunology

* **G0473** Face-to-face behavioral counseling for obesity, group (2-10), 30 minutes Qp Qh S

* **G0475** HIV antigen/antibody, combination assay, screening Qp Qh A

Laboratory Certification: Virology, General immunology

* **G0476** Infectious agent detection by nucleic acid (DNA or RNA); human papillomavirus (HPV), high-risk types (e.g., 16, 18, 31, 33, 35, 39, 45, 51, 52, 56, 58, 59, 68) for cervical cancer screening, must be performed in addition to pap test Qp Qh A

Laboratory Certification: Virology

Drug Tests

* **G0480** Drug test(s), definitive, utilizing drug identification methods able to identify individual drugs and distinguish between structural isomers (but not necessarily stereoisomers), including, but not limited to GC/MS (any type, single or tandem) and LC/MS (any type, single or tandem and excluding immunoassays (e.g., IA, EIA, ELISA, EMIT, FPIA) and enzymatic methods (e.g., alcohol dehydrogenase)); qualitative or quantitative, all sources(s), includes specimen validity testing, per day, 1-7 drug class(es), including metabolite(s) if performed Qp Qh Q4

Coding Clinic: 2018, Q1, P5

* **G0481** Drug test(s), definitive, utilizing drug identification methods able to identify individual drugs and distinguish between structural isomers (but not necessarily stereoisomers), including, but not limited to GC/MS (any type, single or tandem) and LC/MS (any type, single or tandem and excluding immunoassays (e.g., IA, EIA, ELISA, EMIT, FPIA) and enzymatic methods (e.g., alcohol dehydrogenase)); qualitative or quantitative, all sources(s), includes specimen validity testing, per day, 8-14 drug class(es), including metabolite(s) if performed Qp Qh Q4

Coding Clinic: 2018, Q1, P5

✻ **G0482** Drug test(s), definitive, utilizing drug identification methods able to identify individual drugs and distinguish between structural isomers (but not necessarily stereoisomers), including, but not limited to GC/MS (any type, single or tandem) and LC/MS (any type, single or tandem and excluding immunoassays (e.g., IA, EIA, ELISA, EMIT, FPIA) and enzymatic methods (e.g., alcohol dehydrogenase)); qualitative or quantitative, all sources(s), includes specimen validity testing, per day, 15-21 drug class(es), including metabolite(s) if performed Ⓑ Qp Qh Q4

Coding Clinic: 2018, Q1, P5

✻ **G0483** Drug test(s), definitive, utilizing drug identification methods able to identify individual drugs and distinguish between structural isomers (but not necessarily stereoisomers), including, but not limited to GC/MS (any type, single or tandem) and LC/MS (any type, single or tandem and excluding immunoassays (e.g., IA, EIA, ELISA, EMIT, FPIA) and enzymatic methods (e.g., alcohol dehydrogenase)); qualitative or quantitative, all sources(s), includes specimen validity testing, per day, 22 or more drug class(es), including metabolite(s) if performed Ⓑ Qp Qh Q4

Coding Clinic: 2018, Q1, P5

Home Health Nursing Visit: Area of Shortage

✻ **G0490** Face-to-face home health nursing visit by a rural health clinic (RHC) or federally qualified health center (FQHC) in an area with a shortage of home health agencies (services limited to RN or LPN only) Ⓑ A

Dialysis Procedure

✻ **G0491** Dialysis procedure at a Medicare certified esrd facility for acute kidney injury without ESRD Ⓑ Qp Qh B

✻ **G0492** Dialysis procedure with single evaluation by a physician or other qualified health care professional for acute kidney injury without ESRD Ⓑ Qp Qh B

Home Health or Hospice: Skilled Services

✻ **G0493** Skilled services of a registered nurse (RN) for the observation and assessment of the patient's condition, each 15 minutes (the change in the patient's condition requires skilled nursing personnel to identify and evaluate the patient's need for possible modification of treatment in the home health or hospice setting) Ⓑ B

✻ **G0494** Skilled services of a licensed practical nurse (LPN) for the observation and assessment of the patient's condition, each 15 minutes (the change in the patient's condition requires skilled nursing personnel to identify and evaluate the patient's need for possible modification of treatment in the home health or hospice setting) Ⓑ B

✻ **G0495** Skilled services of a registered nurse (RN), in the training and/or education of a patient or family member, in the home health or hospice setting, each 15 minutes Ⓑ B

✻ **G0496** Skilled services of a licensed practical nurse (LPN), in the training and/or education of a patient or family member, in the home health or hospice setting, each 15 minutes Ⓑ B

Chemotherapy Administration

✻ **G0498** Chemotherapy administration, intravenous infusion technique; initiation of infusion in the office/clinic setting using office/clinic pump/ supplies, with continuation of the infusion in the community setting (e.g., home, domiciliary, rest home or assisted living) using a portable pump provided by the office/clinic, includes follow up office/clinic visit at the conclusion of the infusion Ⓑ Qp Qh S

Hepatitis B Screening

⮌ ✻ **G0499** Hepatitis B screening in non-pregnant, high risk individual includes hepatitis B surface antigen (HBsAG), antibodies to HBsAG (anti-HBs) and antibodies to hepatitis B core antigen (anti-hbc), and is followed by a neutralizing confirmatory test, when performed, only for an initially reactive HBsAG result Ⓑ Qp Qh A

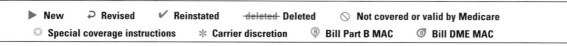

Laboratory Certification: Virology

Moderate Sedation Services

✻ **G0500** Moderate sedation services provided by the same physician or other qualified health care professional performing a gastrointestinal endoscopic service that sedation supports, requiring the presence of an independent trained observer to assist in the monitoring of the patient's level of consciousness and physiological status; initial 15 minutes of intra-service time; patient age 5 years or older (additional time may be reported with 99153, as appropriate) Qp Qh N

Resource-Intensive Service

✻ **G0501** Resource-intensive services for patients for whom the use of specialized mobility-assistive technology (such as adjustable height chairs or tables, patient lift, and adjustable padded leg supports) is medically necessary and used during the provision of an office/ outpatient, evaluation and management visit (list separately in addition to primary service) N

Psychiatric Care Management

✻ **G0506** Comprehensive assessment of and care planning for patients requiring chronic care management services (list separately in addition to primary monthly care management service) Qp Qh N

Critical Care Telehealth Consultation

✻ **G0508** Telehealth consultation, critical care, initial , physicians typically spend 60 minutes communicating with the patient and providers via telehealth Qp Qh B

✻ **G0509** Telehealth consultation, critical care, subsequent, physicians typically spend 50 minutes communicating with the patient and providers via telehealth Qp Qh B

Rural Health Clinic: Management and Care

G0511 Rural health clinic or federally qualified health center (RHC or FQHC) only, general care management, 20 minutes or more of clinical staff time for chronic care management services or behavioral health integration services directed by an RHC or FQHC practitioner (physician, NP, PA, or CNM), per calendar month A

G0512 Rural health clinic or federally qualified health center (RHC/FQHC) only, psychiatric collaborative care model (psychiatric CoCM), 60 minutes or more of clinical staff time for psychiatric CoCM services directed by an RHC or FQHC practitioner (physician, NP, PA, or CNM) and including services furnished by a behavioral health care manager and consultation with a psychiatric consultant, per calendar month A

Prolonged Preventive Services

✻ **G0513** Prolonged preventive service(s) (beyond the typical service time of the primary procedure), in the office or other outpatient setting requiring direct patient contact beyond the usual service; first 30 minutes (list separately in addition to code for preventive service) N

✻ **G0514** Prolonged preventive service(s) (beyond the typical service time of the primary procedure), in the office or other outpatient setting requiring direct patient contact beyond the usual service; each additional 30 minutes (list separately in addition to code G0513 for additional 30 minutes of preventive service) N

Cognitive Development

✻ **G0515** Development of cognitive skills to improve attention, memory, problem solving (includes compensatory training), direct (one-on-one) patient contact, each 15 minutes A

Non-biodegradable Drug Delivery Implants: Removal and Insertion

* * **G0516** Insertion of non-biodegradable drug delivery implants, 4 or more (services for subdermal rod implant) Q1
* * **G0517** Removal of non-biodegradable drug delivery implants, 4 or more (services for subdermal implants) Q1
* * **G0518** Removal with reinsertion, non-biodegradable drug delivery implants, 4 or more (services for subdermal implants) Q1

Drug Test

* * **G0659** Drug test(s), definitive, utilizing drug identification methods able to identify individual drugs and distinguish between structural isomers (but not necessarily stereoisomers), including but not limited to GC/MS (any type, single or tandem) and LC/MS (any type, single or tandem), excluding immunoassays (e.g., IA, EIA, ELISA, EMIT, FPIA) and enzymatic methods (e.g., alcohol dehydrogenase), performed without method or drug-specific calibration, without matrix-matched quality control material, or without use of stable isotope or other universally recognized internal standard(s) for each drug, drug metabolite or drug class per specimen; qualitative or quantitative, all sources, includes specimen validity testing, per day, any number of drug classes Q4

Quality Care Measures: Cataract Surgery

* * **G0913** Improvement in visual function achieved within 90 days following cataract surgery Ⓑ M
* * **G0914** Patient care survey was not completed by patient Ⓑ M
* * **G0915** Improvement in visual function not achieved within 90 days following cataract surgery Ⓑ M
* * **G0916** Satisfaction with care achieved within 90 days following cataract surgery Ⓑ M
* * **G0917** Patient satisfaction survey was not completed by patient Ⓑ M
* * **G0918** Satisfaction with care not achieved within 90 days following cataract surgery Ⓑ M

Therapy, Evaluation and Assessment

* ▶ * **G2000** Blinded administration of convulsive therapy procedure, either electroconvulsive therapy (ECT, current covered gold standard) or magnetic seizure therapy (MST, non-covered experimental therapy), performed in an approved IDE-based clinical trial, per treatment session S
* ▶ * **G2010** Remote evaluation of recorded video and/or images submitted by an established patient (e.g., store and forward), including interpretation with follow-up with the patient within 24 business hours, not originating from a related E/M service provided within the previous 7 days nor leading to an E/M service or procedure within the next 24 hours or soonest available appointment M
* ▶ * **G2011** Alcohol and/or substance (other than tobacco) abuse structured assessment (e.g., AUDIT, DAST), and brief intervention, 5-14 minutes S
* ▶ * **G2012** Brief communication technology-based service, e.g., virtual check-in, by a physician or other qualified health care professional who can report evaluation and management services, provided to an established patient, not originating from a related E/M service provided within the previous 7 days nor leading to an E/M service or procedure within the next 24 hours or soonest available appointment; 5-10 minutes of medical discussion M

Guidance

* **G6001** Ultrasonic guidance for placement of radiation therapy fields Ⓑ Qp Qh B
* * **G6002** Stereoscopic x-ray guidance for localization of target volume for the delivery of radiation therapy Ⓑ Qp Qh B

Radiation Treatment

* * **G6003** Radiation treatment delivery, single treatment area, single port or parallel opposed ports, simple blocks or no blocks: up to 5 mev Ⓑ Qp Qh B
* * **G6004** Radiation treatment delivery, single treatment area, single port or parallel opposed ports, simple blocks or no blocks: 6-10 mev Ⓑ Qp Qh B

▶ New ↩ Revised ✔ Reinstated ~~deleted~~ Deleted ⊘ Not covered or valid by Medicare
Special coverage instructions * Carrier discretion Ⓑ Bill Part B MAC Ⓓ Bill DME MAC

✻ **G6005** Radiation treatment delivery, single treatment area, single port or parallel opposed ports, simple blocks or no blocks: 11-19 mev Ⓑ Qp Qh B

✻ **G6006** Radiation treatment delivery, single treatment area, single port or parallel opposed ports, simple blocks or no blocks: 20 mev or greater Ⓑ Qp Qh B

✻ **G6007** Radiation treatment delivery, 2 separate treatment areas, 3 or more ports on a single treatment area, use of multiple blocks: up to 5 mev Ⓑ Qp Qh B

✻ **G6008** Radiation treatment delivery, 2 separate treatment areas, 3 or more ports on a single treatment area, use of multiple blocks: 6-10 mev Ⓑ Qp Qh B

✻ **G6009** Radiation treatment delivery, 2 separate treatment areas, 3 or more ports on a single treatment area, use of multiple blocks: 11-19 mev Ⓑ Qp Qh B

✻ **G6010** Radiation treatment delivery, 2 separate treatment areas, 3 or more ports on a single treatment area, use of multiple blocks: 20 mev or greater Ⓑ Qp Qh B

✻ **G6011** Radiation treatment delivery, 3 or more separate treatment areas, custom blocking, tangential ports, wedges, rotational beam, compensators, electron beam; up to 5 mev Ⓑ Qp Qh B

✻ **G6012** Radiation treatment delivery, 3 or more separate treatment areas, custom blocking, tangential ports, wedges, rotational beam, compensators, electron beam; 6-10 mev Ⓑ Qp Qh B

✻ **G6013** Radiation treatment delivery, 3 or more separate treatment areas, custom blocking, tangential ports, wedges, rotational beam, compensators, electron beam; 11-19 mev Ⓑ Qp Qh B

✻ **G6014** Radiation treatment delivery, 3 or more separate treatment areas, custom blocking, tangential ports, wedges, rotational beam, compensators, electron beam; 20 mev or greater Ⓑ Qp Qh B

✻ **G6015** Intensity modulated treatment delivery, single or multiple fields/arcs, via narrow spatially and temporally modulated beams, binary, dynamic MLC, per treatment session Ⓑ Qp Qh B

✻ **G6016** Compensator-based beam modulation treatment delivery of inverse planned treatment using 3 or more high resolution (milled or cast) compensator, convergent beam modulated fields, per treatment session Ⓑ Qp Qh B

✻ **G6017** Intra-fraction localization and tracking of target or patient motion during delivery of radiation therapy (e.g., 3D positional tracking, gating, 3D surface tracking), each fraction of treatment Ⓑ Qp Qh B

Quality Measures

✻ **G8395** Left ventricular ejection fraction (LVEF)>=40% or documentation as normal or mildly depressed left ventricular systolic function Ⓑ M

✻ **G8396** Left ventricular ejection fraction (LVEF) not performed or documented Ⓑ M

MIPS ✻ **G8397** Dilated macular or fundus exam performed, including documentation of the presence or absence of macular edema and level of severity of retinopathy Ⓑ M

MIPS ✻ **G8398** Dilated macular or fundus exam not performed Ⓑ M

MIPS ✻ **G8399** Patient with documented results of a central dual-energy x-ray absorptiometry (DXA) ever being performed Ⓑ M

MIPS ✻ **G8400** Patient with central dual-energy x-ray absorptiometry (DXA) results not documented Ⓑ M

MIPS ✻ **G8404** Lower extremity neurological exam performed and documented Ⓑ M

MIPS ✻ **G8405** Lower extremity neurological exam not performed Ⓑ M

MIPS ✻ **G8410** Footwear evaluation performed and documented Ⓑ M

MIPS ✻ **G8415** Footwear evaluation was not performed Ⓑ M

MIPS ✻ **G8416** Clinician documented that patient was not an eligible candidate for footwear evaluation measure Ⓑ M

MIPS ✻ **G8417** BMI is documented above normal parameters and a follow-up plan is documented Ⓑ M

MIPS ✻ **G8418** BMI is documented below normal parameters and a follow-up plan is documented Ⓑ M

MIPS ✻ **G8419** BMI is documented outside normal parameters, no follow-up plan documented, no reason given Ⓑ M

* G8420 BMI is documented within normal parameters and no follow-up plan is required M
* G8421 BMI not documented and no reason is given M
* G8422 BMI not documented, documentation the patient is not eligible for BMI calculation M
* G8427 Eligible clinician attests to documenting in the medical record they obtained, updated, or reviewed the patient's current medications M
* G8428 Current list of medications not documented as obtained, updated, or reviewed by the eligible clinician, reason not given M
* G8430 Eligible clinician attests to documenting in the medical record the patient is not eligible for a current list of medications being obtained, updated, or reviewed by the eligible clinician M
* G8431 Screening for depression is documented as being positive and a follow-up plan is documented M
* G8432 Depression screening not documented, reason not given M
* G8433 Screening for depression not completed, documented reason M
* G8442 Pain assessment not documented as being performed, documentation the patient is not eligible for a pain assessment using a standardized tool at the time of the encounter M
* G8450 Beta-blocker therapy prescribed M
* G8451 beta therapy for LVEF < 40% not prescribed for reasons documented by the clinician (e.g., low blood pressure, fluid overload, asthma, patients recently treated with an intravenous positive inotropic agent, allergy, intolerance, other medical reasons, patient declined, other patient reasons or other reasons attributable to the healthcare system) M
* G8452 Beta-blocker therapy not prescribed M
* G8465 High or very high risk of recurrence of prostate cancer ♂ M
* G8473 Angiotensin converting enzyme (ACE) inhibitor or angiotensin receptor blocker (ARB) therapy prescribed M
* G8474 Angiotensin converting enzyme (ACE) inhibitor or angiotensin receptor blocker (ARB) therapy not prescribed for reasons documented by the clinician (e.g., allergy, intolerance, pregnancy, renal failure due to ACE inhibitor, diseases of the aortic or mitral valve, other medical reasons) or (e.g., patient declined, other patient reasons) or (e.g., lack of drug availability, other reasons attributable to the health care system) M
* G8475 Angiotensin converting enzyme (ACE) inhibitor or angiotensin receptor blocker (ARB) therapy not prescribed, reason not given M
* G8476 Most recent blood pressure has a systolic measurement of < 140 mmHg and a diastolic measurement of <90 mmHg M
* G8477 Most recent blood pressure has a systolic measurement of > = 140 mmHg and/or a diastolic measurement of >=90 mmHg M
* G8478 Blood pressure measurement not performed or documented, reason not given M
* G8482 Influenza immunization administered or previously received M
* G8483 Influenza immunization was not administered for reasons documented by clinician (e.g., patient allergy or other medical reasons, patient declined or other patient reasons, vacine not available or other system reasons) M
* G8484 Influenza immunization was not administered, reason not given M
* G8506 Patient receiving angiotensin converting enzyme (ACE) inhibitor or angiotensin receptor blocker (ARB) therapy M
* G8509 Pain assessment documented as positive using a standardized tool, follow-up plan not documented, reason not given M
* G8510 Screening for depression is documented as negative, a follow-up plan is not required M
* G8511 Screening for depression documented as positive, follow up plan not documented, reason not given M
* G8535 Elder maltreatment screen not documented; documentation that patient is not eligible for the elder maltreatment screen at the time of the encounter A M

▶ New ↩ Revised ✔ Reinstated ~~deleted~~ Deleted ⊘ Not covered or valid by Medicare
Special coverage instructions * Carrier discretion Ⓑ Bill Part B MAC Ⓓ Bill DME MAC

* G8536 No documentation of an elder maltreatment screen, reason not given A M
* G8539 Functional outcome assessment documented as positive using a standardized tool and a care plan based on identified deficiencies on the date of functional outcome assessment is documented M
* G8540 Functional outcome assessment not documented as being performed, documentation the patient is not eligible for a functional outcome assessment using a standardized tool at the time of the encounter M
* G8541 Functional outcome assessment using a standardized tool not documented, reason not given M
* G8542 Functional outcome assessment using a standardized tool is documented; no functional deficiencies identified, care plan not required M
* G8543 Documentation of a positive functional outcome assessment using a standardized tool; care plan not documented, reason not given M
* G8559 Patient referred to a physician (preferably a physician with training in disorders of the ear) for an otologic evaluation M
* G8560 Patient has a history of active drainage from the ear within the previous 90 days M
* G8561 Patient is not eligible for the referral for otologic evaluation for patients with a history of active drainage measure M
* G8562 Patient does not have a history of active drainage from the ear within the previous 90 days M
* G8563 Patient not referred to a physician (preferably a physician with training in disorders of the ear) for an otologic evaluation, reason not given M
* G8564 Patient was referred to a physician (preferably a physician with training in disorders of the ear) for an otologic evaluation, reason not specified M
* G8565 Verification and documentation of sudden or rapidly progressive hearing loss M
* G8566 Patient is not eligible for the "referral for otologic evaluation for sudden or rapidly progressive hearing loss" measure M
* G8567 Patient does not have verification and documentation of sudden or rapidly progressive hearing loss M
* G8568 Patient was not referred to a physician (preferably a physician with training in disorders of the ear) for an otologic evaluation, reason not given M
* G8569 Prolonged postoperative intubation (>24 hrs) required M
* G8570 Prolonged postoperative intubation (>24 hrs) not required M
* G8571 Development of deep sternal wound infection/mediastinitis within 30 days postoperatively M
* G8572 No deep sternal wound infection/ mediastinitis M
* G8573 Stroke following isolated CABG surgery M
* G8574 No stroke following isolated CABG surgery M
* G8575 Developed postoperative renal failure or required dialysis M
* G8576 No postoperative renal failure/dialysis not required M
* G8577 Re-exploration required due to mediastinal bleeding with or without tamponade, graft occlusion, valve disfunction, or other cardiac reason M
* G8578 Re-exploration not required due to mediastinal bleeding with or without tamponade, graft occlusion, valve dysfunction, or other cardiac reason M
* G8598 Aspirin or another antiplatelet therapy used M
* G8599 Aspirin or another antiplatelet therapy not used, reason not given M
* G8600 IV T-PA initiated within three hours (<=180 minutes) of time last known well M
* G8601 IV T-PA not initiated within three hours (<=180 minutes) of time last known well for reasons documented by clinician M
* G8602 IV T-PA not initiated within three hours (<=180 minutes) of time last known well, reason not given M
* G8627 Surgical procedure performed within 30 days following cataract surgery for major complications (e.g., retained nuclear fragments, endophthalmitis, dislocated or wrong power IOL, retinal detachment, or wound dehiscence) M

* G8628 Surgical procedure not performed within 30 days following cataract surgery for major complications (e.g., retained nuclear fragments, endophthalmitis, dislocated or wrong power IOL, retinal detachment, or wound dehiscence) Ⓑ M

* G8633 Pharmacologic therapy (other than minierals/vitamins) for osteoporosis prescribed Ⓑ M

* G8635 Pharmacologic therapy for osteoporosis was not prescribed, reason not given Ⓑ M

* G8647 Risk-adjusted functional status change residual score for the knee impairment successfully calculated and the score was equal to zero (0) or greater than zero (>0) Ⓑ M

* G8648 Risk-adjusted functional status change residual score for the knee impairment successfully calculated and the score was less than zero (<0) Ⓑ M

* G8649 Risk-adjusted functional status change residual scores for the knee impairment not measured because the patient did not complete FOTO'S status survey near discharge, not appropriate Ⓑ M

* G8650 Risk-adjusted functional status change residual scores for the knee impairment not measured because the patient did not complete FOTO'S functional intake on admission and/or follow up status survey near discharge, reason not given Ⓑ M

* G8651 Risk-adjusted functional status change residual score for the hip impairment successfully calculated and the score was equal to zero (0) or greater than zero (>0) Ⓑ M

* G8652 Risk-adjusted functional status change residual score for the hip impairment successfully calculated and the score was less than zero (<0) Ⓑ M

* G8653 Risk-adjusted functional status change residual scores for the hip impairment not measured because the patient did not complete follow up status survey near discharge, patient not appropriate Ⓑ M

* G8654 Risk-adjusted functional status change residual scores for the hip impairment not measured because the patient did not complete FOTO'S functional intake on admission and/or follow up status survey near discharge, reason not given Ⓑ M

* G8655 Risk-adjusted functional status change residual score for the foot or ankle impairment successfully calculated and the score was equal to zero (0) or greater than zero (>0) Ⓑ M

* G8656 Risk-adjusted functional status change residual score for the foot or ankle impairment successfully calculated and the score was less than zero (<0) Ⓑ M

* G8657 Risk-adjusted functional status change residual scores for the foot or ankle impairment not measured because the patient did not complete FOTO'S status survey near discharge, patient not appropriate Ⓑ M

* G8658 Risk-adjusted functional status change residual scores for the foot or ankle impairment not measured because the patient did not complete FOTO'S functional intake on admission and/or follow up status survey near discharge, reason not given Ⓑ M

* G8659 Risk-adjusted functional status change residual score for the low back impairment successfully calculated and the score was equal to zero (0) or greater than zero (>0) Ⓑ M

* G8660 Risk-adjusted functional status change residual score for the low back impairment successfully calculated and the score was less than zero (<0) Ⓑ M

* G8661 Risk-adjusted functional status change residual scores for the low back impairment not measured because the patient did not complete FOTO'S status survey near discharge, patient not appropriate Ⓑ M

* G8662 Risk-adjusted functional status change residual scores for the low back impairment not measured because the patient did not complete FOTO'S functional intake on admission and/or follow up status survey near discharge, reason not given Ⓑ M

* G8663 Risk-adjusted functional status change residual score for the shoulder impairment successfully calculated and the score was equal to zero (0) or greater than zero (>0) Ⓑ M

* G8664 Risk-adjusted functional status change residual score for the shoulder impairment successfully calculated and the score was less than zero (<0) Ⓑ M

* G8665 Risk-adjusted functional status change residual scores for the shoulder impairment not measured because the patient did not complete FOTO'S functional status survey near discharge, patient not appropriate Ⓑ M

* G8666 Risk-adjusted functional status change residual scores for the shoulder impairment not measured because the patient did not complete FOTO'S functional intake on admission and/or follow up status survey near discharge, reason not given M
* G8667 Risk-adjusted functional status change residual score for the elbow, wrist or hand impairment successfully calculated and the score was equal to zero (0) or greater than zero (>0) M
* G8668 Risk-adjusted functional status change residual score for the elbow, wrist or hand impairment successfully calculated and the score was less than zero (<0) M
* G8669 Risk-adjusted functional status change residual scores for the elbow, wrist or hand impairment not measured because the patient did not complete the FS status survey near discharge, patient not appropriate M
* G8670 Risk-adjusted functional status change residual scores for the elbow, wrist or hand impairment not measured because the patient did not complete the FS intake on admission and/or follow up status survey near discharge, reason not given M
* G8671 Risk-adjusted functional status change residual score for the neck, cranium, mandible, thoracic spine, ribs, or other general orthopaedic impairment successfully calculated and the score was equal to zero (0) or greater than zero (>0) M
* G8672 Risk-adjusted functional status change residual score for the neck, cranium, mandible, thoracic spine, ribs, or other general orthopaedic impairment successfully calculated and the score was less than zero (<0) M
* G8673 Risk-adjusted functional status change residual scores for the neck, cranium, mandible, thoracic spine, ribs, or other general orthopaedic impairment not measured because the patient did not complete the FS status survey near discharge, patient not appropriate M
* G8674 Risk-adjusted functional status change residual scores for the neck, cranium, mandible, thoracic spine, ribs, or other general orthopaedic impairment not measured because the patient did not complete the FS intake on admission and/or follow up status survey near discharge, reason not given M
* G8694 Left ventriucular ejection fraction (LVEF) <40% M
* G8708 Patient not prescribed or dispensed antibiotic M
* G8709 Patient prescribed or dispensed antibiotic for documented medical reason(s) within three days after the initial diagnosis of URI (e.g., intestinal infection, pertussis, bacterial infection, Lyme disease, otitis media, acute sinusitis, acute pharyngitis, acute tonsillitis, chronic sinusitis, infection of the pharynx/larynx/tonsils/adenoids, prostatitis, cellulitis, mastoiditis, or bone infections, acute lymphadenitis, impetigo, skin staph infections, pneumonia/gonococcal infections, venereal disease [syphilis, chlamydia, inflammatory diseases (female reproductive organs)], infections of the kidney, cystitis or UTI, and acne) M
* G8710 Patient prescribed or dispensed antibiotic M
* G8711 Prescribed or dispensed antibiotic M
* G8712 Antibiotic not prescribed or dispensed M
* G8721 PT category (primary tumor), PN category (regional lymph nodes), and histologic grade were documented in pathology report M
* G8722 Documentation of medical reason(s) for not including the PT category, the PN category or the histologic grade in the pathology report (e.g., re-excision without residual tumor; non-carcinomasanal canal) M
* G8723 Specimen site is other than anatomic location of primary tumor M
* G8724 PT category, PN category and histologic grade were not documented in the pathology report, reason not given M
* G8730 Pain assessment documented as positive using a standardized tool and a follow-up plan is documented M
* G8731 Pain assessment using a standardized tool is documented as negative, no follow-up plan required M
* G8732 No documentation of pain assessment, reason not given M
* G8733 Elder maltreatment screen documented as positive and a follow-up plan is documented A M
* G8734 Elder maltreatment screen documented as negative, no follow-up required A M

MIPS | Qp Quantity Physician | Qh Quantity Hospital | ♀ Female only | ♂ Male only | A Age | DMEPOS | A2-Z3 ASC Payment Indicator | A-Y ASC Status Indicator | Coding Clinic

* G8735 Elder maltreatment screen documented as positive, follow-up plan not documented, reason not given Ⓑ A M
⊋* G8749 Absence of signs of melanoma (tenderness, jaundice, localized neurologic signs such as weakness, or any other sign suggesting systemic spread) or absence of symptoms of melanoma (cough, dyspnea, pain, paresthesia, or any other symptom suggesting the possibility of systemic spread of melanoma) Ⓑ M
* G8752 Most recent systolic blood pressure <140 mmhg Ⓑ M
* G8753 Most recent systolic blood pressure >=140 mmhg Ⓑ M
* G8754 Most recent diastolic blood pressure <90 mmhg Ⓑ M
* G8755 Most recent diastolic blood pressure >=90 mmhg Ⓑ M
* G8756 No documentation of blood pressure measurement, reason not given Ⓑ M
* G8783 Normal blood pressure reading documented, follow-up not required Ⓑ M
* G8785 Blood pressure reading not documented, reason not given Ⓑ M
* G8797 Specimen site other than anatomic location of esophagus Ⓑ M
* G8798 Specimen site other than anatomic location of prostate Ⓑ M
⊋* G8806 Performance of trans-abdominal or trans-vaginal ultrasound and pregnancy location documented Ⓑ M
* G8807 Trans-abdominal or trans-vaginal ultrasound not performed for reasons documented by clinician (e.g., patient has visited the ED multiple times within 72 hours, patient has a documented intrauterine pregnancy [IUP]) Ⓑ M
* G8808 Trans-abdominal or trans-vaginal ultrasound not performed, reason not given Ⓑ M
* G8809 Rh-immunoglobulin (RhoGAM) ordered Ⓑ M
* G8810 Rh-immunoglobulin (RhoGAM) not ordered for reasons documented by clinician (e.g., patient had prior documented report of RhoGAM within 12 weeks, patient refusal) Ⓑ M
* G8811 Documentation RH-immunoglobulin (RhoGAM) was not ordered, reason not given Ⓑ M
* G8815 Documented reason in the medical records for why the statin therapy was not prescribed (i.e., lower extremity bypass was for a patient with non-artherosclerotic disease) Ⓑ M
* G8816 Statin medication prescribed at discharge Ⓑ M
* G8817 Statin therapy not prescribed at discharge, reason not given Ⓑ M
* G8818 Patient discharge to home no later than post-operative day #7 Ⓑ M
* G8825 Patient not discharged to home by post-operative day #7 Ⓑ M
* G8826 Patient discharge to home no later than post-operative day #2 following EVAR Ⓑ M
* G8833 Patient not discharged to home by post-operative day #2 following EVAR Ⓑ M
* G8834 Patient discharged to home no later than post-operative day #2 following CEA Ⓑ M
* G8838 Patient not discharged to home by post-operative day #2 following CEA Ⓑ M
* G8839 Sleep apnea symptoms assessed, including presence or absence of snoring and daytime sleepiness Ⓑ M
* G8840 Documentation of reason(s) for not documenting an assessment of sleep symptoms (e.g., patient didn't have initial daytime sleepiness, patient visited between initial testing and initiation of therapy) Ⓑ M
* G8841 Sleep apnea symptoms not assessed, reason not given Ⓑ M
* G8842 Apnea Hypopnea Index (AHI) or Respiratory Disturbance Index (RDI) measured at the time of initial diagnosis Ⓑ M
* G8843 Documentation of reason(s) for not measuring an Apnea Hypopnea Index (AHI) or a Respiratory Disturbance Index (RDI) at the time of initial diagnosis (e.g., psychiatric disease, dementia, patient declined, financial, insurance coverage, test ordered but not yet completed) Ⓑ M

▶ New ⊋ Revised ✔ Reinstated ~~deleted~~ Deleted ⊘ Not covered or valid by Medicare
Special coverage instructions * Carrier discretion Ⓑ Bill Part B MAC Ⓓ Bill DME MAC

MIPS * **G8844** Apnea Hypopnea Index (AHI) or Respiratory Disturbance Index (RDI) not measured at the time of initial diagnosis, reason not given B M

MIPS * **G8845** Positive airway pressure therapy prescribed B M

MIPS * **G8846** Moderate or severe obstructive sleep apnea (Apnea Hypopnea Index (AHI) or Respiratory Disturbance Index (RDI) of 15 or greater) B M

MIPS * **G8849** Documentation of reason(s) for not prescribing positive airway pressure therapy (e.g., patient unable to tolerate, alternative therapies use, patient declined, financial, insurance coverage) B M

MIPS * **G8850** Positive airway pressure therapy not prescribed, reason not given B M

MIPS * **G8851** Objective measurement of adherence to positive airway pressure therapy, documented B M

MIPS * **G8852** Positive airway pressure therapy prescribed B M

MIPS * **G8854** Documentation of reason(s) for not objectively measuring adherence to positive airway pressure therapy (e.g., patient didn't bring data from continuous positive airway pressure [CPAP], therapy was not yet initiated, not available on machine) B M

MIPS * **G8855** Objective measurement of adherence to positive airway pressure therapy not performed, reason not given B M

MIPS * **G8856** Referral to a physician for an otologic evaluation performed B M

MIPS * **G8857** Patient is not eligible for the referral for otologic evaluation measure (e.g., patients who are already under the care of a physician for acute or chronic dizziness) B M

MIPS * **G8858** Referral to a physician for an otologic evaluation not performed, reason not given B M

MIPS * **G8861** Within the past 2 years, central dual-energy x-ray absorptiometry (DXA) ordered and documented, review of systems and medication history or pharmacologic therapy (other than minerals/vitamins) for osteoporosis prescribed B M

* **G8863** Patients not assessed for risk of bone loss, reason not given B M

* **G8864** Pneumococcal vaccine administered or previously received B M

* **G8865** Documentation of medical reason(s) for not administering or previously receiving pneumococcal vaccine (e.g., patient allergic reaction, potential adverse drug reaction) B M

* **G8866** Documentation of patient reason(s) for not administering or previously receiving pneumococcal vaccine (e.g., patient refusal) B M

* **G8867** Pneumococcal vaccine not administered or previously received, reason not given B M

MIPS * **G8869** Patient has documented immunity to hepatitis B and initiating anti-TNF therapy B M

MIPS * **G8872** Excised tissue evaluated by imaging intraoperatively to confirm successful inclusion of targeted lesion B M

MIPS * **G8873** Patients with needle localization specimens which are not amenable to intraoperative imaging such as MRI needle wire localization, or targets which are tentatively identified on mammogram or ultrasound which do not contain a biopsy marker but which can be verified on intraoperative inspection or pathology (e.g., needle biopsy site where the biopsy marker is remote from the actual biopsy site) B M

MIPS * **G8874** Excised tissue not evaluated by imaging intraoperatively to confirm successful inclusion of targeted lesion B M

MIPS * **G8875** Clinician diagnosed breast cancer preoperatively by a minimally invasive biopsy method B M

MIPS * **G8876** Documentation of reason(s) for not performing minimally invasive biopsy to diagnose breast cancer preoperatively (e.g., lesion too close to skin, implant, chest wall, etc., lesion could not be adequately visualized for needle biopsy, patient condition prevents needle biopsy [weight, breast thickness, etc.], duct excision without imaging abnormality, prophylactic mastectomy, reduction mammoplasty, excisional biopsy performed by another physician) B M

MIPS * **G8877** Clinician did not attempt to achieve the diagnosis of breast cancer preoperatively by a minimally invasive biopsy method, reason not given B M

* G8878 Sentinel lymph node biopsy procedure performed M
* G8880 Documentation of reason(s) sentinel lymph node biopsy not performed (e.g., reasons could include but not limited to; non-invasive cancer, incidental discovery of breast cancer on prophylactic mastectomy, incidental discovery of breast cancer on reduction mammoplasty, pre-operative biopsy proven lymph node (LN) metastases, inflammatory carcinoma, stage 3 locally advanced cancer, recurrent invasive breast cancer, clinically node positive after neoadjuvant systemic therapy, patient refusal after informed consent; patient with significant age, comorbidities, or limited life expectancy and favorable tumor; adjuvant systemic therapy unlikely to change) M
* G8881 Stage of breast cancer is greater than T1N0M0 or T2N0M0 M
* G8882 Sentinel lymph node biopsy procedure not performed, reason not given M
* G8883 Biopsy results reviewed, communicated, tracked and documented M
* G8884 Clinician documented reason that patient's biopsy results were not reviewed M
* G8885 Biopsy results not reviewed, communicated, tracked or documented M
* G8907 Patient documented not to have experienced any of the following events: a burn prior to discharge; a fall within the facility; wrong site/side/patient/procedure/implant event; or a hospital transfer or hospital admission upon discharge from the facility M
* G8908 Patient documented to have received a burn prior to discharge M
* G8909 Patient documented not to have received a burn prior to discharge M
* G8910 Patient documented to have experienced a fall within ASC M
* G8911 Patient documented not to have experienced a fall within ambulatory surgical center M
* G8912 Patient documented to have experienced a wrong site, wrong side, wrong patient, wrong procedure or wrong implant event M
* G8913 Patient documented not to have experienced a wrong site, wrong side, wrong patient, wrong procedure or wrong implant event M
* G8914 Patient documented to have experienced a hospital transfer or hospital admission upon discharge from ASC M
* G8915 Patient documented not to have experienced a hospital transfer or hospital admission upon discharge from ASC M
* G8916 Patient with preoperative order for IV antibiotic surgical site infection (SSI) prophylaxis, antibiotic initiated on time M
* G8917 Patient with preoperative order for IV antibiotic surgical site infection (SSI) prophylaxis, antibiotic not initiated on time M
* G8918 Patient without preoperative order for IV antibiotic surgical site infection(SSI) prophylaxis M
* G8923 Left ventricular ejection fraction (LVEF) <40% or documentation of moderately or severely depressed left ventricular systolic function M
* G8924 Spirometry test results demonstrate FEV1/FVC <70%, FEV <60% predicted and patient has COPD symptoms (e.g., dyspnea, cough/sputum, wheezing) M
* G8925 Spirometry test results demonstrate FEV1>=60% FEV1/FVC>=70%, predicted or patient does not have COPD symptoms M
* G8926 Spirometry test not performed or documented, reason not given M
* G8934 Left ventricular ejection fraction (LVEF) <40% or documentation of moderately or severely depressed left ventricular systolic function M
* G8935 Clinician prescribed angiotensin converting enzyme (ACE) inhibitor or angiotensin receptor blocker (ARB) therapy M
* G8936 Clinician documented that patient was not an eligible candidate for angiotensin converting enzyme (ACE) inhibitor or angiotensin receptor blocker (ARB) therapy (e.g., allergy, intolerance, pregnancy, renal failure due to ace inhibitor, diseases of the aortic or mitral valve, other medical reasons) or (e.g., patient declined, other patient reasons) or (e.g., lack of drug availability, other reasons attributable to the health care system) M

* **G8937** Clinician did not prescribe angiotensin converting enzyme (ACE) inhibitor or angiotensin receptor blocker (ARB) therapy, reason not given M
* **G8938** BMI is documented as being outside of normal limits, follow-up plan is not documented, documentation the patient is not eligible M
* **G8939** Pain assessment documented as positive, follow-up plan not documented, documentation the patient is not eligible at the time of the encounter at the time of the encounter M
* **G8941** Elder maltreatment screen documented as positive, follow-up plan not documented, documentation the patient is not eligible for follow-up plan at the time of the encounter A M
* **G8942** Functional outcomes assessment using a standardized tool is documented within the previous 30 days and care plan, based on identified deficiencies on the date of the functional outcome assessment, is documented M
* **G8944** AJCC melanoma cancer stage 0 through IIC melanoma M
* **G8946** Minimally invasive biopsy method attempted but not diagnostic of breast cancer (e.g., high risk lesion of breast such as atypical ductal hyperplasia, lobular neoplasia, atypical lobular hyperplasia, lobular carcinoma in situ, atypical columnar hyperplasia, flat epithelial atypia, radial scar, complex sclerosing lesion, papillary lesion, or any lesion with spindle cells) M
* **G8950** Pre-hypertensive or hypertensive blood pressure reading documented, and the indicated follow-up documented M
* **G8952** Pre-hypertensive or hypertensive blood pressure reading documented, indicated follow-up not documented, reason not given M
* **G8955** Most recent assessment of adequacy of volume management documented M
* **G8956** Patient receiving maintenance hemodialysis in an outpatient dialysis facility M
* **G8958** Assessment of adequacy of volume management not documented, reason not given M
* **G8959** Clinician treating major depressive disorder communicates to clinician treating comorbid condition M
* **G8960** Clinician treating major depressive disorder did not communicate to clinician treating comorbid condition, reason not given M
* **G8961** Cardiac stress imaging test primarily performed on low-risk surgery patient for preoperative evaluation within 30 days preceding this surgery M
* **G8962** Cardiac stress imaging test performed on patient for any reason including those who did not have low risk surgery or test that was performed more than 30 days preceding low risk surgery M
* **G8963** Cardiac stress imaging performed primarily for monitoring of asymptomatic patient who had PCI within 2 years M
* **G8964** Cardiac stress imaging test performed primarily for any other reason than monitoring of asymptomatic patient who had PCI within 2 years (e.g., symptomatic patient, patient greater than 2 years since PCI, initial evaluation, etc.) M
* **G8965** Cardiac stress imaging test primarily performed on low CHD risk patient for initial detection and risk assessment M
* **G8966** Cardiac stress imaging test performed on symptomatic or higher than low CHD risk patient or for any reason other than initial detection and risk assessment M
* **G8967** Warfarin or another FDA-approved oral anticoagulant is prescribed M
* **G8968** Documentation of medical reason(s) for not prescribing warfarin or another FDA-approved anticoagulant (e.g., atrial appendage device in place) M
* **G8969** Documentation of patient reason(s) for not prescribing warfarin or another FDA-approved oral anticoagulant that is FDA approved for the prevention of thromboembolism (e.g., patient choice of having atrial appendage device placed) M
* **G8970** No risk factors or one moderate risk factor for thromboembolism M
* **G8973** Most recent hemoglobin (Hgb) level <10 g/dl M

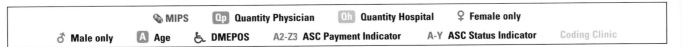

MIPS | Qp Quantity Physician | Qh Quantity Hospital | ♀ Female only | ♂ Male only | A Age | DMEPOS | A2-Z3 ASC Payment Indicator | A-Y ASC Status Indicator | Coding Clinic

* G8974 Hemoglobin level measurement not documented, reason not given (B) M

* G8975 Documentation of medical reason(s) for patient having a hemoglobin level <10 g/dl (e.g., patients who have non-renal etiologies of anemia [e.g., sickle cell anemia or other hemoglobinopathies, hypersplenism, primary bone marrow disease, anemia related to chemotherapy for diagnosis of malignancy, postoperative bleeding, active bloodstream or peritoneal infection], other medical reasons) (B) M

* G8976 Most recent hemoglobin (Hgb) level >=10 g/dl (B) M

Functional Limitation

* G8978 Mobility: walking & moving around functional limitation, current status, at therapy episode outset and at reporting intervals (B) E1

* G8979 Mobility: walking & moving around functional limitation, projected goal status, at therapy episode outset, at reporting intervals, and at discharge or to end reporting (B) E1

* G8980 Mobility: walking & moving around functional limitation, discharge status, at discharge from therapy or to end reporting (B) E1

* G8981 Changing and maintaining body position functional limitation, current status, at therapy episode outset and at reporting intervals (B) E1

* G8982 Changing and maintaining body position functional limitation, projected goal status, at therapy episode outset, at reporting intervals, and at discharge or to end reporting (B) E1

* G8983 Changing and maintaining body position functional limitation, discharge status, at discharge from therapy or to end reporting (B) E1

* G8984 Carrying, moving and handling objects functional limitation, current status, at therapy episode outset and at reporting intervals (B) E1

* G8985 Carrying, moving and handling objects, projected goal status, at therapy episode outset, at reporting intervals, and at discharge or to end reporting (B) E1

* G8986 Carrying, moving & handling objects functional limitation, discharge status, at discharge from therapy or to end reporting (B) E1

* G8987 Self-care functional limitation, current status, at therapy episode outset and at reporting intervals (B) E1

* G8988 Self-care functional limitation, projected goal status, at therapy episode outset, at reporting intervals, and at discharge or to end reporting (B) E1

* G8989 Self-care functional limitation, discharge status, at discharge from therapy or to end reporting (B) E1

* G8990 Other physical or occupational therapy primary functional limitation, current status, at therapy episode outset and at reporting intervals (B) E1

* G8991 Other physical or occupational therapy primary functional limitation, projected goal status, at therapy episode outset, at reporting intervals, and at discharge or to end reporting (B) E1

* G8992 Other physical or occupational therapy primary functional limitation, discharge status, at discharge from therapy or to end reporting (B) E1

* G8993 Other physical or occupational therapy subsequent functional limitation, current status, at therapy episode outset and at reporting intervals (B) E1

* G8994 Other physical or occupational therapy subsequent functional limitation, projected goal status, at therapy episode outset, at reporting intervals, and at discharge or to end reporting (B) E1

* G8995 Other physical or occupational therapy subsequent functional limitation, discharge status, at discharge from therapy or to end reporting (B) E1

* G8996 Swallowing functional limitation, current status at therapy episode outset and at reporting intervals (B) E1

* G8997 Swallowing functional limitation, projected goal status, at therapy episode outset, at reporting intervals, and at discharge or to end reporting (B) E1

* G8998 Swallowing functional limitation, discharge status, at discharge from therapy or to end reporting (B) E1

* G8999 Motor speech functional limitation, current status at therapy episode outset and at reporting intervals (B) E1

Coordinated Care

G9001 Coordinated care fee, initial rate B

G9002 Coordinated care fee, maintenance rate B

G9003 Coordinated care fee, risk adjusted high, initial B

G9004 Coordinated care fee, risk adjusted low, initial B

G9005 Coordinated care fee, risk adjusted maintenance B

G9006 Coordinated care fee, home monitoring B

G9007 Coordinated care fee, scheduled team conference B

G9008 Coordinated care fee, physician coordinated care oversight services B

G9009 Coordinated care fee, risk adjusted maintenance, level 3 B

G9010 Coordinated care fee, risk adjusted maintenance, level 4 B

G9011 Coordinated care fee, risk adjusted maintenance, level 5 B

G9012 Other specified case management services not elsewhere classified B

Demonstration Project

G9013 ESRD demo basic bundle Level I E1

G9014 ESRD demo expanded bundle including venous access and related services E1

G9016 Smoking cessation counseling, individual, in the absence of or in addition to any other evaluation and management service, per session (6-10 minutes) [demo project code only] E1

* **G9017** Amantadine hydrochloride, oral, per 100 mg (for use in a Medicare-approved demonstration project) A

* **G9018** Zanamivir, inhalation powder, administered through inhaler, per 10 mg (for use in a Medicare-approved demonstration project) A

* **G9019** Oseltamivir phosphate, oral, per 75 mg (for use in a Medicare-approved demonstration project) A

* **G9020** Rimantadine hydrochloride, oral, per 100 mg (for use in a Medicare-approved demonstration project) A

* **G9033** Amantadine hydrochloride, oral brand, per 100 mg (for use in a Medicare-approved demonstration project) A

* **G9034** Zanamivir, inhalation powder, administered through inhaler, brand, per 10 mg (for use in a Medicare-approved demonstration project) A

* **G9035** Oseltamivir phosphate, oral, brand, per 75 mg (for use in a Medicare-approved demonstration project) A

* **G9036** Rimantadine hydrochloride, oral, brand, per 100 mg (for use in a Medicare-approved demonstration project) A

G9050 Oncology; primary focus of visit; work-up, evaluation, or staging at the time of cancer diagnosis or recurrence (for use in a Medicare-approved demonstration project) E1

G9051 Oncology; primary focus of visit; treatment decision-making after disease is staged or restaged, discussion of treatment options, supervising/ coordinating active cancer directed therapy or managing consequences of cancer directed therapy (for use in a Medicare-approved demonstration project) E1

G9052 Oncology; primary focus of visit; surveillance for disease recurrence for patient who has completed definitive cancer-directed therapy and currently lacks evidence of recurrent disease; cancer directed therapy might be considered in the future (for use in a Medicare-approved demonstration project) E1

G9053 Oncology; primary focus of visit; expectant management of patient with evidence of cancer for whom no cancer directed therapy is being administered or arranged at present; cancer directed therapy might be considered in the future (for use in a Medicare-approved demonstration project) E1

⃠ **G9054** Oncology; primary focus of visit; supervising, coordinating or managing care of patient with terminal cancer or for whom other medical illness prevents further cancer treatment; includes symptom management, end-of-life care planning, management of palliative therapies (for use in a Medicare-approved demonstration project) Ⓑ E1

⃠ **G9055** Oncology; primary focus of visit; other, unspecified service not otherwise listed (for use in a Medicare-approved demonstration project) Ⓑ E1

⃠ **G9056** Oncology; practice guidelines; management adheres to guidelines (for use in a Medicare-approved demonstration project) Ⓑ E1

⃠ **G9057** Oncology; practice guidelines; management differs from guidelines as a result of patient enrollment in an institutional review board approved clinical trial (for use in a Medicare-approved demonstration project) Ⓑ E1

⃠ **G9058** Oncology; practice guidelines; management differs from guidelines because the treating physician disagrees with guideline recommendations (for use in a Medicare-approved demonstration project) Ⓑ E1

⃠ **G9059** Oncology; practice guidelines; management differs from guidelines because the patient, after being offered treatment consistent with guidelines, has opted for alternative treatment or management, including no treatment (for use in a Medicare-approved demonstration project) Ⓑ E1

⃠ **G9060** Oncology; practice guidelines; management differs from guidelines for reason(s) associated with patient comorbid illness or performance status not factored into guidelines (for use in a Medicare-approved demonstration project) Ⓑ E1

⃠ **G9061** Oncology; practice guidelines; patient's condition not addressed by available guidelines (for use in a Medicare-approved demonstration project) Ⓑ E1

⃠ **G9062** Oncology; practice guidelines; management differs from guidelines for other reason(s) not listed (for use in a Medicare-approved demonstration project) Ⓑ E1

* **G9063** Oncology; disease status; limited to non-small cell lung cancer; extent of disease initially established as stage I (prior to neo-adjuvant therapy, if any) with no evidence of disease progression, recurrence, or metastases (for use in a Medicare-approved demonstration project) Ⓑ M

* **G9064** Oncology; disease status; limited to non-small cell lung cancer; extent of disease initially established as stage II (prior to neo-adjuvant therapy, if any) with no evidence of disease progression, recurrence, or metastases (for use in a Medicare-approved demonstration project) Ⓑ M

* **G9065** Oncology; disease status; limited to non-small cell lung cancer; extent of disease initially established as stage IIIA (prior to neo-adjuvant therapy, if any) with no evidence of disease progression, recurrence, or metastases (for use in a Medicare-approved demonstration project) Ⓑ M

* **G9066** Oncology; disease status; limited to non-small cell lung cancer; stage IIIB-IV at diagnosis, metastatic, locally recurrent, or progressive (for use in a Medicare-approved demonstration project) Ⓑ M

* **G9067** Oncology; disease status; limited to non-small cell lung cancer; extent of disease unknown, staging in progress, or not listed (for use in a Medicare-approved demonstration project) Ⓑ M

* **G9068** Oncology; disease status; limited to small cell and combined small cell/non-small cell; extent of disease initially established as limited with no evidence of disease progression, recurrence, or metastases (for use in a Medicare-approved demonstration project) Ⓑ M

* **G9069** Oncology; disease status; small cell lung cancer, limited to small cell and combined small cell/non-small cell; extensive stage at diagnosis, metastatic, locally recurrent, or progressive (for use in a Medicare-approved demonstration project) Ⓑ M

✻ **G9070** Oncology; disease status; small cell lung cancer, limited to small cell and combined small cell/non-small cell; extent of disease unknown, staging in progress, or not listed (for use in a Medicare-approved demonstration project) Ⓑ M

✻ **G9071** Oncology; disease status; invasive female breast cancer (does not include ductal carcinoma in situ); adenocarcinoma as predominant cell type; stage I or stage IIA-IIB; or T3, N1, M0; and ER and/or PR positive; with no evidence of disease progression, recurrence, or metastases (for use in a Medicare-approved demonstration project) Ⓑ ♀ M

✻ **G9072** Oncology; disease status; invasive female breast cancer (does not include ductal carcinoma in situ); adenocarcinoma as predominant cell type; stage I, or stage IIA-IIB; or T3, N1, M0; and ER and PR negative; with no evidence of disease progression, recurrence, or metastases (for use in a Medicare-approved demonstration project) Ⓑ ♀ M

✻ **G9073** Oncology; disease status; invasive female breast cancer (does not include ductal carcinoma in situ); adenocarcinoma as predominant cell type; stage IIIA-IIIB; and not T3, N1, M0; and ER and/or PR positive; with no evidence of disease progression, recurrence, or metastases (for use in a Medicare-approved demonstration project) Ⓑ ♀ M

✻ **G9074** Oncology; disease status; invasive female breast cancer (does not include ductal carcinoma in situ); adenocarcinoma as predominant cell type; stage IIIA-IIIB; and not T3, N1, M0; and ER and PR negative; with no evidence of disease progression, recurrence, or metastases (for use in a Medicare-approved demonstration project) Ⓑ ♀ M

✻ **G9075** Oncology; disease status; invasive female breast cancer (does not include ductal carcinoma in situ); adenocarcinoma as predominant cell type; M1 at diagnosis, metastatic, locally recurrent, or progressive (for use in a Medicare-approved demonstration project) Ⓑ ♀ M

✻ **G9077** Oncology; disease status; prostate cancer, limited to adenocarcinoma as predominant cell type; T1-T2c and Gleason 2-7 and PSA < or equal to 20 at diagnosis with no evidence of disease progression, recurrence, or metastases (for use in a Medicare-approved demonstration project) Ⓑ ♂ M

✻ **G9078** Oncology; disease status; prostate cancer, limited to adenocarcinoma as predominant cell type; T2 or T3a Gleason 8-10 or PSA >20 at diagnosis with no evidence of disease progression, recurrence, or metastases (for use in a Medicare-approved demonstration project) Ⓑ ♂ M

✻ **G9079** Oncology; disease status; prostate cancer, limited to adenocarcinoma as predominant cell type; T3b-T4, any N; any T, N1 at diagnosis with no evidence of disease progression, recurrence, or metastases (for use in a Medicare-approved demonstration project) Ⓑ ♂ M

✻ **G9080** Oncology; disease status; prostate cancer, limited to adenocarcinoma; after initial treatment with rising PSA or failure of PSA decline (for use in a Medicare-approved demonstration project) Ⓑ ♂ M

✻ **G9083** Oncology; disease status; prostate cancer, limited to adenocarcinoma; extent of disease unknown, staging in progress, or not listed (for use in a Medicare-approved demonstration project) Ⓑ ♂ M

✻ **G9084** Oncology; disease status; colon cancer, limited to invasive cancer, adenocarcinoma as predominant cell type; extent of disease initially established as T1-3, N0, M0 with no evidence of disease progression, recurrence, or metastases (for use in a Medicare-approved demonstration project) Ⓑ M

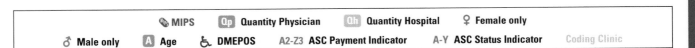

✻ **G9085** Oncology; disease status; colon cancer, limited to invasive cancer, adenocarcinoma as predominant cell type; extent of disease initially established as T4, N0, M0 with no evidence of disease progression, recurrence, or metastases (for use in a Medicare-approved demonstration project) Ⓑ M

✻ **G9086** Oncology; disease status; colon cancer, limited to invasive cancer, adenocarcinoma as predominant cell type; extent of disease initially established as T1-4, N1-2, M0 with no evidence of disease progression, recurrence, or metastases (for use in a Medicare-approved demonstration project) Ⓑ M

✻ **G9087** Oncology; disease status; colon cancer, limited to invasive cancer, adenocarcinoma as predominant cell type; M1 at diagnosis, metastatic, locally recurrent, or progressive with current clinical, radiologic, or biochemical evidence of disease (for use in a Medicare-approved demonstration project) Ⓑ M

✻ **G9088** Oncology; disease status; colon cancer, limited to invasive cancer, adenocarcinoma as predominant cell type; M1 at diagnosis, metastatic, locally recurrent, or progressive without current clinical, radiologic, or biochemical evidence of disease (for use in a Medicare-approved demonstration project) Ⓑ M

✻ **G9089** Oncology; disease status; colon cancer, limited to invasive cancer, adenocarcinoma as predominant cell type; extent of disease unknown, staging in progress, or not listed (for use in a Medicare-approved demonstration project) Ⓑ M

✻ **G9090** Oncology; disease status; rectal cancer, limited to invasive cancer, adenocarcinoma as predominant cell type; extent of disease initially established as T1-2, N0, M0 (prior to neo-adjuvant therapy, if any) with no evidence of disease progression, recurrence, or metastases (for use in a Medicare-approved demonstration project) Ⓑ M

✻ **G9091** Oncology; disease status; rectal cancer, limited to invasive cancer, adenocarcinoma as predominant cell type; extent of disease initially established as T3, N0, M0 (prior to neo-adjuvant therapy, if any) with no evidence of disease progression, recurrence, or metastases (for use in a Medicare-approved demonstration project) Ⓑ M

✻ **G9092** Oncology; disease status; rectal cancer, limited to invasive cancer, adenocarcinoma as predominant cell type; extent of disease initially established as T1-3, N1-2, M0 (prior to neo-adjuvant therapy, if any) with no evidence of disease progression, recurrence or metastases (for use in a Medicare-approved demonstration project) Ⓑ M

✻ **G9093** Oncology; disease status; rectal cancer, limited to invasive cancer, adenocarcinoma as predominant cell type; extent of disease initially established as T4, any N, M0 (prior to neo-adjuvant therapy, if any) with no evidence of disease progression, recurrence, or metastases (for use in a Medicare-approved demonstration project) Ⓑ M

✻ **G9094** Oncology; disease status; rectal cancer, limited to invasive cancer, adenocarcinoma as predominant cell type; M1 at diagnosis, metastatic, locally recurrent, or progressive (for use in a Medicare-approved demonstration project) Ⓑ M

✻ **G9095** Oncology; disease status; rectal cancer, limited to invasive cancer, adenocarcinoma as predominant cell type; extent of disease unknown, staging in progress, or not listed (for use in a Medicare-approved demonstration project) Ⓑ M

✻ **G9096** Oncology; disease status; esophageal cancer, limited to adenocarcinoma or squamous cell carcinoma as predominant cell type; extent of disease initially established as T1-T3, N0-N1 or NX (prior to neo-adjuvant therapy, if any) with no evidence of disease progression, recurrence, or metastases (for use in a Medicare-approved demonstration project) Ⓑ M

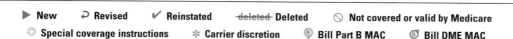

✻ **G9097** Oncology; disease status; esophageal cancer, limited to adenocarcinoma or squamous cell carcinoma as predominant cell type; extent of disease initially established as T4, any N, M0 (prior to neo-adjuvant therapy, if any) with no evidence of disease progression, recurrence, or metastases (for use in a Medicare-approved demonstration project) Ⓑ M

✱ **G9098** Oncology; disease status; esophageal cancer, limited to adenocarcinoma or squamous cell carcinoma as predominant cell type; M1 at diagnosis, meta-static, locally recurrent, or progressive (for use in a Medicare-approved demonstration project) Ⓑ M

✱ **G9099** Oncology; disease status; esophageal cancer, limited to adenocarcinoma or squamous cell carcinoma as predominant cell type; extent of disease unknown, staging in progress, or not listed (for use in a Medicare-approved demonstration project) Ⓑ M

✱ **G9100** Oncology; disease status; gastric cancer, limited to adenocarcinoma as predominant cell type; post R0 resection (with or without neoadjuvant therapy) with no evidence of disease recurrence, progression, or metastases (for use in a Medicare-approved demonstration project) Ⓑ M

✱ **G9101** Oncology; disease status; gastric cancer, limited to adenocarcinoma as predominant cell type; post R1 or R2 resection (with or without neoadjuvant therapy) with no evidence of disease progression, or metastases (for use in a Medicare-approved demonstration project) Ⓑ M

✱ **G9102** Oncology; disease status; gastric cancer, limited to adenocarcinoma as predominant cell type; clinical or pathologic M0, unresectable with no evidence of disease progression, or metastases (for use in a Medicare-approved demonstration project Ⓑ M

✱ **G9103** Oncology; disease status; gastric cancer, limited to adenocarcinoma as predominant cell type; clinical or pathologic M1 at diagnosis, metastatic, locally recurrent, or progressive (for use in a Medicare-approved demonstration project) Ⓑ M

✱ **G9104** Oncology; disease status; gastric cancer, limited to adenocarcinoma as predominant cell type; extent of disease unknown, staging in progress, or not listed (for use in a Medicare-approved demonstration project Ⓑ M

✱ **G9105** Oncology; disease status; pancreatic cancer, limited to adenocarcinoma as predominant cell type; post R0 resection without evidence of disease progression, recurrence, or metastases (for use in a Medicare-approved demonstration project) Ⓑ M

✱ **G9106** Oncology; disease status; pancreatic cancer, limited to adenocarcinoma; post R1 or R2 resection with no evidence of disease progression or metastases (for use in a Medicare-approved demonstration project) Ⓑ M

✱ **G9107** Oncology; disease status; pancreatic cancer, limited to adenocarcinoma; unresectable at diagnosis, M1 at diagnosis, metastatic, locally recurrent, or progressive (for use in a Medicare-approved demonstration project) Ⓑ M

✱ **G9108** Oncology; disease status; pancreatic cancer, limited to adenocarcinoma; extent of disease unknown, staging in progress, or not listed (for use in a Medicare-approved demonstration project) Ⓑ M

✱ **G9109** Oncology; disease status; head and neck cancer, limited to cancers of oral cavity, pharynx and larynx with squamous cell as predominant cell type; extent of disease initially established as T1-T2 and N0, M0 (prior to neo-adjuvant therapy, if any) with no evidence of disease progression, recurrence, or metastases (for use in a Medicare-approved demonstration project) Ⓑ M

✱ **G9110** Oncology; disease status; head and neck cancer, limited to cancers of oral cavity, pharynx, and larynx with squamous cell as predominant cell type; extent of disease initially established as T3-4 and/ or N1-3, M0 (prior to neo-adjuvant therapy, if any) with no evidence of disease progression, recurrence, or metastases (for use in a Medicare-approved demonstration project) Ⓑ M

✱ **G9111** Oncology; disease status; head and neck cancer, limited to cancers of oral cavity, pharynx and larynx with squamous cell as predominant cell type; M1 at diagnosis, metastatic, locally recurrent, or progressive (for use in a Medicare-approved demonstration project) Ⓑ M

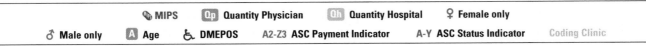

✱ **G9112** Oncology; disease status; head and neck cancer, limited to cancers of oral cavity, pharynx and larynx with squamous cell as predominant cell type; extent of disease unknown, staging in progress, or not listed (for use in a Medicare-approved demonstration project) Ⓑ M

✻ **G9113** Oncology; disease status; ovarian cancer, limited to epithelial cancer; pathologic stage IA-B (grade 1) without evidence of disease progression, recurrence, or metastases (for use in a Medicare-approved demonstration project) Ⓑ ♀ M

✻ **G9114** Oncology; disease status; ovarian cancer, limited to epithelial cancer; pathologic stage IA-B (grade 2-3); or stage IC (all grades); or stage II; without evidence of disease progression, recurrence, or metastases (for use in a Medicare-approved demonstration project) Ⓑ ♀ M

✻ **G9115** Oncology; disease status; ovarian cancer, limited to epithelial cancer; pathologic stage III-IV; without evidence of progression, recurrence, or metastases (for use in a Medicare-approved demonstration project) Ⓑ ♀ M

✻ **G9116** Oncology; disease status; ovarian cancer, limited to epithelial cancer; evidence of disease progression, or recurrence and/or platinum resistance (for use in a Medicare-approved demonstration project) Ⓑ ♀ M

✻ **G9117** Oncology; disease status; ovarian cancer, limited to epithelial cancer; extent of disease unknown, staging in progress, or not listed (for use in a Medicare-approved demonstration project) Ⓑ ♀ M

✻ **G9123** Oncology; disease status; chronic myelogenous leukemia, limited to Philadelphia chromosome positive and/or BCR-ABL positive; chronic phase not in hematologic, cytogenetic, or molecular remission (for use in a Medicare-approved demonstration project) Ⓑ M

✻ **G9124** Oncology; disease status; chronic myelogenous leukemia, limited to Philadelphia chromosome positive and/or BCR-ABL positive; accelerated phase not in hematologic cytogenetic, or molecular remission (for use in a Medicare-approved demonstration project) Ⓑ M

✻ **G9125** Oncology; disease status; chronic myelogenous leukemia, limited to Philadelphia chromosome positive and/or BCR-ABL positive; blast phase not in hematologic, cytogenetic, or molecular remission (for use in a Medicare-approved demonstration project) Ⓑ M

✻ **G9126** Oncology; disease status; chronic myelogenous leukemia, limited to Philadelphia chromosome positive and/or BCR-ABL positive; in hematologic, cytogenetic, or molecular remission (for use in a Medicare-approved demonstration project) Ⓑ M

✻ **G9128** Oncology: disease status; limited to multiple myeloma, systemic disease; smouldering, stage I (for use in a Medicare-approved demonstration project) Ⓑ M

✻ **G9129** Oncology; disease status; limited to multiple myeloma, systemic disease; stage II or higher (for use in a Medicare-approved demonstration project) Ⓑ M

✻ **G9130** Oncology; disease status; limited to multiple myeloma, systemic disease; extent of disease unknown, staging in progress, or not listed (for use in a Medicare-approved demonstration project) Ⓑ M

✻ **G9131** Oncology; disease status; invasive female breast cancer (does not include ductal carcinoma in situ); adenocarcinoma as predominant cell type; extent of disease unknown, staging in progress, or not listed (for use in a Medicare-approved demonstration project) Ⓑ ♀ M

✻ **G9132** Oncology; disease status; prostate cancer, limited to adenocarcinoma; hormone-refractory/androgen-independent (e.g., rising PSA on anti-androgen therapy or post-orchiectomy); clinical metastases (for use in a Medicare-approved demonstration project) Ⓑ ♂ M

✻ **G9133** Oncology; disease status; prostate cancer, limited to adenocarcinoma; hormone-responsive; clinical metastases or M1 at diagnosis (for use in a Medicare-approved demonstration project) Ⓑ ♂ M

✻ **G9134** Oncology; disease status; non-Hodgkin's lymphoma, any cellular classification; stage I, II at diagnosis, not relapsed, not refractory (for use in a Medicare-approved demonstration project) Ⓑ M

✻ **G9135** Oncology; disease status; non-Hodgkin's lymphoma, any cellular classification; stage III, IV, not relapsed, not refractory (for use in a Medicare-approved demonstration project) Ⓑ M

* **G9136** Oncology; disease status; non-Hodgkin's lymphoma, transformed from original cellular diagnosis to a second cellular classification (for use in a Medicare-approved demonstration project) Ⓑ M
* **G9137** Oncology; disease status; non-Hodgkin's lymphoma, any cellular classification; relapsed/refractory (for use in a Medicare-approved demonstration project) Ⓑ M
* **G9138** Oncology; disease status; non-Hodgkin's lymphoma, any cellular classification; diagnostic evaluation, stage not determined, evaluation of possible relapse or non-response to therapy, or not listed (for use in a Medicare-approved demonstration project) Ⓑ M
* **G9139** Oncology; disease status; chronic myelogenous leukemia, limited to Philadelphia chromosome positive and/or BCR-ABL positive; extent of disease unknown, staging in progress, not listed (for use in a Medicare-approved demonstration project) Ⓑ M
* **G9140** Frontier extended stay clinic demonstration; for a patient stay in a clinic approved for the CMS demonstration project; the following measures should be present: the stay must be equal to or greater than 4 hours; weather or other conditions must prevent transfer or the case falls into a category of monitoring and observation cases that are permitted by the rules of the demonstration; there is a maximum frontier extended stay clinic (FESC) visit of 48 hours, except in the case when weather or other conditions prevent transfer; payment is made on each period up to 4 hours, after the first 4 hours Ⓑ A

Warfarin Responsiveness Testing

* **G9143** Warfarin responsiveness testing by genetic technique using any method, any number of specimen(s) Ⓑ Qp Qh N

  This would be a once-in-a-lifetime test unless there is a reason to believe that the patient's personal genetic characteristics would change over time. (https://www.cms.gov/ContractorLearningResources/downloads/JA6715.pdf)

  Laboratory Certification: General immunology, Hematology

  Coding Clinic: 2010, Q2, P10

Outpatient IV Insulin Treatment

⊘ **G9147** Outpatient intravenous insulin treatment (OIVIT) either pulsatile or continuous, by any means, guided by the results of measurements for: respiratory quotient; and/or, urine urea nitrogen (UUN); and/or, arterial, venous or capillary glucose; and/or potassium concentration Ⓑ E1

  On December 23, 2009, CMS issued a national non-coverage decision on the use of OIVIT. CR 6775.

  Not covered on Physician Fee Schedule

  Coding Clinic: 2010, Q2, P10

Quality Assurance

* **G9148** National committee for quality assurance - level 1 medical home Ⓑ M
* **G9149** National committee for quality assurance - level 2 medical home Ⓑ M
* **G9150** National committee for quality assurance - level 3 medical home Ⓑ M
* **G9151** MAPCP demonstration - state provided services Ⓑ M
* **G9152** MAPCP demonstration - community health teams Ⓑ M
* **G9153** MAPCP demonstration - physician incentive pool Ⓑ M

Wheelchair Evaluation

* **G9156** Evaluation for wheelchair requiring face to face visit with physician Ⓑ Qp Qh M

Cardiac Monitoring

* **G9157** Transesophageal doppler measurement of cardiac output (including probe placement, image acquisition, and interpretation per course of treatment) for monitoring purposes Ⓑ Qp Qh B

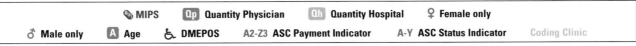

MIPS | Qp Quantity Physician | Qh Quantity Hospital | ♀ Female only | ♂ Male only | A Age | DMEPOS | A2-Z3 ASC Payment Indicator | A-Y ASC Status Indicator | Coding Clinic

Functional Limitation

* ✻ **G9158** Motor speech functional limitation, discharge status, at discharge from therapy or to end reporting Ⓑ E1
* ✻ **G9159** Spoken language comprehension functional limitation, current status at therapy episode outset and at reporting intervals Ⓑ E1
* ✻ **G9160** Spoken language comprehension functional limitation, projected goal status at therapy episode outset, at reporting intervals, and at discharge or to end reporting Ⓑ E1
* ✻ **G9161** Spoken language comprehension functional limitation, discharge status at discharge from therapy or to end reporting Ⓑ E1
* ✻ **G9162** Spoken language expression functional limitation, current status at therapy episode outset and at reporting intervals Ⓑ E1
* ✻ **G9163** Spoken language expression functional limitation, projected goal status at therapy episode outset, at reporting intervals, and at discharge or to end reporting Ⓑ E1
* ✻ **G9164** Spoken language expression functional limitation, discharge status at discharge from therapy or to end reporting Ⓑ E1
* ✻ **G9165** Attention functional limitation, current status at therapy episode outset and at reporting intervals Ⓑ E1
* ✻ **G9166** Attention functional limitation, projected goal status at therapy episode outset, at reporting intervals, and at discharge or to end reporting Ⓑ E1
* ✻ **G9167** Attention functional limitation, discharge status at discharge from therapy or to end reporting Ⓑ E1
* ✻ **G9168** Memory functional limitation, current status at therapy episode outset and at reporting intervals Ⓑ E1
* ✻ **G9169** Memory functional limitation, projected goal status at therapy episode outset, at reporting intervals, and at discharge or to end reporting Ⓑ E1
* ✻ **G9170** Memory functional limitation, discharge status at discharge from therapy or to end reporting Ⓑ E1
* ✻ **G9171** Voice functional limitation, current status at therapy episode outset and at reporting intervals Ⓑ E1
* ✻ **G9172** Voice functional limitation, projected goal status at therapy episode outset, at reporting intervals, and at discharge or to end reporting Ⓑ E1
* ✻ **G9173** Voice functional limitation, discharge status at discharge from therapy or to end reporting Ⓑ E1
* ✻ **G9174** Other speech language pathology functional limitation, current status at therapy episode outset and at reporting intervals Ⓑ E1
* ✻ **G9175** Other speech language pathology functional limitation, projected goal status at therapy episode outset, at reporting intervals, and at discharge or to end reporting Ⓑ E1
* ✻ **G9176** Other speech language pathology functional limitation, discharge status at discharge from therapy or to end reporting Ⓑ E1
* ✻ **G9186** Motor speech functional limitation, projected goal status at therapy episode outset, at reporting intervals, and at discharge or to end reporting Ⓑ E1

Bundled Payment Care Improvement

* ✻ **G9187** Bundled payments for care improvement initiative home visit for patient assessment performed by a qualified health care professional for individuals not considered homebound including, but not limited to, assessment of safety, falls, clinical status, fluid status, medication reconciliation/management, patient compliance with orders/plan of care, performance of activities of daily living, appropriateness of care setting; (for use only in the Medicare-approved bundled payments for care improvement initiative); may not be billed for a 30-day period covered by a transitional care management code Ⓑ Qp Qh E1

Quality Measures: Miscellaneous

* ✻ **G9188** Beta-blocker therapy not prescribed, reason not given Ⓑ M
* ✻ **G9189** Beta-blocker therapy prescribed or currently being taken Ⓑ M
* ✻ **G9190** Documentation of medical reason(s) for not prescribing beta-blocker therapy (e.g., allergy, intolerance, other medical reasons) Ⓑ M

▶ New ⮐ Revised ✔ Reinstated ~~deleted~~ Deleted ⃠ Not covered or valid by Medicare
Special coverage instructions ✻ Carrier discretion Ⓑ Bill Part B MAC Ⓓ Bill DME MAC

* **G9191** Documentation of patient reason(s) for not prescribing beta-blocker therapy (e.g., patient declined, other patient reasons) M
* **G9192** Documentation of system reason(s) for not prescribing beta-blocker therapy (e.g., other reasons attributable to the health care system) M
* **G9196** Documentation of medical reason(s) for not ordering a first or second generation cephalosporin for antimicrobial prophylaxis (e.g., patients enrolled in clinical trials, patients with documented infection prior to surgical procedure of interest, patients who were receiving antibiotics more than 24 hours prior to surgery [except colon surgery patients taking oral prophylactic antibiotics], patients who were receiving antibiotics within 24 hours prior to arrival [except colon surgery patients taking oral prophylactic antibiotics], other medical reason(s)) M
* **G9197** Documentation of order for first or second generation cephalosporin for antimicrobial prophylaxis M
* **G9198** Order for first or second generation cephalosporin for antimicrobial prophylaxis was not documented, reason not given M
* **G9212** DSM-IVTM criteria for major depressive disorder documented at the initial evaluation M
* **G9213** DSM-IV-TR criteria for major depressive disorder not documented at the initial evaluation, reason not otherwise specified M
* **G9223** Pneumocystis jiroveci pneumonia prophylaxis prescribed within 3 months of low CD4+ cell count below 500 cells/mm3 or a CD4 percentage below 15% M
* **G9225** Foot exam was not performed, reason not given M
* **G9226** Foot examination performed (includes examination through visual inspection, sensory exam with 10-g monofilament plus testing any one of the following: vibration using 128-hz tuning fork, pinprick sensation, ankle reflexes, or vibration perception threshold, and pulse exam; report when all of the 3 components are completed) M
* **G9227** Functional outcome assessment documented, care plan not documented, documentation the patient is not eligible for a care plan at the time of the encounter M
* **G9228** Chlamydia, gonorrhea and syphilis screening results documented (report when results are present for all of the 3 screenings) M
* **G9229** Chlamydia, gonorrhea, and syphilis screening results not documented (patient refusal is the only allowed exception) M
* **G9230** Chlamydia, gonorrhea, and syphilis not screened, reason not given M
* **G9231** Documentation of end stage renal disease (ESRD), dialysis, renal transplant before or during the measurement period or pregnancy during the measurement period M
* **G9232** Clinician treating major depressive disorder did not communicate to clinician treating comorbid condition for specified patient reason (e.g., patient is unable to communicate the diagnosis of a comorbid condition; the patient is unwilling to communicate the diagnosis of a comorbid condition; or the patient is unaware of the comorbid condition, or any other specified patient reason) M
* **G9239** Documentation of reasons for patient initiating maintenance hemodialysis with a catheter as the mode of vascular access (e.g., patient has a maturing AVF/AVG, time-limited trial of hemodialysis, other medical reasons, patient declined AVF/AVG, other patient reasons, patient followed by reporting nephrologist for fewer than 90 days, other system reasons) M
* **G9240** Patient whose mode of vascular access is a catheter at the time maintenance hemodialysis is initiated M
* **G9241** Patient whose mode of vascular access is not a catheter at the time maintenance hemodialysis is initiated M
* **G9242** Documentation of viral load equal to or greater than 200 copies/ml or viral load not performed M
* **G9243** Documentation of viral load less than 200 copies/ml M
* **G9246** Patient did not have at least one medical visit in each 6 month period of the 24 month measurement period, with a minimum of 60 days between medical visits M

MIPS | Qp Quantity Physician | Qh Quantity Hospital | ♀ Female only | ♂ Male only | A Age | DMEPOS | A2-Z3 ASC Payment Indicator | A-Y ASC Status Indicator | Coding Clinic

* G9247 Patient had at least one medical visit in each 6 month period of the 24 month measurement period, with a minimum of 60 days between medical visits Ⓑ M

* G9250 Documentation of patient pain brought to a comfortable level within 48 hours from initial assessment Ⓑ M

* G9251 Documentation of patient with pain not brought to a comfortable level within 48 hours from initial assessment Ⓑ M

* G9254 Documentation of patient discharged to home later than post-operative day 2 following CAS Ⓑ M

* G9255 Documentation of patient discharged to home no later than post operative day 2 following CAS Ⓑ M

* G9256 Documentation of patient death following CAS Ⓑ M

* G9257 Documentation of patient stroke following CAS Ⓑ M

* G9258 Documentation of patient stroke following CEA Ⓑ M

* G9259 Documentation of patient survival and absence of stroke following CAS Ⓑ M

* G9260 Documentation of patient death following CEA Ⓑ M

* G9261 Documentation of patient survival and absence of stroke following CEA Ⓑ M

* G9262 Documentation of patient death in the hospital following endovascular AAA repair Ⓑ M

* G9263 Documentation of patient discharged alive following endovascular AAA repair Ⓑ M

* G9264 Documentation of patient receiving maintenance hemodialysis for greater than or equal to 90 days with a catheter for documented reasons (e.g., other medical reasons, patient declined AVF/AVG, other patient reasons) Ⓑ M

* G9265 Patient receiving maintenance hemodialysis for greater than or equal to 90 days with a catheter as the mode of vascular access Ⓑ M

* G9266 Patient receiving maintenance hemodialysis for greater than or equal to 90 days without a catheter as the mode of vascular access Ⓑ M

* G9267 Documentation of patient with one or more complications or mortality within 30 days Ⓑ M

* G9268 Documentation of patient with one or more complications within 90 days Ⓑ M

* G9269 Documentation of patient without one or more complications and without mortality within 30 days Ⓑ M

* G9270 Documentation of patient without one or more complications within 90 days Ⓑ M

* G9273 Blood pressure has a systolic value of <140 and a diastolic value of <90 Ⓑ M

* G9274 Blood pressure has a systolic value of = 140 and a diastolic value of = 90 or systolic value <140 and diastolic value = 90 or systolic value = 140 and diastolic value <90 Ⓑ M

* G9275 Documentation that patient is a current non-tobacco user Ⓑ M

* G9276 Documentation that patient is a current tobacco user Ⓑ M

* G9277 Documentation that the patient is on daily aspirin or anti-platelet or has documentation of a valid contraindication or exception to aspirin/anti-platelet; contraindications/exceptions include anti-coagulant use, allergy to aspirin or anti-platelets, history of gastrointestinal bleed and bleeding disorder; additionally, the following exceptions documented by the physician as a reason for not taking daily aspirin or anti-platelet are acceptable (use of non-steroidal anti-inflammatory agents, documented risk for drug interaction, uncontrolled hypertension defined as >180 systolic or >110 diastolic or gastroesophageal reflux) Ⓑ M

* G9278 Documentation that the patient is not on daily aspirin or anti-platelet regimen Ⓑ M

* G9279 Pneumococcal screening performed and documentation of vaccination received prior to discharge Ⓑ M

* G9280 Pneumococcal vaccination not administered prior to discharge, reason not specified Ⓑ M

* G9281 Screening performed and documentation that vaccination not indicated/patient refusal Ⓑ M

* G9282 Documentation of medical reason(s) for not reporting the histological type or NSCLC-NOS classification with an explanation (e.g., biopsy taken for other purposes in a patient with a history of non-small cell lung cancer or other documented medical reasons) Ⓑ M

▶ New ↩ Revised ✔ Reinstated ~~deleted~~ Deleted ⊘ Not covered or valid by Medicare
Special coverage instructions * Carrier discretion Ⓑ Bill Part B MAC Ⓓ Bill DME MAC

* **G9283** Non small cell lung cancer biopsy and cytology specimen report documents classification into specific histologic type or classified as NSCLC-NOS with an explanation Ⓑ M
* **G9284** Non small cell lung cancer biopsy and cytology specimen report does not document classification into specific histologic type or classified as NSCLC-NOS with an explanation Ⓑ M
* **G9285** Specimen site other than anatomic location of lung or is not classified as non small cell lung cancer Ⓑ M
* **G9286** Antibiotic regimen prescribed within 10 days after onset of symptoms Ⓑ M
* **G9287** Antibiotic regimen not prescribed within 10 days after onset of symptoms Ⓑ M
* **G9288** Documentation of medical reason(s) for not reporting the histological type or NSCLC-NOS classification with an explanation (e.g., a solitary fibrous tumor in a person with a history of non-small cell carcinoma or other documented medical reasons) Ⓑ M
* **G9289** Non-small cell lung cancer biopsy and cytology specimen report documents classification into specific histologic type or classified as NSCLC-NOS with an explanation Ⓑ M
* **G9290** Non-small cell lung cancer biopsy and cytology specimen report does not document classification into specific histologic type or classified as NSCLC-NOS with an explanation Ⓑ M
* **G9291** Specimen site other than anatomic location of lung, is not classified as non small cell lung cancer or classified as NSCLC-NOS Ⓑ M
* **G9292** Documentation of medical reason(s) for not reporting PT category and a statement on thickness and ulceration and for PT1, mitotic rate (e.g., negative skin biopsies in a patient with a history of melanoma or other documented medical reasons) Ⓑ M
* **G9293** Pathology report does not include the PT category and a statement on thickness and ulceration and for PT1, mitotic rate Ⓑ M
* **G9294** Pathology report includes the PT category and a statement on thickness and ulceration and for PT1, mitotic rate Ⓑ M
* **G9295** Specimen site other than anatomic cutaneous location Ⓑ M
* **G9296** Patients with documented shared decision-making including discussion of conservative (non-surgical) therapy (e.g., NSAIDs, analgesics, weight loss, exercise, injections) prior to the procedure Ⓑ M
* **G9297** Shared decision-making including discussion of conservative (non-surgical) therapy (e.g., NSAIDs, analgesics, weight loss, exercise, injections) prior to the procedure not documented, reason not given Ⓑ M
* **G9298** Patients who are evaluated for venous thromboembolic and cardiovascular risk factors within 30 days prior to the procedure (e.g., history of DVT, PE, MI, arrhythmia and stroke) Ⓑ M
* **G9299** Patients who are not evaluated for venous thromboembolic and cardiovascular risk factors within 30 days prior to the procedure (e.g., history of DVT, PE, MI, arrhythmia and stroke, reason not given) Ⓑ M
* **G9300** Documentation of medical reason(s) for not completely infusing the prophylactic antibiotic prior to the inflation of the proximal tourniquet (e.g., a tourniquet was not used) Ⓑ M
* **G9301** Patients who had the prophylactic antibiotic completely infused prior to the inflation of the proximal tourniquet Ⓑ M
* **G9302** Prophylactic antibiotic not completely infused prior to the inflation of the proximal tourniquet, reason not given Ⓑ M
* **G9303** Operative report does not identify the prosthetic implant specifications including the prosthetic implant manufacturer, the brand name of the prosthetic implant and the size of each prosthetic implant, reason not given Ⓑ M
* **G9304** Operative report identifies the prosthetic implant specifications including the prosthetic implant manufacturer, the brand name of the prosthetic implant and the size of each prosthetic implant Ⓑ M
* **G9305** Intervention for presence of leak of endoluminal contents through an anastomosis not required Ⓑ M
* **G9306** Intervention for presence of leak of endoluminal contents through an anastomosis required Ⓑ M

MIPS | Qp Quantity Physician | Qh Quantity Hospital | ♀ Female only
♂ Male only | A Age | DMEPOS | A2-Z3 ASC Payment Indicator | A-Y ASC Status Indicator | Coding Clinic

* **G9307** No return to the operating room for a surgical procedure, for complications of the principal operative procedure, within 30 days of the principal operative procedure Ⓑ M
* **G9308** Unplanned return to the operating room for a surgical procedure, for complications of the principal operative procedure, within 30 days of the principal operative procedure Ⓑ M
* **G9309** No unplanned hospital readmission within 30 days of principal procedure Ⓑ M
* **G9310** Unplanned hospital readmission within 30 days of principal procedure Ⓑ M
* **G9311** No surgical site infection Ⓑ M
* **G9312** Surgical site infection Ⓑ M
* **G9313** Amoxicillin, with or without clavulanate, not prescribed as first line antibiotic at the time of diagnosis for documented reason Ⓑ M
* **G9314** Amoxicillin, with or without clavulanate, not prescribed as first line antibiotic at the time of diagnosis, reason not given Ⓑ M
* **G9315** Documentation amoxicillin, with or without clavulanate, prescribed as a first line antibiotic at the time of diagnosis Ⓑ M
* **G9316** Documentation of patient-specific risk assessment with a risk calculator based on multi-institutional clinical data, the specific risk calculator used, and communication of risk assessment from risk calculator with the patient or family Ⓑ M
* **G9317** Documentation of patient-specific risk assessment with a risk calculator based on multi-institutional clinical data, the specific risk calculator used, and communication of risk assessment from risk calculator with the patient or family not completed Ⓑ M
* **G9318** Imaging study named according to standardized nomenclature Ⓑ M
* **G9319** Imaging study not named according to standardized nomenclature, reason not given Ⓑ M
* **G9321** Count of previous CT (any type of CT) and cardiac nuclear medicine (myocardial perfusion) studies documented in the 12-month period prior to the current study Ⓑ M
* **G9322** Count of previous CT and cardiac nuclear medicine (myocardial perfusion) studies not documented in the 12-month period prior to the current study, reason not given Ⓑ M
* **G9326** CT studies performed not reported to a radiation dose index registry that is capable of collecting at a minimum all necessary data elements, reason not given Ⓑ M
* **G9327** CT studies performed reported to a radiation dose index registry that is capable of collecting at a minimum all necessary data elements Ⓑ M
* **G9329** DICOM format image data available to non-affiliated external healthcare facilities or entities on a secure, media free, reciprocally searchable basis with patient authorization for at least a 12-month period after the study not documented in final report, reason not given Ⓑ M
* **G9340** Final report documented that DICOM format image data available to non-affiliated external healthcare facilities or entities on a secure, media free, reciprocally searchable basis with patient authorization for at least a 12-month period after the study Ⓑ M
* **G9341** Search conducted for prior patient CT studies completed at non-affiliated external healthcare facilities or entities within the past 12-months and are available through a secure, authorized, media-free, shared archive prior to an imaging study being performed Ⓑ M
* **G9342** Search not conducted prior to an imaging study being performed for prior patient CT studies completed at non-affiliated external healthcare facilities or entities within the past 12-months and are available through a secure, authorized, media-free, shared archive, reason not given Ⓑ M
* **G9344** Due to system reasons search not conducted for DICOM format images for prior patient CT imaging studies completed at non-affiliated external healthcare facilities or entities within the past 12 months that are available through a secure, authorized, media-free, shared archive (e.g., non-affiliated external healthcare facilities or entities does not have archival abilities through a shared archival system) Ⓑ M

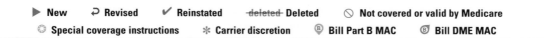

▶ New ⤾ Revised ✔ Reinstated ~~deleted~~ Deleted ⃠ Not covered or valid by Medicare
Special coverage instructions * Carrier discretion Ⓑ Bill Part B MAC Ⓔ Bill DME MAC

* **G9345** Follow-up recommendations documented according to recommended guidelines for incidentally detected pulmonary nodules (e.g., follow-up CT imaging studies needed or that no follow-up is needed) based at a minimum on nodule size and patient risk factors M

* **G9347** Follow-up recommendations not documented according to recommended guidelines for incidentally detected pulmonary nodules, reason not given M

* **G9348** CT scan of the paranasal sinuses ordered at the time of diagnosis for documented reasons M

* **G9349** Documentation of a CT scan of the paranasal sinuses ordered at the time of diagnosis or received within 28 days after date of diagnosis M

* **G9350** CT scan of the paranasal sinuses not ordered at the time of diagnosis or received within 28 days after date of diagnosis M

* **G9351** More than one CT scan of the paranasal sinuses ordered or received within 90 days after diagnosis M

* **G9352** More than one CT scan of the paranasal sinuses ordered or received within 90 days after the date of diagnosis, reason not given M

* **G9353** More than one CT scan of the paranasal sinuses ordered or received within 90 days after the date of diagnosis for documented reasons (e.g., patients with complications, second CT obtained prior to surgery, other medical reasons) M

* **G9354** One CT scan or no CT scan of the paranasal sinuses ordered within 90 days after the date of diagnosis M

* **G9355** Elective delivery or early induction not performed M

* **G9356** Elective delivery or early induction performed M

* **G9357** Post-partum screenings, evaluations and education performed M

* **G9358** Post-partum screenings, evaluations and education not performed M

* **G9359** Documentation of negative or managed positive TB screen with further evidence that TB is not active within one year of patient visit M

* **G9360** No documentation of negative or managed positive TB screen M

* **G9361** Medical indication for induction [documentation of reason(s) for elective delivery (c-section) or early induction (e.g., hemorrhage and placental complications, hypertension, preeclampsia and eclampsia, rupture of membranes-premature or prolonged, maternal conditions complicating pregnancy/delivery, fetal conditions complicating pregnancy/delivery, late pregnancy, prior uterine surgery, or participation in clinical trial)] M

* **G9364** Sinusitis caused by, or presumed to be caused by, bacterial infection M

* **G9365** One high-risk medication ordered M

* **G9366** One high-risk medication not ordered M

* **G9367** At least two different high-risk medications ordered M

* **G9368** At least two different high-risk medications not ordered M

* **G9380** Patient offered assistance with end of life issues during the measurement period M

* **G9382** Patient not offered assistance with end of life issues during the measurement period M

* **G9383** Patient received screening for HCV infection within the 12 month reporting period M

* **G9384** Documentation of medical reason(s) for not receiving annual screening for HCV infection (e.g., decompensated cirrhosis indicating advanced disease [i.e., ascites, esophageal variceal bleeding, hepatic encephalopathy], hepatocellular carcinoma, waitlist for organ transplant, limited life expectancy, other medical reasons) M

* **G9385** Documentation of patient reason(s) for not receiving annual screening for HCV infection (e.g., patient declined, other patient reasons) M

* **G9386** Screening for HCV infection not received within the 12 month reporting period, reason not given M

* **G9389** Unplanned rupture of the posterior capsule requiring vitrectomy during cataract surgery M

* **G9390** No unplanned rupture of the posterior capsule requiring vitrectomy during cataract surgery M

✻ **G9393** Patient with an initial PHQ-9 score greater than nine who achieves remission at 12 months as demonstrated by a 12 month (+/- 30 days) PHQ-9 score of less than five Ⓑ M

✻ **G9394** Patient who had a diagnosis of bipolar disorder or personality disorder, death, permanent nursing home resident or receiving hospice or palliative care any time during the measurement or assessment period Ⓑ M

✻ **G9395** Patient with an initial PHQ-9 score greater than nine who did not achieve remission at 12 months as demonstrated by a 12 month (+/- 30 days) PHQ-9 score greater than or equal to five Ⓑ M

✻ **G9396** Patient with an initial PHQ-9 score greater than nine who was not assessed for remission at 12 months (+/- 30 days) Ⓑ M

✻ **G9399** Documentation in the patient record of a discussion between the physician/ clinician and the patient that includes all of the following: treatment choices appropriate to genotype, risks and benefits, evidence of effectiveness, and patient preferences toward the outcome of the treatment Ⓑ M

✻ **G9400** Documentation of medical or patient reason(s) for not discussing treatment options; medical reasons: patient is not a candidate for treatment due to advanced physical or mental health comorbidity (including active substance use); currently receiving antiviral treatment; successful antiviral treatment (with sustained virologic response) prior to reporting period; other documented medical reasons; patient reasons: patient unable or unwilling to participate in the discussion or other patient reasons Ⓑ M

✻ **G9401** No documentation of a discussion in the patient record of a discussion between the physician or other qualified health care professional and the patient that includes all of the following: treatment choices appropriate to genotype, risks and benefits, evidence of effectiveness, and patient preferences toward treatment Ⓑ M

✻ **G9402** Patient received follow-up on the date of discharge or within 30 days after discharge Ⓑ M

✻ **G9403** Clinician documented reason patient was not able to complete 30 day follow-up from acute inpatient setting discharge (e.g., patient death prior to follow-up visit, patient non-compliant for visit follow-up) Ⓑ M

✻ **G9404** Patient did not receive follow-up on the date of discharge or within 30 days after discharge Ⓑ M

✻ **G9405** Patient received follow-up within 7 days from discharge Ⓑ M

✻ **G9406** Clinician documented reason patient was not able to complete 7 day follow-up from acute inpatient setting discharge (i.e patient death prior to follow-up visit, patient non-compliance for visit follow-up) Ⓑ M

✻ **G9407** Patient did not receive follow-up on or within 7 days after discharge Ⓑ M

✻ **G9408** Patients with cardiac tamponade and/ or pericardiocentesis occurring within 30 days Ⓑ M

✻ **G9409** Patients without cardiac tamponade and/or pericardiocentesis occurring within 30 days Ⓑ M

✻ **G9410** Patient admitted within 180 days, status post CIED implantation, replacement, or revision with an infection requiring device removal or surgical revision Ⓑ M

✻ **G9411** Patient not admitted within 180 days, status post CIED implantation, replacement, or revision with an infection requiring device removal or surgical revision Ⓑ M

✻ **G9412** Patient admitted within 180 days, status post CIED implantation, replacement, or revision with an infection requiring device removal or surgical revision Ⓑ M

✻ **G9413** Patient not admitted within 180 days, status post CIED implantation, replacement, or revision with an infection requiring device removal or surgical revision Ⓑ M

✻ **G9414** Patient had one dose of meningococcal vaccine on or between the patient's 11th and 13th birthdays Ⓑ M

✻ **G9415** Patient did not have one dose of meningococcal vaccine on or between the patient's 11th and 13th birthdays Ⓑ M

✻ **G9416** Patient had one tetanus, diphtheria toxoids and acellular pertussis vaccine (Tdap) or one tetanus, diphtheria toxoids vaccine (Td) on or between the patient's 10th and 13th birthdays Ⓑ M

▶ New ↩ Revised ✔ Reinstated ~~deleted~~ Deleted ⊘ Not covered or valid by Medicare
Special coverage instructions ✻ Carrier discretion Ⓑ Bill Part B MAC Ⓓ Bill DME MAC

* G9417 Patient did not have one tetanus, diphtheria toxoids and acellular pertussis vaccine (Tdap) on or between the patient's 10th and 13th birthdays M
* G9418 Primary non-small cell lung cancer biopsy and cytology specimen report documents classification into specific histologic type or classified as NSCLC-NOS with an explanation M
* G9419 Documentation of medical reason(s) for not including the histological type or NSCLC-NOS classification with an explanation (e.g., biopsy taken for other purposes in a patient with a history of primary non-small cell lung cancer or other documented medical reasons) M
* G9420 Specimen site other than anatomic location of lung or is not classified as primary non-small cell lung cancer M
* G9421 Primary non-small cell lung cancer biopsy and cytology specimen report does not document classification into specific histologic type or classified as NSCLC-NOS with an explanation M
* G9422 Primary lung carcinoma resection report documents pT category, pN category and for non-small cell lung cancer, histologic type (squamous cell carcinoma, adenocarcinoma and not nsclc-nos) M
* G9423 Documentation of medical reason for not including pT category, pN category and histologic type [for patient with appropriate exclusion criteria (e.g., metastatic disease, benign tumors, malignant tumors other than carcinomas, inadequate surgical specimens)] M
* G9424 Specimen site other than anatomic location of lung, or classified as NSCLC-NOS M
* G9425 Primary lung carcinoma resection report does not document pT category, pN category and for non-small cell lung cancer, histologic type (squamous cell carcinoma,adenocarcinoma) M
* G9426 Improvement in median time from ED arrival to initial ED oral or parenteral pain medication administration performed for ED admitted patients M
* G9427 Improvement in median time from ED arrival to initial ED oral or parenteral pain medication administration not performed for ED admitted patients M
* G9428 Pathology report includes the pT category and a statement on thickness, ulceration and mitotic rate M
* G9429 Documentation of medical reason(s) for not including pT category and a statement on thickness, ulceration and mitotic rate (e.g., negative skin biopsies in a patient with a history of melanoma or other documented medical reasons) M
* G9430 Specimen site other than anatomic cutaneous location M
* G9431 Pathology report does not include the pT category and a statement on thickness, ulceration and mitotic rate M
* G9432 Asthma well-controlled based on the ACT, C-ACT, ACQ, or ATAQ score and results documented M
* G9434 Asthma not well-controlled based on the ACT, C-ACT, ACQ, or ATAQ score, or specified asthma control tool not used, reason not given M
* G9448 Patients who were born in the years 1945-1965 M
* G9449 History of receiving blood transfusions prior to 1992 M
* G9450 History of injection drug use M
* G9451 Patient received one-time screening for HCV infection M
* G9452 Documentation of medical reason(s) for not receiving one-time screening for HCV infection (e.g., decompensated cirrhosis indicating advanced disease [i.e., ascites, esophageal variceal bleeding, hepatic encephalopathy], hepatocellular carcinoma, waitlist for organ transplant, limited life expectancy, other medical reasons) M
* G9453 Documentation of patient reason(s) for not receiving one-time screening for HCV infection (e.g., patient declined, other patient reasons) M
* G9454 One-time screening for HCV infection not received within 12 month reporting period and no documentation of prior screening for HCV infection, reason not given M
* G9455 Patient underwent abdominal imaging with ultrasound, contrast enhanced CT or contrast MRI for HCC M

* **G9456** Documentation of medical or patient reason(s) for not ordering or performing screening for HCC. medical reason: comorbid medical conditions with expected survival <5 years, hepatic decompensation and not a candidate for liver transplantation, or other medical reasons; patient reasons: patient declined or other patient reasons (e.g., cost of tests, time related to accessing testing equipment) ⑧ **M**

↻ * **G9457** Patient did not undergo abdominal imaging and did not have a documented reason for not undergoing abdominal imaging in the submission period ⑧ **M**

* **G9458** Patient documented as tobacco user and received tobacco cessation intervention (must include at least one of the following: advice given to quit smoking or tobacco use, counseling on the benefits of quitting smoking or tobacco use, assistance with or referral to external smoking or tobacco cessation support programs, or current enrollment in smoking or tobacco use cessation program) if identified as a tobacco user ⑧ **M**

* **G9459** Currently a tobacco non-user ⑧ **M**

* **G9460** Tobacco assessment or tobacco cessation intervention not performed, reason not given ⑧ **M**

* **G9468** Patient not receiving corticosteroids greater than or equal to 10 mg/day of prednisone equivalents for 60 or greater consecutive days or a single prescription equating to 600 mg prednisone or greater for all fills ⑧ **M**

* **G9469** Patients who have received or are receiving corticosteroids greater than or equal to 10 mg/day of prednisone equivalents for 60 or greater consecutive days or a single prescription equating to 600 mg prednisone or greater for all fills ⑧ **M**

* **G9470** Patients not receiving corticosteroids greater than or equal to 10 mg/day of prednisone equivalents for 60 or greater consecutive days or a single prescription equating to 600 mg prednisone or greater for all fills ⑧ **M**

* **G9471** Within the past 2 years, central dual-energy x-ray absorptiometry (DXA) not ordered or documented ⑧ **M**

* **G9472** Within the past 2 years, central dual-energy x-ray absorptiometry (DXA) not ordered and documented, no review of systems and no medication history or pharmacologic therapy (other than minerals/vitamins) for osteoporosis prescribed ⑧ **M**

* **G9473** Services performed by chaplain in the hospice setting, each 15 minutes ⑧ **B**

* **G9474** Services performed by dietary counselor in the hospice setting, each 15 minutes ⑧ **B**

* **G9475** Services performed by other counselor in the hospice setting, each 15 minutes ⑧ **B**

* **G9476** Services performed by volunteer in the hospice setting, each 15 minutes ⑧ **B**

* **G9477** Services performed by care coordinator in the hospice setting, each 15 minutes ⑧ **B**

* **G9478** Services performed by other qualified therapist in the hospice setting, each 15 minutes ⑧ **B**

* **G9479** Services performed by qualified pharmacist in the hospice setting, each 15 minutes ⑧ **B**

* **G9480** Admission to Medicare Care Choice Model program (MCCM) ⑧ **Qp** **Qh** **B**

▶ **New** ↻ **Revised** ✔ **Reinstated** ~~deleted~~ **Deleted** ⊘ **Not covered or valid by Medicare**

* **G9481** Remote in-home visit for the evaluation and management of a new patient for use only in the Medicare-approved comprehensive care for joint replacement model, which requires these 3 key components: a problem focused history; a problem focused examination; and straightforward medical decision making, furnished in real time using interactive audio and video technology. Counseling and coordination of care with other physicians, other qualified health care professionals or agencies are provided consistent with the nature of the problem(s) and the needs of the patient or the family or both. Usually, the presenting problem(s) are self limited or minor. Typically, 10 minutes are spent with the patient or family or both via real time, audio and video intercommunications technology ⑧ **B**

* **G9482** Remote in-home visit for the evaluation and management of a new patient for use only in the Medicare-approved comprehensive care for joint replacement model, which requires these 3 key components: an expanded problem focused history; an expanded problem focused examination; straightforward medical decision making, furnished in real time using interactive audio and video technology. Counseling and coordination of care with other physicians, other qualified health care professionals or agencies are provided consistent with the nature of the problem(s) and the needs of the patient or the family or both. Usually, the presenting problem(s) are of low to moderate severity. Typically, 20 minutes are spent with the patient or family or both via real time, audio and video intercommunications technology B

* **G9483** Remote in-home visit for the evaluation and management of a new patient for use only in the Medicare-approved comprehensive care for joint replacement model, which requires these 3 key components: a detailed history; a detailed examination; medical decision making of low complexity, furnished in real time using interactive audio and video technology. Counseling and coordination of care with other physicians, other qualified health care professionals or agencies are provided consistent with the nature of the problem(s) and the needs of the patient or the family or both. Usually, the presenting problem(s) are of moderate severity. Typically, 30 minutes are spent with the patient or family or both via real time, audio and video intercommunications technology B

* **G9484** Remote in-home visit for the evaluation and management of a new patient for use only in the Medicare-approved comprehensive care for joint replacement model, which requires these 3 key components: a comprehensive history; a comprehensive examination; medical decision making of moderate complexity, furnished in real time using interactive audio and video technology. Counseling and coordination of care with other physicians, other qualified health care professionals or agencies are provided consistent with the nature of the problem(s) and the needs of the patient or the family or both. Usually, the presenting problem(s) are of moderate to high severity. Typically, 45 minutes are spent with the patient or family or both via real time, audio and video intercommunications technology B

* **G9485** Remote in-home visit for the evaluation and management of a new patient for use only in the Medicare-approved comprehensive care for joint replacement model, which requires these 3 key components: a comprehensive history; a comprehensive examination; medical decision making of high complexity, furnished in real time using interactive audio and video technology. Counseling and coordination of care with other physicians, other qualified health care professionals or agencies are provided consistent with the nature of the problem(s) and the needs of the patient or the family or both. Usually, the presenting problem(s) are of moderate to high severity. Typically, 60 minutes are spent with the patient or family or both via real time, audio and video intercommunications technology B

* **G9486** Remote in-home visit for the evaluation and management of an established patient for use only in the Medicare-approved comprehensive care for joint replacement model, which requires at least 2 of the following 3 key components: a problem focused history; a problem focused examination; straightforward medical decision making, furnished in real time using interactive audio and video technology. Counseling and coordination of care with other physicians, other qualified health care professionals or agencies are provided consistent with the nature of the problem(s) and the needs of the patient or the family or both. Usually, the presenting problem(s) are self limited or minor. Typically, 10 minutes are spent with the patient or family or both via real time, audio and video intercommunications technology Ⓑ B

* **G9487** Remote in-home visit for the evaluation and management of an established patient for use only in the Medicare-approved comprehensive care for joint replacement model, which requires at least 2 of the following 3 key components: an expanded problem focused history; an expanded problem focused examination; medical decision making of low complexity, furnished in real time using interactive audio and video technology. Counseling and coordination of care with other physicians, other qualified health care professionals or agencies are provided consistent with the nature of the problem(s) and the needs of the patient or the family or both. Usually, the presenting problem(s) are of low to moderate severity. Typically, 15 minutes are spent with the patient or family or both via real time, audio and video intercommunications technology Ⓑ B

* **G9488** Remote in-home visit for the evaluation and management of an established patient for use only in the Medicare-approved comprehensive care for joint replacement model, which requires at least 2 of the following 3 key components: a detailed history; a detailed examination; medical decision making of moderate complexity, furnished in real time using interactive audio and video technology. Counseling and coordination of care with other physicians, other qualified health care professionals or agencies are provided consistent with the nature of the problem(s) and the needs of the patient or the family or both. Usually, the presenting problem(s) are of moderate to high severity. Typically, 25 minutes are spent with the patient or family or both via real time, audio and video intercommunications technology Ⓑ B

* **G9489** Remote in-home visit for the evaluation and management of an established patient for use only in the Medicare-approved comprehensive care for joint replacement model, which requires at least 2 of the following 3 key components: a comprehensive history; a comprehensive examination; medical decision making of high complexity, furnished in real time using interactive audio and video technology. Counseling and coordination of care with other physicians, other qualified health care professionals or agencies are provided consistent with the nature of the problem(s) and the needs of the patient or the family or both. Usually, the presenting problem(s) are of moderate to high severity. Typically, 40 minutes are spent with the patient or family or both via real time, audio and video intercommunications technology Ⓑ B

✻ **G9490** Comprehensive care for joint replacement model, home visit for patient assessment performed by clinical staff for an individual not considered homebound, including, but not necessarily limited to patient assessment of clinical status, safety/fall prevention, functional status/ ambulation, medication reconciliation/ management, compliance with orders/ plan of care, performance of activities of daily living, and ensuring beneficiary connections to community and other services. (for use only in the Medicare-approved CJR model); may not be billed for a 30 day period covered by a transitional care management code B

✻ **G9497** Received instruction from the anesthesiologist or proxy prior to the day of surgery to abstain from smoking on the day of surgery M

✻ **G9498** Antibiotic regimen prescribed M

✻ **G9500** Radiation exposure indices, or exposure time and number of fluorographic images in final report for procedures using fluoroscopy, documented M

✻ **G9501** Radiation exposure indices, or exposure time and number of fluorographic images not documented in final report for procedure using fluoroscopy, reason not given M

✻ **G9502** Documentation of medical reason for not performing foot exam (i.e., patients who have had either a bilateral amputation above or below the knee, or both a left and right amputation above or below the knee before or during the measurement period) M

✻ **G9503** Patient taking tamsulosin hydrochloride M

✻ **G9504** Documented reason for not assessing Hepatitis B virus (HBV) status (e.g. patient not initiating anti-TNF therapy, patient declined) prior to initiating anti-TNF therapy M

✻ **G9505** Antibiotic regimen prescribed within 10 days after onset of symptoms for documented medical reason M

✻ **G9506** Biologic immune response modifier prescribed M

✻ **G9507** Documentation that the patient is on a statin medication or has documentation of a valid contraindication or exception to statin medications; contraindications/exceptions that can be defined by diagnosis codes include pregnancy during the measurement period, active liver disease, rhabdomyolysis, end stage renal disease on dialysis and heart failure; provider documented contraindications/ exceptions include breastfeeding during the measurement period, woman of child-bearing age not actively taking birth control, allergy to statin, drug interaction (HIV protease inhibitors, nefazodone, cyclosporine, gemfibrozil, and danazol) and intolerance (with supporting documentation of trying a statin at least once within the last 5 years or diagnosis codes for myostitis or toxic myopathy related to drugs) M

✻ **G9508** Documentation that the patient is not on a statin medication M

✻ **G9509** Adult patients 18 years of age or older with major depression or dysthymia who reached remission at 12 months as demonstrated by a 12 month (+/-60 days) PHQ-9 or PHQ-9m score of less than 5 M

✻ **G9510** Remission at 12 months not demonstrated by a 12 month (+/-30 days) PHQ-9 score of less than five; either PHQ-9 score was not assessed or is greater than or equal to 5 M

✻ **G9511** Index event date PHQ-9 score greater than 9 documented during the 12 month denominator identification period M

✻ **G9512** Individual had a PDC of 0.8 or greater M

✻ **G9513** Individual did not have a PDC of 0.8 or greater M

✻ **G9514** Patient required a return to the operating room within 90 days of surgery M

✻ **G9515** Patient did not require a return to the operating room within 90 days of surgery M

✻ **G9516** Patient achieved an improvement in visual acuity, from their preoperative level, within 90 days of surgery M

✻ **G9517** Patient did not achieve an improvement in visual acuity, from their preoperative level, within 90 days of surgery, reason not given M

* G9518 Documentation of active injection drug use M
* G9519 Patient achieves final refraction (spherical equivalent) +/-0.5 diopters of their planned refraction within 90 days of surgery M
* G9520 Patient does not achieve final refraction (spherical equivalent) +/-0.5 diopters of their planned refraction within 90 days of surgery M
* G9521 Total number of emergency department visits and inpatient hospitalizations less than two in the past 12 months M
* G9522 Total number of emergency department visits and inpatient hospitalizations equal to or greater than two in the past 12 months or patient not screened, reason not given M
* G9523 Patient discontinued from hemodialysis or peritoneal dialysis M
* G9524 Patient was referred to hospice care M
* G9525 Documentation of patient reason(s) for not referring to hospice care (e.g., patient declined, other patient reasons) M
* G9526 Patient was not referred to hospice care, reason not given M
* G9529 Patient with minor blunt head trauma had an appropriate indication(s) for a head CT M
* G9530 Patient presented within a minor blunt head trauma and had a head CT ordered for trauma by an emergency care provider M
* G9531 Patient has documentation of ventricular shunt, brain tumor, multisystem trauma, pregnancy, or is currently taking an antiplatelet medication including: abciximab, cangrelor, cilostazol, clopidogrel, eptifibatide, prasugrel, ticlopidine, ticagrelor, tirofiban, or vorapaxar M
* G9532 Patient had a head CT for trauma ordered by someone other than an emergency care provider, or was ordered for a reason other than trauma M
* G9533 Patient with minor blunt head trauma did not have an appropriate indication(s) for a head CT M

~~G9534 Advanced brain imaging (CTA, CT, MRA or MRI) was not ordered~~ ✖

~~G9535 Patients with a normal neurological examination~~ ✖

~~G9536 Documentation of medical reason(s) for ordering an advanced brain imaging study (i.e., patient has an abnormal neurological examination; patient has the coexistence of seizures, or both; recent onset of severe headache; change in the type of headache; signs of increased intracranial pressure (e.g., papilledema, absent venous pulsations on funduscopic examination, altered mental status, focal neurologic deficits, signs of meningeal irritation); HIV-positive patients with a new type of headache; immunocompromised patient with unexplained headache symptoms; patient on coagulopathy/anti-coagulation or anti-platelet therapy; very young patients with unexplained headache symptoms)~~ ✖

* G9537 Documentation of system reason(s) for obtaining imaging of the head (CT or MRI) (i.e., needed as part of a clinical trial; other clinician ordered the study) M

~~G9538 Advanced brain imaging (CTA, CT, MRA or MRI) was ordered~~ ✖

* G9539 Intent for potential removal at time of placement M
* G9540 Patient alive 3 months post procedure M
* G9541 Filter removed within 3 months of placement M
* G9542 Documented re-assessment for the appropriateness of filter removal within 3 months of placement M
* G9543 Documentation of at least two attempts to reach the patient to arrange a clinical re-assessment for the appropriateness of filter removal within 3 months of placement M
* G9544 Patients that do not have the filter removed, documented re-assessment for the appropriateness of filter removal, or documentation of at least two attempts to reach the patient to arrange a clinical re-assessment for the appropriateness of filter removal within 3 months of placement M
* G9547 Incidental finding: liver lesion <=0.5 cm, cystic kidney lesion <1.0 cm or adrenal lesion <=1.0 cm M
* G9548 Final reports for abdominal imaging studies with follow-up imaging recommended M

✻ **G9549** Documentation of medical reason(s) that follow-up imaging is indicated (e.g., patient has a known malignancy that can metastasize, other medical reason(s) such as fever in an immunocompromised patient) M

✻ **G9550** Final reports for abdominal imaging studies with follow-up imaging not recommended M

✻ **G9551** Final reports for abdominal imaging studies without an incidentally found lesion noted: liver lesion <=0.5 cm, cystic kidney lesion <1.0 cm or adrenal lesion <=1.0 cm noted or no lesion found M

✻ **G9552** Incidental thyroid nodule <1.0 cm noted in report M

✻ **G9553** Prior thyroid disease diagnosis M

✻ **G9554** Final reports for CT, CTA, MRI or MRA of the chest or neck or ultrasound of the neck with follow-up imaging recommended M

✻ **G9555** Documentation of medical reason(s) for recommending follow up imaging (e.g., patient has multiple endocrine neoplasia, patient has cervical lymphadenopathy, other medical reason(s)) M

✻ **G9556** Final reports for CT, CTA, MRI or MRA of the chest or neck or ultrasound of the neck with follow-up imaging not recommended M

✻ **G9557** Final reports for CT, CTA, MRI or MRA studies of the chest or neck or ultrasound of the neck without an incidentally found thyroid nodule <1.0 cm noted or no nodule found M

✻ **G9558** Patient treated with a beta-lactam antibiotic as definitive therapy M

✻ **G9559** Documentation of medical reason(s) for not prescribing a beta-lactam antibiotic (e.g., allergy, intolerance to beta-lactam antibiotics) M

✻ **G9560** Patient not treated with a beta-lactam antibiotic as definitive therapy, reason not given M

✻ **G9561** Patients prescribed opiates for longer than six weeks M

✻ **G9562** Patients who had a follow-up evaluation conducted at least every three months during opioid therapy M

✻ **G9563** Patients who did not have a follow-up evaluation conducted at least every three months during opioid therapy M

✻ **G9573** Adult patients 18 years of age or older with major depression or dysthymia who did not reach remission at six months as demonstrated by a six month (+/-60 days) PHQ-9 or PHQ-9m score of less than five M

✻ **G9574** Adult patients 18 years of age or older with major depression or dysthymia who did not reach remission at six months as demonstrated by a six month (+/-60 days) PHQ-9 or PHQ-9m score of less than five; either PHQ-9 or PHQ-9m score was not assessed or is greater than or equal to five M

✻ **G9577** Patients prescribed opiates for longer than six weeks M

✻ **G9578** Documentation of signed opioid treatment agreement at least once during opioid therapy M

✻ **G9579** No documentation of signed an opioid treatment agreement at least once during opioid therapy M

✻ **G9580** Door to puncture time of less than 2 hours M

✻ **G9582** Door to puncture time of greater than 2 hours, no reason given M

✻ **G9583** Patients prescribed opiates for longer than 6 weeks M

✻ **G9584** Patient evaluated for risk of misuse of opiates by using a brief validated instrument (e.g., opioid risk tool, SOAPP-R) or patient interviewed at least once during opioid therapy M

✻ **G9585** Patient not evaluated for risk of misuse of opiates by using a brief validated instrument (e.g., opioid risk tool, SOAPP-R) or patient not interviewed at least once during opioid therapy M

✻ **G9593** Pediatric patient with minor blunt head trauma classified as low risk according to the pecarn Prediction Rules A M

✻ **G9594** Patient presented with a minor blunt head trauma and had a head CT ordered for trauma by an emergency care provider M

✻ **G9595** Patient has documentation of ventricular shunt, brain tumor, coagulopathy, including thrombocytopenia M

✻ **G9596** Pediatric patient had a head CT for trauma ordered by someone other than an emergency care provider, or was ordered for a reason other than trauma A M

MIPS | Qp Quantity Physician | Qh Quantity Hospital | ♀ Female only
♂ Male only | A Age | DMEPOS | A2-Z3 ASC Payment Indicator | A-Y ASC Status Indicator | Coding Clinic

* G9597 Pediatric patient with minor blunt head trauma not classified as low risk according to the pecarn Prediction Rules Ⓑ A M
* G9598 Aortic aneurysm 5.5-5.9 cm maximum diameter on centerline formatted CT or minor diameter on axial formatted CT Ⓑ M
* G9599 Aortic aneurysm 6.0 cm or greater maximum diameter on centerline formatted CT or minor diameter on axial formatted CT Ⓑ M
* G9600 Symptomatic AAAS that required urgent/emergent (non-elective) repair Ⓑ M
* G9601 Patient discharge to home no later than post-operative day #7 Ⓑ M
* G9602 Patient not discharged to home by post-operative day #7 Ⓑ M
* G9603 Patient survey score improved from baseline following treatment Ⓑ M
* G9604 Patient survey results not available Ⓑ M
* G9605 Patient survey score did not improve from baseline following treatment Ⓑ M
* G9606 Intraoperative cystoscopy performed to evaluate for lower tract injury Ⓑ M
* G9607 Documented medical reasons for not performing intraoperative cystoscopy (e.g., urethral pathology precluding cystoscopy, any patient who has a congenital or acquired absence of the urethra) or in the case of patient death Ⓑ M
* G9608 Intraoperative cystoscopy not performed to evaluate for lower tract injury Ⓑ M
* G9609 Documentation of an order for anti-platelet agents Ⓑ M
* G9610 Documentation of medical reason(s) in the patient's record for not ordering anti-platelet agents Ⓑ M
* G9611 Order for anti-platelet agents was not documented in the patient's record, reason not given Ⓑ M
* ⊋ G9612 Photodocumentation of two or more cecal landmarks to establish a complete examination Ⓑ M
* G9613 Documentation of post-surgical anatomy (e.g., right hemicolectomy, ileocecal resection, etc.) Ⓑ M
* ⊋ G9614 Photodocumentation of less than two cecal landmarks (i.e., no cecal landmarks or only one cecal landmark) to establish a complete examination Ⓑ M
* G9615 Preoperative assessment documented Ⓑ M
* G9616 Documentation of reason(s) for not documenting a preoperative assessment (e.g., patient with a gynecologic or other pelvic malignancy noted at the time of surgery) Ⓑ M
* G9617 Preoperative assessment not documented, reason not given Ⓑ M
* G9618 Documentation of screening for uterine malignancy or those that had an ultrasound and/or endometrial sampling of any kind Ⓑ M
* G9620 Patient not screened for uterine malignancy, or those that have not had an ultrasound and/or endometrial sampling of any kind, reason not given Ⓑ M
* G9621 Patient identified as an unhealthy alcohol user when screened for unhealthy alcohol use using a systematic screening method and received brief counseling Ⓑ M
* G9622 Patient not identified as an unhealthy alcohol user when screened for unhealthy alcohol use using a systematic screening method Ⓑ M
* G9623 Documentation of medical reason(s) for not screening for unhealthy alcohol use (e.g., limited life expectancy, other medical reasons) Ⓑ M
* G9624 Patient not screened for unhealthy alcohol use using a systematic screening method or patient did not receive brief counseling if identified as an unhealthy alcohol user, reason not given Ⓑ M
* ⊋ G9625 Patient sustained bladder injury at the time of surgery or discovered subsequently up to 30 days post-surgery Ⓑ M
* G9626 Documented medical reason for reporting bladder injury (e.g., gynecologic or other pelvic malignancy documented, concurrent surgery involving bladder pathology, injury that occurs during urinary incontinence procedure, patient death from non-medical causes not related to surgery, patient died during procedure without evidence of bladder injury) Ⓑ M
* ⊋ G9627 Patient did not sustain bladder injury at the time of surgery nor discovered subsequently up to 30 days post-surgery Ⓑ M

* **G9628** Patient sustained bowel injury at the time of surgery or discovered subsequently up to 30 days post-surgery M
* **G9629** Documented medical reasons for not reporting bowel injury (e.g., gynecologic or other pelvic malignancy documented, planned (e.g., not due to an unexpected bowel injury) resection and/or re-anastomosis of bowel, or patient death from non-medical causes not related to surgery, patient died during procedure without evidence of bowel injury) M
* **G9630** Patient did not sustain a bowel injury at the time of surgery nor discovered subsequently up to 30 days post-surgery M
* **G9631** Patient sustained ureter injury at the time of surgery or discovered subsequently up to 30 days post-surgery M
* **G9632** Documented medical reasons for not reporting ureter injury (e.g., gynecologic or other pelvic malignancy documented, concurrent surgery involving bladder pathology, injury that occurs during a urinary incontinence procedure, patient death from non-medical causes not related to surgery, patient died during procedure without evidence of ureter injury) M
* **G9633** Patient did not sustain ureter injury at the time of surgery nor discovered subsequently up to 30 days post-surgery M
* **G9634** Health-related quality of life assessed with tool during at least two visits and quality of life score remained the same or improved M
* **G9635** Health-related quality of life not assessed with tool for documented reason(s) (e.g., patient has a cognitive or neuropsychiatric impairment that impairs his/her ability to complete the HRQOL survey, patient has the inability to read and/or write in order to complete the HRQOL questionnaire) M
* **G9636** Health-related quality of life not assessed with tool during at least two visits or quality of life score declined M
* **G9637** At least two orders for the same high-risk medications M
* **G9638** At least two orders for the same high-risk medications not ordered M
* **G9639** Major amputation or open surgical bypass not required within 48 hours of the index endovascular lower extremity revascularization procedure M
* **G9640** Documentation of planned hybrid or staged procedure M
* **G9641** Major amputation or open surgical bypass required within 48 hours of the index endovascular lower extremity revascularization procedure M
* **G9642** Current smokers (e.g., cigarette, cigar, pipe, e-cigarette or marijuana) M
* **G9643** Elective surgery M
* **G9644** Patients who abstained from smoking prior to anesthesia on the day of surgery or procedure M
* **G9645** Patients who did not abstain from smoking prior to anesthesia on the day of surgery or procedure M
* **G9646** Patients with 90 day MRS score of 0 to 2 M
* **G9647** Patients in whom MRS score could not be obtained at 90 day follow-up M
* **G9648** Patients with 90 day MRS score greater than 2 M
* **G9649** Psoriasis assessment tool documented meeting any one of the specified benchmarks (e.g., PGA; 5-point or 6-point scale), body surface area (BSA), psoriasis area and severity index (PASI) and/or dermatology life quality index) (DLQI)) M
* **G9651** Psoriasis assessment tool documented not meeting any one of the specified benchmarks (e.g., (pga; 5-point or 6-point scale), body surface area (bsa), psoriasis area and severity index (pasi) and/or dermatology life quality index) (dlqi)) or psoriasis assessment tool not documented M
* **G9654** Monitored anesthesia care (mac) M
* **G9655** A transfer of care protocol or handoff tool/checklist that includes the required key handoff elements is used M
* **G9656** Patient transferred directly from anesthetizing location to PACU or other non-ICU location M
* **G9658** A transfer of care protocol or handoff tool/checklist that includes the required key handoff elements is not used M

MIPS | Op Quantity Physician | Oh Quantity Hospital | ♀ Female only | ♂ Male only | A Age | DMEPOS | A2-Z3 ASC Payment Indicator | A-Y ASC Status Indicator | Coding Clinic

* **G9659** Patients greater than 85 years of age who did not have a history of colorectal cancer or valid medical reason for the colonoscopy, including: iron deficiency anemia, lower gastrointestinal bleeding, Crohn's Disease (i.e., regional enteritis), familial adenomatous polyposis, lynch syndrome (i.e., hereditary non-polyposis colorectal cancer), inflammatory bowel disease, ulcerative colitis, abnormal finding of gastrointestinal tract, or changes in bowel habits M

* **G9660** Documentation of medical reason(s) for a colonoscopy performed on a patient greater than 85 years of age (e.g., last colonoscopy incomplete, last colonoscopy had inadequate prep, iron deficiency anemia, lower gastrointestinal bleeding, Crohn's Disease (i.e., regional enteritis), familial history of adenomatous polyposis, lynch syndrome (i.e., hereditary non-polyposis colorectal cancer), inflammatory bowel disease, ulcerative colitis, abnormal finding of gastrointestinal tract, or changes in bowel habits) M

* **G9661** Patients greater than 85 years of age who received a routine colonoscopy for a reason other than the following: an assessment of signs/symptoms of GI tract illness, and/or the patient is considered high risk, and/or to follow-up on previously diagnosed advance lesions M

* **G9662** Previously diagnosed or have an active diagnosis of clinical ascvd M

* **G9663** Any fasting or direct ldl-c laboratory test result = 190 mg/dL M

* **G9664** Patients who are currently statin therapy users or received an order (prescription) for statin therapy M

* **G9665** Patients who are not currently statin therapy users or did not receive an order (prescription) for statin therapy M

* **G9666** The highest fasting or direct ldl-c laboratory test result of 70-189 mg/dL in the measurement period or two years prior to the beginning of the measurement period M

* **G9674** Patients with clinical ascvd diagnosis M

* **G9675** Patients who have ever had a fasting or direct laboratory result of ldl-c = 190 mg/dl M

* **G9676** Patients aged 40 to 75 years at the beginning of the measurement period with type 1 or type 2 diabetes and with an ldl-c result of 70-189 mg/dl recorded as the highest fasting or direct laboratory test result in the measurement year or during the two years prior to the beginning of the measurement period M

* **G9678** Oncology care model (OCM) monthly enhanced oncology services (MEOS) payment for OCM enhanced services. G9678 payments may only be made to OCM practitioners for ocm beneficiaries for the furnishment of enhanced services as defined in the OCM participation agreement Qp Qh B

* **G9679** This code is for onsite acute care treatment of a nursing facility resident with pneumonia; may only be billed once per day per beneficiary B

* **G9680** This code is for onsite acute care treatment of a nursing facility resident with CHF; may only be billed once per day per beneficiary B

* **G9681** This code is for onsite acute care treatment of a resident with COPD or asthma; may only be billed once per day per beneficiary B

* **G9682** This code is for the onsite acute care treatment a nursing facility resident with a skin infection; may only be billed once per day per beneficiary B

* **G9683** Facility service(s) for the onsite acute care treatment of a nursing facility resident with fluid or electrolyte disorder. (May only be billed once per day per beneficiary). This service is for a demonstration project. B

* **G9684** This code is for the onsite acute care treatment of a nursing facility resident for a UTI; may only be billed once per day per beneficiary B

* **G9685** Physician service or other qualified health care professional for the evaluation and management of a beneficiary's acute change in condition in a nursing facility. This service is for a demonstration project. M

~~G9686 Onsite nursing facility conference, that is separate and distinct from an evaluation and management visit, including qualified practitioner and at least one member of the nursing facility interdisciplinary care team~~ ✖

* **G9687** Hospice services provided to patient any time during the measurement period M

▶ New ↻ Revised ✔ Reinstated ~~deleted~~ Deleted ⊘ Not covered or valid by Medicare
Special coverage instructions * Carrier discretion Bill Part B MAC Bill DME MAC

* ✻ **G9688** Patients using hospice services any time during the measurement period M
* ✻ **G9689** Patient admitted for performance of elective carotid intervention M
* ✻ **G9690** Patient receiving hospice services any time during the measurement period M
* ✻ **G9691** Patient had hospice services any time during the measurement period M
* ✻ **G9692** Hospice services received by patient any time during the measurement period M
* ✻ **G9693** Patient use of hospice services any time during the measurement period M
* ✻ **G9694** Hospice services utilized by patient any time during the measurement period M
* ✻ **G9695** Long-acting inhaled bronchodilator prescribed M
* ✻ **G9696** Documentation of medical reason(s) for not prescribing a long-acting inhaled bronchodilator M
* ✻ **G9697** Documentation of patient reason(s) for not prescribing a long-acting inhaled bronchodilator M
* ✻ **G9698** Documentation of system reason(s) for not prescribing a long-acting inhaled bronchodilator M
* ✻ **G9699** Long-acting inhaled bronchodilator not prescribed, reason not otherwise specified M
* ✻ **G9700** Patients who use hospice services any time during the measurement period M
* ✻ **G9701** Children who are taking antibiotics in the 30 days prior to the date of the encounter during which the diagnosis was established M
* ✻ **G9702** Patients who use hospice services any time during the measurement period M
* ✻ **G9703** Children who are taking antibiotics in the 30 days prior to the diagnosis of pharyngitis M
* ✻ **G9704** AJCC breast cancer stage I: T1 mic or T1a documented M
* ✻ **G9705** AJCC breast cancer stage I: T1b (tumor >0.5 cm but <=1 cm in greatest dimension) documented M
* ✻ **G9706** Low (or very low) risk of recurrence, prostate cancer M
* ✻ **G9707** Patient received hospice services any time during the measurement period M
* ✻ **G9708** Women who had a bilateral mastectomy or who have a history of a bilateral mastectomy or for whom there is evidence of a right and a left unilateral mastectomy M
* ✻ **G9709** Hospice services used by patient any time during the measurement period M
* ✻ **G9710** Patient was provided hospice services any time during the measurement period M
* ✻ **G9711** Patients with a diagnosis or past history of total colectomy or colorectal cancer M
* ✻ **G9712** Documentation of medical reason(s) for prescribing or dispensing antibiotic (e.g., intestinal infection, pertussis, bacterial infection, Lyme disease, otitis media, acute sinusitis, acute pharyngitis, acute tonsillitis, chronic sinusitis, infection of the pharynx/larynx/tonsils/adenoids, prostatitis, cellulitis/ mastoiditis/bone infections, acute lymphadenitis, impetigo, skin staph infections, pneumonia, gonococcal infections/venereal disease/ syphilis, chlamydia, inflammatory diseases, female reproductive organs), infections of the kidney, cystitis/UTI, acne, HIV disease/asymptomatic HIV, cystic fibrosis, disorders of the immune system, malignancy neoplasms, chronic bronchitis, emphysema, bronchiectasis, extrinsic allergic alveolitis, chronic airway obstruction, chronic obstructive asthma, pneumoconiosis and other lung disease due to external agents, other diseases of the respiratory system, and tuberculosis M
* ✻ **G9713** Patients who use hospice services any time during the measurement period M
* ✻ **G9714** Patient is using hospice services any time during the measurement period M
* ✻ **G9715** Patients who use hospice services any time during the measurement period M
* ✻ **G9716** BMI is documented as being outside of normal limits, follow-up plan is not completed for documented reason M
* ✻ **G9717** Documentation stating the patient has an active diagnosis of depression or has a diagnosed bipolar disorder, therefore screening or follow-up not required M
* ✻ **G9718** Hospice services for patient provided any time during the measurement period M

* **G9719** Patient is not ambulatory, bed ridden, immobile, confined to chair, wheelchair bound, dependent on helper pushing wheelchair, independent in wheelchair or minimal help in wheelchair Ⓑ M

* **G9720** Hospice services for patient occurred any time during the measurement period Ⓑ M

* **G9721** Patient not ambulatory, bed ridden, immobile, confined to chair, wheelchair bound, dependent on helper pushing wheelchair, independent in wheelchair or minimal help in wheelchair Ⓑ M

* **G9722** Documented history of renal failure or baseline serum creatinine = 4.0 mg/dl; renal transplant recipients are not considered to have preoperative renal failure, unless, since transplantation the CR has been or is 4.0 or higher Ⓑ M

* **G9723** Hospice services for patient received any time during the measurement period Ⓑ M

* **G9724** Patients who had documentation of use of anticoagulant medications overlapping the measurement year Ⓑ M

* **G9725** Patients who use hospice services any time during the measurement period Ⓑ M

* **G9726** Patient refused to participate Ⓑ M

↩ * **G9727** Patient unable to complete the knee FS prom at admission and discharge due to blindness, illiteracy, severe mental incapacity or language incompatibility and an adequate proxy is not available Ⓑ M

* **G9728** Patient refused to participate Ⓑ M

↩ * **G9729** Patient unable to complete the hip FS prom at admission and discharge due to blindness, illiteracy, severe mental incapacity or language incompatibility and an adequate proxy is not available Ⓑ M

* **G9730** Patient refused to participate Ⓑ M

↩ * **G9731** Patient unable to complete the foot/ankle FS prom at admission and discharge due to blindness, illiteracy, severe mental incapacity or language incompatibility and an adequate proxy is not available Ⓑ M

* **G9732** Patient refused to participate Ⓑ M

↩ * **G9733** Patient unable to complete the low back FS prom at admission and discharge due to blindness, illiteracy, severe mental incapacity or language incompatibility and an adequate proxy is not available Ⓑ M

* **G9734** Patient refused to participate Ⓑ M

↩ * **G9735** Patient unable to complete the shoulder FS prom at admission and discharge due to blindness, illiteracy, severe mental incapacity or language incompatibility and an adequate proxy is not available Ⓑ M

* **G9736** Patient refused to participate Ⓑ M

↩ * **G9737** Patient unable to complete the elbow/wrist/hand FS prom at admission and discharge due to blindness, illiteracy, severe mental incapacity or language incompatibility and an adequate proxy is not available Ⓑ M

* **G9738** Patient refused to participate Ⓑ M

↩ * **G9739** Patient unable to complete the general orthopedic FS prom at admission and discharge due to blindness, illiteracy, severe mental incapacity or language incompatibility and an adequate proxy is not available Ⓑ M

* **G9740** Hospice services given to patient any time during the measurement period Ⓑ M

* **G9741** Patients who use hospice services any time during the measurement period Ⓑ M

* **G9742** Psychiatric symptoms assessed Ⓑ M

* **G9743** Psychiatric symptoms not assessed, reason not otherwise specified Ⓑ M

* **G9744** Patient not eligible due to active diagnosis of hypertension Ⓑ M

* **G9745** Documented reason for not screening or recommending a follow-up for high blood pressure Ⓑ M

* **G9746** Patient has mitral stenosis or prosthetic heart valves or patient has transient or reversible cause of AF (e.g., pneumonia, hyperthyroidism, pregnancy, cardiac surgery) Ⓑ M

* **G9747** Patient is undergoing palliative dialysis with a catheter Ⓑ M

* **G9748** Patient approved by a qualified transplant program and scheduled to receive a living donor kidney transplant Ⓑ M

* **G9749** Patient is undergoing palliative dialysis with a catheter Ⓑ M

* **G9750** Patient approved by a qualified transplant program and scheduled to receive a living donor kidney transplant Ⓑ M

* **G9751** Patient died at any time during the 24-month measurement period Ⓑ M

* **G9752** Emergency surgery Ⓑ M

▶ New ↩ Revised ✔ Reinstated ~~deleted~~ Deleted ⊘ Not covered or valid by Medicare
Special coverage instructions * Carrier discretion Ⓑ Bill Part B MAC Ⓓ Bill DME MAC

* G9753 Documentation of medical reason for not conducting a search for DICOM format images for prior patient CT imaging studies completed at non-affiliated external healthcare facilities or entities within the past 12 months that are available through a secure, authorized, media-free, shared archive (e.g., trauma, acute myocardial infarction, stroke, aortic aneurysm where time is of the essence) M
* G9754 A finding of an incidental pulmonary nodule M
* G9755 Documentation of medical reason(s) for not including a recommended interval and modality for follow-up or for no follow-up, and source of recommendations (e.g., patients with unexplained fever, immunocompromised patients who are at risk for infection) M
* G9756 Surgical procedures that included the use of silicone oil M
* G9757 Surgical procedures that included the use of silicone oil M
* G9758 Patient in hospice at any time during the measurement period M
* G9759 History of preoperative posterior capsule rupture M
* G9760 Patients who use hospice services any time during the measurement period M
* G9761 Patients who use hospice services any time during the measurement period M
* G9762 Patient had at least two HPV vaccines (with at least 146 days between the two) or three HPV vaccines on or between the patient's 9th and 13th birthdays M
* G9763 Patient did not have at least two HPV vaccines (with at least 146 days between the two) or three HPV vaccines on or between the patient's 9th and 13th birthdays M
* G9764 Patient has been treated with systemic medication for psoriasis vulgaris M
* G9765 Documentation that the patient declined change in medication or alternative therapies were unavailable, has documented contraindications, or has not been treated with systemic for at least six consecutive months (e.g., experienced adverse effects or lack of efficacy with all other therapy options) in order to achieve better disease control as measured by PGA, BSA, PASI, or DLQI M
* G9766 Patients who are transferred from one institution to another with a known diagnosis of CVA for endovascular stroke treatment M
* G9767 Hospitalized patients with newly diagnosed CVA considered for endovascular stroke treatment M
* G9768 Patients who utilize hospice services any time during the measurement period M
* G9769 Patient had a bone mineral density test in the past two years or received osteoporosis medication or therapy in the past 12 months M
* G9770 Peripheral nerve block (PNB) M
* G9771 At least 1 body temperature measurement equal to or greater than 35.5 degrees Celsius (or 95.9 degrees Fahrenheit) achieved within the 30 minutes immediately before or the 15 minutes immediately after anesthesia end time M
* G9772 Documentation of one of the following medical reason(s) for not achieving at least 1 body temperature measurement equal to or greater than 35.5 degrees Celsius (or 95.9 degrees Fahrenheit) within the 30 minutes immediately before or the 15 minutes immediately after anesthesia end time (e.g., emergency cases, intentional hypothermia, etc.) M
* G9773 At least 1 body temperature measurement equal to or greater than 35.5 degrees Celsius (or 95.9 degrees Fahrenheit) not achieved within the 30 minutes immediately before or the 15 minutes immediately after anesthesia end time, reason not given M
* G9774 Patients who have had a hysterectomy M
* G9775 Patient received at least 2 prophylactic pharmacologic anti-emetic agents of different classes preoperatively and/or intraoperatively M
* G9776 Documentation of medical reason for not receiving at least 2 prophylactic pharmacologic anti-emetic agents of different classes preoperatively and/or intraoperatively (e.g., intolerance or other medical reason) M
* G9777 Patient did not receive at least 2 prophylactic pharmacologic anti-emetic agents of different classes preoperatively and/or intraoperatively M

MIPS | Qp Quantity Physician | Qh Quantity Hospital | ♀ Female only
♂ Male only | A Age | DMEPOS | A2-Z3 ASC Payment Indicator | A-Y ASC Status Indicator | Coding Clinic

* G9778 Patients who have a diagnosis of pregnancy M
* G9779 Patients who are breastfeeding M
* G9780 Patients who have a diagnosis of rhabdomyolysis M
* G9781 Documentation of medical reason(s) for not currently being a statin therapy user or receive an order (prescription) for statin therapy (e.g., patient with adverse effect, allergy or intolerance to statin medication therapy, patients who are receiving palliative care, patients with active liver disease or hepatic disease or insufficiency, and patients with end stage renal disease [ESRD]) M
* G9782 History of or active diagnosis of familial or pure hypercholesterolemia M
* G9783 Documentation of patients with diabetes who have a most recent fasting or direct LDL-C laboratory test result <70 mg/dl and are not taking statin therapy M
* G9784 Pathologists/dermatopathologists providing a second opinion on a biopsy M
* G9785 Pathology report diagnosing cutaneous basal cell carcinoma or squamous cell carcinoma (to include in situ disease) sent from the pathologist/ dermatopathologist to the biopsying clinician for review within 7 days from the time when the tissue specimen was received by the pathologist M
* G9786 Pathology report diagnosing cutaneous basal cell carcinoma or squamous cell carcinoma (to include in situ disease) was not sent from the pathologist/ dermatopathologist to the biopsying clinician for review within 7 days from the time when the tissue specimen was received by the pathologist M
* G9787 Patient alive as of the last day of the measurement year M
* G9788 Most recent bp is less than or equal to 140/90 mm hg M
* G9789 Blood pressure recorded during inpatient stays, emergency room visits, urgent care visits, and patient self-reported BP's (home and health fair BP results) M
* G9790 Most recent BP is greater than 140/90 mm hg, or blood pressure not documented M
* G9791 Most recent tobacco status is tobacco free M
* G9792 Most recent tobacco status is not tobacco free M
* G9793 Patient is currently on a daily aspirin or other antiplatelet M
* G9794 Documentation of medical reason(s) for not on a daily aspirin or other antiplatelet (e.g., history of gastrointestinal bleed, intra-cranial bleed, idiopathic thrombocytopenic purpura (ITP), gastric bypass or documentation of active anticoagulant use during the measurement period) M
* G9795 Patient is not currently on a daily aspirin or other antiplatelet M
* G9796 Patient is currently on a statin therapy M
* G9797 Patient is not on a statin therapy M
* G9798 Discharge(s) for AMI between July 1 of the year prior measurement year to June 30 of the measurement period M
* G9799 Patients with a medication dispensing event indicator of a history of asthma any time during the patient's history through the end of the measure period M
* G9800 Patients who are identified as having an intolerance or allergy to beta-blocker therapy M
* G9801 Hospitalizations in which the patient was transferred directly to a non-acute care facility for any diagnosis M
* G9802 Patients who use hospice services any time during the measurement period M
* G9803 Patient prescribed at least a 135 day treatment within the 180-day course of treatment with beta-blockers post discharge for AMI M
* G9804 Patient was not prescribed at least a 135 day treatment within the 180-day course of treatment with beta-blockers post discharge for AMI M
* G9805 Patients who use hospice services any time during the measurement period M
* G9806 Patients who received cervical cytology or an HPV test M
* G9807 Patients who did not receive cervical cytology or an HPV test M
* G9808 Any patients who had no asthma controller medications dispensed during the measurement year M
* G9809 Patients who use hospice services any time during the measurement period M

▶ New ⤾ Revised ✔ Reinstated ~~deleted~~ Deleted ⊘ Not covered or valid by Medicare
Special coverage instructions * Carrier discretion Ⓑ Bill Part B MAC Ⓓ Bill DME MAC

* G9810 Patient achieved a pDC of at least 75% for their asthma controller medication M
* G9811 Patient did not achieve a pDC of at least 75% for their asthma controller medication M
* G9812 Patient died including all deaths occurring during the hospitalization in which the operation was performed, even if after 30 days, and those deaths occurring after discharge from the hospital, but within 30 days of the procedure M
* G9813 Patient did not die within 30 days of the procedure or during the index hospitalization M
* G9814 Death occurring during the index acute care hospitalization M
* G9815 Death did not occur during the index acute care hospitalization M
* G9816 Death occurring after discharge from the hospital but within 30 days post procedure M
* G9817 Death did not occur after discharge from the hospital within 30 days post procedure M
* G9818 Documentation of sexual activity M
* G9819 Patients who use hospice services any time during the measurement period M
* G9820 Documentation of a chlamydia screening test with proper follow-up M
* G9821 No documentation of a chlamydia screening test with proper follow-up M
* G9822 Women who had an endometrial ablation procedure during the year prior to the index date (exclusive of the index date) M
* G9823 Endometrial sampling or hysteroscopy with biopsy and results documented M
* G9824 Endometrial sampling or hysteroscopy with biopsy and results not documented M
* G9825 HER-2/neu negative or undocumented/unknown M
* G9826 Patient transferred to practice after initiation of chemotherapy M
* G9827 HER2-targeted therapies not administered during the initial course of treatment M
* G9828 HER2-targeted therapies administered during the initial course of treatment M
* G9829 Breast adjuvant chemotherapy administered M
* G9830 HER-2/neu positive M
* G9831 AJCC stage at breast cancer diagnosis = II or III M
* G9832 AJCC stage at breast cancer diagnosis = I (Ia or Ib) and T-stage at breast cancer diagnosis does not equal = T1, T1a, T1b M
* G9833 Patient transfer to practice after initiation of chemotherapy M
* G9834 Patient has metastatic disease at diagnosis M
* G9835 Trastuzumab administered within 12 months of diagnosis M
* G9836 Reason for not administering trastuzumab documented (e.g., patient declined, patient died, patient transferred, contraindication or other clinical exclusion, neoadjuvant chemotherapy or radiation not complete) M
* G9837 Trastuzumab not administered within 12 months of diagnosis M
* G9838 Patient has metastatic disease at diagnosis M
* G9839 Anti-EGFR monoclonal antibody therapy M
* G9840 Ras (KRas and NRas) gene mutation testing performed before initiation of anti-EGFR MoAb M
* G9841 Ras (KRas and NRas) gene mutation testing not performed before initiation of anti-EGFR MoAb M
* G9842 Patient has metastatic disease at diagnosis M
* G9843 Ras (KRas and NRas) gene mutation M
* G9844 Patient did not receive anti-EGFR monoclonal antibody therapy M
* G9845 Patient received anti-EGFR monoclonal antibody therapy M
* G9846 Patients who died from cancer M
* G9847 Patient received chemotherapy in the last 14 days of life M
* G9848 Patient did not receive chemotherapy in the last 14 days of life M
* G9849 Patients who died from cancer M
* G9850 Patient had more than one emergency department visit in the last 30 days of life M
* G9851 Patient had one or less emergency department visits in the last 30 days of life M

MIPS | Qp Quantity Physician | Qh Quantity Hospital | ♀ Female only
♂ Male only | A Age | DMEPOS | A2-Z3 ASC Payment Indicator | A-Y ASC Status Indicator | Coding Clinic

* * **G9852** Patients who died from cancer Ⓑ M
* * **G9853** Patient admitted to the ICU in the last 30 days of life Ⓑ M
* * **G9854** Patient was not admitted to the ICU in the last 30 days of life Ⓑ M
* * **G9855** Patients who died from cancer Ⓑ M
* * **G9856** Patient was not admitted to hospice Ⓑ M
* * **G9857** Patient admitted to hospice Ⓑ M
* * **G9858** Patient enrolled in hospice Ⓑ M
* * **G9859** Patients who died from cancer Ⓑ M
* * **G9860** Patient spent less than three days in hospice care Ⓑ M
* * **G9861** Patient spent greater than or equal to three days in hospice care Ⓑ M
* * **G9862** Documentation of medical reason(s) for not recommending at least a 10 year follow-up interval (e.g., inadequate prep, familial or personal history of colonic polyps, patient had no adenoma and age is = 66 years old, or life expectancy <10 years old, other medical reasons) Ⓑ M

▶ * **G9873** First Medicare diabetes prevention program (MDPP) core session was attended by an MDPP beneficiary under the MDPP expanded model (EM). A core session is an MDPP service that: (1) is furnished by an MDPP supplier during months 1 through 6 of the MDPP services period; (2) is approximately 1 hour in length; and (3) adheres to a CDC-approved DPP curriculum for core sessions. M

▶ * **G9874** Four total Medicare diabetes prevention program (MDPP) core sessions were attended by an MDPP beneficiary under the mdpp expanded model (EM). A core session is an MDPP service that: (1) is furnished by an MDPP supplier during months 1 through 6 of the MDPP services period; (2) is approximately 1 hour in length; and (3) adheres to a CDC-approved DPP curriculum for core sessions. M

▶ * **G9875** Nine total Medicare diabetes prevention program (MDPP) core sessions were attended by an MDPP beneficiary under the MDPP expanded model (EM). A core session is an MDPP service that: (1) is furnished by an MDPP supplier during months 1 through 6 of the MDPP services period; (2) is approximately 1 hour in length; and (3) adheres to a CDC-approved DPP curriculum for core sessions. M

▶ * **G9876** Two Medicare diabetes prevention program (MDPP) core maintenance sessions (MS) were attended by an MDPP beneficiary in months (mo) 7-9 under the mdpp expanded model (EM). A core maintenance session is an MDPP service that: (1) is furnished by an MDPP supplier during months 7 through 12 of the MDPP services period; (2) is approximately 1 hour in length; and (3) adheres to a CDC-approved DPP curriculum for maintenance sessions. The beneficiary did not achieve at least 5% weight loss (WL) from his/her baseline weight, as measured by at least one in-person weight measurement at a core maintenance session in months 7-9. M

▶ * **G9877** Two Medicare diabetes prevention program (MDPP) core maintenance sessions (MS) were attended by an MDPP beneficiary in months (mo) 10-12 under the MDPP expanded model (EM). A core maintenance session is an MDPP service that: (1) is furnished by an MDPP supplier during months 7 through 12 of the MDPP services period; (2) is approximately 1 hour in length; and (3) adheres to a CDC-approved DPP curriculum for maintenance sessions. The beneficiary did not achieve at least 5% weight loss (WL) from his/her baseline weight, as measured by at least one in-person weight measurement at a core maintenance session in months 10-12. M

▶ * **G9878** Two Medicare diabetes prevention program (MDPP) core maintenance sessions (MS) were attended by an MDPP beneficiary in months (mo) 7-9 under the MDPP expanded model (EM). A core maintenance session is an MDPP service that: (1) is furnished by an MDPP supplier during months 7 through 12 of the MDPP services period; (2) is approximately 1 hour in length; and (3) adheres to a CDC-approved DPP curriculum for maintenance sessions. The beneficiary achieved at least 5% weight loss (WL) from his/her baseline weight, as measured by at least one in-person weight measurement at a core maintenance session in months 7-9. M

▶ New ↩ Revised ✔ Reinstated ~~deleted~~ Deleted ⊘ Not covered or valid by Medicare
Special coverage instructions * Carrier discretion Ⓑ Bill Part B MAC Ⓓ Bill DME MAC

▶ ✻ **G9879** Two Medicare diabetes prevention program (MDPP) core maintenance sessions (MS) were attended by an MDPP beneficiary in months (mo) 10-12 under the MDPP expanded model (EM). A core maintenance session is an MDPP service that: (1) is furnished by an MDPP supplier during months 7 through 12 of the MDPP services period; (2) is approximately 1 hour in length; and (3) adheres to a CDC-approved DPP curriculum for maintenance sessions. The beneficiary achieved at least 5% weight loss (WL) from his/her baseline weight, as measured by at least one in-person weight measurement at a core maintenance session in months 10-12. M

▶ ✻ **G9880** The MDPP beneficiary achieved at least 5% weight loss (WL) from his/her baseline weight in months 1-12 of the MDPP services period under the MDPP expanded model (EM). This is a one-time payment available when a beneficiary first achieves at least 5% weight loss from baseline as measured by an in-person weight measurement at a core session or core maintenance session. M

▶ ✻ **G9881** The MDPP beneficiary achieved at least 9% weight loss (WL) from his/her baseline weight in months 1-24 under the MDPP expanded model (EM). This is a one-time payment available when a beneficiary first achieves at least 9% weight loss from baseline as measured by an in-person weight measurement at a core session, core maintenance session, or ongoing maintenance session. M

▶ ✻ **G9882** Two Medicare diabetes prevention program (MDPP) ongoing maintenance sessions (MS) were attended by an MDPP beneficiary in months (mo) 13-15 under the MDPP expanded model (EM). An ongoing maintenance session is an MDPP service that: (1) is furnished by an MDPP supplier during months 13 through 24 of the MDPP services period; (2) is approximately 1 hour in length; and (3) adheres to a CDC-approved DPP curriculum for maintenance sessions. The beneficiary maintained at least 5% weight loss (WL) from his/her baseline weight, as measured by at least one in-person weight measurement at an ongoing maintenance session in months 13-15. M

▶ ✻ **G9883** Two Medicare diabetes prevention program (MDPP) ongoing maintenance sessions (MS) were attended by an MDPP beneficiary in months (mo) 16-18 under the MDPP expanded model (EM). An ongoing maintenance session is an MDPP service that: (1) is furnished by an MDPP supplier during months 13 through 24 of the MDPP services period; (2) is approximately 1 hour in length; and (3) adheres to a CDC-approved DPP curriculum for maintenance sessions. The beneficiary maintained at least 5% weight loss (WL) from his/her baseline weight, as measured by at least one in-person weight measurement at an ongoing maintenance session in months 16-18. M

▶ ✻ **G9884** Two Medicare diabetes prevention program (MDPP) ongoing maintenance sessions (MS) were attended by an MDPP beneficiary in months (mo) 19-21 under the MDPP expanded model (EM). An ongoing maintenance session is an MDPP service that: (1) is furnished by an MDPP supplier during months 13 through 24 of the MDPP services period; (2) is approximately 1 hour in length; and (3) adheres to a CDC-approved DPP curriculum for maintenance sessions. The beneficiary maintained at least 5% weight loss (WL) from his/her baseline weight, as measured by at least one in-person weight measurement at an ongoing maintenance session in months 19-21. M

▶ ✻ **G9885** Two Medicare diabetes prevention program (MDPP) ongoing maintenance sessions (MS) were attended by an MDPP beneficiary in months (mo) 22-24 under the MDPP expanded model (EM). An ongoing maintenance session is an MDPP service that: (1) is furnished by an MDPP supplier during months 13 through 24 of the MDPP services period; (2) is approximately 1 hour in length; and (3) adheres to a CDC-approved DPP curriculum for maintenance sessions. The beneficiary maintained at least 5% weight loss (WL) from his/her baseline weight, as measured by at least one in-person weight measurement at an ongoing maintenance session in months 22-24. M

* **G9943** Back pain was not measured by the visual analog scale (VAS) within three months preoperatively and at three months (6-20 weeks) postoperatively Ⓑ M
* **G9944** Back pain was measured by the visual analog scale (VAS) within three months preoperatively and at one year (9 to 15 months) postoperatively Ⓑ M
* **G9945** Patient had cancer, fracture or infection related to the lumbar spine or patient had idiopathic or congenital scoliosis Ⓑ M
* **G9946** Back pain was not measured by the visual analog scale (VAS) within three months preoperatively and at one year (9 to 15 months) postoperatively Ⓑ M
* **G9947** Leg pain was measured by the visual analog scale (VAS) within three months preoperatively and at three months (6 to 20 weeks) postoperatively Ⓑ M
* **G9948** Patient had any additional spine procedures performed on the same date as the lumbar discectomy/laminotomy Ⓑ M
* **G9949** Leg pain was not measured by the visual analog scale (VAS) within three months preoperatively and at three months (6 to 20 weeks) postoperatively Ⓑ M
* **G9954** Patient exhibits 2 or more risk factors for post-operative vomiting Ⓑ M
* **G9955** Cases in which an inhalational anesthetic is used only for induction Ⓑ M
* **G9956** Patient received combination therapy consisting of at least two prophylactic pharmacologic anti-emetic agents of different classes preoperatively and/or intraoperatively Ⓑ M
* **G9957** Documentation of medical reason for not receiving combination therapy consisting of at least two prophylactic pharmacologic anti-emetic agents of different classes preoperatively and/or intraoperatively (e.g., intolerance or other medical reason) Ⓑ M
* **G9958** Patient did not receive combination therapy consisting of at least two prophylactic pharmacologic anti-emetic agents of different classes preoperatively and/or intraoperatively Ⓑ M
* **G9959** Systemic antimicrobials not prescribed Ⓑ M
* **G9960** Documentation of medical reason(s) for prescribing systemic antimicrobials Ⓑ M
* **G9961** Systemic antimicrobials prescribed Ⓑ M
* **G9962** Embolization endpoints are documented separately for each embolized vessel and ovarian artery angiography or embolization performed in the presence of variant uterine artery anatomy Ⓑ M
* **G9963** Embolization endpoints are not documented separately for each embolized vessel or ovarian artery angiography or embolization not performed in the presence of variant uterine artery anatomy Ⓑ M
* **G9964** Patient received at least one well-child visit with a PCP during the performance period Ⓑ M
* **G9965** Patient did not receive at least one well-child visit with a PCP during the performance period Ⓑ M
* **G9966** Children who were screened for risk of developmental, behavioral and social delays using a standardized tool with interpretation and report Ⓑ M
* **G9967** Children who were not screened for risk of developmental, behavioral and social delays using a standardized tool with interpretation and report Ⓑ M
* **G9968** Patient was referred to another provider or specialist during the performance period Ⓑ M
* **G9969** Provider who referred the patient to another provider received a report from the provider to whom the patient was referred Ⓑ M
* **G9970** Provider who referred the patient to another provider did not receive a report from the provider to whom the patient was referred Ⓑ M
* **G9974** Dilated macular exam performed, including documentation of the presence or absence of macular thickening or geographic atrophy or hemorrhage and the level of macular degeneration severity Ⓑ M
* **G9975** Documentation of medical reason(s) for not performing a dilated macular examination Ⓑ M
* **G9976** Documentation of patient reason(s) for not performing a dilated macular examination Ⓑ M
* **G9977** Dilated macular exam was not performed, reason not otherwise specified Ⓑ M

▶ ✻ **G9978** Remote in-home visit for the evaluation and management of a new patient for use only in a Medicare-approved bundled payments for care improvement advanced (BCPI advanced) model episode of care, which requires these 3 key components: a problem focused history; a problem focused examination; and straightforward medical decision making, furnished in real time using interactive audio and video technology. Counseling and coordination of care with other physicians, other qualified health care professionals or agencies are provided consistent with the nature of the problem(s) and the needs of the patient or the family or both. Usually, the presenting problem(s) are self limited or minor. Typically, 10 minutes are spent with the patient or family or both via real time, audio and video intercommunications technology. B

▶ ✻ **G9979** Remote in-home visit for the evaluation and management of a new patient for use only in a Medicare-approved bundled payments for care improvement advanced (BCPI advanced) model episode of care, which requires these 3 key components: an expanded problem focused history; an expanded problem focused examination; straightforward medical decision making, furnished in real time using interactive audio and video technology. Counseling and coordination of care with other physicians, other qualified health care professionals or agencies are provided consistent with the nature of the problem(s) and the needs of the patient or the family or both. Usually, the presenting problem(s) are of low to moderate severity. Typically, 20 minutes are spent with the patient or family or both via real time, audio and video intercommunications technology. B

▶ ✻ **G9980** Remote in-home visit for the evaluation and management of a new patient for use only in a Medicare-approved bundled payments for care improvement advanced (BCPI advanced) model episode of care, which requires these 3 key components: a detailed history; a detailed examination; medical decision making of low complexity, furnished in real time using interactive audio and video technology. Counseling and coordination of care with other physicians, other qualified health care professionals or agencies are provided consistent with the nature of the problem(s) and the needs of the patient or the family or both. Usually, the presenting problem(s) are of moderate severity. Typically, 30 minutes are spent with the patient or family or both via real time, audio and video intercommunications technology. B

▶ ✻ **G9981** Remote in-home visit for the evaluation and management of a new patient for use only in a Medicare-approved bundled payments for care improvement advanced (BCPI advanced) model episode of care, which requires these 3 key components: a comprehensive history; a comprehensive examination; medical decision making of moderate complexity, furnished in real time using interactive audio and video technology. Counseling and coordination of care with other physicians, other qualified health care professionals or agencies are provided consistent with the nature of the problem(s) and the needs of the patient or the family or both. Usually, the presenting problem(s) are of moderate to high severity. Typically, 45 minutes are spent with the patient or family or both via real time, audio and video intercommunications technology. B

▶ ✻ **G9982** Remote in-home visit for the evaluation and management of a new patient for use only in a Medicare-approved bundled payments for care improvement advanced (BCPI advanced) model episode of care, which requires these 3 key components: a comprehensive history; a comprehensive examination; medical decision making of high complexity, furnished in real time using interactive audio and video technology. Counseling and coordination of care with other physicians, other qualified health care professionals or agencies are provided consistent with the nature of the problem(s) and the needs of the patient or the family or both. Usually, the presenting problem(s) are of moderate to high severity. Typically, 60 minutes are spent with the patient or family or both via real time, audio and video intercommunications technology. B

▶ ✻ **G9983** Remote in-home visit for the evaluation and management of an established patient for use only in a Medicare-approved bundled payments for care improvement advanced (BCPI advanced) model episode of care, which requires at least 2 of the following 3 key components: a problem focused history; a problem focused examination; straightforward medical decision making, furnished in real time using interactive audio and video technology. Counseling and coordination of care with other physicians, other qualified health care professionals or agencies are provided consistent with the nature of the problem(s) and the needs of the patient or the family or both. Usually, the presenting problem(s) are self limited or minor. Typically, 10 minutes are spent with the patient or family or both via real time, audio and video intercommunications technology. B

▶ ✻ **G9984** Remote in-home visit for the evaluation and management of an established patient for use only in a Medicare-approved bundled payments for care improvement advanced (BCPI advanced) model episode of care, which requires at least 2 of the following 3 key components: an expanded problem focused history; an expanded problem focused examination; medical decision making of low complexity, furnished in real time using interactive audio and video technology. Counseling and coordination of care with other physicians, other qualified health care professionals or agencies are provided consistent with the nature of the problem(s) and the needs of the patient or the family or both. Usually, the presenting problem(s) are of low to moderate severity. Typically, 15 minutes are spent with the patient or family or both via real time, audio and video intercommunications technology. B

▶ ✻ **G9985** Remote in-home visit for the evaluation and management of an established patient for use only in a Medicare-approved bundled payments for care improvement advanced (BCPI advanced) model episode of care, which requires at least 2 of the following 3 key components: a detailed history; a detailed examination; medical decision making of moderate complexity, furnished in real time using interactive audio and video technology. Counseling and coordination of care with other physicians, other qualified health care professionals or agencies are provided consistent with the nature of the problem(s) and the needs of the patient or the family or both. Usually, the presenting problem(s) are of moderate to high severity. Typically, 25 minutes are spent with the patient or family or both via real time, audio and video intercommunications technology. B

▶ ✻ **G9986** Remote in-home visit for the evaluation and management of an established patient for use only in a Medicare-approved bundled payments for care improvement advanced (BCPI advanced) model episode of care, which requires at least 2 of the following 3 key components: a comprehensive history; a comprehensive examination; medical decision making of high complexity, furnished in real time using interactive audio and video technology. Counseling and coordination of care with other physicians, other qualified health care professionals or agencies are provided consistent with the nature of the problem(s) and the needs of the patient or the family or both. Usually, the presenting problem(s) are of moderate to high severity. Typically, 40 minutes are spent with the patient or family or both via real time, audio and video intercommunications technology. B

▶ ✻ **G9987** Bundled payments for care improvement advanced (BCPI advanced) model home visit for patient assessment performed by clinical staff for an individual not considered homebound, including, but not necessarily limited to patient assessment of clinical status, safety/fall prevention, functional status/ambulation, medication reconciliation/management, compliance with orders/plan of care, performance of activities of daily living, and ensuring beneficiary connections to community and other services; for use only for a BCPI advanced model episode of care; may not be billed for a 30-day period covered by a transitional care management code. B

BEHAVIORAL HEALTH AND/OR SUBSTANCE ABUSE TREATMENT SERVICES (H0001-H9999)

Note: Used by Medicaid state agencies because no national code exists to meet the reporting needs of these agencies.

⃠ **H0001** Alcohol and/or drug assessment

⃠ **H0002** Behavioral health screening to determine eligibility for admission to treatment program

⃠ **H0003** Alcohol and/or drug screening; laboratory analysis of specimens for presence of alcohol and/or drugs

⃠ **H0004** Behavioral health counseling and therapy, per 15 minutes

⃠ **H0005** Alcohol and/or drug services; group counseling by a clinician

⃠ **H0006** Alcohol and/or drug services; case management

⃠ **H0007** Alcohol and/or drug services; crisis intervention (outpatient)

⃠ **H0008** Alcohol and/or drug services; sub-acute detoxification (hospital inpatient)

⃠ **H0009** Alcohol and/or drug services; acute detoxification (hospital inpatient)

⃠ **H0010** Alcohol and/or drug services; sub-acute detoxification (residential addiction program inpatient)

⃠ **H0011** Alcohol and/or drug services; acute detoxification (residential addiction program inpatient)

⃠ **H0012** Alcohol and/or drug services; sub-acute detoxification (residential addiction program outpatient)

⃠ **H0013** Alcohol and/or drug services; acute detoxification (residential addiction program outpatient)

⃠ **H0014** Alcohol and/or drug services; ambulatory detoxification

⃠ **H0015** Alcohol and/or drug services; intensive outpatient (treatment program that operates at least 3 hours/day and at least 3 days/week and is based on an individualized treatment plan), including assessment, counseling; crisis intervention, and activity therapies or education

⃠ **H0016** Alcohol and/or drug services; medical/somatic (medical intervention in ambulatory setting)

⃠ **H0017** Behavioral health; residential (hospital residential treatment program), without room and board, per diem

⃠ **H0018** Behavioral health; short-term residential (non-hospital residential treatment program), without room and board, per diem

⃠ **H0019** Behavioral health; long-term residential (non-medical, non-acute care in a residential treatment program where stay is typically longer than 30 days), without room and board, per diem

⃠ **H0020** Alcohol and/or drug services; methadone administration and/or service (provision of the drug by a licensed program)

⃠ **H0021** Alcohol and/or drug training service (for staff and personnel not employed by providers)

⃠ **H0022** Alcohol and/or drug intervention service (planned facilitation)

⃠ **H0023** Behavioral health outreach service (planned approach to reach a targeted population)

⃠ **H0024** Behavioral health prevention information dissemination service (one-way direct or non-direct contact with service audiences to affect knowledge and attitude)

⃠ **H0025** Behavioral health prevention education service (delivery of services with target population to affect knowledge, attitude and/or behavior)

⃠ **H0026** Alcohol and/or drug prevention process service, community-based (delivery of services to develop skills of impactors)

⃠ **H0027** Alcohol and/or drug prevention environmental service (broad range of external activities geared toward modifying systems in order to mainstream prevention through policy and law)

⃠ **H0028** Alcohol and/or drug prevention problem identification and referral service (e.g., student assistance and employee assistance programs), does not include assessment

⃠ **H0029** Alcohol and/or drug prevention alternatives service (services for populations that exclude alcohol and other drug use, e.g., alcohol-free social events)

⃠ **H0030** Behavioral health hotline service

⃠ **H0031** Mental health assessment, by non-physician

⃠ **H0032** Mental health service plan development by non-physician

⃠ **H0033** Oral medication administration, direct observation

- MIPS ⊘ **H0034** Medication training and support, per 15 minutes
- MIPS ⊘ **H0035** Mental health partial hospitalization, treatment, less than 24 hours
- MIPS ⊘ **H0036** Community psychiatric supportive treatment, face-to-face, per 15 minutes
- MIPS ⊘ **H0037** Community psychiatric supportive treatment program, per diem
- ⊘ **H0038** Self-help/peer services, per 15 minutes
- MIPS ⊘ **H0039** Assertive community treatment, face-to-face, per 15 minutes
- MIPS ⊘ **H0040** Assertive community treatment program, per diem
- ⊘ **H0041** Foster care, child, non-therapeutic, per diem A
- ⊘ **H0042** Foster care, child, non-therapeutic, per month A
- ⊘ **H0043** Supported housing, per diem
- ⊘ **H0044** Supported housing, per month
- ⊘ **H0045** Respite care services, not in the home, per diem
- ⊘ **H0046** Mental health services, not otherwise specified
- ⊘ **H0047** Alcohol and/or other drug abuse services, not otherwise specified
- ⊘ **H0048** Alcohol and/or other drug testing: collection and handling only, specimens other than blood
- ⊘ **H0049** Alcohol and/or drug screening
- ⊘ **H0050** Alcohol and/or drug services, brief intervention, per 15 minutes
- ⊘ **H1000** Prenatal care, at-risk assessment ♀
- ⊘ **H1001** Prenatal care, at-risk enhanced service; antepartum management ♀
- ⊘ **H1002** Prenatal care, at-risk enhanced service; care coordination ♀
- ⊘ **H1003** Prenatal care, at-risk enhanced service; education ♀
- ⊘ **H1004** Prenatal care, at-risk enhanced service; follow-up home visit ♀
- ⊘ **H1005** Prenatal care, at-risk enhanced service package (includes H1001-H1004) ♀
- ⊘ **H1010** Non-medical family planning education, per session
- ⊘ **H1011** Family assessment by licensed behavioral health professional for state defined purposes
- MIPS ⊘ **H2000** Comprehensive multidisciplinary evaluation
- MIPS ⊘ **H2001** Rehabilitation program, per 1/2 day
- MIPS ⊘ **H2010** Comprehensive medication services, per 15 minutes
- MIPS ⊘ **H2011** Crisis intervention service, per 15 minutes
- MIPS ⊘ **H2012** Behavioral health day treatment, per hour
- MIPS ⊘ **H2013** Psychiatric health facility service, per diem
- MIPS ⊘ **H2014** Skills training and development, per 15 minutes
- MIPS ⊘ **H2015** Comprehensive community support services, per 15 minutes
- MIPS ⊘ **H2016** Comprehensive community support services, per diem
- MIPS ⊘ **H2017** Psychosocial rehabilitation services, per 15 minutes
- MIPS ⊘ **H2018** Psychosocial rehabilitation services, per diem
- MIPS ⊘ **H2019** Therapeutic behavioral services, per 15 minutes
- MIPS ⊘ **H2020** Therapeutic behavioral services, per diem
- ⊘ **H2021** Community-based wrap-around services, per 15 minutes
- ⊘ **H2022** Community-based wrap-around services, per diem
- ⊘ **H2023** Supported employment, per 15 minutes
- ⊘ **H2024** Supported employment, per diem
- ⊘ **H2025** Ongoing support to maintain employment, per 15 minutes
- ⊘ **H2026** Ongoing support to maintain employment, per diem
- ⊘ **H2027** Psychoeducational service, per 15 minutes
- ⊘ **H2028** Sexual offender treatment service, per 15 minutes
- ⊘ **H2029** Sexual offender treatment service, per diem
- ⊘ **H2030** Mental health clubhouse services, per 15 minutes
- ⊘ **H2031** Mental health clubhouse services, per diem
- ⊘ **H2032** Activity therapy, per 15 minutes
- ⊘ **H2033** Multisystemic therapy for juveniles, per 15 minutes A
- ⊘ **H2034** Alcohol and/or drug abuse halfway house services, per diem
- ⊘ **H2035** Alcohol and/or other drug treatment program, per hour
- ⊘ **H2036** Alcohol and/or other drug treatment program, per diem
- ⊘ **H2037** Developmental delay prevention activities, dependent child of client, per 15 minutes A

DRUGS OTHER THAN CHEMOTHERAPY DRUGS (J0100-J8999)

Injection

J0120 Injection, tetracycline, up to 250 mg — N1 N
Other: Achromycin
IOM: 100-02, 15, 50

* **J0129** Injection, abatacept, 10 mg (code may be used for medicare when drug administered under the direct supervision of a physician, not for use when drug is self-administered) — K2 K
Other: Orencia

J0130 Injection, abciximab, 10 mg — N1 N
Other: ReoPro
IOM: 100-02, 15, 50

* **J0131** Injection, acetaminophen, 10 mg — N1 N
Other: Ofirmev
Coding Clinic: 2012, Q1, P9

* **J0132** Injection, acetylcysteine, 100 mg — N1 N
Other: Acetadote

* **J0133** Injection, acyclovir, 5 mg — N1 N

* **J0135** Injection, adalimumab, 20 mg — K2 K
Other: Humira
IOM: 100-02, 15, 50

J0153 Injection, adenosine, 1 mg (not to be used to report any adenosine phosphate compounds) — N1 N
Other: Adenocard, Adenoscan

J0171 Injection, adrenalin, epinephrine, 0.1 mg — N1 N
Other: AUVI-Q, Sus-Phrine
IOM: 100-02, 15, 50
Coding Clinic: 2011, Q1, P8

* **J0178** Injection, aflibercept, 1 mg — K2 K
Other: Eylea

* **J0180** Injection, agalsidase beta, 1 mg — K2 K
Other: Fabrazyme
IOM: 100-02, 15, 50

▶ * **J0185** Injection, aprepitant, 1 mg — G
Other: Emend

J0190 Injection, biperiden lactate, per 5 mg — E2
Other: Akineton
IOM: 100-02, 15, 50

J0200 Injection, alatrofloxacin mesylate, 100 mg — E2
Other: Trovan
IOM: 100-02, 15, 50

* **J0202** Injection, alemtuzumab, 1 mg — K2 K
Other: Lemtrada

J0205 Injection, alglucerase, per 10 units — E2
Other: Ceredase
IOM: 100-02, 15, 50

J0207 Injection, amifostine, 500 mg — K2 K
Other: Ethyol
IOM: 100-02, 15, 50

J0210 Injection, methyldopate HCL, up to 250 mg — N1 N
Other: Aldomet
IOM: 100-02, 15, 50

* **J0215** Injection, alefacept, 0.5 mg — E2

* **J0220** Injection, alglucosidase alfa, not otherwise specified, 10 mg — K2 K
Coding Clinic: 2013: Q2, P5; 2012, Q1, P9

* **J0221** Injection, alglucosidase alfa, (lumizyme), 10 mg — K2 K
Coding Clinic: 2013: Q2, P5

J0256 Injection, alpha 1-proteinase inhibitor (human), not otherwise specified, 10 mg — K2 K
Other: Prolastin, Zemaira
IOM: 100-02, 15, 50
Coding Clinic: 2012, Q1, P9

J0257 Injection, alpha 1 proteinase inhibitor (human), (glassia), 10 mg — K2 K
IOM: 100-02, 15, 50
Coding Clinic: 2012, Q1, P8

J0270 Injection, alprostadil, per 1.25 mcg (Code may be used for Medicare when drug administered under the direct supervision of a physician, not for use when drug is self-administered) Qp Qh B

Other: Caverject, Prostaglandin E1, Prostin VR Pediatric

IOM: 100-02, 15, 50

J0275 Alprostadil urethral suppository (Code may be used for Medicare when drug administered under the direct supervision of a physician, not for use when drug is self-administered) Qp Qh B

Other: Muse

IOM: 100-02, 15, 50

* **J0278** Injection, amikacin sulfate, 100 mg Qp Qh N1 N

J0280 Injection, aminophylline, up to 250 mg Qp Qh N1 N

IOM: 100-02, 15, 50

J0282 Injection, amiodarone hydrochloride, 30 mg Qp Qh N1 N

Other: Cordarone

IOM: 100-02, 15, 50

J0285 Injection, amphotericin B, 50 mg Qp Qh N1 N

Other: ABLC, Amphocin, Fungizone

IOM: 100-02, 15, 50

J0287 Injection, amphotericin B lipid complex, 10 mg Qp Qh K2 K

Other: Abelcet

IOM: 100-02, 15, 50

J0288 Injection, amphotericin B cholesteryl sulfate complex, 10 mg Qp Qh E2

IOM: 100-02, 15, 50

J0289 Injection, amphotericin B liposome, 10 mg Qp Qh K2 K

Other: AmBisome

IOM: 100-02, 15, 50

J0290 Injection, ampicillin sodium, 500 mg Qp Qh N1 N

Other: Omnipen-N, Polycillin-N, Totacillin-N

IOM: 100-02, 15, 50

J0295 Injection, ampicillin sodium/sulbactam sodium, per 1.5 gm Qp Qh N1 N

Other: Omnipen-N, Polycillin-N, Totacillin-N, Unasyn

IOM: 100-02, 15, 50

J0300 Injection, amobarbital, up to 125 mg Qp Qh K2 K

Other: Amytal

IOM: 100-02, 15, 50

J0330 Injection, succinylcholine chloride, up to 20 mg Qp Qh N1 N

Other: Anectine, Quelicin, Surostrin

IOM: 100-02, 15, 50

* **J0348** Injection, anidulafungin, 1 mg Qp Qh N1 N

Other: Eraxis

J0350 Injection, anistreplase, per 30 units Qp Qh E2

Other: Eminase

IOM: 100-02, 15, 50

J0360 Injection, hydralazine hydrochloride, up to 20 mg Qp Qh N1 N

Other: Apresoline

IOM: 100-02, 15, 50

* **J0364** Injection, apomorphine hydrochloride, 1 mg Qp Qh E2

J0365 Injection, aprotinin, 10,000 KIU Qp Qh E2

IOM: 100-02, 15, 50

J0380 Injection, metaraminol bitartrate, per 10 mg Qp Qh N1 N

Other: Aramine

IOM: 100-02, 15, 50

J0390 Injection, chloroquine hydrochloride, up to 250 mg Qp Qh N1 N

Benefit only for diagnosed malaria or amebiasis

Other: Aralen

IOM: 100-02, 15, 50

J0395 Injection, arbutamine HCL, 1 mg Qp Qh E2

IOM: 100-02, 15, 50

* **J0400** Injection, aripiprazole, intramuscular, 0.25 mg Qp Qh K2 K

MIPS | Qp Quantity Physician | Qh Quantity Hospital | ♀ Female only
♂ Male only | A Age | DMEPOS | A2-Z3 ASC Payment Indicator | A-Y ASC Status Indicator | Coding Clinic

* **J0401** Injection, aripiprazole, extended release, 1 mg Ⓑ Ⓔ Qp Qh K2 K
  Other: Abilify Maintena
* **J0456** Injection, azithromycin, 500 mg Ⓑ Ⓔ Qp Qh N1 N
  Other: Zithromax
  IOM: 100-02, 15, 50
* **J0461** Injection, atropine sulfate, 0.01 mg Ⓑ Ⓔ Qp Qh N1 N
  IOM: 100-02, 15, 50
* **J0470** Injection, dimercaprol, per 100 mg Ⓑ Ⓔ Qp Qh K2 K
  Other: BAL In Oil
  IOM: 100-02, 15, 50
* **J0475** Injection, baclofen, 10 mg Ⓑ Ⓔ Qp Qh K2 K
  Other: Gablofen, Lioresal
  IOM: 100-02, 15, 50
* **J0476** Injection, baclofen 50 mcg for intrathecal trial Ⓑ Ⓔ Qp Qh K2 K
  Other: Gablofen, Lioresal
  IOM: 100-02, 15, 50
* **J0480** Injection, basiliximab, 20 mg Ⓑ Ⓔ Qp Qh K2 K
  Other: Simulect
  IOM: 100-02, 15, 50
* **J0485** Injection, belatacept, 1 mg Ⓑ Ⓔ Qp Qh K2 K
  Other: Nulojix
* **J0490** Injection, belimumab, 10 mg Ⓑ Ⓔ Qp Qh K2 K
  Other: Benlysta
  Coding Clinic: 2012, Q1, P9
* **J0500** Injection, dicyclomine HCL, up to 20 mg Ⓑ Ⓔ Qp Qh N1 N
  Other: Antispas, Bentyl, Dibent, Dilomine, Di-Spaz, Neoquess, Or-Tyl, Spasmoject
  IOM: 100-02, 15, 50
* **J0515** Injection, benztropine mesylate, per 1 mg Ⓑ Ⓔ Qp Qh N1 N
  Other: Cogentin
  IOM: 100-02, 15, 50
* ▶ **J0517** Injection, benralizumab, 1 mg G
  Other: Fasenra
* **J0520** Injection, bethanechol chloride, myotonachol or urecholine, up to 5 mg Ⓑ Ⓔ Qp Qh E2
  IOM: 100-02, 15, 50
* **J0558** Injection, penicillin G benzathine and penicillin G procaine,100,000 units Ⓑ Ⓔ Qp Qh N1 N
  Other: Bicillin C-R
  Coding Clinic: 2011, Q1, P8
* **J0561** Injection, penicillin G benzathine, 100,000 units Ⓑ Ⓔ Qp Qh K2 K
  Other: Bicillin L-A, Permapen
  IOM: 100-02, 15, 50
  Coding Clinic: 2013: Q2, P3; 2011, Q1, P8
* **J0565** Injection, bezlotoxumab, 10 mg K2 G
* ▶ **J0567** Injection, cerliponase alfa, 1 mg G
  Other: Brineura
* **J0570** Buprenorphine implant, 74.2 mg Qp Qh K2 G
  Other: Probuphine System Kit
  Coding Clinic: 2017, Q1, P9
* **J0571** Buprenorphine, oral, 1 mg Ⓑ Ⓔ Qp Qh E1
* **J0572** Buprenorphine/naloxone, oral, less than or equal to 3 mg buprenorphine Ⓑ Ⓔ Qp Qh E1
* **J0573** Buprenorphine/naloxone, oral, greater than 3 mg, but less than or equal to 6 mg buprenorphine Ⓑ Ⓔ Qp Qh E1
* **J0574** Buprenorphine/naloxone, oral, greater than 6 mg, but less than or equal to 10 mg buprenorphine Ⓑ Ⓔ Qp Qh E1
* **J0575** Buprenorphine/naloxone, oral, greater than 10 mg buprenorphine Ⓑ Ⓔ Qp Qh E1
* **J0583** Injection, bivalirudin, 1 mg Ⓑ Ⓔ Qp Qh N1 N
  Other: Angiomax
* ▶ **J0584** Injection, burosumab-twza 1 mg K
  Other: Crysvita
* **J0585** Injection, onabotulinumtoxinaA, 1 unit Ⓑ Ⓔ Qp Qh K2 K
  Other: Botox, Botox Cosmetic, Oculinum
  IOM: 100-02, 15, 50
* **J0586** Injection, abobotulinumtoxinaA, 5 units Ⓑ Ⓔ Qp Qh K2 K
* **J0587** Injection, rimabotulinumtoxinB, 100 units Ⓑ Ⓔ Qp Qh K2 K
  Other: Myobloc, Nplate
  IOM: 100-02, 15, 50
* **J0588** Injection, incobotulinumtoxin A, 1 unit Ⓑ Ⓔ Qp Qh K2 K
  Other: Xeomin
  Coding Clinic: 2012, Q1, P9

▶ New ⮌ Revised ✔ Reinstated ~~deleted~~ Deleted ⊘ Not covered or valid by Medicare
Special coverage instructions * Carrier discretion Ⓑ Bill Part B MAC Ⓔ Bill DME MAC

J0592 Injection, buprenorphine hydrochloride, 0.1 mg Qp Qh N1 N
Other: Buprenex
IOM: 100-02, 15, 50

* J0594 Injection, busulfan, 1 mg Qp Qh K2 K
Other: Myleran

* J0595 Injection, butorphanol tartrate, 1 mg Qp Qh N1 N

* J0596 Injection, C1 esterase inhibitor (recombinant), ruconest, 10 units Qp Qh K2 K

* J0597 Injection, C-1 esterase inhibitor (human), Berinert, 10 units Qp Qh K2 K
Coding Clinic: 2011, Q1, P7

* J0598 Injection, C1 esterase inhibitor (human), cinryze, 10 units Qp Qh K2 K

▶ * J0599 Injection, c-1 esterase inhibitor (human), (haegarda), 10 units G
Other: Berinert

J0600 Injection, edetate calcium disodium, up to 1000 mg Qp Qh K2 K
Other: Calcium Disodium Versenate
IOM: 100-02, 15, 50

J0604 Cinacalcet, oral, 1 mg, (for ESRD on dialysis) B

J0606 Injection, etelcalcetide, 0.1 mg K2 K

J0610 Injection, calcium gluconate, per 10 ml Qp Qh N1 N
Other: Kaleinate
IOM: 100-02, 15, 50

J0620 Injection, calcium glycerophosphate and calcium lactate, per 10 ml Qp Qh N1 N
Other: Calphosan
MCM: 2049
IOM: 100-02, 15, 50

J0630 Injection, calcitonin (salmon), up to 400 units Qp Qh K2 K
Other: Calcimar, Calcitonin-salmon, Miacalcin
IOM: 100-02, 15, 50

J0636 Injection, calcitriol, 0.1 mcg Qp Qh N1 N
Non-dialysis use
Other: Calcijex
IOM: 100-02, 15, 50

* J0637 Injection, caspofungin acetate, 5 mg Qp Qh K2 K
Other: Cancidas, Caspofungin

* J0638 Injection, canakinumab, 1 mg Qp Qh K2 K
Other: Ilaris

J0640 Injection, leucovorin calcium, per 50 mg Qp Qh N1 N
Other: Wellcovorin
IOM: 100-02, 15, 50
Coding Clinic: 2009, Q1, P10

J0641 Injection, levoleucovorin calcium, 0.5 mg Qp Qh K2 K
Part of treatment regimen for osteosarcoma

J0670 Injection, mepivacaine HCL, per 10 ml Qp Qh N1 N
Other: Carbocaine, Isocaine HCl, Polocaine
IOM: 100-02, 15, 50

J0690 Injection, cefezolin sodium, 500 mg Qp Qh N1 N
Other: Ancef, Kefzol, Zolicef
IOM: 100-02, 15, 50

* J0692 Injection, cefepime HCL, 500 mg Qp Qh N1 N
Other: Maxipime

J0694 Injection, cefoxitin sodium, 1 gm Qp Qh N1 N
Other: Mefoxin
IOM: 100-02, 15, 50,
Cross Reference Q0090

* J0695 Injection, ceftolozane 50 mg and tazobactam25 mg Qp Qh K2 K
Other: Zerbaxa

J0696 Injection, ceftriaxone sodium, per 250 mg Qp Qh N1 N
Other: Rocephin
IOM: 100-02, 15, 50

J0697 Injection, sterile cefuroxime sodium, per 750 mg Qp Qh N1 N
Other: Kefurox, Zinacef
IOM: 100-02, 15, 50

J0698 Injection, cefotaxime sodium, per gm Qp Qh N1 N
Other: Claforan
IOM: 100-02, 15, 50

J0702 Injection, betamethasone acetate 3 mg and betamethasone sodium phosphate 3 mg Qp Qh N1 N
Other: Betameth, Celestone Soluspan, Selestoject
IOM: 100-02, 15, 50

MIPS | Qp Quantity Physician | Qh Quantity Hospital | ♀ Female only
♂ Male only | A Age | DMEPOS | A2-Z3 ASC Payment Indicator | A-Y ASC Status Indicator | Coding Clinic

* J0706 Injection, caffeine citrate, 5 mg Qp Qh N1 N
  Other: Cafcit, Cipro IV, Ciprofloxacin

J0710 Injection, cephapirin sodium, up to 1 gm Qp Qh E2
  Other: Cefadyl
  IOM: 100-02, 15, 50

* J0712 Injection, ceftaroline fosamil, 10 mg Qp Qh K2 K
  Other: Teflaro
  Coding Clinic: 2012, Q1, P9

J0713 Injection, ceftazidime, per 500 mg Qp Qh N1 N
  Other: Fortaz, Tazicef
  IOM: 100-02, 15, 50

* J0714 Injection, ceftazidime and avibactam, 0.5 g/0.125 g Qp Qh K2 K

J0715 Injection, ceftizoxime sodium, per 500 mg Qp Qh N1 N
  IOM: 100-02, 15, 50

* J0716 Injection, centruroides immune F(ab)2, up to 120 milligrams Qp Qh K2 K
  Other: Anascorp

* J0717 Injection, certolizumab pegol, 1 mg (code may be used for Medicare when drug administered under the direct supervision of a physician, not for use when drug is self-administered) Qp Qh K2 K
  Other: Cimzia

J0720 Injection, chloramphenicol sodium succinate, up to 1 gm Qp Qh N1 N
  Other: Chloromycetin Sodium Succinate
  IOM: 100-02, 15, 50

J0725 Injection, chorionic gonadotropin, per 1,000 USP units Qp Qh N1 N
  Other: A.P.L., Chorex-5, Chorex-10, Chorignon, Choron-10, Chorionic Gonadotropin, Choron 10, Corgonject-5, Follutein, Glukor, Gonic, Novarel, Pregnyl, Profasi HP
  IOM: 100-02, 15, 50

J0735 Injection, clonidine hydrochloride (HCL), 1 mg Qp Qh N1 N
  Other: Duraclon
  IOM: 100-02, 15, 50

J0740 Injection, cidofovir, 375 mg Qp Qh K2 K
  Other: Vistide
  IOM: 100-02, 15, 50

J0743 Injection, cilastatin sodium; imipenem, per 250 mg Qp Qh N1 N
  Other: Primaxin
  IOM: 100-02, 15, 50

* J0744 Injection, ciprofloxacin for intravenous infusion, 200 mg Qp Qh N1 N

J0745 Injection, codeine phosphate, per 30 mg Qp Qh N1 N
  IOM: 100-02, 15, 50

J0770 Injection, colistimethate sodium, up to 150 mg Qp Qh N1 N
  Other: Coly-Mycin M
  IOM: 100-02, 15, 50

* J0775 Injection, collagenase, clostridium histolyticum, 0.01 mg Qp Qh K2 K
  Other: Xiaflex
  Coding Clinic: 2011, Q1, P7

J0780 Injection, prochlorperazine, up to 10 mg Qp Qh N1 N
  Other: Compa-Z, Compazine, Cotranzine, Ultrazine-10
  IOM: 100-02, 15, 50

J0795 Injection, corticorelin ovine triflutate, 1 mcg Qp Qh K2 K
  Other: Acthrel
  IOM: 100-02, 15, 50

J0800 Injection, corticotropin, up to 40 units Qp Qh K2 K
  Other: ACTH, Acthar
  IOM: 100-02, 15, 50

~~J0833 Injection, cosyntropin, not otherwise specified, 0.25 mg~~ ✖

↩ * J0834 Injection, cosyntropin, 0.25 mg Qp Qh N1 N

* J0840 Injection, crotalidae polyvalent immune fab (ovine), up to 1 gram Qp Qh K2 K
  Other: Crofab
  Coding Clinic: 2012, Q1, P9

▶ * J0841 Injection, crotalidae immune f(ab')2 (equine), 120 mg K
  Other: Anavip

J0850 Injection, cytomegalovirus immune globulin intravenous (human), per vial Qp Qh K2 K
  Prophylaxis to prevent cytomegalovirus disease associated with transplantation of kidney, lung, liver, pancreas, and heart.
  Other: Cytogam
  IOM: 100-02, 15, 50

▶ New ↩ Revised ✔ Reinstated ~~deleted~~ Deleted ⃠ Not covered or valid by Medicare
Special coverage instructions * Carrier discretion Bill Part B MAC Bill DME MAC

✻ **J0875** Injection, dalbavancin, 5 mg Ⓑ Ⓢ Qp Qh K2 K
Other: Dalvance

✻ **J0878** Injection, daptomycin, 1 mg Ⓑ Ⓢ Qp Qh K2 K
Other: Cubicin

◎ **J0881** Injection, darbepoetin alfa, 1 mcg (non-ESRD use) Ⓑ Ⓢ Qp Qh K2 K
Other: Aranesp

◎ **J0882** Injection, darbepoetin alfa, 1 mcg (for ESRD on dialysis) Ⓑ Ⓢ Qp Qh K2 K
Other: Aranesp
IOM: 100-02, 6, 10; 100-04, 4, 240

◎ **J0883** Injection, argatroban, 1 mg (for non-ESRD use) Qp Qh K2 K
IOM: 100-02, 15, 50

◎ **J0884** Injection, argatroban, 1 mg (for ESRD on dialysis) Qp Qh K2 K
IOM: 100-02, 15, 50

◎ **J0885** Injection, epoetin alfa, (for non-ESRD use), 1000 units Ⓑ Ⓢ Qp Qh K2 K
Other: Epogen, Procrit
IOM: 100-02, 15, 50
Coding Clinic: 2006, Q2, P5

◎ **J0887** Injection, epoetin beta, 1 mcg, (for ESRD on dialysis) Ⓑ Ⓢ Qp Qh N1 N
Other: Mircera

◎ **J0888** Injection, epoetin beta, 1 mcg, (for non ESRD use) Ⓑ Ⓢ Qp Qh K2 K
Other: Mircera

✻ **J0890** Injection, peginesatide, 0.1 mg (for ESRD on dialysis) Ⓑ Ⓢ Qp Qh E1
Other: Omontys

✻ **J0894** Injection, decitabine, 1 mg Ⓑ Ⓢ Qp Qh K2 K
Indicated for treatment of myelodysplastic syndromes (MDS)
Other: Dacogen

◎ **J0895** Injection, deferoxamine mesylate, 500 mg Ⓑ Ⓢ Qp Qh N1 N
Other: Desferal, Desferal mesylate
IOM: 100-02, 15, 50,
Cross Reference Q0087

✻ **J0897** Injection, denosumab, 1 mg Ⓑ Ⓢ Qp Qh K2 K
Other: Prolia, Xgeva
Coding Clinic: 2016, Q1, P5; 2012, Q1, P9

◎ **J0945** Injection, brompheniramine maleate, per 10 mg Ⓑ Ⓢ Qp Qh N1 N
Other: Codimal-A, Cophene-B, Dehist, Histaject, Nasahist B, ND Stat, Oraminic II, Sinusol-B
IOM: 100-02, 15, 50

◎ **J1000** Injection, depo-estradiol cypionate, up to 5 mg Ⓑ Ⓢ Qp Qh N1 N
Other: DepGynogen, Depogen, Dura-Estrin, Estra-D, Estro-Cyp, Estroject LA, Estronol-LA
IOM: 100-02, 15, 50

◎ **J1020** Injection, methylprednisolone acetate, 20 mg Ⓑ Ⓢ Qp Qh N1 N
Other: DepMedalone, Depoject, Depo-Medrol, Depopred, D-Med 80, Duralone, Medralone, M-Prednisol, Rep-Pred
IOM: 100-02, 15, 50
Coding Clinic: 2005, Q3, P10

◎ **J1030** Injection, methylprednisolone acetate, 40 mg Ⓑ Ⓢ Qp Qh N1 N
Other: DepMedalone, Depoject, Depo-Medrol, Depropred, D-Med 80, Duralone, Medralone, M-Prednisol, Rep-Pred
IOM: 100-02, 15, 50
Coding Clinic: 2005, Q3, P10

◎ **J1040** Injection, methylprednisolone acetate, 80 mg Ⓑ Ⓢ Qp Qh N1 N
Other: DepMedalone, Depoject, Depo-Medrol, Depropred, D-Med 80, Duralone, Medralone, M-Prednisol, Rep-Pred
IOM: 100-02, 15, 50

✻ **J1050** Injection, medroxyprogesterone acetate, 1 mg Ⓑ Ⓢ Qp Qh N1 N
Other: Depo-Provera Contraceptive

◎ **J1071** Injection, testosterone cypionate, 1 mg Qp Qh N1 N
Other: Andro-Cyp, Andro/Fem, Andronaq-LA, Andronate, De-Comberol, DepAndro, DepAndrogyn, Depotest, Depo-Testadiol, Depo-Testosterone, Depotestrogen, Duratest, Duratestrin, Menoject LA, Testa-C, Testadiate-Depo, Testaject-LA, Test-Estro Cypionates, Testoject-LA,
Coding Clinic: 2015, Q2, P7

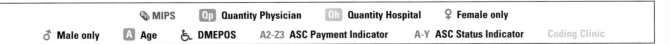

J1094 Injection, dexamethasone acetate, 1 mg Qp Qh N1 N
Other: Dalalone LA, Decadron LA, Decaject LA, Dexacen-LA-8, Dexasone L.A., Dexone-LA, Solurex LA
IOM: 100-02, 15, 50

▶ **J1095** Injection, dexamethasone 9%

J1100 Injection, dexamethasone sodium phosphate, 1 mg Qp Qh N1 N
Other: Dalalone, Decadron Phosphate, Decaject, Dexacen-4, Dexone, Hexadrol Phosphate, Solurex
IOM: 100-02, 15, 50

J1110 Injection, dihydroergotamine mesylate, per 1 mg Qp Qh K2 K
Other: D.H.E. 45
IOM: 100-02, 15, 50

J1120 Injection, acetazolamide sodium, up to 500 mg Qp Qh N1 N
Other: Diamox
IOM: 100-02, 15, 50

✻ **J1130** Injection, diclofenac sodium, 0.5 mg Qp Qh K2 K
Coding Clinic: 2017, Q1, P9

J1160 Injection, digoxin, up to 0.5 mg Qp Qh N1 N
Other: Lanoxin
IOM: 100-02, 15, 50

J1162 Injection, digoxin immune Fab (ovine), per vial Qp Qh K2 K
Other: DigiFab
IOM: 100-02, 15, 50

J1165 Injection, phenytoin sodium, per 50 mg Qp Qh N1 N
Other: Dilantin
IOM: 100-02, 15, 50

J1170 Injection, hydromorphone, up to 4 mg Qp Qh N1 N
Other: Dilaudid
IOM: 100-02, 15, 50

J1180 Injection, dyphylline, up to 500 mg Qp Qh E2
Other: Dilor, Lufyllin
IOM: 100-02, 15, 50

J1190 Injection, dexrazoxane hydrochloride, per 250 mg Qp Qh K2 K
Other: Totect, Zinecard
IOM: 100-02, 15, 50

J1200 Injection, diphenhydramine HCL, up to 50 mg Qp Qh N1 N
Other: Bena-D, Benadryl, Benahist, Ben-Allergin, Benoject, Chlorothiazide sodium, Dihydrex, Diphenacen-50, Hyrexin-50, Nordryl, Wehdryl
IOM: 100-02, 15, 50

J1205 Injection, chlorothiazide sodium, per 500 mg Qp Qh N1 N
Other: Diuril
IOM: 100-02, 15, 50

J1212 Injection, DMSO, dimethyl sulfoxide, 50%, 50 ml Qp Qh K2 K
Other: Rimso-50
IOM: 100-02, 15, 50; 100-03, 4, 230.12

J1230 Injection, methadone HCL, up to 10 mg Qp Qh N1 N
Other: Dolophine HCl
MCM: 2049
IOM: 100-02, 15, 50

J1240 Injection, dimenhydrinate, up to 50 mg Qp Qh N1 N
Other: Dinate, Dommanate, Dramamine, Dramanate, Dramilin, Dramocen, Dramoject, Dymenate, Hydrate, Marmine, Wehamine
IOM: 100-02, 15, 50

J1245 Injection, dipyridamole, per 10 mg Qp Qh N1 N
Other: Persantine
IOM: 100-04, 15, 50; 100-04, 12, 30.6

J1250 Injection, dobutamine HCL, per 250 mg Qp Qh N1 N
Other: Dobutrex
IOM: 100-02, 15, 50

J1260 Injection, dolasetron mesylate, 10 mg Qp Qh N1 N
Other: Anzemet
IOM: 100-02, 15, 50

✻ **J1265** Injection, dopamine HCL, 40 mg Qp Qh N1 N

✻ **J1267** Injection, doripenem, 10 mg Qp Qh N1 N
Other: Donbax, Doribax

✻ **J1270** Injection, doxercalciferol, 1 mcg Qp Qh N1 N
Other: Hectorol

▶ New ⮐ Revised ✔ Reinstated ~~deleted~~ Deleted ⃠ Not covered or valid by Medicare
Special coverage instructions ✻ Carrier discretion Bill Part B MAC Bill DME MAC

* **J1290** Injection, ecallantide, 1 mg Qp Qh K2 K
Other: Kalbitor
Coding Clinic: 2011, Q1, P7

* **J1300** Injection, eculizumab, 10 mg Qp Qh K2 K
Other: Soliris

▶ * **J1301** Injection, edaravone, 1 mg G
Other: Radicava

J1320 Injection, amitriptyline HCL, up to 20 mg Qp Qh N1 N
Other: Elavil, Enovil
IOM: 100-02, 15, 50

* **J1322** Injection, elosulfase alfa, 1 mg Qp Qh K2 K

* **J1324** Injection, enfuvirtide, 1 mg Qp Qh E2

J1325 Injection, epoprostenol, 0.5 mg Qp Qh N1 N
Other: Flolan, Veletri
IOM: 100-02, 15, 50

J1327 Injection, eptifibatide, 5 mg Qp Qh K2 K
Other: Integrilin
IOM: 100-02, 15, 50

J1330 Injection, ergonovine maleate, up to 0.2 mg Qp Qh N1 N
Benefit limited to obstetrical diagnosis
IOM: 100-02, 15, 50

* **J1335** Injection, ertapenem sodium, 500 mg Qp Qh N1 N
Other: Invanz

J1364 Injection, erythromycin lactobionate, per 500 mg Qp Qh K2 K
IOM: 100-02, 15, 50

J1380 Injection, estradiol valerate, up to 10 mg Qp Qh N1 N
Other: Delestrogen, Dioval, Duragen, Estra-L, Gynogen L.A., L.A.E. 20, Valergen
IOM: 100-02, 15, 50
Coding Clinic: 2011, Q1, P8

J1410 Injection, estrogen conjugated, per 25 mg Qp Qh K2 K
Other: Premarin
IOM: 100-02, 15, 50

* **J1428** Injection, eteplirsen, 10 mg K2 G

J1430 Injection, ethanolamine oleate, 100 mg Qp Qh K2 K
Other: Ethamolin
IOM: 100-02, 15, 50

J1435 Injection, estrone, per 1 mg Qp Qh E2
Other: Estronol, Kestrone 5, Theelin Aqueous
IOM: 100-02, 15, 50

J1436 Injection, etidronate disodium, per 300 mg Qp Qh E1
Other: Didronel
IOM: 100-02, 15, 50

J1438 Injection, etanercept, 25 mg (Code may be used for Medicare when drug administered under the direct supervision of a physician, not for use when drug is self-administered.) Qp Qh K2 K
Other: Enbrel
IOM: 100-02, 15, 50

* **J1439** Injection, ferric carboxymaltose, 1 mg Qp Qh K2 K
Other: Injectafer

J1442 Injection, filgrastim (G-CSF), excludes biosimilars, 1 mcg Qp Qh K2 K
Other: Neupogen

* **J1443** Injection, ferric pyrophosphate citrate solution, 0.1 mg of iron Qp Qh N1 N

J1447 Injection, TBO-filgrastim, 1 mcg Qp Qh K2 K
Other: GRANIX
IOM: 100-02, 15, 50

J1450 Injection, fluconazole, 200 mg Qp Qh N1 N
Other: Diflucan
IOM: 100-02, 15, 50

J1451 Injection, fomepizole, 15 mg Qp Qh K2 K
IOM: 100-02, 15, 50

J1452 Injection, fomivirsen sodium, intraocular, 1.65 mg Qp Qh E2
IOM: 100-02, 15, 50

* **J1453** Injection, fosaprepitant, 1 mg Qp Qh K2 K
Prevents chemotherapy-induced nausea and vomiting
Other: Emend

▶ * **J1454** Injection, fosnetupitant 235 mg and palonosetron 0.25 mg G
Other: Akynzeo and Aloxi

J1455 Injection, foscarnet sodium, per 1000 mg Qp Qh K2 K
Other: Foscavir
IOM: 100-02, 15, 50

* J1457 Injection, gallium nitrate, 1 mg Qp Qh E2

* J1458 Injection, galsulfase, 1 mg Qp Qh K2 K
Other: Naglazyme

* J1459 Injection, immune globulin (Privigen), intravenous, non-lyophilized (e.g., liquid), 500 mg Qp Qh K2 K

J1460 Injection, gamma globulin, intramuscular, 1 cc Qp Qh K2 K
Other: Gammar, GamaSTAN
IOM: 100-02, 15, 50
Coding Clinic: 2011, Q1, P8

* J1555 Injection, immune globulin (cuvitru), 100 mg K2 K

* J1556 Injection, immune globulin (Bivigam), 500 mg Qp Qh K2 K

* J1557 Injection, immune globulin, (gammaplex), intravenous, non-lyophilized (e.g., liquid), 500 mg Qp Qh K2 K
Coding Clinic: 2012, Q1, P9

* J1559 Injection, immune globulin (hizentra), 100 mg Qp Qh K2 K
Coding Clinic: 2011, Q1, P6

J1560 Injection, gamma globulin, intramuscular, over 10 cc Qp Qh K2 K
Other: Gammar, GamaSTAN
IOM: 100-02, 15, 50

J1561 Injection, immune globulin, (Gamunex-C/Gammaked), non-lyophilized (e.g., liquid), 500 mg Qp Qh K2 K
IOM: 100-02, 15, 50
Coding Clinic: 2012, Q1, P9

* J1562 Injection, immune globulin (Vivaglobin), 100 mg Qp Qh E2

J1566 Injection, immune globulin, intravenous, lyophilized (e.g., powder), not otherwise specified, 500 mg Qp Qh K2 K
Other: Carimune, Gammagard S/D, Polygam
IOM: 100-02, 15, 50

* J1568 Injection, immune globulin, (Octagam), intravenous, non-lyophilized (e.g., liquid), 500 mg Qp Qh K2 K

J1569 Injection, immune globulin, (Gammagard Liquid), non-lyophilized (e.g., liquid), 500 mg Qp Qh K2 K
IOM: 100-02, 15, 50

J1570 Injection, ganciclovir sodium, 500 mg Qp Qh N1 N
Other: Cytovene
IOM: 100-02, 15, 50

J1571 Injection, hepatitis B immune globulin (HepaGam B), intramuscular, 0.5 ml Qp Qh K2 K
IOM: 100-02, 15, 50
Coding Clinic: 2008, Q3, P7-8

J1572 Injection, immune globulin, (flebogamma/flebogamma DIF) intravenous, non-lyophilized (e.g., liquid), 500 mg Qp Qh K2 K
IOM: 100-02, 15, 50

* J1573 Injection, hepatitis B immune globulin (HepaGam B), intravenous, 0.5 ml Qp Qh K2 K
Coding Clinic: 2008, Q3, P8

* J1575 Injection, immune globulin/ hyaluronidase (HYQVIA), 100 mg immunoglobulin Qp Qh K2 K

J1580 Injection, Garamycin, gentamicin, up to 80 mg Qp Qh N1 N
Other: Gentamicin Sulfate, Jenamicin
IOM: 100-02, 15, 50

J1595 Injection, glatiramer acetate, 20 mg Qp Qh K2 K
Other: Copaxone
IOM: 100-02, 15, 50

* J1599 Injection, immune globulin, intravenous, non-lyophilized (e.g., liquid), not otherwise specified, 500 mg Qp Qh N1 N
Coding Clinic: 2011, P1, Q6

J1600 Injection, gold sodium thiomalate, up to 50 mg Qp Qh E2
Other: Myochrysine
IOM: 100-02, 15, 50

* J1602 Injection, golimumab, 1 mg,for intravenous use Qp Qh K2 K
Other: Simponi Aria

J1610 Injection, glucagon hydrochloride, per 1 mg Qp Qh K2 K
Other: GlucaGen, Glucagon Emergency
IOM: 100-02, 15, 50

J1620 Injection, gonadorelin hydrochloride, per 100 mcg Qp Qh E2
Other: Factrel
IOM: 100-02, 15, 50

▶ New ↻ Revised ✔ Reinstated ~~deleted~~ Deleted ⊘ Not covered or valid by Medicare
Special coverage instructions * Carrier discretion Bill Part B MAC Bill DME MAC

J1626 Injection, granisetron hydrochloride, 100 mcg Qp Qh N1 N
Other: Kytril
IOM: 100-02, 15, 50

* **J1627** Injection, granisetron, extended-release, 0.1 mg K2 G

▶ * **J1628** Injection, guselkumab, 1 mg G
Other: Tremfya

J1630 Injection, haloperidol, up to 5 mg Qp Qh N1 N
Other: Haldol, Haloperidol Lactate
IOM: 100-02, 15, 50

J1631 Injection, haloperidol decanoate, per 50 mg Qp Qh N1 N
IOM: 100-02, 15, 50

J1640 Injection, hemin, 1 mg Qp Qh K2 K
Other: Panhematin
IOM: 100-02, 15, 50

J1642 Injection, heparin sodium, (heparin lock flush), per 10 units Qp Qh N1 N
Other: Hep-Lock U/P, Vasceze
IOM: 100-02, 15, 50

J1644 Injection, heparin sodium, per 1000 units Qp Qh N1 N
Other: Heparin Sodium (Porcine), Liquaemin Sodium
IOM: 100-02, 15, 50

J1645 Injection, dalteparin sodium, per 2500 IU Qp Qh N1 N
Other: Fragmin
IOM: 100-02, 15, 50

* **J1650** Injection, enoxaparin sodium, 10 mg Qp Qh N1 N
Other: Lovenox

J1652 Injection, fondaparinux sodium, 0.5 mg Qp Qh N1 N
Other: Arixtra
IOM: 100-02, 15, 50

* **J1655** Injection, tinzaparin sodium, 1000 IU Qp Qh N1 N
Other: Innohep

J1670 Injection, tetanus immune globulin, human, up to 250 units Qp Qh K2 K
Indicated for transient protection against tetanus post-exposure to tetanus (V03.7).
Other: Hyper-Tet
IOM: 100-02, 15, 50

J1675 Injection, histrelin acetate, 10 mcg Qp Qh B
IOM: 100-02, 15, 50

J1700 Injection, hydrocortisone acetate, up to 25 mg Qp Qh N1 N
Other: Hydrocortone Acetate
IOM: 100-02, 15, 50

J1710 Injection, hydrocortisone sodium phosphate, up to 50 mg Qp Qh N1 N
Other: A-hydroCort, Hydrocortone phosphate, Solu-Cortef
IOM: 100-02, 15, 50

J1720 Injection, hydrocortisone sodium succinate, up to 100 mg Qp Qh N1 N
Other: A-HydroCort, Solu-Cortef
IOM: 100-02, 15, 50

* **J1726** Injection, hydroxyprogesterone caproate (makena), 10 mg K2 K

* **J1729** Injection, hydroxyprogesterone caproate, not otherwise specified, 10 mg N1 N

J1730 Injection, diazoxide, up to 300 mg Qp Qh E2
Other: Hyperstat
IOM: 100-02, 15, 50

* **J1740** Injection, ibandronate sodium, 1 mg Qp Qh K2 K
Other: Boniva

* **J1741** Injection, ibuprofen, 100 mg Qp Qh N1 N
Other: Caldolor

J1742 Injection, ibutilide fumarate, 1 mg Qp Qh K2 K
Other: Corvert
IOM: 100-02, 15, 50

* **J1743** Injection, idursulfase, 1 mg Qp Qh K2 K
Other: Elaprase

* **J1744** Injection, icatibant, 1 mg Qp Qh K2 K
Other: Firazyr

J1745 Injection, infliximab, excludes biosimilar, 10 mg Qp Qh K2 K
Report total number of 10 mg increments administered
For biosimilar, Inflectra, report Q5102
Other: Remicade
IOM: 100-02, 15, 50

▶ ✻ **J1746** Injection, ibalizumab-uiyk, 10 mg K
Other: Trogarzo

◎ **J1750** Injection, iron dextran, 50 mg Ⓑ Ⓓ Qp Qh K2 K
Other: Dexferrum, Imferon, Infed
IOM: 100-02, 15, 50

✻ **J1756** Injection, iron sucrose, 1 mg Ⓑ Ⓓ Qp Qh N1 N
Other: Venofer

◎ **J1786** Injection, imiglucerase, 10 units Ⓑ Ⓓ Qp Qh K2 K
Other: Cerezyme
IOM: 100-02, 15, 50
Coding Clinic: 2011, Q1, P8

◎ **J1790** Injection, droperidol, up to 5 mg Ⓑ Ⓓ Qp Qh N1 N
Other: Inapsine
IOM: 100-02, 15, 50

◎ **J1800** Injection, propranolol HCL, up to 1 mg Ⓑ Ⓓ Qp Qh N1 N
Other: Inderal
IOM: 100-02, 15, 50

◎ **J1810** Injection, droperidol and fentanyl citrate, up to 2 ml ampule Ⓑ Ⓓ Qp Qh E1
Other: Innovar
IOM: 100-02, 15, 50

◎ **J1815** Injection, insulin, per 5 units Ⓑ Ⓓ Qp Qh N1 N
Other: Humalog, Humulin, Lantus, Novolin, Novolog
IOM: 100-02, 15, 50; 100-03, 4, 280.14

✻ **J1817** Insulin for administration through DME (i.e., insulin pump) per 50 units Ⓑ Ⓓ Qp Qh N1 N
Other: Apidra Solostar, Insulin Lispro, Humalog, Humulin, Novolin, Novolog

✻ **J1826** Injection, interferon beta-1a, 30 mcg Ⓑ Ⓓ K2 K
Other: Avonex
Coding Clinic: 2011, Q2, P9; Q1, P8

◎ **J1830** Injection, interferon beta-1b, 0.25 mg (Code may be used for Medicare when drug administered under the direct supervision of a physician, not for use when drug is self-administered) Ⓑ Ⓓ Qp Qh K2 K
Other: Betaseron
IOM: 100-02, 15, 50

✻ **J1833** Injection, isavuconazonium, 1 mg Ⓑ Ⓓ Qp Qh K2 K

✻ **J1835** Injection, itraconazole, 50 mg Ⓑ Ⓓ Qp Qh E2
Other: Sporanox

◎ **J1840** Injection, kanamycin sulfate, up to 500 mg Ⓑ Ⓓ Qp Qh N1 N
Other: Kantrex, Klebcil
IOM: 100-02, 15, 50

◎ **J1850** Injection, kanamycin sulfate, up to 75 mg Ⓑ Ⓓ Qp Qh N1 N
Other: Kantrex, Klebcil
IOM: 100-02, 15, 50
Coding Clinic: 2013: Q2, P3

◎ **J1885** Injection, ketorolac tromethamine, per 15 mg Ⓑ Ⓓ Qp Qh N1 N
Other: Toradol
IOM: 100-02, 15, 50

◎ **J1890** Injection, cephalothin sodium, up to 1 gram Ⓑ Ⓓ Qp Qh N1 N
Other: Keflin
IOM: 100-02, 15, 50

✻ **J1930** Injection, lanreotide, 1 mg Ⓑ Ⓓ Qp Qh K2 K
Treats acromegaly and symptoms caused by neuroendocrine tumors
Other: Somatuline Depot

✻ **J1931** Injection, laronidase, 0.1 mg Ⓑ Ⓓ Qp Qh K2 K
Other: Aldurazyme

◎ **J1940** Injection, furosemide, up to 20 mg Ⓑ Ⓓ Qp Qh N1 N
Other: Furomide M.D., Lasix
MCM: 2049
IOM: 100-02, 15, 50

✻ **J1942** Injection, aripiprazole lauroxil, 1 mg Qp Qh K2 G
Other: Aristada

◎ **J1945** Injection, lepirudin, 50 mg Ⓑ Ⓓ Qp Qh E2
IOM: 100-02, 15, 50

◎ **J1950** Injection, leuprolide acetate (for depot suspension), per 3.75 mg Ⓑ Ⓓ Qp Qh K2 K
Other: Lupron, Lupron Depot, Lupron Depot-Ped
IOM: 100-02, 15, 50

▶ New ↩ Revised ✔ Reinstated ~~deleted~~ Deleted ⊘ Not covered or valid by Medicare
◎ Special coverage instructions ✻ Carrier discretion Ⓑ Bill Part B MAC Ⓓ Bill DME MAC

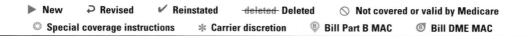

✻ **J1953** Injection, levetiracetam, 10 mg Qp Qh N1 N
Other: Keppra

J1955 Injection, levocarnitine, per 1 gm Qp Qh B
Other: Carnitor
IOM: 100-02, 15, 50

J1956 Injection, levofloxacin, 250 mg Qp Qh N1 N
Other: Levaquin
IOM: 100-02, 15, 50

J1960 Injection, levorphanol tartrate, up to 2 mg Qp Qh N1 N
Other: Levo-Dromoran
MCM: 2049
IOM: 100-02, 15, 50

J1980 Injection, hyoscyamine sulfate, up to 0.25 mg Qp Qh N1 N
Other: Levsin
IOM: 100-02, 15, 50

J1990 Injection, chlordiazepoxide HCL, up to 100 mg Qp Qh N1 N
Other: Librium
IOM: 100-02, 15, 50

J2001 Injection, lidocaine HCL for intravenous infusion, 10 mg Qp Qh N1 N
Other: Caine-1, Caine-2, Dilocaine, L-Caine, Lidocaine in D5W, Lidoject, Nervocaine, Nulicaine, Xylocaine
IOM: 100-02, 15, 50

J2010 Injection, lincomycin HCL, up to 300 mg Qp Qh N1 N
Other: Lincocin
IOM: 100-02, 15, 50

✻ **J2020** Injection, linezolid, 200 mg Qp Qh N1 N
Other: Zyvox

J2060 Injection, lorazepam, 2 mg Qp Qh N1 N
Other: Ativan
IOM: 100-02, 15, 50

▶ ✻ **J2062** Loxapine for inhalation, 1 mg K
Other: Adasuve

J2150 Injection, mannitol, 25% in 50 ml Qp Qh N1 N
Other: Aridol
MCM: 2049
IOM: 100-02, 15, 50

✻ **J2170** Injection, mecasermin, 1 mg Qp Qh N1 N
Other: Increlex

J2175 Injection, meperidine hydrochloride, per 100 mg Qp Qh N1 N
Other: Demerol
IOM: 100-02, 15, 50

J2180 Injection, meperidine and promethazine HCL, up to 50 mg Qp Qh N1 N
Other: Mepergan
IOM: 100-02, 15, 50

✻ **J2182** Injection, mepolizumab, 1 mg Qp Qh K2 G

✻ **J2185** Injection, meropenem, 100 mg Qp Qh N1 N
Other: Merrem

▶ ✻ **J2186** Inj., meropenem, vaborbactam G
Other: Vabomere
Medicare Statute 1833(t)

J2210 Injection, methylergonovine maleate, up to 0.2 mg Qp Qh N1 N
Benefit limited to obstetrical diagnoses for prevention and control of post-partum hemorrhage
Other: Methergine
IOM: 100-02, 15, 50

✻ **J2212** Injection, methylnaltrexone, 0.1 mg Qp Qh N1 N
Other: Relistor

✻ **J2248** Injection, micafungin sodium, 1 mg Qp Qh N1 N
Other: Mycamine

J2250 Injection, midazolam hydrochloride, per 1 mg Qp Qh N1 N
Other: Versed
IOM: 100-02, 15, 50

J2260 Injection, milrinone lactate, 5 mg Qp Qh N1 N
Other: Primacor
IOM: 100-02, 15, 50

✻ **J2265** Injection, minocycline hydrochloride, 1 mg Qp Qh K2 K
Other: Minocine

J2270 Injection, morphine sulfate, up to 10 mg Qp Qh N1 N
Other: Astramorph PF, Duramorph
IOM: 100-02, 15, 50
Coding Clinic: 2013, Q2, P4

MIPS | Qp Quantity Physician | Qh Quantity Hospital | ♀ Female only | ♂ Male only | A Age | DMEPOS | A2-Z3 ASC Payment Indicator | A-Y ASC Status Indicator | Coding Clinic

J2274 Injection, morphine sulfate, preservative-free for epidural or intrathecal use, 10 mg Ⓑ Ⓔ Qp Qh N1 N
Other: Duramorph, Infumorph
IOM: 100-03, 4, 280.1; 100-02, 15, 50

J2278 Injection, ziconotide, 1 mcg Ⓑ Ⓔ Qp Qh K2 K
Other: Prialt

* J2280 Injection, moxifloxacin, 100 mg Ⓑ Ⓔ Qp Qh N1 N
Other: Avelox

J2300 Injection, nalbuphine hydrochloride, per 10 mg Ⓑ Ⓔ Qp Qh N1 N
Other: Nubain
IOM: 100-02, 15, 50

J2310 Injection, naloxone hydrochloride, per 1 mg Ⓑ Ⓔ Qp Qh N1 N
Other: Narcan
IOM: 100-02, 15, 50

* J2315 Injection, naltrexone, depot form, 1 mg Ⓑ Ⓔ Qp Qh K2 K
Other: Vivitrol

J2320 Injection, nandrolone decanoate, up to 50 mg Ⓑ Ⓔ Qp Qh K2 K
Other: Anabolin LA 100, Androlone, Deca-Durabolin, Decolone, Hybolin Decanoate, Nandrobolic LA, Neo-Durabolic
IOM: 100-02, 15, 50
Coding Clinic: 2011, Q1, P8

* J2323 Injection, natalizumab, 1 mg Ⓑ Ⓔ Qp Qh K2 K
Other: Tysabri

J2325 Injection, nesiritide, 0.1 mg Ⓑ Ⓔ Qp Qh K2 K
Other: Natrecor
IOM: 100-02, 15, 50

* J2326 Injection, nusinersen, 0.1 mg K2 G

* J2350 Injection, ocrelizumab, 1 mg K2 G

* J2353 Injection, octreotide, depot form for intramuscular injection, 1 mg Ⓑ Ⓔ Qp Qh K2 K
Other: Sandostatin LAR Depot

* J2354 Injection, octreotide, non-depot form for subcutaneous or intravenous injection, 25 mcg Ⓑ Ⓔ Qp Qh N1 N
Other: Sandostatin LAR Depot

J2355 Injection, oprelvekin, 5 mg Ⓑ Ⓔ Qp Qh K2 K
Other: Neumega
IOM: 100-02, 15, 50

* J2357 Injection, omalizumab, 5 mg Ⓑ Ⓔ Qp Qh K2 K
Other: Xolair

* J2358 Injection, olanzapine, long-acting, 1 mg Ⓑ Ⓔ Qp Qh N1 N
Other: Zyprexa Relprevv
Coding Clinic: 2011, Q1, P6

J2360 Injection, orphenadrine citrate, up to 60 mg Ⓑ Ⓔ Qp Qh N1 N
Other: Antiflex, Banflex, Flexoject, Flexon, K-Flex, Myolin, Neocyten, Norflex, O-Flex, Orphenate
IOM: 100-02, 15, 50

J2370 Injection, phenylephrine HCL, up to 1 ml Ⓑ Ⓔ Qp Qh N1 N
Other: Neo-Synephrine
IOM: 100-02, 15, 50

J2400 Injection, chloroprocaine hydrochloride, per 30 ml Ⓑ Ⓔ Qp Qh N1 N
Other: Nesacaine, Nesacaine-MPF
IOM: 100-02, 15, 50

J2405 Injection, ondansetron hydrochloride, per 1 mg Ⓑ Ⓔ Qp Qh N1 N
Other: Zofran
IOM: 100-02, 15, 50

J2407 Injection, oritavancin, 10 mg Ⓑ Ⓔ Qp Qh K2 K
Other: Orbactiv
IOM: 100-02, 15, 50

J2410 Injection, oxymorphone HCL, up to 1 mg Ⓑ Ⓔ Qp Qh N1 N
Other: Numorphan, Opana
IOM: 100-02, 15, 50

* J2425 Injection, palifermin, 50 mcg Ⓑ Ⓔ Qp Qh K2 K
Other: Kepivance

* J2426 Injection, paliperidone palmitate extended release, 1 mg Ⓑ Ⓔ Qp Qh K2 K
Other: Invega Sustenna
Coding Clinic: 2011, Q1, P7

▶ New ↻ Revised ✔ Reinstated ~~deleted~~ Deleted ⊘ Not covered or valid by Medicare
Special coverage instructions * Carrier discretion Ⓑ Bill Part B MAC Ⓔ Bill DME MAC

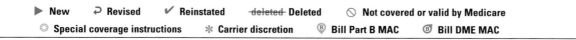

J2430 Injection, pamidronate disodium, per 30 mg Qp Qh N1 N
Other: Aredia
IOM: 100-02, 15, 50

J2440 Injection, papaverine HCL, up to 60 mg Qp Qh N1 N
IOM: 100-02, 15, 50

J2460 Injection, oxytetracycline HCL, up to 50 mg Qp Qh E2
Other: Terramycin IM
IOM: 100-02, 15, 50

* **J2469** Injection, palonosetron HCL, 25 mcg Qp Qh K2 K
Example: 0.25 mgm dose = 10 units Example of use is acute, delayed, nausea and vomiting due to chemotherapy
Other: Aloxi

J2501 Injection, paricalcitol, 1 mcg Qp Qh N1 N
Other: Zemplar
IOM: 100-02, 15, 50

* **J2502** Injection, pasireotide long acting, 1 mg Qp Qh K2 K
Other: Signifor LAR

* **J2503** Injection, pegaptanib sodium, 0.3 mg Qp Qh K2 K
Other: Macugen

J2504 Injection, pegademase bovine, 25 IU Qp Qh K2 K
Other: Adagen
IOM: 100-02, 15, 50

* **J2505** Injection, pegfilgrastim, 6 mg Qp Qh K2 K
Report 1 unit per 6 mg.
Other: Neulasta

* **J2507** Injection, pegloticase, 1 mg Qp Qh K2 K
Other: Krystexxa
Coding Clinic: 2012, Q1, P9

J2510 Injection, penicillin G procaine, aqueous, up to 600,000 units Qp Qh N1 N
Other: Crysticillin, Duracillin AS, Pfizerpen AS, Wycillin
IOM: 100-02, 15, 50

J2513 Injection, pentastarch, 10% solution, 100 ml Qp Qh E2
IOM: 100-02, 15, 50

J2515 Injection, pentobarbital sodium, per 50 mg Qp Qh K2 K
Other: Nembutal sodium solution
IOM: 100-02, 15, 50

J2540 Injection, penicillin G potassium, up to 600,000 units Qp Qh N1 N
Other: Pfizerpen-G
IOM: 100-02, 15, 50

J2543 Injection, piperacillin sodium/tazobactam sodium, 1 gram/0.125 grams (1.125 grams) Qp Qh N1 N
Other: Zosyn
IOM: 100-02, 15, 50

J2545 Pentamidine isethionate, inhalation solution, FDA-approved final product, non-compounded, administered through DME, unit dose form, per 300 mg Qp Qh B
Other: Nebupent

* **J2547** Injection, peramivir, 1 mg Qp Qh K2 K

J2550 Injection, promethazine HCL, up to 50 mg Qp Qh N1 N
Administration of phenergan suppository considered part of E/M encounter
Other: Anergan, Phenazine, Phenergan, Prorex, Prothazine, V-Gan
IOM: 100-02, 15, 50

J2560 Injection, phenobarbital sodium, up to 120 mg Qp Qh N1 N
Other: Luminal Sodium
IOM: 100-02, 15, 50

* **J2562** Injection, plerixafor, 1 mg Qp Qh K2 K
FDA approved for non-Hodgkin lymphoma and multiple myeloma in 2008.
Other: Mozobil

J2590 Injection, oxytocin, up to 10 units Qp Qh N1 N
Other: Pitocin, Syntocinon
IOM: 100-02, 15, 50

J2597 Injection, desmopressin acetate, per 1 mcg Qp Qh K2 K
Other: DDAVP
IOM: 100-02, 15, 50

J2650 Injection, prednisolone acetate, up to 1 ml Qp Qh N1 N
Other: Key-Pred, Predalone, Predcor, Predicort, Predoject
IOM: 100-02, 15, 50

J2670 Injection, tolazoline HCL, up to 25 mg Qp Qh N1 N
Other: Priscoline HCl
IOM: 100-02, 15, 50

J2675 Injection, progesterone, per 50 mg Qp Qh N1 N
Other: Gesterol 50, Progestaject
IOM: 100-02, 15, 50

J2680 Injection, fluphenazine decanoate, up to 25 mg Qp Qh N1 N
Other: Prolixin Decanoate
MCM: 2049
IOM: 100-02, 15, 50

J2690 Injection, procainamide HCL, up to 1 gm Qp Qh ♀ N1 N
Benefit limited to obstetrical diagnoses
Other: Pronestyl, Prostaphlin
IOM: 100-02, 15, 50

J2700 Injection, oxacillin sodium, up to 250 mg Qp Qh N1 N
Other: Bactocill
IOM: 100-02, 15, 50

* J2704 Injection, propofol, 10 mg Qp Qh N1 N
Other: Diprivan

J2710 Injection, neostigmine methylsulfate, up to 0.5 mg Qp Qh N1 N
Other: Prostigmin
IOM: 100-02, 15, 50

J2720 Injection, protamine sulfate, per 10 mg Qp Qh N1 N
IOM: 100-02, 15, 50

* J2724 Injection, protein C concentrate, intravenous, human, 10 IU Qp Qh K2 K
Other: Ceprotin

J2725 Injection, protirelin, per 250 mcg Qp Qh E2
Other: Relefact TRH, Thypinone
IOM: 100-02, 15, 50

J2730 Injection, pralidoxime chloride, up to 1 gm Qp Qh N1 N
Other: Protopam Chloride
IOM: 100-02, 15, 50

J2760 Injection, phentolamine mesylate, up to 5 mg Qp Qh K2 K
Other: Regitine
IOM: 100-02, 15, 50

J2765 Injection, metoclopramide HCL, up to 10 mg Qp Qh N1 N
Other: Reglan
IOM: 100-02, 15, 50

J2770 Injection, quinupristin/dalfopristin, 500 mg (150/350) Qp Qh K2 K
Other: Synercid
IOM: 100-02, 15, 50

* J2778 Injection, ranibizumab, 0.1 mg Qp Qh K2 K
May be reported for exudative senile macular degeneration (wet AMD) with 67028 (RT or LT)
Other: Lucentis

J2780 Injection, ranitidine hydrochloride, 25 mg Qp Qh N1 N
Other: Zantac
IOM: 100-02, 15, 50

* J2783 Injection, rasburicase, 0.5 mg Qp Qh K2 K
Other: Elitek

* J2785 Injection, regadenoson, 0.1 mg Qp Qh N1 N
One billing unit equal to 0.1 mg of regadenoson
Other: Lexiscan

* J2786 Injection, reslizumab, 1 mg Qp Qh K2 G
Coding Clinic: 2016, Q4, P9

▶ * J2787 Riboflavin 5'-phosphate, ophthalmic solution, up to 3 mL
Other: Photrexa Viscous

J2788 Injection, Rho D immune globulin, human, minidose, 50 mcg (250 IU) Qp Qh N1 N
Other: HypRho-D, MicRhoGAM, Rhesonativ, RhoGam
IOM: 100-02, 15, 50

J2790 Injection, Rho D immune globulin, human, full dose, 300 mcg (1500 IU) Qp Qh N1 N
Administered to pregnant female to prevent hemolistic disease of newborn. Report 90384 to private payer
Other: Gamulin Rh, Hyperrho S/D, HypRho-D, Rhesonativ, RhoGAM
IOM: 100-02, 15, 50

▶ New ↻ Revised ✓ Reinstated ~~deleted~~ Deleted ⊘ Not covered or valid by Medicare
Special coverage instructions * Carrier discretion Ⓑ Bill Part B MAC Ⓓ Bill DME MAC

J2791 Injection, Rho(D) immune globulin (human), (Rhophylac), intramuscular or intravenous, 100 IU Qp Qh N1 N

Agent must be billed per 100 IU in both physician office and hospital outpatient settings

Other: HypRho-D

IOM: 100-02, 15, 50

J2792 Injection, Rho D immune globulin intravenous, human, solvent detergent, 100 IU Qp Qh K2 K

Other: Gamulin Rh, Hyperrho S/D, WinRHo-SDF

IOM: 100-02, 15, 50

J2793 Injection, rilonacept, 1 mg Qp Qh K2 K

Other: Arcalyst

IOM: 100-02, 15, 50

* **J2794** Injection, risperidone, long acting, 0.5 mg Qp Qh K2 K

Other: Risperdal Costa

* **J2795** Injection, ropivacaine hydrochloride, 1 mg Qp Qh N1 N

Other: Naropin

* **J2796** Injection, romiplostim, 10 mcg Qp Qh K2 K

Stimulates bone marrow megakarocytes to produce platelets (i.e., ITP)

Other: Nplate

▶ **J2797** Injection, rolapitant, 0.5 mg G

Other: Varubi

J2800 Injection, methocarbamol, up to 10 ml Qp Qh N1 N

Other: Robaxin

IOM: 100-02, 15, 50

* **J2805** Injection, sincalide, 5 mcg Qp Qh N1 N

Other: Kinevac

J2810 Injection, theophylline, per 40 mg Qp Qh N1 N

IOM: 100-02, 15, 50

J2820 Injection, sargramostim (GM-CSF), 50 mcg Qp Qh K2 K

Other: Leukine, Prokine

IOM: 100-02, 15, 50

* **J2840** Injection, sebelipase alfa, 1 mg Qp Qh K2 G

J2850 Injection, secretin, synthetic, human, 1 mcg Qp Qh K2 K

Other: Chirhostim

IOM: 100-02, 15, 50

* **J2860** Injection, siltuximab, 10 mg Qp Qh K2 K

J2910 Injection, aurothioglucose, up to 50 mg Qp Qh E2

Other: Solganal

IOM: 100-02, 15, 50

J2916 Injection, sodium ferric gluconate complex in sucrose injection, 12.5 mg Qp Qh N1 N

Other: Ferrlecit, Nulecit

IOM: 100-02, 15, 50

J2920 Injection, methylprednisolone sodium succinate, up to 40 mg Qp Qh N1 N

Other: A-MethaPred, Solu-Medrol

IOM: 100-02, 15, 50

J2930 Injection, methylprednisolone sodium succinate, up to 125 mg Qp Qh N1 N

Other: A-MethaPred, Solu-Medrol

IOM: 100-02, 15, 50

J2940 Injection, somatrem, 1 mg Qp Qh E2

IOM: 100-02, 15, 50, Medicare Statute 1861s2b

J2941 Injection, somatropin, 1 mg Qp Qh K2 K

Other: Genotropin, Humatrope, Nutropin, Omnitrope, Saizen, Serostim, Zorbtive

IOM: 100-02, 15, 50, Medicare Statute 1861s2b

J2950 Injection, promazine HCL, up to 25 mg Qp Qh N1 N

Other: Prozine-50, Sparine

IOM: 100-02, 15, 50

J2993 Injection, reteplase, 18.1 mg Qp Qh K2 K

Other: Retavase

IOM: 100-02, 15, 50

J2995 Injection, streptokinase, per 250,000 IU Qp Qh N1 N

Bill 1 unit for each 250,000 IU

Other: Kabikinase, Streptase

IOM: 100-02, 15, 50

◎ **J2997** Injection, alteplase recombinant, 1 mg Ⓑ Ⓔ Qp Qh K2 K

Thrombolytic agent, treatment of occluded catheters. Bill units of 1 mg administered.

Other: Activase, Cathflo Activase

IOM: 100-02, 15, 50

Coding Clinic: 2014, Q1, P4

◎ **J3000** Injection, streptomycin, up to 1 gm Ⓑ Ⓔ Qp Qh N1 N

IOM: 100-02, 15, 50

◎ **J3010** Injection, fentanyl citrate, 0.1 mg Ⓑ Ⓔ Qp Qh N1 N

Other: Sublimaze

IOM: 100-02, 15, 50

◎ **J3030** Injection, sumatriptan succinate, 6 mg (Code may be used for Medicare when drug administered under the direct supervision of a physician, not for use when drug is self-administered) Ⓑ Ⓔ Qp Qh N1 N

Other: Imitrex, Sumarel Dosepro

IOM: 100-02, 15, 150

* **J3060** Injection, taliglucerase alfa, 10 units Ⓑ Ⓔ Qp Qh K2 K

Other: Elelyso

◎ **J3070** Injection, pentazocine, 30 mg Ⓑ Ⓔ Qp Qh K2 K

Other: Talwin

IOM: 100-02, 15, 50

* **J3090** Injection, tedizolid phosphate, 1 mg Ⓑ Ⓔ Qp Qh K2 K

Other: Sivextro

* **J3095** Injection, televancin, 10 mg Ⓑ Ⓔ Qp Qh K2 K

Prescribed for the treatment of adults with complicated skin and skin structure infections (cSSSI) of the following Gram-positive microorganisms: Staphylococcus aureus; Streptococcus pyogenes, Streptococcus agalactiae, Streptococcus anginosusgroup. Separately payable under the ASC payment system.

Other: Vibativ

Coding Clinic: 2011, Q1, P7

* **J3101** Injection, tenecteplase, 1 mg Ⓑ Ⓔ Qp Qh K2 K

Other: TNKase

◎ **J3105** Injection, terbutaline sulfate, up to 1 mg Ⓑ Ⓔ Qp Qh N1 N

Other: Brethine

IOM: 100-02, 15, 50

◎ **J3110** Injection, teriparatide, 10 mcg Ⓑ Ⓔ Qp Qh B

◎ **J3121** Injection, testosterone enanthate, 1 mg Ⓑ Ⓔ Qp Qh N1 N

Other: Andrest 90-4, Andro L.A. 200, Andro-Estro 90-4, Androgyn L.A, Andropository 100, Andryl 200, Deladumone, Deladumone OB, Delatest, Delatestadiol, Delatestryl, Ditate-DS, Dua-Gen L.A., Duoval P.A., Durathate-200, Estra-Testrin, Everone, TEEV, Testadiate, Testone LA, Testradiol 90/4, Testrin PA, Valertest

◎ **J3145** Injection, testosterone undecanoate, 1 mg Ⓑ Ⓔ Qp Qh K2 K

◎ **J3230** Injection, chlorpromazine HCL, up to 50 mg Ⓑ Ⓔ Qp Qh N1 N

Other: Ormazine, Thorazine

IOM: 100-02, 15, 50

◎ **J3240** Injection, thyrotropin alfa, 0.9 mg provided in 1.1 mg vial Ⓑ Ⓔ Qp Qh K2 K

Other: Thyrogen

IOM: 100-02, 15, 50

* **J3243** Injection, tigecycline, 1 mg Ⓑ Ⓔ Qp Qh K2 K

▶ * **J3245** Injection, tildrakizumab, 1 mg E2

Other: Ilumya

* **J3246** Injection, tirofiban HCL, 0.25 mg Ⓑ Ⓔ Qp Qh K2 K

Other: Aggrastat

◎ **J3250** Injection, trimethobenzamide HCL, up to 200 mg Ⓑ Ⓔ Qp Qh N1 N

Other: Arrestin, Ticon, Tigan, Tiject 20

IOM: 100-02, 15, 50

◎ **J3260** Injection, tobramycin sulfate, up to 80 mg Ⓑ Ⓔ Qp Qh N1 N

Other: Nebcin

IOM: 100-02, 15, 50

* **J3262** Injection, tocilizumab, 1 mg Ⓑ Ⓔ Qp Qh K2 K

Indicated for the treatment of adult patients with moderately to severely active rheumatoid arthritis (RA) who have had an inadequate response to one or more tumor necrosis factor (TNF) antagonist therapies.

Other: Actemra

Coding Clinic: 2011, Q1, P7

J3265 Injection, torsemide, 10 mg/ml Qp Qh N1 N

Other: Demadex

IOM: 100-02, 15, 50

J3280 Injection, thiethylperazine maleate, up to 10 mg Qp Qh E2

Other: Norzine, Torecan

IOM: 100-02, 15, 50

✻ **J3285** Injection, treprostinil, 1 mg Qp Qh K2 K

Other: Remodulin

J3300 Injection, triamcinolone acetonide, preservative free, 1 mg Qp Qh K2 K

Other: Cenacort A-40, Kenaject-40, Kenalog, Triam-A, Triesence, Tri-Kort, Trilog

J3301 Injection, triamcinolone acetonide, not otherwise specified, 10 mg Qp Qh N1 N

Other: Cenacort A-40, Kenaject-40, Kenalog, Triam A, Triesence, Tri-Kort, Trilog

IOM: 100-02, 15, 50

Coding Clinic: 2013, Q2, P4

J3302 Injection, triamcinolone diacetate, per 5 mg Qp Qh N1 N

Other: Amcort, Aristocort , Cenacort Forte, Trilone

IOM: 100-02, 15, 50

J3303 Injection, triamcinolone hexacetonide, per 5 mg Qp Qh N1 N

Other: Aristospan

IOM: 100-02, 15, 50

▶ **J3304** Injection, triamcinolone acetonide, preservative-free, extended-release, microsphere formulation, 1 mg G

Other: Zilretta

J3305 Injection, trimetrexate glucuronate, per 25 mg Qp Qh E2

Other: NeuTrexin

IOM: 100-02, 15, 50

J3310 Injection, perphenazine, up to 5 mg Qp Qh N1 N

Other: Trilafon

IOM: 100-02, 15, 50

J3315 Injection, triptorelin pamoate, 3.75 mg Qp Qh K2 K

Other: Trelstar

IOM: 100-02, 15, 50

▶ **J3316** Injection, triptorelin, extended-release, 3.75 mg G

Other: Trelstar, Trelstar Depot, Trelstar LA

J3320 Injection, spectinomycin dihydrochloride, up to 2 gm Qp Qh E2

Other: Trobicin

IOM: 100-02, 15, 50

J3350 Injection, urea, up to 40 gm Qp Qh N1 N

Other: Ureaphil

IOM: 100-02, 15, 50

J3355 Injection, urofollitropin, 75 IU Qp Qh E2

Other: Bravelle, Metrodin

IOM: 100-02, 15, 50

✻ **J3357** Ustekinumab, for subcutaneous injection, 1 mg Qp Qh K2 K

Other: Stelara

Coding Clinic: 2017, Q1, P3; 2016, Q4, P10; 2011, Q1, P7

✻ **J3358** Ustekinumab, for intravenous injection, 1 mg K2 G

Cross Reference Q9989

J3360 Injection, diazepam, up to 5 mg Qp Qh N1 N

Other: Valium, Zetran

IOM: 100-02, 15, 50

Coding Clinic: 2007, Q2, P6-7

J3364 Injection, urokinase, 5000 IU vial Qp Qh N1 N

Other: Abbokinase

IOM: 100-02, 15, 50

J3365 Injection, IV, urokinase, 250,000 IU vial Qp Qh E2

Other: Abbokinase

IOM: 100-02, 15, 50,

Cross Reference Q0089

J3370 Injection, vancomycin HCL, 500 mg Qp Qh N1 N

Other: Vancocin, Vancoled

IOM: 100-02, 15, 50; 100-03, 4, 280.14

J3380 Injection, vedolizumab, 1 mg Qp Qh K2 K

Other: Entyvio

MIPS | Qp Quantity Physician | Qh Quantity Hospital | ♀ Female only
♂ Male only | A Age | DMEPOS | A2-Z3 ASC Payment Indicator | A-Y ASC Status Indicator | Coding Clinic

✻ **J3385** Injection, velaglucerase alfa, 100 units Ⓑ Ⓖ Qp Qh K2 K

Enzyme replacement therapy in Gaucher Disease that results from a specific enzyme deficiency in the body, caused by a genetic mutation received from both parents. Type 1 is the most prevalent Ashkenazi Jewish genetic disease, occurring in one in every 1,000.

Other: VPRIV

Coding Clinic: 2011, Q1, P7

⊙ **J3396** Injection, verteporfin, 0.1 mg Ⓑ Ⓖ Qp Qh K2 K

Other: Visudyne

IOM: 100-03, 1, 80.2; 100-03, 1, 80.3

▶ ✻ **J3397** Injection, vestronidase alfa-vjbk, 1 mg K

Other: Mepsevii

▶ ✻ **J3398** Injection, voretigene neparvovec-rzyl, 1 billion vector genomes G

Other: Luxturna

⊙ **J3400** Injection, triflupromazine HCL, up to 20 mg Ⓑ Ⓖ Qp Qh E2

Other: Vesprin

IOM: 100-02, 15, 50

⊙ **J3410** Injection, hydroxyzine HCL, up to 25 mg Ⓑ Ⓖ Qp Qh N1 N

Other: Hyzine-50, Vistaject 25, Vistaril

IOM: 100-02, 15, 50

✻ **J3411** Injection, thiamine HCL, 100 mg Ⓑ Ⓖ Qp Qh N1 N

✻ **J3415** Injection, pyridoxine HCL, 100 mg Ⓑ Ⓖ Qp Qh N1 N

⊙ **J3420** Injection, vitamin B-12 cyanocobalamin, up to 1000 mcg Ⓑ Ⓖ Qp Qh N1 N

Medicare carriers may have local coverage decisions regarding vitamin B12 injections that provide reimbursement only for patients with certain types of anemia and other conditions.

Other: Berubigen, Betalin 12, Cobex, Redisol, Rubramin PC, Sytobex

IOM: 100-02, 15, 50; 100-03, 2, 150.6

⊙ **J3430** Injection, phytonadione (vitamin K), per 1 mg Ⓑ Ⓖ Qp Qh N1 N

Other: AquaMephyton, Konakion, Menadione, Synkavite, Vitamin K1

IOM: 100-02, 15, 50

⊙ **J3465** Injection, voriconazole, 10 mg Ⓑ Ⓖ Qp Qh K2 K

Other: VFEND

IOM: 100-02, 15, 50

⊙ **J3470** Injection, hyaluronidase, up to 150 units Ⓑ Ⓖ Qp Qh N1 N

Other: Amphadase, Wydase

IOM: 100-02, 15, 50

⊙ **J3471** Injection, hyaluronidase, ovine, preservative free, per 1 USP unit (up to 999 USP units) Ⓑ Ⓖ Qp Qh N1 N

Other: Vitrase

⊙ **J3472** Injection, hyaluronidase, ovine, preservative free, per 1000 USP units Ⓑ Ⓖ Qp Qh N1 N

⊙ **J3473** Injection, hyaluronidase, recombinant, 1 USP unit Ⓑ Ⓖ Qp Qh N1 N

Other: Hylenex

IOM: 100-02, 15, 50

⊙ **J3475** Injection, magnesium sulfate, per 500 mg Ⓑ Ⓖ Qp Qh N1 N

IOM: 100-02, 15, 50

⊙ **J3480** Injection, potassium chloride, per 2 meq Ⓑ Ⓖ Qp Qh N1 N

IOM: 100-02, 15, 50

⊙ **J3485** Injection, zidovudine, 10 mg Ⓑ Ⓖ Qp Qh N1 N

Other: Retrovir

IOM: 100-02, 15, 50

✻ **J3486** Injection, ziprasidone mesylate, 10 mg Ⓑ Ⓖ Qp Qh N1 N

Other: Geodon

✻ **J3489** Injection, zoledronic acid, 1 mg Ⓑ Ⓖ Qp Qh N1 N

Other: Reclast, Zometra

⊙ **J3490** Unclassified drugs Ⓑ Ⓖ N1 N

Bill on paper. Bill one unit. Identify drug and total dosage in "Remarks" field.

Other: Acthib, Aminocaproic Acid, Baciim, Bacitracin, Benzocaine, Bumetanide, Bupivacaine, Cefotetan, Ciprofloxacin, Cleocin Phosphate, Clindamycin, Cortisone Acetate Micronized, Definity, Diprivan, Doxy, Engerix-B, Ethanolamine, Famotidine, Ganirelix, Gonal-F, Hyaluronic Acid, Marcaine, Metronidazole, Nafcillin, Naltrexone, Ovidrel, Pegasys, Peg-Intron, Penicillin G Sodium, Propofol, Protonix, Recombivax, Rifadin, Rifampin, Sensorcaine-MPF, Smz-TMP, Sufentanil Citrate, Testopel Pellets, Testosterone, Treanda, Valcyte, Veritas Collagen Matrix

IOM: 100-02, 15, 50

Coding Clinic: 2017, Q1, P1-3, P8; 2014, Q2, P6; 2013, Q2, P3-4

▶ New ⤺ Revised ✔ Reinstated ~~deleted~~ Deleted ⊘ Not covered or valid by Medicare
⊙ Special coverage instructions ✻ Carrier discretion Ⓑ Bill Part B MAC Ⓖ Bill DME MAC

⊘ **J3520** Edetate disodium, per 150 mg Qp Qh E1

Other: Chealamide, Disotate, Endrate ethylenediamine-tetra-acetic

IOM: 100-03, 1, 20.21; 100-03, 1, 20.22

J3530 Nasal vaccine inhalation Qp Qh N1 N

IOM: 100-02, 15, 50

⊘ **J3535** Drug administered through a metered dose inhaler E1

Other: Ipratropium bromide

IOM: 100-02, 15, 50

⊘ **J3570** Laetrile, amygdalin, vitamin B-17 E1

IOM: 100-03, 1, 30.7

* **J3590** Unclassified biologics N1 N

Bill on paper. Bill one unit. Identify drug and total dosage in "Remarks" field.

Coding Clinic: 2017, Q1, P1-3; 2016, Q4, P10

▶ * **J3591** Unclassified drug or biological used for ESRD on dialysis B

J7030 Infusion, normal saline solution, 1000 cc Qp Qh N1 N

Other: Sodium Chloride

IOM: 100-02, 15, 50

J7040 Infusion, normal saline solution, sterile (500 ml = 1 unit) Qp Qh N1 N

Other: Sodium Chloride

IOM: 100-02, 15, 50

J7042 5% dextrose/normal saline (500 ml = 1 unit) Qp Qh N1 N

Other: Dextrose-Nacl

IOM: 100-02, 15, 50

J7050 Infusion, normal saline solution, 250 cc Qp Qh N1 N

Other: Sodium Chloride

IOM: 100-02, 15, 50

J7060 5% dextrose/water (500 ml = 1 unit) Qp Qh N1 N

IOM: 100-02, 15, 50

J7070 Infusion, D 5 W, 1000 cc Qp Qh N1 N

Other: Dextrose

IOM: 100-02, 15, 50

J7100 Infusion, dextran 40, 500 ml Qp Qh N1 N

Other: Gentran, LMD, Rheomacrodex

IOM: 100-02, 15, 50

J7110 Infusion, dextran 75, 500 ml Qp Qh N1 N

Other: Gentran 75

IOM: 100-02, 15, 50

J7120 Ringer's lactate infusion, up to 1000 cc Qp Qh N1 N

Replacement fluid or electrolytes.

Other: Potassium Chloride

IOM: 100-02, 15, 50

J7121 5% dextrose in lactated ringers infusion, up to 1000 cc Qp Qh N1 N

IOM: 100-02, 15, 50

J7131 Hypertonic saline solution, 1 ml Qp Qh N1 N

IOM: 100-02, 15, 50

Coding Clinic: 2012, Q1, P9

Clotting Factors

▶ * **J7170** Injection, emicizumab-kxwh, 0.5 mg G

Other: Hemlibra

* **J7175** Injection, Factor X, (human), 1 IU Qp Qh K2 K

Coding Clinic: 2017, Q1, P9

▶ * **J7177** Injection, human fibrinogen concentrate (fibryga), 1 mg K

↩ * **J7178** Injection, human fibrinogen concentrate, not otherwise specified, 1 mg Qp Qh K2 K

Other: Riastap

J7179 Injection, von Willebrand factor (recombinant), (vonvendi), 1 IU VWF:RCo Qp Qh K2 G

Coding Clinic: 2017, Q1, P9

* **J7180** Injection, factor XIII (antihemophilic factor, human), 1 IU Qp Qh K2 K

Other: Corifact

Coding Clinic: 2012, Q1, P8

* **J7181** Injection, factor XIII a-subunit, (recombinant), per IU Qp Qh K2 K

* **J7182** Injection, factor VIII, (antihemophilic factor, recombinant), (novoeight), per IU Qp Qh K2 K

J7183 Injection, von Willebrand factor complex (human), wilate, 1 IU VWF:RCo Qp Qh K2 K

IOM: 100-02, 15, 50

Coding Clinic: 2012, Q1, P9

✻ **J7185** Injection, Factor VIII (antihemophilic factor, recombinant) (Xyntha), per IU Ⓑ Qp Qh K2 K

◌ **J7186** Injection, anti-hemophilic factor VIII/von Willebrand factor complex (human), per factor VIII IU Ⓑ Qp Qh K2 K

Other: Alphanate

IOM: 100-02, 15, 50

◌ **J7187** Injection, von Willebrand factor complex (HUMATE-P), per IU VWF:RCo Ⓑ Qp Qh K2 K

Other: Humate-P Low Dilutent

IOM: 100-02, 15, 50

◌ **J7188** Injection, factor VIII (antihemophilic factor, recombinant), (obizur), per IU Ⓑ Qp Qh K2 K

IOM: 100-02, 15, 50

◌ **J7189** Factor VIIa (anti-hemophilic factor, recombinant), per 1 mcg Ⓑ Qp Qh K2 K

Other: NovoSeven

IOM: 100-02, 15, 50

◌ **J7190** Factor VIII anti-hemophilic factor, human, per IU Ⓑ Qp Qh K2 K

Other: Alphanate/von Willebrand factor complex, Hemofil M, Koate DVI, Koate-HP, Kogenate, Monoclate-P, Recombinate

IOM: 100-02, 15, 50

◌ **J7191** Factor VIII, anti-hemophilic factor (porcine), per IU Ⓑ Qp Qh E2

Other: Hyate:C, Koate-HP, Kogenate, Monoclate-P, Recombinate

IOM: 100-02, 15, 50

◌ **J7192** Factor VIII (anti-hemophilic factor, recombinant) per IU, not otherwise specified Ⓑ Qp Qh K2 K

Other: Advate, Helixate FS, Kogenate FS, Koate-HP, Recombinate, Xyntha

IOM: 100-02, 15, 50

◌ **J7193** Factor IX (anti-hemophilic factor, purified, non-recombinant) per IU Ⓑ Qp Qh K2 K

Other: AlphaNine SD, Mononine, Proplex

IOM: 100-02, 15, 50

◌ **J7194** Factor IX, complex, per IU Ⓑ Qp Qh K2 K

Other: Bebulin, Konyne-80, Profilnine Heat-treated, Profilnine SD, Proplex SX-T, Proplex T

IOM: 100-02, 15, 50

◌ **J7195** Injection, Factor IX (anti-hemophilic factor, recombinant) per IU, not otherwise specified Ⓑ Qp Qh K2 K

Other: Benefix, Profiline, Proplex T

IOM: 100-02, 15, 50

✻ **J7196** Injection, antithrombin recombinant, 50 IU Ⓑ Qp Qh E2

Other: ATryn, Feiba VH Immuno

Coding Clinic: 2011, Q1, P6

◌ **J7197** Anti-thrombin III (human), per IU Ⓑ Qp Qh K2 K

Other: Thrombate III

IOM: 100-02, 15, 50

◌ **J7198** Anti-inhibitor, per IU Ⓑ Qp Qh K2 K

Diagnosis examples: 286.0 Congenital Factor VIII disorder; 286.1 Congenital Factor IX disorder; 286.4 VonWillebrand's disease

Other: Autoplex T, Feiba NF, Hemophilia clotting factors

IOM: 100-02, 15, 50; 100-03, 2, 110.3

◌ **J7199** Hemophilia clotting factor, not otherwise classified Ⓑ B

Other: Autoplex T

IOM: 100-02, 15, 50; 100-03, 2, 110.3

◌ **J7200** Injection, factor IX, (antihemophilic factor, recombinant), rixubis, per IU Ⓑ Qp Qh K2 K

IOM: 100-02, 15, 50

◌ **J7201** Injection, factor IX, fc fusion protein (recombinant), alprolix, 1 IU Ⓑ Qp Qh K2 K

IOM: 100-02, 15, 50

◌ **J7202** Injection, Factor IX, albumin fusion protein, (recombinant), idelvion, 1 IU Qp Qh K2 G

Coding Clinic: 2016, Q4, P9

▶ ◌ **J7203** Injection factor ix, (antihemophilic factor, recombinant), glycopegylated, (rebinyn), 1 iu G

Other: Profilnine SD, Bebulin VH, Bebulin, Proplex T

◌ **J7205** Injection, factor VIII Fc fusion protein (recombinant), per IU Ⓑ Qp Qh K2 K

Other: Eloctate

◌ **J7207** Injection, Factor VIII, (antihemophilic factor, recombinant), PEGylated, 1 IU Qp Qh K2 G

Other: Adynovate

▶ New ↩ Revised ✔ Reinstated ~~deleted~~ Deleted ⊘ Not covered or valid by Medicare
◌ Special coverage instructions ✻ Carrier discretion Ⓑ Bill Part B MAC ⓔ Bill DME MAC

* **J7209** Injection, Factor VIII, (antihemophilic factor, recombinant), (Nuwiq), 1 IU Qp Qh K2 G
* **J7210** Injection, Factor VIII, (antihemophilic factor, recombinant), (afstyla), 1 i.u. B K2 G
* **J7211** Injection, Factor VIII, (antihemophilic factor, recombinant), (kovaltry), 1 i.u. B K2 K

Contraceptives

⦸ **J7296** Levonorgestrel-releasing intrauterine contraceptive system, (kyleena), 19.5 mg B E1

Medicare Statute 1862(a)(1)

Cross Reference Q9984

⦸ **J7297** Levonorgestrel-releasing intrauterine contraceptive system (liletta), 52 mg B Qp Qh E1

Medicare Statute 1862(a)(1)

⦸ **J7298** Levonorgestrel-releasing intrauterine contraceptive system (mirena), 52 mg B Qp Qh E1

Medicare Statute 1862(a)(1)

⦸ **J7300** Intrauterine copper contraceptive B E1

Report IUD insertion with 58300. Bill usual and customary charge.

Other: Paragard T 380 A

Medicare Statute 1862a1

⦸ **J7301** Levonorgestrel-releasing intrauterine contraceptive system (skyla), 13.5 mg B Qp Qh E1

Medicare Statute 1862(a)(1)

⦸ **J7303** Contraceptive supply, hormone containing vaginal ring, each B ♀ E1

Medicare Statute 1862.1

⦸ **J7304** Contraceptive supply, hormone containing patch, each B ♀ E1

Only billed by Family Planning Clinics

Medicare Statute 1862.1

⦸ **J7306** Levonorgestrel (contraceptive) implant system, including implants and supplies B E1

⦸ **J7307** Etonogestrel (contraceptive) implant system, including implant and supplies B E1

Aminolevulinic Acid HCL

* **J7308** Aminolevulinic acid HCL for topical administration, 20%, single unit dosage form (354 mg) B Qp Qh K2 K

Other: Levulan Kerastick

○ **J7309** Methyl aminolevulinate (MAL) for topical administration, 16.8%, 1 gram B Qp Qh N1 N

Other: Metvixia

Coding Clinic: 2011, Q1, P6

Ganciclovir

○ **J7310** Ganciclovir, 4.5 mg, long-acting implant B Qp Qh E2

IOM: 100-02, 15, 50

Ophthalmic Drugs

* **J7311** Fluocinolone acetonide, intravitreal implant B Qp Qh K2 K

Treatment of chronic noninfectious posterior segment uveitis

Other: Retisert

* **J7312** Injection, dexamethasone, intravitreal implant, 0.1 mg B Qp Qh K2 K

To bill for Ozurdex services submit the following codes: J7312 and 67028 with the modifier -22 (for the increased work difficulty and increased risk). Indicated for the treatment of macular edema occurring after branch retinal vein occlusion (BRVO) or central retinal vein occlusion (CRVO) and non-infectious uveitis affecting the posterior segment of the eye.

Other: Ozurdex

Coding Clinic: 2011, Q1, P7

* **J7313** Injection, fluocinolone acetonide, intravitreal implant, 0.01 mg B Qp Qh K2 K

Other: Iluvien

* **J7315** Mitomycin, ophthalmic, 0.2 mg B Qp Qh N1 N

Other: Mitosol, Mutamycin

Coding Clinic: 2016, Q4, P8; 2014, Q2, P6

* **J7316** Injection, ocriplasmin, 0.125 mg B Qp Qh K2 K

Other: Jetrea

Hyaluronan

▶ * **J7318** Hyaluronan or derivative, durolane, for intra-articular injection, 1 mg G

Other: Morisu

* **J7320** Hyaluronan or derivitive, genvisc 850, for intra-articular injection, 1 mg Ⓑ Qp Qh K2 K

* **J7321** Hyaluronan or derivative, Hyalgan, Supartz or Visco-3, for intra-articular injection, per dose Ⓑ Qp Qh K2 K

Therapeutic goal is to restore visco-elasticity of synovial hyaluronan, thereby decreasing pain, improving mobility and restoring natural protective functions of hyaluronan in joint

* **J7322** Hyaluronan or derivative, hymovis, for intra-articular injection, 1 mg Ⓑ Qp Qh K2 G

* **J7323** Hyaluronan or derivative, Euflexxa, for intra-articular injection, per dose Ⓑ Qp Qh K2 K

* **J7324** Hyaluronan or derivative, Orthovisc, for intra-articular injection, per dose Ⓑ Qp Qh K2 K

* **J7325** Hyaluronan or derivative, Synvisc or Synvisc-One, for intra-articular injection, 1 mg Ⓑ Qp Qh K2 K

* **J7326** Hyaluronan or derivative, Gel-One, for intra-articular injection, per dose Ⓑ Qp Qh K2 K

Coding Clinic: 2012, Q1, P8

* **J7327** Hyaluronan or derivative, monovisc, for intra-articular injection, per dose Ⓑ Qp Qh K2 K

* **J7328** Hyaluronan or derivative, gelsyn-3, for intra-articular injection, 0.1 mg Ⓑ Qp Qh K2 G

▶ * **J7329** Hyaluronan or derivative, trivisc, for intra-articular injection, 1 mg E2

Miscellaneous Drugs

* **J7330** Autologous cultured chondrocytes, implant Ⓑ Qp Qh B

Other: Carticel

Coding Clinic: 2010, Q4, P3

* **J7336** Capsaicin 8% patch, per square centimeter Ⓑ Qp Qh K2 K

Other: Qutenza

* **J7340** Carbidopa 5 mg/levodopa 20 mg enteral suspension, 100 ml Ⓑ Ⓓ Qp Qh K2 K

Other: Duopa

* **J7342** Instillation, ciprofloxacin otic suspension, 6 mg Ⓑ Qp Qh K2 G

○ **J7345** Aminolevulinic acid hcl for topical administration, 10% gel, 10 mg Ⓑ K2 G

Immunosuppressive Drugs (Includes Non-injectibles)

○ **J7500** Azathioprine, oral, 50 mg Ⓑ Ⓓ Qp Qh N1 N

Other: Azasan, Imuran

IOM: 100-02, 15, 50

○ **J7501** Azathioprine, parenteral, 100 mg Ⓑ Ⓓ Qp Qh K2 K

Other: Imuran

IOM: 100-02, 15, 50

○ **J7502** Cyclosporine, oral, 100 mg Ⓑ Ⓓ Qp Qh N1 N

Other: Gengraf, Neoral, Sandimmune

IOM: 100-02, 15, 50

○ **J7503** Tacrolimus, extended release, (Envarsus XR), oral, 0.25 mg Ⓑ Ⓓ Qp Qh K2 G

IOM: 100-02, 15, 50

○ **J7504** Lymphocyte immune globulin, antithymocyte globulin, equine, parenteral, 250 mg Ⓑ Ⓓ Qp Qh K2 K

Other: Atgam

IOM: 100-02, 15, 50; 100-03, 2, 110.3

○ **J7505** Muromonab-CD3, parenteral, 5 mg Ⓑ Ⓓ Qp Qh K2 K

Other: Monoclonal antibodies (parenteral)

IOM: 100-02, 15, 50

○ **J7507** Tacrolimus, immediate release, oral, 1 mg Ⓑ Ⓓ Qp Qh N1 N

Other: Prograf

IOM: 100-02, 15, 50

○ **J7508** Tacrolimus, extended release, (Astagraf XL), oral, 0.1 mg Ⓑ Ⓓ Qp Qh N1 N

IOM: 100-02, 15, 50

○ **J7509** Methylprednisolone oral, per 4 mg Ⓑ Ⓓ Qp Qh N1 N

Other: Medrol

IOM: 100-02, 15, 50

○ **J7510** Prednisolone oral, per 5 mg Ⓑ Ⓓ Qp Qh N1 N

Other: Delta-Cortef, Flo-Pred, Orapred

IOM: 100-02, 15, 50

* **J7511** Lymphocyte immune globulin, antithymocyte globulin, rabbit, parenteral, 25 mg Ⓑ Ⓓ Qp Qh K2 K

Other: Thymoglobulin

▶ New ↩ Revised ✔ Reinstated ~~deleted~~ Deleted ⊘ Not covered or valid by Medicare
○ Special coverage instructions * Carrier discretion Ⓑ Bill Part B MAC Ⓓ Bill DME MAC

J7512 Prednisone, immediate release or delayed release, oral, 1 mg Qp Qh N1 N

Other: Cyclosporine

IOM: 100-02, 15, 50

J7513 Daclizumab, parenteral, 25 mg Qp Qh E2

Other: Zenapax

IOM: 100-02, 15, 50

* J7515 Cyclosporine, oral, 25 mg Qp Qh N1 N

Other: Gengraf, Neoral, Sandimmune

* J7516 Cyclosporin, parenteral, 250 mg Qp Qh N1 N

Other: Sandimmune

* J7517 Mycophenolate mofetil, oral, 250 mg Qp Qh N1 N

Other: CellCept

J7518 Mycophenolic acid, oral, 180 mg Qp Qh N1 N

Other: Myfortic

IOM: 100-04, 4, 240; 100-4, 17, 80.3.1

J7520 Sirolimus, oral, 1 mg Qp Qh N1 N

Other: Rapamune

IOM: 100-02, 15, 50

J7525 Tacrolimus, parenteral, 5 mg Qp Qh K2 K

Other: Prograf

IOM: 100-02, 15, 50

J7527 Everolimus, oral, 0.25 mg Qp Qh N1 N

Other: Zortress

IOM: 100-02, 15, 50

J7599 Immunosuppressive drug, not otherwise classified N1 N

Bill on paper. Bill one unit. Identify drug and total dosage in "Remarks" field.

IOM: 100-02, 15, 50

Inhalation Solutions

* J7604 Acetylcysteine, inhalation solution, compounded product, administered through DME, unit dose form, per gram Qp Qh M

Other: Mucomyst (unit dose form), Mucosol

* J7605 Arformoterol, inhalation solution, FDA approved final product, non-compounded, administered through DME, unit dose form, 15 mcg Qp Qh M

Maintenance treatment of bronchoconstriction in patients with chronic obstructive pulmonary disease (COPD).

Other: Brovana

* J7606 Formoterol fumarate, inhalation solution, FDA approved final product, non-compounded, administered through DME, unit dose form, 20 mcg Qp Qh M

Other: Perforomist

* J7607 Levalbuterol, inhalation solution, compounded product, administered through DME, concentrated form, 0.5 mg Qp Qh M

J7608 Acetylcysteine, inhalation solution, FDA-approved final product, non-compounded, administered through DME, unit dose form, per gram Qp Qh M

Other: Mucomyst, Mucosol

* J7609 Albuterol, inhalation solution, compounded product, administered through DME, unit dose, 1 mg Qp Qh M

Patient's home, medications—such as a albuterol when administered through a nebulizer—are considered DME and are payable under Part B.

Other: Proventil, Ventolin, Xopenex

* J7610 Albuterol, inhalation solution, compounded product, administered through DME, concentrated form, 1 mg Qp Qh M

Other: Proventil, Ventolin, Xopenex

J7611 Albuterol, inhalation solution, FDA-approved final product, non-compounded, administered through DME, concentrated form, 1 mg Qp Qh M

Report once for each milligram administered. For example, 2 mg of concentrated albuterol (usually diluted with saline), reported with J7611×2.

Other: Proventil, Ventolin, Xopenex

J7612 Levalbuterol, inhalation solution, FDA-approved final product, non-compounded, administered through DME, concentrated form, 0.5 mg Qp Qh M

Other: Xopenex

J7613 Albuterol, inhalation solution, FDA-approved final product, non-compounded, administered through DME, unit dose, 1 mg Ⓑ Ⓔ Qp Qh M

Other: Accuneb, Proventil, Ventolin, Xopenex

J7614 Levalbuterol, inhalation solution, FDA-approved final product, non-compounded, administered through DME, unit dose, 0.5 mg Ⓑ Ⓔ Qp Qh M

Other: Xopenex

* **J7615** Levalbuterol, inhalation solution, compounded product, administered through DME, unit dose, 0.5 mg Ⓑ Ⓔ Qp Qh M

J7620 Albuterol, up to 2.5 mg and ipratropium bromide, up to 0.5 mg,FDA-approved final product, non-compounded, administered through DME Ⓑ Ⓔ Qp Qh M

Other: DuoNeb

* **J7622** Beclomethasone, inhalation solution, compounded product, administered through DME, unit dose form, per mg Ⓑ Ⓔ Qp Qh M

* **J7624** Betamethasone, inhalation solution, compounded product, administered through DME, unit dose form, per mg Ⓑ Ⓔ Qp Qh M

* **J7626** Budesonide inhalation solution, FDA-approved final product, non-compounded, administered through DME, unit dose form, up to 0.5 mg Ⓑ Ⓔ Qp Qh M

Other: Pulmicort

* **J7627** Budesonide, inhalation solution, compounded product, administered through DME, unit dose form, up to 0.5 mg Ⓑ Ⓔ Qp Qh M

Other: Pulmicort Respules

J7628 Bitolterol mesylate, inhalation solution, compounded product, administered through DME, concentrated form, per milligram Ⓑ Ⓔ Qp Qh M

Other: Tornalate

J7629 Bitolterol mesylate, inhalation solution, compounded product, administered through DME, unit dose form, per milligram Ⓑ Ⓔ Qp Qh M

Other: Tornalate

J7631 Cromolyn sodium, inhalation solution, FDA-approved final product, non-compounded, administered through DME, unit dose form, per 10 mg Ⓑ Ⓔ Qp Qh M

Other: Intal

* **J7632** Cromolyn sodium, inhalation solution, compounded product, administered through DME, unit dose form, per 10 mg Ⓑ Ⓔ Qp Qh M

Other: Intal

* **J7633** Budesonide, inhalation solution, FDA-approved final product, non-compounded, administered through DME, concentrated form, per 0.25 mg Ⓑ Ⓔ Qp Qh M

Other: Pulmicort Respules

* **J7634** Budesonide, inhalation solution, compounded product, administered through DME, concentrated form, per 0.25 mg Ⓑ Ⓔ Qp Qh M

Other: Pulmicort Respules

J7635 Atropine, inhalation solution, compounded product, administered through DME, concentrated form, per milligram Ⓑ Ⓔ Qp Qh M

J7636 Atropine, inhalation solution, compounded product, administered through DME, unit dose form, per milligram Ⓑ Ⓔ Qp Qh M

J7637 Dexamethasone, inhalation solution, compounded product, administered through DME, concentrated form, per milligram Ⓑ Ⓔ Qp Qh M

J7638 Dexamethasone, inhalation solution, compounded product, administered through DME, unit dose form, per milligram Ⓑ Ⓔ Qp Qh M

J7639 Dornase alfa, inhalation solution, FDA-approved final product, non-compounded, administered through DME, unit dose form, per milligram Ⓑ Ⓔ Qp Qh M

Other: Pulmozyme

* **J7640** Formoterol, inhalation solution, compounded product, administered through DME, unit dose form, 12 mcg Ⓑ Ⓔ Qp Qh E1

* **J7641** Flunisolide, inhalation solution, compounded product, administered through DME, unit dose, per milligram Ⓑ Ⓔ Qp Qh M

J7642 Glycopyrrolate, inhalation solution, compounded product, administered through DME, concentrated form, per milligram Ⓑ Ⓔ Qp Qh M

▶ New ⤴ Revised ✔ Reinstated ~~deleted~~ Deleted ⊘ Not covered or valid by Medicare
Special coverage instructions * Carrier discretion Ⓑ Bill Part B MAC Ⓔ Bill DME MAC

J7643 Glycopyrrolate, inhalation solution, compounded product, administered through DME, unit dose form, per milligram Qp Qh M

J7644 Ipratropium bromide, inhalation solution, FDA-approved final product, non-compounded, administered through DME, unit dose form, per milligram Qp Qh M

Other: Atrovent

J7645 Ipratropium bromide, inhalation solution, compounded product, administered through DME, unit dose form, per milligram Qp Qh M

Other: Atrovent

J7647 Isoetharine HCL, inhalation solution, compounded product, administered through DME, concentrated form, per milligram Qp Qh M

Other: Bronkosol

J7648 Isoetharine HCL, inhalation solution, FDA-approved final product, non-compounded, administered through DME, concentrated form, per milligram Qp Qh M

Other: Bronkosol

J7649 Isoetharine HCL, inhalation solution, FDA-approved final product, non-compounded, administered through DME, unit dose form, per milligram Qp Qh M

Other: Bronkosol

J7650 Isoetharine HCL, inhalation solution, compounded product, administered through DME, unit dose form, per milligram Qp Qh M

Other: Bronkosol

J7657 Isoproterenol HCL, inhalation solution, compounded product, administered through DME, concentrated form, per milligram Qp Qh M

Other: Isuprel

J7658 Isoproterenol HCL inhalation solution, FDA-approved final product, non-compounded, administered through DME, concentrated form, per milligram Qp Qh M

Other: Isuprel

J7659 Isoproterenol HCL, inhalation solution, FDA-approved final product, non-compounded, administered through DME, unit dose form, per milligram Qp Qh M

Other: Isuprel

J7660 Isoproterenol HCL, inhalation solution, compounded product, administered through DME, unit dose form, per milligram Qp Qh M

Other: Isuprel

J7665 Mannitol, administered through an inhaler, 5 mg Qp Qh N1 N

Other: Aridol

J7667 Metaproterenol sulfate, inhalation solution, compounded product, concentrated form, per 10 mg Qp Qh M

Other: Alupent, Metaprel

J7668 Metaproterenol sulfate, inhalation solution, FDA-approved final product, non-compounded, administered through DME, concentrated form, per 10 mg Qp Qh M

Other: Alupent, Metaprel

J7669 Metaproterenol sulfate, inhalation solution, FDA-approved final product, non-compounded, administered through DME, unit dose form, per 10 mg Qp Qh M

Other: Alupent, Metaprel

J7670 Metaproterenol sulfate, inhalation solution, compounded product, administered through DME, unit dose form, per 10 mg Qp Qh M

Other: Alupent, Metaprel

J7674 Methacholine chloride administered as inhalation solution through a nebulizer, per 1 mg Qp Qh N1 N

Other: Provocholine

J7676 Pentamidine isethionate, inhalation solution, compounded product, administered through DME, unit dose form, per 300 mg Qp Qh M

Other: NebuPent, Pentam

J7680 Terbutaline sulfate, inhalation solution, compounded product, administered through DME, concentrated form, per milligram Qp Qh M

Other: Brethine

J7681 Terbutaline sulfate, inhalation solution, compounded product, administered through DME, unit dose form, per milligram Qp Qh M

Other: Brethine

MIPS | Qp Quantity Physician | Qh Quantity Hospital | ♀ Female only | ♂ Male only | A Age | DMEPOS | A2-Z3 ASC Payment Indicator | A-Y ASC Status Indicator | Coding Clinic

J7682 Tobramycin, inhalation solution, FDA-approved final product, non-compounded unit dose form, administered through DME, per 300 mg Qp Qh M

Other: Bethkis, Kitabis PAK, Tobi

J7683 Triamcinolone, inhalation solution, compounded product, administered through DME, concentrated form, per milligram Qp Qh M

J7684 Triamcinolone, inhalation solution, compounded product, administered through DME, unit dose form, per milligram Qp Qh M

Other: Triamcinolone acetonide

* **J7685** Tobramycin, inhalation solution, compounded product, administered through DME, unit dose form, per 300 mg Qp Qh M

Other: Tobi

* **J7686** Treprostinil, inhalation solution, FDA-approved final product, non-compounded, administered through DME, unit dose form, 1.74 mg Qp Qh M

Other: Tyvaso

Not Otherwise Classified/Specified

J7699 NOC drugs, inhalation solution administered through DME M

Other: Gentamicin Sulfate

J7799 NOC drugs, other than inhalation drugs, administered through DME N1 N

Bill on paper. Bill one unit and identify drug and total dosage in the "Remark" field.

Other: Cuvitru, Epinephrine, Mannitol, Osmitrol, Phenylephrine, Resectisol, Sodium chloride

IOM: 100-02, 15, 110.3

J7999 Compounded drug, not otherwise classified N1 N

Coding Clinic: 2017, Q1, P1-2; 2016, Q4, P8

J8498 Antiemetic drug, rectal/suppository, not otherwise specified B

Other: Compazine, Compro, Phenadoz, Phenergan, Prochlorperazine, Promethazine, Promethegan

Medicare Statute 1861(s)2t

J8499 Prescription drug, oral, non chemotherapeutic, NOS E1

Other: Acyclovir, Calcitrol, Cromolyn Sodium, OFEV, Valganciclovir HCL, Zovirax

IOM: 100-02, 15, 50

Coding Clinic: 2013, Q2, P4

Oral Anti-Cancer Drugs

J8501 Aprepitant, oral, 5 mg Qp Qh K2 K

Other: Emend

J8510 Busulfan; oral, 2 mg Qp Qh N1 N

Other: Myleran

IOM: 100-02, 15, 50; 100-04, 4, 240; 100-04, 17, 80.1.1

J8515 Cabergoline, oral, 0.25 mg E1

IOM: 100-02, 15, 50; 100-04, 4, 240

J8520 Capecitabine, oral, 150 mg Qp Qh N1 N

Other: Xeloda

IOM: 100-02, 15, 50; 100-04, 4, 240; 100-04, 17, 80.1.1

J8521 Capecitabine, oral, 500 mg Qp Qh N1 N

Other: Xeloda

IOM: 100-02, 15, 50; 100-04, 4, 240; 100-04, 17, 80.1.1

J8530 Cyclophosphamide; oral, 25 mg Qp Qh N1 N

Other: Cytoxan

IOM: 100-02, 15, 50; 100-04, 4, 240; 100-04, 17, 80.1.1

J8540 Dexamethasone, oral, 0.25 mg Qp Qh N1 N

Other: Decadron, Dexone, Dexpak, Locort

Medicare Statute 1861(s)2t

J8560 Etoposide; oral, 50 mg Qp Qh K2 K

Other: VePesid

IOM: 100-02, 15, 50; 100-04, 4, 230.1; 100-04, 4, 240; 100-04, 17, 80.1.1

* **J8562** Fludarabine phosphate, oral, 10 mg Qp Qh E2

Other: Fludara, Oforta

Coding Clinic: 2011, Q1, P9

J8565 Gefitinib, oral, 250 mg E2

Other: Iressa

▶ New ↩ Revised ✔ Reinstated ~~deleted~~ Deleted ⊘ Not covered or valid by Medicare
Special coverage instructions * Carrier discretion Bill Part B MAC Bill DME MAC

J8597 Antiemetic drug, oral, not otherwise specified N1 N

Medicare Statute 1861(s)2t

J8600 Melphalan; oral, 2 mg Qp Qh N1 N

Other: Alkeran

IOM: 100-02, 15, 50; 100-04, 4, 240; 100-04, 17, 80.1.1

J8610 Methotrexate; oral, 2.5 mg Qp Qh N1 N

Other: Rheumatrex, Trexall

IOM: 100-02, 15, 50; 100-04, 4, 240; 100-04, 17, 80.1.1

J8650 Nabilone, oral, 1 mg Qp Qh E2

J8655 Netupitant 300 mg and palonosetron 0.5 mg, oral Qp Qh K2 K

Other: Akynzeo

Coding Clinic: 2015, Q4, P4

J8670 Rolapitant, oral, 1 mg Qp Qh K2 K

Other: Varubi

J8700 Temozolomide, oral, 5 mg Qp Qh N1 N

Other: Temodar

IOM: 100-02, 15, 50; 100-04, 4, 240

J8705 Topotecan, oral, 0.25 mg Qp Qh K2 K

Treatment for ovarian and lung cancers, etc. Report J9350 (Topotecan, 4 mg) for intravenous version

Other: Hycamtin

J8999 Prescription drug, oral, chemotherapeutic, NOS B

Other: Anastrozole, Arimidex, Aromasin, Droxia, Erivedge, Flutamide, Gleevec, Hydrea, Hydroxyurea, Leukeran, Matulane, Megestrol Acetate, Mercaptopurine, Nolvadex, Tamoxifen Citrate

IOM: 100-02, 15, 50; 100-04, 4, 250; 100-04, 17, 80.1.1; 100-04, 17, 80.1.2

CHEMOTHERAPY DRUGS (J9000-J9999)

NOTE: These codes cover the cost of the chemotherapy drug only, not to include the administration

J9000 Injection, doxorubicin hydrochloride, 10 mg Qp Qh N1 N

Other: Adriamycin, Rubex

IOM: 100-02, 15, 50

Coding Clinic: 2007, Q4, P5

J9015 Injection, aldesleukin, per single use vial Qp Qh K2 K

Other: Proleukin

IOM: 100-02, 15, 50

J9017 Injection, arsenic trioxide, 1 mg Qp Qh K2 K

Other: Trisenox

J9019 Injection, asparaginase (Erwinaze), 1,000 IU Qp Qh K2 K

IOM: 100-02, 15, 50

J9020 Injection, asparaginase, not otherwise specified 10,000 units Qp Qh N1 N

IOM: 100-02, 15, 50

J9022 Injection, atezolizumab, 10 mg K2 G

J9023 Injection, avelumab, 10 mg K2 G

J9025 Injection, azacitidine, 1 mg Qp Qh K2 K

J9027 Injection, clofarabine, 1 mg Qp Qh K2 K

Other: Clolar

J9031 BCG (intravesical), per instillation Qp Qh K2 K

Other: TheraCys, Tice BCG

IOM: 100-02, 15, 50

J9032 Injection, belinostat, 10 mg Qp Qh K2 K

Other: Beleodaq

J9033 Injection, bendamustine HCL (treanda), 1 mg Qp Qh K2 K

Treatment for form of non-Hodgkin's lymphoma; standard administration time is as an intravenous infusion over 30 minutes

Other: Treanda

J9034 Injection, bendamustine hcl (bendeka), 1 mg Qp Qh K2 G

Coding Clinic: 2017, Q1, P10

J9035 Injection, bevacizumab, 10 mg Qp Qh K2 K

For malignant neoplasm of breast, considered J9207.

Other: Avastin

Coding Clinic: 2013, Q3, P9, Q2, P8

J9039 Injection, blinatumomab, 1 mcg Qp Qh K2 K

Other: Blincyto

MIPS | Qp Quantity Physician | Qh Quantity Hospital | ♀ Female only | ♂ Male only | A Age | DMEPOS | A2-Z3 ASC Payment Indicator | A-Y ASC Status Indicator | Coding Clinic

J9040 Injection, bleomycin sulfate, 15 units Qp Qh N1 N
Other: Blenoxane
IOM: 100-02, 15, 50

J9041 Injection, bortezomib (velcade), 0.1 mg Qp Qh K2 K
Other: Velcade

J9042 Injection, brentuximab vedotin, 1 mg Qp Qh K2 K
Other: Adcetris

J9043 Injection, cabazitaxel, 1 mg Qp Qh K2 K
Other: Jevtana
Coding Clinic: 2012, Q1, P9

J9044 Injection, bortezomib, not otherwise specified, 0.1 mg K
Other: Velcade

J9045 Injection, carboplatin, 50 mg Qp Qh N1 N
Other: Paraplatin
IOM: 100-02, 15, 50

J9047 Injection, carfilzomib, 1 mg Qp Qh K2 K
Other: Kyprolis

J9050 Injection, carmustine, 100 mg Qp Qh K2 K
Other: BiCNU
IOM: 100-02, 15, 50

J9055 Injection, cetuximab, 10 mg Qp Qh K2 K
Other: Erbitux

J9057 Injection, copanlisib, 1 mg G
Other: Aliqopa

J9060 Injection, cisplatin, powder or solution, 10 mg Qp Qh N1 N
Other: Plantinol AQ
IOM: 100-02, 15, 50
Coding Clinic: 2013, Q2, P6; 2011, Q1, P8

J9065 Injection, cladribine, per 1 mg Qp Qh K2 K
Other: Leustatin
IOM: 100-02, 15, 50

J9070 Cyclophosphamide, 100 mg Qp Qh K2 K
Other: Cytoxan, Neosar
IOM: 100-02, 15, 50
Coding Clinic: 2011, Q1, P8-9

J9098 Injection, cytarabine liposome, 10 mg Qp Qh K2 K
Other: DepoCyt

J9100 Injection, cytarabine, 100 mg Qp Qh N1 N
Other: Cytosar-U
IOM: 100-02, 15, 50
Coding Clinic: 2011, Q1, P9

J9120 Injection, dactinomycin, 0.5 mg Qp Qh K2 K
Other: Cosmegen
IOM: 100-02, 15, 50

J9130 Dacarbazine, 100 mg Qp Qh N1 N
Other: DTIC-Dome
IOM: 100-02, 15, 50
Coding Clinic: 2011, Q1, P9

J9145 Injection, daratumumab, 10 mg Qp Qh K2 G
Other: Darzalex
IOM: 100-02, 15, 50

J9150 Injection, daunorubicin, 10 mg Qp Qh K2 K
Other: Cerubidine
IOM: 100-02, 15, 50

J9151 Injection, daunorubicin citrate, liposomal formulation, 10 mg Qp Qh E2
Other: Daunoxome
IOM: 100-02, 15, 50

J9153 njection, liposomal, 1 mg daunorubicin and 2.27 mg cytarabine G
Other: Vyxeos

J9155 Injection, degarelix, 1 mg Qp Qh K2 K
Report 1 unit for every 1 mg.
Other: Firmagon

J9160 Injection, denileukin diftitox, 300 mcg Qp Qh E2

J9165 Injection, diethylstilbestrol diphosphate, 250 mg Qp Qh E2
Other: Stilphostrol
IOM: 100-02, 15, 50

J9171 Injection, docetaxel, 1 mg Qp Qh K2 K
Report 1 unit for every 1 mg.
Other: Docefrez, Taxotere
IOM: 100-02, 15, 50
Coding Clinic: 2012, Q1, P9

▶ New ⤺ Revised ✔ Reinstated ~~deleted~~ Deleted ⊘ Not covered or valid by Medicare
Special coverage instructions * Carrier discretion Bill Part B MAC Bill DME MAC

▶ * **J9173** Injection, durvalumab, 10 mg G
Other: Imfinzi

J9175 Injection, Elliott's B solution, 1 ml Qp Qh N1 N
IOM: 100-02, 15, 50

* **J9176** Injection, elotuzumab, 1 mg Qp Qh K2 G
Other: Empliciti

* **J9178** Injection, epirubicin HCL, 2 mg Qp Qh N1 N
Other: Ellence

* **J9179** Injection, eribulin mesylate, 0.1 mg Qp Qh K2 K
Other: Halaven

J9181 Injection, etoposide, 10 mg Qp Qh N1 N
Other: Etopophos, Toposar

J9185 Injection, fludarabine phosphate, 50 mg Qp Qh K2 K
Other: Fludara
IOM: 100-02, 15, 50

J9190 Injection, fluorouracil, 500 mg Qp Qh N1 N
Other: Adrucil
IOM: 100-02, 15, 50

J9200 Injection, floxuridine, 500 mg Qp Qh N1 N
Other: FUDR
IOM: 100-02, 15, 50

J9201 Injection, gemcitabine hydrochloride, 200 mg Qp Qh N1 N
Other: Gemzar
IOM: 100-02, 15, 50

J9202 Goserelin acetate implant, per 3.6 mg Qp Qh K2 K
Other: Zoladex
IOM: 100-02, 15, 50

* **J9203** Injection, gemtuzumab ozogamicin, 0.1 mg K2 G

J9205 Injection, irinotecan liposome, 1 mg Qp Qh K2 G
Other: ONIVYDE
IOM: 100-02, 15, 50

J9206 Injection, irinotecan, 20 mg Qp Qh N1 N
Other: Camptosar
IOM: 100-02, 15, 50

* **J9207** Injection, ixabepilone, 1 mg Qp Qh K2 K
Other: Ixempra Kit

J9208 Injection, ifosfamide, 1 gm Qp Qh N1 N
Other: Ifex
IOM: 100-02, 15, 50

J9209 Injection, mesna, 200 mg Qp Qh N1 N
Other: Mesnex
IOM: 100-02, 15, 50

J9211 Injection, idarubicin hydrochloride, 5 mg Qp Qh K2 K
Other: Idamycin PFS
IOM: 100-02, 15, 50

J9212 Injection, interferon alfacon-1, recombinant, 1 mcg Qp Qh N1 N
Other: Amgen, Infergen
IOM: 100-02, 15, 50

J9213 Injection, interferon, alfa-2a, recombinant, 3 million units Qp Qh N1 N
Other: Roferon-A
IOM: 100-02, 15, 50

J9214 Injection, interferon, alfa-2b, recombinant, 1 million units Qp Qh K2 K
Other: Intron-A
IOM: 100-02, 15, 50

J9215 Injection, interferon, alfa-n3 (human leukocyte derived), 250,000 IU Qp Qh E2
Other: Alferon N
IOM: 100-02, 15, 50

J9216 Injection, interferon, gamma-1B, 3 million units Qp Qh K2 K
Other: Actimmune
IOM: 100-02, 15, 50

J9217 Leuprolide acetate (for depot suspension), 7.5 mg Qp Qh K2 K
Other: Eligard, Lupron Depot
IOM: 100-02, 15, 50
Coding Clinic: 2015, Q3, P3

J9218 Leuprolide acetate, per 1 mg Qp Qh K2 K
Other: Lupron
IOM: 100-02, 15, 50
Coding Clinic: 2015, Q3, P3

⊙ **J9219** Leuprolide acetate implant, 65 mg Ⓑ Ⓓ Qp Qh E2

Other: Viadur

IOM: 100-02, 15, 50

⊙ **J9225** Histrelin implant (Vantas), 50 mg Ⓑ Ⓓ Qp Qh K2 K

IOM: 100-02, 15, 50

⊙ **J9226** Histrelin implant (Supprelin LA), 50 mg Ⓑ Ⓓ Qp Qh K2 K

Other: Vantas

IOM: 100-02, 15, 50

* **J9228** Injection, ipilimumab, 1 mg Ⓑ Ⓓ Qp Qh K2 K

Other: Yervoy

Coding Clinic: 2012, Q1, P9

▶ * **J9229** Injection, inotuzumab ozogamicin, 0.1 mg G

Other: Besponsa

⊙ **J9230** Injection, mechlorethamine hydrochloride, (nitrogen mustard), 10 mg Ⓑ Ⓓ Qp Qh K2 K

Other: Mustargen

IOM: 100-02, 15, 50

⊙ **J9245** Injection, melphalan hydrochloride, 50 mg Ⓑ Ⓓ Qp Qh K2 K

Other: Alkeran, Evomela

IOM: 100-02, 15, 50

⊙ **J9250** Methotrexate sodium, 5 mg Ⓑ Ⓓ Qp Qh N1 N

Other: Folex

IOM: 100-02, 15, 50

⊙ **J9260** Methotrexate sodium, 50 mg Ⓑ Ⓓ Qp Qh N1 N

Other: Folex

IOM: 100-02, 15, 50

* **J9261** Injection, nelarabine, 50 mg Ⓑ Ⓓ Qp Qh K2 K

Other: Arranon

* **J9262** Injection, omacetaxine mepesuccinate, 0.01 mg Ⓑ Ⓓ Qp Qh K2 K

Other: Synribo

* **J9263** Injection, oxaliplatin, 0.5 mg Ⓑ Ⓓ Qp Qh N1 N

Eloxatin, platinum-based anticancer drug that destroys cancer cells

Other: Eloxatin

Coding Clinic: 2009, Q1, P10

* **J9264** Injection, paclitaxel protein-bound particles, 1 mg Ⓑ Ⓓ K2 K

Other: Abraxane

⊙ **J9266** Injection, pegaspargase, per single dose vial Ⓑ Ⓓ Qp Qh K2 K

Other: Oncaspar

IOM: 100-02, 15, 50

⊙ **J9267** Injection, paclitaxel, 1 mg Ⓑ Ⓓ Qp Qh N1 N

Other: Taxol

⊙ **J9268** Injection, pentostatin, 10 mg Ⓑ Ⓓ Qp Qh K2 K

Other: Nipent

IOM: 100-02, 15, 50

⊙ **J9270** Injection, plicamycin, 2.5 mg Ⓑ Ⓓ Qp Qh N1 N

Other: Mithracin

IOM: 100-02, 15, 50

* **J9271** Injection, pembrolizumab, 1 mg Ⓑ Ⓓ Qp Qh K2 K

Other: Keytruda

⊙ **J9280** Injection, mitomycin, 5 mg Ⓑ Ⓓ Qp Qh K2 K

Other: Mitosol, Mutamycin

IOM: 100-02, 15, 50

Coding Clinic: 2016, Q4, P8; 2014, Q2, P6; 2011, Q1, P9

* **J9285** Injection, olaratumab, 10 mg K2 G

⊙ **J9293** Injection, mitoxantrone hydrochloride, per 5 mg Ⓑ Ⓓ Qp Qh K2 K

Other: Novantrone

IOM: 100-02, 15, 50

* **J9295** Injection, necitumumab, 1 mg Qp Qh K2 G

Other: Portrazza

⊙ **J9299** Injection, nivolumab, 1 mg Ⓑ Ⓓ Qp Qh K2 K

Other: Opdivo

* **J9301** Injection, obinutuzumab, 10 mg Ⓑ Ⓓ Qp Qh K2 K

Other: Gazyva

* **J9302** Injection, ofatumumab, 10 mg Ⓑ Ⓓ Qp Qh K2 K

Other: Arzerra

Coding Clinic: 2011, Q1, P7

* **J9303** Injection, panitumumab, 10 mg Ⓑ Ⓓ Qp Qh K2 K

Other: Vectibix

* **J9305** Injection, pemetrexed, 10 mg Ⓑ Ⓓ Qp Qh K2 K

Other: Alimta

▶ New ↩ Revised ✔ Reinstated ~~deleted~~ Deleted ⊘ Not covered or valid by Medicare
⊙ Special coverage instructions * Carrier discretion Ⓑ Bill Part B MAC Ⓓ Bill DME MAC

* J9306 Injection, pertuzumab, 1 mg Qp Qh K2 K
  Other: Perjeta

* J9307 Injection, pralatrexate, 1 mg Qp Qh K2 K
  Other: Folotyn
  Coding Clinic: 2011, Q1, P7

* J9308 Injection, ramucirumab, 5 mg Qp Qh K2 K
  Other: Cyramza

~~J9310 Injection, rituximab, 100 mg~~ ✖

▶ J9311 Injection, rituximab 10 mg and hyaluronidase G
  Other: Rituxan

▶ J9312 Injection, rituximab, 10 mg K
  Other: Rituxan

* J9315 Injection, romidepsin, 1 mg Qp Qh K2 K
  Other: Istodax
  Coding Clinic: 2011, Q1, P7

J9320 Injection, streptozocin, 1 gram Qp Qh K2 K
  Other: Zanosar
  IOM: 100-02, 15, 50

* J9325 Injection, talimogene laherparepvec, per 1 million plaque forming units Qp Qh K2 G
  Other: Imlygic

* J9328 Injection, temozolomide, 1 mg Qp Qh K2 K
  Intravenous formulation, not for oral administration
  Other: Temodar

* J9330 Injection, temsirolimus, 1 mg Qp Qh K2 K
  Treatment for advanced renal cell carcinoma; standard administration is intravenous infusion greater than 30-60 minutes
  Other: Torisel

J9340 Injection, thiotepa, 15 mg Qp Qh K2 K
  Other: Tepadina, Triethylene thio Phosphoramide/T
  IOM: 100-02, 15, 50

* J9351 Injection, topotecan, 0.1 mg Qp Qh N1 N
  Other: Hycamtin
  Coding Clinic: 2011, Q1, P9

* J9352 Injection, trabectedin, 0.1 mg Qp Qh K2 G
  Other: Yondelis

* J9354 Injection, ado-trastuzumab emtansine, 1 mg Qp Qh K2 K
  Other: Kadcyla

* J9355 Injection, trastuzumab, 10 mg Qp Qh K2 K
  Other: Herceptin

J9357 Injection, valrubicin, intravesical, 200 mg Qp Qh K2 K
  Other: Valstar
  IOM: 100-02, 15, 50

J9360 Injection, vinblastine sulfate, 1 mg Qp Qh N1 N
  Other: Alkaban-AQ, Velban, Velsar
  IOM: 100-02, 15, 50

J9370 Vincristine sulfate, 1 mg Qp Qh N1 N
  Other: Oncovin, Vincasar PFS
  IOM: 100-02, 15, 50
  Coding Clinic: 2011, Q1, P9

* J9371 Injection, vincristine sulfate liposome, 1 mg Qp Qh K2 K

J9390 Injection, vinorelbine tartrate, 10 mg Qp Qh N1 N
  Other: Navelbine
  IOM: 100-02, 15, 50

* J9395 Injection, fulvestrant, 25 mg Qp Qh K2 K
  Other: Faslodex

* J9400 Injection, ziv-aflibercept, 1 mg Qp Qh K2 K
  Other: Zaltrap

J9600 Injection, porfimer sodium, 75 mg Qp Qh K2 K
  Other: Photofrin
  IOM: 100-02, 15, 50

J9999 Not otherwise classified, antineoplastic drugs N1 N
  Bill on paper, bill one unit, and identify drug and total dosage in "Remarks" field. Include invoice of cost or NDC number in "Remarks" field.
  Other: Imlygic, Yondelis
  IOM: 100-02, 15, 50; 100-03, 2, 110.2
  Coding Clinic: 2017, Q1, P3; 2013, Q2, P3

TEMPORARY CODES ASSIGNED TO DME REGIONAL CARRIERS (K0000-K9999)

NOTE: This section contains national codes assigned by CMS on a temporary basis and for the exclusive use of the durable medical equipment regional carriers (DMERC).

Wheelchairs and Accessories

* **K0001** Standard wheelchair Ⓔ Qp Qh ♿ Y
  Capped rental
* **K0002** Standard hemi (low seat) wheelchair Ⓔ Qp Qh ♿ Y
  Capped rental
* **K0003** Lightweight wheelchair Ⓔ Qp Qh ♿ Y
  Capped rental
* **K0004** High strength, lightweight wheelchair Ⓔ Qp Qh ♿ Y
  Capped rental
* **K0005** Ultralightweight wheelchair Ⓔ Qp Qh ♿ Y
  Capped rental. Inexpensive and routinely purchased DME
* **K0006** Heavy duty wheelchair Ⓔ Qp Qh ♿ Y
  Capped rental
* **K0007** Extra heavy duty wheelchair Ⓔ Qp Qh ♿ Y
  Capped rental
* **K0008** Custom manual wheelchair/base Ⓑ Qh Y
* **K0009** Other manual wheelchair/base Ⓑ Qp Qh ♿ Y
  Not otherwise classified
* **K0010** Standard - weight frame motorized/power wheelchair Ⓔ ♿ Y
  Capped rental. Codes K0010-K0014 are not for manual wheelchairs with add-on power packs. Use the appropriate code for the manual wheelchair base provided (K0001-K0009) and code K0460.
* **K0011** Standard - weight frame motorized/power wheelchair with programmable control parameters for speed adjustment, tremor dampening, acceleration control and braking Ⓑ ♿ Y
  Capped rental. A patient who requires a power wheelchair usually is totally nonambulatory and has severe weakness of the upper extremities due to a neurologic or muscular disease/condition.
* **K0012** Lightweight portable motorized/power wheelchair Ⓑ ♿ Y
  Capped rental
* **K0013** Custom motorized/power wheelchair base Ⓑ Qh Y
* **K0014** Other motorized/power wheelchair base Ⓑ Y
  Capped rental
* **K0015** Detachable, non-adjustable height armrest, replacement only, each Ⓔ Qp Qh ♿ Y
  Inexpensive and routinely purchased DME
* **K0017** Detachable, adjustable height armrest, base, replacement only, each Ⓔ Qp Qh ♿ Y
  Inexpensive and routinely purchased DME
* **K0018** Detachable, adjustable height armrest, upper portion, replacement only, each Ⓔ Qp Qh ♿ Y
  Inexpensive and routinely purchased DME
* **K0019** Arm pad, replacement only, each Ⓔ Qp Qh ♿ Y
  Inexpensive and routinely purchased DME
* **K0020** Fixed, adjustable height armrest, pair Ⓑ Qp Qh ♿ Y
  Inexpensive and routinely purchased DME
* ⤾ **K0037** High mount flip-up footrest, each Ⓔ Qp Qh ♿ Y
  Inexpensive and routinely purchased DME
* **K0038** Leg strap, each Ⓑ Qp Qh ♿ Y
  Inexpensive and routinely purchased DME
* **K0039** Leg strap, H style, each Ⓑ Qp Qh ♿ Y
  Inexpensive and routinely purchased DME

▶ New ⤾ Revised ✔ Reinstated ~~deleted~~ Deleted ⊘ Not covered or valid by Medicare
Special coverage instructions * Carrier discretion Ⓑ Bill Part B MAC Ⓔ Bill DME MAC

* **K0040** Adjustable angle footplate, each Ⓑ Qp Qh ♿ Y
  Inexpensive and routinely purchased DME
* **K0041** Large size footplate, each Ⓑ Qp Qh ♿ Y
  Inexpensive and routinely purchased DME
* **K0042** Standard size footplate, replacement only, each Ⓑ Qp Qh ♿ Y
  Inexpensive and routinely purchased DME
* **K0043** Footrest, lower extension tube, replacement only, each Ⓑ Qp Qh ♿ Y
  Inexpensive and routinely purchased DME
* **K0044** Footrest, upper hanger bracket, replacement only, each Ⓑ Qp Qh ♿ Y
  Inexpensive and routinely purchased DME
* **K0045** Footrest, complete assembly, replacement only, each Ⓑ Qp Qh ♿ Y
  Inexpensive and routinely purchased DME
* **K0046** Elevating legrest, lower extension tube, replacement only, each Ⓑ Qp Qh ♿ Y
  Inexpensive and routinely purchased DME
* **K0047** Elevating legrest, upper hanger bracket, replacement only, each Ⓑ Qp Qh ♿ Y
  Inexpensive and routinely purchased DME
* **K0050** Ratchet assembly, replacement only Ⓑ Qp Qh ♿ Y
  Inexpensive and routinely purchased DME
* **K0051** Cam release assembly, footrest or legrests, replacement only, each Ⓑ Qp Qh ♿ Y
  Inexpensive and routinely purchased DME
* **K0052** Swing-away, detachable footrests, replacement only, each Ⓑ Qp Qh ♿ Y
  Inexpensive and routinely purchased DME
* **K0053** Elevating footrests, articulating (telescoping), each Ⓑ Qp Qh ♿ Y
  Inexpensive and routinely purchased DME
* **K0056** Seat height less than 17" or equal to or greater than 21" for a high strength, lightweight, or ultralightweight wheelchair Ⓑ Qp Qh ♿ Y
  Inexpensive and routinely purchased DME
* **K0065** Spoke protectors, each Ⓑ Qp Qh ♿ Y
  Inexpensive and routinely purchased DME
* **K0069** Rear wheel assembly, complete, with solid tire, spokes or molded, replacement only, each Ⓑ Qp Qh ♿ Y
  Inexpensive and routinely purchased DME
* **K0070** Rear wheel assembly, complete, with pneumatic tire, spokes or molded, replacement only, each Ⓑ Qp Qh ♿ Y
  Inexpensive and routinely purchased DME
* **K0071** Front caster assembly, complete, with pneumatic tire, replacement only, each Ⓑ Qp Qh ♿ Y
  Caster assembly includes a caster fork (E2396), wheel rim, and tire. Inexpensive and routinely purchased DME
* **K0072** Front caster assembly, complete, with semi-pneumatic tire, replacement only, each Ⓑ Qp Qh ♿ Y
  Inexpensive and routinely purchased DME
* **K0073** Caster pin lock, each Ⓑ Qp Qh ♿ Y
  Inexpensive and routinely purchased DME
* **K0077** Front caster assembly, complete, with solid tire, replacement only, each Ⓑ Qp Qh ♿ Y
* **K0098** Drive belt for power wheelchair, replacement only Ⓑ ♿ Y
  Inexpensive and routinely purchased DME
* **K0105** IV hanger, each Ⓑ Qp Qh ♿ Y
  Inexpensive and routinely purchased DME
* **K0108** Wheelchair component or accessory, not otherwise specified Ⓑ Y

○ **K0195** Elevating leg rests, pair (for use with capped rental wheelchair base) Ⓑ Qp Qh ♿ Y
  Medically necessary replacement items are covered if rollabout chair or transport chair covered
  IOM: 100-03, 4, 280.1

MIPS	Qp Quantity Physician	Qh Quantity Hospital	♀ Female only	
♂ Male only	A Age	♿ DMEPOS	A2-Z3 ASC Payment Indicator	A-Y ASC Status Indicator	Coding Clinic

Infusion Pump, Supplies, and Batteries

◌ **K0455** Infusion pump used for uninterrupted parenteral administration of medication (e.g., epoprostenol or treprostinol) Ⓑ Qp Qh ♿ Y

An EIP may also be referred to as an external insulin pump, ambulatory pump, or mini-infuser. CMN/DIF required. Frequent and substantial service DME.

IOM: 100-03, 1, 50.3

◌ **K0462** Temporary replacement for patient owned equipment being repaired, any type Ⓑ Qp Qh Y

Only report for maintenance and service for an item for which initial claim was paid. The term power mobility device (PMD) includes power operated vehicles (POVs) and power wheelchairs (PWCs). Not Otherwise Classified.

IOM: 100-04, 20, 40.1

◌ **K0552** Supplies for external non-insulin drug infusion pump, syringe type cartridge, sterile, each Ⓑ Qh ♿ Y

Supplies

IOM: 100-03, 1, 50.3

◌ **K0553** Supply allowance for therapeutic continuous glucose monitor (CGM), includes all supplies and accessories, 1 month supply = 1 unit of service Ⓑ ♿ Y

◌ **K0554** Receiver (monitor), dedicated, for use with therapeutic glucose continuous monitor system Ⓑ ♿ Y

* **K0601** Replacement battery for external infusion pump owned by patient, silver oxide, 1.5 volt, each Ⓑ Qh ♿ Y

Inexpensive and routinely purchased DME

* **K0602** Replacement battery for external infusion pump owned by patient, silver oxide, 3 volt, each Ⓑ Qp Qh ♿ Y

Inexpensive and routinely purchased DME

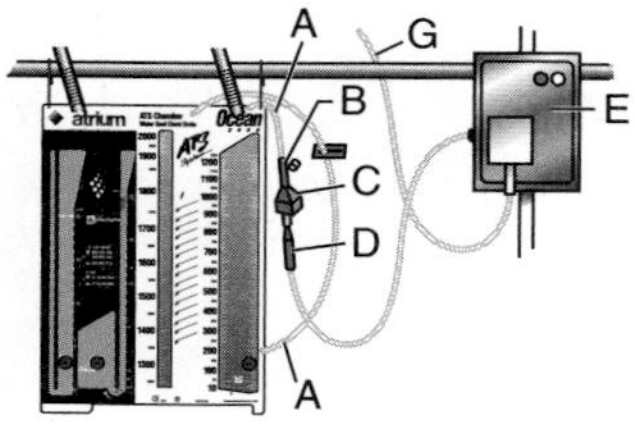
A
G
B
C
D
E
A

Figure 18 Infusion pump.

* **K0603** Replacement battery for external infusion pump owned by patient, alkaline, 1.5 volt, each Ⓑ Qh ♿ Y

Inexpensive and routinely purchased DME

* **K0604** Replacement battery for external infusion pump owned by patient, lithium, 3.6 volt, each Ⓑ Qh ♿ Y

Inexpensive and routinely purchased DME

* **K0605** Replacement battery for external infusion pump owned by patient, lithium, 4.5 volt, each Ⓑ Qp Qh ♿ Y

Inexpensive and routinely purchased DME

Defibrillator and Accessories

* **K0606** Automatic external defibrillator, with integrated electrocardiogram analysis, garment type Ⓑ Qp Qh ♿ Y

Capped rental

* **K0607** Replacement battery for automated external defibrillator, garment type only, each Ⓑ Qp Qh ♿ Y

Inexpensive and routinely purchased DME

* **K0608** Replacement garment for use with automated external defibrillator, each Ⓑ Qp Qh ♿ Y

Inexpensive and routinely purchased DME

* **K0609** Replacement electrodes for use with automated external defibrillator, garment type only, each Ⓑ Qp Qh ♿ Y

Supplies

Miscellaneous

* **K0669** Wheelchair accessory, wheelchair seat or back cushion, does not meet specific code criteria or no written coding verification from DME PDAC Ⓑ Y

Inexpensive and routinely purchased DME

* **K0672** Addition to lower extremity orthosis, removable soft interface, all components, replacement only, each Ⓑ Qp ♿ A

Prosthetics/Orthotics

▶ New ⮌ Revised ✔ Reinstated ~~deleted~~ Deleted ⊘ Not covered or valid by Medicare
◌ Special coverage instructions * Carrier discretion Ⓑ Bill Part B MAC Ⓑ Bill DME MAC

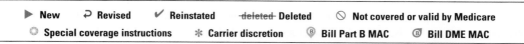

* **K0730** Controlled dose inhalation drug delivery system Ⓑ Qp Qh DMEPOS — Y
  Inexpensive and routinely purchased DME
* **K0733** Power wheelchair accessory, 12 to 24 amp hour sealed lead acid battery, each (e.g., gel cell, absorbed glassmat) Ⓑ Qp Qh DMEPOS — Y
  Inexpensive and routinely purchased DME
* **K0738** Portable gaseous oxygen system, rental; home compressor used to fill portable oxygen cylinders; includes portable containers, regulator, flowmeter, humidifier, cannula or mask, and tubing Ⓑ Qp Qh DMEPOS — Y
  Oxygen and oxygen equipment
* **K0739** Repair or nonroutine service for durable medical equipment other than oxygen equipment requiring the skill of a technician, labor component, per 15 minutes Ⓑ — Y
* ⃠ **K0740** Repair or nonroutine service for oxygen equipment requiring the skill of a technician, labor component, per 15 minutes Ⓑ Qp Qh — E1
* **K0743** Suction pump, home model, portable, for use on wounds Ⓑ Qp Qh — Y
* **K0744** Absorptive wound dressing for use with suction pump, home model, portable, pad size 16 square inches or less Ⓑ Qp — A
* **K0745** Absorptive wound dressing for use with suction pump, home model, portable, pad size more than 16 square inches but less than or equal to 48 square inches Ⓑ Qp — A
* **K0746** Absorptive wound dressing for use with suction pump, home model, portable, pad size greater than 48 square inches Ⓑ Qp — A

Power Mobility Devices

* **K0800** Power operated vehicle, group 1 standard, patient weight capacity up to and including 300 pounds Ⓑ Qp Qh DMEPOS — Y
  Power mobility device (PMD) includes power operated vehicles (POVs) and power wheelchairs (PWCs). Inexpensive and routinely purchased DME
* **K0801** Power operated vehicle, group 1 heavy duty, patient weight capacity 301 to 450 pounds Ⓑ Qp Qh DMEPOS — Y
  Inexpensive and routinely purchased DME
* **K0802** Power operated vehicle, group 1 very heavy duty, patient weight capacity 451 to 600 pounds Ⓑ Qp Qh DMEPOS — Y
  Inexpensive and routinely purchased DME
* **K0806** Power operated vehicle, group 2 standard, patient weight capacity up to and including 300 pounds Ⓑ Qp Qh DMEPOS — Y
  Inexpensive and routinely purchased DME
* **K0807** Power operated vehicle, group 2 heavy duty, patient weight capacity 301 to 450 pounds Ⓑ Qp Qh DMEPOS — Y
  Inexpensive and routinely purchased DME
* **K0808** Power operated vehicle, group 2 very heavy duty, patient weight capacity 451 to 600 pounds Ⓑ Qp Qh DMEPOS — Y
  Inexpensive and routinely purchased DME
* **K0812** Power operated vehicle, not otherwise classified Ⓑ Qp Qh — Y
  Not Otherwise Classified.
* **K0813** Power wheelchair, group 1 standard, portable, sling/solid seat and back, patient weight capacity up to and including 300 pounds Ⓑ Qp Qh DMEPOS — Y
  Capped rental
* **K0814** Power wheelchair, group 1 standard, portable, captains chair, patient weight capacity up to and including 300 pounds Ⓑ Qp Qh DMEPOS — Y
  Capped rental
* **K0815** Power wheelchair, group 1 standard, sling/solid seat and back, patient weight capacity up to and including 300 pounds Ⓑ Qp Qh DMEPOS — Y
  Capped rental
* **K0816** Power wheelchair, group 1 standard, captains chair, patient weight capacity up to and including 300 pounds Ⓑ Qp Qh DMEPOS — Y
  Capped rental

* **K0820** Power wheelchair, group 2 standard, portable, sling/solid seat/back, patient weight capacity up to and including 300 pounds Ⓑ Qp Qh ♿ Y
  Capped rental
* **K0821** Power wheelchair, group 2 standard, portable, captains chair, patient weight capacity up to and including 300 pounds Ⓑ Qp Qh ♿ Y
  Capped rental
* **K0822** Power wheelchair, group 2 standard, sling/solid seat/back, patient weight capacity up to and including 300 pounds Ⓑ Qp Qh ♿ Y
  Capped rental
* **K0823** Power wheelchair, group 2 standard, captains chair, patient weight capacity up to and including 300 pounds Ⓑ Qp Qh ♿ Y
  Capped rental
* **K0824** Power wheelchair, group 2 heavy duty, sling/solid seat/back, patient weight capacity 301 to 450 pounds Ⓑ Qp Qh ♿ Y
  Capped rental
* **K0825** Power wheelchair, group 2 heavy duty, captains chair, patient weight capacity 301 to 450 pounds Ⓑ Qp Qh ♿ Y
  Capped rental
* **K0826** Power wheelchair, group 2 very heavy duty, sling/solid seat/back, patient weight capacity 451 to 600 pounds Ⓑ Qp Qh ♿ Y
  Capped rental
* **K0827** Power wheelchair, group 2 very heavy duty, captains chair, patient weight capacity 451 to 600 pounds Ⓑ Qp Qh ♿ Y
  Capped rental
* **K0828** Power wheelchair, group 2 extra heavy duty, sling/solid seat/back, patient weight capacity 601 pounds or more Ⓑ Qp Qh ♿ Y
  Capped rental
* **K0829** Power wheelchair, group 2 extra heavy duty, captains chair, patient weight 601 pounds or more Ⓑ Qp Qh ♿ Y
  Capped rental
* **K0830** Power wheelchair, group 2 standard, seat elevator, sling/solid seat/back, patient weight capacity up to and including 300 pounds Ⓑ Qp Qh Y
  Capped rental
* **K0831** Power wheelchair, group 2 standard, seat elevator, captains chair, patient weight capacity up to and including 300 pounds Ⓑ Qp Qh Y
* **K0835** Power wheelchair, group 2 standard, single power option, sling/solid seat/back, patient weight capacity up to and including 300 pounds Ⓑ Qp Qh ♿ Y
  Capped rental
* **K0836** Power wheelchair, group 2 standard, single power option, captains chair, patient weight capacity up to and including 300 pounds Ⓑ Qp Qh ♿ Y
  Capped rental
* **K0837** Power wheelchair, group 2 heavy duty, single power option, sling/solid seat/back, patient weight capacity 301 to 450 pounds Ⓑ Qp Qh ♿ Y
  Capped rental
* **K0838** Power wheelchair, group 2 heavy duty, single power option, captains chair, patient weight capacity 301 to 450 pounds Ⓑ Qp Qh ♿ Y
  Capped rental
* **K0839** Power wheelchair, group 2 very heavy duty, single power option, sling/solid seat/back, patient weight capacity 451 to 600 pounds Ⓑ Qp Qh ♿ Y
  Capped rental
* **K0840** Power wheelchair, group 2 extra heavy duty, single power option, sling/solid seat/back, patient weight capacity 601 pounds or more Ⓑ Qp Qh ♿ Y
  Capped rental
* **K0841** Power wheelchair, group 2 standard, multiple power option, sling/solid seat/back, patient weight capacity up to and including 300 pounds Ⓑ Qp Qh ♿ Y
  Capped rental
* **K0842** Power wheelchair, group 2 standard, multiple power option, captains chair, patient weight capacity up to and including 300 pounds Ⓑ Qp Qh ♿ Y
  Capped rental
* **K0843** Power wheelchair, group 2 heavy duty, multiple power option, sling/solid seat/back, patient weight capacity 301 to 450 pounds Ⓑ Qp Qh ♿ Y
  Capped rental
* **K0848** Power wheelchair, group 3 standard, sling/solid seat/back, patient weight capacity up to and including 300 pounds Ⓑ Qp Qh ♿ Y
  Capped rental

▶ New ↩ Revised ✔ Reinstated ~~deleted~~ Deleted ⊘ Not covered or valid by Medicare
Special coverage instructions * Carrier discretion Ⓑ Bill Part B MAC Ⓑ Bill DME MAC

✻ **K0849** Power wheelchair, group 3 standard, captains chair, patient weight capacity up to and including 300 pounds Ⓑ Qp Qh ♿ Y
Capped rental

✻ **K0850** Power wheelchair, group 3 heavy duty, sling/solid seat/back, patient weight capacity 301 to 450 pounds Ⓑ Qp Qh ♿ Y
Capped rental

✻ **K0851** Power wheelchair, group 3 heavy duty, captains chair, patient weight capacity 301 to 450 pounds Ⓑ Qp Qh ♿ Y
Capped rental

✻ **K0852** Power wheelchair, group 3 very heavy duty, sling/solid seat/back, patient weight capacity 451 to 600 pounds Ⓑ Qp Qh ♿ Y
Capped rental

✻ **K0853** Power wheelchair, group 3 very heavy duty, captains chair, patient weight capacity 451 to 600 pounds Ⓑ Qp Qh ♿ Y
Capped rental

✻ **K0854** Power wheelchair, group 3 extra heavy duty, sling/solid seat/back, patient weight capacity 601 pounds or more Ⓑ Qp Qh ♿ Y
Capped rental

✻ **K0855** Power wheelchair, group 3 extra heavy duty, captains chair, patient weight capacity 601 pounds or more Ⓑ Qp Qh ♿ Y
Capped rental

✻ **K0856** Power wheelchair, group 3 standard, single power option, sling/solid seat/back, patient weight capacity up to and including 300 pounds Ⓑ Qp Qh ♿ Y
Capped rental

✻ **K0857** Power wheelchair, group 3 standard, single power option, captains chair, patient weight capacity up to and including 300 pounds Ⓑ Qp Qh ♿ Y
Capped rental

✻ **K0858** Power wheelchair, group 3 heavy duty, single power option, sling/solid seat/back, patient weight 301 to 450 pounds Ⓑ Qp Qh ♿ Y
Capped rental

✻ **K0859** Power wheelchair, group 3 heavy duty, single power option, captains chair, patient weight capacity 301 to 450 pounds Ⓑ Qp Qh ♿ Y
Capped rental

✻ **K0860** Power wheelchair, group 3 very heavy duty, single power option, sling/solid seat/back, patient weight capacity 451 to 600 pounds Ⓑ Qp Qh ♿ Y
Capped rental

✻ **K0861** Power wheelchair, group 3 standard, multiple power option, sling/solid seat/back, patient weight capacity up to and including 300 pounds Ⓑ Qp Qh ♿ Y
Capped rental

✻ **K0862** Power wheelchair, group 3 heavy duty, multiple power option, sling/solid seat/back, patient weight capacity 301 to 450 pounds Ⓑ Qp Qh ♿ Y
Capped rental

✻ **K0863** Power wheelchair, group 3 very heavy duty, multiple power option, sling/solid seat/back, patient weight capacity 451 to 600 pounds Ⓑ Qp Qh ♿ Y
Capped rental

✻ **K0864** Power wheelchair, group 3 extra heavy duty, multiple power option, sling/solid seat/back, patient weight capacity 601 pounds or more Ⓑ Qp Qh ♿ Y
Capped rental

✻ **K0868** Power wheelchair, group 4 standard, sling/solid seat/back, patient weight capacity up to and including 300 pounds Ⓑ Qp Qh Y
Capped rental

✻ **K0869** Power wheelchair, group 4 standard, captains chair, patient weight capacity up to and including 300 pounds Ⓑ Qp Qh Y
Capped rental

✻ **K0870** Power wheelchair, group 4 heavy duty, sling/solid seat/back, patient weight capacity 301 to 450 pounds Ⓑ Qp Qh Y
Capped rental

✻ **K0871** Power wheelchair, group 4 very heavy duty, sling/solid seat/back, patient weight capacity 451 to 600 pounds Ⓑ Qp Qh Y
Capped rental

✻ **K0877** Power wheelchair, group 4 standard, single power option, sling/solid seat/back, patient weight capacity up to and including 300 pounds Ⓑ Qp Qh Y
Capped rental

✻ **K0878** Power wheelchair, group 4 standard, single power option, captains chair, patient weight capacity up to and including 300 pounds Ⓔ Qp Qh Y

Capped rental

✻ **K0879** Power wheelchair, group 4 heavy duty, single power option, sling/solid seat/back, patient weight capacity 301 to 450 pounds Ⓔ Qp Qh Y

Capped rental

✻ **K0880** Power wheelchair, group 4 very heavy duty, single power option, sling/solid seat/back, patient weight 451 to 600 pounds Ⓔ Qp Qh Y

Capped rental

✻ **K0884** Power wheelchair, group 4 standard, multiple power option, sling/solid seat/back, patient weight capacity up to and including 300 pounds Ⓔ Qp Qh Y

Capped rental

✻ **K0885** Power wheelchair, group 4 standard, multiple power option, captains chair, patient weight capacity up to and including 300 pounds Ⓔ Qp Qh Y

Capped rental

✻ **K0886** Power wheelchair, group 4 heavy duty, multiple power option, sling/solid seat/back, patient weight capacity 301 to 450 pounds Ⓔ Qp Qh Y

Capped rental

✻ **K0890** Power wheelchair, group 5 pediatric, single power option, sling/solid seat/back, patient weight capacity up to and including 125 pounds Ⓔ Qp Qh A Y

Capped rental

✻ **K0891** Power wheelchair, group 5 pediatric, multiple power option, sling/solid seat/back, patient weight capacity up to and including 125 pounds Ⓔ Qp Qh A Y

Capped rental

✻ **K0898** Power wheelchair, not otherwise classified Ⓔ Qp Qh Y

✻ **K0899** Power mobility device, not coded by DME PDAC or does not meet criteria Ⓔ Y

Customized DME: Other than Wheelchair

◌ **K0900** Customized durable medical equipment, other than wheelchair Ⓔ Qp Qh Y

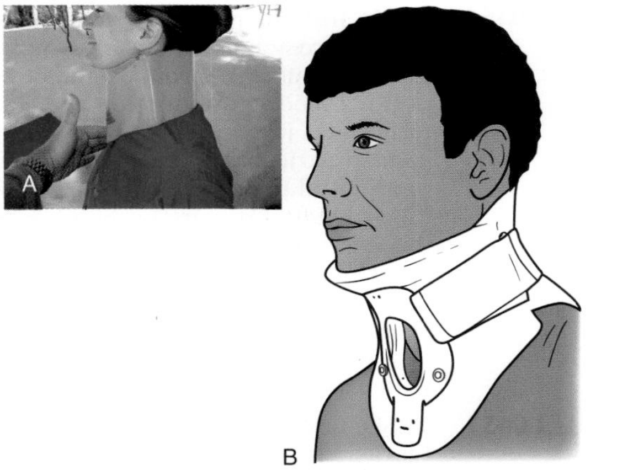
A
B

Figure 19 (A) Flexible cervical collar. (B) Adjustable cervical collar.

ORTHOTICS (L0100-L4999)

Note: DMEPOS fee schedule https://www.cms.gov/Medicare/Medicare-Fee-for-Service-Payment/DMEPOSFeeSched/DMEPOS-Fee-Schedule.html

Cervical Orthotics

* **L0112** Cranial cervical orthosis, congenital torticollis type, with or without soft interface material, adjustable range of motion joint, custom fabricated Ⓑ Qp Qh ♿ A
* **L0113** Cranial cervical orthosis, torticollis type, with or without joint, with or without soft interface material, prefabricated, includes fitting and adjustment Ⓑ Qp Qh ♿ A
* **L0120** Cervical, flexible, non-adjustable, prefabricated, off-the-shelf (foam collar) Ⓑ Qp Qh ♿ A

  Cervical orthoses, including soft and rigid devices may be used as nonoperative management for cervical trauma
* **L0130** Cervical, flexible, thermoplastic collar, molded to patient Ⓑ Qp Qh ♿ A
* **L0140** Cervical, semi-rigid, adjustable (plastic collar) Ⓑ Qp Qh ♿ A
* **L0150** Cervical, semi-rigid, adjustable molded chin cup (plastic collar with mandibular/occipital piece) Ⓑ Qp Qh ♿ A
* **L0160** Cervical, semi-rigid, wire frame occipital/mandibular support, prefabricated, off-the-shelf Ⓑ Qp Qh ♿ A
* **L0170** Cervical, collar, molded to patient model Ⓑ Qp Qh ♿ A
* **L0172** Cervical, collar, semi-rigid thermoplastic foam, two-piece, prefabricated, off-the-shelf Ⓑ Qp Qh ♿ A
* **L0174** Cervical, collar, semi-rigid, thermoplastic foam, two piece with thoracic extension, prefabricated, off-the-shelf Ⓑ Qp Qh ♿ A

Multiple Post Collar: Cervical

* **L0180** Cervical, multiple post collar, occipital/mandibular supports, adjustable Ⓑ Qp Qh ♿ A
* **L0190** Cervical, multiple post collar, occipital/mandibular supports, adjustable cervical bars (SOMI, Guilford, Taylor types) Ⓑ Qp Qh ♿ A
* **L0200** Cervical, multiple post collar, occipital/mandibular supports, adjustable cervical bars, and thoracic extension Ⓑ Qp Qh ♿ A

Thoracic Rib Belt

* **L0220** Thoracic, rib belt, custom fabricated Ⓑ Qp Qh ♿ A

Thoracic-Lumbar-Sacral Orthotics

* **L0450** TLSO, flexible, provides trunk support, upper thoracic region, produces intracavitary pressure to reduce load on the intervertebral disks with rigid stays or panel(s), includes shoulder straps and closures, prefabricated, off-the-shelf Ⓑ Qp Qh ♿ A

  Used to immobilize specified area of spine, and is generally worn under clothing
* **L0452** TLSO, flexible, provides trunk support, upper thoracic region, produces intracavitary pressure to reduce load on the intervertebral disks with rigid stays or panel(s), includes shoulder straps and closures, custom fabricated Ⓑ Qp Qh ♿ A

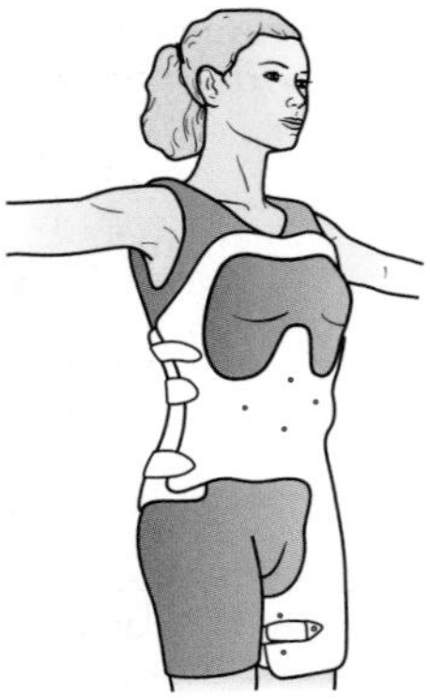

Figure 20 Thoracic-Lumbar-Sacral Orthosis (TLSO).

✻ **L0454** TLSO flexible, provides trunk support, extends from sacrococcygeal junction to above T-9 vertebra, restricts gross trunk motion in the sagittal plane, produces intracavitary pressure to reduce load on the intervertebral disks with rigid stays or panel(s), includes shoulder straps and closures, prefabricated item that has been trimmed, bent, molded, assembled, or otherwise customized to fit a specific patient by an individual with expertise Ⓑ Qp Qh ♿ A

Used to immobilize specified areas of spine; and is generally designed to be worn under clothing; not specifically designed for patients in wheelchairs

✻ **L0455** TLSO, flexible, provides trunk support, extends from sacrococcygeal junction to above T-9 vertebra, restricts gross trunk motion in the sagittal plane, produces intracavitary pressure to reduce load on the intervertebral disks with rigid stays or panel(s), includes shoulder straps and closures, prefabricated, off-the-shelf Ⓑ Qp Qh ♿ A

✻ **L0456** TLSO, flexible, provides trunk support, thoracic region, rigid posterior panel and soft anterior apron, extends from the sacrococcygeal junction and terminates just inferior to the scapular spine, restricts gross trunk motion in the sagittal plane, produces intracavitary pressure to reduce load on the intervertebral disks, includes straps and closures, prefabricated item that has been trimmed, bent, molded, assembled, or otherwise customized to fit a specific patient by an individual with expertise Ⓑ Qp Qh ♿ A

✻ **L0457** TLSO, flexible, provides trunk support, thoracic region, rigid posterior panel and soft anterior apron, extends from the sacrococcygeal junction and terminates just inferior to the scapular spine, restricts gross trunk motion in the sagittal plane, produces intracavitary pressure to reduce load on the intervertebral disks, includes straps and closures, prefabricated, off-the-shelf Ⓑ Qp Qh ♿ A

✻ **L0458** TLSO, triplanar control, modular segmented spinal system, two rigid plastic shells, posterior extends from the sacrococcygeal junction and terminates just inferior to the scapular spine, anterior extends from the symphysis pubis to the xiphoid, soft liner, restricts gross trunk motion in the sagittal, coronal, and transverse planes, lateral strength is provided by overlapping plastic and stabilizing closures, includes straps and closures, prefabricated, includes fitting and adjustment Ⓑ Qp Qh ♿ A

To meet Medicare's definition of body jacket, orthosis has to have rigid plastic shell that circles trunk with overlapping edges and stabilizing closures, and entire circumference of shell must be made of same rigid material.

✻ **L0460** TLSO, triplanar control, modular segmented spinal system, two rigid plastic shells, posterior extends from the sacrococcygeal junction and terminates just inferior to the scapular spine, anterior extends from the symphysis pubis to the sternal notch, soft liner, restricts gross trunk motion in the sagittal, coronal, and transverse planes, lateral strength is provided by overlapping plastic and stabilizing closures, includes straps and closures, prefabricated item that has been trimmed, bent, molded, assembled, or otherwise customized to fit a specific patient by an individual with expertise Ⓑ Qp Qh ♿ A

✻ **L0462** TLSO, triplanar control, modular segmented spinal system, three rigid plastic shells, posterior extends from the sacrococcygeal junction and terminates just inferior to the scapular spine, anterior extends from the symphysis pubis to the sternal notch, soft liner, restricts gross trunk motion in the sagittal, coronal, and transverse planes, lateral strength is provided by overlapping plastic and stabilizing closures, includes straps and closures, prefabricated, includes fitting and adjustment Ⓑ Qp Qh ♿ A

✻ **L0464** TLSO, triplanar control, modular segmented spinal system, four rigid plastic shells, posterior extends from sacrococcygeal junction and terminates just inferior to scapular spine, anterior extends from symphysis pubis to the sternal notch, soft liner, restricts gross trunk motion in sagittal, coronal, and transverse planes, lateral strength is provided by overlapping plastic and stabilizing closures, includes straps and closures, prefabricated, includes fitting and adjustment Ⓑ Qp Qh ♿ A

✻ **L0466** TLSO, sagittal control, rigid posterior frame and flexible soft anterior apron with straps, closures and padding, restricts gross trunk motion in sagittal plane, produces intracavitary pressure to reduce load on intervertebral disks, prefabricated item that has been trimmed, bent, molded, assembled, or otherwise customized to fit a specific patient by an individual with expertise Ⓑ Qp Qh ♿ A

✻ **L0467** TLSO, sagittal control, rigid posterior frame and flexible soft anterior apron with straps, closures and padding, restricts gross trunk motion in sagittal plane, produces intracavitary pressure to reduce load on intervertebral disks, prefabricated, off-the-shelf Ⓑ Qp Qh ♿ A

✻ **L0468** TLSO, sagittal-coronal control, rigid posterior frame and flexible soft anterior apron with straps, closures and padding, extends from sacrococcygeal junction over scapulae, lateral strength provided by pelvic, thoracic, and lateral frame pieces, restricts gross trunk motion in sagittal, and coronal planes, produces intracavitary pressure to reduce load on intervertebral disks, prefabricated item that has been trimmed, bent, molded, assembled, or otherwise customized to fit a specific patient by an individual with expertise Ⓑ Qp Qh ♿ A

✻ **L0469** TLSO, sagittal-coronal control, rigid posterior frame and flexible soft anterior apron with straps, closures and padding, extends from sacrococcygeal junction over scapulae, lateral strength provided by pelvic, thoracic, and lateral frame pieces, restricts gross trunk motion in sagittal and coronal planes, produces intracavitary pressure to reduce load on intervertebral disks, prefabricated, off-the-shelf Ⓑ Qp Qh ♿ A

MIPS | Qp Quantity Physician | Qh Quantity Hospital | ♀ Female only
♂ Male only | A Age | ♿ DMEPOS | A2-Z3 ASC Payment Indicator | A-Y ASC Status Indicator | Coding Clinic

323

ORTHOTICS L0460 – L0469

* **L0470** TLSO, triplanar control, rigid posterior frame and flexible soft anterior apron with straps, closures and padding, extends from sacrococcygeal junction to scapula, lateral strength provided by pelvic, thoracic, and lateral frame pieces, rotational strength provided by subclavicular extensions, restricts gross trunk motion in sagittal, coronal, and transverse planes, provides intracavitary pressure to reduce load on the intervertebral disks, includes fitting and shaping the frame, prefabricated, includes fitting and adjustment Ⓓ Qp Qh ♿ A

* **L0472** TLSO, triplanar control, hyperextension, rigid anterior and lateral frame extends from symphysis pubis to sternal notch with two anterior components (one pubic and one sternal), posterior and lateral pads with straps and closures, limits spinal flexion, restricts gross trunk motion in sagittal, coronal, and transverse planes, includes fitting and shaping the frame, prefabricated, includes fitting and adjustment Ⓓ Qp Qh ♿ A

* **L0480** TLSO, triplanar control, one piece rigid plastic shell without interface liner, with multiple straps and closures, posterior extends from sacrococcygeal junction and terminates just inferior to scapular spine, anterior extends from symphysis pubis to sternal notch, anterior or posterior opening, restricts gross trunk motion in sagittal, coronal, and transverse planes, includes a carved plaster or CAD-CAM model, custom fabricated Ⓓ Qp Qh ♿ A

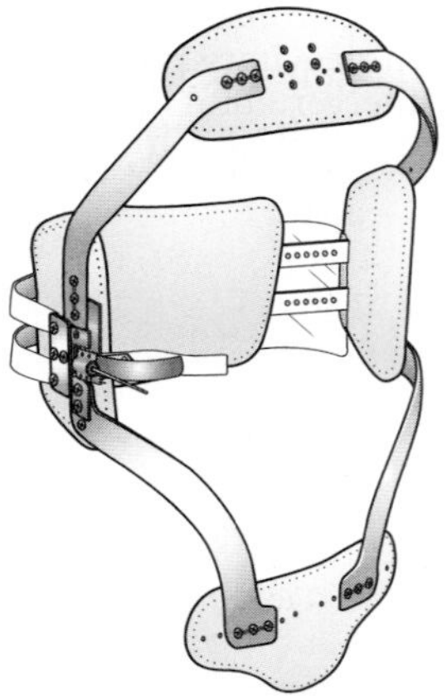

Figure 21 Thoracic-lumbar-sacral orthosis (TLSO) Jewett flexion control.

* **L0482** TLSO, triplanar control, one piece rigid plastic shell with interface liner, multiple straps and closures, posterior extends from sacrococcygeal junction and terminates just inferior to scapular spine, anterior extends from symphysis pubis to sternal notch, anterior or posterior opening, restricts gross trunk motion in sagittal, coronal, and transverse planes, includes a carved plaster or CAD-CAM model, custom fabricated Ⓓ Qp Qh ♿ A

* **L0484** TLSO, triplanar control, two piece rigid plastic shell without interface liner, with multiple straps and closures, posterior extends from sacrococcygeal junction and terminates just inferior to scapular spine, anterior extends from symphysis pubis to sternal notch, lateral strength is enhanced by overlapping plastic, restricts gross trunk motion in the sagittal, coronal, and transverse planes, includes a carved plaster or CAD-CAM model, custom fabricated Ⓓ Qp Qh ♿ A

* **L0486** TLSO, triplanar control, two piece rigid plastic shell with interface liner, multiple straps and closures, posterior extends from sacrococcygeal junction and terminates just inferior to scapular spine, anterior extends from symphysis pubis to sternal notch, lateral strength is enhanced by overlapping plastic, restricts gross trunk motion in the sagittal, coronal, and transverse planes, includes a carved plaster or CAD-CAM model, custom fabricated Ⓓ Qp Qh ♿ A

* **L0488** TLSO, triplanar control, one piece rigid plastic shell with interface liner, multiple straps and closures, posterior extends from sacrococcygeal junction and terminates just inferior to scapular spine, anterior extends from symphysis pubis to sternal notch, anterior or posterior opening, restricts gross trunk motion in sagittal, coronal, and transverse planes, prefabricated, includes fitting and adjustment Ⓓ Qp Qh ♿ A

* **L0490** TLSO, sagittal-coronal control, one piece rigid plastic shell, with overlapping reinforced anterior, with multiple straps and closures, posterior extends from sacrococcygeal junction and terminates at or before the T-9 vertebra, anterior extends from symphysis pubis to xiphoid, anterior opening, restricts gross trunk motion in sagittal and coronal planes, prefabricated, includes fitting and adjustment Ⓑ Qp Qh ♿ A

* **L0491** TLSO, sagittal-coronal control, modular segmented spinal system, two rigid plastic shells, posterior extends from the sacrococcygeal junction and terminates just inferior to the scapular spine, anterior extends from the symphysis pubis to the xiphoid, soft liner, restricts gross trunk motion in the sagittal and coronal planes, lateral strength is provided by overlapping plastic and stabilizing closures, includes straps and closures, prefabricated, includes fitting and adjustment Ⓑ Qp Qh ♿ A

* **L0492** TLSO, sagittal-coronal control, modular segmented spinal system, three rigid plastic shells, posterior extends from the sacrococcygeal junction and terminates just inferior to the scapular spine, anterior extends from the symphysis pubis to the xiphoid, soft liner, restricts gross trunk motion in the sagittal and coronal planes, lateral strength is provided by overlapping plastic and stabilizing closures, includes straps and closures, prefabricated, includes fitting and adjustment Ⓑ Qp Qh ♿ A

Sacroilliac Orthotics

* **L0621** Sacroiliac orthosis, flexible, provides pelvic-sacral support, reduces motion about the sacroiliac joint, includes straps, closures, may include pendulous abdomen design, prefabricated, off-the-shelf Ⓑ Qp Qh ♿ A

* **L0622** Sacroiliac orthosis, flexible, provides pelvic-sacral support, reduces motion about the sacroiliac joint, includes straps, closures, may include pendulous abdomen design, custom fabricated Ⓑ Qp Qh ♿ A

  Type of custom-fabricated device for which impression of specific body part is made (e.g., by means of plaster cast, or CAD-CAM [computer-aided design] technology); impression then used to make specific patient model

* **L0623** Sacroiliac orthosis, provides pelvic-sacral support, with rigid or semi-rigid panels over the sacrum and abdomen, reduces motion about the sacroiliac joint, includes straps, closures, may include pendulous abdomen design, prefabricated, off-the-shelf Ⓑ Qp Qh ♿ A

* **L0624** Sacroiliac orthosis, provides pelvic-sacral support, with rigid or semi-rigid panels placed over the sacrum and abdomen, reduces motion about the sacroiliac joint, includes straps, closures, may include pendulous abdomen design, custom fabricated Ⓑ Qp Qh ♿ A

  Custom fitted

Lumbar Orthotics

* **L0625** Lumbar orthosis, flexible, provides lumbar support, posterior extends from L-1 to below L-5 vertebra, produces intracavitary pressure to reduce load on the intervertebral discs, includes straps, closures, may include pendulous abdomen design, shoulder straps, stays, prefabricated, off-the-shelf Ⓑ Qp Qh ♿ A

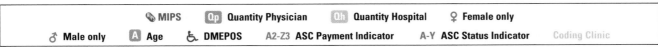

* **L0626** Lumbar orthosis, sagittal control, with rigid posterior panel(s), posterior extends from L-1 to below L-5 vertebra, produces intracavitary pressure to reduce load on the intervertebral discs, includes straps, closures, may include padding, stays, shoulder straps, pendulous abdomen design, prefabricated item that has been trimmed, bent, molded, assembled, or otherwise customized to fit a specific patient by an individual with expertise Ⓑ Qp Qh ♿ A

✻ **L0627** Lumbar orthosis, sagittal control, with rigid anterior and posterior panels, posterior extends from L-1 to below L-5 vertebra, produces intracavitary pressure to reduce load on the intervertebral discs, includes straps, closures, may include padding, shoulder straps, pendulous abdomen design, prefabricated item that has been trimmed, bent, molded, assembled, or otherwise customized to fit a specific patient by an individual with expertise Ⓓ Qp Qh ♿ A

Lumbar-Sacral Orthotics

✻ **L0628** Lumbar-sacral orthosis, flexible, provides lumbo-sacral support, posterior extends from sacrococcygeal junction to T-9 vertebra, produces intracavitary pressure to reduce load on the intervertebral discs, includes straps, closures, may include stays, shoulder straps, pendulous abdomen design, prefabricated, off-the-shelf Ⓓ Qp Qh ♿ A

✻ **L0629** Lumbar-sacral orthosis, flexible, provides lumbo-sacral support, posterior extends from sacrococcygeal junction to T-9 vertebra, produces intracavitary pressure to reduce load on the intervertebral discs, includes straps, closures, may include stays, shoulder straps, pendulous abdomen design, custom fabricated Ⓓ Qp Qh ♿ A

Custom fitted

✻ **L0630** Lumbar-sacral orthosis, sagittal control, with rigid posterior panel(s), posterior extends from sacrococcygeal junction to T-9 vertebra, produces intracavitary pressure to reduce load on the intervertebral discs, includes straps, closures, may include padding, stays, shoulder straps, pendulous abdomen design, prefabricated item that has been trimmed, bent, molded, assembled, or otherwise customized to fit a specific patient by an individual with expertise Ⓓ Qp Qh ♿ A

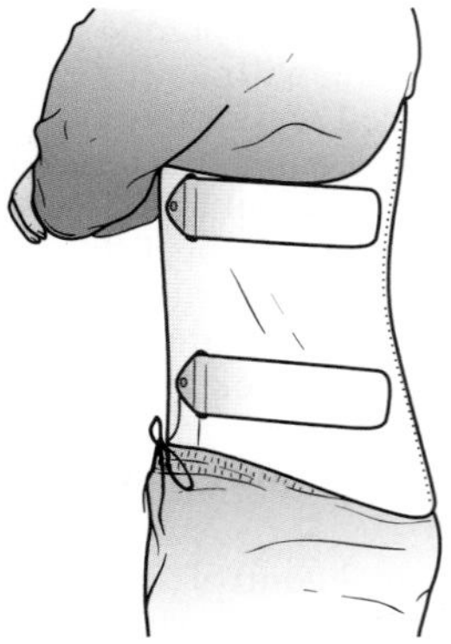

Figure 22 Lumbar-sacral orthosis.

✻ **L0631** Lumbar-sacral orthosis, sagittal control, with rigid anterior and posterior panels, posterior extends from sacrococcygeal junction to T-9 vertebra, produces intracavitary pressure to reduce load on the intervertebral discs, includes straps, closures, may include padding, shoulder straps, pendulous abdomen design, prefabricated item that has been trimmed, bent, molded, assembled, or otherwise customized to fit a specific patient by an individual with expertise Ⓓ Qp Qh ♿ A

✻ **L0632** Lumbar-sacral orthosis, sagittal control, with rigid anterior and posterior panels, posterior extends from sacrococcygeal junction to T-9 vertebra, produces intracavitary pressure to reduce load on the intervertebral discs, includes straps, closures, may include padding, shoulder straps, pendulous abdomen design, custom fabricated Ⓓ Qp Qh ♿ A

Custom fitted

✻ **L0633** Lumbar-sacral orthosis, sagittal-coronal control, with rigid posterior frame/panel(s), posterior extends from sacrococcygeal junction to T-9 vertebra, lateral strength provided by rigid lateral frame/panels, produces intracavitary pressure to reduce load on intervertebral discs, includes straps, closures, may include padding, stays, shoulder straps, pendulous abdomen design, prefabricated item that has been trimmed, bent, molded, assembled, or otherwise customized to fit a specific patient by an individual with expertise Ⓓ Qp Qh ♿ A

* **L0634** Lumbar-sacral orthosis, sagittal-coronal control, with rigid posterior frame/panel(s), posterior extends from sacrococcygeal junction to T-9 vertebra, lateral strength provided by rigid lateral frame/panel(s), produces intracavitary pressure to reduce load on intervertebral discs, includes straps, closures, may include padding, stays, shoulder straps, pendulous abdomen design, custom fabricated Ⓑ Qp Qh ♿ A

Custom fitted

* **L0635** Lumbar-sacral orthosis, sagittal-coronal control, lumbar flexion, rigid posterior frame/panel(s), lateral articulating design to flex the lumbar spine, posterior extends from sacrococcygeal junction to T-9 vertebra, lateral strength provided by rigid lateral frame/panel(s), produces intracavitary pressure to reduce load on intervertebral discs, includes straps, closures, may include padding, anterior panel, pendulous abdomen design, prefabricated, includes fitting and adjustment Ⓑ Qp Qh ♿ A

* **L0636** Lumbar sacral orthosis, sagittal-coronal control, lumbar flexion, rigid posterior frame/panels, lateral articulating design to flex the lumbar spine, posterior extends from sacrococcygeal junction to T-9 vertebra, lateral strength provided by rigid lateral frame/panels, produces intracavitary pressure to reduce load on intervertebral discs, includes straps, closures, may include padding, anterior panel, pendulous abdomen design, custom fabricated Ⓑ Qp Qh ♿ A

Custom fitted

* **L0637** Lumbar-sacral orthosis, sagittal-coronal control, with rigid anterior and posterior frame/panels, posterior extends from sacrococcygeal junction to T-9 vertebra, lateral strength provided by rigid lateral frame/panels, produces intracavitary pressure to reduce load on intervertebral discs, includes straps, closures, may include padding, shoulder straps, pendulous abdomen design, prefabricated item that has been trimmed, bent, molded, assembled, or otherwise customized to fit a specific patient by an individual with expertise Ⓑ Qp Qh ♿ A

* **L0638** Lumbar-sacral orthosis, sagittal-coronal control, with rigid anterior and posterior frame/panels, posterior extends from sacrococcygeal junction to T-9 vertebra, lateral strength provided by rigid lateral frame/panels, produces intracavitary pressure to reduce load on intervertebral discs, includes straps, closures, may include padding, shoulder straps, pendulous abdomen design, custom fabricated Ⓑ Qp Qh ♿ A

* **L0639** Lumbar-sacral orthosis, sagittal-coronal control, rigid shell(s)/panel(s), posterior extends from sacrococcygeal junction to T-9 vertebra, anterior extends from symphysis pubis to xyphoid, produces intracavitary pressure to reduce load on the intervertebral discs, overall strength is provided by overlapping rigid material and stabilizing closures, includes straps, closures, may include soft interface, pendulous abdomen design, prefabricated item that has been trimmed, bent, molded, assembled, or otherwise customized to fit a specific patient by an individual with expertise Ⓑ Qp Qh ♿ A

Characterized by rigid plastic shell that encircles trunk with overlapping edges and stabilizing closures and provides high degree of immobility

* **L0640** Lumbar-sacral orthosis, sagittal-coronal control, rigid shell(s)/panel(s), posterior extends from sacrococcygeal junction to T-9 vertebra, anterior extends from symphysis pubis to xyphoid, produces intracavitary pressure to reduce load on the intervertebral discs, overall strength is provided by overlapping rigid material and stabilizing closures, includes straps, closures, may include soft interface, pendulous abdomen design, custom fabricated Ⓑ Qp Qh ♿ A

Custom fitted

Lumbar Orthotics

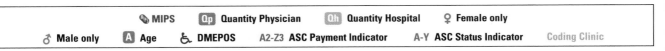

* **L0641** Lumbar orthosis, sagittal control, with rigid posterior panel(s), posterior extends from L-1 to below L-5 vertebra, produces intracavitary pressure to reduce load on the intervertebral discs, includes straps, closures, may include padding, stays, shoulder straps, pendulous abdomen design, prefabricated, off-the-shelf Ⓑ Qp Qh ♿ A

✻ **L0642** Lumbar orthosis, sagittal control, with rigid anterior and posterior panels, posterior extends from L-1 to below L-5 vertebra, produces intracavitary pressure to reduce load on the intervertebral discs, includes straps, closures, may include padding, shoulder straps, pendulous abdomen design, prefabricated, off-the-shelf Ⓔ Qp Qh ♿ A

Lumbar-Sacral Orthotics

✻ **L0643** Lumbar-sacral orthosis, sagittal control, with rigid posterior panel(s), posterior extends from sacrococcygeal junction to T-9 vertebra, produces intracavitary pressure to reduce load on the intervertebral discs, includes straps, closures, may include padding, stays, shoulder straps, pendulous abdomen design, prefabricated, off-the-shelf Ⓔ Qp Qh ♿ A

✻ **L0648** Lumbar-sacral orthosis, sagittal control, with rigid anterior and posterior panels, posterior extends from sacrococcygeal junction to T-9 vertebra, produces intracavitary pressure to reduce load on the intervertebral discs, includes straps, closures, may include padding, shoulder straps, pendulous abdomen design, prefabricated, off-the-shelf Ⓔ Qp Qh ♿ A

✻ **L0649** Lumbar-sacral orthosis, sagittal-coronal control, with rigid posterior frame/panel(s), posterior extends from sacrococcygeal junction to T-9 vertebra, lateral strength provided by rigid lateral frame/panels, produces intracavitary pressure to reduce load on intervertebral discs, includes straps, closures, may include padding, stays, shoulder straps, pendulous abdomen design, prefabricated, off-the-shelf Ⓔ Qp Qh ♿ A

✻ **L0650** Lumbar-sacral orthosis, sagittal-coronal control, with rigid anterior and posterior frame/panel(s), posterior extends from sacrococcygeal junction to T-9 vertebra, lateral strength provided by rigid lateral frame/panel(s), produces intracavitary pressure to reduce load on intervertebral discs, includes straps, closures, may include padding, shoulder straps, pendulous abdomen design, prefabricated, off-the-shelf Ⓔ Qp Qh ♿ A

✻ **L0651** Lumbar-sacral orthosis, sagittal-coronal control, rigid shell(s)/panel(s), posterior extends from sacrococcygeal junction to T-9 vertebra, anterior extends from symphysis pubis to xyphoid, produces intracavitary pressure to reduce load on the intervertebral discs, overall strength is provided by overlapping rigid material and stabilizing closures, includes straps, closures, may include soft interface, pendulous abdomen design, prefabricated, off-the-shelf Ⓔ Qp Qh ♿ A

Cervical-Thoracic-Lumbar-Sacral

✻ **L0700** Cervical-thoracic-lumbar-sacral-orthoses (CTLSO), anterior-posterior-lateral control, molded to patient model (Minerva type) Ⓔ Qp Qh ♿ A

✻ **L0710** CTLSO, anterior-posterior-lateral-control, molded to patient model, with interface material (Minerva type) Ⓔ Qp Qh ♿ A

HALO Procedure

✻ **L0810** HALO procedure, cervical halo incorporated into jacket vest Ⓔ Qp Qh ♿ A

✻ **L0820** HALO procedure, cervical halo incorporated into plaster body jacket Ⓔ Qp Qh ♿ A

✻ **L0830** HALO procedure, cervical halo incorporated into Milwaukee type orthosis Ⓔ Qp Qh ♿ A

✻ **L0859** Addition to HALO procedure, magnetic resonance image compatible systems, rings and pins, any material Ⓔ Qp Qh ♿ A

✻ **L0861** Addition to HALO procedure, replacement liner/interface material Ⓔ Qp Qh ♿ A

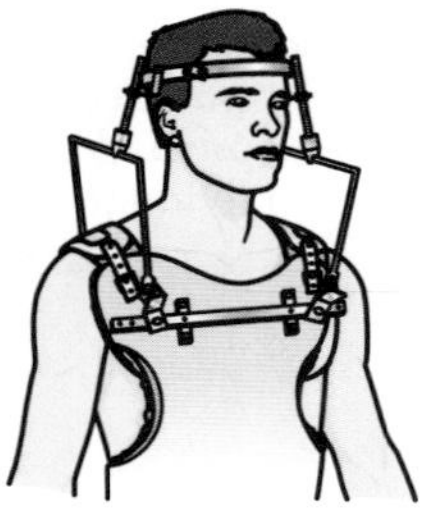

Figure 23 Halo device.

Additions to Spinal Orthotics

Note: TLSO - Thoraci-lumbar-sacral orthoses/ Spinal orthoses may be prefabricated, prefitted, or custom fabricated. Conservative treatment for back pain may include the use of spinal orthoses.

* **L0970** TLSO, corset front Qp Qh A
* **L0972** LSO, corset front Qp Qh A
* **L0974** TLSO, full corset Qp Qh A
* **L0976** LSO, full corset Qp Qh A
* **L0978** Axillary crutch extension Qp Qh A
* **L0980** Peroneal straps, prefabricated, off-the-shelf, pair Qp Qh A
* **L0982** Stocking supporter grips, prefabricated, off-the-shelf, set of four (4) Qp Qh A
  Convenience item
* **L0984** Protective body sock, prefabricated, off-the-shelf, each Qp Qh A
  Garment made of cloth or similar material that is worn under spinal orthosis and is not primarily medical in nature
* **L0999** Addition to spinal orthosis, not otherwise specified A

Orthotic Devices: Scoliosis Procedures

Note: Orthotic care of scoliosis differs from other orthotic care in that the treatment is more dynamic in nature and uses ongoing continual modification of the orthosis to the patient's changing condition. This coding structure uses the proper names, or eponyms, of the procedures because they have historic and universal acceptance in the profession. It should be recognized that variations to the basic procedures described by the founders/ developers are accepted in various medical and orthotic practices throughout the country. All procedures include a model of patient when indicated.

* **L1000** Cervical-thoracic-lumbar-sacral orthosis (CTLSO) (Milwaukee), inclusive of furnishing initial orthosis, including model Qp Qh A
* **L1001** Cervical thoracic lumbar sacral orthosis, immobilizer, infant size, prefabricated, includes fitting and adjustment Qp Qh A

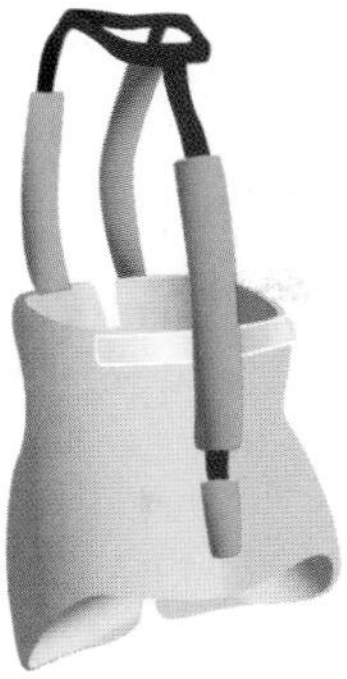

Figure 24 Milwaukee CTLSO.

* **L1005** Tension based scoliosis orthosis and accessory pads, includes fitting and adjustment Qp Qh A
* **L1010** Addition to cervical-thoracic-lumbar-sacral orthosis (CTLSO) or scoliosis orthosis, axilla sling Qp Qh A
* **L1020** Addition to CTLSO or scoliosis orthosis, kyphosis pad Qp Qh A
* **L1025** Addition to CTLSO or scoliosis orthosis, kyphosis pad, floating Qp Qh A
* **L1030** Addition to CTLSO or scoliosis orthosis, lumbar bolster pad Qp Qh A
* **L1040** Addition to CTLSO or scoliosis orthosis, lumbar or lumbar rib pad Qp Qh A
* **L1050** Addition to CTLSO or scoliosis orthosis, sternal pad Qp Qh A
* **L1060** Addition to CTLSO or scoliosis orthosis, thoracic pad Qp Qh A
* **L1070** Addition to CTLSO or scoliosis orthosis, trapezius sling Qp Qh A
* **L1080** Addition to CTLSO or scoliosis orthosis, outrigger Qp Qh A
* **L1085** Addition to CTLSO or scoliosis orthosis, outrigger, bilateral with vertical extensions Qp Qh A
* **L1090** Addition to CTLSO or scoliosis orthosis, lumbar sling Qp Qh A
* **L1100** Addition to CTLSO or scoliosis orthosis, ring flange, plastic or leather Qp Qh A
* **L1110** Addition to CTLSO or scoliosis orthosis, ring flange, plastic or leather, molded to patient model Qp Qh A
* **L1120** Addition to CTLSO, scoliosis orthosis, cover for upright, each Qp Qh A

MIPS | Qp Quantity Physician | Qh Quantity Hospital | ♀ Female only
♂ Male only | A Age | DMEPOS | A2-Z3 ASC Payment Indicator | A-Y ASC Status Indicator | Coding Clinic

Thoracic-Lumbar-Sacral (Low Profile)

* L1200 Thoracic-lumbar-sacral-orthosis (TLSO), inclusive of furnishing initial orthosis only Ⓑ Qp Qh ♿ A
* L1210 Addition to TLSO, (low profile), lateral thoracic extension Ⓑ Qp Qh ♿ A
* L1220 Addition to TLSO, (low profile), anterior thoracic extension Ⓑ Qp Qh ♿ A
* L1230 Addition to TLSO, (low profile), Milwaukee type superstructure Ⓑ Qp Qh ♿ A
* L1240 Addition to TLSO, (low profile), lumbar derotation pad Ⓑ Qp Qh ♿ A
* L1250 Addition to TLSO, (low profile), anterior ASIS pad Ⓑ Qp Qh ♿ A
* L1260 Addition to TLSO, (low profile), anterior thoracic derotation pad Ⓑ Qp Qh ♿ A
* L1270 Addition to TLSO, (low profile), abdominal pad Ⓑ Qp Qh ♿ A
* L1280 Addition to TLSO, (low profile), rib gusset (elastic), each Ⓑ Qp Qh ♿ A
* L1290 Addition to TLSO, (low profile), lateral trochanteric pad Ⓑ Qp Qh ♿ A

Other Scoliosis Procedures

* L1300 Other scoliosis procedure, body jacket molded to patient model Ⓑ Qp Qh ♿ A
* L1310 Other scoliosis procedure, postoperative body jacket Ⓑ Qp Qh ♿ A
* L1499 Spinal orthosis, not otherwise specified Ⓑ Qp Qh A

Orthotic Devices: Lower Limb (L1600-L3649)

Note: the procedures in L1600-L2999 are considered as base or basic proceduresand may be modified by listing procedure from the Additions Sections and adding them to the base procedure.

Hip: Flexible

* L1600 Hip orthosis, abduction control of hip joints, flexible, frejka type with cover, prefabricated item that has been trimmed, bent, molded, assembled, or otherwise customized to fit a specific patient by an individual with expertise Ⓑ Qp Qh ♿ A
* L1610 Hip orthosis, abduction control of hip joints, flexible, (frejka cover only), prefabricated item that has been trimmed, bent, molded, assembled, or otherwise customized to fit a specific patient by an individual with expertise Ⓑ Qp Qh ♿ A
* L1620 Hip orthosis, abduction control of hip joints, flexible, (Pavlik harness), prefabricated item that has been trimmed, bent, molded, assembled, or otherwise customized to fit a specific patient by an individual with expertise Ⓑ Qp Qh ♿ A
* L1630 Hip orthosis, abduction control of hip joints, semi-flexible (Von Rosen type), custom-fabricated Ⓑ Qp Qh ♿ A
* L1640 Hip orthosis, abduction control of hip joints, static, pelvic band or spreader bar, thigh cuffs, custom-fabricated Ⓑ Qp Qh ♿ A
* L1650 Hip orthosis, abduction control of hip joints, static, adjustable, (Ilfled type), prefabricated, includes fitting and adjustment Ⓑ Qp Qh ♿ A
* L1652 Hip orthosis, bilateral thigh cuffs with adjustable abductor spreader bar, adult size, prefabricated, includes fitting and adjustment, any type Ⓑ Qp Qh A ♿ A
* L1660 Hip orthosis, abduction control of hip joints, static, plastic, prefabricated, includes fitting and adjustment Ⓑ Qp Qh ♿ A
* L1680 Hip orthosis, abduction control of hip joints, dynamic, pelvic control, adjustable hip motion control, thigh cuffs (Rancho hip action type), custom fabrication Ⓑ Qp Qh ♿ A
* L1685 Hip orthosis, abduction control of hip joint, postoperative hip abduction type, custom fabricated Ⓑ Qp Qh ♿ A
* L1686 Hip orthosis, abduction control of hip joint, postoperative hip abduction type, prefabricated, includes fitting and adjustment Ⓑ Qp Qh ♿ A
* L1690 Combination, bilateral, lumbo-sacral, hip, femur orthosis providing adduction and internal rotation control, prefabricated, includes fitting and adjustment Ⓑ Qp Qh ♿ A

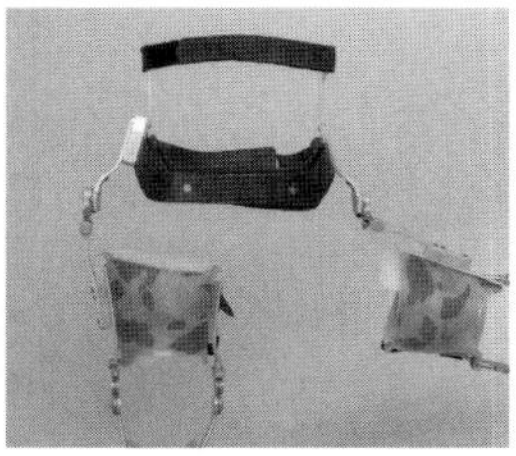

Figure 25 Thoracic-hip-knee-ankle orthosis (THKAO).

Legg Perthes

* **L1700** Legg-Perthes orthosis, (Toronto type), custom-fabricated Ⓑ Qp Qh ♿ A
* **L1710** Legg-Perthes orthosis, (Newington type), custom-fabricated Ⓑ Qp Qh ♿ A
* **L1720** Legg-Perthes orthosis, trilateral, (Tachdjian type), custom-fabricated Ⓑ Qp Qh ♿ A
* **L1730** Legg-Perthes orthosis, (Scottish Rite type), custom-fabricated Ⓑ Qp Qh ♿ A
* **L1755** Legg-Perthes orthosis, (Patten bottom type), custom-fabricated Ⓑ Qp Qh ♿ A

Knee (KO)

* **L1810** Knee orthosis, elastic with joints, prefabricated item that has been trimmed, bent, molded, assembled, or otherwise customized to fit a specific patient by an individual with expertise Ⓑ Qp Qh ♿ A
* **L1812** Knee orthosis, elastic with joints, prefabricated, off-the-shelf Ⓑ Qp Qh ♿ A
* **L1820** Knee orthosis, elastic with condylar pads and joints, with or without patellar control, prefabricated, includes fitting and adjustment Ⓑ Qp Qh ♿ A

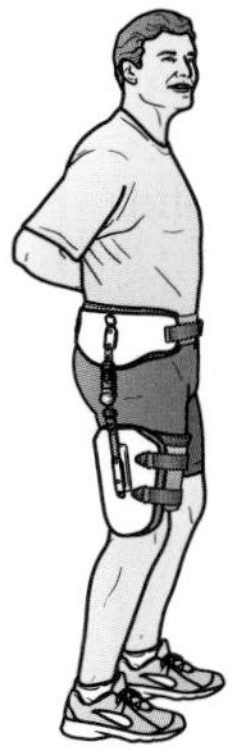

Figure 26 Hip orthosis.

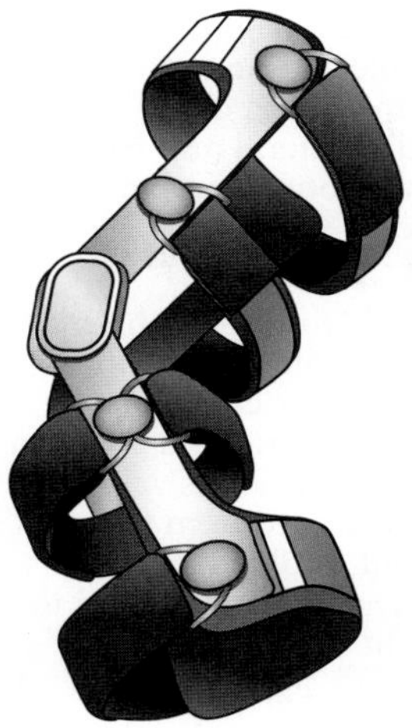

Figure 27 Knee orthosis.

* **L1830** Knee orthosis, immobilizer, canvas longitudinal, prefabricated, off-the-shelf Ⓑ Qp Qh ♿ A
* **L1831** Knee orthosis, locking knee joint(s), positional orthosis, prefabricated, includes fitting and adjustment Ⓑ Qp Qh ♿ A
* **L1832** Knee orthosis, adjustable knee joints (unicentric or polycentric), positional orthosis, rigid support, prefabricated item that has been trimmed, bent, molded, assembled, or otherwise customized to fit a specific patient by an individual with expertise Ⓑ Qp Qh ♿ A
* **L1833** Knee orthosis, adjustable knee joints (unicentric or polycentric), positional orthosis, rigid support, prefabricated, off-the-shelf Ⓑ Qp Qh ♿ A
* **L1834** Knee orthosis, without knee joint, rigid, custom-fabricated Ⓑ Qp Qh ♿ A
* **L1836** Knee orthosis, rigid, without joint(s), includes soft interface material, prefabricated, off-the-shelf Ⓑ Qp Qh ♿ A
* **L1840** Knee orthosis, derotation, medial-lateral, anterior cruciate ligament, custom fabricated Ⓑ Qp Qh ♿ A
* **L1843** Knee orthosis, single upright, thigh and calf, with adjustable flexion and extension joint (unicentric or polycentric), medial-lateral and rotation control, with or without varus/valgus adjustment, prefabricated item that has been trimmed, bent, molded, assembled, or otherwise customized to fit a specific patient by an individual with expertise Ⓑ Qp Qh ♿ A

MIPS | Qp Quantity Physician | Qh Quantity Hospital | ♀ Female only
♂ Male only | A Age | ♿ DMEPOS | A2-Z3 ASC Payment Indicator | A-Y ASC Status Indicator | Coding Clinic

* **L1844** Knee orthosis, single upright, thigh and calf, with adjustable flexion and extension joint (unicentric or polycentric), medial-lateral and rotation control, with or without varus/ valgus adjustment, custom fabricated Ⓔ Qp Qh ♿ A

* **L1845** Knee orthosis, double upright, thigh and calf, with adjustable flexion and extension joint (unicentric or polycentric), medial-lateral and rotation control, with or without varus/valgus adjustment, prefabricated item that has been trimmed, bent, molded, assembled, or otherwise customized to fit a specific patient by an individual with expertise Ⓔ Qp Qh ♿ A

* **L1846** Knee orthrosis, double upright, thigh and calf, with adjustable flexion and extension joint (unicentric or polycentric), medial-lateral and rotation control, with or without varus/ valgus adjustment, custom fabricated Ⓔ Qp Qh ♿ A

* **L1847** Knee orthosis, double upright with adjustable joint, with inflatable air support chamber(s), prefabricated item that has been trimmed, bent, molded, assembled, or otherwise customized to fit a specific patient by an individual with expertise Ⓔ Qp Qh ♿ A

* **L1848** Knee orthosis, double upright with adjustable joint, with inflatable air support chamber(s), prefabricated, off-the-shelf Ⓔ Qp Qh ♿ A

* **L1850** Knee orthosis, Swedish type, prefabricated, off-the-shelf Ⓔ Qp Qh ♿ A

* **L1851** Knee orthosis (KO), single upright, thigh and calf, with adjustable flexion and extension joint (unicentric or polycentric), medial-lateral and rotation control, with or without varus/valgus adjustment, prefabricated, off-the-shelf Qp Qh ♿ A

* **L1852** Knee orthosis (KO), double upright, thigh and calf, with adjustable flexion and extension joint (unicentric or polycentric), medial-lateral and rotation control, with or without varus/valgus adjustment, prefabricated, off-the-shelf Qp Qh ♿ A

* **L1860** Knee orthosis, modification of supracondylar prosthetic socket, custom fabricated (SK) Ⓔ Qp Qh ♿ A

Ankle-Foot (AFO)

* **L1900** Ankle foot orthosis (AFO), spring wire, dorsiflexion assist calf band, custom-fabricated Ⓔ Qp Qh ♿ A

* **L1902** Ankle orthosis, ankle gauntlet or similiar, with or without joints, prefabricated, off-the-shelf Ⓔ Qp Qh ♿ A

* **L1904** Ankle orthosis, ankle gauntlet or similiar, with or without joints, custom fabricated Ⓔ Qp Qh ♿ A

* **L1906** Ankle foot orthosis, multiligamentus ankle support, prefabricated, off-the-shelf Ⓔ Qp Qh ♿ A

* **L1907** Ankle orthosis, supramalleolar with straps, with or without interface/pads, custom fabricated Ⓔ Qp Qh ♿ A

* **L1910** Ankle foot orthosis, posterior, single bar, clasp attachment to shoe counter, prefabricated, includes fitting and adjustment Ⓔ Qp Qh ♿ A

* **L1920** Ankle foot orthosis, single upright with static or adjustable stop (Phelps or Perlstein type), custom fabricated Ⓔ Qp Qh ♿ A

* **L1930** Ankle-foot orthosis, plastic or other material, prefabricated, includes fitting and adjustment Ⓔ Qp Qh ♿ A

* **L1932** AFO, rigid anterior tibial section, total carbon fiber or equal material, prefabricated, includes fitting and adjustment Ⓔ Qp Qh ♿ A

* **L1940** Ankle foot orthosis, plastic or other material, custom fabricated Ⓔ Qp Qh ♿ A

* **L1945** Ankle foot orthosis, plastic, rigid anterior tibial section (floor reaction), custom fabricated Ⓔ Qp Qh ♿ A

* **L1950** Ankle foot orthosis, spiral, (Institute of Rehabilitation Medicine type), plastic, custom fabricated Ⓔ Qp Qh ♿ A

* **L1951** Ankle foot orthosis, spiral, (Institute of Rehabilitative Medicine type), plastic or other material, prefabricated, includes fitting and adjustment Ⓔ Qp Qh ♿ A

* **L1960** Ankle foot orthosis, posterior solid ankle, plastic, custom fabricated Ⓔ Qp Qh ♿ A

* **L1970** Ankle foot orthosis, plastic, with ankle joint, custom fabricated Ⓔ Qp Qh ♿ A

* **L1971** Ankle foot orthosis, plastic or other material with ankle joint, prefabricated, includes fitting and adjustment Ⓔ Qp Qh ♿ A

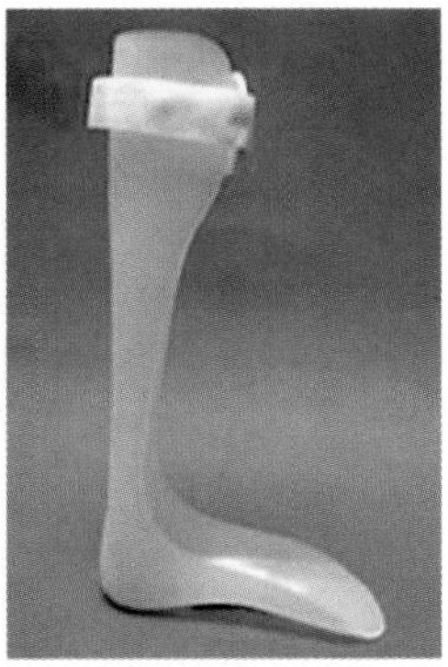

Figure 28 Ankle-foot orthosis (AFO).

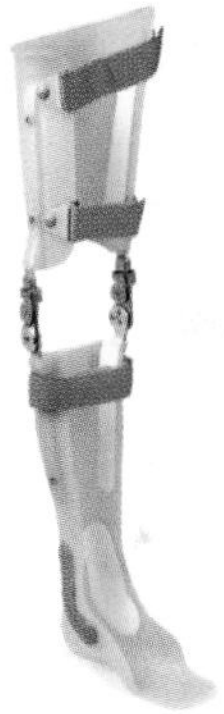

Figure 29 Knee-ankle-foot orthosis (KAFO).

✻ **L1980** Ankle foot orthosis, single upright free plantar dorsiflexion, solid stirrup, calf band/cuff (single bar 'BK' orthosis), custom fabricated Qp Qh A

✻ **L1990** Ankle foot orthosis, double upright free plantar dorsiflexion, solid stirrup, calf band/cuff (double bar 'BK' orthosis), custom fabricated Qp Qh A

Hip-Knee-Ankle-Foot (or Any Combination)

NOTE: L2000, L2020, and L2036 are base procedures to be used with any knee joint. L2010 and L2030 are to be used only with no knee joint.

✻ **L2000** Knee ankle foot orthosis, single upright, free knee, free ankle, solid stirrup, thigh and calf bands/cuffs (single bar 'AK' orthosis), custom-fabricated Qp Qh A

✻ **L2005** Knee ankle foot orthosis, any material, single or double upright, stance control, automatic lock and swing phase release, any type activation; includes ankle joint, any type, custom fabricated Qp Qh A

✻ **L2010** Knee ankle foot orthosis, single upright, free ankle, solid stirrup, thigh and calf bands/cuffs (single bar 'AK' orthosis), without knee joint, custom-fabricated Qp Qh A

✻ **L2020** Knee ankle foot orthosis, double upright, free knee, free ankle, solid stirrup, thigh and calf bands/cuffs (double bar 'AK' orthosis), custom fabricated Qp Qh A

✻ **L2030** Knee ankle foot orthosis, double upright, free ankle, solid stirrup, thigh and calf bands/cuffs (double bar 'AK' orthosis), without knee joint, custom fabricated Qp Qh A

✻ **L2034** Knee ankle foot orthosis, full plastic, single upright, with or without free motion knee, medial lateral rotation control, with or without free motion ankle, custom fabricated Qp Qh A

✻ **L2035** Knee ankle foot orthosis, full plastic, static (pediatric size), without free motion ankle, prefabricated, includes fitting and adjustment Qp Qh A A

✻ **L2036** Knee ankle foot orthosis, full plastic, double upright, with or without free motion knee, with or without free motion ankle, custom fabricated Qp Qh A

✻ **L2037** Knee ankle foot orthosis, full plastic, single upright, with or without free motion knee, with or without free motion ankle, custom fabricated Qp Qh A

✻ **L2038** Knee ankle foot orthosis, full plastic, with or without free motion knee, multi-axis ankle, custom fabricated Qp Qh A

Torsion Control: Hip-Knee-Ankle-Foot (TLSO)

✻ **L2040** Hip knee ankle foot orthosis, torsion control, bilateral rotation straps, pelvic band/belt, custom fabricated Qp Qh A

✻ **L2050** Hip knee ankle foot orthosis, torsion control, bilateral torsion cables, hip joint, pelvic band/belt, custom fabricated Qp Qh A

✻ **L2060** Hip knee ankle foot orthosis, torsion control, bilateral torsion cables, ball bearing hip joint, pelvic band/belt, custom fabricated Qp Qh A

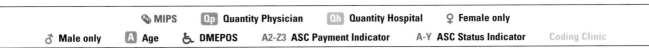

MIPS | Qp Quantity Physician | Qh Quantity Hospital | ♀ Female only
♂ Male only | A Age | DMEPOS | A2-Z3 ASC Payment Indicator | A-Y ASC Status Indicator | Coding Clinic

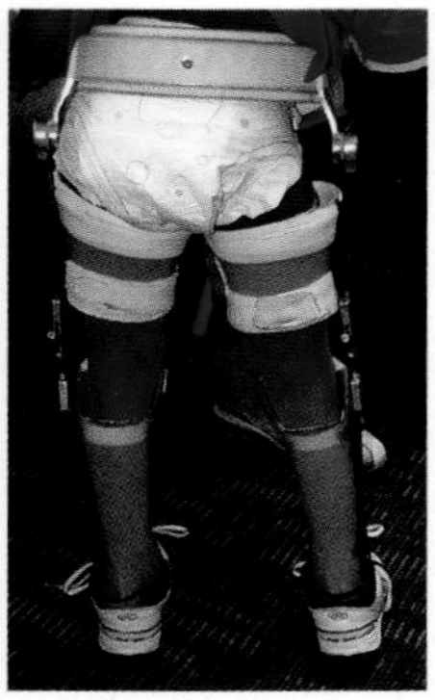

Figure 30 Hip-knee-ankle-foot orthosis (HKAFO).

* **L2070** Hip knee ankle foot orthosis, torsion control, unilateral rotation straps, pelvic band/belt, custom fabricated Ⓑ Qp Qh ᕱ A

* **L2080** Hip knee ankle foot orthosis, torsion control, unilateral torsion cable, hip joint, pelvic band/belt, custom fabricated Ⓑ Qp Qh ᕱ A

* **L2090** Hip knee ankle foot orthosis, torsion control, unilateral torsion cable, ball bearing hip joint, pelvic band/belt, custom fabricated Ⓑ Qp Qh ᕱ A

Fracture Orthotics: Ankle-Foot and Knee-Ankle-Foot

* **L2106** Ankle foot orthosis, fracture orthosis, tibial fracture cast orthosis, thermoplastic type casting material, custom fabricated Ⓑ Qp Qh ᕱ A

* **L2108** Ankle foot orthosis, fracture orthosis, tibial fracture cast orthosis, custom fabricated Ⓑ Qp Qh ᕱ A

* **L2112** Ankle foot orthosis, fracture orthosis, tibial fracture orthosis, soft, prefabricated, includes fitting and adjustment Ⓑ Qp Qh ᕱ A

* **L2114** Ankle foot orthosis, fracture orthosis, tibial fracture orthosis, semi-rigid, prefabricated, includes fitting and adjustment Ⓑ Qp Qh ᕱ A

* **L2116** Ankle foot orthosis, fracture orthosis, tibial fracture orthosis, rigid, prefabricated, includes fitting and adjustment Ⓑ Qp Qh ᕱ A

* **L2126** Knee ankle foot orthosis, fracture orthosis, femoral fracture cast orthosis, thermoplastic type casting material, custom fabricated Ⓑ Qp Qh ᕱ A

* **L2128** Knee ankle foot orthosis, fracture orthosis, femoral fracture cast orthosis, custom fabricated Ⓑ Qp Qh ᕱ A

* **L2132** KAFO, femoral fracture cast orthosis, soft, prefabricated, includes fitting and adjustment Ⓑ Qp Qh ᕱ A

* **L2134** KAFO, femoral fracture cast orthosis, semi-rigid, prefabricated, includes fitting and adjustment Ⓑ Qp Qh ᕱ A

* **L2136** KAFO, fracture orthosis, femoral fracture cast orthosis, rigid, prefabricated, includes fitting and adjustment Ⓑ Qp Qh ᕱ A

Additions to Fracture Orthotics

* **L2180** Addition to lower extremity fracture orthosis, plastic shoe insert with ankle joints Ⓑ Qp Qh ᕱ A

* **L2182** Addition to lower extremity fracture orthosis, drop lock knee joint Ⓑ Qp Qh ᕱ A

* **L2184** Addition to lower extremity fracture orthosis, limited motion knee joint Ⓑ Qp Qh ᕱ A

* **L2186** Addition to lower extremity fracture orthosis, adjustable motion knee joint, Lerman type Ⓑ Qp Qh ᕱ A

* **L2188** Addition to lower extremity fracture orthosis, quadrilateral brim Ⓑ Qp Qh ᕱ A

* **L2190** Addition to lower extremity fracture orthosis, waist belt Ⓑ Qp Qh ᕱ A

* **L2192** Addition to lower extremity fracture orthosis, hip joint, pelvic band, thigh flange, and pelvic belt Ⓑ Qp Qh ᕱ A

Additions to Lower Extremity Orthotics

* **L2200** Addition to lower extremity, limited ankle motion, each joint Ⓑ Qp Qh ᕱ A

* **L2210** Addition to lower extremity, dorsiflexion assist (plantar flexion resist), each joint Ⓑ Qp Qh ᕱ A

* **L2220** Addition to lower extremity, dorsiflexion and plantar flexion assist/resist, each joint Ⓑ Qp Qh ᕱ A

* **L2230** Addition to lower extremity, split flat caliper stirrups and plate attachment Ⓑ Qp Qh ᕱ A

* **L2232** Addition to lower extremity orthosis, rocker bottom for total contact ankle foot orthosis, for custom fabricated orthosis only Ⓑ Qp Qh ᕱ A

▶ **New** ⮌ **Revised** ✔ **Reinstated** ~~deleted~~ **Deleted** ⊘ **Not covered or valid by Medicare**

 ⊛ **Special coverage instructions** * **Carrier discretion** Ⓑ **Bill Part B MAC** Ⓑ **Bill DME MAC**

* **L2240** Addition to lower extremity, round caliper and plate attachment Ⓑ Qp Qh ᕱ A

* L2250 Addition to lower extremity, foot plate, molded to patient model, stirrup attachment Ⓑ Qp Qh ♿ A

* L2260 Addition to lower extremity, reinforced solid stirrup (Scott-Craig type) Ⓑ Qp Qh ♿ A

* L2265 Addition to lower extremity, long tongue stirrup Ⓑ Qp Qh ♿ A

* L2270 Addition to lower extremity, varus/ valgus correction ('T') strap, padded/ lined or malleolus pad Ⓑ Qp Qh ♿ A

* L2275 Addition to lower extremity, varus/ valgus correction, plastic modification, padded/lined Ⓑ Qp Qh ♿ A

* L2280 Addition to lower extremity, molded inner boot Ⓑ Qp Qh ♿ A

* L2300 Addition to lower extremity, abduction bar (bilateral hip involvement), jointed, adjustable Ⓑ Qp Qh ♿ A

* L2310 Addition to lower extremity, abduction bar-straight Ⓑ Qp Qh ♿ A

* L2320 Addition to lower extremity, non-molded lacer, for custom fabricated orthosis only Ⓑ Qp Qh ♿ A

* L2330 Addition to lower extremity, lacer molded to patient model, for custom fabricated orthosis only Ⓑ Qp Qh ♿ A

  Used whether closure is lacer or Velcro

* L2335 Addition to lower extremity, anterior swing band Ⓑ Qp Qh ♿ A

* L2340 Addition to lower extremity, pre-tibial shell, molded to patient model Ⓑ Qp Qh ♿ A

* L2350 Addition to lower extremity, prosthetic type, (BK) socket, molded to patient model, (used for 'PTB' and 'AFO' orthoses) Ⓑ Qp Qh ♿ A

* L2360 Addition to lower extremity, extended steel shank Ⓑ Qp Qh ♿ A

* L2370 Addition to lower extremity, Patten bottom Ⓑ Qp Qh ♿ A

* L2375 Addition to lower extremity, torsion control, ankle joint and half solid stirrup Ⓑ Qp Qh ♿ A

* L2380 Addition to lower extremity, torsion control, straight knee joint, each joint Ⓑ Qp Qh ♿ A

* L2385 Addition to lower extremity, straight knee joint, heavy duty, each joint Ⓑ Qp ♿ A

* L2387 Addition to lower extremity, polycentric knee joint, for custom fabricated knee ankle foot orthosis, each joint Ⓑ Qp ♿ A

* L2390 Addition to lower extremity, offset knee joint, each joint Ⓑ Qp ♿ A

* L2395 Addition to lower extremity, offset knee joint, heavy duty, each joint Ⓑ Qp ♿ A

* L2397 Addition to lower extremity orthosis, suspension sleeve Ⓑ Qp ♿ A

Additions to Straight Knee or Offset Knee Joints

* L2405 Addition to knee joint, drop lock, each Ⓑ Qp ♿ A

* L2415 Addition to knee lock with integrated release mechanism (bail, cable, or equal), any material, each joint Ⓑ Qp ♿ A

* L2425 Addition to knee joint, disc or dial lock for adjustable knee flexion, each joint Ⓑ Qp ♿ A

* L2430 Addition to knee joint, ratchet lock for active and progressive knee extension, each joint Ⓑ Qp ♿ A

* L2492 Addition to knee joint, lift loop for drop lock ring Ⓑ Qp ♿ A

Additions to Thigh/Weight Bearing Gluteal/Ischial Weight Bearing

* L2500 Addition to lower extremity, thigh/ weight bearing, gluteal/ischial weight bearing, ring Ⓑ Qp Qh ♿ A

* L2510 Addition to lower extremity, thigh/ weight bearing, quadri-lateral brim, molded to patient model Ⓑ Qp Qh ♿ A

* L2520 Addition to lower extremity, thigh/ weight bearing, quadri-lateral brim, custom fitted Ⓑ Qp Qh ♿ A

* L2525 Addition to lower extremity, thigh/ weight bearing, ischial containment/ narrow M-L brim molded to patient model Ⓑ Qp Qh ♿ A

* L2526 Addition to lower extremity, thigh/ weight bearing, ischial containment/ narrow M-L brim, custom fitted Ⓑ Qp Qh ♿ A

* L2530 Addition to lower extremity, thigh-weight bearing, lacer, non-molded Ⓑ Qp Qh ♿ A

* L2540 Addition to lower extremity, thigh/ weight bearing, lacer, molded to patient model Ⓑ Qp Qh ♿ A

* L2550 Addition to lower extremity, thigh/ weight bearing, high roll cuff Ⓑ Qp Qh ♿ A

Additions to Pelvic and Thoracic Control

* L2570 Addition to lower extremity, pelvic control, hip joint, Clevis type two position joint, each Ⓔ Qp Qh ♿ A
* L2580 Addition to lower extremity, pelvic control, pelvic sling Ⓔ Qp Qh ♿ A
* L2600 Addition to lower extremity, pelvic control, hip joint, Clevis type, or thrust bearing, free, each Ⓔ Qp Qh ♿ A
* L2610 Addition to lower extremity, pelvic control, hip joint, Clevis or thrust bearing, lock, each Ⓔ Qp Qh ♿ A
* L2620 Addition to lower extremity, pelvic control, hip joint, heavy duty, each Ⓔ Qp Qh ♿ A
* L2622 Addition to lower extremity, pelvic control, hip joint, adjustable flexion, each Ⓔ Qp Qh ♿ A
* L2624 Addition to lower extremity, pelvic control, hip joint, adjustable flexion, extension, abduction control, each Ⓔ Qp Qh ♿ A
* L2627 Addition to lower extremity, pelvic control, plastic, molded to patient model, reciprocating hip joint and cables Ⓔ Qp Qh ♿ A
* L2628 Addition to lower extremity, pelvic control, metal frame, reciprocating hip joint and cables Ⓔ Qp Qh ♿ A
* L2630 Addition to lower extremity, pelvic control, band and belt, unilateral Ⓔ Qp Qh ♿ A
* L2640 Addition to lower extremity, pelvic control, band and belt, bilateral Ⓔ Qp Qh ♿ A
* L2650 Addition to lower extremity, pelvic and thoracic control, gluteal pad, each Ⓔ Qp Qh ♿ A
* L2660 Addition to lower extremity, thoracic control, thoracic band Ⓔ Qp Qh ♿ A
* L2670 Addition to lower extremity, thoracic control, paraspinal uprights Ⓔ Qp Qh ♿ A
* L2680 Addition to lower extremity, thoracic control, lateral support uprights Ⓔ Qp Qh ♿ A

General Additions

* L2750 Addition to lower extremity orthosis, plating chrome or nickel, per bar Ⓔ Qp ♿ A
* L2755 Addition to lower extremity orthosis, high strength, lightweight material, all hybrid lamination/prepreg composite, per segment, for custom fabricated orthosis only Ⓔ Qp ♿ A
* L2760 Addition to lower extremity orthosis, extension, per extension, per bar (for lineal adjustment for growth) Ⓔ Qp ♿ A
* L2768 Orthotic side bar disconnect device, per bar Ⓔ Qp ♿ A
* L2780 Addition to lower extremity orthosis, non-corrosive finish, per bar Ⓔ Qp ♿ A
* L2785 Addition to lower extremity orthosis, drop lock retainer, each Ⓔ Qp ♿ A
* L2795 Addition to lower extremity orthosis, knee control, full kneecap Ⓔ Qp Qh ♿ A
* L2800 Addition to lower extremity orthosis, knee control, knee cap, medial or lateral pull, for use with custom fabricated orthosis only Ⓔ Qp Qh ♿ A
* L2810 Addition to lower extremity orthosis, knee control, condylar pad Ⓔ Qp ♿ A
* L2820 Addition to lower extremity orthosis, soft interface for molded plastic, below knee section Ⓔ Qp Qh ♿ A

  Only report if soft interface provided, either leather or other material
* L2830 Addition to lower extremity orthosis, soft interface for molded plastic, above knee section Ⓔ Qp Qh ♿ A
* L2840 Addition to lower extremity orthosis, tibial length sock, fracture or equal, each Ⓔ Qp ♿ A
* L2850 Addition to lower extremity orthosis, femoral length sock, fracture or equal, each Ⓔ Qp ♿ A

⃠ L2861 Addition to lower extremity joint, knee or ankle, concentric adjustable torsion style mechanism for custom fabricated orthotics only, each Ⓔ Qp Qh E1

* L2999 Lower extremity orthoses, not otherwise specified Ⓔ A

► New ↻ Revised ✓ Reinstated ~~deleted~~ Deleted ⃠ Not covered or valid by Medicare
Special coverage instructions * Carrier discretion Ⓑ Bill Part B MAC Ⓔ Bill DME MAC

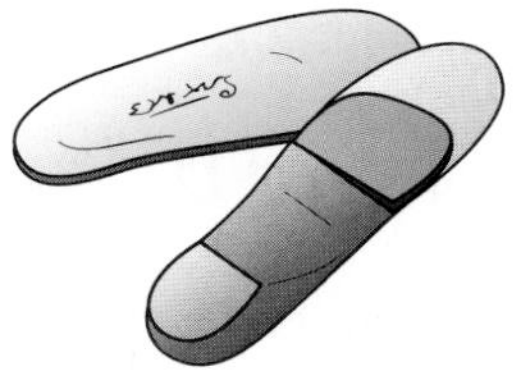

Figure 31 Foot inserts.

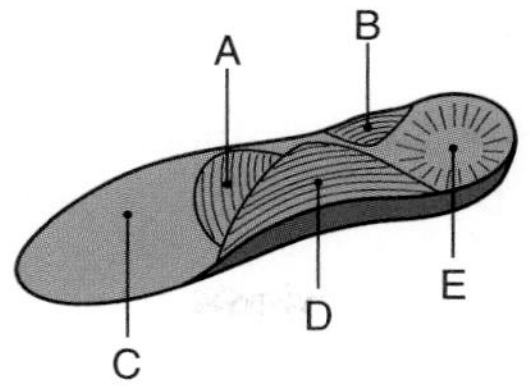
A
B
C
D
E

Figure 32 Arch support.

Foot (Orthopedic Shoes) (L3000-L3649)

Inserts

L3000 Foot, insert, removable, molded to patient model, 'UCB' type, Berkeley shell, each Qp Qh A

If both feet casted and supplied with an orthosis, bill L3000-LT and L3000-RT

IOM: 100-02, 15, 290

L3001 Foot, insert, removable, molded to patient model, Spenco, each Qp Qh A

IOM: 100-02, 15, 290

L3002 Foot, insert, removable, molded to patient model, Plastazote or equal, each Qp Qh A

IOM: 100-02, 15, 290

L3003 Foot, insert, removable, molded to patient model, silicone gel, each Qp Qh A

IOM: 100-02, 15, 290

L3010 Foot, insert, removable, molded to patient model, longitudinal arch support, each Qp Qh A

IOM: 100-02, 15, 290

L3020 Foot, insert, removable, molded to patient model, longitudinal/metatarsal support, each Qp Qh A

IOM: 100-02, 15, 290

L3030 Foot, insert, removable, formed to patient foot, each Qp Qh A

IOM: 100-02, 15, 290

* **L3031** Foot, insert/plate, removable, addition to lower extremity orthosis, high strength, lightweight material, all hybrid lamination/prepreg composite, each Qp Qh A

Arch Support, Removable, Premolded

L3040 Foot, arch support, removable, premolded, longitudinal, each Qp Qh A

IOM: 100-02, 15, 290

L3050 Foot, arch support, removable, premolded, metatarsal, each Qp Qh A

IOM: 100-02, 15, 290

L3060 Foot, arch support, removable, premolded, longitudinal/metatarsal, each Qp Qh A

IOM: 100-02, 15, 290

Arch Support, Non-removable, Attached to Shoe

L3070 Foot, arch support, non-removable attached to shoe, longitudinal, each Qp Qh A

IOM: 100-02, 15, 290

L3080 Foot, arch support, non-removable attached to shoe, metatarsal, each Qp Qh A

IOM: 100-02, 15, 290

L3090 Foot, arch support, non-removable attached to shoe, longitudinal/metatarsal, each Qp Qh A

IOM: 100-02, 15, 290

L3100 Hallus-valgus night dynamic splint, prefabricated, off-the-shelf Qp Qh A

IOM: 100-02, 15, 290

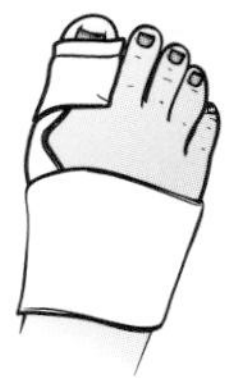

Figure 33 Hallux valgus splint.

Abduction and Rotation Bars

L3140 Foot, abduction rotation bar, including shoes Qp Qh — A
IOM: 100-02, 15, 290

L3150 Foot, abduction rotation bar, without shoes Qp Qh — A
IOM: 100-02, 15, 290

* **L3160** Foot, adjustable shoe-styled positioning device Qp Qh — A

L3170 Foot, plastic, silicone or equal, heel stabilizer, prefabricated, off-the-shelf, each Qp Qh — A
IOM: 100-02, 15, 290

Orthopedic Footwear

L3201 Orthopedic shoe, oxford with supinator or pronator, infant A — A
IOM: 100-02, 15, 290

L3202 Orthopedic shoe, oxford with supinator or pronator, child A — A
IOM: 100-02, 15, 290

L3203 Orthopedic shoe, oxford with supinator or pronator, junior A — A
IOM: 100-02, 15, 290

L3204 Orthopedic shoe, hightop with supinator or pronator, infant A — A
IOM: 100-02, 15, 290

L3206 Orthopedic shoe, hightop with supinator or pronator, child A — A
IOM: 100-02, 15, 290

L3207 Orthopedic shoe, hightop with supinator or pronator, junior A — A
IOM: 100-02, 15, 290

L3208 Surgical boot, infant, each A — A
IOM: 100-02, 15, 100

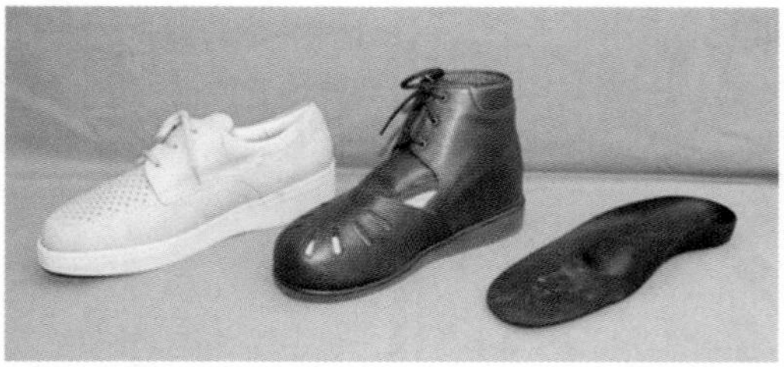

Figure 34 Molded custom shoe.

L3209 Surgical boot, each, child A — A
IOM: 100-02, 15, 100

L3211 Surgical boot, each, junior A — A
IOM: 100-02, 15, 100

L3212 Benesch boot, pair, infant A — A
IOM: 100-02, 15, 100

L3213 Benesch boot, pair, child A — A
IOM: 100-02, 15, 100

L3214 Benesch boot, pair, junior A — A
IOM: 100-02, 15, 100

⃠ **L3215** Orthopedic footwear, ladies shoe, oxford, each Qp Qh ♀ — E1
Medicare Statute 1862a8

⃠ **L3216** Orthopedic footwear, ladies shoe, depth inlay, each Qp Qh ♀ — E1
Medicare Statute 1862a8

⃠ **L3217** Orthopedic footwear, ladies shoe, hightop, depth inlay, each Qp Qh ♀ — E1
Medicare Statute 1862a8

⃠ **L3219** Orthopedic footwear, mens shoe, oxford, each Qp Qh ♂ — E1
Medicare Statute 1862a8

⃠ **L3221** Orthopedic footwear, mens shoe, depth inlay, each Qp Qh ♂ — E1
Medicare Statute 1862a8

⃠ **L3222** Orthopedic footwear, mens shoe, hightop, depth inlay, each Qp Qh ♂ — E1
Medicare Statute 1862a8

L3224 Orthopedic footwear, ladies shoe, oxford, used as an integral part of a brace (orthosis) Qp Qh ♀ — A
IOM: 100-02, 15, 290

L3225 Orthopedic footwear, mens shoe, oxford, used as an integral part of a brace (orthosis) Qp Qh ♀ — A
IOM: 100-02, 15, 290

L3230 Orthopedic footwear, custom shoe, depth inlay, each Qp Qh — A
IOM: 100-02, 15, 290

L3250 Orthopedic footwear, custom molded shoe, removable inner mold, prosthetic shoe, each Qp Qh — A
IOM: 100-02, 15, 290

L3251 Foot, shoe molded to patient model, silicone shoe, each Qp Qh — A
IOM: 100-02, 15, 290

L3252 Foot, shoe molded to patient model, Plastazote (or similar), custom fabricated, each Qp Qh A
IOM: 100-02, 15, 290

L3253 Foot, molded shoe Plastazote (or similar), custom fitted, each Qp Qh A
IOM: 100-02, 15, 290

L3254 Non-standard size or width A
IOM: 100-02, 15, 290

L3255 Non-standard size or length A
IOM: 100-02, 15, 290

L3257 Orthopedic footwear, additional charge for split size A
IOM: 100-02, 15, 290

L3260 Surgical boot/shoe, each E1
IOM: 100-02, 15, 100

* L3265 Plastazote sandal, each A

Shoe Lifts

L3300 Lift, elevation, heel, tapered to metatarsals, per inch Qp A
IOM: 100-02, 15, 290

L3310 Lift, elevation, heel and sole, Neoprene, per inch Qp A
IOM: 100-02, 15, 290

L3320 Lift, elevation, heel and sole, cork, per inch Qp A
IOM: 100-02, 15, 290

L3330 Lift, elevation, metal extension (skate) Qp Qh A
IOM: 100-02, 15, 290

L3332 Lift, elevation, inside shoe, tapered, up to one-half inch Qp Qh A
IOM: 100-02, 15, 290

L3334 Lift, elevation, heel, per inch Qp A
IOM: 100-02, 15, 290

Shoe Wedges

L3340 Heel wedge, SACH Qp Qh A
IOM: 100-02, 15, 290

L3350 Heel wedge Qp Qh A
IOM: 100-02, 15, 290

L3360 Sole wedge, outside sole Qp Qh A
IOM: 100-02, 15, 290

L3370 Sole wedge, between sole Qp Qh A
IOM: 100-02, 15, 290

L3380 Clubfoot wedge Qp Qh A
IOM: 100-02, 15, 290

L3390 Outflare wedge Qp Qh A
IOM: 100-02, 15, 290

L3400 Metatarsal bar wedge, rocker Qp Qh A
IOM: 100-02, 15, 290

L3410 Metatarsal bar wedge, between sole Qp Qh A
IOM: 100-02, 15, 290

L3420 Full sole and heel wedge, between sole Qp Qh A
IOM: 100-02, 15, 290

Shoe Heels

L3430 Heel, counter, plastic reinforced Qp Qh A
IOM: 100-02, 15, 290

L3440 Heel, counter, leather reinforced Qp Qh A
IOM: 100-02, 15, 290

L3450 Heel, SACH cushion type Qp Qh A
IOM: 100-02, 15, 290

L3455 Heel, new leather, standard Qp Qh A
IOM: 100-02, 15, 290

L3460 Heel, new rubber, standard Qp Qh A
IOM: 100-02, 15, 290

L3465 Heel, Thomas with wedge Qp Qh A
IOM: 100-02, 15, 290

L3470 Heel, Thomas extended to ball Qp Qh A
IOM: 100-02, 15, 290

L3480 Heel, pad and depression for spur Qp Qh A
IOM: 100-02, 15, 290

L3485 Heel, pad, removable for spur Qp Qh A
IOM: 100-02, 15, 290

Orthopedic Shoe Additions: Other

L3500 Orthopedic shoe addition, insole, leather Qp Qh A
IOM: 100-02, 15, 290

MIPS | Qp Quantity Physician | Qh Quantity Hospital | ♀ Female only
♂ Male only | A Age | DMEPOS | A2-Z3 ASC Payment Indicator | A-Y ASC Status Indicator | Coding Clinic

L3510 Orthopedic shoe addition, insole, rubber Ⓔ Qp Qh ♿ A
IOM: 100-02, 15, 290

L3520 Orthopedic shoe addition, insole, felt covered with leather Ⓔ Qp Qh ♿ A
IOM: 100-02, 15, 290

L3530 Orthopedic shoe addition, sole, half Ⓔ Qp Qh ♿ A
IOM: 100-02, 15, 290

L3540 Orthopedic shoe addition, sole, full Ⓔ Qp Qh ♿ A
IOM: 100-02, 15, 290

L3550 Orthopedic shoe addition, toe tap standard Ⓔ Qp Qh ♿ A
IOM: 100-02, 15, 290

L3560 Orthopedic shoe addition, toe tap, horseshoe Ⓔ Qp Qh ♿ A
IOM: 100-02, 15, 290

L3570 Orthopedic shoe addition, special extension to instep (leather with eyelets) Ⓔ Qp Qh ♿ A
IOM: 100-02, 15, 290

L3580 Orthopedic shoe addition, convert instep to Velcro closure Ⓔ Qp Qh ♿ A
IOM: 100-02, 15, 290

L3590 Orthopedic shoe addition, convert firm shoe counter to soft counter Ⓔ Qp Qh ♿ A
IOM: 100-02, 15, 290

L3595 Orthopedic shoe addition, March bar Ⓔ Qp Qh ♿ A
IOM: 100-02, 15, 290

Transfer or Replacement

L3600 Transfer of an orthosis from one shoe to another, caliper plate, existing Ⓔ Qp Qh ♿ A
IOM: 100-02, 15, 290

L3610 Transfer of an orthosis from one shoe to another, caliper plate, new Ⓔ Qp Qh ♿ A
IOM: 100-02, 15, 290

L3620 Transfer of an orthosis from one shoe to another, solid stirrup, existing Ⓔ Qp Qh ♿ A
IOM: 100-02, 15, 290

L3630 Transfer of an orthosis from one shoe to another, solid stirrup, new Ⓔ Qp Qh ♿ A
IOM: 100-02, 15, 290

L3640 Transfer of an orthosis from one shoe to another, Dennis Browne splint (Riveton), both shoes Ⓔ Qp Qh ♿ A
IOM: 100-02, 15, 290

L3649 Orthopedic shoe, modification, addition or transfer, not otherwise specified Ⓔ A
IOM: 100-02, 15, 290

Orthotic Devices: Upper Limb

Note: The procedures in this section are considered as base or basic procedures and may be modified by listing procedures from the Additions section and adding them to the base procedure.

Shoulder

* **L3650** Shoulder orthosis, figure of eight design abduction restrainer, prefabricated, off-the-shelf Ⓔ Qp Qh ♿ A

* **L3660** Shoulder orthosis, figure of eight design abduction restrainer, canvas and webbing, prefabricated, off-the-shelf Ⓔ Qp Qh ♿ A

* **L3670** Shoulder orthosis, acromio/clavicular (canvas and webbing type), prefabricated, off-the-shelf Ⓔ Qp Qh ♿ A

* **L3671** Shoulder orthosis, shoulder joint design, without joints, may include soft interface, straps, custom fabricated, includes fitting and adjustment Ⓔ Qp Qh ♿ A

* **L3674** Shoulder orthosis, abduction positioning (airplane design), thoracic component and support bar, with or without nontorsion joint/turnbuckle, may include soft interface, straps, custom fabricated, includes fitting and adjustment Ⓔ Qp Qh ♿ A

* **L3675** Shoulder orthosis, vest type abduction restrainer, canvas webbing type or equal, prefabricated, off-the-shelf Ⓔ Qp Qh ♿ A

L3677 Shoulder orthosis, shoulder joint design, without joints, may include soft interface, straps, prefabricated item that has been trimmed, bent, molded, assembled, or otherwise customized to fit a specific patient by an individual with expertise Ⓔ Qp Qh A

* **L3678** Shoulder orthosis, shoulder joint design, without joints, may include soft interface, straps, prefabricated, off-the-shelf Ⓔ Qp Qh A

▶ New ↻ Revised ✔ Reinstated ~~deleted~~ Deleted ⃠ Not covered or valid by Medicare
Special coverage instructions * Carrier discretion Ⓑ Bill Part B MAC Ⓔ Bill DME MAC

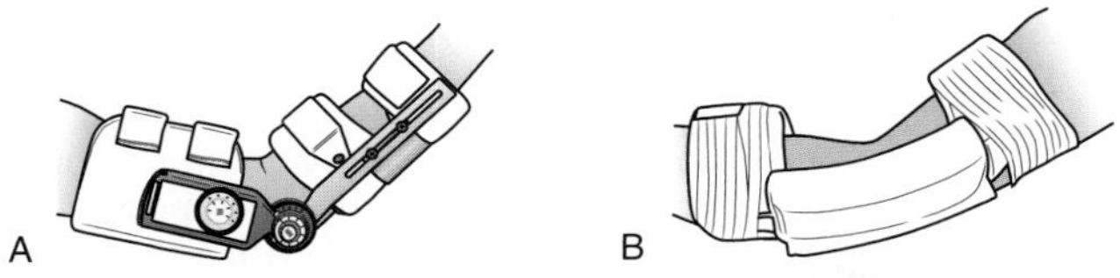
A
B

Figure 35 Elbow orthoses.

Elbow

✻ **L3702** Elbow orthosis, without joints, may include soft interface, straps, custom fabricated, includes fitting and adjustment Ⓑ Qp Qh ♿ A

✻ **L3710** Elbow orthosis, elastic with metal joints, prefabricated, off-the-shelf Ⓑ Qp Qh ♿ A

✻ **L3720** Elbow orthosis, double upright with forearm/arm cuffs, free motion, custom fabricated Ⓑ Qp Qh ♿ A

✻ **L3730** Elbow orthosis, double upright with forearm/arm cuffs, extension/flexion assist, custom fabricated Ⓑ Qp Qh ♿ A

✻ **L3740** Elbow orthosis, double upright with forearm/arm cuffs, adjustable position lock with active control, custom fabricated Ⓑ Qp Qh ♿ A

✻**L3760** Elbow orthosis (EO), with adjustable position locking joint(s), prefabricated, item that has been trimmed, bent, molded, assembled, or otherwise customized to fit a specific patient by an individual with expertise Ⓑ Qp Qh ♿ A

✻ **L3761** Elbow orthosis (EO), with adjustable position locking joint(s), prefabricated, off-the-shelf A

✻ **L3762** Elbow orthosis, rigid, without joints, includes soft interface material, prefabricated, off-the-shelf Ⓑ Qp Qh ♿ A

✻ **L3763** Elbow wrist hand orthosis, rigid, without joints, may include soft interface, straps, custom fabricated, includes fitting and adjustment Ⓑ Qp Qh ♿ A

✻ **L3764** Elbow wrist hand orthosis, includes one or more nontorsion joints, elastic bands, turnbuckles, may include soft interface, straps, custom fabricated, includes fitting and adjustment Ⓑ Qp Qh ♿ A

✻ **L3765** Elbow wrist hand finger orthosis, rigid, without joints, may include soft interface, straps, custom fabricated, includes fitting and adjustment Ⓑ Qp Qh ♿ A

✻ **L3766** Elbow wrist hand finger orthosis, includes one or more nontorsion joints, elastic bands, turnbuckles, may include soft interface, straps, custom fabricated, includes fitting and adjustment Ⓑ Qp Qh ♿ A

Wrist-Hand-Finger Orthosis (WHFO)

✻ **L3806** Wrist hand finger orthosis, includes one or more nontorsion joint(s), turnbuckles, elastic bands/springs, may include soft interface material, straps, custom fabricated, includes fitting and adjustment Ⓑ Qp Qh ♿ A

✻ **L3807** Wrist hand finger orthosis, without joint(s), prefabricated item that has been trimmed, bent, molded, assembled, or otherwise customized to fit a specific patient by an individual with expertise Ⓑ Qp Qh ♿ A

✻ **L3808** Wrist hand finger orthosis, rigid without joints, may include soft interface material; straps, custom fabricated, includes fitting and adjustment Ⓑ Qp Qh ♿ A

✻ **L3809** Wrist hand finger orthosis, without joint(s), prefabricated, off-the-shelf, any type Ⓑ Qp Qh ♿ A

⃠ **L3891** Addition to upper extremity joint, wrist or elbow, concentric adjustable torsion style mechanism for custom fabricated orthotics only, each Ⓑ Qp Qh E1

✻ **L3900** Wrist hand finger orthosis, dynamic flexor hinge, reciprocal wrist extension/flexion, finger flexion/extension, wrist or finger driven, custom fabricated Ⓑ Qp Qh ♿ A

✻ **L3901** Wrist hand finger orthosis, dynamic flexor hinge, reciprocal wrist extension/flexion, finger flexion/extension, cable driven, custom fabricated Ⓑ Qp Qh ♿ A

✻ **L3904** Wrist hand finger orthosis, external powered, electric, custom fabricated Ⓑ Qp Qh ♿ A

Other Upper Extremity Orthotics

* **L3905** Wrist hand orthosis, includes one or more nontorsion joints, elastic bands, turnbuckles, may include soft interface, straps, custom fabricated, includes fitting and adjustment Ⓔ Qp Qh ♿ A
* **L3906** Wrist hand orthosis, without joints, may include soft interface, straps, custom fabricated, includes fitting and adjustment Ⓔ Qp Qh ♿ A
* **L3908** Wrist hand orthosis, wrist extension control cock-up, non-molded, prefabricated, off-the-shelf Ⓔ Qp Qh ♿ A
* **L3912** Hand finger orthosis (HFO), flexion glove with elastic finger control, prefabricated, off-the-shelf Ⓔ Qp Qh ♿ A
* **L3913** Hand finger orthosis, without joints, may include soft interface, straps, custom fabricated, includes fitting and adjustment Ⓔ Qp Qh ♿ A
* **L3915** Wrist hand orthosis, includes one or more nontorsion joint(s), elastic bands, turnbuckles, may include soft interface, straps, prefabricated item that has been trimmed, bent, molded, assembled, or otherwise customized to fit a specific patient by an individual with expertise Ⓔ Qp Qh ♿ A
* **L3916** Wrist hand orthosis, includes one or more nontorsion joint(s), elastic bands, turnbuckles, may include soft interface, straps, prefabricated, off-the-shelf Ⓔ Qp Qh ♿ A
* **L3917** Hand orthosis, metacarpal fracture orthosis, prefabricated item that has been trimmed, bent, molded, assembled, or otherwise customized to fit a specific patient by an individual with expertise Ⓔ Qp Qh ♿ A
* **L3918** Hand orthosis, metacarpal fracture orthosis, prefabricated, off-the-shelf Ⓔ Qp Qh ♿ A
* **L3919** Hand orthosis, without joints, may include soft interface, straps, custom fabricated, includes fitting and adjustment Ⓔ Qp Qh ♿ A
* **L3921** Hand finger orthosis, includes one or more nontorsion joints, elastic bands, turnbuckles, may include soft interface, straps, custom fabricated, includes fitting and adjustment Ⓔ Qp Qh ♿ A
* **L3923** Hand finger orthosis, without joints, may include soft interface, straps, prefabricated item that has been trimmed, bent, molded, assembled, or otherwise customized to fit a specific patient by an individual with expertise Ⓔ Qp Qh ♿ A
* **L3924** Hand finger orthosis, without joints, may include soft interface, straps, prefabricated, off-the-shelf Ⓔ Qp Qh ♿ A
* **L3925** Finger orthosis, proximal interphalangeal (PIP)/distal interphalangeal (DIP), non torsion joint/spring, extension/flexion, may include soft interface material, prefabricated, off-the-shelf Ⓔ Qp Qh ♿ A
* **L3927** Finger orthosis, proximal interphalangeal (PIP)/distal interphalangeal (DIP), without joint/spring, extension/flexion (e.g., static or ring type), may include soft interface material, prefabricated, off-the-shelf Ⓔ Qp Qh ♿ A
* **L3929** Hand finger orthosis, includes one or more nontorsion joint(s), turnbuckles, elastic bands/springs, may include soft interface material, straps, prefabricated item that has been trimmed, bent, molded, assembled, or otherwise customized to fit a specific patient by an individual with expertise Ⓔ Qp Qh ♿ A
* **L3930** Hand finger orthosis, includes one or more nontorsion joint(s), turnbuckles, elastic bands/springs, may include soft interface material, straps, prefabricated, off-the-shelf Ⓔ Qp Qh ♿ A
* **L3931** Wrist hand finger orthosis, includes one or more nontorsion joint(s), turnbuckles, elastic bands/springs, may include soft interface material, straps, prefabricated, includes fitting and adjustment Ⓔ Qp Qh ♿ A
* **L3933** Finger orthosis, without joints, may include soft interface, custom fabricated, includes fitting and adjustment Ⓔ Qp Qh ♿ A
* **L3935** Finger orthosis, nontorsion joint, may include soft interface, custom fabricated, includes fitting and adjustment Ⓔ Qp Qh ♿ A
* **L3956** Addition of joint to upper extremity orthosis, any material, per joint Ⓔ Qp ♿ A

Shoulder-Elbow-Wrist-Hand Orthotics (SEWHO) (L3960-L3973)

✻ **L3960** Shoulder elbow wrist hand orthosis, abduction positioning, airplane design, prefabricated, includes fitting and adjustment Ⓑ Qp Qh ♿ A

✻ **L3961** Shoulder elbow wrist hand orthosis, shoulder cap design, without joints, may include soft interface, straps, custom fabricated, includes fitting and adjustment Ⓑ Qp Qh ♿ A

✻ **L3962** Shoulder elbow wrist hand orthosis, abduction positioning, Erb's palsy design, prefabricated, includes fitting and adjustment Ⓑ Qp Qh ♿ A

✻ **L3967** Shoulder elbow wrist hand orthosis, abduction positioning (airplane design), thoracic component and support bar, without joints, may include soft interface, straps, custom fabricated, includes fitting and adjustment Ⓑ Qp Qh ♿ A

✻ **L3971** Shoulder elbow wrist hand orthosis, shoulder cap design, includes one or more nontorsion joints, elastic bands, turnbuckles, may include soft interface, straps, custom fabricated, includes fitting and adjustment Ⓑ Qp Qh ♿ A

✻ **L3973** Shoulder elbow wrist hand orthosis, abduction positioning (airplane design), thoracic component and support bar, includes one or more nontorsion joints, elastic bands, turnbuckles, may include soft interface, straps, custom fabricated, includes fitting and adjustment Ⓑ Qp Qh ♿ A

Shoulder-Elbow-Wrist-Hand-Finger Orthotics

✻ **L3975** Shoulder elbow wrist hand finger orthosis, shoulder cap design, without joints, may include soft interface, straps, custom fabricated, includes fitting and adjustment Ⓑ Qp Qh ♿ A

✻ **L3976** Shoulder elbow wrist hand finger orthosis, abduction positioning (airplane design), thoracic component and support bar, without joints, may include soft interface, straps, custom fabricated, includes fitting and adjustment Ⓑ Qp Qh ♿ A

✻ **L3977** Shoulder elbow wrist hand finger orthosis, shoulder cap design, includes one or more nontorsion joints, elastic bands, turnbuckles, may include soft interface, straps, custom fabricated, includes fitting and adjustment Ⓑ Qp Qh ♿ A

✻ **L3978** Shoulder elbow wrist hand finger orthosis, abduction positioning (airplane design), thoracic component and support bar, includes one or more nontorsion joints, elastic bands, turnbuckles, may include soft interface, straps, custom fabricated, includes fitting and adjustment Ⓑ Qp Qh ♿ A

Fracture Orthorics

✻ **L3980** Upper extremity fracture orthosis, humeral, prefabricated, includes fitting and adjustment Ⓑ Qp Qh ♿ A

✻ **L3981** Upper extremity fracture orthosis, humeral, prefabricated, includes shoulder cap design, with or without joints, forearm section, may include soft interface, straps, includes fitting and adjustments Ⓑ Qp Qh ♿ A

✻ **L3982** Upper extremity fracture orthosis, radius/ulnar, prefabricated, includes fitting and adjustment Ⓑ Qp Qh ♿ A

✻ **L3984** Upper extremity fracture orthosis, wrist, prefabricated, includes fitting and adjustment Ⓑ Qp Qh ♿ A

✻ **L3995** Addition to upper extremity orthosis, sock, fracture or equal, each Ⓑ Qp ♿ A

✻ **L3999** Upper limb orthosis, not otherwise specified Ⓑ A

Repairs

✻ **L4000** Replace girdle for spinal orthosis (CTLSO or SO) Ⓑ Qp Qh ♿ A

✻ **L4002** Replacement strap, any orthosis, includes all components, any length, any type Ⓑ Qp ♿ A

✻ **L4010** Replace trilateral socket brim Ⓑ Qp Qh ♿ A

✻ **L4020** Replace quadrilateral socket brim, molded to patient model Ⓑ Qp Qh ♿ A

✻ **L4030** Replace quadrilateral socket brim, custom fitted Ⓑ Qp Qh ♿ A

✻ **L4040** Replace molded thigh lacer, for custom fabricated orthosis only Ⓑ Qp Qh ♿ A

✻ **L4045** Replace non-molded thigh lacer, for custom fabricated orthosis only Ⓑ Qp Qh ♿ A

✻ **L4050** Replace molded calf lacer, for custom fabricated orthosis only Ⓑ Qp Qh ♿ A

* **L4055** Replace non-molded calf lacer, for custom fabricated orthosis only Qp Qh A
* **L4060** Replace high roll cuff Qp Qh A
* **L4070** Replace proximal and distal upright for KAFO Qp Qh A
* **L4080** Replace metal bands KAFO, proximal thigh Qp Qh A
* **L4090** Replace metal bands KAFO-AFO, calf or distal thigh Qp A
* **L4100** Replace leather cuff KAFO, proximal thigh Qp Qh A
* **L4110** Replace leather cuff KAFO-AFO, calf or distal thigh Qp A
* **L4130** Replace pretibial shell Qp Qh A
* **L4205** Repair of orthotic device, labor component, per 15 minutes Qp A

  IOM: 100-02, 15, 110.2

* **L4210** Repair of orthotic device, repair or replace minor parts Qp Qh A

  IOM: 100-02, 15, 110.2; 100-02, 15, 120

Ancillary Orthotic Services

* **L4350** Ankle control orthosis, stirrup style, rigid, includes any type interface (e.g., pneumatic, gel), prefabricated, off-the-shelf Qp Qh A
* **L4360** Walking boot, pneumatic and/or vacuum, with or without joints, with or without interface material, prefabricated item that has been trimmed, bent, molded, assembled, or otherwise customized to fit a specific patient by an individual with expertise Qp Qh A

  Noncovered when walking boots used primarily to relieve pressure, especially on sole of foot, or are used for patients with foot ulcers

* **L4361** Walking boot, pneumatic and/or vacuum, with or without joints, with or without interface material, prefabricated, off-the-shelf Qp Qh A
* **L4370** Pneumatic full leg splint, prefabricated, off-the-shelf Qp Qh A
* **L4386** Walking boot, non-pneumatic, with or without joints, with or without interface material, prefabricated item that has been trimmed, bent, molded, assembled, or otherwise customized to fit a specific patient by an individual with expertise Qp Qh A
* **L4387** Walking boot, non-pneumatic, with or without joints, with or without interface material, prefabricated, off-the-shelf Qp Qh A
* **L4392** Replacement, soft interface material, static AFO Qp Qh A
* **L4394** Replace soft interface material, foot drop splint Qp Qh A
* **L4396** Static or dynamic ankle foot orthosis, including soft interface material, adjustable for fit, for positioning, may be used for minimal ambulation, prefabricated item that has been trimmed, bent, molded, assembled, or otherwise customized to fit a specific patient by an individual with expertise Qp Qh A
* **L4397** Static or dynamic ankle foot orthosis, including soft interface material, adjustable for fit, for positioning, may be used for minimal ambulation, prefabricated, off-the-shelf Qp Qh A
* **L4398** Foot drop splint, recumbent positioning device, prefabricated, off-the-shelf Qp Qh A
* **L4631** Ankle foot orthosis, walking boot type, varus/valgus correction, rocker bottom, anterior tibial shell, soft interface, custom arch support, plastic or other material, includes straps and closures, custom fabricated Qp Qh A

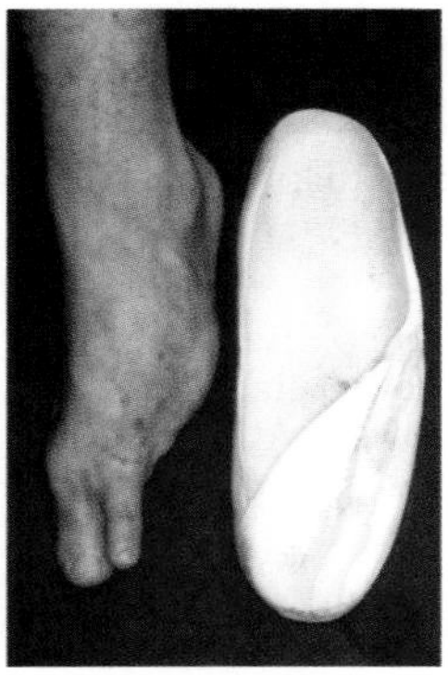

Figure 36 Partial foot.

PROSTHETICS (L5000-L9999)

Lower Limb (L5000-L5999)

NOTE: The procedures in this section are considered as base or basic proceduresand may be modified by listing items/procedures or special materials from the Additions section and adding them to the base procedure.

Partial Foot

L5000 Partial foot, shoe insert with longitudinal arch, toe filler Ⓑ Qp Qh ♿ A
IOM: 100-02, 15, 290

L5010 Partial foot, molded socket, ankle height, with toe filler Ⓑ Qp Qh ♿ A
IOM: 100-02, 15, 290

L5020 Partial foot, molded socket, tibial tubercle height, with toe filler Ⓑ Qp Qh ♿ A
IOM: 100-02, 15, 290

Ankle

* **L5050** Ankle, Symes, molded socket, SACH foot Ⓑ Qp Qh ♿ A

* **L5060** Ankle, Symes, metal frame, molded leather socket, articulated ankle/foot Ⓑ Qp Qh ♿ A

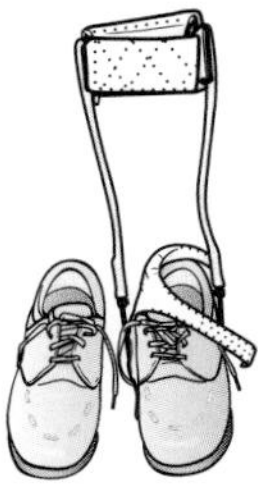

Figure 37 Ankle Symes.

Below Knee

* **L5100** Below knee, molded socket, shin, SACH foot Ⓑ Qp Qh ♿ A

* **L5105** Below knee, plastic socket, joints and thigh lacer, SACH foot Ⓑ Qp Qh ♿ A

Knee Disarticulation

* **L5150** Knee disarticulation (or through knee), molded socket, external knee joints, shin, SACH foot Ⓑ Qp Qh ♿ A

* **L5160** Knee disarticulation (or through knee), molded socket, bent knee configuration, external knee joints, shin, SACH foot Ⓑ Qp Qh ♿ A

Above Knee

* **L5200** Above knee, molded socket, single axis constant friction knee, shin, SACH foot Ⓑ Qp Qh ♿ A

* **L5210** Above knee, short prosthesis, no knee joint ('stubbies'), with foot blocks, no ankle joints, each Ⓑ Qp Qh ♿ A

* **L5220** Above knee, short prosthesis, no knee joint ('stubbies'), with articulated ankle/foot, dynamically aligned, each Ⓑ Qp Qh ♿ A

* **L5230** Above knee, for proximal femoral focal deficiency, constant friction knee, shin, SACH foot Ⓑ Qp Qh ♿ A

Hip Disarticulation

* **L5250** Hip disarticulation, Canadian type; molded socket, hip joint, single axis constant friction knee, shin, SACH foot Ⓑ Qp Qh ♿ A

* **L5270** Hip disarticulation, tilt table type; molded socket, locking hip joint, single axis constant friction knee, shin, SACH foot Ⓑ Qp Qh ♿ A

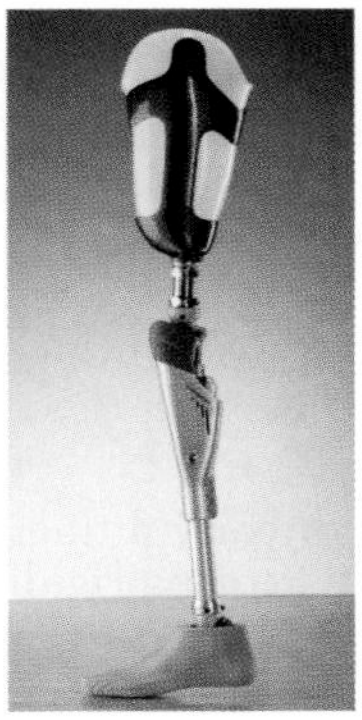

Figure 38 Above knee.

Hemipelvectomy

* **L5280** Hemipelvectomy, Canadian type; molded socket, hip joint, single axis constant friction knee, shin, SACH foot Ⓑ Qp Qh ♿ A

Endoskeletal

* **L5301** Below knee, molded socket, shin, SACH foot, endoskeletal system Ⓑ Qp Qh ♿ A
* **L5312** Knee disarticulation (or through knee), molded socket, single axis knee, pylon, sach foot, endoskeletal system Ⓑ Qp Qh ♿ A
* **L5321** Above knee, molded socket, open end, SACH foot, endoskeletal system, single axis knee Ⓑ Qp Qh ♿ A
* **L5331** Hip disarticulation, Canadian type, molded socket, endoskeletal system, hip joint, single axis knee, SACH foot Ⓑ Qp Qh ♿ A
* **L5341** Hemipelvectomy, Canadian type, molded socket, endoskeletal system, hip joint, single axis knee, SACH foot Ⓑ Qp Qh ♿ A

Immediate Postsurgical or Early Fitting Procedures

* **L5400** Immediate post surgical or early fitting, application of initial rigid dressing, including fitting, alignment, suspension, and one cast change, below knee Ⓑ Qp Qh ♿ A
* **L5410** Immediate post surgical or early fitting, application of initial rigid dressing, including fitting, alignment and suspension, below knee, each additional cast change and realignment Ⓑ Qp Qh ♿ A
* **L5420** Immediate post surgical or early fitting, application of initial rigid dressing, including fitting, alignment and suspension and one cast change 'AK' or knee disarticulation Ⓑ Qp Qh ♿ A
* **L5430** Immediate postsurgical or early fitting, application of initial rigid dressing, including fitting, alignment, and suspension, 'AK' or knee disarticulation, each additional cast change and realignment Ⓑ Qp Qh ♿ A
* **L5450** Immediate post surgical or early fitting, application of non-weight bearing rigid dressing, below knee Ⓑ Qp Qh ♿ A
* **L5460** Immediate post surgical or early fitting, application of non-weight bearing rigid dressing, above knee Ⓑ Qp Qh ♿ A

Initial Prosthesis

* **L5500** Initial, below knee 'PTB' type socket, non-alignable system, pylon, no cover, SACH foot, plaster socket, direct formed Ⓑ Qp Qh ♿ A
* **L5505** Initial, above knee-knee disarticulation, ischial level socket, non-alignable system, pylon, no cover, SACH foot, plaster socket, direct formed Ⓑ Qp Qh ♿ A

Preparatory Prosthesis

* **L5510** Preparatory, below knee 'PTB' type socket, non-alignable system, pylon, no cover, SACH foot, plaster socket, molded to model Ⓑ Qp Qh ♿ A
* **L5520** Preparatory, below knee 'PTB' type socket, non-alignable system, pylon, no cover, SACH foot, thermoplastic or equal, direct formed Ⓑ Qp Qh ♿ A
* **L5530** Preparatory, below knee 'PTB' type socket, non-alignable system, pylon, no cover, SACH foot, thermoplastic or equal, molded to model Ⓑ Qp Qh ♿ A
* **L5535** Preparatory, below knee 'PTB' type socket, non-alignable system, no cover, SACH foot, prefabricated, adjustable open end socket Ⓑ Qp Qh ♿ A
* **L5540** Preparatory, below knee 'PTB' type socket, non-alignable system, pylon, no cover, SACH foot, laminated socket, molded to model Ⓑ Qp Qh ♿ A
* **L5560** Preparatory, above knee - knee disarticulation, ischial level socket, non-alignable system, pylon, no cover, SACH foot, plaster socket, molded to model Ⓑ Qp Qh ♿ A
* **L5570** Preparatory, above knee - knee disarticulation, ischial level socket, non-alignable system, pylon, no cover, SACH foot, thermoplastic or equal, direct formed Ⓑ Qp Qh ♿ A
* **L5580** Preparatory, above knee - knee disarticulation, ischial level socket, non-alignable system, pylon, no cover, SACH foot, thermoplastic or equal, molded to model Ⓑ Qp Qh ♿ A
* **L5585** Preparatory, above knee - knee disarticulation, ischial level socket, non-alignable system, pylon, no cover, SACH foot, prefabricated adjustable open end socket Ⓑ Qp Qh ♿ A

▶ New ⤻ Revised ✔ Reinstated ~~deleted~~ Deleted ⊘ Not covered or valid by Medicare
◌ Special coverage instructions * Carrier discretion Ⓑ Bill Part B MAC Ⓑ Bill DME MAC

* L5590 Preparatory, above knee - knee disarticulation, ischial level socket, non-alignable system, pylon, no cover, SACH foot, laminated socket, molded to model Ⓑ Qp Qh ♿ A
* L5595 Preparatory, hip disarticulation-hemipelvectomy, pylon, no cover, SACH foot, thermoplastic or equal, molded to patient model Ⓑ Qp Qh ♿ A
* L5600 Preparatory, hip disarticulation-hemipelvectomy, pylon, no cover, SACH foot, laminated socket, molded to patient model Ⓑ Qp Qh ♿ A

Additions to Lower Extremity

* L5610 Addition to lower extremity, endoskeletal system, above knee, hydracadence system Ⓑ Qp Qh ♿ A
* L5611 Addition to lower extremity, endoskeletal system, above knee-knee disarticulation, 4 bar linkage, with friction swing phase control Ⓑ Qp Qh ♿ A
* L5613 Addition to lower extremity, endoskeletal system, above knee-knee disarticulation, 4 bar linkage, with hydraulic swing phase control Ⓑ Qp Qh ♿ A
* L5614 Addition to lower extremity, exoskeletal system, above knee-knee disarticulation, 4 bar linkage, with pneumatic swing phase control Ⓑ Qp Qh ♿ A
* L5616 Addition to lower extremity, endoskeletal system, above knee, universal multiplex system, friction swing phase control Ⓑ Qp Qh ♿ A
* L5617 Addition to lower extremity, quick change self-aligning unit, above knee or below knee, each Ⓑ Qp Qh ♿ A

Additions to Test Sockets

* L5618 Addition to lower extremity, test socket, Symes Ⓑ Qp ♿ A
* L5620 Addition to lower extremity, test socket, below knee Ⓑ Qp ♿ A
* L5622 Addition to lower extremity, test socket, knee disarticulation Ⓑ Qp ♿ A
* L5624 Addition to lower extremity, test socket, above knee Ⓑ Qp ♿ A
* L5626 Addition to lower extremity, test socket, hip disarticulation Ⓑ Qp ♿ A
* L5628 Addition to lower extremity, test socket, hemipelvectomy Ⓑ Qp Qh ♿ A

Additions to Socket Variations

* L5629 Addition to lower extremity, below knee, acrylic socket Ⓑ Qp Qh ♿ A
* L5630 Addition to lower extremity, Symes type, expandable wall socket Ⓑ Qp Qh ♿ A
* L5631 Addition to lower extremity, above knee or knee disarticulation, acrylic socket Ⓑ Qp Qh ♿ A
* L5632 Addition to lower extremity, Symes type, 'PTB' brim design socket Ⓑ Qp Qh ♿ A
* L5634 Addition to lower extremity, Symes type, posterior opening (Canadian) socket Ⓑ Qp Qh ♿ A
* L5636 Addition to lower extremity, Symes type, medial opening socket Ⓑ Qp Qh ♿ A
* L5637 Addition to lower extremity, below knee, total contact Ⓑ Qp Qh ♿ A
* L5638 Addition to lower extremity, below knee, leather socket Ⓑ Qp Qh ♿ A
* L5639 Addition to lower extremity, below knee, wood socket Ⓑ Qp Qh ♿ A
* L5640 Addition to lower extremity, knee disarticulation, leather socket Ⓑ Qp Qh ♿ A
* L5642 Addition to lower extremity, above knee, leather socket Ⓑ Qp Qh ♿ A
* L5643 Addition to lower extremity, hip disarticulation, flexible inner socket, external frame Ⓑ Qp Qh ♿ A
* L5644 Addition to lower extremity, above knee, wood socket Ⓑ Qp Qh ♿ A
* L5645 Addition to lower extremity, below knee, flexible inner socket, external frame Ⓑ Qp Qh ♿ A
* L5646 Addition to lower extremity, below knee, air, fluid, gel or equal, cushion socket Ⓑ Qp Qh ♿ A
* L5647 Addition to lower extremity, below knee, suction socket Ⓑ Qp Qh ♿ A
* L5648 Addition to lower extremity, above knee, air, fluid, gel or equal, cushion socket Ⓑ Qp Qh ♿ A
* L5649 Addition to lower extremity, ischial containment/narrow M-L socket Ⓑ Qp Qh ♿ A
* L5650 Additions to lower extremity, total contact, above knee or knee disarticulation socket Ⓑ Qp Qh ♿ A

* **L5651** Addition to lower extremity, above knee, flexible inner socket, external frame Ⓑ Qp Qh ♿ A

* **L5652** Addition to lower extremity, suction suspension, above knee or knee disarticulation socket Ⓑ Qp Qh ♿ A

* **L5653** Addition to lower extremity, knee disarticulation, expandable wall socket Ⓑ Qp Qh ♿ A

Additions to Socket Insert and Suspension

* **L5654** Addition to lower extremity, socket insert, Symes, (Kemblo, Pelite, Aliplast, Plastazote or equal) Ⓑ Qp Qh ♿ A

* **L5655** Addition to lower extremity, socket insert, below knee (Kemblo, Pelite, Aliplast, Plastazote or equal) Ⓑ Qp Qh ♿ A

* **L5656** Addition to lower extremity, socket insert, knee disarticulation (Kemblo, Pelite, Aliplast, Plastazote or equal) Ⓑ Qp Qh ♿ A

* **L5658** Addition to lower extremity, socket insert, above knee (Kemblo, Pelite, Aliplast, Plastazote or equal) Ⓑ Qp Qh ♿ A

* **L5661** Addition to lower extremity, socket insert, multi-durometer Symes Ⓑ Qp Qh ♿ A

* **L5665** Addition to lower extremity, socket insert, multi-durometer, below knee Ⓑ Qp Qh ♿ A

* **L5666** Addition to lower extremity, below knee, cuff suspension Ⓑ Qp Qh ♿ A

* **L5668** Addition to lower extremity, below knee, molded distal cushion Ⓑ Qp Qh ♿ A

* **L5670** Addition to lower extremity, below knee, molded supracondylar suspension ('PTS' or similar) Ⓑ Qp Qh ♿ A

* **L5671** Addition to lower extremity, below knee/above knee suspension locking mechanism (shuttle, lanyard or equal), excludes socket insert Ⓑ Qp Qh ♿ A

* **L5672** Addition to lower extremity, below knee, removable medial brim suspension Ⓑ Qp Qh ♿ A

* **L5673** Addition to lower extremity, below knee/above knee, custom fabricated from existing mold or prefabricated, socket insert, silicone gel, elastomeric or equal, for use with locking mechanism Ⓑ Qp ♿ A

* **L5676** Additions to lower extremity, below knee, knee joints, single axis, pair Ⓑ Qp Qh ♿ A

* **L5677** Additions to lower extremity, below knee, knee joints, polycentric, pair Ⓑ Qp Qh ♿ A

* **L5678** Additions to lower extremity, below knee, joint covers, pair Ⓑ Qp Qh ♿ A

* **L5679** Addition to lower extremity, below knee/above knee, custom fabricated from existing mold or prefabricated, socket insert, silicone gel, elastomeric or equal, not for use with locking mechanism Ⓑ Qp ♿ A

* **L5680** Addition to lower extremity, below knee, thigh lacer, non-molded Ⓑ Qp Qh ♿ A

* **L5681** Addition to lower extremity, below knee/above knee, custom fabricated socket insert for congenital or atypical traumatic amputee, silicone gel, elastomeric or equal, for use with or without locking mechanism, initial only (for other than initial, use code L5673 or L5679) Ⓑ Qp Qh ♿ A

* **L5682** Addition to lower extremity, below knee, thigh lacer, gluteal/ischial, molded Ⓑ Qp Qh ♿ A

* **L5683** Addition to lower extremity, below knee/above knee, custom fabricated socket insert for other than congenital or atypical traumatic amputee, silicone gel, elastomeric, or equal, for use with or without locking mechanism, initial only (for other than initial, use code L5673 or L5679) Ⓑ Qp Qh ♿ A

* **L5684** Addition to lower extremity, below knee, fork strap Ⓑ Qp Qh ♿ A

* **L5685** Addition to lower extremity prosthesis, below knee, suspension/sealing sleeve, with or without valve, any material, each Ⓑ Qp ♿ A

* **L5686** Addition to lower extremity, below knee, back check (extension control) Ⓑ Qp Qh ♿ A

* **L5688** Addition to lower extremity, below knee, waist belt, webbing Ⓑ Qp Qh ♿ A

* **L5690** Addition to lower extremity, below knee, waist belt, padded and lined Ⓑ Qp Qh ♿ A

* **L5692** Addition to lower extremity, above knee, pelvic control belt, light Ⓑ Qp Qh ♿ A

* **L5694** Addition to lower extremity, above knee, pelvic control belt, padded and lined Ⓑ Qp Qh ♿ A

✻ **L5695** Addition to lower extremity, above knee, pelvic control, sleeve suspension, neoprene or equal, each Ⓑ Qp Qh ♿ A

✻ **L5696** Addition to lower extremity, above knee or knee disarticulation, pelvic joint Ⓑ Qp Qh ♿ A

✻ **L5697** Addition to lower extremity, above knee or knee disarticulation, pelvic band Ⓑ Qp Qh ♿ A

✻ **L5698** Addition to lower extremity, above knee or knee disarticulation, Silesian bandage Ⓑ Qp Qh ♿ A

✻ **L5699** All lower extremity prostheses, shoulder harness Ⓑ Qp Qh ♿ A

Replacement Sockets

✻ **L5700** Replacement, socket, below knee, molded to patient model Ⓑ Qp Qh ♿ A

✻ **L5701** Replacement, socket, above knee/knee disarticulation, including attachment plate, molded to patient model Ⓑ Qp Qh ♿ A

✻ **L5702** Replacement, socket, hip disarticulation, including hip joint, molded to patient model Ⓑ Qp Qh ♿ A

✻ **L5703** Ankle, Symes, molded to patient model, socket without solid ankle cushion heel (SACH) foot, replacement only Ⓑ Qp Qh ♿ A

Protective Covers

✻ **L5704** Custom shaped protective cover, below knee Ⓑ Qp Qh ♿ A

✻ **L5705** Custom shaped protective cover, above knee Ⓑ Qp Qh ♿ A

✻ **L5706** Custom shaped protective cover, knee disarticulation Ⓑ Qp Qh ♿ A

✻ **L5707** Custom shaped protective cover, hip disarticulation Ⓑ Qp Qh ♿ A

Additions to Exoskeletal–Knee-Shin System

✻ **L5710** Addition, exoskeletal knee-shin system, single axis, manual lock Ⓑ Qp Qh ♿ A

✻ **L5711** Additions exoskeletal knee-shin system, single axis, manual lock, ultra-light material Ⓑ Qp Qh ♿ A

✻ **L5712** Addition, exoskeletal knee-shin system, single axis, friction swing and stance phase control (safety knee) Ⓑ Qp Qh ♿ A

✻ **L5714** Addition, exoskeletal knee-shin system, single axis, variable friction swing phase control Ⓑ Qp Qh ♿ A

✻ **L5716** Addition, exoskeletal knee-shin system, polycentric, mechanical stance phase lock Ⓑ Qp Qh ♿ A

✻ **L5718** Addition, exoskeletal knee-shin system, polycentric, friction swing and stance phase control Ⓑ Qp Qh ♿ A

✻ **L5722** Addition, exoskeletal knee-shin system, single axis, pneumatic swing, friction stance phase control Ⓑ Qp Qh ♿ A

✻ **L5724** Addition, exoskeletal knee-shin system, single axis, fluid swing phase control Ⓑ Qp Qh ♿ A

✻ **L5726** Addition, exoskeletal knee-shin system, single axis, external joints, fluid swing phase control Ⓑ Qp Qh ♿ A

✻ **L5728** Addition, exoskeletal knee-shin system, single axis, fluid swing and stance phase control Ⓑ Qp Qh ♿ A

✻ **L5780** Addition, exoskeletal knee-shin system, single axis, pneumatic/hydra pneumatic swing phase control Ⓑ Qp Qh ♿ A

Vacuum Pumps

✻ **L5781** Addition to lower limb prosthesis, vacuum pump, residual limb volume management and moisture evacuation system Ⓑ Qp Qh ♿ A

✻ **L5782** Addition to lower limb prosthesis, vacuum pump, residual limb volume management and moisture evacuation system, heavy duty Ⓑ Qp Qh ♿ A

Component Modification

✻ **L5785** Addition, exoskeletal system, below knee, ultra-light material (titanium, carbon fiber, or equal) Ⓑ Qp Qh ♿ A

✻ **L5790** Addition, exoskeletal system, above knee, ultra-light material (titanium, carbon fiber, or equal) Ⓑ Qp Qh ♿ A

✻ **L5795** Addition, exoskeletal system, hip disarticulation, ultra-light material (titanium, carbon fiber, or equal) Ⓑ Qp Qh ♿ A

Endoskeletal

✻ **L5810** Addition, endoskeletal knee-shin system, single axis, manual lock Ⓑ Qp Qh ♿ A

✻ **L5811** Addition, endoskeletal knee-shin system, single axis, manual lock, ultralight material Ⓑ Qp Qh ♿ A

* **L5812** Addition, endoskeletal knee-shin system, single axis, friction swing and stance phase control (safety knee) Ⓑ Qp Qh ♿ A

* **L5814** Addition, endoskeletal knee-shin system, polycentric, hydraulic swing phase control, mechanical stance phase lock Ⓑ Qp Qh ♿ A

* **L5816** Addition, endoskeletal knee-shin system, polycentric, mechanical stance phase lock Ⓑ Qp Qh ♿ A

* **L5818** Addition, endoskeletal knee-shin system, polycentric, friction swing, and stance phase control Ⓑ Qp Qh ♿ A

* **L5822** Addition, endoskeletal knee-shin system, single axis, pneumatic swing, friction stance phase control Ⓑ Qp Qh ♿ A

* **L5824** Addition, endoskeletal knee-shin system, single axis, fluid swing phase control Ⓑ Qp Qh ♿ A

* **L5826** Addition, endoskeletal knee-shin system, single axis, hydraulic swing phase control, with miniature high activity frame Ⓑ Qp Qh ♿ A

* **L5828** Addition, endoskeletal knee-shin system, single axis, fluid swing and stance phase control Ⓑ Qp Qh ♿ A

* **L5830** Addition, endoskeletal knee-shin system, single axis, pneumatic/swing phase control Ⓑ Qp Qh ♿ A

* **L5840** Addition, endoskeletal knee/shin system, 4-bar linkage or multiaxial, pneumatic swing phase control Ⓑ Qp Qh ♿ A

* **L5845** Addition, endoskeletal, knee-shin system, stance flexion feature, adjustable Ⓑ Qp Qh ♿ A

* **L5848** Addition to endoskeletal, knee-shin system, fluid stance extension, dampening feature, with or without adjustability Ⓑ Qp Qh ♿ A

* **L5850** Addition, endoskeletal system, above knee or hip disarticulation, knee extension assist Ⓑ Qp Qh ♿ A

* **L5855** Addition, endoskeletal system, hip disarticulation, mechanical hip extension assist Ⓑ Qp Qh ♿ A

* **L5856** Addition to lower extremity prosthesis, endoskeletal knee-shin system, microprocessor control feature, swing and stance phase; includes electronic sensor(s), any type Ⓑ Qp Qh ♿ A

* **L5857** Addition to lower extremity prosthesis, endoskeletal knee-shin system, microprocessor control feature, swing phase only; includes electronic sensor(s), any type Ⓑ Qp Qh ♿ A

* **L5858** Addition to lower extremity prosthesis, endoskeletal knee shin system, microprocessor control feature, stance phase only, includes electronic sensor(s), any type Ⓑ Qp Qh ♿ A

* **L5859** Addition to lower extremity prosthesis, endoskeletal knee-shin system, powered and programmable flexion/extension assist control, includes any type motor(s) Ⓑ Qp Qh ♿ A

* **L5910** Addition, endoskeletal system, below knee, alignable system Ⓑ Qp Qh ♿ A

* **L5920** Addition, endoskeletal system, above knee or hip disarticulation, alignable system Ⓑ Qp Qh ♿ A

* **L5925** Addition, endoskeletal system, above knee, knee disarticulation or hip disarticulation, manual lock Ⓑ Qp Qh ♿ A

* **L5930** Addition, endoskeletal system, high activity knee control frame Ⓑ Qp Qh ♿ A

* **L5940** Addition, endoskeletal system, below knee, ultra-light material (titanium, carbon fiber or equal) Ⓑ Qp Qh ♿ A

* **L5950** Addition, endoskeletal system, above knee, ultra-light material (titanium, carbon fiber or equal) Ⓑ Qp Qh ♿ A

* **L5960** Addition, endoskeletal system, hip disarticulation, ultra-light material (titanium, carbon fiber, or equal) Ⓑ Qp Qh ♿ A

* **L5961** Addition, endoskeletal system, polycentric hip joint, pneumatic or hydraulic control, rotation control, with or without flexion, and/or extension control Ⓑ Qp Qh ♿ A

* **L5962** Addition, endoskeletal system, below knee, flexible protective outer surface covering system Ⓑ Qp Qh ♿ A

* **L5964** Addition, endoskeletal system, above knee, flexible protective outer surface covering system Ⓑ Qp Qh ♿ A

▶ New	↻ Revised	✔ Reinstated	~~deleted~~ Deleted	⊘ Not covered or valid by Medicare
✪ Special coverage instructions		✳ Carrier discretion	Ⓑ Bill Part B MAC	Ⓓ Bill DME MAC

* **L5966** Addition, endoskeletal system, hip disarticulation, flexible protective outer surface covering system Ⓑ Qp Qh ♿ A

Additions to Ankle and/or Foot

* **L5968** Addition to lower limb prosthesis, multiaxial ankle with swing phase active dorsiflexion feature Qp Qh A
* **L5969** Addition, endoskeletal ankle-foot or ankle system, power assist, includes any type motor(s) Qp Qh A
* **L5970** All lower extremity prostheses, foot, external keel, SACH foot Qp Qh A
* **L5971** All lower extremity prosthesis, solid ankle cushion keel (SACH) foot, replacement only Qp Qh A
* **L5972** All lower extremity prostheses (foot, flexible keel) Qp Qh A
* **L5973** Endoskeletal ankle foot system, microprocessor controlled feature, dorsiflexion and/or plantar flexion control, includes power source Qh A
* **L5974** All lower extremity prostheses, foot, single axis ankle/foot Qp Qh A
* **L5975** All lower extremity prostheses, combination single axis ankle and flexible keel foot Qp Qh A
* **L5976** All lower extremity prostheses, energy storing foot (Seattle Carbon Copy II or equal) Qp Qh A
* **L5978** All lower extremity prostheses, foot, multiaxial ankle/foot Qp Qh A
* **L5979** All lower extremity prostheses, multiaxial ankle, dynamic response foot, one piece system Qp Qh A
* **L5980** All lower extremity prostheses, flex foot system Qp Qh A
* **L5981** All lower extremity prostheses, flexwalk system or equal Qp Qh A
* **L5982** All exoskeletal lower extremity prostheses, axial rotation unit Qp Qh A
* **L5984** All endoskeletal lower extremity prostheses, axial rotation unit, with or without adjustability Qp Qh A
* **L5985** All endoskeletal lower extremity prostheses, dynamic prosthetic pylon Qp Qh A
* **L5986** All lower extremity prostheses, multiaxial rotation unit ('MCP' or equal) Qp Qh A
* **L5987** All lower extremity prostheses, shank foot system with vertical loading pylon Qp Qh A
* **L5988** Addition to lower limb prosthesis, vertical shock reducing pylon feature Qp Qh A
* **L5990** Addition to lower extremity prosthesis, user adjustable heel height Qp Qh A
* **L5999** Lower extremity prosthesis, not otherwise specified A

Upper Limb (L6000-L7600)

Note: The procedures in L6000-L6599 are considered as base or basic procedures and may be modified by listing procedures from the additions sections. The base procedures include only standard friction wrist and control cable system unless otherwise specified.

Partial Hand

* **L6000** Partial hand, thumb remaining Qp Qh A
* **L6010** Partial hand, little and/or ring finger remaining Qp Qh A
* **L6020** Partial hand, no finger remaining Qp Qh A
* **L6026** Transcarpal/metacarpal or partial hand disarticulation prosthesis, external power, self-suspended, inner socket with removable forearm section, electrodes and cables, two batteries, charger, myoelectric control of terminal device, excludes terminal device(s) Qp Qh A

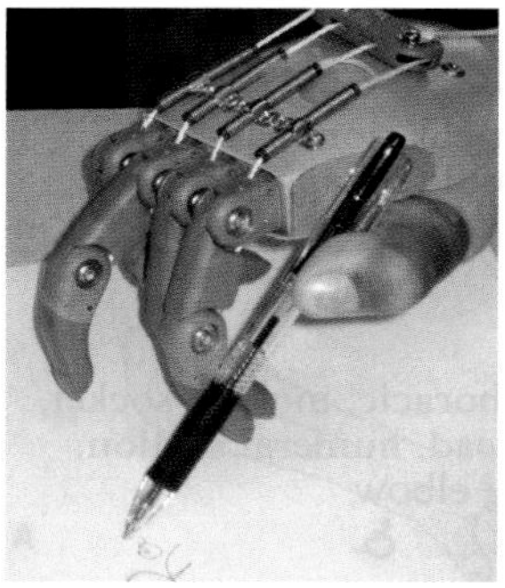

Figure 39 Partial hand.

MIPS | Qp Quantity Physician | Qh Quantity Hospital | ♀ Female only | ♂ Male only | A Age | DMEPOS | A2-Z3 ASC Payment Indicator | A-Y ASC Status Indicator | Coding Clinic

2019 HCPCS LEVEL II NATIONAL CODES

Breast Prosthetics

L8000 Breast prosthesis, mastectomy bra, without integrated breast prosthesis form, any size, any type Ⓑ Qp ♀ ♿ A
IOM: 100-02, 15, 120

L8001 Breast prosthesis, mastectomy bra, with integrated breast prosthesis form, unilateral, any size, any type Ⓑ Qp ♀ ♿ A
IOM: 100-02, 15, 120

L8002 Breast prosthesis, mastectomy bra, with integrated breast prosthesis form, bilateral, any size, any type Ⓑ Qp ♀ ♿ A
IOM: 100-02, 15, 120

L8010 Breast prosthesis, mastectomy sleeve Ⓑ ♀ A
IOM: 100-02, 15, 120

L8015 External breast prosthesis garment, with mastectomy form, post mastectomy Ⓑ Qp ♀ ♿ A
IOM: 100-02, 15, 120

L8020 Breast prosthesis, mastectomy form Ⓑ Qp ♀ ♿ A
IOM: 100-02, 15, 120

L8030 Breast prosthesis, silicone or equal, without integral adhesive Ⓑ Qp Qh ♀ ♿ A
IOM: 100-02, 15, 120

L8031 Breast prosthesis, silicone or equal, with integral adhesive Ⓑ Qp Qh ♿ A
IOM: 100-02, 15, 120

* **L8032** Nipple prosthesis, reusable, any type, each Ⓑ Qp Qh ♿ A

L8035 Custom breast prosthesis, post mastectomy, molded to patient model Ⓑ Qp Qh ♀ ♿ A
IOM: 100-02, 15, 120

* **L8039** Breast prosthesis, not otherwise specified Ⓑ Qp Qh ♀ A

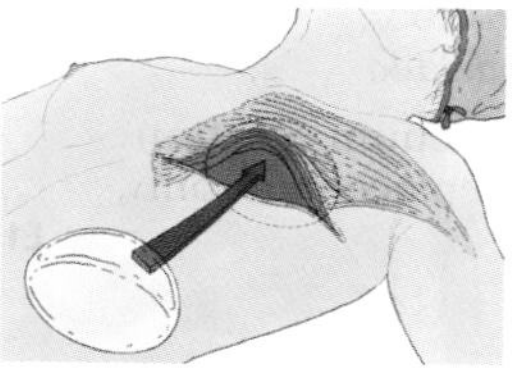

Figure 43 Implant breast prosthesis.

Nasal, Orbital, Auricular Prosthetics

* **L8040** Nasal prosthesis, provided by a non-physician Ⓑ Qp Qh ♿ A

* **L8041** Midfacial prosthesis, provided by a non-physician Ⓑ Qp Qh ♿ A

* **L8042** Orbital prosthesis, provided by a non-physician Ⓑ Qp Qh ♿ A

* **L8043** Upper facial prosthesis, provided by a non-physician Ⓑ Qp Qh ♿ A

* **L8044** Hemi-facial prosthesis, provided by a non-physician Ⓑ Qp Qh ♿ A

* **L8045** Auricular prosthesis, provided by a non-physician Ⓑ Qp Qh ♿ A

* **L8046** Partial facial prosthesis, provided by a non-physician Ⓑ Qp Qh ♿ A

* **L8047** Nasal septal prosthesis, provided by a non-physician Ⓑ Qp Qh ♿ A

* **L8048** Unspecified maxillofacial prosthesis, by report, provided by a non-physician Ⓑ Qp Qh A

* **L8049** Repair or modification of maxillofacial prosthesis, labor component, 15 minute increments, provided by a non-physician Ⓑ Qp A

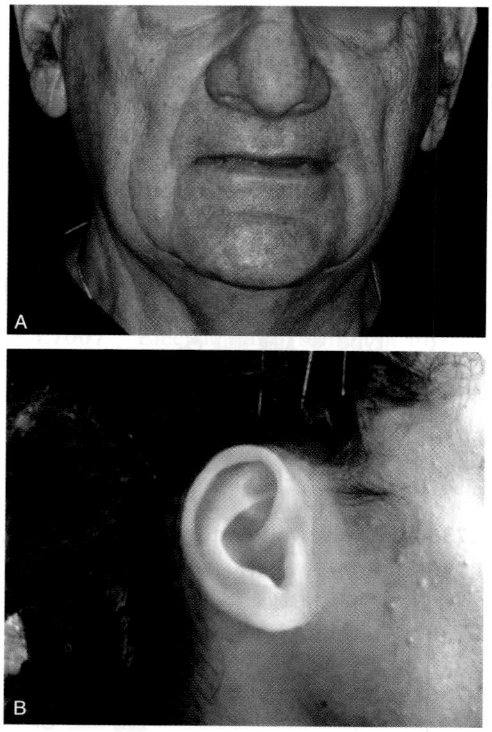
A
B

Figure 44 (A) Nasal prosthesis, (B) Auricular prosthesis.

▶ New ⤾ Revised ✔ Reinstated ~~deleted~~ Deleted ⊘ Not covered or valid by Medicare
Special coverage instructions * Carrier discretion Ⓑ Bill Part B MAC Ⓑ Bill DME MAC

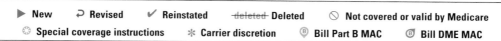

Trusses

L8300 Truss, single with standard pad Qp Qh A

IOM: 100-02, 15, 120; 100-03, 4, 280.11; 100-03, 4, 280.12; 100-04, 4, 240

L8310 Truss, double with standard pads Qp Qh A

IOM: 100-02, 15, 120; 100-03, 4, 280.11; 100-03, 4, 280.12; 100-04, 4, 240

L8320 Truss, addition to standard pad, water pad Qp Qh A

IOM: 100-02, 15, 120; 100-03, 4, 280.11; 100-03, 4, 280.12; 100-04, 4, 240

L8330 Truss, addition to standard pad, scrotal pad Qp Qh ♂ A

IOM: 100-02, 15, 120; 100-03, 4, 280.11; 100-03, 4, 280.12; 100-04, 4, 240

Prosthetic Socks

L8400 Prosthetic sheath, below knee, each Qp A

IOM: 100-02, 15, 200

L8410 Prosthetic sheath, above knee, each Qp A

IOM: 100-02, 15, 200

L8415 Prosthetic sheath, upper limb, each Qp A

IOM: 100-02, 15, 200

* L8417 Prosthetic sheath/sock, including a gel cushion layer, below knee or above knee, each Qp A

L8420 Prosthetic sock, multiple ply, below knee, each Qp A

IOM: 100-02, 15, 200

L8430 Prosthetic sock, multiple ply, above knee, each Qp A

IOM: 100-02, 15, 200

L8435 Prosthetic sock, multiple ply, upper limb, each Qp A

IOM: 100-02, 15, 200

L8440 Prosthetic shrinker, below knee, each Qp A

IOM: 100-02, 15, 200

L8460 Prosthetic shrinker, above knee, each Qp A

IOM: 100-02, 15, 200

L8465 Prosthetic shrinker, upper limb, each Qp A

IOM: 100-02, 15, 200

L8470 Prosthetic sock, single ply, fitting, below knee, each Qp A

IOM: 100-02, 15, 200

L8480 Prosthetic sock, single ply, fitting, above knee, each Qp A

IOM: 100-02, 15, 200

L8485 Prosthetic sock, single ply, fitting, upper limb, each Qp A

IOM: 100-02, 15, 200

Unlisted

* L8499 Unlisted procedure for miscellaneous prosthetic services A

Prosthetic Implants (L8500-L9900)

Larynx, Tracheoesophageal

L8500 Artificial larynx, any type Qp Qh A

IOM: 100-02, 15, 120; 100-03, 1, 50.2; 100-04, 4, 240

L8501 Tracheostomy speaking valve Qp Qh A

IOM: 100-03, 1, 50.4

* L8505 Artificial larynx replacement battery/accessory, any type A

* L8507 Tracheo-esophageal voice prosthesis, patient inserted, any type, each Qp Qh A

* L8509 Tracheo-esophageal voice prosthesis, inserted by a licensed health care provider, any type Qp Qh A

L8510 Voice amplifier Qp Qh A

IOM: 100-03, 1, 50.2

* L8511 Insert for indwelling tracheoesophageal prosthesis, with or without valve, replacement only, each Qp Qh A

* L8512 Gelatin capsules or equivalent, for use with tracheoesophageal voice prosthesis, replacement only, per 10 A

* L8513 Cleaning device used with tracheoesophageal voice prosthesis, pipet, brush, or equal, replacement only, each A

✻ **L8514** Tracheoesophageal puncture dilator, replacement only, each Ⓑ Ⓓ Qp Qh ♿ A

✻ **L8515** Gelatin capsule, application device for use with tracheoesophageal voice prosthesis, each Ⓑ Ⓓ Qp Qh ♿ A

Breast

L8600 Implantable breast prosthesis, silicone or equal Ⓑ Qp Qh ♀ ♿ N1 N

IOM: 100-02, 15, 120; 100-3, 2, 140.2

Bulking Agents

L8603 Injectable bulking agent, collagen implant, urinary tract, 2.5 ml syringe, includes shipping and necessary supplies Ⓑ ♿ N1 N

Bill on paper, acquisition cost invoice required

IOM: 100-03, 4, 280.1

✻ **L8604** Injectable bulking agent, dextranomer/hyaluronic acid copolymer implant, urinary tract, 1 ml, includes shipping and necessary supplies Ⓑ Qp Qh N1 N

✻ **L8605** Injectable bulking agent, dextranomer/hyaluronic acid copolymer implant, anal canal, 1 ml, includes shipping and necessary supplies Ⓑ Qp Qh ♿ N1 N

L8606 Injectable bulking agent, synthetic implant, urinary tract, 1 ml syringe, includes shipping and necessary supplies Ⓑ Qp Qh ♿ N1 N

Bill on paper, acquisition cost invoice required

IOM: 100-03, 4, 280.1

L8607 Injectable bulking agent for vocal cord medialization, 0.1 ml, includes shipping and necessary supplies Ⓑ Qp Qh ♿ N1 N

IOM: 100-03, 4, 280.1

Eye and Ear

▶ ✻ **L8608** Miscellaneous external component, supply or accessory for use with the Argus II retinal prosthesis system N

✻ **L8609** Artificial cornea Ⓑ Qp Qh ♿ N1 N

L8610 Ocular implant Ⓑ Qp Qh ♿ N1 N

IOM: 100-02, 15, 120

L8612 Aqueous shunt Ⓑ Qp Qh ♿ N1 N

IOM: 100-02, 15, 120

Cross Reference Q0074

L8613 Ossicula implant Ⓑ Qp Qh ♿ N1 N

IOM: 100-02, 15, 120

L8614 Cochlear device, includes all internal and external components Ⓑ Qp Qh ♿ N1 N

IOM: 100-02, 15, 120; 100-03, 1, 50.3

L8615 Headset/headpiece for use with cochlear implant device, replacement Ⓑ Qp Qh ♿ A

IOM: 100-03, 1, 50.3

L8616 Microphone for use with cochlear implant device, replacement Ⓑ Qp Qh ♿ A

IOM: 100-03, 1, 50.3

L8617 Transmitting coil for use with cochlear implant device, replacement Ⓑ Qp Qh ♿ A

IOM: 100-03, 1, 50.3

L8618 Transmitter cable for use with cochlear implant device or auditory osseointegrated device, replacement Ⓑ Qp Qh ♿ A

IOM: 100-03, 1, 50.3

L8619 Cochlear implant, external speech processor and controller, integrated system, replacement Ⓑ Qp Qh ♿ A

IOM: 100-03, 1, 50.3

✻ **L8621** Zinc air battery for use with cochlear implant device and auditory osseointegrated sound processors, replacement, each Ⓑ Qp Qh ♿ A

✻ **L8622** Alkaline battery for use with cochlear implant device, any size, replacement, each Ⓑ Qp Qh ♿ A

✻ **L8623** Lithium ion battery for use with cochlear implant device speech processor, other than ear level, replacement, each Ⓑ ♿ A

✻ **L8624** Lithium ion battery for use with cochlear implant or auditory osseointegrated device speech processor, ear level, replacement, each Ⓑ ♿ A

L8625 External recharging system for battery for use with cochlear implant or auditory osseointegrated device, replacement only, each A

IOM: 103-03, PART 1, 50.3

L8627 Cochlear implant, external speech processor, component, replacement Ⓑ Qp Qh ♿ A

IOM: 103-03, PART 1, 50.3

L8628 Cochlear implant, external controller component, replacement Ⓑ Qp Qh ♿ A

IOM: 103-03, PART 1, 50.3

▶ New ⤺ Revised ✔ Reinstated ~~deleted~~ Deleted ⊘ Not covered or valid by Medicare
Special coverage instructions ✻ Carrier discretion Ⓑ Bill Part B MAC Ⓓ Bill DME MAC

L8629 Transmitting coil and cable, integrated, for use with cochlear implant device, replacement Qp Qh A

IOM: 103-03, PART 1, 50.3

Hand and Foot

L8630 Metacarpophalangeal joint implant N1 N

IOM: 100-02, 15, 120

L8631 Metacarpal phalangeal joint replacement, two or more pieces, metal (e.g., stainless steel or cobalt chrome), ceramic-like material (e.g., pyrocarbon), for surgical implantation (all sizes, includes entire system) Qp Qh N1 N

IOM: 100-02, 15, 120

L8641 Metatarsal joint implant Qp Qh N1 N

IOM: 100-02, 15, 120

L8642 Hallux implant Qp Qh N1 N

May be billed by ambulatory surgical center or surgeon

IOM: 100-02, 15, 120

Cross Reference Q0073

L8658 Interphalangeal joint spacer, silicone or equal, each Qp Qh N1 N

IOM: 100-02, 15, 120

L8659 Interphalangeal finger joint replacement, 2 or more pieces, metal (e.g., stainless steel or cobalt chrome), ceramic-like material (e.g., pyrocarbon) for surgical implantation, any size Qp Qh N1 N

IOM: 100-02, 15, 120

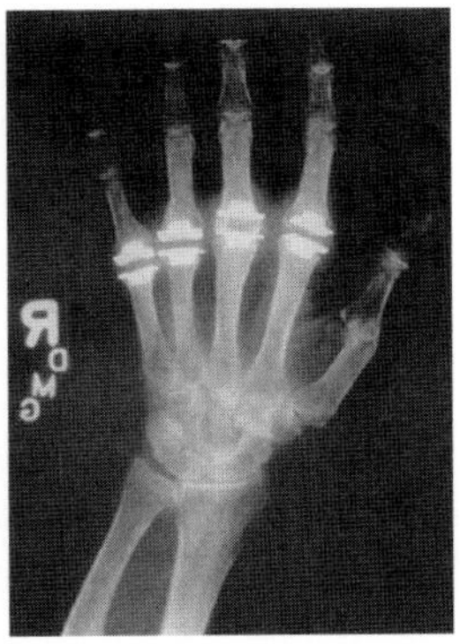

Figure 45 Metacarpophalangeal implant.

Vascular

L8670 Vascular graft material, synthetic, implant Qp Qh N1 N

IOM: 100-02, 15, 120

Neurostimulator

L8679 Implantable neurostimulator, pulse generator, any type Qp Qh N1 N

IOM: 100-03, 4, 280.4

L8680 Implantable neurostimulator electrode, each Qh E1

Related CPT codes: 43647, 63650, 63655, 64553, 64555, 64560, 64561, 64565, 64573, 64575, 64577, 64580, 64581.

L8681 Patient programmer (external) for use with implantable programmable neurostimulator pulse generator, replacement only Qp Qh A

IOM: 100-03, 4, 280.4

L8682 Implantable neurostimulator radiofrequency receiver Qp Qh N1 N

IOM: 100-03, 4, 280.4

L8683 Radiofrequency transmitter (external) for use with implantable neurostimulator radiofrequency receiver Qp Qh A

IOM: 100-03, 4, 280.4

L8684 Radiofrequency transmitter (external) for use with implantable sacral root neurostimulator receiver for bowel and bladder management, replacement Qp Qh A

IOM: 100-03, 4, 280.4

L8685 Implantable neurostimulator pulse generator, single array, rechargeable, includes extension Qp Qh E1

Related CPT codes: 61885, 64590, 63685.

L8686 Implantable neurostimulator pulse generator, single array, non-rechargeable, includes extension Qp Qh E1

Related CPT codes: 61885, 64590, 63685.

L8687 Implantable neurostimulator pulse generator, dual array, rechargeable, includes extension Qp Qh E1

Related CPT codes: 64590, 63685, 61886.

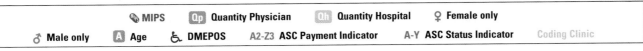

⊘ **L8688** Implantable neurostimulator pulse generator, dual array, non-rechargeable, includes extension ⑬ Qp Qh E1

Related CPT codes: 61885, 64590, 63685.

⊛ **L8689** External recharging system for battery (internal) for use with implantable neurostimulator, replacement only ⑬ Qp Qh ♿ A

IOM: 100-03, 4, 280.4

Miscellaneous Orthotic and Prosthetic Components, Services, and Supplies

∗ **L8690** Auditory osseointegrated device, includes all internal and external components ⑬ Qp Qh ♿ N1 N

Related CPT codes: 69714, 69715, 69717, 69718.

∗ **L8691** Auditory osseointegrated device, external sound processor, excludes transducer/actuator, replacement only, each ⑬ Qp Qh ♿ A

⊘ **L8692** Auditory osseointegrated device, external sound processor, used without osseointegration, body worn, includes headband or other means of external attachment ⑬ Qp Qh E1

Medicare Statute 1862(a)(7)

∗ **L8693** Auditory osseointegrated device abutment, any length, replacement only ⑨ Qp Qh ♿ A

∗ **L8694** Auditory osseointegrated device, transducer/actuator, replacement only, each A

⊛ **L8695** External recharging system for battery (external) for use with implantable neurostimulator, replacement only ⑬ Qp Qh ♿ A

IOM: 100-03, 4, 280.4

⊛ **L8696** Antenna (external) for use with implantable diaphragmatic/phrenic nerve stimulation device, replacement, each ⑬ Qp Qh ♿ A

▶ ⊛ **L8698** Miscellaneous component, supply or accessory for use with total artificial heart system A

∗ **L8699** Prosthetic implant, not otherwise specified ⑬ N1 N

▶ ∗ **L8701** Powered upper extremity range of motion assist device, elbow, wrist, hand with single or double upright(s), includes microprocessor, sensors, all components and accessories, custom fabricated A

▶ ∗ **L8702** Powered upper extremity range of motion assist device, elbow, wrist, hand, finger, single or double upright(s), includes microprocessor, sensors, all components and accessories, custom fabricated A

∗ **L9900** Orthotic and prosthetic supply, accessory, and/or service component of another HCPCS "L" code ⑨ ⑬ N1 N

▶ **New** ↻ **Revised** ✔ **Reinstated** ~~deleted~~ **Deleted** ⊘ **Not covered or valid by Medicare**
⊛ **Special coverage instructions** ∗ **Carrier discretion** ⑬ **Bill Part B MAC** ⑬ **Bill DME MAC**

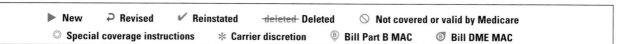

OTHER MEDICAL SERVICES (M0000-M0301)

▶ ✻ **M1000** Pain screened as moderate to severe M

▶ ✻ **M1001** Plan of care to address moderate to severe pain documented on or before the date of the second visit with a clinician M

▶ ✻ **M1002** Plan of care for moderate to severe pain not documented on or before the date of the second visit with a clinician, reason not given M

▶ ✻ **M1003** TB screening performed and results interpreted within twelve months prior to initiation of first-time biologic disease modifying anti-rheumatic drug therapy for RA M

▶ ✻ **M1004** Documentation of medical reason for not screening for TB or interpreting results (i.e., patient positive for TB and documentation of past treatment; patient who has recently completed a course of anti-TB therapy) M

▶ ✻ **M1005** TB screening not performed or results not interpreted, reason not given M

▶ ✻ **M1006** Disease activity not assessed, reason not given M

▶ ✻ **M1007** >=50% of total number of a patient's outpatient RA encounters assessed M

▶ ✻ **M1008** <50% of total number of a patient's outpatient RA encounters assessed M

▶ ✻ **M1009** Patient treatment and final evaluation complete M

▶ ✻ **M1010** Patient treatment and final evaluation complete M

▶ ✻ **M1011** Patient treatment and final evaluation complete M

▶ ✻ **M1012** Patient treatment and final evaluation complete M

▶ ✻ **M1013** Patient treatment and final evaluation complete M

▶ ✻ **M1014** Patient treatment and final evaluation complete M

▶ ✻ **M1015** Patient treatment and final evaluation complete M

▶ ✻ **M1016** Female patients unable to bear children M

▶ ✻ **M1017** Patient admitted to palliative care services M

▶ ✻ **M1018** Patients with an active diagnosis or history of cancer (except basal cell and squamous cell skin carcinoma), patients who are heavy tobacco smokers, lung cancer screening patients M

▶ ✻ **M1019** Adolescent patients 12 to 17 years of age with major depression or dysthymia who reached remission at twelve months as demonstrated by a twelve month (+/-60 days) PHQ-9 or PHQ-9m score of less than five M

▶ ✻ **M1020** Adolescent patients 12 to 17 years of age with major depression or dysthymia who did not reach remission at twelve months as demonstrated by a twelve month (+/-60 days) PHQ-9 or PHQ-9m score of less than 5. Either PHQ-9 or PHQ-9m score was not assessed or is greater than or equal to 5 M

▶ ✻ **M1021** Patient had only urgent care visits during the performance period M

▶ ✻ **M1022** Patients who were in hospice at any time during the performance period M

▶ ✻ **M1023** Adolescent patients 12 to 17 years of age with major depression or dysthymia who reached remission at six months as demonstrated by a six month (+/-60 days) PHQ-9 or PHQ-9m score of less than five M

▶ ✻ **M1024** Adolescent patients 12 to 17 years of age with major depression or dysthymia who did not reach remission at six months as demonstrated by a six month (+/-60 days) PHQ-9 or PHQ-9m score of less than five. Either PHQ-9 or PHQ-9m score was not assessed or is greater than or equal to five M

▶ ✻ **M1025** Patients who were in hospice at any time during the performance period M

▶ ✻ **M1026** Patients who were in hospice at any time during the performance period M

▶ ✻ **M1027** Imaging of the head (CT or MRI) was obtained M

▶ ✻ **M1028** Documentation of patients with primary headache diagnosis and imaging other than CT or MRI obtained M

▶ ✻ **M1029** Imaging of the head (CT or MRI) was not obtained, reason not given M

▶ ✻ **M1030** Patients with clinical indications for imaging of the head M

▶ ✻ **M1031** Patients with no clinical indications for imaging of the head M

▶ ✻ **M1032** Adults currently taking pharmacotherapy for OUD M

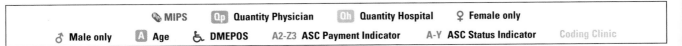

▶ ✻ **M1033** Pharmacotherapy for OUD initiated after June 30th of performance period M

▶ ✻ **M1034** Adults who have at least 180 days of continuous pharmacotherapy with a medication prescribed for OUD without a gap of more than seven days M

▶ ✻ **M1035** Adults who are deliberately phased out of medication assisted treatment (MAT) prior to 180 days of continuous treatment M

▶ ✻ **M1036** Adults who have not had at least 180 days of continuous pharmacotherapy with a medication prescribed for oud without a gap of more than seven days M

▶ ✻ **M1037** Patients with a diagnosis of lumbar spine region cancer at the time of the procedure M

▶ ✻ **M1038** Patients with a diagnosis of lumbar spine region fracture at the time of the procedure M

▶ ✻ **M1039** Patients with a diagnosis of lumbar spine region infection at the time of the procedure M

▶ ✻ **M1040** Patients with a diagnosis of lumbar idiopathic or congenital scoliosis M

▶ ✻ **M1041** Patient had cancer, fracture or infection related to the lumbar spine or patient had idiopathic or congenital scoliosis M

▶ ✻ **M1042** Functional status measurement with score was obtained utilizing the Oswestry Disability Index (ODI version 2.1a) patient reported outcome tool within three months preoperatively and at one year (9 to 15 months) postoperatively M

▶ ✻ **M1043** Functional status measurement with score was not obtained utilizing the Oswestry Disability Index (ODI version 2.1a) patient reported outcome tool within three months preoperatively and at one year (9 to 15 months) postoperatively M

▶ ✻ **M1044** Functional status was measured by the Oswestry Disability Index (ODI version 2.1a) patient reported outcome tool within three months preoperatively and at one year (9 to 15 months) postoperatively M

▶ ✻ **M1045** Functional status measurement with score was obtained utilizing the Oxford Knee Score (OKS) patient reported outcome tool within three months preoperatively and at one year (9 to 15 months) postoperatively M

▶ ✻ **M1046** Functional status measurement with score was not obtained utilizing the Oxford Knee Score (OKS) patient reported outcome tool within three months preoperatively and at one year (9 to 15 months) postoperatively M

▶ ✻ **M1047** Functional status was measured by the Oxford Knee Score (OKS) patient reported outcome tool within three months preoperatively and at one year (9 to 15 months) postoperatively M

▶ ✻ **M1048** Functional status measurement with score was obtained utilizing the Oswestry Disability Index (ODI version 2.1a) patient reported outcome tool within three months preoperatively and at three months (6 to 20 weeks) postoperatively M

▶ ✻ **M1049** Functional status measurement with score was not obtained utilizing the Oswestry Disability Index (ODI version 2.1a) patient reported outcome tool within three months preoperatively and at three months (6 to 20 weeks) postoperatively M

▶ ✻ **M1050** Functional status was measured by the Oswestry Disability Index (ODI version 2.1a) patient reported outcome tool within three months preoperatively and at three months (6 to 20 weeks) postoperatively M

▶ ✻ **M1051** Patient had cancer, fracture or infection related to the lumbar spine or patient had idiopathic or congenital scoliosis M

▶ ✻ **M1052** Leg pain was not measured by the visual analog scale (VAS) within three months preoperatively and at one year (9 to 15 months) postoperatively M

▶ ✻ **M1053** Leg pain was measured by the visual analog scale (VAS) within three months preoperatively and at one year (9 to 15 months) postoperatively M

▶ ✻ **M1054** Patient had only urgent care visits during the performance period M

▶ ✻ **M1055** Aspirin or another antiplatelet therapy used M

▶ ✻ **M1056** Prescribed anticoagulant medication during the performance period, history of gi bleeding, history of intracranial bleeding, bleeding disorder and specific provider documented reasons: allergy to aspirin or anti-platelets, use of non-steroidal anti-inflammatory agents, drug-drug interaction, uncontrolled hypertension >180/110 mmhg or gastroesophageal reflux disease M

▶ ✻ **M1057** Aspirin or another antiplatelet therapy not used, reason not given M

▶ ✻ **M1058** Patient was a permanent nursing home resident at any time during the performance period M

▶ ✻ **M1059** Patient was in hospice or receiving palliative care at any time during the performance period M

▶ ✻ **M1060** Patient died prior to the end of the performance period M

▶ ✻ **M1061** Patient pregnancy M

▶ ✻ **M1062** Patient immunocompromised M

▶ ✻ **M1063** Patients receiving high doses of immunosuppressive therapy M

▶ ✻ **M1064** Shingrix vaccine documented as administered or previously received M

▶ ✻ **M1065** Shingrix vaccine was not administered for reasons documented by clinician (e.g., patient administered vaccine other than shingrix, patient allergy or other medical reasons, patient declined or other patient reasons, vaccine not available or other system reasons) M

▶ ✻ **M1066** Shingrix vaccine not documented as administered, reason not given M

▶ ✻ **M1067** Hospice services for patient provided any time during the measurement period M

▶ ✻ **M1068** Adults who are not ambulatory M

▶ ✻ **M1069** Patient screened for future fall risk M

▶ ✻ **M1070** Patient not screened for future fall risk, reason not given M

▶ ✻ **M1071** Patient had any additional spine procedures performed on the same date as the lumbar discectomy/laminotomy M

⊘ **M0075** Cellular therapy Ⓑ E1

⊘ **M0076** Prolotherapy Ⓑ E1

Prolotherapy stimulates production of new ligament tissue. Not covered by Medicare.

⊘ **M0100** Intragastric hypothermia using gastric freezing Ⓑ E1

⊘ **M0300** IV chelation therapy (chemical endarterectomy) Ⓑ E1

⊘ **M0301** Fabric wrapping of abdominal aneurysm Ⓑ E1

Treatment for abdominal aneurysms that involves wrapping aneurysms with cellophane or fascia lata. Fabric wrapping of abdominal aneurysms is not a covered Medicare procedure.

LABORATORY SERVICES (P0000-P9999)

Chemistry and Toxicology Tests

P2028 Cephalin floculation, blood Ⓑ Qp Qh A

This code appears on a CMS list of codes that represent obsolete and unreliable tests and procedures. Verify before reporting.

IOM: 100-03, 4, 300.1

P2029 Congo red, blood Ⓑ Qp Qh A

This code appears on a CMS list of codes that represent obsolete and unreliable tests and procedures. Verify before reporting.

IOM: 100-03, 4, 300.1

⊘ **P2031** Hair analysis (excluding arsenic) Ⓑ E1

IOM: 100-03, 4, 300.1

P2033 Thymol turbidity, blood Ⓑ Qp Qh A

This code appears on a CMS list of codes that represent obsolete and unreliable tests and procedures. Verify before reporting.

IOM: 100-03, 4, 300.1

P2038 Mucoprotein, blood (seromucoid) (medical necessity procedure) Ⓑ Qp Qh A

This code appears on a CMS list of codes that represent obsolete and unreliable tests and procedures. Verify before reporting.

IOM: 100-03, 4, 300.1

Pathology Screening Tests

P3000 Screening Papanicolaou smear, cervical or vaginal, up to three smears, by technician under physician supervision Ⓑ Qp Qh ♀ A

Co-insurance and deductible waived

Assign for Pap smear ordered for screening purposes only, conventional method, performed by technician

IOM: 100-03, 3, 190.2,

Laboratory Certification: Cytology

P3001 Screening Papanicolaou smear, cervical or vaginal, up to three smears, requiring interpretation by physician Ⓑ Qp Qh ♀ B

Co-insurance and deductible waived

Report professional component for Pap smears requiring physician interpretation. There are CPT codes assigned for diagnostic Paps, such as, 88141; HCPCS are for screening Paps.

IOM: 100-03, 3, 190.2

Laboratory Certification: Cytology

Microbiology Tests

⊘ **P7001** Culture, bacterial, urine; quantitative, sensitivity study Ⓑ E1

Cross Reference CPT

Laboratory Certification: Bacteriology

Miscellaneous Pathology

P9010 Blood (whole), for transfusion, per unit Ⓑ Qp Qh R

Blood furnished on an outpatient basis, subject to Medicare Part B blood deductible; applicable to first 3 pints of whole blood or equivalent units of packed red cells in calendar year

IOM: 100-01, 3, 20.5; 100-02, 1, 10

P9011 Blood, split unit Ⓑ Qp Qh R

Reports all splitting activities of any blood component

IOM: 100-01, 3, 20.5; 100-02, 1, 10

P9012 Cryoprecipitate, each unit Ⓑ Qp Qh R

IOM: 100-01, 3, 20.5; 100-02, 1, 10

P9016 Red blood cells, leukocytes reduced, each unit Ⓑ Qp Qh R

IOM: 100-01, 3, 20.5; 100-02, 1, 10

P9017 Fresh frozen plasma (single donor), frozen within 8 hours of collection, each unit Ⓑ Qp Qh R

IOM: 100-01, 3, 20.5; 100-02, 1, 10

P9019 Platelets, each unit Ⓑ Qp Qh R

IOM: 100-01, 3, 20.5; 100-02, 1, 10

P9020 Platelet rich plasma, each unit Ⓑ Qp Qh R

IOM: 100-01, 3, 20.5; 100-02, 1, 10

P9021 Red blood cells, each unit Ⓑ Qp Qh R

IOM: 100-01, 3, 20.5; 100-02, 1, 10

▶ New ↩ Revised ✔ Reinstated ~~deleted~~ Deleted ⊘ Not covered or valid by Medicare
Special coverage instructions ✻ Carrier discretion Ⓑ Bill Part B MAC Ⓔ Bill DME MAC

○ **P9022** Red blood cells, washed, each unit Ⓑ Qp Qh R
IOM: 100-01, 3, 20.5; 100-02, 1, 10

○ **P9023** Plasma, pooled multiple donor, solvent/detergent treated, frozen, each unit Ⓑ Qp Qh R
IOM: 100-01, 3, 20.5; 100-02, 1, 10

○ **P9031** Platelets, leukocytes reduced, each unit Ⓑ Qp Qh R
IOM: 100-01, 3, 20.5; 100-02, 1, 10

○ **P9032** Platelets, irradiated, each unit Ⓑ Qp Qh R
IOM: 100-01, 3, 20.5; 100-02, 1, 10

○ **P9033** Platelets, leukocytes reduced, irradiated, each unit Ⓑ Qp Qh R
IOM: 100-01, 3, 20.5; 100-02, 1, 10

○ **P9034** Platelets, pheresis, each unit Ⓑ Qp Qh R
IOM: 100-01, 3, 20.5; 100-02, 1, 10

○ **P9035** Platelets, pheresis, leukocytes reduced, each unit Ⓑ Qp Qh R
IOM: 100-01, 3, 20.5; 100-02, 1, 10

○ **P9036** Platelets, pheresis, irradiated, each unit Ⓑ Qp Qh R
IOM: 100-01, 3, 20.5; 100-02, 1, 10

○ **P9037** Platelets, pheresis, leukocytes reduced, irradiated, each unit Ⓑ Qp Qh R
IOM: 100-01, 3, 20.5; 100-02, 1, 10

○ **P9038** Red blood cells, irradiated, each unit Ⓑ Qp Qh R
IOM: 100-01, 3, 20.5; 100-02, 1, 10

○ **P9039** Red blood cells, deglycerolized, each unit Ⓑ Qp Qh R
IOM: 100-01, 3, 20.5; 100-02, 1, 10

○ **P9040** Red blood cells, leukocytes reduced, irradiated, each unit Ⓑ Qp Qh R
IOM: 100-01, 3, 20.5; 100-02, 1, 10

* **P9041** Infusion, albumin (human), 5%, 50 ml Ⓑ Qp Qh K2 K

○ **P9043** Infusion, plasma protein fraction (human), 5%, 50 ml Ⓑ Qp Qh R
IOM: 100-01, 3, 20.5; 100-02, 1, 10

○ **P9044** Plasma, cryoprecipitate reduced, each unit Ⓑ Qp Qh R
IOM: 100-01, 3, 20.5; 100-02, 1, 10

* **P9045** Infusion, albumin (human), 5%, 250 ml Ⓑ Qp Qh K2 K

* **P9046** Infusion, albumin (human), 25%, 20 ml Ⓑ Qp Qh K2 K

* **P9047** Infusion, albumin (human), 25%, 50 ml Ⓑ Qp Qh K2 K

* **P9048** Infusion, plasma protein fraction (human), 5%, 250 ml Ⓑ Qp Qh R

* **P9050** Granulocytes, pheresis, each unit Ⓑ Qp Qh E2

○ **P9051** Whole blood or red blood cells, leukocytes reduced, CMV-negative, each unit Ⓑ Qp Qh R
Medicare Statute 1833(t)

○ **P9052** Platelets, HLA-matched leukocytes reduced, apheresis/pheresis, each unit Ⓑ Qp Qh R
Medicare Statute 1833(t)

○ **P9053** Platelets, pheresis, leukocytes reduced, CMV-negative, irradiated, each unit Ⓑ Qp Qh R
Freezing and thawing are reported separately, see Transmittal 1487 (Hospital outpatient)
Medicare Statute 1833(t)

○ **P9054** Whole blood or red blood cells, leukocytes reduced, frozen, deglycerol, washed, each unit Ⓑ Qp Qh R
Medicare Statute 1833(t)

○ **P9055** Platelets, leukocytes reduced, CMV-negative, apheresis/pheresis, each unit Ⓑ Qp Qh R
Medicare Statute 1833(t)

○ **P9056** Whole blood, leukocytes reduced, irradiated, each unit Ⓑ Qp Qh R
Medicare Statute 1833(t)

○ **P9057** Red blood cells, frozen/deglycerolized/washed, leukocytes reduced, irradiated, each unit Ⓑ Qp Qh R
Medicare Statute 1833(t)

○ **P9058** Red blood cells, leukocytes reduced, CMV-negative, irradiated, each unit Ⓑ Qp Qh R
Medicare Statute 1833(t)

○ **P9059** Fresh frozen plasma between 8-24 hours of collection, each unit Ⓑ Qp Qh R
Medicare Statute 1833(t)

○ **P9060** Fresh frozen plasma, donor retested, each unit Ⓑ Qp Qh R
Medicare Statute 1833(t)

○ **P9070** Plasma, pooled multiple donor, pathogen reduced, frozen, each unit Ⓑ Qp Qh R
Medicare Statute 1833(T)

MIPS | Qp Quantity Physician | Qh Quantity Hospital | ♀ Female only | ♂ Male only | A Age | DMEPOS | A2-Z3 ASC Payment Indicator | A-Y ASC Status Indicator | Coding Clinic

P9071 Plasma (single donor), pathogen reduced, frozen, each unit Qp Qh R

IOM: 100-01, 3, 20.5; 100-02, 1, 10

Medicare Statute 1833T

P9073 Platelets, pheresis, pathogen-reduced, each unit R

IOM: 100-01, 3, 20.5; 100-02, 1, 10

Medicare Statute 1833T

P9100 Pathogen(s) test for platelets S

IOM: 100-03, 4, 300.1

Travel Allowance for Specimen Collection

P9603 Travel allowance one way in connection with medically necessary laboratory specimen collection drawn from home bound or nursing home bound patient; prorated miles actually traveled Qp Qh A

Fee for clinical laboratory travel (P9603) is $1.025 per mile for CY2015.

IOM: 100-04, 16, 60

P9604 Travel allowance one way in connection with medically necessary laboratory specimen collection drawn from home bound or nursing home bound patient; prorated trip charge Qp Qh A

For CY2010, the fee for clinical laboratory travel is $10.30 per flat rate trip for CY2015.

IOM: 100-04, 16, 60

Catheterization for Specimen Collection

P9612 Catheterization for collection of specimen, single patient, all places of service Qp Qh A

NCCI edits indicate that when 51701 is comprehensive or is a Column 1 code, P9612 cannot be reported. When the catheter insertion is a component of another procedure, do not report straight catheterization separately.

IOM: 100-04, 16, 60

Coding Clinic: 2007, Q3, P7

P9615 Catheterization for collection of specimen(s) (multiple patients) Qp Qh N

IOM: 100-04, 16, 60

TEMPORARY CODES ASSIGNED BY CMS (Q0000-Q9999)

Cardiokymography

Q0035 Cardiokymography Qp Qh Q1

Report modifier 26 if professional component only

IOM: 100-03, 1, 20.24

Infusion Therapy

Q0081 Infusion therapy, using other than chemotherapeutic drugs, per visit Qh B

IV piggyback only assigned one time per patient encounter per day. Report for hydration or the intravenous administration of antibiotics, anti-emetics, or analgesics. Bill on paper. Requires a report.

IOM: 100-03, 4, 280.14

Coding Clinic: 2004, Q2, P11; Q1, P5, 8; 2002, Q2, P10; Q1, P7

Chemotherapy Administration

* **Q0083** Chemotherapy administration by other than infusion technique only (e.g., subcutaneous, intramuscular, push), per visit Qh B

Coding Clinic: 2002, Q1, P7

Q0084 Chemotherapy administration by infusion technique only, per visit Qh B

IOM: 100-03, 4, 280.14

Coding Clinic: 2004, Q2, P11; 2002, Q1, P7

* **Q0085** Chemotherapy administration by both infusion technique and other technique(s) (e.g., subcutaneous, intramuscular, push), per visit Qh B

Coding Clinic: 2002, Q1, P7

Smear Preparation

Q0091 Screening Papanicolaou smear; obtaining, preparing and conveyance of cervical or vaginal smear to laboratory Qp Qh ♀ S

Medicare does not cover comprehensive preventive medicine services; however, services described by G0101 and Q0091 (only for Medicare patients) are covered. Includes the services necessary to procure and transport the specimen to the laboratory.

IOM: 100-03, 3, 190.2

Coding Clinic: 2002, Q4, P8

Portable X-ray Setup

Q0092 Set-up portable x-ray equipment N

IOM: 100-04, 13, 90

Miscellaneous Lab Services

* **Q0111** Wet mounts, including preparations of vaginal, cervical or skin specimens Qp Qh A

Laboratory Certification: Bacteriology,Mycology,Parasitology

* **Q0112** All potassium hydroxide (KOH) preparations Qp Qh A

Laboratory Certification: Mycology

* **Q0113** Pinworm examinations Qp Qh A

Laboratory Certification: Parasitology

* **Q0114** Fern test Qp Qh ♀ A

Laboratory Certification: Routine chemistry

* **Q0115** Post-coital direct, qualitative examinations of vaginal or cervical mucous Qp Qh ♀ A

Laboratory Certification: Hematology

Drugs

* **Q0138** Injection, ferumoxytol, for treatment of iron deficiency anemia, 1 mg (non-ESRD use) Qp Qh K2 K

Feraheme is FDA approved for chronic kidney disease.

Other: Feraheme

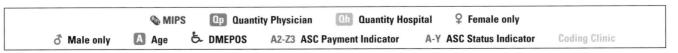

MIPS | Qp Quantity Physician | Qh Quantity Hospital | ♀ Female only
♂ Male only | A Age | DMEPOS | A2-Z3 ASC Payment Indicator | A-Y ASC Status Indicator | Coding Clinic

✻ **Q0139** Injection, ferumoxytol, for treatment of iron deficiency anemia, 1 mg (for ESRD on dialysis) Ⓑ Qp Qh K2 K

Other: Feraheme

⊘ **Q0144** Azithromycin dihydrate, oral, capsules/powder, 1 gm Ⓑ Ⓔ Qp Qh E1

Other: Zithromax, Zmax

✻ **Q0161** Chlorpromazine hydrochloride, 5 mg, oral, FDA approved prescription anti-emetic, for use as a complete therapeutic substitute for an IV anti-emetic at the time of chemotherapy treatment, not to exceed a 48 hour dosage regimen Ⓔ Qp Qh N1 N

◌ **Q0162** Ondansetron 1 mg, oral, FDA-approved prescription anti-emetic, for use as a complete therapeutic substitute for an iv anti-emetic at the time of chemotherapy treatment, not to exceed a 48 hour dosage regimen Ⓔ Qp Qh N1 N

Other: Zofran

Medicare Statute 4557

Coding Clinic: 2012, Q1, P9

◌ **Q0163** Diphenhydramine hydrochloride, 50 mg, oral, FDA approved prescription anti-emetic, for use as a complete therapeutic substitute for an IV anti-emetic at time of chemotherapy treatment not to exceed a 48 hour dosage regimen Ⓔ Qp Qh N1 N

Other: Alercap, Alertab, Allergy Relief Medicine, Allermax, Anti-Hist, Antihistamine, Banophen, Complete Allergy Medication, Complete Allergy medicine, Diphedryl, Diphenhist, Diphenhydramine, Dormin Sleep Aid, Genahist, Geridryl, Good Sense Antihistamine Allergy Relief, Good Sense Nighttime Sleep Aid, Mediphedryl, Night Time Sleep Aid, Nytol Quickcaps, Nytol Quickgels maximum strength, Quality Choice Sleep Aid, Quality Choice Rest Simply, Rapidpaq Dicopanol, Rite Aid Allergy, Serabrina La France, Siladryl Allergy, Silphen, Simply Sleep, Sleep Tabs, Sleepinal, Sominex, Twilite, Valu-Dryl Allergy

Medicare Statute 4557

Coding Clinic: 2012, Q2, P10

◌ **Q0164** Prochlorperazine maleate, 5 mg, oral, FDA approved prescription anti-emetic, for use as a complete therapeutic substitute for an IV anti-emetic at the time of chemotherapy treatment, not to exceed a 48 hour dosage regimen Ⓔ Qp Qh N1 N

Other: Compazine

Medicare Statute 4557

Coding Clinic: 2012, Q2, P10

◌ **Q0166** Granisetron hydrochloride, 1 mg, oral, FDA approved prescription anti-emetic, for use as a complete therapeutic substitute for an IV anti-emetic at the time of chemotherapy treatment, not to exceed a 24 hour dosage regimen Ⓔ Qp Qh N1 N

Other: Kytril

Medicare Statute 4557

Coding Clinic: 2012, Q2, P10

◌ **Q0167** Dronabinol, 2.5 mg, oral, FDA approved prescription anti-emetic, for use as a complete therapeutic substitute for an IV anti-emetic at the time of chemotherapy treatment, not to exceed a 48 hour dosage regimen Ⓔ Qp Qh N1 N

Other: Marinol

Medicare Statute 4557

Coding Clinic: 2012, Q2, P10

◌ **Q0169** Promethazine hydrochloride, 12.5 mg, oral, FDA approved prescription anti-emetic, for use as a complete therapeutic substitute for an IV anti-emetic at the time of chemotherapy treatment, not to exceed a 48 hour dosage regimen Ⓔ Qp Qh N1 N

Other: Anergan, Chlorpromazine, Hydroxyzine Pamoate, Phenazine, Phenergan, Prorex, Prothazine, V-Gan

Medicare Statute 4557

Coding Clinic: 2012, Q2, P10

◌ **Q0173** Trimethobenzamide hydrochloride, 250 mg, oral, FDA approved prescription anti-emetic, for use as a complete therapeutic substitute for an IV anti-emetic at the time of chemotherapy treatment, not to exceed a 48 hour dosage regimen Ⓔ Qp Qh N1 N

Other: Arrestin, Ticon, Tigan, Tiject

Medicare Statute 4557

Coding Clinic: 2012, Q2, P10

▶ New ↩ Revised ✔ Reinstated ~~deleted~~ Deleted ⊘ Not covered or valid by Medicare
◌ Special coverage instructions ✻ Carrier discretion Ⓑ Bill Part B MAC Ⓔ Bill DME MAC

Q0174 Thiethylperazine maleate, 10 mg, oral, FDA approved prescription anti-emetic, for use as a complete therapeutic substitute for an IV anti-emetic at the time of chemotherapy treatment, not to exceed a 48 hour dosage regimen Qp Qh E2

Other: Torecan

Medicare Statute 4557

Coding Clinic: 2012, Q2, P10

Q0175 Perphenazine, 4 mg, oral, FDA approved prescription anti-emetic, for use as a complete therapeutic substitute for an IV anti-emetic at the time of chemotherapy treatment, not to exceed a 48 hour dosage regimen Qp Qh N1 N

Medicare Statute 4557

Coding Clinic: 2012, Q2, P10

Q0177 Hydroxyzine pamoate, 25 mg, oral, FDA approved prescription anti-emetic, for use as a complete therapeutic substitute for an IV anti-emetic at the time of chemotherapy treatment, not to exceed a 48 hour dosage regimen Qp Qh N1 N

Other: Vistaril

Medicare Statute 4557

Coding Clinic: 2012, Q2, P10

Q0180 Dolasetron mesylate, 100 mg, oral, FDA approved prescription anti-emetic, for use as a complete therapeutic substitute for an IV anti-emetic at the time of chemotherapy treatment, not to exceed a 24 hour dosage regimen Qp Qh N1 N

Other: Anzemet

Medicare Statute 4557

Coding Clinic: 2012, Q2, P10

Q0181 Unspecified oral dosage form, FDA approved prescription anti-emetic, for use as a complete therapeutic substitute for a IV anti-emetic at the time of chemotherapy treatment, not to exceed a 48 hour dosage regimen N1 N

Medicare Statute 4557

Coding Clinic: 2012, Q2, P10

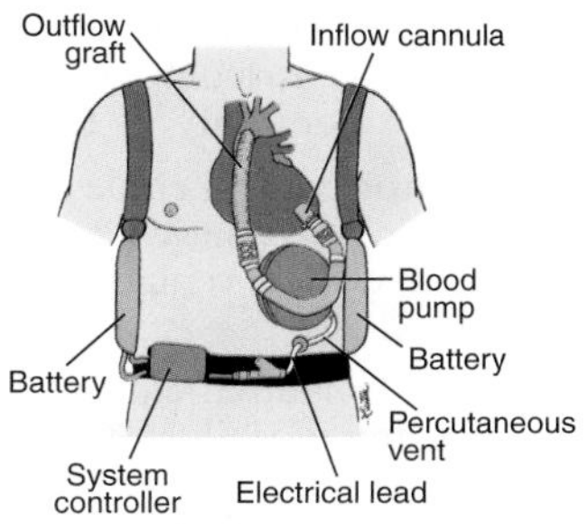

Outflow graft
Inflow cannula
Blood pump
Battery
Battery
Percutaneous vent
System controller
Electrical lead

Figure 46 Ventricular assist device.

Ventricular Assist Devices

Q0477 Power module patient cable for use with electric or electric/pneumatic ventricular assist device, replacement only A

Q0478 Power adapter for use with electric or electric/pneumatic ventricular assist device, vehicle type Qp Qh A

CMS has determined the reasonable useful lifetime is one year. Add modifier RA to claims to report when battery is replaced because it was lost, stolen, or irreparably damaged.

Q0479 Power module for use with electric or electric/pneumatic ventricular assist device, replacemment only Qp Qh A

CMS has determined the reasonable useful lifetime is one year. Add modifier RA in cases where the battery is being replaced because it was lost, stolen, or irreparably damaged.

Q0480 Driver for use with pneumatic ventricular assist device, replacement only Qp Qh A

Q0481 Microprocessor control unit for use with electric ventricular assist device, replacement only Qp Qh A

Q0482 Microprocessor control unit for use with electric/pneumatic combination ventricular assist device, replacement only Qp Qh A

Q0483 Monitor/display module for use with electric ventricular assist device, replacement only Qp Qh A

Q0484 Monitor/display module for use with electric or electric/pneumatic ventricular assist device, replacement only Qp Qh A

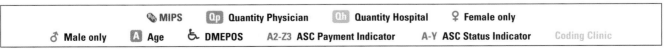

MIPS | Qp Quantity Physician | Qh Quantity Hospital | ♀ Female only | ♂ Male only | A Age | DMEPOS | A2-Z3 ASC Payment Indicator | A-Y ASC Status Indicator | Coding Clinic

Q0485 Monitor control cable for use with electric ventricular assist device, replacement only Qp Qh A

Q0486 Monitor control cable for use with electric/pneumatic ventricular assist device, replacement only Qp Qh A

Q0487 Leads (pneumatic/electrical) for use with any type electric/pneumatic ventricular assist device, replacement only Qp Qh A

Q0488 Power pack base for use with electric ventricular assist device, replacement only Qp Qh A

Q0489 Power pack base for use with electric/pneumatic ventricular assist device, replacement only Qp Qh A

Q0490 Emergency power source for use with electric ventricular assist device, replacement only Qp Qh A

Q0491 Emergency power source for use with electric/pneumatic ventricular assist device, replacement only Qp Qh A

Q0492 Emergency power supply cable for use with electric ventricular assist device, replacement only Qp Qh A

Q0493 Emergency power supply cable for use with electric/pneumatic ventricular assist device, replacement only Qp Qh A

Q0494 Emergency hand pump for use with electric or electric/pneumatic ventricular assist device, replacement only Qp Qh A

Q0495 Battery/power pack charger for use with electric or electric/pneumatic ventricular assist device, replacement only Qp Qh A

Q0496 Battery, other than lithium-ion, for use with electric or electric/pneumatic ventricular assist device, replacement only A

Reasonable useful lifetime is 6 months (CR3931).

Q0497 Battery clips for use with electric or electric/pneumatic ventricular assist device, replacement only Qp Qh A

Q0498 Holster for use with electric or electric/pneumatic ventricular assist device, replacement only Qp Qh A

Q0499 Belt/vest/bag for use to carry external peripheral components of any type ventricular assist device, replacement only Qp Qh A

Q0500 Filters for use with electric or electric/pneumatic ventricular assist device, replacement only A

Q0501 Shower cover for use with electric or electric/pneumatic ventricular assist device, replacement only Qp Qh A

Q0502 Mobility cart for pneumatic ventricular assist device, replacement only Qp Qh A

Q0503 Battery for pneumatic ventricular assist device, replacement only, each Qp Qh A

Reasonable useful lifetime is 6 months (CR3931).

Q0504 Power adapter for pneumatic ventricular assist device, replacement only, vehicle type Qp Qh A

Q0506 Battery, lithium-ion, for use with electric or electric/pneumatic, ventricular assist device, replacement only Qp Qh A

Reasonable useful lifetime is 12 months. Add -RA for replacement if lost, stolen, or irreparable damage.

Q0507 Miscellaneous supply or accessory for use with an external ventricular assist device Qp Qh A

Q0508 Miscellaneous supply or accessory for use with an implanted ventricular assist device Qp Qh A

Q0509 Miscellaneous supply or accessory for use with any implanted ventricular assist device for which payment was not made under Medicare Part A Qp Qh A

Pharmacy: Supply and Dispensing Fee

Q0510 Pharmacy supply fee for initial immunosuppressive drug(s), first month following transplant Qp Qh B

Q0511 Pharmacy supply fee for oral anti-cancer, oral anti-emetic or immunosuppressive drug(s); for the first prescription in a 30-day period Qp Qh B

Q0512 Pharmacy supply fee for oral anti-cancer, oral anti-emetic or immunosuppressive drug(s); for a subsequent prescription in a 30-day period Qp Qh B

New | Revised | Reinstated | ~~deleted~~ Deleted | Not covered or valid by Medicare | Special coverage instructions | Carrier discretion | Bill Part B MAC | Bill DME MAC

Q0513 Pharmacy dispensing fee for inhalation drug(s); per 30 days Qp Qh B

Q0514 Pharmacy dispensing fee for inhalation drug(s); per 90 days Qp Qh B

Sermorelin Acetate

Q0515 Injection, sermorelin acetate, 1 microgram Qp Qh E2

IOM: 100-02, 15, 50

New Technology: Intraocular Lens

Q1004 New technology intraocular lens category 4 as defined in Federal Register notice Qp Qh E1

Q1005 New technology intraocular lens category 5 as defined in Federal Register notice Qp Qh E1

Solutions and Drugs

Q2004 Irrigation solution for treatment of bladder calculi, for example renacidin, per 500 ml Qp Qh N1 N

IOM: 100-02, 15, 50

Medicare Statute 1861S2B

Q2009 Injection, fosphenytoin, 50 mg phenytoin equivalent Qp Qh K2 K

IOM: 100-02, 15, 50

Medicare Statute 1861S2B

Q2017 Injection, teniposide, 50 mg Qp Qh K2 K

IOM: 100-02, 15, 50

Medicare Statute 1861S2B

Q2026 Injection, radiesse, 0.1 ml Qp Qh E2

Coding Clinic: 2010, Q3, P8

Q2028 Injection, sculptra, 0.5 mg Qp Qh E2

Q2034 Influenza virus vaccine, split virus, for intramuscular use (Agriflu) Sipuleucel-t, minimum of 50 million autologous CD54+ cells activated with PAP-GM-CSF, including leukapheresis and all other preparatory procedures, per infusion Qp Qh L1 L

IOM: 100-02, 15, 50

Q2035 Influenza virus vaccine, split virus, when administered to individuals 3 years of age and older, for intramuscular use (Afluria) Qp Qh A L1 L

Preventive service; no deductible

IOM: 100-02, 15, 50

Coding Clinic: 2011, Q1, P7; 2010, Q4, P8-9

Q2036 Influenza virus vaccine, split virus, when administered to individuals 3 years of age and older, for intramuscular use (Flulaval) Qp Qh A L1 L

Preventive service; no deductible

IOM: 100-02, 15, 50

Coding Clinic: 2011, Q1, P7; 2010, Q4, P8-9

Q2037 Influenza virus vaccine, split virus, when administered to individuals3 years of age and older, for intramuscular use (Fluvirin) Qp Qh A L1 L

Preventive service; no deductible

IOM: 100-02, 15, 50

Coding Clinic: 2011, Q1, P7; 2010, Q4, P8-9

Q2038 Influenza virus vaccine, split virus, when administered to individuals 3 years of age or older, for intramuscular use (Fluzone) Qp Qh A L1 L

Preventive service; no deductible

IOM: 100-02, 15, 50

Coding Clinic: 2011, Q1, P7; 2010, Q4, P8-9

Q2039 Influenza virus vaccine, not otherwise specified Qp Qh A L1 L

Preventive service; no deductible

IOM: 100-02, 15, 50

Coding Clinic: 2011, Q1, P7; 2010, Q4, P8-9

~~Q2040 Tisagenlecleucel, up to 250 million car-positive viable T cells, including leukapheresis and dose preparation procedures, per infusion~~ ✖

▶ **Q2041** Axicabtagene ciloleucel, up to 200 million autologous anti-CD 19 CAR-positive viable T cells, including leukapheresis and dose preparation procedures, per therapeutic dose G

▶ **Q2042** Tisagenlecleucel, up to 600 million CAR-positive viable T cells, including leukapheresis and dose preparation procedures, per therapeutic dose G

MIPS | Qp Quantity Physician | Qh Quantity Hospital | ♀ Female only | ♂ Male only | A Age | DMEPOS | A2-Z3 ASC Payment Indicator | A-Y ASC Status Indicator | Coding Clinic

Q2043 Sipuleucel-T, minimum of 50 million autologous CD54+ cells activated with PAP-GM-CSF, including leukapheresis and all other preparatory procedures, per infusion Qp Qh K2 K

Other: Provenge

Coding Clinic: 2012, Q2, P7; Q1, P7, 9; 2011, Q3, P9

* **Q2049** Injection, doxorubicin hydrochloride, liposomal, imported lipodox, 10 mg Qp Qh K2 K

Coding Clinic: 2012, Q3, P10

Q2050 Injection, doxorubicin hydrochloride, liposomal, not otherwise specified, 10 mg Qp Qh K2 K

Other: Doxil

IOM: 100-02, 15, 50

Q2052 Services, supplies and accessories used in the home under the Medicare intravenous immune globulin (IVIG) demonstration Qp Qh E1

Coding Clinic: 2014, Q2, P6

Brachytherapy Radioelements

Q3001 Radioelements for brachytherapy, any type, each B

IOM: 100-04, 12, 70; 100-04, 13, 20

Telehealth

* **Q3014** Telehealth originating site facility fee Qp Qh A

Effective January of each year, the fee for telehealth services is increased by the Medicare Economic Index (MEI). The telehealth originating facility site fee (HCPCS code Q3014) for 2011 was 80 percent of the lesser of the actual charge or $24.10.

Drugs

Q3027 Injection, interferon beta-1a, 1 mcg for intramuscular use Qp Qh K2 K

Other: Avonex

IOM: 100-02, 15, 50

⃠ **Q3028** Injection, interferon beta-1a, 1 mcg for subcutaneous use Qp Qh E1

Skin Test

Q3031 Collagen skin test Qp Qh N1 N

IOM: 100-03, 4, 280.1

Supplies: Cast

Q4001-Q4051: Payment on a reasonable charge basis is required for splints, casts by regulations contained in 42 CFR 405.501.

* **Q4001** Casting supplies, body cast adult, with or without head, plaster Qp Qh A B

* **Q4002** Cast supplies, body cast adult, with or without head, fiberglass Qp Qh A B

* **Q4003** Cast supplies, shoulder cast, adult (11 years +), plaster Qp Qh A B

* **Q4004** Cast supplies, shoulder cast, adult (11 years +), fiberglass Qp Qh A B

* **Q4005** Cast supplies, long arm cast, adult (11 years +), plaster A B

* **Q4006** Cast supplies, long arm cast, adult (11 years +), fiberglass A B

* **Q4007** Cast supplies, long arm cast, pediatric (0-10 years), plaster A B

* **Q4008** Cast supplies, long arm cast, pediatric (0-10 years), fiberglass A B

* **Q4009** Cast supplies, short arm cast, adult (11 years +), plaster A B

* **Q4010** Cast supplies, short arm cast, adult (11 years +), fiberglass A B

* **Q4011** Cast supplies, short arm cast, pediatric (0-10 years), plaster A B

* **Q4012** Cast supplies, short arm cast, pediatric (0-10 years), fiberglass A B

* **Q4013** Cast supplies, gauntlet cast (includes lower forearm and hand), adult (11 years +), plaster A B

* **Q4014** Cast supplies, gauntlet cast (includes lower forearm and hand), adult (11 years +), fiberglass A B

* **Q4015** Cast supplies, gauntlet cast (includes lower forearm and hand), pediatric (0-10 years), plaster A B

* **Q4016** Cast supplies, gauntlet cast (includes lower forearm and hand), pediatric (0-10 years), fiberglass A B

* **Q4017** Cast supplies, long arm splint, adult (11 years +), plaster A B

▶ New ⤻ Revised ✔ Reinstated ~~deleted~~ Deleted ⃠ Not covered or valid by Medicare
Special coverage instructions * Carrier discretion Ⓑ Bill Part B MAC Ⓓ Bill DME MAC

✻ **Q4018** Cast supplies, long arm splint, adult (11 years +), fiberglass A B

✻ **Q4019** Cast supplies, long arm splint, pediatric (0-10 years), plaster A B

✻ **Q4020** Cast supplies, long arm splint, pediatric (0-10 years), fiberglass A B

✻ **Q4021** Cast supplies, short arm splint, adult (11 years +), plaster A B

✻ **Q4022** Cast supplies, short arm splint, adult (11 years +), fiberglass A B

✻ **Q4023** Cast supplies, short arm splint, pediatric (0-10 years), plaster A B

✻ **Q4024** Cast supplies, short arm splint, pediatric (0-10 years), fiberglass A B

✻ **Q4025** Cast supplies, hip spica (one or both legs), adult (11 years +), plaster Qp Qh A B

✻ **Q4026** Cast supplies, hip spica (one or both legs), adult (11 years +), fiberglass Qp Qh A B

✻ **Q4027** Cast supplies, hip spica (one or both legs), pediatric (0-10 years), plaster Qp Qh A B

✻ **Q4028** Cast supplies, hip spica (one or both legs), pediatric (0-10 years), fiberglass Qp Qh A B

✻ **Q4029** Cast supplies, long leg cast, adult (11 years +), plaster A B

✻ **Q4030** Cast supplies, long leg cast, adult (11 years +), fiberglass A B

✻ **Q4031** Cast supplies, long leg cast, pediatric (0-10 years), plaster A B

✻ **Q4032** Cast supplies, long leg cast, pediatric (0-10 years), fiberglass A B

✻ **Q4033** Cast supplies, long leg cylinder cast, adult (11 years +), plaster A B

✻ **Q4034** Cast supplies, long leg cylinder cast, adult (11 years +), fiberglass A B

✻ **Q4035** Cast supplies, long leg cylinder cast, pediatric (0-10 years), plaster A B

✻ **Q4036** Cast supplies, long leg cylinder cast, pediatric (0-10 years), fiberglass A B

✻ **Q4037** Cast supplies, short leg cast, adult (11 years +), plaster A B

✻ **Q4038** Cast supplies, short leg cast, adult (11 years +), fiberglass A B

✻ **Q4039** Cast supplies, short leg cast, pediatric (0-10 years), plaster A B

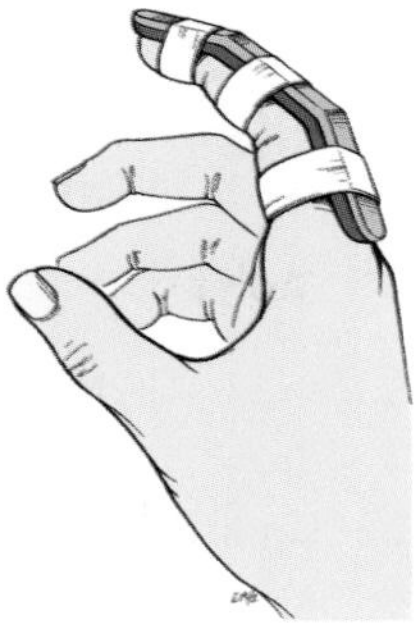

Figure 47 Finger splint.

✻ **Q4040** Cast supplies, short leg cast, pediatric (0-10 years), fiberglass A B

✻ **Q4041** Cast supplies, long leg splint, adult (11 years +), plaster A B

✻ **Q4042** Cast supplies, long leg splint, adult (11 years +), fiberglass A B

✻ **Q4043** Cast supplies, long leg splint, pediatric (0-10 years), plaster A B

✻ **Q4044** Cast supplies, long leg splint, pediatric (0-10 years), fiberglass A B

✻ **Q4045** Cast supplies, short leg splint, adult (11 years +), plaster A B

✻ **Q4046** Cast supplies, short leg splint, adult (11 years +), fiberglass A B

✻ **Q4047** Cast supplies, short leg splint, pediatric (0-10 years), plaster A B

✻ **Q4048** Cast supplies, short leg splint, pediatric (0-10 years), fiberglass A B

✻ **Q4049** Finger splint, static B

✻ **Q4050** Cast supplies, for unlisted types and materials of casts B

✻ **Q4051** Splint supplies, miscellaneous (includes thermoplastics, strapping, fasteners, padding and other supplies) B

Drugs

✻ **Q4074** Iloprost, inhalation solution, FDA-approved final product, non-compounded, administered through DME, unit dose form, up to 20 micrograms Qp Qh Y

Other: Ventavis

Q4081 Injection, epoetin alfa, 100 units (for ESRD on dialysis) Qp Qh N

Other: Epogen, Procrit

✻ **Q4082** Drug or biological, not otherwise classified, Part B drug competitive acquisition program (CAP) B

MIPS | Qp Quantity Physician | Qh Quantity Hospital | ♀ Female only
♂ Male only | A Age | DMEPOS | A2-Z3 ASC Payment Indicator | A-Y ASC Status Indicator | Coding Clinic

Skin Substitutes

* * Q4100 Skin substitute, not otherwise specified N1 N
  Coding Clinic: 2018, Q2, P3; 2012, Q2, P7
* * Q4101 Apligraf, per square centimeter Qp Qh N1 N
  Coding Clinic: 2012, Q2, P7; 2011, Q1, P9
* * Q4102 Oasis Wound Matrix, per square centimeter Qp Qh N1 N
  Coding Clinic: 2012, Q3, P8; Q2, P7; 2011, Q1, P9
* * Q4103 Oasis Burn Matrix, per square centimeter Qp Qh N1 N
  Coding Clinic: 2012, Q2, P7; 2011, Q1, P9
* * Q4104 Integra Bilayer Matrix Wound Dressing (BMWD), per square centimeter Qp Qh N1 N
  Coding Clinic: 2012, Q2, P7; 2011, Q1, P9; 2010, Q2, P8
* * Q4105 Integra Dermal Regeneration Template (DRT,) or integra omnigraft dermal regeneration matrix, per square centimeter Qp Qh N1 N
  Coding Clinic: 2012, Q2, P7; 2011, Q1, P9; 2010, Q2, P8
* * Q4106 Dermagraft, per square centimeter Qp Qh N1 N
  Coding Clinic: 2012, Q2, P7; 2011, Q1, P9
* * Q4107 Graftjacket, per square centimeter Qp Qh N1 N
  Coding Clinic: 2012, Q2, P7; 2011, Q1, P9
* * Q4108 Integra Matrix, per square centimeter Qp Qh N1 N
  Coding Clinic: 2012, Q2, P7; 2011, Q1, P9; 2010, Q2, P8
* * Q4110 Primatrix, per square centimeter Qp Qh N1 N
  Coding Clinic: 2012, Q2, P7; 2011, Q1, P9
* * Q4111 GammaGraft, per square centimeter Qp Qh N1 N
  Coding Clinic: 2012, Q2, P7; 2011, Q1, P9
* * Q4112 Cymetra, injectable, 1 cc Qp Qh N1 N
  Coding Clinic: 2012, Q2, P7; 2011, Q1, P9
* * Q4113 GraftJacket Xpress, injectable, 1 cc Qp Qh N1 N
  Coding Clinic: 2012, Q2, P7; 2011, Q1, P9
* * Q4114 Integra Flowable Wound Matrix, injectable, 1 cc Qp Qh N1 N
  Coding Clinic: 2012, Q2, P7; 2010, Q2, P8
* * Q4115 Alloskin, per square centimeter Qp Qh N1 N
  Coding Clinic: 2012, Q2, P7; 2011, Q1, P9
* * Q4116 Alloderm, per square centimeter Qp Qh N1 N
  Coding Clinic: 2012, Q2, P7; 2011, Q1, P9
* * Q4117 Hyalomatrix, per square centimeter Qp Qh N1 N
  IOM: 100-02, 15, 50
* * Q4118 Matristem micromatrix, 1 mg Qp Qh N1 N
  Coding Clinic: 2013, Q4, P2; 2012, Q2, P7; 2011, Q1, P6
* * Q4121 Theraskin, per square centimeter Qp Qh N1 N
  Coding Clinic: 2012, Q2, P7; 2011, Q1, P6
* * Q4122 Dermacell, per square centimeter Qp Qh N1 N
  Coding Clinic: 2012, Q2, P7; Q1, P8
* * Q4123 AlloSkin RT, per square centimeter Qp Qh N1 N
* * Q4124 Oasis Ultra Tri-layer Wound Matrix, per square centimeter Qp Qh N1 N
  Coding Clinic: 2012, Q2, P7; Q1, P9
* * Q4125 Arthroflex, per square centimeter Qp Qh N1 N
* * Q4126 Memoderm, dermaspan, tranzgraft or integuply, per square centimeter Qp Qh N1 N
* * Q4127 Talymed, per square centimeter Qp Qh N1 N
* * Q4128 FlexHD, Allopatch HD, or Matrix HD, per square centimeter Qp Qh N1 N
* * Q4130 Strattice TM, per square centimeter Qp Qh N1 N
  Coding Clinic: 2012, Q2, P7
* ~~Q4131 Epifix, per square centimeter~~ ✖
* * Q4132 Grafix core and GrafixPL core, per square centimeter Qp Qh N1 N
* ↩ * Q4133 Grafix prime, GrafixPL prime, stravix and stravixpl, per square centimeter Qp Qh N1 N
* * Q4134 Hmatrix, per square centimeter Qp Qh N1 N
* * Q4135 Mediskin, per square centimeter Qp Qh N1 N
* * Q4136 Ez-derm, per square centimeter Qp Qh N1 N
* ↩ * Q4137 Amnioexcel, amnioexcel plus or biodexcel, per square centimeter Qp Qh N1 N
* * Q4138 Biodfence dryflex, per square centimeter Qp Qh N1 N

▶ New ↩ Revised ✔ Reinstated ~~deleted~~ Deleted ⊘ Not covered or valid by Medicare
Special coverage instructions * Carrier discretion Ⓑ Bill Part B MAC Ⓓ Bill DME MAC

✻ **Q4139** Amniomatrix or biodmatrix, injectable, 1 cc Qp Qh N1 N

✻ **Q4140** Biodfence, per square centimeter Qp Qh N1 N

✻ **Q4141** Alloskin ac, per square centimeter Qp Qh N1 N

✻ **Q4142** XCM biologic tissue matrix, per square centimeter Qp Qh N1 N

✻ **Q4143** Repriza, per square centimeter Qp Qh N1 N

✻ **Q4145** Epifix, injectable, 1 mg Qp Qh N1 N

✻ **Q4146** Tensix, per square centimeter Qp Qh N1 N

✻ **Q4147** Architect, architect PX, or architect FX, extracellular matrix, per square centimeter Qp Qh N1 N

✻ **Q4148** Neox cord 1K, Neox cord RT, or Clarix cord 1K, per square centimeter Qp Qh N1 N

✻ **Q4149** Excellagen, 0.1 cc Qp Qh N1 N

✻ **Q4150** AlloWrap DS or dry, per square centimeter Qp Qh N1 N

✻ **Q4151** Amnioband or guardian, per square centimeter Qp Qh N1 N

✻ **Q4152** DermaPure, per square centimeter Qp Qh N1 N

✻ **Q4153** Dermavest and Plurivest, per square centimeter Qp Qh N1 N

✻ **Q4154** Biovance, per square centimeter Qp Qh N1 N

✻ **Q4155** Neoxflo or clarixflo, 1 mg Qp Qh N1 N

✻ **Q4156** Neox 100 or Clarix 100, per square centimeter Qp Qh N1 N

✻ **Q4157** Revitalon, per square centimeter Qp Qh N1 N

✻ **Q4158** Kerecis Omega3, per square centimeter Qp Qh N1 N

✻ **Q4159** Affinity, per square centimeter Qp Qh N1 N

✻ **Q4160** Nushield, per square centimeter Qp Qh N1 N

✻ **Q4161** Bio-ConneKt Wound Matrix, per square centimeter Qp Qh N1 N

✻ **Q4162** Woundex flow, BioSkin flow 0.5 cc Qp Qh N1 N

✻ **Q4163** Woundex, BioSkin per square centimeter Qp Qh N1 N

✻ **Q4164** Helicoll, per square centimeter Qp Qh N1 N

✻ **Q4165** Keramatrix, per square centimeter Qp Qh N1 N

✻ **Q4166** Cytal, per square centimeter Qp Qh N1 N

Coding Clinic: 2017, Q1, P10

✻ **Q4167** TruSkin, per square centimeter Qp Qh N1 N

Coding Clinic: 2017, Q1, P10

✻ **Q4168** AmnioBand, 1 mg Qp Qh N1 N

Coding Clinic: 2017, Q1, P10

✻ **Q4169** Artacent wound, per square centimeter Qp Qh N1 N

Coding Clinic: 2017, Q1, P10

✻ **Q4170** Cygnus, per square centimeter Qp Qh N1 N

Coding Clinic: 2017, Q1, P10

✻ **Q4171** Interfyl, 1 mg Qp Qh N1 N

Coding Clinic: 2017, Q1, P10

~~Q4172 Puraply or puraply am, per square centimeter~~ ✖

✻ **Q4173** PalinGen or PalinGen XPlus, per square centimeter Qp Qh N1 N

Coding Clinic: 2017, Q1, P10

✻ **Q4174** PalinGen or ProMatrX, 0.36 mg per 0.25 cc Qp Qh N1 N

Coding Clinic: 2017, Q1, P10

✻ **Q4175** Miroderm, per square centimeter Qp Qh N1 N

Coding Clinic: 2017, Q1, P10

✻ **Q4176** Neopatch, per square centimeter N1 N

✻ **Q4177** Floweramnioflo, 0.1 cc N1 N

✻ **Q4178** Floweramniopatch, per square centimeter N1 N

✻ **Q4179** Flowerderm, per square centimeter N1 N

✻ **Q4180** Revita, per square centimeter N1 N

✻ **Q4181** Amnio wound, per square centimeter N1 N

✻ **Q4182** Transcyte, per square centimeter N1 N

▶ ✻ **Q4183** Surgigraft, per square centimeter N

▶ ✻ **Q4184** Cellesta, per square centimeter N

▶ ✻ **Q4185** Cellesta flowable amnion (25 mg per cc); per 0.5 cc N

▶ ✻ **Q4186** Epifix, per square centimeter N

▶ ✻ **Q4187** Epicord, per square centimeter N

▶ ✻ **Q4188** Amnioarmor, per square centimeter N

▶ ✻ **Q4189** Artacent ac, 1 mg N

▶ ✻ **Q4190** Artacent ac, per square centimeter N

MIPS | Qp Quantity Physician | Qh Quantity Hospital | ♀ Female only
♂ Male only | A Age | DMEPOS | A2-Z3 ASC Payment Indicator | A-Y ASC Status Indicator | Coding Clinic

▶ ✻ **Q4191** Restorigin, per square centimeter N

▶ ✻ **Q4192** Restorigin, 1 cc N

▶ ✻ **Q4193** Coll-e-derm, per square centimeter N

▶ ✻ **Q4194** Novachor, per square centimeter N

▶ ✻ **Q4195** Puraply, per square centimeter G

▶ ✻ **Q4196** Puraply am, per square centimeter G

▶ ✻ **Q4197** Puraply xt, per square centimeter N

▶ ✻ **Q4198** Genesis amniotic membrane, per square centimeter N

▶ ✻ **Q4200** Skin te, per square centimeter N

▶ ✻ **Q4201** Matrion, per square centimeter N

▶ ✻ **Q4202** Keroxx (2.5g/cc), 1cc N

▶ ✻ **Q4203** Derma-gide, per square centimeter N

▶ ✻ **Q4204** Xwrap, per square centimeter N

Hospice Care

Q5001 Hospice or home health care provided in patient's home/residence B

Q5002 Hospice or home health care provided in assisted living facility B

Q5003 Hospice care provided in nursing long term care facility (LTC) or non-skilled nursing facility (NF) B

Q5004 Hospice care provided in skilled nursing facility (SNF) B

Q5005 Hospice care provided in inpatient hospital B

Q5006 Hospice care provided in inpatient hospice facility B

Hospice care provided in an inpatient hospice facility. These are residential facilities, which are places for patients to live while receiving routine home care or continuous home care. These hospice residential facilities are not certified by Medicare or Medicaid for provision of General Inpatient (GIP) or respite care, and regulations at 42 CFR 418.202(e) do not allow provision of GIP or respite care at hospice residential facilities.

Q5007 Hospice care provided in long term care facility B

Q5008 Hospice care provided in inpatient psychiatric facility B

Q5009 Hospice or home health care provided in place not otherwise specified (NOS) B

Q5010 Hospice home care provided in a hospice facility B

Biosimilar Drugs

↩ **Q5101** Injection, filgrastim-sndz, biosimilar, (zarxio), 1 microgram Qp Qh K2 G

Other: Zarxio

~~Q5102 Injection, infliximab, biosimilar, 10 mg~~ ✖

▶ **Q5103** Injection, infliximab-dyyb, biosimilar, (inflectra), 10 mg G

Other: Remicade, Inflectra, Renflexis

▶ **Q5104** Injection, infliximab-abda, biosimilar, (renflexis), 10 mgn K2 G

Other: Remicade

▶ **Q5105** Injection, epoetin alfa, biosimilar, (retacrit) (for ESRD on dialysis), 100 units K2 G

Other: Retacrit

▶ **Q5106** Injection, epoetin alfa, biosimilar, (retacrit) (for non-ESRD use), 1000 units G

Other: Retacrit

▶ **Q5107** Injection, bevacizumab-awwb, biosimilar, (mvasi), 10 mg E2

Other: Avastin

▶ **Q5108** Injection, pegfilgrastim-jmdb, biosimilar, (fulphila), 0.5 mg K

Other: Neulasta

▶ **Q5109** Injection, infliximab-qbtx, biosimilar, (ixifi), 10 mg E2

Other: Remicade, Inflectra, Renflexis

▶ **Q5110** Injection, filgrastim-aafi, biosimilar, (nivestym), 1 microgram K

Other: Nivestym

Contrast Agents

✻ **Q9950** Injection, sulfur hexafluoride lipid microspheres, per ml Qp Qh N1 N

Other: Lumason

Q9951 Low osmolar contrast material, 400 or greater mg/ml iodine concentration, per ml Qp Qh N1 N

IOM: 100-04, 12, 70; 100-04, 13, 20; 100-04, 13, 90

Coding Clinic: 2012, Q3, P8

Q9953 Injection, iron-based magnetic resonance contrast agent, per ml Qp Qh N1 N

IOM: 100-04, 12, 70; 100-04, 13, 20; 100-04, 13, 90

Coding Clinic: 2012, Q3, P8

▶ New ↩ Revised ✔ Reinstated ~~deleted~~ Deleted ⊘ Not covered or valid by Medicare
Special coverage instructions ✻ Carrier discretion Bill Part B MAC Bill DME MAC

Q9954 Oral magnetic resonance contrast agent, per 100 ml Qp Qh N1 N

IOM: 100-04, 12, 70; 100-04, 13, 20; 100-04, 13, 90

Coding Clinic: 2012, Q3, P8

* **Q9955** Injection, perflexane lipid microspheres, per ml Qp Qh N1 N

Coding Clinic: 2012, Q3, P8

* **Q9956** Injection, octafluoropropane microspheres, per ml Qp Qh N1 N

Other: Optison

Coding Clinic: 2012, Q3, P8

* **Q9957** Injection, perflutren lipid microspheres, per ml Qp Qh N1 N

Other: Definity

Coding Clinic: 2012, Q3, P8

Q9958 High osmolar contrast material, up to 149 mg/ml iodine concentration, per ml Qp Qh N1 N

Other: Conray 30, Cysto-Conray II, Cystografin

IOM: 100-04, 12, 70; 100-04, 13, 20; 100-04, 13, 90

Coding Clinic: 2012, Q3, P8; 2007, Q1, P6

Q9959 High osmolar contrast material, 150-199 mg/ml iodine concentration, per ml Qp Qh N1 N

IOM: 100-04, 12, 70; 100-04, 13, 20; 100-04, 13, 90

Coding Clinic: 2012, Q3, P8; 2007, Q1, P6

Q9960 High osmolar contrast material, 200-249 mg/mliodine concentration, per ml Qp Qh N1 N

Other: Conray 43

IOM: 100-04, 12, 70; 100-04, 13, 20; 100-04, 13, 90

Coding Clinic: 2012, Q3, P8; 2007, Q1, P6

Q9961 High osmolar contrast material, 250-299 mg/mliodine concentration, per ml Qp Qh N1 N

Other: Conray, Cholografin Meglumine

IOM: 100-04, 12, 70; 100-04, 13, 20; 100-04, 13, 90

Coding Clinic: 2012, Q3, P8; 2007, Q1, P6

Q9962 High osmolar contrast material, 300-349 mg/ml iodine concentration, per ml Qp Qh N1 N

IOM: 100-04, 12, 70; 100-04, 13, 20; 100-04, 13, 90

Coding Clinic: 2012, Q3, P8; 2007, Q1, P6

Q9963 High osmolar contrast material, 350-399 mg/ml iodine concentration, per ml Qp Qh N1 N

Other: Gastrografin, MD-76R, MD Gastroview, Sinografin

IOM: 100-04, 12, 70; 100-04, 13, 20; 100-04, 13, 90

Coding Clinic: 2012, Q3, P8; 2007, Q1, P6

Q9964 High osmolar contrast material, 400 or greater mg/ml iodine concentration, per ml Qp Qh N1 N

IOM: 100-04, 12, 70; 100-04, 13, 20; 100-04, 13, 90

Coding Clinic: 2012, Q3, P8; 2007, Q1, P6

Q9965 Low osmolar contrast material, 100-199 mg/ml iodine concentration, per ml N1 N

Other: Omnipaque

IOM: 100-04, 12, 70; 100-04, 13, 20; 100-04, 13, 90

Coding Clinic: 2012, Q3, P8

Q9966 Low osmolar contrast material, 200-299 mg/ml iodine concentration, per ml Qp Qh N1 N

Other: Isovue, Omnipaque, Optiray, Ultravist 240, Visipaque

IOM: 100-04, 12, 70; 100-04, 13, 20; 100-04, 13, 90

Coding Clinic: 2012, Q3, P8

Q9967 Low osmolar contrast material, 300-399 mg/ml iodine concentration, per ml Qp Qh N1 N

Other: Hexabrix 320, Isovue, Omnipaque, Optiray, Oxilan, Ultravist, Vispaque

IOM: 100-04, 12, 70; 100-04, 13, 20; 100-04, 13, 90

Coding Clinic: 2012, Q3, P8

* **Q9968** Injection, non-radioactive, non-contrast, visualization adjunct (e.g., Methylene Blue, Isosulfan Blue), 1 mg K2 K

Q9969 Tc-99m from non-highly enriched uranium source, full cost recovery add-on, per study dose Qp Qh K

Radiopharmaceuticals

◎ **Q9982** Flutemetamol F18, diagnostic, per study dose, up to 5 millicuries Ⓑ Qp Qh K2 G

Other: Vizamyl

◎ **Q9983** Florbetaben F18, diagnostic, per study dose, up to 8.1 millicuries Ⓑ Qp Qh K2 G

Other: Neuraceq

▶ * **Q9991** Injection, buprenorphine extended-release (sublocade), less than or equal to 100 mg G

Other: Subutex, Buprenex, Belbuca, Probuphine, Butrans

▶ * **Q9992** Injection, buprenorphine extended-release (sublocade), greater than 100 mg G

Other: Subutex, Buprenex, Belbuca, Probuphine, Butrans

DIAGNOSTIC RADIOLOGY SERVICES (R0000-R9999)

Transportation/Setup of Portable Equipment

R0070 Transportation of portable x-ray equipment and personnel to home or nursing home, per trip to facility or location, one patient seen Qp Qh B

CMS Transmittal B03-049; specific instructions to contractors on pricing

IOM: 100-04, 13, 90; 100-04, 13, 90.3

R0075 Transportation of portable x-ray equipment and personnel to home or nursing home, per trip to facility or location, more than one patient seen Qp Qh B

This code would not apply to the x-ray equipment if stored at the location where the x-ray was performed (e.g., a nursing home).

IOM: 100-04, 13, 90; 100-04, 13, 90.3

R0076 Transportation of portable ECG to facility or location, per patient Qp Qh B

EKG procedure code 93000 or 93005 must be submitted on same claim as transportation code. Bundled status on physician fee schedule

IOM: 100-01, 5, 90.2; 100-02, 15, 80; 100-03, 1, 20.15; 100-04, 13, 90; 100-04, 16, 10; 100-04, 16, 110.4

TEMPORARY NATIONAL CODES ESTABLISHED BY PRIVATE PAYERS (S0000-S9999)

NOTE: Medicare and other federal payers do not recognize "S" codes; however, S codes may be useful for claims to some private insurers.

Non-Medicare Drugs

⃠ **S0012** Butorphanol tartrate, nasal spray, 25 mg

⃠ **S0014** Tacrine hydrochloride, 10 mg

⃠ **S0017** Injection, aminocaproic acid, 5 grams

⃠ **S0020** Injection, bupivacaine hydrochloride, 30 ml

⃠ **S0021** Injection, cefoperazone sodium, 1 gram

⃠ **S0023** Injection, cimetidine hydrochloride, 300 mg

⃠ **S0028** Injection, famotidine, 20 mg

⃠ **S0030** Injection, metronidazole, 500 mg

⃠ **S0032** Injection, nafcillin sodium, 2 grams

⃠ **S0034** Injection, ofloxacin, 400 mg

⃠ **S0039** Injection, sulfamethoxazole and trimethoprim, 10 ml

⃠ **S0040** Injection, ticarcillin disodium and clavulanate potassium, 3.1 grams

⃠ **S0073** Injection, aztreonam, 500 mg

⃠ **S0074** Injection, cefotetan disodium, 500 mg

⃠ **S0077** Injection, clindamycin phosphate, 300 mg

⃠ **S0078** Injection, fosphenytoin sodium, 750 mg

⃠ **S0080** Injection, pentamidine isethionate, 300 mg

⃠ **S0081** Injection, piperacillin sodium, 500 mg

⃠ **S0088** Imatinib, 100 mg

⃠ **S0090** Sildenafil citrate, 25 mg A

⃠ **S0091** Granisetron hydrochloride, 1 mg (for circumstances falling under the Medicare Statute, use Q0166)

⃠ **S0092** Injection, hydromorphone hydrochloride, 250 mg (loading dose for infusion pump)

⃠ **S0093** Injection, morphine sulfate, 500 mg (loading dose for infusion pump)

⃠ **S0104** Zidovudine, oral, 100 mg

⃠ **S0106** Bupropion HCl sustained release tablet, 150 mg, per bottle of 60 tablets

⃠ **S0108** Mercaptopurine, oral, 50 mg

⃠ **S0109** Methadone, oral, 5 mg

⃠ **S0117** Tretinoin, topical, 5 grams

⃠ **S0119** Ondansetron, oral, 4 mg (for circumstances falling under the Medicare statute, use HCPCS Q code)

⃠ **S0122** Injection, menotropins, 75 IU

⃠ **S0126** Injection, follitropin alfa, 75 IU

⃠ **S0128** Injection, follitropin beta, 75 IU

⃠ **S0132** Injection, ganirelix acetate, 250 mcg

⃠ **S0136** Clozapine, 25 mg

⃠ **S0137** Didanosine (DDI), 25 mg

⃠ **S0138** Finasteride, 5 mg

⃠ **S0139** Minoxidil, 10 mg

⃠ **S0140** Saquinavir, 200 mg

⃠ **S0142** Colistimethate sodium, inhalation solution administered through DME, concentrated form, per mg

⃠ **S0145** Injection, pegylated interferon alfa-2a, 180 mcg per ml

⃠ **S0148** Injection, pegylated interferon ALFA-2b, 10 mcg

⃠ **S0155** Sterile dilutant for epoprostenol, 50 ml

⃠ **S0156** Exemestane, 25 mg

⃠ **S0157** Becaplermin gel 0.01%, 0.5 gm

⃠ **S0160** Dextroamphetamine sulfate, 5 mg

⃠ **S0164** Injection, pantoprazole sodium, 40 mg

⃠ **S0166** Injection, olanzapine, 2.5 mg

⃠ **S0169** Calcitrol, 0.25 microgram

⃠ **S0170** Anastrozole, oral, 1 mg

⃠ **S0171** Injection, bumetanide, 0.5 mg

⃠ **S0172** Chlorambucil, oral, 2 mg

⃠ **S0174** Dolasetron mesylate, oral 50 mg (for circumstances falling under the Medicare Statute, use Q0180)

⃠ **S0175** Flutamide, oral, 125 mg

⃠ **S0176** Hydroxyurea, oral, 500 mg

⃠ **S0177** Levamisole hydrochloride, oral, 50 mg

⃠ **S0178** Lomustine, oral, 10 mg

⃠ **S0179** Megestrol acetate, oral, 20 mg

⃠ **S0182** Procarbazine hydrochloride, oral, 50 mg

⃠ **S0183** Prochlorperazine maleate, oral, 5 mg (for circumstances falling under the Medicare Statute, use Q0164)

⃠ **S0187** Tamoxifen citrate, oral, 10 mg

▶ New ↻ Revised ✔ Reinstated ~~deleted~~ Deleted ⃠ Not covered or valid by Medicare
Special coverage instructions ✻ Carrier discretion Ⓑ Bill Part B MAC Ⓑ Bill DME MAC

⊘ **S0189** Testosterone pellet, 75 mg

⊘ **S0190** Mifepristone, oral, 200 mg

⊘ **S0191** Misoprostol, oral 200 mcg

⊘ **S0194** Dialysis/stress vitamin supplement, oral, 100 capsules

⊘ **S0197** Prenatal vitamins, 30-day supply ♀

Provider Services

⊘ **S0199** Medically induced abortion by oral ingestion of medication including all associated services and supplies (e.g., patient counseling, office visits, confirmation of pregnancy by HCG, ultrasound to confirm duration of pregnancy, ultrasound to confirm completion of abortion) except drugs ♀

MIPS ⊘ **S0201** Partial hospitalization services, less than 24 hours, per diem

⊘ **S0207** Paramedic intercept, non-hospital-based ALS service (non-voluntary), non-transport

⊘ **S0208** Paramedic intercept, hospital-based ALS service (non-voluntary), non-transport

⊘ **S0209** Wheelchair van, mileage, per mile

⊘ **S0215** Non-emergency transportation; mileage per mile

⊘ **S0220** Medical conference by a physician with interdisciplinary team of health professionals or representatives of community agencies to coordinate activities of patient care (patient is present); approximately 30 minutes

⊘ **S0221** Medical conference by a physician with interdisciplinary team of health professionals or representatives of community agencies to coordinate activities of patient care (patient is present); approximately 60 minutes

⊘ **S0250** Comprehensive geriatric assessment and treatment planning performed by assessment team A

⊘ **S0255** Hospice referral visit (advising patient and family of care options) performed by nurse, social worker, or other designated staff

⊘ **S0257** Counseling and discussion regarding advance directives or end of life care planning and decisions, with patient and/or surrogate (list separately in addition to code for appropriate evaluation and management service)

⊘ **S0260** History and physical (outpatient or office) related to surgical procedure (list separately in addition to code for appropriate evaluation and management service)

⊘ **S0265** Genetic counseling, under physician supervision, each 15 minutes

⊘ **S0270** Physician management of patient home care, standard monthly case rate (per 30 days)

⊘ **S0271** Physician management of patient home care, hospice monthly case rate (per 30 days)

⊘ **S0272** Physician management of patient home care, episodic care monthly case rate (per 30 days)

⊘ **S0273** Physician visit at member's home, outside of a capitation arrangement

⊘ **S0274** Nurse practitioner visit at member's home, outside of a capitation arrangement

⊘ **S0280** Medical home program, comprehensive care coordination and planning, initial plan

⊘ **S0281** Medical home program, comprehensive care coordination and planning, maintenance of plan

⊘ **S0285** Colonoscopy consultation performed prior to a screening colonoscopy procedure

⊘ **S0302** Completed Early Periodic Screening Diagnosis and Treatment (EPSDT) service (list in addition to code for appropriate evaluation and management service) A

⊘ **S0310** Hospitalist services (list separately in addition to code for appropriate evaluation and management service)

⊘ **S0311** Comprehensive management and care coordination for advanced illness, per calendar month

⊘ **S0315** Disease management program; initial assessment and initiation of the program

⊘ **S0316** Disease management program; follow-up/reassessment

⊘ **S0317** Disease management program; per diem

⊘ **S0320** Telephone calls by a registered nurse to a disease management program member for monitoring purposes; per month

⃠ **S0340** Lifestyle modification program for management of coronary artery disease, including all supportive services; first quarter/stage

⃠ **S0341** Lifestyle modification program for management of coronary artery disease, including all supportive services; second or third quarter/stage

⃠ **S0342** Lifestyle modification program for management of coronary artery disease, including all supportive services; fourth quarter/stage

⃠ **S0353** Treatment planning and care coordination management for cancer, initial treatment

⃠ **S0354** Treatment planning and care coordination management for cancer, established patient with a change of regimen

⃠ **S0390** Routine foot care; removal and/or trimming of corns, calluses and/or nails and preventive maintenance in specific medical conditions (e.g., diabetes), per visit

⃠ **S0395** Impression casting of a foot performed by a practitioner other than the manufacturer of the orthotic

⃠ **S0400** Global fee for extracorporeal shock wave lithotripsy treatment of kidney stone(s)

Vision Supplies

⃠ **S0500** Disposable contact lens, per lens

⃠ **S0504** Single vision prescription lens (safety, athletic, or sunglass), per lens

⃠ **S0506** Bifocal vision prescription lens (safety, athletic, or sunglass), per lens

⃠ **S0508** Trifocal vision prescription lens (safety, athletic, or sunglass), per lens

⃠ **S0510** Non-prescription lens (safety, athletic, or sunglass), per lens

⃠ **S0512** Daily wear specialty contact lens, per lens

⃠ **S0514** Color contact lens, per lens

⃠ **S0515** Scleral lens, liquid bandage device, per lens

⃠ **S0516** Safety eyeglass frames

⃠ **S0518** Sunglasses frames

⃠ **S0580** Polycarbonate lens (list this code in addition to the basic code for the lens)

⃠ **S0581** Nonstandard lens (list this code in addition to the basic code for the lens)

⃠ **S0590** Integral lens service, miscellaneous services reported separately

⃠ **S0592** Comprehensive contact lens evaluation

⃠ **S0595** Dispensing new spectacle lenses for patient supplied frame

⃠ **S0596** Phakic intraocular lens for correction of refractive error

Screening and Examinations

⃠ **S0601** Screening proctoscopy

⃠ **S0610** Annual gynecological examination, new patient ♀

⃠ **S0612** Annual gynecological examination, established patient ♀

⃠ **S0613** Annual gynecological examination; clinical breast examination without pelvic evaluation ♀

⃠ **S0618** Audiometry for hearing aid evaluation to determine the level and degree of hearing loss

⃠ **S0620** Routine ophthalmological examination including refraction; new patient

Many non-Medicare vision plans may require code for routine encounter, no complaints

⃠ **S0621** Routine ophthalmological examination including refraction; established patient

Many non-Medicare vision plans may require code for routine encounter, no complaints

⃠ **S0622** Physical exam for college, new or established patient (list separately) in addition to appropriate evaluation and management code A

Provider Services and Supplies

⃠ **S0630** Removal of sutures; by a physician other than the physician who originally closed the wound

⃠ **S0800** Laser in situ keratomileusis (LASIK)

▶ New ↩ Revised ✔ Reinstated ~~deleted~~ Deleted ⃠ Not covered or valid by Medicare
Special coverage instructions ✻ Carrier discretion Ⓑ Bill Part B MAC Ⓑ Bill DME MAC

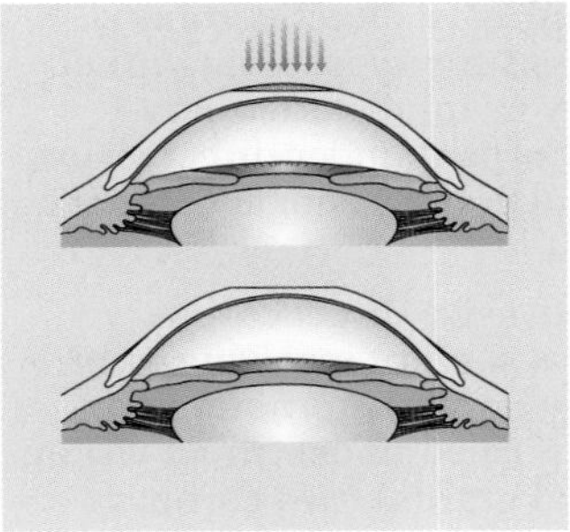

Figure 48 Phototherapeutic keratectomy (PRK).

⊘ **S0810** Photorefractive keratectomy (PRK)

⊘ **S0812** Phototherapeutic keratectomy (PTK)

⊘ **S1001** Deluxe item, patient aware (list in addition to code for basic item)

⊘ **S1002** Customized item (list in addition to code for basic item)

⊘ **S1015** IV tubing extension set

⊘ **S1016** Non-PVC (polyvinyl chloride) intravenous administration set, for use with drugs that are not stable in PVC (e.g., paclitaxel)

⊘ **S1030** Continuous noninvasive glucose monitoring device, purchase (for physician interpretation of data, use CPT code)

⊘ **S1031** Continuous noninvasive glucose monitoring device, rental, including sensor, sensor replacement, and download to monitor (for physician interpretation of data, use CPT code)

⊘ **S1034** Artificial pancreas device system (e.g., low glucose suspend (LGS) feature) including continuous glucose monitor, blood glucose device, insulin pump and computer algorithm that communicates with all of the devices

⊘ **S1035** Sensor; invasive (e.g., subcutaneous), disposable, for use with artificial pancreas device system

⊘ **S1036** Transmitter; external, for use with artificial pancreas device system

⊘ **S1037** Receiver (monitor); external, for use with artificial pancreas device system

⊘ **S1040** Cranial remolding orthosis, pediatric, rigid, with soft interface material, custom fabricated, includes fitting and adjustment(s) A

⊘ **S1090** Mometasone furoate sinus implant, 370 micrograms

⊘ **S2053** Transplantation of small intestine and liver allografts

⊘ **S2054** Transplantation of multivisceral organs

⊘ **S2055** Harvesting of donor multivisceral organs, with preparation and maintenance of allografts; from cadaver donor

⊘ **S2060** Lobar lung transplantation

⊘ **S2061** Donor lobectomy (lung) for transplantation, living donor

⊘ **S2065** Simultaneous pancreas kidney transplantation

⊘ **S2066** Breast reconstruction with gluteal artery perforator (GAP) flap, including harvesting of the flap, microvascular transfer, closure of donor site and shaping the flap into a breast, unilateral ♀

⊘ **S2067** Breast reconstruction of a single breast with "stacked" deep inferior epigastric perforator (DIEP) flap(s) and/or gluteal artery perforator (GAP) flap(s), including harvesting of the flap(s), microvascular transfer, closure of donor site(s) and shaping the flap into a breast, unilateral ♀

⊘ **S2068** Breast reconstruction with deep inferior epigastric perforator (DIEP) flap, or superficial inferior epigastric artery (SIEA) flap, including harvesting of the flap, microvascular transfer, closure of donor site and shaping the flap into a breast, unilateral ♀

⊘ **S2070** Cystourethroscopy, with ureteroscopy and/or pyeloscopy; with endoscopic laser treatment of ureteral calculi (includes ureteral catheterization)

⊘ **S2079** Laparoscopic esophagomyotomy (Heller type)

⊘ **S2080** Laser-assisted uvulopalatoplasty (LAUP)

⊘ **S2083** Adjustment of gastric band diameter via subcutaneous port by injection or aspiration of saline

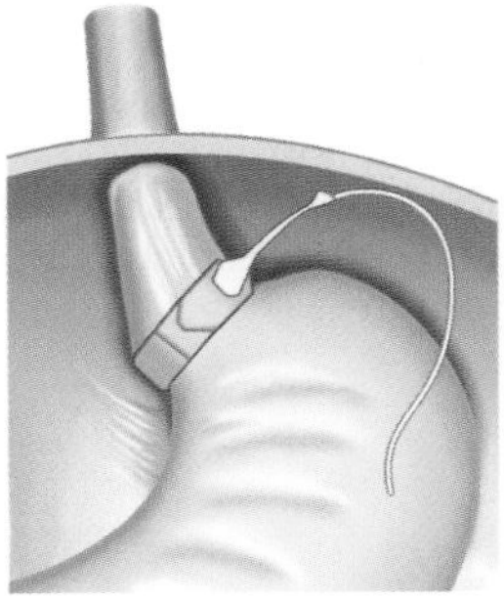

Figure 49 Gastric band.

⃠ **S2095** Transcatheter occlusion or embolization for tumor destruction, percutaneous, any method, using yttrium-90 microspheres

⃠ **S2102** Islet cell tissue transplant from pancreas; allogeneic

⃠ **S2103** Adrenal tissue transplant to brain

⃠ **S2107** Adoptive immunotherapy i.e. development of specific anti-tumor reactivity (e.g., tumor-infiltrating lymphocyte therapy) per course of treatment

⃠ **S2112** Arthroscopy, knee, surgical for harvesting of cartilage (chondrocyte cells)

⃠ **S2115** Osteotomy, periacetabular, with internal fixation

⃠ **S2117** Arthroereisis, subtalar

⃠ **S2118** Metal-on-metal total hip resurfacing, including acetabular and femoral components

⃠ **S2120** Low density lipoprotein (LDL) apheresis using heparin-induced extracorporeal LDL precipitation

⃠ **S2140** Cord blood harvesting for transplantation, allogeneic

⃠ **S2142** Cord blood-derived stem cell transplantation, allogeneic

⃠ **S2150** Bone marrow or blood-derived stem cells (peripheral or umbilical), allogeneic or autologous, harvesting, transplantation, and related complications; including: pheresis and cell preparation/storage; marrow ablative therapy; drugs, supplies, hospitalization with outpatient follow-up; medical/surgical, diagnostic, emergency, and rehabilitative services; and the number of days of pre- and post-transplant care in the global definition

⃠ **S2152** Solid organ(s), complete or segmental, single organ or combination of organs; deceased or living donor(s), procurement, transplantation, and related complications; including: drugs; supplies; hospitalization with outpatient follow-up; medical/surgical, diagnostic, emergency, and rehabilitative services, and the number of days of pre- and post-transplant care in the global definition

⃠ **S2202** Echosclerotherapy

⃠ **S2205** Minimally invasive direct coronary artery bypass surgery involving mini-thoracotomy or mini-sternotomy surgery, performed under direct vision; using arterial graft(s), single coronary arterial graft

⃠ **S2206** Minimally invasive direct coronary artery bypass surgery involving mini-thoracotomy or mini-sternotomy surgery, performed under direct vision; using arterial graft(s), two coronary arterial grafts

⃠ **S2207** Minimally invasive direct coronary artery bypass surgery involving mini-thoracotomy or mini-sternotomy surgery, performed under direct vision; using venous graft only, single coronary venous graft

⃠ **S2208** Minimally invasive direct coronary artery bypass surgery involving mini-thoracotomy or mini-sternotomy surgery, performed under direct vision; using single arterial and venous graft(s), single venous graft

⃠ **S2209** Minimally invasive direct coronary artery bypass surgery involving mini-thoracotomy or mini-sternotomy surgery, performed under direct vision; using two arterial grafts and single venous graft

⃠ **S2225** Myringotomy, laser-assisted

⃠ **S2230** Implantation of magnetic component of semi-implantable hearing device on ossicles in middle ear

⃠ **S2235** Implantation of auditory brain stem implant

⃠ **S2260** Induced abortion, 17 to 24 weeks ♀

⃠ **S2265** Induced abortion, 25 to 28 weeks ♀

⃠ **S2266** Induced abortion, 29 to 31 weeks ♀

⃠ **S2267** Induced abortion, 32 weeks or greater ♀

⃠ **S2300** Arthroscopy, shoulder, surgical; with thermally-induced capsulorrhaphy

⃠ **S2325** Hip core decompression

Coding Clinic: 2017, Q3, P1

⃠ **S2340** Chemodenervation of abductor muscle(s) of vocal cord

⃠ **S2341** Chemodenervation of adductor muscle(s) of vocal cord

⃠ **S2342** Nasal endoscopy for post-operative debridement following functional endoscopic sinus surgery, nasal and/or sinus cavity(s), unilateral or bilateral

▶ New ↩ Revised ✔ Reinstated ~~deleted~~ Deleted ⃠ Not covered or valid by Medicare
Special coverage instructions ✻ Carrier discretion Ⓑ Bill Part B MAC Ⓓ Bill DME MAC

⃠ **S2348** Decompression procedure, percutaneous, of nucleus pulpous of intervertebral disc, using radiofrequency energy, single or multiple levels, lumbar

⃠ **S2350** Diskectomy, anterior, with decompression of spinal cord and/or nerve root(s), including osteophytectomy; lumbar, single interspace

⃠ **S2351** Diskectomy, anterior, with decompression of spinal cord and/or nerve root(s) including osteophytectomy; lumbar, each additional interspace (list separately in addition to code for primary procedure)

⃠ **S2400** Repair, congenital diaphragmatic hernia in the fetus using temporary tracheal occlusion, procedure performed in utero ♀ A

⃠ **S2401** Repair, urinary tract obstruction in the fetus, procedure performed in utero ♀ A

⃠ **S2402** Repair, congenital cystic adenomatoid malformation in the fetus, procedure performed in utero ♀ A

⃠ **S2403** Repair, extralobar pulmonary sequestration in the fetus, procedure performed in utero ♀ A

⃠ **S2404** Repair, myelomeningocele in the fetus, procedure performed in utero ♀ A

⃠ **S2405** Repair of sacrococcygeal teratoma in the fetus, procedure performed in utero ♀ A

⃠ **S2409** Repair, congenital malformation of fetus, procedure performed in utero, not otherwise classified ♀ A

⃠ **S2411** Fetoscopic laser therapy for treatment of twin-to-twin transfusion syndrome A

⃠ **S2900** Surgical techniques requiring use of robotic surgical system (list separately in addition to code for primary procedure)

Coding Clinic: 2010, Q2, P6

⃠ **S3000** Diabetic indicator; retinal eye exam, dilated, bilateral

⃠ **S3005** Performance measurement, evaluation of patient self assessment, depression

⃠ **S3600** STAT laboratory request (situations other than S3601)

⃠ **S3601** Emergency STAT laboratory charge for patient who is homebound or residing in a nursing facility

S3620 Newborn metabolic screening panel, includes test kit, postage and the laboratory tests specified by the state for inclusion in this panel (e.g., galactose; hemoglobin, electrophoresis; hydroxyprogesterone, 17-D; phenylalanine (PKU); and thyroxine, total) A

⃠ **S3630** Eosinophil count, blood, direct

⃠ **S3645** HIV-1 antibody testing of oral mucosal transudate

⃠ **S3650** Saliva test, hormone level; during menopause ♀

⃠ **S3652** Saliva test, hormone level; to assess preterm labor risk ♀

⃠ **S3655** Antisperm antibodies test (immunobead) ♀

⃠ **S3708** Gastrointestinal fat absorption study

⃠ **S3722** Dose optimization by area under the curve (AUC) analysis, for infusional 5-fluorouracil

Genetic Testing

⃠ **S3800** Genetic testing for amyotrophic lateral sclerosis (ALS)

⃠ **S3840** DNA analysis for germline mutations of the RET proto-oncogene for susceptibility to multiple endocrine neoplasia type 2

⃠ **S3841** Genetic testing for retinoblastoma

⃠ **S3842** Genetic testing for von Hippel-Lindau disease

⃠ **S3844** DNA analysis of the connexin 26 gene (GJB2) for susceptibility to congenital, profound deafness

⃠ **S3845** Genetic testing for alpha-thalassemia

⃠ **S3846** Genetic testing for hemoglobin E beta-thalassemia

⃠ **S3849** Genetic testing for Niemann-Pick disease

⃠ **S3850** Genetic testing for sickle cell anemia

⃠ **S3852** DNA analysis for APOE epilson 4 allele for susceptibility to Alzheimer's disease

⃠ **S3853** Genetic testing for myotonic muscular dystrophy

⃠ **S3854** Gene expression profiling panel for use in the management of breast cancer treatment ♀

⃠ **S3861** Genetic testing, sodium channel, voltage-gated, type V, alpha subunit (SCN5A) and variants for suspected Brugada syndrome

⃠ **S3865** Comprehensive gene sequence analysis for hypertrophic cardiomyopathy

⃠ **S3866** Genetic analysis for a specific gene mutation for hypertrophic cardiomyopathy (HCM) in an individual with a known HCM mutation in the family

⃠ **S3870** Comparative genomic hybridization (CGH) microarray testing for developmental delay, autism spectrum disorder and/or intellectual disability

Other Tests

⃠ **S3900** Surface electromyography (EMG)

⃠ **S3902** Ballistrocardiogram

⃠ **S3904** Masters two step

Bill on paper. Requires a report.

Obstetric and Fertility Services

⃠ **S4005** Interim labor facility global (labor occurring but not resulting in delivery) ♀

⃠ **S4011** In vitro fertilization; including but not limited to identification and incubation of mature oocytes, fertilization with sperm, incubation of embryo(s), and subsequent visualization for determination of development ♀

⃠ **S4013** Complete cycle, gamete intrafallopian transfer (GIFT), case rate ♀

⃠ **S4014** Complete cycle, zygote intrafallopian transfer (ZIFT), case rate ♀

⃠ **S4015** Complete in vitro fertilization cycle, not otherwise specified, case rate ♀

⃠ **S4016** Frozen in vitro fertilization cycle, case rate ♀

⃠ **S4017** Incomplete cycle, treatment cancelled prior to stimulation, case rate ♀

⃠ **S4018** Frozen embryo transfer procedure cancelled before transfer, case rate ♀

⃠ **S4020** In vitro fertilization procedure cancelled before aspiration, case rate ♀

⃠ **S4021** In vitro fertilization procedure cancelled after aspiration, case rate ♀

⃠ **S4022** Assisted oocyte fertilization, case rate ♀

⃠ **S4023** Donor egg cycle, incomplete, case rate ♀

⃠ **S4025** Donor services for in vitro fertilization (sperm or embryo), case rate

⃠ **S4026** Procurement of donor sperm from sperm bank ♂

⃠ **S4027** Storage of previously frozen embryos ♀

⃠ **S4028** Microsurgical epididymal sperm aspiration (MESA) ♂

⃠ **S4030** Sperm procurement and cryopreservation services; initial visit ♂

⃠ **S4031** Sperm procurement and cryopreservation services; subsequent visit ♂

⃠ **S4035** Stimulated intrauterine insemination (IUI), case rate ♀

⃠ **S4037** Cryopreserved embryo transfer, case rate ♀

⃠ **S4040** Monitoring and storage of cryopreserved embryos, per 30 days ♀

⃠ **S4042** Management of ovulation induction (interpretation of diagnostic tests and studies, non-face-to-face medical management of the patient), per cycle ♀

⃠ **S4981** Insertion of levonorgestrel-releasing intrauterine system ♀

⃠ **S4989** Contraceptive intrauterine device (e.g., Progestasert IUD), including implants and supplies ♀

Therapeutic Substances and Medications

⃠ **S4990** Nicotine patches, legend

⃠ **S4991** Nicotine patches, non-legend

⃠ **S4993** Contraceptive pills for birth control ♀

Only billed by Family Planning Clinics

⃠ **S4995** Smoking cessation gum

⃠ **S5000** Prescription drug, generic

⃠ **S5001** Prescription drug, brand name

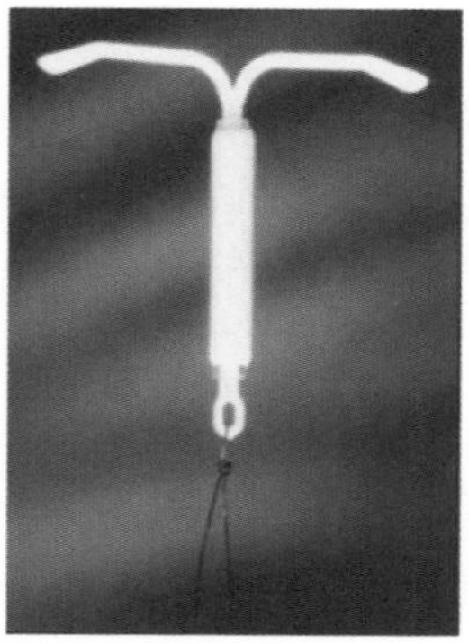

Figure 50 IUD.

⃠ **S5010** 5% dextrose and 0.45% normal saline, 1000 ml

⃠ **S5012** 5% dextrose with potassium chloride, 1000 ml

⃠ **S5013** 5% dextrose/0.45% normal saline with potassium chloride and magnesium sulfate, 1000 ml

⃠ **S5014** 5% dextrose/0.45% normal saline with potassium chloride and magnesium sulfate, 1500 ml

Home Care Services

⃠ **S5035** Home infusion therapy, routine service of infusion device (e.g., pump maintenance)

⃠ **S5036** Home infusion therapy, repair of infusion device (e.g., pump repair)

⃠ **S5100** Day care services, adult; per 15 minutes A

⃠ **S5101** Day care services, adult; per half day A

⃠ **S5102** Day care services, adult; per diem A

⃠ **S5105** Day care services, center-based; services not included in program fee, per diem

⃠ **S5108** Home care training to home care client, per 15 minutes

⃠ **S5109** Home care training to home care client, per session

⃠ **S5110** Home care training, family; per 15 minutes

⃠ **S5111** Home care training, family; per session

⃠ **S5115** Home care training, non-family; per 15 minutes

⃠ **S5116** Home care training, non-family; per session

⃠ **S5120** Chore services; per 15 minutes

⃠ **S5121** Chore services; per diem

⃠ **S5125** Attendant care services; per 15 minutes

⃠ **S5126** Attendant care services; per diem

⃠ **S5130** Homemaker service, NOS; per 15 minutes

⃠ **S5131** Homemaker service, NOS; per diem

⃠ **S5135** Companion care, adult (e.g., IADL/ ADL); per 15 minutes A

⃠ **S5136** Companion care, adult (e.g., IADL/ ADL); per diem A

⃠ **S5140** Foster care, adult; per diem A

⃠ **S5141** Foster care, adult; per month A

⃠ **S5145** Foster care, therapeutic, child; per diem A

⃠ **S5146** Foster care, therapeutic, child; per month A

⃠ **S5150** Unskilled respite care, not hospice; per 15 minutes

⃠ **S5151** Unskilled respite care, not hospice; per diem

⃠ **S5160** Emergency response system; installation and testing

⃠ **S5161** Emergency response system; service fee, per month (excludes installation and testing)

⃠ **S5162** Emergency response system; purchase only

⃠ **S5165** Home modifications; per service

⃠ **S5170** Home delivered meals, including preparation; per meal

⃠ **S5175** Laundry service, external, professional; per order

⃠ **S5180** Home health respiratory therapy, initial evaluation

⃠ **S5181** Home health respiratory therapy, NOS, per diem

⃠ **S5185** Medication reminder service, non-face-to-face; per month

⃠ **S5190** Wellness assessment, performed by non-physician

⃠ **S5199** Personal care item, NOS, each

Home Infusion Therapy

⃠ **S5497** Home infusion therapy, catheter care/ maintenance, not otherwise classified; includes administrative services, professional pharmacy services, care coordination, and all necessary supplies and equipment (drugs and nursing visits coded separately), per diem

⃠ **S5498** Home infusion therapy, catheter care/ maintenance, simple (single lumen), includes administrative services, professional pharmacy services, care coordination and all necessary supplies and equipment, (drugs and nursing visits coded separately), per diem

⃠ **S5501** Home infusion therapy, catheter care/ maintenance, complex (more than one lumen), includes administrative services, professional pharmacy services, care coordination, and all necessary supplies and equipment (drugs and nursing visits coded separately), per diem

⊘ **S5502** Home infusion therapy, catheter care/maintenance, implanted access device, includes administrative services, professional pharmacy services, care coordination, and all necessary supplies and equipment, (drugs and nursing visits coded separately), per diem (use this code for interim maintenance of vascular access not currently in use)

⊘ **S5517** Home infusion therapy, all supplies necessary for restoration of catheter patency or declotting

⊘ **S5518** Home infusion therapy, all supplies necessary for catheter repair

⊘ **S5520** Home infusion therapy, all supplies (including catheter) necessary for a peripherally inserted central venous catheter (PICC) line insertion

Bill on paper. Requires a report.

⊘ **S5521** Home infusion therapy, all supplies (including catheter) necessary for a midline catheter insertion

⊘ **S5522** Home infusion therapy, insertion of peripherally inserted central venous catheter (PICC), nursing services only (no supplies or catheter included)

⊘ **S5523** Home infusion therapy, insertion of midline central venous catheter, nursing services only (no supplies or catheter included)

Insulin Services

⊘ **S5550** Insulin, rapid onset, 5 units

⊘ **S5551** Insulin, most rapid onset (Lispro or Aspart); 5 units

⊘ **S5552** Insulin, intermediate acting (NPH or Lente); 5 units

⊘ **S5553** Insulin, long acting; 5 units

⊘ **S5560** Insulin delivery device, reusable pen; 1.5 ml size

⊘ **S5561** Insulin delivery device, reusable pen; 3 ml size

⊘ **S5565** Insulin cartridge for use in insulin delivery device other than pump; 150 units

⊘ **S5566** Insulin cartridge for use in insulin delivery device other than pump; 300 units

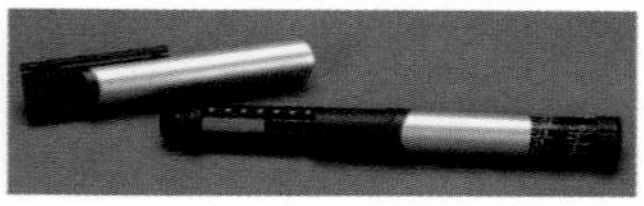

Figure 51 Nova pen.

⊘ **S5570** Insulin delivery device, disposable pen (including insulin); 1.5 ml size

⊘ **S5571** Insulin delivery device, disposable pen (including insulin); 3 ml size

Imaging

⊘ **S8030** Scleral application of tantalum ring(s) for localization of lesions for proton beam therapy

⊘ **S8035** Magnetic source imaging

⊘ **S8037** Magnetic resonance cholangiopancreatography (MRCP)

⊘ **S8040** Topographic brain mapping

⊘ **S8042** Magnetic resonance imaging (MRI), low-field

⊘ **S8055** Ultrasound guidance for multifetal pregnancy reduction(s), technical component (only to be used when the physician doing the reduction procedure does not perform the ultrasound, guidance is included in the CPT code for multifetal pregnancy reduction - 59866) ♀

⊘ **S8080** Scintimammography (radioimmunoscintigraphy of the breast), unilateral, including supply of radiopharmaceutical ♀

⊘ **S8085** Fluorine-18 fluorodeoxyglucose (F-18 FDG) imaging using dual-head coincidence detection system (non-dedicated PET scan)

⊘ **S8092** Electron beam computed tomography (also known as ultrafast CT, cine CT)

Assistive Breathing Supplies

⊘ **S8096** Portable peak flow meter

⊘ **S8097** Asthma kit (including but not limited to portable peak expiratory flow meter, instructional video, brochure, and/or spacer)

⊘ **S8100** Holding chamber or spacer for use with an inhaler or nebulizer; without mask

⊘ **S8101** Holding chamber or spacer for use with an inhaler or nebulizer; with mask

⊘ **S8110** Peak expiratory flow rate (physician services)

⊘ **S8120** Oxygen contents, gaseous, 1 unit equals 1 cubic foot

⊘ **S8121** Oxygen contents, liquid, 1 unit equals 1 pound

⃠ **S8130** Interferential current stimulator, 2 channel

⃠ **S8131** Interferential current stimulator, 4 channel

⃠ **S8185** Flutter device

⃠ **S8186** Swivel adapter

⃠ **S8189** Tracheostomy supply, not otherwise classified

⃠ **S8210** Mucus trap

Miscellaneous Supplies and Services

⃠ **S8265** Haberman feeder for cleft lip/palate

⃠ **S8270** Enuresis alarm, using auditory buzzer and/or vibration device

⃠ **S8301** Infection control supplies, not otherwise specified

⃠ **S8415** Supplies for home delivery of infant A

⃠ **S8420** Gradient pressure aid (sleeve and glove combination), custom made

⃠ **S8421** Gradient pressure aid (sleeve and glove combination), ready made

⃠ **S8422** Gradient pressure aid (sleeve), custom made, medium weight

⃠ **S8423** Gradient pressure aid (sleeve), custom made, heavy weight

⃠ **S8424** Gradient pressure aid (sleeve), ready made

⃠ **S8425** Gradient pressure aid (glove), custom made, medium weight

⃠ **S8426** Gradient pressure aid (glove), custom made, heavy weight

⃠ **S8427** Gradient pressure aid (glove), ready made

⃠ **S8428** Gradient pressure aid (gauntlet), ready made

⃠ **S8429** Gradient pressure exterior wrap

⃠ **S8430** Padding for compression bandage, roll

⃠ **S8431** Compression bandage, roll

⃠ **S8450** Splint, prefabricated, digit (specify digit by use of modifier)

⃠ **S8451** Splint, prefabricated, wrist or ankle

⃠ **S8452** Splint, prefabricated, elbow

⃠ **S8460** Camisole, post-mastectomy

⃠ **S8490** Insulin syringes (100 syringes, any size)

⃠ **S8930** Electrical stimulation of auricular acupuncture points; each 15 minutes of personal one-on-one contact with the patient

⃠ **S8940** Equestrian/Hippotherapy, per session

⃠ **S8948** Application of a modality (requiring constant provider attendance) to one or more areas; low-level laser; each 15 minutes

⃠ **S8950** Complex lymphedema therapy, each 15 minutes

⃠ **S8990** Physical or manipulative therapy performed for maintenance rather than restoration

⃠ **S8999** Resuscitation bag (for use by patient on artificial respiration during power failure or other catastrophic event)

⃠ **S9001** Home uterine monitor with or without associated nursing services ♀

⃠ **S9007** Ultrafiltration monitor

⃠ **S9024** Paranasal sinus ultrasound

⃠ **S9025** Omnicardiogram/cardiointegram

⃠ **S9034** Extracorporeal shockwave lithotripsy for gall stones (if performed with ERCP, use 43265)

⃠ **S9055** Procuren or other growth factor preparation to promote wound healing

⃠ **S9056** Coma stimulation per diem

⃠ **S9061** Home administration of aerosolized drug therapy (e.g., pentamidine); administrative services, professional pharmacy services, care coordination, all necessary supplies and equipment (drugs and nursing visits coded separately), per diem

⃠ **S9083** Global fee urgent care centers

⃠ **S9088** Services provided in an urgent care center (list in addition to code for service)

⃠ **S9090** Vertebral axial decompression, per session

⃠ **S9097** Home visit for wound care

⃠ **S9098** Home visit, phototherapy services (e.g., Bili-Lite), including equipment rental, nursing services, blood draw, supplies, and other services, per diem

⃠ **S9110** Telemonitoring of patient in their home, including all necessary equipment; computer system, connections, and software; maintenance; patient education and support; per month

⃠ **S9117** Back school, per visit

⃠ **S9122** Home health aide or certified nurse assistant, providing care in the home; per hour

⦸ **S9123** Nursing care, in the home; by registered nurse, per hour (use for general nursing care only, not to be used when CPT codes 99500-99602 can be used)

⦸ **S9124** Nursing care, in the home; by licensed practical nurse, per hour

⦸ **S9125** Respite care, in the home, per diem

⦸ **S9126** Hospice care, in the home, per diem

⦸ **S9127** Social work visit, in the home, per diem

⦸ **S9128** Speech therapy, in the home, per diem

⦸ **S9129** Occupational therapy, in the home, per diem

⦸ **S9131** Physical therapy; in the home, per diem

⦸ **S9140** Diabetic management program, follow-up visit to non-MD provider

⦸ **S9141** Diabetic management program, follow-up visit to MD provider

⦸ **S9145** Insulin pump initiation, instruction in initial use of pump (pump not included)

⦸ **S9150** Evaluation by ocularist

⦸ **S9152** Speech therapy, re-evaluation

Home Management of Pregnancy

⦸ **S9208** Home management of preterm labor, including administrative services, professional pharmacy services, care coordination, and all necessary supplies or equipment (drugs and nursing visits coded separately), per diem (do not use this code with any home infusion per diem code) ♀

⦸ **S9209** Home management of preterm premature rupture of membranes (PPROM), including administrative services, professional pharmacy services, care coordination, and all necessary supplies or equipment (drugs and nursing visits coded separately), per diem (do not use this code with any home infusion per diem code) ♀

⦸ **S9211** Home management of gestational hypertension, includes administrative services, professional pharmacy services, care coordination, and all necessary supplies and equipment (drugs and nursing visits coded separately); per diem (do not use this code with any home infusion per diem code) ♀

⦸ **S9212** Home management of postpartum hypertension, includes administrative services, professional pharmacy services, care coordination, and all necessary supplies and equipment (drugs and nursing visits coded separately), per diem (do not use this code with any home infusion per diem code) ♀

⦸ **S9213** Home management of preeclampsia, includes administrative services, professional pharmacy services, care coordination, and all necessary supplies and equipment (drugs and nursing services coded separately); per diem (do not use this code with any home infusion per diem code) ♀

⦸ **S9214** Home management of gestational diabetes, includes administrative services, professional pharmacy services, care coordination, and all necessary supplies and equipment (drugs and nursing visits coded separately); per diem (do not use this code with any home infusion per diem code) ♀

Home Infusion Therapy

⦸ **S9325** Home infusion therapy, pain management infusion; administrative services, professional pharmacy services, care coordination, and all necessary supplies and equipment, (drugs and nursing visits coded separately), per diem (do not use this code with S9326, S9327 or S9328)

⦸ **S9326** Home infusion therapy, continuous (twenty-four hours or more) pain management infusion; administrative services, professional pharmacy services, care coordination, and all necessary supplies and equipment (drugs and nursing visits coded separately), per diem

⦸ **S9327** Home infusion therapy, intermittent (less than twenty-four hours) pain management infusion; administrative services, professional pharmacy services, care coordination, and all necessary supplies and equipment (drugs and nursing visits coded separately), per diem

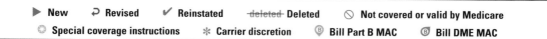

⃠ **S9328** Home infusion therapy, implanted pump pain management infusion; administrative services, professional pharmacy services, care coordination, and all necessary supplies and equipment (drugs and nursing visits coded separately), per diem

⃠ **S9329** Home infusion therapy, chemotherapy infusion; administrative services, professional pharmacy services, care coordination, and all necessary supplies and equipment (drugs and nursing visits coded separately), per diem (do not use this code with S9330 or S9331)

⃠ **S9330** Home infusion therapy, continuous (twenty-four hours or more) chemotherapy infusion; administrative services, professional pharmacy services, care coordination, and all necessary supplies and equipment (drugs and nursing visits coded separately), per diem

⃠ **S9331** Home infusion therapy, intermittent (less than twenty-four hours) chemotherapy infusion; administrative services, professional pharmacy services, care coordination, and all necessary supplies and equipment (drugs and nursing visits coded separately), per diem

⃠ **S9335** Home therapy, hemodialysis; administrative services, professional pharmacy services, care coordination, and all necessary supplies and equipment (drugs and nursing services coded separately), per diem

⃠ **S9336** Home infusion therapy, continuous anticoagulant infusion therapy (e.g., heparin), administrative services, professional pharmacy services, care coordination, and all necessary supplies and equipment (drugs and nursing visits coded separately), per diem

⃠ **S9338** Home infusion therapy, immunotherapy, administrative services, professional pharmacy services, care coordination, and all necessary supplies and equipment (drug and nursing visits coded separately), per diem

⃠ **S9339** Home therapy; peritoneal dialysis, administrative services, professional pharmacy services, care coordination and all necessary supplies and equipment (drugs and nursing visits coded separately), per diem

⃠ **S9340** Home therapy; enteral nutrition; administrative services, professional pharmacy services, care coordination, and all necessary supplies and equipment (enteral formula and nursing visits coded separately), per diem

⃠ **S9341** Home therapy; enteral nutrition via gravity; administrative services, professional pharmacy services, care coordination, and all necessary supplies and equipment (enteral formula and nursing visits coded separately), per diem

⃠ **S9342** Home therapy; enteral nutrition via pump; administrative services, professional pharmacy services, care coordination, and all necessary supplies and equipment (enteral formula and nursing visits coded separately), per diem

⃠ **S9343** Home therapy; enteral nutrition via bolus; administrative services, professional pharmacy services, care coordination, and all necessary supplies and equipment (enteral formula and nursing visits coded separately), per diem

⃠ **S9345** Home infusion therapy, anti-hemophilic agent infusion therapy (e.g., Factor VIII); administrative services, professional pharmacy services, care coordination, and all necessary supplies and equipment (drugs and nursing visits coded separately), per diem

⃠ **S9346** Home infusion therapy, alpha-1-proteinase inhibitor (e.g., Prolastin); administrative services, professional pharmacy services, care coordination, and all necessary supplies and equipment (drugs and nursing visits coded separately), per diem

⃠ **S9347** Home infusion therapy, uninterrupted, long-term, controlled rate intravenous or subcutaneous infusion therapy (e.g., Epoprostenol); administrative services, professional pharmacy services, care coordination, and all necessary supplies and equipment (drugs and nursing visits coded separately), per diem

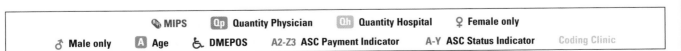

⃠ **S9348** Home infusion therapy, sympathomimetic/inotropic agent infusion therapy (e.g., Dobutamine); administrative services, professional pharmacy services, care coordination, all necessary supplies and equipment (drugs and nursing visits coded separately), per diem

⃠ **S9349** Home infusion therapy, tocolytic infusion therapy; administrative services, professional pharmacy services, care coordination, and all necessary supplies and equipment (drugs and nursing visits coded separately), per diem

⃠ **S9351** Home infusion therapy, continuous or intermittent anti-emetic infusion therapy; administrative services, professional pharmacy services, care coordination, and all necessary supplies and equipment (drugs and visits coded separately), per diem

⃠ **S9353** Home infusion therapy, continuous insulin infusion therapy; administrative services, professional pharmacy services, care coordination, and all necessary supplies and equipment (drugs and nursing visits coded separately), per diem

⃠ **S9355** Home infusion therapy, chelation therapy; administrative services, professional pharmacy services, care coordination, and all necessary supplies and equipment (drugs and nursing visits coded separately), per diem

⃠ **S9357** Home infusion therapy, enzyme replacement intravenous therapy (e.g., Imiglucerase); administrative services, professional pharmacy services, care coordination, and all necessary supplies and equipment (drugs and nursing visits coded separately), per diem

⃠ **S9359** Home infusion therapy, anti-tumor necrosis factor intravenous therapy (e.g., Infliximab); administrative services, professional pharmacy services, care coordination, and all necessary supplies and equipment (drugs and nursing visits coded separately), per diem

⃠ **S9361** Home infusion therapy, diuretic intravenous therapy; administrative services, professional pharmacy services, care coordination, and all necessary supplies and equipment (drugs and nursing visits coded separately), per diem

⃠ **S9363** Home infusion therapy, anti-spasmotic therapy; administrative services, professional pharmacy services, care coordination, and all necessary supplies and equipment (drugs and nursing visits coded separately), per diem

⃠ **S9364** Home infusion therapy, total parenteral nutrition (TPN); administrative services, professional pharmacy services, care coordination, and all necessary supplies and equipment including standard TPN formula (lipids, specialty amino acid formulas, drugs other than in standard formula, and nursing visits coded separately) per diem (do not use with home infusion codes S9365-S9368 using daily volume scales)

⃠ **S9365** Home infusion therapy, total parenteral nutrition (TPN); one liter per day, administrative services, professional pharmacy services, care coordination, and all necessary supplies and equipment including standard TPN formula (lipids, specialty amino acid formulas, drugs other than in standard formula and nursing visits coded separately), per diem

⃠ **S9366** Home infusion therapy, total parenteral nutrition (TPN); more than one liter but no more than two liters per day, administrative services, professional pharmacy services, care coordination, and all necessary supplies and equipment including standard TPN formula (lipids, specialty amino acid formulas, drugs other than in standard formula and nursing visits coded separately), per diem

⃠ **S9367** Home infusion therapy, total parenteral nutrition (TPN); more than two liters but no more than three liters per day, administrative services, professional pharmacy services, care coordination, and all necessary supplies and equipment including standard TPN formula (lipids, specialty amino acid formulas, drugs other than in standard formula and nursing visits coded separately), per diem

⃠ **S9368** Home infusion therapy, total parenteral nutrition (TPN); more than three liters per day, administrative services, professional pharmacy services, care coordination, and all necessary supplies and equipment (including standard TPN formula; lipids, specialty amino acid formulas, drugs other than in standard formula and nursing visits coded separately), per diem

⊘ **S9370** Home therapy, intermittent anti-emetic injection therapy; administrative services, professional pharmacy services, care coordination, and all necessary supplies and equipment (drugs and nursing visits coded separately), per diem

⊘ **S9372** Home therapy; intermittent anticoagulant injection therapy (e.g., heparin); administrative services, professional pharmacy services, care coordination, and all necessary supplies and equipment (drugs and nursing visits coded separately), per diem (do not use this code for flushing of infusion devices with heparin to maintain patency)

⊘ **S9373** Home infusion therapy, hydration therapy; administrative services, professional pharmacy services, care coordination, and all necessary supplies and equipment (drugs and nursing visits coded separately), per diem (do not use with hydration therapy codes S9374-S9377 using daily volume scales)

⊘ **S9374** Home infusion therapy, hydration therapy; one liter per day, administrative services, professional pharmacy services, care coordination, and all necessary supplies and equipment (drugs and nursing visits coded separately), per diem

⊘ **S9375** Home infusion therapy, hydration therapy; more than one liter but no more than two liters per day, administrative services, professional pharmacy services, care coordination, and all necessary supplies and equipment (drugs and nursing visits coded separately), per diem

⊘ **S9376** Home infusion therapy, hydration therapy; more than two liters but no more than three liters per day, administrative services, professional pharmacy services, care coordination, and all necessary supplies and equipment (drugs and nursing visits coded separately), per diem

⊘ **S9377** Home infusion therapy, hydration therapy; more than three liters per day, administrative services, professional pharmacy services, care coordination, and all necessary supplies (drugs and nursing visits coded separately), per diem

⊘ **S9379** Home infusion therapy, infusion therapy, not otherwise classified; administrative services, professional pharmacy services, care coordination, and all necessary supplies and equipment (drugs and nursing visits coded separately), per diem

Miscellaneous Supplies and Services

⊘ **S9381** Delivery or service to high risk areas requiring escort or extra protection, per visit

⊘ **S9401** Anticoagulation clinic, inclusive of all services except laboratory tests, per session

⊘ **S9430** Pharmacy compounding and dispensing services

⊘ **S9433** Medical food nutritionally complete, administered orally, providing 100% of nutritional intake

⊘ **S9434** Modified solid food supplements for inborn errors of metabolism

⊘ **S9435** Medical foods for inborn errors of metabolism

⊘ **S9436** Childbirth preparation/Lamaze classes, non-physician provider, per session ♀

⊘ **S9437** Childbirth refresher classes, non-physician provider, per session ♀

⊘ **S9438** Cesarean birth classes, non-physician provider, per session ♀

⊘ **S9439** VBAC (vaginal birth after cesarean) classes, non-physician provider, per session ♀

⊘ **S9441** Asthma education, non-physician provider, per session

⊘ **S9442** Birthing classes, non-physician provider, per session ♀

⊘ **S9443** Lactation classes, non-physician provider, per session ♀

⊘ **S9444** Parenting classes, non-physician provider, per session

⊘ **S9445** Patient education, not otherwise classified, non-physician provider, individual, per session

⊘ **S9446** Patient education, not otherwise classified, non-physician provider, group, per session

⊘ **S9447** Infant safety (including CPR) classes, non-physician provider, per session

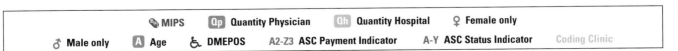

⊘ **S9449** Weight management classes, non-physician provider, per session

⃠ **S9451** Exercise classes, non-physician provider, per session

⃠ **S9452** Nutrition classes, non-physician provider, per session

⃠ **S9453** Smoking cessation classes, non-physician provider, per session

⃠ **S9454** Stress management classes, non-physician provider, per session

⃠ **S9455** Diabetic management program, group session

⃠ **S9460** Diabetic management program, nurse visit

⃠ **S9465** Diabetic management program, dietitian visit

⃠ **S9470** Nutritional counseling, dietitian visit

⃠ **S9472** Cardiac rehabilitation program, non-physician provider, per diem

⃠ **S9473** Pulmonary rehabilitation program, non-physician provider, per diem

⃠ **S9474** Enterostomal therapy by a registered nurse certified in enterostomal therapy, per diem

⃠ **S9475** Ambulatory setting substance abuse treatment or detoxification services, per diem

⃠ **S9476** Vestibular rehabilitation program, non-physician provider, per diem

⃠ **S9480** Intensive outpatient psychiatric services, per diem

⃠ **S9482** Family stabilization services, per 15 minutes

⃠ **S9484** Crisis intervention mental health services, per hour

⃠ **S9485** Crisis intervention mental health services, per diem

Home Therapy Services

⃠ **S9490** Home infusion therapy, corticosteroid infusion; administrative services, professional pharmacy services, care coordination, and all necessary supplies and equipment (drugs and nursing visits coded separately), per diem

⃠ **S9494** Home infusion therapy, antibiotic, antiviral, or antifungal therapy; administrative services, professional pharmacy services, care coordination, and all necessary supplies and equipment (drugs and nursing visits coded separately) per diem (do not use this code with home infusion codes for hourly dosing schedules S9497-S9504)

⃠ **S9497** Home infusion therapy, antibiotic, antiviral, or antifungal therapy; once every 3 hours; administrative services, professional pharmacy services, care coordination, and all necessary supplies and equipment (drugs and nursing visits coded separately), per diem

⃠ **S9500** Home infusion therapy, antibiotic, antiviral, or antifungal therapy; once every 24 hours; administrative services, professional pharmacy services, care coordination, and all necessary supplies and equipment (drugs and nursing visits coded separately), per diem

⃠ **S9501** Home infusion therapy, antibiotic, antiviral, or antifungal therapy; once every 12 hours; administrative services, professional pharmacy services, care coordination, and all necessary supplies and equipment (drugs and nursing visits coded separately), per diem

⃠ **S9502** Home infusion therapy, antibiotic, antiviral, or antifungal therapy; once every 8 hours, administrative services, professional pharmacy services, care coordination, and all necessary supplies and equipment (drugs and nursing visits coded separately), per diem

⃠ **S9503** Home infusion therapy, antibiotic, antiviral, or antifungal; once every 6 hours; administrative services, professional pharmacy services, care coordination, and all necessary supplies and equipment (drugs and nursing visits coded separately), per diem

⃠ **S9504** Home infusion therapy, antibiotic, antiviral, or antifungal; once every 4 hours; administrative services, professional pharmacy services, care coordination, and all necessary supplies and equipment (drugs and nursing visits coded separately), per diem

⃠ **S9529** Routine venipuncture for collection of specimen(s), single home bound, nursing home, or skilled nursing facility patient

⃠ **S9537** Home therapy; hematopoietic hormone injection therapy (e.g., erythropoietin, G-CSF, GM-CSF); administrative services, professional pharmacy services, care coordination, and all necessary supplies and equipment (drugs and nursing visits coded separately), per diem

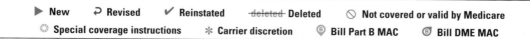

⊘ **S9538** Home transfusion of blood product(s); administrative services, professional pharmacy services, care coordination, and all necessary supplies and equipment (blood products, drugs, and nursing visits coded separately), per diem

⊘ **S9542** Home injectable therapy; not otherwise classified, including administrative services, professional pharmacy services, care coordination, and all necessary supplies and equipment (drugs and nursing visits coded separately), per diem

⊘ **S9558** Home injectable therapy; growth hormone, including administrative services, professional pharmacy services, care coordination, and all necessary supplies and equipment (drugs and nursing visits coded separately), per diem

⊘ **S9559** Home injectable therapy; interferon, including administrative services, professional pharmacy services, care coordination, and all necessary supplies and equipment (drugs and nursing visits coded separately), per diem

⊘ **S9560** Home injectable therapy; hormonal therapy (e.g., Leuprolide, Goserelin), including administrative services, professional pharmacy services, care coordination, and all necessary supplies and equipment (drugs and nursing visits coded separately), per diem

⊘ **S9562** Home injectable therapy, palivizumab, including administrative services, professional pharmacy services, care coordination, and all necessary supplies and equipment (drugs and nursing visits coded separately), per diem

⊘ **S9590** Home therapy, irrigation therapy (e.g., sterile irrigation of an organ or anatomical cavity); including administrative services, professional pharmacy services, care coordination, and all necessary supplies and equipment (drugs and nursing visits coded separately), per diem

⊘ **S9810** Home therapy; professional pharmacy services for provision of infusion, specialty drug administration, and/or disease state management, not otherwise classified, per hour (do not use this code with any per diem code)

Other Services and Fees

⊘ **S9900** Services by journal-listed Christian Science Practitioner for the purpose of healing, per diem

⊘ **S9901** Services by a journal-listed Christian Science nurse, per hour

⊘ **S9960** Ambulance service, conventional air service, nonemergency transport, one way (fixed wing)

⊘ **S9961** Ambulance service, conventional air service, nonemergency transport, one way (rotary wing)

⊘ **S9970** Health club membership, annual

⊘ **S9975** Transplant related lodging, meals and transportation, per diem

⊘ **S9976** Lodging, per diem, not otherwise classified

⊘ **S9977** Meals, per diem, not otherwise specified

⊘ **S9981** Medical records copying fee, administrative

⊘ **S9982** Medical records copying fee, per page

⊘ **S9986** Not medically necessary service (patient is aware that service not medically necessary)

⊘ **S9988** Services provided as part of a Phase I clinical trial

⊘ **S9989** Services provided outside of the United States of America (list in addition to code(s) for services(s))

⊘ **S9990** Services provided as part of a Phase II clinical trial

⊘ **S9991** Services provided as part of a Phase III clinical trial

⊘ **S9992** Transportation costs to and from trial location and local transportation costs (e.g., fares for taxicab or bus) for clinical trial participant and one caregiver/companion

⊘ **S9994** Lodging costs (e.g., hotel charges) for clinical trial participant and one caregiver/companion

⊘ **S9996** Meals for clinical trial participant and one caregiver/companion

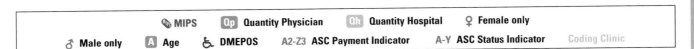

⊘ **S9999** Sales tax

TEMPORARY NATIONAL CODES ESTABLISHED BY MEDICAID (T1000-T9999)

Not Valid For Medicare

⃠ **T1000** Private duty/independent nursing service(s) - licensed, up to 15 minutes

⃠ **T1001** Nursing assessment/evaluation

⃠ **T1002** RN services, up to 15 minutes

⃠ **T1003** LPN/LVN services, up to 15 minutes

⃠ **T1004** Services of a qualified nursing aide, up to 15 minutes

⃠ **T1005** Respite care services, up to 15 minutes

⃠ **T1006** Alcohol and/or substance abuse services, family/couple counseling

⃠ **T1007** Alcohol and/or substance abuse services, treatment plan development and/or modification

⃠ **T1009** Child sitting services for children of the individual receiving alcohol and/or substance abuse services A

⃠ **T1010** Meals for individuals receiving alcohol and/or substance abuse services (when meals not included in the program)

⃠ **T1012** Alcohol and/or substance abuse services, skills development

⃠ **T1013** Sign language or oral interpretive services, per 15 minutes

⃠ **T1014** Telehealth transmission, per minute, professional services bill separately

⃠ **T1015** Clinic visit/encounter, all-inclusive

⃠ **T1016** Case Management, each 15 minutes

⃠ **T1017** Targeted Case Management, each 15 minutes

⃠ **T1018** School-based individualized education program (IEP) services, bundled

⃠ **T1019** Personal care services, per 15 minutes, not for an inpatient or resident of a hospital, nursing facility, ICF/MR or IMD, part of the individualized plan of treatment (code may not be used to identify services provided by home health aide or certified nurse assistant)

⃠ **T1020** Personal care services, per diem, not for an inpatient or resident of a hospital, nursing facility, ICF/MR or IMD, part of the individualized plan of treatment (code may not be used to identify services provided by home health aide or certified nurse assistant)

⃠ **T1021** Home health aide or certified nurse assistant, per visit

⃠ **T1022** Contracted home health agency services, all services provided under contract, per day

⃠ **T1023** Screening to determine the appropriateness of consideration of an individual for participation in a specified program, project or treatment protocol, per encounter

⃠ **T1024** Evaluation and treatment by an integrated, specialty team contracted to provide coordinated care to multiple or severely handicapped children, per encounter A

⃠ **T1025** Intensive, extended multidisciplinary services provided in a clinic setting to children with complex medical, physical, mental and psychosocial impairments, per diem A

⃠ **T1026** Intensive, extended multidisciplinary services provided in a clinic setting to children with complex medical, physical, medical and psychosocial impairments, per hour A

⃠ **T1027** Family training and counseling for child development, per 15 minutes A

⃠ **T1028** Assessment of home, physical and family environment, to determine suitability to meet patient's medical needs

⃠ **T1029** Comprehensive environmental lead investigation, not including laboratory analysis, per dwelling

⃠ **T1030** Nursing care, in the home, by registered nurse, per diem

⃠ **T1031** Nursing care, in the home, by licensed practical nurse, per diem

⃠ **T1040** Medicaid certified community behavioral health clinic services, per diem

⃠ **T1041** Medicaid certified community behavioral health clinic services, per month

⃠ **T1502** Administration of oral, intramuscular and/or subcutaneous medication by health care agency/professional, per visit

⃠ **T1503** Administration of medication, other than oral and/or injectable, by a health care agency/professional, per visit

⃠ **T1505** Electronic medication compliance management device, includes all components and accessories, not otherwise classified

▶ New ⤾ Revised ✔ Reinstated ~~deleted~~ Deleted ⃠ Not covered or valid by Medicare
Special coverage instructions ✻ Carrier discretion Bill Part B MAC Bill DME MAC

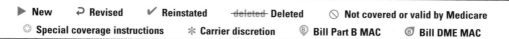

⃠ **T1999** Miscellaneous therapeutic items and supplies, retail purchases, not otherwise classified; identify product in "remarks"

⃠ **T2001** Non-emergency transportation; patient attendant/escort

⃠ **T2002** Non-emergency transportation; per diem

⃠ **T2003** Non-emergency transportation; encounter/trip

⃠ **T2004** Non-emergency transport; commercial carrier, multi-pass

⃠ **T2005** Non-emergency transportation: stretcher van

⃠ **T2007** Transportation waiting time, air ambulance and non-emergency vehicle, one-half (1/2) hour increments

⃠ **T2010** Preadmission screening and resident review (PASRR) level I identification screening, per screen

⃠ **T2011** Preadmission screening and resident review (PASRR) level II evaluation, per evaluation

⃠ **T2012** Habilitation, educational, waiver; per diem

⃠ **T2013** Habilitation, educational, waiver; per hour

⃠ **T2014** Habilitation, prevocational, waiver; per diem

⃠ **T2015** Habilitation, prevocational, waiver; per hour

⃠ **T2016** Habilitation, residential, waiver; per diem

⃠ **T2017** Habilitation, residential, waiver; 15 minutes

⃠ **T2018** Habilitation, supported employment, waiver; per diem

⃠ **T2019** Habilitation, supported employment, waiver; per 15 minutes

⃠ **T2020** Day habilitation, waiver; per diem

⃠ **T2021** Day habilitation, waiver; per 15 minutes

⃠ **T2022** Case management, per month

⃠ **T2023** Targeted case management; per month

⃠ **T2024** Service assessment/plan of care development, waiver

⃠ **T2025** Waiver services; not otherwise specified (NOS)

⃠ **T2026** Specialized childcare, waiver; per diem

⃠ **T2027** Specialized childcare, waiver; per 15 minutes

⃠ **T2028** Specialized supply, not otherwise specified, waiver

⃠ **T2029** Specialized medical equipment, not otherwise specified, waiver

⃠ **T2030** Assisted living, waiver; per month

⃠ **T2031** Assisted living; waiver, per diem

⃠ **T2032** Residential care, not otherwise specified (NOS), waiver; per month

⃠ **T2033** Residential care, not otherwise specified (NOS), waiver; per diem

⃠ **T2034** Crisis intervention, waiver; per diem

⃠ **T2035** Utility services to support medical equipment and assistive technology/devices, waiver

⃠ **T2036** Therapeutic camping, overnight, waiver; each session

⃠ **T2037** Therapeutic camping, day, waiver; each session

⃠ **T2038** Community transition, waiver; per service

⃠ **T2039** Vehicle modifications, waiver; per service

⃠ **T2040** Financial management, self-directed, waiver; per 15 minutes

⃠ **T2041** Supports brokerage, self-directed, waiver; per 15 minutes

⃠ **T2042** Hospice routine home care; per diem

⃠ **T2043** Hospice continuous home care; per hour

⃠ **T2044** Hospice inpatient respite care; per diem

⃠ **T2045** Hospice general inpatient care; per diem

⃠ **T2046** Hospice long term care, room and board only; per diem

⃠ **T2048** Behavioral health; long-term care residential (non-acute care in a residential treatment program where stay is typically longer than 30 days), with room and board, per diem

⃠ **T2049** Non-emergency transportation; stretcher van, mileage; per mile

⃠ **T2101** Human breast milk processing, storage and distribution only ♀

⃠ **T4521** Adult sized disposable incontinence product, brief/diaper, small, each A

IOM: 100-03, 4, 280.1

⃠ **T4522** Adult sized disposable incontinence product, brief/diaper, medium, each A

IOM: 100-03, 4, 280.1

MIPS | Qp Quantity Physician | Qh Quantity Hospital | ♀ Female only
♂ Male only | A Age | DMEPOS | A2-Z3 ASC Payment Indicator | A-Y ASC Status Indicator | Coding Clinic

⊘ **T4523** Adult sized disposable incontinence product, brief/diaper, large, each A

IOM: 100-03, 4, 280.1

⊘ **T4524** Adult sized disposable incontinence product, brief/diaper, extra large, each A

IOM: 100-03, 4, 280.1

⊘ **T4525** Adult sized disposable incontinence product, protective underwear/pull-on, small size, each A

IOM: 100-03, 4, 280.1

⊘ **T4526** Adult sized disposable incontinence product, protective underwear/pull-on, medium size, each A

IOM: 100-03, 4, 280.1

⊘ **T4527** Adult sized disposable incontinence product, protective underwear/pull-on, large size, each A

IOM: 100-03, 4, 280.1

⊘ **T4528** Adult sized disposable incontinence product, protective underwear/pull-on, extra large size, each A

IOM: 100-03, 4, 280.1

⊘ **T4529** Pediatric sized disposable incontinence product, brief/diaper, small/medium size, each A

IOM: 100-03, 4, 280.1

⊘ **T4530** Pediatric sized disposable incontinence product, brief/diaper, large size, each A

IOM: 100-03, 4, 280.1

⊘ **T4531** Pediatric sized disposable incontinence product, protective underwear/pull-on, small/medium size, each A

IOM: 100-03, 4, 280.1

⊘ **T4532** Pediatric sized disposable incontinence product, protective underwear/pull-on, large size, each A

IOM: 100-03, 4, 280.1

⊘ **T4533** Youth sized disposable incontinence product, brief/diaper, each A

IOM: 100-03, 4, 280.1

⊘ **T4534** Youth sized disposable incontinence product, protective underwear/pull-on, each A

IOM: 100-03, 4, 280.1

⊘ **T4535** Disposable liner/shield/guard/pad/undergarment, for incontinence, each

IOM: 100-03, 4, 280.1

⊘ **T4536** Incontinence product, protective underwear/pull-on, reusable, any size, each

IOM: 100-03, 4, 280.1

⊘ **T4537** Incontinence product, protective underpad, reusable, bed size, each

IOM: 100-03, 4, 280.1

⊘ **T4538** Diaper service, reusable diaper, each diaper

IOM: 100-03, 4, 280.1

⊘ **T4539** Incontinence product, diaper/brief, reusable, any size, each

IOM: 100-03, 4, 280.1

⊘ **T4540** Incontinence product, protective underpad, reusable, chair size, each

IOM: 100-03, 4, 280.1

⊘ **T4541** Incontinence product, disposable underpad, large, each

⊘ **T4542** Incontinence product, disposable underpad, small size, each

⊘ **T4543** Adult sized disposable incontinence product, protective brief/diaper, above extra large, each A

IOM: 100-03, 4, 280.1

⊘ **T4544** Adult sized disposable incontinence product, protective underwear/pull-on, above extra large, each A

IOM: 100-03, 4, 280.1

▶ ⊘ **T4545** Incontinence product, disposable, penile wrap, each ♂

⊘ **T5001** Positioning seat for persons with special orthopedic needs, supply, not otherwise specified

⊘ **T5999** Supply, not otherwise specified

▶ **New** ⮐ **Revised** ✔ **Reinstated** ~~deleted~~ **Deleted** ⊘ **Not covered or valid by Medicare**
⊛ **Special coverage instructions** ✻ **Carrier discretion** Ⓑ **Bill Part B MAC** Ⓑ **Bill DME MAC**

VISION SERVICES (V0000-V2999)

Frames

V2020 Frames, purchases A

Includes cost of frame/replacement and dispensing fee. One unit of service represents one pair of eyeglass frames.

IOM: 100-02, 15, 120

V2025 Deluxe frame E1

Not a benefit. Billing deluxe frames-submit V2020 on one line; V2025 on second line.

IOM: 100-04, 1, 30.3.5

If a CPT procedure code for supply of spectacles or a permanent prosthesis is reported, recode with the specific lens type listed below.

Single Vision Lenses

* V2100 Sphere, single vision, plano to plus or minus 4.00, per lens A
* V2101 Sphere, single vision, plus or minus 4.12 to plus or minus 7.00d, per lens A
* V2102 Sphere, single vision, plus or minus 7.12 to plus or minus 20.00d, per lens A
* V2103 Spherocylinder, single vision, plano to plus or minus 4.00d sphere, .12 to 2.00d cylinder, per lens A
* V2104 Spherocylinder, single vision, plano to plus or minus 4.00d sphere, 2.12 to 4.00d cylinder, per lens A
* V2105 Spherocylinder, single vision, plano to plus or minus 4.00d sphere, 4.25 to 6.00d cylinder, per lens A
* V2106 Spherocylinder, single vision, plano to plus or minus 4.00d sphere, over 6.00d cylinder, per lens A
* V2107 Spherocylinder, single vision, plus or minus 4.25 to plus or minus 7.00 sphere, .12 to 2.00d cylinder, per lens A
* V2108 Spherocylinder, single vision, plus or minus 4.25d to plus or minus 7.00d sphere, 2.12 to 4.00d cylinder, per lens A
* V2109 Spherocylinder, single vision, plus or minus 4.25 to plus or minus 7.00d sphere, 4.25 to 6.00d cylinder, per lens A
* V2110 Sperocylinder, single vision, plus or minus 4.25 to 7.00d sphere, over 6.00d cylinder, per lens A
* V2111 Spherocylinder, single vision, plus or minus 7.25 to plus or minus 12.00d sphere, .25 to 2.25d cylinder, per lens A
* V2112 Spherocylinder, single vision, plus or minus 7.25 to plus or minus 12.00d sphere, 2.25d to 4.00d cylinder, per lens A
* V2113 Spherocylinder, single vision, plus or minus 7.25 to plus or minus 12.00d sphere, 4.25 to 6.00d cylinder, per lens A
* V2114 Spherocylinder, single vision, sphere over plus or minus 12.00d, per lens A
* V2115 Lenticular, (myodisc), per lens, single vision A
* V2118 Aniseikonic lens, single vision A

V2121 Lenticular lens, per lens, single A

IOM: 100-02, 15, 120; 100-04, 3, 10.4

* V2199 Not otherwise classified, single vision lens A

Bill on paper. Requires report of type of single vision lens and optical lab invoice.

Bifocal Lenses

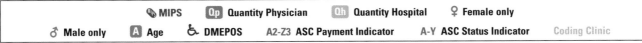

* V2200 Sphere, bifocal, plano to plus or minus 4.00d, per lens A
* V2201 Sphere, bifocal, plus or minus 4.12 to plus or minus 7.00d, per lens A
* V2202 Sphere, bifocal, plus or minus 7.12 to plus or minus 20.00d, per lens A
* V2203 Spherocylinder, bifocal, plano to plus or minus 4.00d sphere, .12 to 2.00d cylinder, per lens A
* V2204 Spherocylinder, bifocal, plano to plus or minus 4.00d sphere, 2.12 to 4.00d cylinder, per lens A
* V2205 Spherocylinder, bifocal, plano to plus or minus 4.00d sphere, 4.25 to 6.00d cylinder, per lens A
* V2206 Spherocylinder, bifocal, plano to plus or minus 4.00d sphere, over 6.00d cylinder, per lens A

* **V2207** Spherocylinder, bifocal, plus or minus 4.25 to plus or minus 7.00d sphere, .12 to 2.00d cylinder, per lens Qp Qh A
* **V2208** Spherocylinder, bifocal, plus or minus 4.25 to plus or minus 7.00d sphere, 2.12 to 4.00d cylinder, per lens Qp Qh A
* **V2209** Spherocylinder, bifocal, plus or minus 4.25 to plus or minus 7.00d sphere, 4.25 to 6.00d cylinder, per lens Qp Qh A
* **V2210** Spherocylinder, bifocal, plus or minus 4.25 to plus or minus 7.00d sphere, over 6.00d cylinder, per lens Qp Qh A
* **V2211** Spherocylinder, bifocal, plus or minus 7.25 to plus or minus 12.00d sphere, .25 to 2.25d cylinder, per lens Qp Qh A
* **V2212** Spherocylinder, bifocal, plus or minus 7.25 to plus or minus 12.00d sphere, 2.25 to 4.00d cylinder, per lens Qp Qh A
* **V2213** Spherocylinder, bifocal, plus or minus 7.25 to plus or minus 12.00d sphere, 4.25 to 6.00d cylinder, per lens Qp Qh A
* **V2214** Spherocylinder, bifocal, sphere over plus or minus 12.00d, per lens Qp Qh A
* **V2215** Lenticular (myodisc), per lens, bifocal Qp Qh A
* **V2218** Aniseikonic, per lens, bifocal Qp Qh A
* **V2219** Bifocal seg width over 28 mm Qp Qh A
* **V2220** Bifocal add over 3.25d Qp Qh A
* **V2221** Lenticular lens, per lens, bifocal Qp Qh A

  IOM: 100-02, 15, 120; 100-04, 3, 10.4
* **V2299** Specialty bifocal (by report) Qp Qh A

  Bill on paper. Requires report of type of specialty bifocal lens and optical lab invoice.

Trifocal Lenses

* **V2300** Sphere, trifocal, plano to plus or minus 4.00d, per lens Qp Qh A
* **V2301** Sphere, trifocal, plus or minus 4.12 to plus or minus 7.00d per lens Qp Qh A
* **V2302** Sphere, trifocal, plus or minus 7.12 to plus or minus 20.00, per lens Qp Qh A
* **V2303** Spherocylinder, trifocal, plano to plus or minus 4.00d sphere, .12 to 2.00d cylinder, per lens Qp Qh A
* **V2304** Spherocylinder, trifocal, plano to plus or minus 4.00d sphere, 2.25-4.00d cylinder, per lens Qp Qh A
* **V2305** Spherocylinder, trifocal, plano to plus or minus 4.00d sphere, 4.25 to 6.00 cylinder, per lens Qp Qh A
* **V2306** Spherocylinder, trifocal, plano to plus or minus 4.00d sphere, over 6.00d cylinder, per lens Qp Qh A
* **V2307** Spherocylinder, trifocal, plus or minus 4.25 to plus or minus 7.00d sphere, .12 to 2.00d cylinder, per lens Qp Qh A
* **V2308** Spherocylinder, trifocal, plus or minus 4.25 to plus or minus 7.00d sphere, 2.12 to 4.00d cylinder, per lens Qp Qh A
* **V2309** Spherocylinder, trifocal, plus or minus 4.25 to plus or minus 7.00d sphere, 4.25 to 6.00d cylinder, per lens Qp Qh A
* **V2310** Spherocylinder, trifocal, plus or minus 4.25 to plus or minus 7.00d sphere, over 6.00d cylinder, per lens Qp Qh A
* **V2311** Spherocylinder, trifocal, plus or minus 7.25 to plus or minus 12.00d sphere, .25 to 2.25d cylinder, per lens Qp Qh A
* **V2312** Spherocylinder, trifocal, plus or minus 7.25 to plus or minus 12.00d sphere, 2.25 to 4.00d cylinder, per lens Qp Qh A
* **V2313** Spherocylinder, trifocal, plus or minus 7.25 to plus or minus 12.00d sphere, 4.25 to 6.00d cylinder, per lens Qp Qh A
* **V2314** Spherocylinder, trifocal, sphere over plus or minus 12.00d, per lens Qp Qh A
* **V2315** Lenticular, (myodisc), per lens, trifocal Qp Qh A
* **V2318** Aniseikonic lens, trifocal Qp Qh A
* **V2319** Trifocal seg width over 28 mm Qp Qh A
* **V2320** Trifocal add over 3.25d Qp Qh A

▶ New ↻ Revised ✓ Reinstated ~~deleted~~ Deleted ⊘ Not covered or valid by Medicare
Special coverage instructions * Carrier discretion Bill Part B MAC Bill DME MAC

V2321 Lenticular lens, per lens, trifocal Op Qh A

IOM: 100-02, 15, 120; 100-04, 3, 10.4

V2399 Specialty trifocal (by report) Op Qh A

Bill on paper. Requires report of type of trifocal lens and optical lab invoice.

Variable Asphericity/Sphericity Lenses

V2410 Variable asphericity lens, single vision, full field, glass or plastic, per lens Op Qh A

V2430 Variable asphericity lens, bifocal, full field, glass or plastic, per lens Op Qh A

V2499 Variable sphericity lens, other type Op Qh A

Bill on paper. Requires report of other ptical lab invoice.

Contact Lenses

If a CPT procedure code for supply of contact lens is reported, recode with specific lens type listed below (per lens).

V2500 Contact lens, PMMA, spherical, per lens Op Qh A

Requires prior authorization for patients under age 21.

V2501 Contact lens, PMMA, toric or prism ballast, per lens Op Qh A

Requires prior authorization for clients under age 21.

V2502 Contact lens, PMMA, bifocal, per lens Op Qh A

Requires prior authorization for clients under age 21. Bill on paper. Requires optical lab invoice.

V2503 Contact lens PMMA, color vision deficiency, per lens Op Qh A

Requires prior authorization for clients under age 21. Bill on paper. Requires optical lab invoice.

V2510 Contact lens, gas permeable, spherical, per lens Op Qh A

Requires prior authorization for clients under age 21.

V2511 Contact lens, gas permeable, toric, prism ballast, per lens Op Qh A

Requires prior authorization for clients under age 21.

V2512 Contact lens, gas permeable, bifocal, per lens Op Qh A

Requires prior authorization for clients under age 21.

V2513 Contact lens, gas permeable, extended wear, per lens Op Qh A

Requires prior authorization for clients under age 21.

V2520 Contact lens, hydrophilic, spherical, per lens Op Qh A

Requires prior authorization for clients under age 21.

IOM: 100-03, 1, 80.1; 100-03, 1, 80.4

V2521 Contact lens, hydrophilic, toric, or prism ballast, per lens Op Qh A

Requires prior authorization for clients under age 21.

IOM: 100-03, 1, 80.1; 100-03, 1, 80.4

V2522 Contact lens, hydrophilic, bifocal, per lens Op Qh A

Requires prior authorization for clients under age 21.

IOM: 100-03, 1, 80.1; 100-03, 1, 80.4

V2523 Contact lens, hydrophilic, extended wear, per lens Op Qh A

Requires prior authorization for clients under age 21.

IOM: 100-03, 1, 80.1; 100-03, 1, 80.4

V2530 Contact lens, scleral, gas impermeable, per lens (for contact lens modification, *see* 92325) Op Qh A

Requires prior authorization for clients under age 21.

V2531 Contact lens, scleral, gas permeable, per lens (for contact lens modification, see 92325) Op Qh A

Requires prior authorization for clients under age 21. Bill on paper. Requires optical lab invoice.

IOM: 100-03, 1, 80.5

V2599 Contact lens, other type Op Qh A

Requires prior authorization for clients under age 21. Bill on paper. Requires report of other type of contact lens and optical invoice.

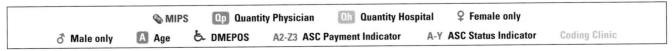

Low Vision Aids

If a CPT procedure code for supply of low vision aid is reported, recode with specific systems listed below.

* **V2600** Hand held low vision aids and other nonspectacle mounted aids Ⓔ Qp Qh A
  Requires prior authorization.
* **V2610** Single lens spectacle mounted low vision aids Ⓔ Qp Qh A
  Requires prior authorization.
* **V2615** Telescopic and other compound lens system, including distance vision telescopic, near vision telescopes and compound microscopic lens system Ⓔ Qp Qh A
  Requires prior authorization. Bill on paper. Requires optical lab invoice.

Prosthetic Eye

V2623 Prosthetic eye, plastic, custom Ⓔ Qp Qh ♿ A
DME regional carrier. Requires prior authorization. Bill on paper. Requires optical lab invoice.

* **V2624** Polishing/resurfacing of ocular prosthesis Ⓔ Qp Qh ♿ A
  Requires prior authorization. Bill on paper. Requires optical lab invoice.
* **V2625** Enlargement of ocular prosthesis Ⓔ Qp Qh ♿ A
  Requires prior authorization. Bill on paper. Requires optical lab invoice.
* **V2626** Reduction of ocular prosthesis Ⓔ Qp Qh ♿ A
  Requires prior authorization. Bill on paper. Requires optical lab invoice.

V2627 Scleral cover shell Ⓔ Qp Qh ♿ A
DME regional carrier
Requires prior authorization. Bill on paper. Requires optical lab invoice.
IOM: 100-03, 4, 280.2

* **V2628** Fabrication and fitting of ocular conformer Ⓔ Qp Qh ♿ A
  Requires prior authorization. Bill on paper. Requires optical lab invoice.
* **V2629** Prosthetic eye, other type Ⓔ Qp Qh A
  Requires prior authorization. Bill on paper. Requires optical lab invoice.

Intraocular Lenses

V2630 Anterior chamber intraocular lens Ⓑ Qp Qh ♿ N1 N
IOM: 100-02, 15, 120

V2631 Iris supported intraocular lens Ⓑ Qp Qh ♿ N1 N
IOM: 100-02, 15, 120

V2632 Posterior chamber intraocular lens Ⓑ Qp Qh ♿ N1 N
IOM: 100-02, 15, 120

Figure 52 Posterior intraocular lens.

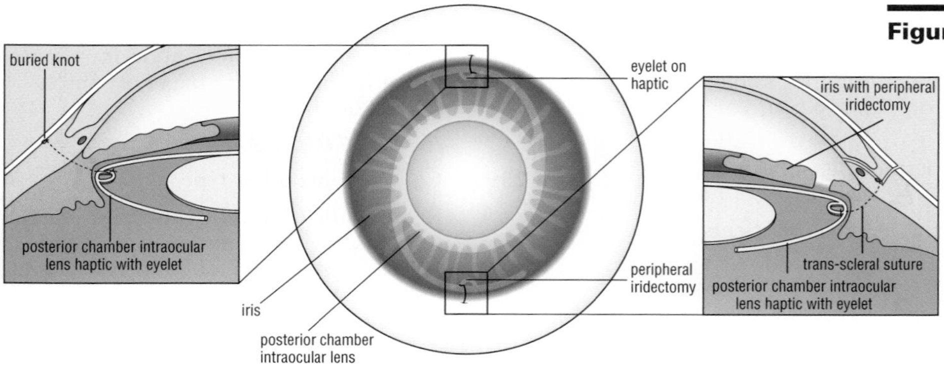

buried knot
posterior chamber intraocular lens haptic with eyelet
iris
posterior chamber intraocular lens
eyelet on haptic
peripheral iridectomy
iris with peripheral iridectomy
trans-scleral suture
posterior chamber intraocular lens haptic with eyelet

▶ New ↻ Revised ✔ Reinstated ~~deleted~~ Deleted ⊘ Not covered or valid by Medicare
Special coverage instructions * Carrier discretion Ⓑ Bill Part B MAC Ⓔ Bill DME MAC

Miscellaneous Vision Services

✻ **V2700** Balance lens, per lens Qp Qh A

⃠ **V2702** Deluxe lens feature Qp Qh E1

IOM: 100-02, 15, 120; 100-04, 3, 10.4

✻ **V2710** Slab off prism, glass or plastic, per lens Qp Qh A

✻ **V2715** Prism, per lens Qp Qh A

✻ **V2718** Press-on lens, Fresnel prism, per lens Qp Qh A

✻ **V2730** Special base curve, glass or plastic, per lens Qp Qh A

V2744 Tint, photochromatic, per lens Qp Qh A

Requires prior authorization.

IOM: 100-02, 15, 120; 100-04, 3, 10.4

V2745 Addition to lens, tint, any color, solid, gradient or equal, excludes photochroatic, any lens material, per lens Qp Qh A

Includes photochromatic lenses (V2744) used as sunglasses, which are prescribed in addition to regular prosthetic lenses for aphakic patient will be denied as not medically necessary.

IOM: 100-02, 15, 120; 100-04, 3, 10.4

V2750 Anti-reflective coating, per lens Qp Qh A

Requires prior authorization.

IOM: 100-02, 15, 120; 100-04, 3, 10.4

V2755 U-V lens, per lens Qp Qh A

IOM: 100-02, 15, 120; 100-04, 3, 10.4

✻ **V2756** Eye glass case Qp Qh E1

✻ **V2760** Scratch resistant coating, per lens Qp Qh E1

V2761 Mirror coating, any type, solid, gradient or equal, any lens material, per lens Qp Qh B

IOM: 100-02, 15, 120; 100-04, 3, 10.4

V2762 Polarization, any lens material, per lens Qp Qh E1

IOM: 100-02, 15, 120; 100-04, 3, 10.4

✻ **V2770** Occluder lens, per lens Qp Qh A

Requires prior authorization.

✻ **V2780** Oversize lens, per lens Qp Qh A

Requires prior authorization.

✻ **V2781** Progressive lens, per lens Qp Qh B

Requires prior authorization.

V2782 Lens, index 1.54 to 1.65 plastic or 1.60 to 1.79 glass, excludes polycarbonate, per lens Qp Qh A

Do not bill in addition to V2784

IOM: 100-02, 15, 120; 100-04, 3, 10.4

V2783 Lens, index greater than or equal to 1.66 plastic or greater than or equal to 1.80 glass, excludes polycarbonate, per lens Qp Qh A

Do not bill in addition to V2784

IOM: 100-02, 15, 120; 100-04, 3, 10.4

V2784 Lens, polycarbonate or equal, any index, per lens Qp Qh A

Covered only for patients with functional vision in one eye-in this situation, an impact-resistant material is covered for both lenses if eyeglasses are covered. Claims with V2784 that do not meet this coverage criterion will be denied as not medically necessary.

IOM: 100-02, 15, 120; 100-04, 3, 10.4

✻ **V2785** Processing, preserving and transporting corneal tissue Qp Qh F4 F

For ASC, bill on paper. Must attach eye bank invoice to claim.

For Hospitals, bill charges for corneal tissue to receive cost based reimbursement.

IOM: 100- 4, 4, 200.1

V2786 Specialty occupational multifocal lens, per lens Qp Qh E1

IOM: 100-02, 15, 120; 100-04, 3, 10.4

V2787 Astigmatism correcting function of intraocular lens E1

Medicare Statute 1862(a)(7)

⃠ **V2788** Presbyopia correcting function of intraocular lens E1

Medicare Statute 1862a7

✻ **V2790** Amniotic membrane for surgical reconstruction, per procedure Qp Qh N1 N

✻ **V2797** Vision supply, accessory and/or service component of another HCPCS vision code Qp Qh E1

✻ **V2799** Vision item or service, miscellaneous A

Bill on paper. Requires report of miscellaneous service and optical lab invoice.

⚕ MIPS	ⓆP Quantity Physician	ⓆH Quantity Hospital	♀ Female only
♂ Male only	Ⓐ Age	⓵ DMEPOS A2-Z3 ASC Payment Indicator	A-Y ASC Status Indicator Coding Clinic

HEARING SERVICES (V5000-V5999)

These codes are for non-physician services.

Assessments and Evaluations

⃠ **V5008** Hearing screening Ⓑ Qp Qh E1
IOM: 100-02, 16, 90

⃠ **V5010** Assessment for hearing aid Ⓑ Qp Qh E1
Medicare Statute 1862a7

⃠ **V5011** Fitting/orientation/checking of hearing aid Ⓑ Qp Qh E1
Medicare Statute 1862a7

⃠ **V5014** Repair/modification of a hearing aid Ⓑ E1
Medicare Statute 1862a7

⃠ **V5020** Conformity evaluation Ⓑ E1
Medicare Statute 1862a7

Monaural Hearing Aid

⃠ **V5030** Hearing aid, monaural, body worn, air conduction Ⓑ E1
Medicare Statute 1862a7

⃠ **V5040** Hearing aid, monaural, body worn, bone conduction Ⓑ E1
Medicare Statute 1862a7

⃠ **V5050** Hearing aid, monaural, in the ear Ⓑ E1
Medicare Statute 1862a7

⃠ **V5060** Hearing aid, monaural, behind the ear Ⓑ E1
Medicare Statute 1862a7

Miscellaneous Services and Supplies

⃠ **V5070** Glasses, air conduction Ⓑ E1
Medicare Statute 1862a7

⃠ **V5080** Glasses, bone conduction Ⓑ E1
Medicare Statute 1862a7

⃠ **V5090** Dispensing fee, unspecified hearing aid Ⓑ E1
Medicare Statute 1862a7

⃠ **V5095** Semi-implantable middle ear hearing prosthesis Ⓑ E1
Medicare Statute 1862a7

⃠ **V5100** Hearing aid, bilateral, body worn Ⓑ E1
Medicare Statute 1862a7

⃠ **V5110** Dispensing fee, bilateral Ⓑ E1
Medicare Statute 1862a7

Hearing Aids

⃠ **V5120** Binaural, body Ⓑ E1
Medicare Statute 1862a7

⃠ **V5130** Binaural, in the ear Ⓑ E1
Medicare Statute 1862a7

⃠ **V5140** Binaural, behind the ear Ⓑ E1
Medicare Statute 1862a7

⃠ **V5150** Binaural, glasses Ⓑ E1
Medicare Statute 1862a7

⃠ **V5160** Dispensing fee, binaural Ⓑ E1
Medicare Statute 1862a7

~~V5170 Hearing aid, CROS, in the ear~~ ✖

▶ ⃠ **V5171** Hearing aid, contralateral routing device, monaural, in the ear (ITE) E1
Medicare Statute 1862a7

▶ ⃠ **V5172** Hearing aid, contralateral routing device, monaural, in the canal (ITC) E1
Medicare Statute 1862a7

~~V5180 Hearing aid, CROS, behind the ear~~ ✖

▶ ⃠ **V5181** Hearing aid, contralateral routing device, monaural, behind the ear (BTE) E1
Medicare Statute 1862a7

↩ ⃠ **V5190** Hearing aid, contralateral routing, monaural, glasses Ⓑ E1
Medicare Statute 1862a7

↩ ⃠ **V5200** Dispensing fee, contralateral, monaural Ⓑ E1
Medicare Statute 1862a7

~~V5210 Hearing aid, BICROS, in the ear~~ ✖

▶ ⃠ **V5211** Hearing aid, contralateral routing system, binaural, ITE/ITE E1
Medicare Statute 1862a7

▶ ⃠ **V5212** Hearing aid, contralateral routing system, binaural, ITE/ITC E1
Medicare Statute 1862a7

▶ ⃠ **V5213** Hearing aid, contralateral routing system, binaural, ITE/BTE E1
Medicare Statute 1862a7

▶ ⃠ **V5214** Hearing aid, contralateral routing system, binaural, ITC/ITC E1
Medicare Statute 1862a7

▶ ⃠ **V5215** Hearing aid, contralateral routing system, binaural, ITC/BTE E1
Medicare Statute 1862a7

~~V5220 Hearing aid, contralateral, monaural, behind the ear~~ ✖

▶ ⃠ **V5221** Hearing aid, contralateral routing system, binaural, BTE/BTE E1
Medicare Statute 1862a7

⃠ **V5230** Hearing aid, contralateral routing system, binaural, glasses E1
Medicare Statute 1862a7

⃠ **V5240** Dispensing fee, contralateral routing system, binaural E1
Medicare Statute 1862a7

⃠ **V5241** Dispensing fee, monaural hearing aid, any type E1
Medicare Statute 1862a7

⃠ **V5242** Hearing aid, analog, monaural, CIC (completely in the ear canal) E1
Medicare Statute 1862a7

⃠ **V5243** Hearing aid, analog, monaural, ITC (in the canal) E1
Medicare Statute 1862a9

⃠ **V5244** Hearing aid, digitally programmable analog, monaural, CIC E1
Medicare Statute 1862a7

⃠ **V5245** Hearing aid, digitally programmable, analog, monaural, ITC E1
Medicare Statute 1862a7

⃠ **V5246** Hearing aid, digitally programmable analog, monaural, ITE (in the ear) E1
Medicare Statute 1862a7

⃠ **V5247** Hearing aid, digitally programmable analog, monaural, BTE (behind the ear) E1
Medicare Statute 1862a7

⃠ **V5248** Hearing aid, analog, binaural, CIC E1
Medicare Statute 1862a7

⃠ **V5249** Hearing aid, analog, binaural, ITC E1
Medicare Statute 1862a7

⃠ **V5250** Hearing aid, digitally programmable analog, binaural, CIC E1
Medicare Statute 1862a7

⃠ **V5251** Hearing aid, digitally programmable analog, binaural, ITC E1
Medicare Statute 1862a7

⃠ **V5252** Hearing aid, digitally programmable, binaural, ITE E1
Medicare Statute 1862a7

⃠ **V5253** Hearing aid, digitally programmable, binaural, BTE E1
Medicare Statute 1862a7

⃠ **V5254** Hearing aid, digital, monaural, CIC E1
Medicare Statute 1862a7

⃠ **V5255** Hearing aid, digital, monaural, ITC E1
Medicare Statute 1862a7

⃠ **V5256** Hearing aid, digital, monaural, ITE E1
Medicare Statute 1862a7

⃠ **V5257** Hearing aid, digital, monaural, BTE E1
Medicare Statute 1862a7

⃠ **V5258** Hearing aid, digital, binaural, CIC E1
Medicare Statute 1862a7

⃠ **V5259** Hearing aid, digital, binaural, ITC E1
Medicare Statute 1862a7

⃠ **V5260** Hearing aid, digital, binaural, ITE E1
Medicare Statute 1862a7

⃠ **V5261** Hearing aid, digital, binaural, BTE E1
Medicare Statute 1862a7

⃠ **V5262** Hearing aid, disposable, any type, monaural E1
Medicare Statute 1862a7

⃠ **V5263** Hearing aid, disposable, any type, binaural E1
Medicare Statute 1862a7

⃠ **V5264** Ear mold/insert, not disposable, any type E1
Medicare Statute 1862a7

⃠ **V5265** Ear mold/insert, disposable, any type E1
Medicare Statute 1862a7

⃠ **V5266** Battery for use in hearing device E1
Medicare Statute 1862a7

⃠ **V5267** Hearing aid or assistive listening device/supplies/accessories, not otherwise specified E1
Medicare Statute 1862a7

MIPS | Qp Quantity Physician | Qh Quantity Hospital | ♀ Female only
♂ Male only | A Age | DMEPOS | A2-Z3 ASC Payment Indicator | A-Y ASC Status Indicator | Coding Clinic

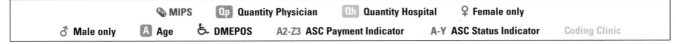

Assistive Listening Devices

⃠ **V5268** Assistive listening device, telephone amplifier, any type Ⓑ E1
Medicare Statute 1862a7

⃠ **V5269** Assistive listening device, alerting, any type Ⓑ E1
Medicare Statute 1862a7

⃠ **V5270** Assistive listening device, television amplifier, any type Ⓑ E1
Medicare Statute 1862a7

⃠ **V5271** Assistive listening device, television caption decoder Ⓑ E1
Medicare Statute 1862a7

⃠ **V5272** Assistive listening device, TDD Ⓑ E1
Medicare Statute 1862a7

⃠ **V5273** Assistive listening device, for use with cochlear implant Ⓑ E1
Medicare Statute 1862a7

⃠ **V5274** Assistive listening device, not otherwise specified Ⓑ Qp Qh E1
Medicare Statute 1862a7

⃠ **V5275** Ear impression, each Ⓑ E1
Medicare Statute 1862a7

⃠ **V5281** Assistive listening device, personal FM/DM system, monaural (1 receiver, transmitter, microphone), any type Ⓑ Qp Qh E1
Medicare Statute 1862a7

⃠ **V5282** Assistive listening device, personal FM/DM system, binaural (2 receivers, transmitter, microphone), any type Ⓑ Qp Qh E1
Medicare Statute 1862a7

⃠ **V5283** Assistive listening device, personal FM/DM neck, loop induction receiver Ⓑ Qp Qh E1
Medicare Statute 1862a7

⃠ **V5284** Assistive listening device, personal FM/DM, ear level receiver Ⓑ Qp Qh E1
Medicare Statute 1862a7

⃠ **V5285** Assistive listening device, personal FM/DM, direct audio input receiver Ⓑ Qp Qh E1
Medicare Statute 1862a7

⃠ **V5286** Assistive listening device, personal blue tooth FM/DM receiver Ⓑ Qp Qh E1
Medicare Statute 1862a7

⃠ **V5287** Assistive listening device, personal FM/DM receiver, not otherwise specified Ⓑ Qp Qh E1
Medicare Statute 1862a7

⃠ **V5288** Assistive listening device, personal FM/DM transmitter assistive listening device Ⓑ Qp Qh E1
Medicare Statute 1862a7

⃠ **V5289** Assistive listening device, personal FM/DM adapter/boot coupling device for receiver, any type Ⓑ Qp Qh E1
Medicare Statute 1862a7

⃠ **V5290** Assistive listening device, transmitter microphone, any type Ⓑ Qp Qh E1
Medicare Statute 1862a7

Other Supllies and Miscellaneous Services

⃠ **V5298** Hearing aid, not otherwise classified Ⓑ E1
Medicare Statute 1862a7

V5299 Hearing service, miscellaneous Ⓑ B
IOM: 100-02, 16, 90

Repair/Modification

⃠ **V5336** Repair/modification of augmentative communicative system or device (excludes adaptive hearing aid) Ⓓ E1
Medicare Statute 1862a7

Speech, Language, and Pathology Screening

These codes are for non-physician services.

⃠ **V5362** Speech screening Ⓑ E1
Medicare Statute 1862a7

⃠ **V5363** Language screening Ⓑ E1
Medicare Statute 1862a7

⃠ **V5364** Dysphagia screening Ⓑ E1
Medicare Statute 1862a7

▶ New ⟲ Revised ✔ Reinstated ~~deleted~~ Deleted ⃠ Not covered or valid by Medicare
Special coverage instructions ✻ Carrier discretion Ⓑ Bill Part B MAC Ⓓ Bill DME MAC

APPENDIX A

Jurisdiction List for DMEPOS HCPCS Codes

Deleted codes are valid for dates of service on or before the date of deletion. The jurisdiction list includes codes that are not payable by Medicare. Please consult the Medicare contractor in whose jurisdiction a claim would be filed in order to determine coverage under Medicare.

NOTE: All Local Carrier language has been changed to Part B MAC

HCPCS	DESCRIPTION	JURISDICTION
A0021 - A0999	Ambulance Services	Part B MAC
A4206 - A4209	Medical, Surgical, and Self- Administered Injection Supplies	Part B MAC if incident to a physician's service (not separately payable). If other, DME MAC.
A4210	Needle Free Injection Device	DME MAC
A4211	Medical, Surgical, and Self-Administered Injection Supplies	Part B MAC if incident to a physician's service (not separately payable). If other, DME MAC.
A4212	Non Coring Needle or Stylet with or without Catheter	Part B MAC
A4213 - A4215	Medical, Surgical, and Self-Administered Injection Supplies	Part B MAC if incident to a physician's service (not separately payable). If other, DME MAC.
A4216 - A4218	Saline	Part B MAC if incident to a physician's service (not separately payable). If other, DME MAC.
A4220	Refill Kit for Implantable Pump	Part B MAC
A4221 - A4236	Self-Administered Injection and Diabetic Supplies	DME MAC
A4244 - A4250	Medical, Surgical, and Self-Administered Injection Supplies	Part B MAC if incident to a physician's service (not separately payable). If other, DME MAC.
A4252 - A4259	Diabetic Supplies	DME MAC
A4261	Cervical Cap for Contraceptive Use	Part B MAC
A4262 - A4263	Lacrimal Duct Implants	Part B MAC
A4264	Contraceptive Implant	Part B MAC
A4265	Paraffin	Part B MAC if incident to a physician's service (not separately payable). If other, DME MAC.
A4266 - A4269	Contraceptives	Part B MAC
A4270	Endoscope Sheath	Part B MAC
A4280	Accessory for Breast Prosthesis	DME MAC
A4281 - A4286	Accessory for Breast Pump	DME MAC
A4290	Sacral Nerve Stimulation Test Lead	Part B MAC
A4300 - A4301	Implantable Catheter	Part B MAC
A4305 - A4306	Disposable Drug Delivery System	Part B MAC if incident to a physician's service (not separately payable). If other, DME MAC.
A4310 - A4358	Incontinence Supplies/ Urinary Supplies	If provided in the physician's office for a temporary condition, the item is incident to the physician's service & billed to the Part B MAC. If provided in the physician's office or other place of service for a permanent condition, the item is a prosthetic device & billed to the DME MAC.
A4360 - A4435	Urinary Supplies	If provided in the physician's office for a temporary condition, the item is incident to the physician's service & billed to the Part B MAC. If provided in the physician's office or other place of service for a permanent condition, the item is a prosthetic device & billed to the DME MAC.
A4450 - A4456	Tape; Adhesive Remover	Part B MAC if incident to a physician's service (not separately payable), or if supply for implanted prosthetic device. If other, DME MAC.
A4458-A4459	Enema Bag/System	DME MAC
A4461-A4463	Surgical Dressing Holders	Part B MAC if incident to a physician's service (not separately payable). If other, DME MAC.
A4465 - A4467	Non-elastic Binder and Garment, Strap, Covering	DME MAC
A4470	Gravlee Jet Washer	Part B MAC
A4480	Vabra Aspirator	Part B MAC
A4481	Tracheostomy Supply	Part B MAC if incident to a physician's service (not separately payable). If other, DME MAC.
A4483	Moisture Exchanger	DME MAC
A4490 - A4510	Surgical Stockings	DME MAC
A4520	Diapers	DME MAC
A4550	Surgical Trays	Part B MAC
A4553 - A4554	Underpads	DME MAC
A4555 - A4558	Electrodes; Lead Wires; Conductive Paste	Part B MAC if incident to a physician's service (not separately payable). If other, DME MAC.
A4559	Coupling Gel	Part B MAC if incident to a physician's service (not separately payable). If other, DME MAC.
A4561 - A4562	Pessary	Part B MAC

HCPCS	DESCRIPTION	JURISDICTION
A4565-A4566	Sling	Part B MAC
A4570	Splint	Part B MAC
A4575	Topical Hyperbaric Oxygen Chamber, Disposable	DME MAC
A4580 - A4590	Casting Supplies & Material	Part B MAC
A4595	TENS Supplies	Part B MAC if incident to a physician's service (not separately payable). If other, DME MAC.
A4600	Sleeve for Intermittent Limb Compression Device	DME MAC
A4601-A4602	Lithium Replacement Batteries	DME MAC
A4604	Tubing for Positive Airway Pressure Device	DME MAC
A4605	Tracheal Suction Catheter	DME MAC
A4606	Oxygen Probe for Oximeter	DME MAC
A4608	Transtracheal Oxygen Catheter	DME MAC
A4611 - A4613	Oxygen Equipment Batteries and Supplies	DME MAC
A4614	Peak Flow Rate Meter	Part B MAC if incident to a physician's service (not separately payable). If other, DME MAC.
A4615 - A4629	Oxygen & Tracheostomy Supplies	Part B MAC if incident to a physician's service (not separately payable). If other, DME MAC.
A4630 - A4640	DME Supplies	DME MAC
A4641 - A4642	Imaging Agent; Contrast Material	Part B MAC
A4648	Tissue Marker, Implanted	Part B MAC
A4649	Miscellaneous Surgical Supplies	Part B MAC if incident to a physician's service (not separately payable), or if supply for implanted prosthetic device or implanted DME. If other, DME MAC.
A4650	Implantable Radiation Dosimeter	Part B MAC
A4651 - A4932	Supplies for ESRD	DME MAC (not separately payable)
A5051 - A5093	Additional Ostomy Supplies	If provided in the physician's office for a temporary condition, the item is incident to the physician's service & billed to the Part B MAC. If provided in the physician's office or other place of service for a permanent condition, the item is a prosthetic device & billed to the DME MAC.

HCPCS	DESCRIPTION	JURISDICTION
A5102 - A5200	Additional Incontinence and Ostomy Supplies	If provided in the physician's office for a temporary condition, the item is incident to the physician's service & billed to the Part B MAC. If provided in the physician's office or other place of service for a permanent condition, the item is a prosthetic device & billed to the DME MAC.
A5500 - A5513	Therapeutic Shoes	DME MAC
A6000	Non-Contact Wound Warming Cover	DME MAC
A6010-A6024	Surgical Dressing	Part B MAC if incident to a physician's service (not separately payable) or if supply for implanted prosthetic device or implanted DME. If other, DME MAC.
A6025	Silicone Gel Sheet	Part B MAC if incident to a physician's service (not separately payable) or if supply for implanted prosthetic device or implanted DME. If other, DME MAC.
A6154 - A6411	Surgical Dressing	Part B MAC if incident to a physician's service (not separately payable) or if supply for implanted prosthetic device or implanted DME. If other, DME MAC.
A6412	Eye Patch	Part B MAC if incident to a physician's service (not separately payable) or if supply for implanted prosthetic device or implanted DME. If other, DME MAC.
A6413	Adhesive Bandage	Part B MAC if incident to a physician's service (not separately payable) or if supply for implanted prosthetic device or implanted DME. If other, DME MAC.
A6441 - A6512	Surgical Dressings	Part B MAC if incident to a physician's service (not separately payable) or if supply for implanted prosthetic device or implanted DME. If other, DME MAC.
A6513	Compression Burn Mask	DME MAC
A6530 - A6549	Compression Gradient Stockings	DME MAC
A6550	Supplies for Negative Pressure Wound Therapy Electrical Pump	DME MAC
A7000 - A7002	Accessories for Suction Pumps	DME MAC
A7003 - A7039	Accessories for Nebulizers, Aspirators and Ventilators	DME MAC
A7040 - A7041	Chest Drainage Supplies	Part B MAC
A7044 - A7047	Respiratory Accessories	DME MAC
A7048	Vacuum Drainage Supply	Part B MAC

HCPCS	DESCRIPTION	JURISDICTION
A7501-A7527	Tracheostomy Supplies	DME MAC
A8000-A8004	Protective Helmets	DME MAC
A9150	Non-Prescription Drugs	Part B MAC
A9152 - A9153	Vitamins	Part B MAC
A9155	Artificial Saliva	Part B MAC
A9180	Lice Infestation Treatment	Part B MAC
A9270	Noncovered Items or Services	DME MAC
A9272	Disposable Wound Suction Pump	DME MAC
A9273	Hot Water Bottles, Ice Caps or Collars, and Heat and/or Cold Wraps	DME MAC
A9274 - A9278	Glucose Monitoring	DME MAC
A9279	Monitoring Feature/ Device	DME MAC
A9280	Alarm Device	DME MAC
A9281	Reaching/Grabbing Device	DME MAC
A9282	Wig	DME MAC
A9283	Foot Off Loading Device	DME MAC
A9284- A9286	Non-electric Spirometer, Inversion Devices and Hygienic Items	DME MAC
A9300	Exercise Equipment	DME MAC
A9500 - A9700	Supplies for Radiology Procedures	Part B MAC
A9900	Miscellaneous DME Supply or Accessory	Part B MAC if used with implanted DME. If other, DME MAC.
A9901	Delivery	DME MAC
A9999	Miscellaneous DME Supply or Accessory	Part B MAC if used with implanted DME. If other, DME MAC.
B4034 - B9999	Enteral and Parenteral Therapy	DME MAC
D0120 - D9999	Dental Procedures	Part B MAC
E0100 - E0105	Canes	DME MAC
E0110 - E0118	Crutches	DME MAC
E0130 - E0159	Walkers	DME MAC
E0160 - E0175	Commodes	DME MAC
E0181 - E0199	Decubitus Care Equipment	DME MAC
E0200 - E0239	Heat/Cold Applications	DME MAC
E0240 - E0248	Bath and Toilet Aids	DME MAC
E0249	Pad for Heating Unit	DME MAC
E0250 - E0304	Hospital Beds	DME MAC
E0305 - E0326	Hospital Bed Accessories	DME MAC
E0328 - E0329	Pediatric Hospital Beds	DME MAC

HCPCS	DESCRIPTION	JURISDICTION
E0350 - E0352	Electronic Bowel Irrigation System	DME MAC
E0370	Heel Pad	DME MAC
E0371 - E0373	Decubitus Care Equipment	DME MAC
E0424 - E0484	Oxygen and Related Respiratory Equipment	DME MAC
E0485 - E0486	Oral Device to Reduce Airway Collapsibility	DME MAC
E0487	Electric Spirometer	DME MAC
E0500	IPPB Machine	DME MAC
E0550 - E0585	Compressors/Nebulizers	DME MAC
E0600	Suction Pump	DME MAC
E0601	CPAP Device	DME MAC
E0602 - E0604	Breast Pump	DME MAC
E0605	Vaporizer	DME MAC
E0606	Drainage Board	DME MAC
E0607	Home Blood Glucose Monitor	DME MAC
E0610 - E0615	Pacemaker Monitor	DME MAC
E0616	Implantable Cardiac Event Recorder	Part B MAC
E0617	External Defibrillator	DME MAC
E0618 - E0619	Apnea Monitor	DME MAC
E0620	Skin Piercing Device	DME MAC
E0621 - E0636	Patient Lifts	DME MAC
E0637 - E0642	Standing Devices/Lifts	DME MAC
E0650 - E0676	Pneumatic Compressor and Appliances	DME MAC
E0691 - E0694	Ultraviolet Light Therapy Systems	DME MAC
E0700	Safety Equipment	DME MAC
E0705	Transfer Board	DME MAC
E0710	Restraints	DME MAC
E0720 - E0745	Electrical Nerve Stimulators	DME MAC
E0746	EMG Device	Part B MAC
E0747 - E0748	Osteogenic Stimulators	DME MAC
E0749	Implantable Osteogenic Stimulators	Part B MAC
E0755- E0770	Stimulation Devices	DME MAC
E0776	IV Pole	DME MAC
E0779 - E0780	External Infusion Pumps	DME MAC
E0781	Ambulatory Infusion Pump	DME MAC
E0782 - E0783	Infusion Pumps, Implantable	Part B MAC
E0784	Infusion Pumps, Insulin	DME MAC

HCPCS	DESCRIPTION	JURISDICTION
E0785 - E0786	Implantable Infusion Pump Catheter	Part B MAC
E0791	Parenteral Infusion Pump	DME MAC
E0830	Ambulatory Traction Device	DME MAC
E0840 - E0900	Traction Equipment	DME MAC
E0910 - E0930	Trapeze/Fracture Frame	DME MAC
E0935 - E0936	Passive Motion Exercise Device	DME MAC
E0940	Trapeze Equipment	DME MAC
E0941	Traction Equipment	DME MAC
E0942 - E0945	Orthopedic Devices	DME MAC
E0946 - E0948	Fracture Frame	DME MAC
E0950 - E1298	Wheelchairs	DME MAC
E1300 - E1310	Whirlpool Equipment	DME MAC
E1352 - E1392	Additional Oxygen Related Equipment	DME MAC
E1399	Miscellaneous DME	Part B MAC if implanted DME. If other, DME MAC.
E1405 - E1406	Additional Oxygen Equipment	DME MAC
E1500 - E1699	Artificial Kidney Machines and Accessories	DME MAC (not separately payable)
E1700 - E1702	TMJ Device and Supplies	DME MAC
E1800 - E1841	Dynamic Flexion Devices	DME MAC
E1902	Communication Board	DME MAC
E2000	Gastric Suction Pump	DME MAC
E2100 - E2101	Blood Glucose Monitors with Special Features	DME MAC
E2120	Pulse Generator for Tympanic Treatment of Inner Ear	DME MAC
E2201 - E2397	Wheelchair Accessories	DME MAC
E2402	Negative Pressure Wound Therapy Pump	DME MAC
E2500 - E2599	Speech Generating Device	DME MAC
E2601 - E2633	Wheelchair Cushions and Accessories	DME MAC
E8000 - E8002	Gait Trainers	DME MAC
G0008 - G0329	Misc. Professional Services	Part B MAC
G0333	Dispensing Fee	DME MAC
G0337 - G0365	Misc. Professional Services	Part B MAC
G0372	Misc. Professional Services	Part B MAC

HCPCS	DESCRIPTION	JURISDICTION
G0378 - G0490 G0491-G9977	Misc. Professional Services	Part B MAC
J0120 - J3570	Injection	Part B MAC if incident to a physician's service or used in an implanted infusion pump. If other, DME MAC.
J3590	Unclassified Biologicals	Part B MAC
J7030 - J7131	Miscellaneous Drugs and Solutions	Part B MAC if incident to a physician's service or used in an implanted infusion pump. If other, DME MAC.
J7175-J7179	Clotting Factors	Part B MAC
J7180 - J7195	Antihemophilic Factor	Part B MAC
J7196 - J7197	Antithrombin III	Part B MAC
J7198	Anti-inhibitor; per I.U.	Part B MAC
J7199 - J7211	Other Hemophilia Clotting Factors	Part B MAC
J7296 - J7307	Contraceptives	Part B MAC
J7308 - J7309	Aminolevulinic Acid HCL	Part B MAC
J7310	Ganciclovir, Long-Acting Implant	Part B MAC
J7311 - J7316	Ophthalmic Drugs	Part B MAC
J7320 - J7328	Hyaluronan	Part B MAC
J7330	Autologous Cultured Chondrocytes, Implant	Part B MAC
J7336	Capsaicin	Part B MAC
J7340	Carbidopa/Levodopa	Part B MAC if incident to a physician's service or used in an implanted infusion pump. If other, DME MAC.
J7342 - J7345	Ciprofloxacin otic & Topical Aminolevulinic Acid	Part B MAC
J7500 - J7599	Immunosuppressive Drugs	Part B MAC if incident to a physician's service or used in an implanted infusion pump. If other, DME MAC.
J7604 - J7699	Inhalation Solutions	Part B MAC if incident to a physician's service. If other, DME MAC.
J7799 -J7999	NOC Drugs, Other than Inhalation Drugs	Part B MAC if incident to a physician's service or used in an implanted infusion pump. If other, DME MAC.
J8498	Anti-emetic Drug	DME MAC
J8499	Prescription Drug, Oral, Non Chemotherapeutic	Part B MAC if incident to a physician's service. If other, DME MAC.
J8501 - J8999	Oral Anti-Cancer Drugs	DME MAC
J9000 - J9999	Chemotherapy Drugs	Part B MAC if incident to a physician's service or used in an implanted infusion pump. If other, DME MAC.
K0001 - K0108	Wheelchairs	DME MAC

HCPCS	DESCRIPTION	JURISDICTION
K0195	Elevating Leg Rests	DME MAC
K0455	Infusion Pump used for Uninterrupted Administration of Epoprostenal	DME MAC
K0462	Loaner Equipment	DME MAC
K0552 - K0605	External Infusion Pump Supplies & Continuous Glucose Monitor	DME MAC
K0606 - K0609	Defibrillator Accessories	DME MAC
K0669	Wheelchair Cushion	DME MAC
K0672	Soft Interface for Orthosis	DME MAC
K0730	Inhalation Drug Delivery System	DME MAC
K0733	Power Wheelchair Accessory	DME MAC
K0738	Oxygen Equipment	DME MAC
K0739	Repair or Nonroutine Service for DME	Part B MAC if implanted DME. If other, DME MAC
K0740	Repair or Nonroutine Service for Oxygen Equipment	DME MAC
K0743 - K0746	Suction Pump and Dressings	DME MAC
K0800 - K0899	Power Mobility Devices	DME MAC
K0900	Custom DME, other than Wheelchair	DME MAC
L0112 - L4631	Orthotics	DME MAC
L5000 - L5999	Lower Limb Prosthetics	DME MAC
L6000 - L7499	Upper Limb Prosthetics	DME MAC
L7510 - L7520	Repair of Prosthetic Device	Part B MAC if repair of implanted prosthetic device. If other, DME MAC.
L7600 - L8485	Prosthetics	DME MAC
L8499	Unlisted Procedure for Miscellaneous Prosthetic Services	Part B MAC if implanted prosthetic device. If other, DME MAC.
L8500 - L8501	Artificial Larynx; Tracheostomy Speaking Valve	DME MAC
L8505	Artificial Larynx Accessory	DME MAC
L8507	Voice Prosthesis, Patient Inserted	DME MAC
L8509	Voice Prosthesis, Inserted by a Licensed Health Care Provider	Part B MAC for dates of service on or after 10/01/2010. DME MAC for dates of service prior to 10/01/2010
L8510	Voice Prosthesis	DME MAC
L8511 - L8515	Voice Prosthesis	Part B MAC if used with tracheoesophageal voice prostheses inserted by a licensed health care provider. If other, DME MAC

HCPCS	DESCRIPTION	JURISDICTION
L8600 - L8699	Prosthetic Implants	Part B MAC
L9900	Miscellaneous Orthotic or Prosthetic Component or Accessory	Part B MAC if used with implanted prosthetic device. If other, DME MAC.
M0075 - M0301	Medical Services	Part B MAC
P2028 - P9615	Laboratory Tests	Part B MAC
Q0035	Cardio-kymography	Part B MAC
Q0081	Infusion Therapy	Part B MAC
Q0083 - Q0085	Chemotherapy Administration	Part B MAC
Q0091	Smear Preparation	Part B MAC
Q0092	Portable X-ray Setup	Part B MAC
Q0111 - Q0115	Miscellaneous Lab Services	Part B MAC
Q0138-Q0139	Ferumoxytol Injection	Part B MAC
Q0144	Azithromycin Dihydrate	Part B MAC if incident to a physician's service. If other, DME MAC.
Q0161 - Q0181	Anti-emetic	DME MAC
Q0477 - Q0509	Ventricular Assist Devices	Part B MAC
Q0510 - Q0514	Drug Dispensing Fees	DME MAC
Q0515	Sermorelin Acetate	Part B MAC
Q1004 - Q1005	New Technology IOL	Part B MAC
Q2004	Irrigation Solution	Part B MAC
Q2009	Fosphenytoin	Part B MAC
Q2017	Teniposide	Part B MAC
Q2026-Q2028	Injectable Dermal Fillers	Part B MAC
Q2034 - Q2039	Influenza Vaccine	Part B MAC
Q2040 - Q2043	Cellular Immunotherapy	Part B MAC
Q2049-Q2050	Doxorubicin	Part B MAC if incident to a physician's service or used in an implanted infusion pump. If other, DME MAC.
Q2052	IVIG Demonstration	DME MAC
Q3001	Supplies for Radiology Procedures	Part B MAC
Q3014	Telehealth Originating Site Facility Fee	Part B MAC
Q3027 - Q3028	Vaccines	Part B MAC
Q3031	Collagen Skin Test	Part B MAC
Q4001 - Q4051	Splints and Casts	Part B MAC
Q4074	Inhalation Drug	Part B MAC if incident to a physician's service. If other, DME MAC.
Q4081	Epoetin	Part B MAC
Q4082	Drug Subject to Competitive Acquisition Program	Part B MAC
Q4100 - Q4182	Skin Substitutes	Part B MAC

HCPCS	DESCRIPTION	JURISDICTION
Q5001 - Q5010	Hospice Services	Part B MAC
Q5101-Q5102	Injection	Part B MAC if incident to a physician's service or used in an implanted infusion pump. If other, DME MAC.
Q9950 - Q9954	Imaging Agents	Part B MAC
Q9955 - Q9957	Microspheres	Part B MAC
Q9958 - Q9969	Imaging Agents	Part B MAC
Q9982-Q9983	Supplies for Radiology Procedures	Part B MAC
R0070 - R0076	Diagnostic Radiology Services	Part B MAC
V2020 - V2025	Frames	DME MAC
V2100 - V2513	Lenses	DME MAC
V2520 - V2523	Hydrophilic Contact Lenses	Part B MAC if incident to a physician's service. If other, DME MAC.
V2530 - V2531	Contact Lenses, Scleral	DME MAC
V2599	Contact Lens, Other Type	Part B MAC if incident to a physician's service. If other, DME MAC.
V2600 - V2615	Low Vision Aids	DME MAC

HCPCS	DESCRIPTION	JURISDICTION
V2623 - V2629	Prosthetic Eyes	DME MAC
V2630 - V2632	Intraocular Lenses	Part B MAC
V2700 - V2780	Miscellaneous Vision Service	DME MAC
V2781	Progressive Lens	DME MAC
V2782 - V2784	Lenses	DME MAC
V2785	Processing—Corneal Tissue	Part B MAC
V2786	Lens	DME MAC
V2787 - V2788	Intraocular Lenses	Part B MAC
V2790	Amniotic Membrane	Part B MAC
V2797	Vision Supply	DME MAC
V2799	Miscellaneous Vision Service	DME MAC
V5008 - V5299	Hearing Services	Part B MAC
V5336	Repair/Modification of Augmentative Communicative System or Device	DME MAC
V5362 - V5364	Speech Screening	Part B MAC

APPENDIX B

GENERAL CORRECT CODING POLICIES FOR NATIONAL CORRECT CODING INITIATIVE POLICY MANUAL FOR MEDICARE SERVICES

Chapter I

Revision Date 1/1/2018

GENERAL CORRECT CODING POLICIES

A. Introduction

Healthcare providers utilize HCPCS/CPT codes to report medical services performed on patients to Medicare Carriers (A/B MACs processing practitioner service claims) and Fiscal Intermediaries (FIs). HCPCS (Healthcare Common Procedure Coding System) consists of Level I CPT (Current Procedural Terminology) codes and Level II codes. CPT codes are defined in the American Medical Association's (AMA) *CPT Manual* which is updated and published annually. HCPCS Level II codes are defined by the Centers for Medicare & Medicaid Services (CMS) and are updated throughout the year as necessary. Changes in CPT codes are approved by the AMA CPT Editorial Panel which meets three times per year.

CPT and HCPCS Level II codes define medical and surgical procedures performed on patients. Some procedure codes are very specific defining a single service (e.g., CPT code 93000 (electrocardiogram)) while other codes define procedures consisting of many services (e.g., CPT code 58263 (vaginal hysterectomy with removal of tube(s) and ovary(s) and repair of enterocele)). Because many procedures can be performed by different approaches, different methods, or in combination with other procedures, there are often multiple HCPCS/CPT codes defining similar or related procedures.

CPT and HCPCS Level II code descriptors usually do not define all services included in a procedure. There are often services inherent in a procedure or group of procedures. For example, anesthesia services include certain preparation and monitoring services.

The CMS developed the NCCI to prevent inappropriate payment of services that should not be reported together. Prior to April 1, 2012, NCCI PTP edits were placed into either the "Column One/Column Two Correct Coding Edit Table" or the "Mutually Exclusive Edit Table." However, on April 1, 2012, the edits in the "Mutually Exclusive Edit Table" were moved to the "Column One/Column Two Correct Coding Edit Table" so that all the NCCI PTP edits are currently contained in this single table. Combining the two tables simplifies researching NCCI edits and online use of NCCI tables. Each edit table contains edits which are pairs of HCPCS/CPT codes that in general should not be reported together. Each edit has a column one and column two HCPCS/CPT code. If a provider reports the two codes of an edit pair, the column two code is denied, and the column one code is eligible for payment. However, if it is clinically appropriate to utilize an NCCI-associated modifier, both the column one and column two codes are eligible for payment. (NCCI-associated modifiers and their appropriate use are discussed elsewhere in this chapter.)

When the NCCI was first established and during its early years, the "Column One/Column Two Correct Coding Edit Table" was termed the "Comprehensive/Component Edit Table." This latter terminology was a misnomer. Although the column two code is often a component of a more comprehensive column one code, this relationship is not true for many edits. In the latter type of edit the code pair edit simply represents two codes that should not be reported together. For example, a provider *shall* not report a vaginal hysterectomy code and total abdominal hysterectomy code together.

In this chapter, Sections B–Q address various issues relating to NCCI PTP edits.

Medically Unlikely Edits (MUEs) prevent payment for an inappropriate number/quantity of the same service on a single day. An MUE for a HCPCS/CPT code is the maximum number of units of service (UOS) under most circumstances reportable by the same provider for the same beneficiary on the same date of service. The ideal MUE value for a HCPCS/CPT code is one that allows the vast majority of appropriately coded claims to pass the MUE. More information concerning MUEs is discussed in Section V of this chapter.

In this Manual many policies are described utilizing the term "physician." Unless indicated differently the usage of this term does not restrict the policies to physicians only but applies to all practitioners, hospitals, providers, or suppliers eligible to bill the relevant HCPCS/CPT codes pursuant to applicable portions of the Social Security Act (SSA) of 1965, the Code of Federal Regulations (CFR), and Medicare rules. In some sections of this Manual, the term "physician" would not include some of these entities because specific rules do not apply to them. For example, Anesthesia Rules [e.g., CMS Internet-only Manual, Publication 100-04 (Medicare Claims Processing Manual), Chapter 12 (Physician/Nonphysician Practitioners), Section 50(Payment for Anesthesiology Services)] and Global Surgery Rules [e.g., CMS Internet-only Manual, Publication 100-04 (Medicare Claims Processing Manual), Chapter 12 (Physician/Nonphysician Practitioners), Section 40 (Surgeons and Global Surgery)] do not apply to hospitals.

Providers reporting services under Medicare's hospital outpatient prospective payment system (OPPS) *shall* report all services in accordance with appropriate Medicare Internet-only Manual (IOM) instructions.

Physicians must report services correctly. This manual discusses general coding principles in Chapter I and principles more relevant to other specific groups of HCPCS/CPT codes in the other chapters. There are certain types of improper coding that physicians must avoid.

Procedures *shall* be reported with the most comprehensive CPT code that describes the services performed. Physicians must not unbundle the services described by a HCPCS/CPT code. Some examples follow:

- A physician *shall* not report multiple HCPCS/CPT codes when a single comprehensive HCPCS/CPT code describes these services. For example if a physician performs a vaginal hysterectomy on a uterus weighing less than 250 grams with bilateral salpingo-oophorectomy, the physician *shall* report CPT code 58262 (Vaginal hysterectomy, for uterus 250 g or less; with removal of tube(s), and/or ovary(s)). The physician *shall* not report CPT code 58260 (Vaginal hysterectomy, for uterus 250 g or less;) plus CPT code 58720 (Salpingo-oophorectomy, complete or partial, unilateral or bilateral (separate procedure)).
- A physician *shall* not fragment a procedure into component parts. For example, if a physician performs an anal endoscopy with biopsy, the physician *shall* report CPT code 46606 (Anoscopy; with biopsy, single or multiple). It is improper to unbundle this procedure and report CPT code 46600(Anoscopy; diagnostic,...) plus CPT code 45100 (Biopsy of anorectal wall, anal approach...). The latter code is not intended to be utilized with an endoscopic procedure code.
- A physician *shall* not unbundle a bilateral procedure code into two unilateral procedure codes. For example if a physician performs bilateral mammography, the physician *shall* report CPT code 77066 (Diagnostic mammography . . . bilateral). The physician *shall* not report CPT code 77065 (Diagnostic mammography . . . unilateral) with two units of service or 77065LT plus 77065RT.
- A physician *shall* not unbundle services that are integral to a more comprehensive procedure. For example, surgical access is integral to a surgical procedure. A physician *shall* not report CPT code 49000 (Exploratory laparotomy,...) when performing an open abdominal procedure such as a total abdominal colectomy (e.g., CPT code 44150).

Physicians must avoid downcoding. If a HCPCS/CPT code exists that describes the services performed, the physician must report this code rather than report a less comprehensive code with other codes describing the services not included in the less comprehensive code. For example if a physician performs a unilateral partial mastectomy with axillary lymphadenectomy, the provider *shall* report CPT code 19302 (Mastectomy, partial...; with axillary lymphadenectomy). A physician *shall* not report CPT code 19301 (Mastectomy, partial...) plus CPT code 38745 (Axillary lymphadenectomy; complete).

Physicians must avoid upcoding. A HCPCS/CPT code may be reported only if all services described by that code have been performed. For example, if a physician performs a superficial axillary lymphadenectomy (CPT code 38740), the physician *shall* not report CPT code 38745 (Axillary lymphadenectomy; complete).

Physicians must report units of service correctly. Each HCPCS/CPT code has a defined unit of service for reporting purposes. A physician *shall* not report units of service for a HCPCS/CPT code using a criterion that differs from the code's defined unit of service. For example, some therapy codes are reported in fifteen minute increments (e.g., CPT codes 97110-97124). Others are reported per session (e.g., CPT codes 92507, 92508). A physician *shall* not report a "per session" code using fifteen minute increments. CPT code 92507 or 92508 should be reported with one unit of service on a single date of service.

MUE and NCCI PTP edits are based on services provided by the same physician to the same beneficiary on the same date of service. Physicians *shall* not inconvenience beneficiaries nor increase risks to beneficiaries by performing services on different dates of service to avoid MUE or NCCI PTP edits.

In 2010 the *CPT Manual* modified the numbering of codes so that the sequence of codes as they appear in the *CPT Manual* does not necessarily correspond to a sequential numbering of codes. In the *National Correct Coding Initiative Policy Manual for Medicare Services,* use of a numerical range of codes reflects all codes that numerically fall within the range regardless of their sequential order in the *CPT Manual*.

This chapter addresses general coding principles, issues, and policies. Many of these principles, issues, and policies are addressed further in subsequent chapters dealing with specific groups of HCPCS/CPT codes. In this chapter examples are often utilized to clarify principles, issues, or policies. The examples do not represent the only codes to which the principles, issues, or policies apply.

B. Coding Based on Standards of Medical/ Surgical Practice

Most HCPCS/CPT code defined procedures include services that are integral to them. Some of these integral services have specific CPT codes for reporting the service when not performed as an integral part of another procedure. (For example, CPT code 36000 (introduction of needle or intracatheter into a vein) is integral to all nuclear medicine procedures requiring injection of a radiopharmaceutical into a vein. CPT code 36000 is not separately reportable with these types of nuclear medicine procedures. However, CPT code 36000 may be reported alone if the only service provided is the introduction of a needle into a vein. Other integral services do not have specific CPT codes. (For example, wound irrigation is integral to the treatment of all wounds and does not have a HCPCS/CPT code.) Services integral to HCPCS/CPT code defined procedures are included in those procedures based on the standards of medical/surgical practice. It is inappropriate to separately report services that are integral to another procedure with that procedure.

Many NCCI PTP edits are based on the standards of medical/surgical practice. Services that are integral to another service are component parts of the more comprehensive service. When integral component services have their own HCPCS/CPT codes, NCCI PTP edits place the comprehensive service in column one and the component service in column two. Since a component service integral to a comprehensive service is not separately reportable, the column two code is not separately reportable with the column one code.

Some services are integral to large numbers of procedures. Other services are integral to a more limited number of procedures. Examples of services integral to a large number of procedures include:

- Cleansing, shaving and prepping of skin
- Draping and positioning of patient
- Insertion of intravenous access for medication administration

- Insertion of urinary catheter
- Sedative administration by the physician performing a procedure (see Chapter II, Anesthesia Services)
- Local, topical or regional anesthesia administered by the physician performing the procedure
- Surgical approach including identification of anatomical landmarks, incision, evaluation of the surgical field, debridement of traumatized tissue, lysis of adhesions, and isolation of structures limiting access to the surgical field such as bone, blood vessels, nerve, and muscles including stimulation for identification or monitoring
- Surgical cultures
- Wound irrigation
- Insertion and removal of drains, suction devices, and pumps into same site
- Surgical closure and dressings
- Application, management, and removal of postoperative dressings and analgesic devices (peri-incisional)
- Application of TENS unit
- Institution of Patient Controlled Anesthesia
- Preoperative, intraoperative and postoperative documentation, including photographs, drawings, dictation, or transcription as necessary to document the services provided
- Surgical supplies, except for specific situations where CMS policy permits separate payment

Although other chapters in this Manual further address issues related to the standards of medical/surgical practice for the procedures covered by that chapter, it is not possible because of space limitations to discuss all NCCI PTP edits based on the principle of the standards of medical/surgical practice. However, there are several general principles that can be applied to the edits as follows:

1. The component service is an accepted standard of care when performing the comprehensive service.
2. The component service is usually necessary to complete the comprehensive service.
3. The component service is not a separately distinguishable procedure when performed with the comprehensive service.

Specific examples of services that are not separately reportable because they are components of more comprehensive services follow:

Medical:

1. Since interpretation of cardiac rhythm is an integral component of the interpretation of an electrocardiogram, a rhythm strip is not separately reportable.
2. Since determination of ankle/brachial indices requires both upper and lower extremity Doppler studies, an upper extremity Doppler study is not separately reportable.
3. Since a cardiac stress test includes multiple electrocardiograms, an electrocardiogram is not separately reportable.

Surgical:

1. Since a myringotomy requires access to the tympanic membrane through the external auditory canal, removal of impacted cerumen from the external auditory canal is not separately reportable.
2. A "scout" bronchoscopy to assess the surgical field, anatomic landmarks, extent of disease, etc., is not separately reportable with an open pulmonary procedure such as a pulmonary lobectomy. By contrast, an initial diagnostic bronchoscopy is separately reportable. If the diagnostic bronchoscopy is performed at the same patient encounter as the open pulmonary procedure and does not duplicate an earlier diagnostic bronchoscopy by the same or another physician, the diagnostic bronchoscopy may be reported with modifier –58 appended to the open pulmonary procedure code to indicate a staged procedure. A cursory examination of the upper airway during a bronchoscopy with the bronchoscope *shall* not be reported separately as a laryngoscopy. However, separate endoscopies of anatomically distinct areas with different endoscopes may be reported separately (e.g., thoracoscopy and mediastinoscopy).
3. If an endoscopic procedure is performed at the same patient encounter as a non-endoscopic procedure to ensure no intraoperative injury occurred or verify the procedure was performed correctly, the endoscopic procedure is not separately reportable with the non-endoscopic procedure.
4. Since a colectomy requires exposure of the colon, the laparotomy and adhesiolysis to expose the colon are not separately reportable.

C. Medical/Surgical Package

Most medical and surgical procedures include pre-procedure, intra-procedure, and post-procedure work. When multiple procedures are performed at the same patient encounter, there is often overlap of the pre-procedure and post-procedure work. Payment methodologies for surgical procedures account for the overlap of the pre-procedure and post-procedure work.

The component elements of the pre-procedure and post-procedure work for each procedure are included component services of that procedure as a standard of medical/surgical practice. Some general guidelines follow:

1. Many invasive procedures require vascular and/or airway access. The work associated with obtaining the required access is included in the pre-procedure or intra-procedure work. The work associated with returning a patient to the appropriate post-procedure state is included in the post-procedure work.

Airway access is necessary for general anesthesia and is not separately reportable. There is no CPT code for elective endotracheal intubation. CPT code 31500 describes an emergency endotracheal intubation and *shall* not be reported for elective endotracheal intubation. Visualization of the airway is a component part of an endotracheal intubation, and CPT codes describing procedures that visualize the airway (e.g., nasal endoscopy, laryngoscopy, bronchoscopy) *shall* not be reported with an endotracheal intubation. These CPT codes describe diagnostic and therapeutic endoscopies, and it is a misuse of these codes to report visualization of the airway for endotracheal intubation.

Intravenous access (e.g., CPT codes 36000, 36400, 36410) is not separately reportable when performed with many types of procedures (e.g., surgical procedures, anesthesia procedures, radiological procedures requiring intravenous contrast, nuclear medicine procedures requiring intravenous radiopharmaceutical).

After vascular access is achieved, the access must be maintained by a slow infusion (e.g., saline) or injection of heparin or saline into a "lock". Since these services are necessary for maintenance of the vascular access, they are not separately reportable with the vascular access CPT codes or procedures requiring vascular access as a standard of medical/surgical practice. CPT codes 37211-37214 (Transcatheter therapy with infusion for thrombolysis) *shall* not be reported for use of an anticoagulant to maintain vascular access.

The global surgical package includes the administration of fluids and drugs during the operative procedure. CPT codes 96360-96377 *shall* not be reported separately *for that operative procedure*. Under OPPS, the administration of fluids and drugs during or for an operative procedure are included services and are not separately reportable (e.g., CPT codes 96360-96377).

When a procedure requires more invasive vascular access services (e.g., central venous access, pulmonary artery access), the more invasive vascular service is separately reportable if it is not typical of the procedure and the work of the more invasive vascular service has not been included in the valuation of the procedure.

Insertion of a central venous access device (e.g., central venous catheter, pulmonary artery catheter) requires passage of a catheter through central venous vessels and, in the case of a pulmonary artery catheter, through the right atrium and ventricle. These services often require the use of fluoroscopic guidance. Separate reporting of CPT codes for right heart catheterization, selective venous catheterization, or pulmonary artery catheterization is not appropriate when reporting a CPT code for insertion of a central venous access device. Since CPT code 77001 describes fluoroscopic guidance for central venous access device procedures, CPT codes for more general fluoroscopy (e.g., 76000, 76001, 77002) *shall* not be reported separately.

2. Medicare Anesthesia Rules prevent separate payment for anesthesia services by the same physician performing a surgical or medical procedure. The physician performing a surgical or medical procedure *shall* not report CPT codes 96360-96377 for the administration of anesthetic agents during the procedure. If it is medically reasonable and necessary that a separate provider (anesthesia practitioner) perform anesthesia services (e.g., monitored anesthesia care) for a surgical or medical procedure, a separate anesthesia service may be reported by the second provider.

Under OPPS, anesthesia for a surgical procedure is an included service and is not separately reportable. For example, a provider *shall* not report CPT codes 96360-96377 for anesthesia services.

When anesthesia services are not separately reportable, physicians and facilities *shall* not unbundle components of anesthesia and report them in lieu of an anesthesia code.

3. If an endoscopic procedure is performed at the same patient encounter as a non-endoscopic procedure to ensure no intraoperative injury occurred or verify the procedure was performed correctly, the endoscopic procedure is not separately reportable with the non-endoscopic procedure.
4. Many procedures require cardiopulmonary monitoring either by the physician performing the procedure or an anesthesia practitioner. Since these services are integral to the procedure, they are not separately reportable. Examples of these services include cardiac monitoring, pulse oximetry, and ventilation management (e.g., 93000-93010, 93040-93042, 94760, 94761, 94770).
5. A biopsy performed at the time of another more extensive procedure (e.g., excision, destruction, removal) is separately reportable under specific circumstances.

If the biopsy is performed on a separate lesion, it is separately reportable. This situation may be reported with anatomic modifiers or modifier -59.

If the biopsy is performed on the same lesion on which a more extensive procedure is performed, it is separately reportable only if the biopsy is utilized for immediate pathologic diagnosis prior to the more extensive procedure, and the decision to proceed with the more extensive procedure is based on the diagnosis established by the pathologic examination. The biopsy is not separately reportable if the pathologic examination at the time of surgery is for the purpose of assessing margins of resection or verifying resectability. When separately reportable modifier -58 may be reported to indicate that the biopsy and the more extensive procedure were planned or staged procedures.

If a biopsy is performed and submitted for pathologic evaluation that will be completed after the more extensive procedure is performed, the biopsy is not separately reportable with the more extensive procedure.

If a single lesion is biopsied multiple times, only one biopsy code may be reported with a single unit of service. If multiple lesions are non-endoscopically biopsied, a biopsy code may be reported for each lesion appending a modifier indicating that each biopsy was performed on a separate lesion. For endoscopic biopsies, multiple biopsies of a single or multiple lesions are reported with one unit of service of the biopsy code. If it is medically reasonable and necessary to submit multiple biopsies of the same or different lesions for separate pathologic examination, the medical record must identify the precise location and separate nature of each biopsy.

6. Exposure and exploration of the surgical field is integral to an operative procedure and is not separately reportable. For example, an exploratory laparotomy (CPT code 49000) is not separately reportable with an intra-abdominal procedure. If exploration of the surgical field results in additional procedures other than the primary procedure, the additional procedures may generally be reported separately. However, a procedure designated by the CPT code descriptor as a "separate procedure" is not separately reportable if performed in a region anatomically related to the other procedure(s) through the same skin incision, orifice, or surgical approach.
7. If a definitive surgical procedure requires access through diseased tissue (e.g., necrotic skin, abscess, hematoma, seroma), a separate service for this access (e.g., debridement, incision and drainage) is not separately reportable. Types of procedures to which this principle applies include, but are not limited to, -ectomy, -otomy, excision, resection, -plasty, insertion, revision, replacement, relocation, removal or closure. For example, debridement of skin and subcutaneous tissue at the site of an abdominal incision made to perform an intra-abdominal procedure is not separately reportable. (See Chapter IV, Section H (General Policy Statements), *Subsection* #11 for guidance on reporting debridement with open fractures and dislocations.)
8. If removal, destruction, or other form of elimination of a lesion requires coincidental elimination of other pathology, only the primary procedure may be reported. For example, if an area of pilonidal disease contains an abscess, incision and drainage of the abscess during the procedure to excise the area of pilonidal disease is not separately reportable.
9. An excision and removal (–ectomy) includes the incision and opening (–otomy) of the organ. A HCPCS/CPT code for an –otomy procedure *shall* not be reported with an –ectomy code for the same organ.
10. Multiple approaches to the same procedure are mutually exclusive of one another and *shall* not be reported separately.

For example, both a vaginal hysterectomy and abdominal hysterectomy should not be reported separately.

11. If a procedure utilizing one approach fails and is converted to a procedure utilizing a different approach, only the completed procedure may be reported. For example, if a laparoscopic hysterectomy is converted to an open hysterectomy, only the open hysterectomy procedure code may be reported.
12. If a laparoscopic procedure fails and is converted to an open procedure, the physician *shall* not report a diagnostic laparoscopy in lieu of the failed laparoscopic procedure. For example, if a laparoscopic cholecystectomy is converted to an open cholecystectomy, the physician *shall* not report the failed laparoscopic cholecystectomy nor a diagnostic laparoscopy.
13. If a diagnostic endoscopy is the basis for and precedes an open procedure, the diagnostic endoscopy may be reported with modifier -58 appended to the open procedure code. However, the medical record must document the medical reasonableness and necessity for the diagnostic endoscopy. A scout endoscopy to assess anatomic landmarks and extent of disease is not separately reportable with an open procedure. When an endoscopic procedure fails and is converted to another surgical procedure, only the completed surgical procedure may be reported. The endoscopic procedure is not separately reportable with the completed surgical procedure.
14. Treatment of complications of primary surgical procedures is separately reportable with some limitations. The global surgical package for an operative procedure includes all intra-operative services that are normally a usual and necessary part of the procedure. Additionally the global surgical package includes all medical and surgical services required of the surgeon during the postoperative period of the surgery to treat complications that do not require return to the operating room. Thus, treatment of a complication of a primary surgical procedure is not separately reportable (1) if it represents usual and necessary care in the operating room during the procedure or (2) if it occurs postoperatively and does not require return to the operating room. For example, control of hemorrhage is a usual and necessary component of a surgical procedure in the operating room and is not separately reportable. Control of postoperative hemorrhage is also not separately reportable unless the patient must be returned to the operating room for treatment. In the latter case, the control of hemorrhage may be separately reportable with modifier -78.

D. Evaluation and Management (E&M) Services

Medicare Global Surgery Rules define the rules for reporting evaluation and management (E&M) services with procedures covered by these rules. This section summarizes some of the rules.

All procedures on the Medicare Physician Fee Schedule are assigned a Global period of 000, 010, 090, XXX, YYY, ZZZ, or MMM. The global concept does not apply to XXX procedures. The global period for YYY procedures is defined by the Carrier (A/B MAC processing practitioner service claims). All procedures with a global period of ZZZ are related to another procedure, and the applicable global period for the ZZZ code is determined by the related procedure. Procedures with a global period of MMM are maternity procedures.

Since NCCI PTP edits are applied to same day services by the same provider to the same beneficiary, certain Global Surgery Rules are applicable to NCCI. An E&M service is separately reportable on the same date of service as a procedure with a global period of 000, 010, or 090 under limited circumstances.

If a procedure has a global period of 090 days, it is defined as a major surgical procedure. If an E&M is performed on the same date of service as a major surgical procedure for the purpose of deciding whether to perform this surgical procedure, the E&M service is separately reportable with modifier –57. Other preoperative E&M services on the same date of service as a major surgical procedure are included in the global payment for the procedure and are not separately reportable. NCCI does not contain edits based on this rule because Medicare Carriers (A/B MACs processing practitioner service claims) have separate edits.

If a procedure has a global period of 000 or 010 days, it is defined as a minor surgical procedure. In general E&M services on the same date of service as the minor surgical procedure are included in the payment for the procedure. The decision to perform a minor surgical procedure is included in the payment for the minor surgical procedure and *shall* not be reported separately as an E&M service. However, a significant and separately identifiable E&M service unrelated to the decision to perform the minor surgical procedure is separately reportable with modifier -25. The E&M service and minor surgical procedure do not require different diagnoses. If a minor surgical procedure is performed on a new patient, the same rules for reporting E&M services apply. The fact that the patient is "new" to the provider is not sufficient alone to justify reporting an E&M service on the same date of service as a minor surgical procedure. NCCI contains many, but not all, possible edits based on these principles.

Example: If a physician determines that a new patient with head trauma requires sutures, confirms the allergy and immunization status, obtains informed consent, and performs the repair, an E&M service is not separately reportable. However, if the physician also performs a medically reasonable and necessary full neurological examination, an E&M service may be separately reportable.

For major and minor surgical procedures, postoperative E&M services related to recovery from the surgical procedure during the postoperative period are included in the global surgical package as are E&M services related to complications of the surgery. Postoperative visits unrelated to the diagnosis for which the surgical procedure was performed unless related to a complication of surgery may be reported separately on the same day as a surgical procedure with modifier 24 ("Unrelated Evaluation and Management Service by the Same Physician or Other Qualified Health Care Professional During a Postoperative Period").

Procedures with a global surgery indicator of "XXX" are not covered by these rules. Many of these "XXX" procedures are performed by physicians and have inherent pre-procedure, intra-procedure, and post-procedure work usually performed each time the procedure is completed. This work *shall not* be reported as a separate E&M code. Other "XXX" procedures are not usually performed by a physician and have no physician work relative value units associated with them. A physician *shall not* report a separate E&M code with these procedures for the supervision of others performing the procedure or for the interpretation of the procedure. With most "XXX" procedures, the physician may, however, perform a significant and separately identifiable E&M service on the same date of service which may be reported by appending modifier -25 to the E&M code. This E&M service may be related to the same diagnosis necessitating performance of the "XXX" procedure but cannot include any work inherent in the "XXX" procedure, supervision of others performing the "XXX" procedure, or time for interpreting the result of the "XXX" procedure. Appending modifier -25 to a significant, separately identifiable E&M service when performed on the same date of service as an "XXX" procedure is correct coding.

E. Modifiers and Modifier Indicators

1. The AMA *CPT Manual* and CMS define modifiers that may be appended to HCPCS/CPT codes to provide additional information about the services rendered. Modifiers consist of two alphanumeric characters.

Modifiers may be appended to HCPCS/CPT codes only if the clinical circumstances justify the use of the modifier. A modifier *shall* not be appended to a HCPCS/CPT code solely to bypass an NCCI PTP edit if the clinical circumstances do not justify its use. If the Medicare program imposes restrictions on the use of a modifier, the modifier may only be used to bypass an NCCI PTP edit if the Medicare restrictions are fulfilled.

Modifiers that may be used under appropriate clinical circumstances to bypass an NCCI edit include:

Anatomic modifiers: E1-E4, FA, F1-F9, TA, T1-T9, LT, RT, LC, LD, RC, LM, RI

Global surgery modifiers: -24, -25, -57, -58, -78, -79

Other modifiers: -27,-59, -91, XE, XS, XP, XU

Modifiers 76 ("repeat procedure or service by same physician") and 77 ("repeat procedure by another physician") are not NCCI-associated modifiers. Use of either of these modifiers does not bypass an NCCI PTP edit.

Each NCCI PTP edit has an assigned modifier indicator. A modifier indicator of "0" indicates that NCCI-associated modifiers cannot be used to bypass the edit. A modifier indicator of "1" indicates that NCCI-associated modifiers may be used to bypass an edit under appropriate circumstances. A modifier indicator of "9" indicates that the edit has been deleted, and the modifier indicator is not relevant.

It is very important that NCCI-associated modifiers only be used when appropriate. In general these circumstances relate to separate patient encounters, separate anatomic sites or separate specimens. (See subsequent discussion of modifiers in this section.) Most edits involving paired organs or structures (e.g., eyes, ears, extremities, lungs, kidneys) have NCCI PTP modifier indicators of "1" because the two codes of the code pair edit may be reported if performed on the contralateral organs or structures. Most of these code pairs should not be reported with NCCI-associated modifiers when performed on the ipsilateral organ or structure unless there is a specific coding rationale to bypass the edit. The existence of the NCCI PTP edit indicates that the two codes generally cannot be reported together unless the two corresponding procedures are performed at two separate patient encounters or two separate anatomic locations. However, if the two corresponding procedures are performed at the same patient encounter and in contiguous structures, NCCI-associated modifiers generally should not be utilized.

The appropriate use of most of these modifiers is straightforward. However, further explanation is provided about modifiers -25, -58, and -59. Although modifier -22 is not a modifier that bypasses an NCCI PTP edit, its use is occasionally relevant to an NCCI PTP edit and is discussed below.

a) **Modifier -22:** Modifier -22 is defined by the *CPT Manual* as "Increased Procedural Services." This modifier *shall* not be reported *unless* the service(s) performed is(are) substantially more extensive than the usual service(s) included in the procedure described by the HCPCS/CPT code reported.

Occasionally a provider may perform two procedures that should not be reported together based on an NCCI PTP edit. If the edit allows use of NCCI-associated modifiers to bypass it and the clinical circumstances justify use of one of these modifiers, both services may be reported with the NCCI-associated modifier. However, if the NCCI PTP edit does not allow use of NCCI-associated modifiers to bypass it and the procedure qualifies as an unusual procedural service, the physician may report the column one HCPCS/CPT code of the NCCI PTP edit with modifier -22. The Carrier (A/B MAC processing practitioner service claims) may then evaluate the unusual procedural service to determine whether additional payment is justified.

For example, CMS limits payment for CPT code 69990 (microsurgical techniques, requiring use of operating microscope . . .) to procedures listed in the Internet-only Manual (IOM) (*Claims Processing Manual,* Publication 100-04, 12-§20.4.5). If a physician reports CPT code 69990 with two other CPT codes and one of the codes is not on this list, an NCCI PTP edit with the code not on the list will prevent payment for CPT code 69990. Claims processing systems do not determine which procedure is linked with CPT code 69990. In situations such as this, the physician may submit his claim to the local carrier (A/B MAC processing practitioner service claims) for readjudication appending modifier 22 to the CPT code. Although the carrier (A/B MAC processing practitioner service claims) cannot override an NCCI PTP edit that does not allow use of NCCI-associated modifiers, the carrier (A/B MAC processing practitioner service claims) has discretion to adjust payment to include use of the operating microscope based on modifier 22.

b) **Modifier -25:** The *CPT Manual* defines modifier -25 as a "significant, separately identifiable evaluation and management service by the same physician or other qualified health care professional on the same day of the procedure or other service." Modifier -25 may be appended to an evaluation and management (E&M) CPT code to indicate that the E&M service is significant and separately identifiable from other services reported on the same date of service. The E&M service may be related to the same or different diagnosis as the other procedure(s).

Modifier -25 may be appended to E&M services reported with minor surgical procedures (global period of 000 or 010 days) or procedures not covered by global surgery rules (global indicator of XXX). Since minor surgical procedures and XXX procedures include pre-procedure, intra-procedure, and post-procedure work inherent in the procedure, the provider *shall* not report an E&M service for this work. Furthermore, Medicare Global

Surgery rules prevent the reporting of a separate E&M service for the work associated with the decision to perform a minor surgical procedure whether the patient is a new or established patient.

c) **Modifier -58:** Modifier -58 is defined by the *CPT Manual* as a "staged or related procedure or service by the same physician or other qualified health care professional during the postoperative period." It may be used to indicate that a procedure was followed by a second procedure during the post-operative period of the first procedure. This situation may occur because the second procedure was planned prospectively, was more extensive than the first procedure, or was therapy after a diagnostic surgical service. Use of modifier -58 will bypass NCCI PTP edits that allow use of NCCI-associated modifiers.

If a diagnostic endoscopic procedure results in the decision to perform an open procedure, both procedures may be reported with modifier -58 appended to the HCPCS/CPT code for the open procedure. However, if the endoscopic procedure preceding an open procedure is a "scout" procedure to assess anatomic landmarks and/or extent of disease, it is not separately reportable.

Diagnostic endoscopy is never separately reportable with another endoscopic procedure of the same organ(s) when performed at the same patient encounter. Similarly, diagnostic laparoscopy is never separately reportable with a surgical laparoscopic procedure of the same body cavity when performed at the same patient encounter.

If a planned laparoscopic procedure fails and is converted to an open procedure, only the open procedure may be reported. The failed laparoscopic procedure is not separately reportable. The NCCI contains many, but not all, edits bundling laparoscopic procedures into open procedures. Since the number of possible code combinations bundling a laparoscopic procedure into an open procedure is much greater than the number of such edits in NCCI, the principle stated in this paragraph is applicable regardless of whether the selected code pair combination is included in the NCCI tables. A provider *shall* not select laparoscopic and open HCPCS/CPT codes to report because the combination is not included in the NCCI tables.

d) Modifier -59: Modifier -59 is an important NCCI-associated modifier that is often used incorrectly. For the NCCI its primary purpose is to indicate that two or more procedures are performed at different anatomic sites or different patient encounters. One function of NCCI PTP edits is to prevent payment for codes that report overlapping services except in those instances where the services are "separate and distinct." Modifier 59 *shall* only be used if no other modifier more appropriately describes the relationships of the two or more procedure codes. The *CPT Manual* defines modifier -59 as follows:

Modifier -59: Distinct Procedural Service: Under certain circumstances, it may be necessary to indicate that a procedure or service was distinct or independent from other non E/M services performed on the same day. Modifier -59 is used to identify procedures/services other than E/M services that are not normally reported together, but are appropriate under the circumstances. Documentation must support a different session, different procedure or surgery, different site or organ system, separate incision/excision, separate lesion, or separate injury (or area of injury in extensive injuries) not ordinarily encountered or performed on the same day by the same individual. However, when another already established modifier is appropriate, it should be used rather than modifier -59. Only if no more descriptive modifier is available, and the use of modifier -59 best explains the circumstances, should modifier -59 be used. Note: Modifier 59 should not be appended to an E/M service. To report a separate and distinct E/M service with a non-E/M service performed on the same date, see modifier 25.

NCCI PTP edits define when two procedure HCPCS/CPT codes may not be reported together except under special circumstances. If an edit allows use of NCCI-associated modifiers, the two procedure codes may be reported together when the two procedures are performed at different anatomic sites or different patient encounters. Carrier (A/B MAC processing practitioner service claims) processing systems utilize NCCI-associated modifiers to allow payment of both codes of an edit. Modifier -59 and other NCCI-associated modifiers *shall* NOT be used to bypass an NCCI PTP edit unless the proper criteria for use of the modifier are met. Documentation in the medical record must satisfy the criteria required by any NCCI-associated modifier used.

Some examples of the appropriate use of modifier -59 are contained in the individual chapter policies.

One of the common misuses of modifier -59 is related to the portion of the definition of modifier -59 allowing its use to describe "different procedure or surgery." The code descriptors of the two codes of a code pair edit usually represent different procedures or surgeries. The edit indicates that the two procedures/surgeries cannot be reported together if performed at the same anatomic site and same patient encounter. The provider cannot use modifier -59 for such an edit based on the two codes being different procedures/surgeries. However, if the two procedures/surgeries are performed at separate anatomic sites or at separate patient encounters on the same date of service, modifier -59 may be appended to indicate that they are different procedures/surgeries on that date of service.

There are several exceptions to this general principle about misuse of modifier -59 that apply to some code pair edits for procedures performed at the same patient encounter.

(1) When a diagnostic procedure precedes a surgical or non-surgical therapeutic procedure and is the basis on which the decision to perform the surgical or non-surgical therapeutic procedure is made, that diagnostic procedure may be considered to be a separate and distinct procedure as long as (a) it occurs before the therapeutic procedure and is not interspersed with services that are required for the therapeutic intervention; (b) it clearly provides the information needed to decide whether to proceed with the therapeutic procedure; and (c) it does not constitute a service that would have otherwise been required during the therapeutic intervention. If the diagnostic procedure is an inherent component of the surgical or non-surgical therapeutic procedure, it *shall not be reported separately.*

(2) When a diagnostic procedure follows a surgical procedure or non-surgical therapeutic procedure, that diagnostic procedure may be considered to be a separate and distinct procedure as long as (a)it occurs after the completion of the therapeutic procedure and is not interspersed with or otherwise commingled with services that are only required for the therapeutic intervention, and (b) it does not constitute a service that would have otherwise been required during the therapeutic intervention. If the post-procedure diagnostic procedure is an inherent component or otherwise included (or not separately payable) post-procedure service of the surgical procedure or non-surgical therapeutic procedure, it *shall* not be reported separately.

(3) There is an appropriate use for modifier 59 that is applicable only to codes for which the unit of service is a measure of time (e.g., per 15 minutes, per hour). If two separate and distinct timed services are provided in separate and distinct time blocks, modifier 59 may be used to identify the services. The separate and distinct time blocks for the two services may be sequential to one another or split. When the two services are split, the time block for one service may be followed by a time block for the second service followed by another time block for the first service. All Medicare rules for reporting timed services are applicable. For example, the total time is calculated for all related timed services performed. The number of reportable units of service is based on the total time, and these units of service are allocated between the HCPCS/CPT codes for the individual services performed. The physician is not permitted to perform multiple services, each for the minimal reportable time, and report each of these as separate units of service. (e.g., A physician or therapist performs eight minutes of neuromuscular reeducation (CPT code 97112) and eight minutes of therapeutic exercises (CPT code 97110). Since the physician or therapist performed 16 minutes of related timed services, only one unit of service may be reported for one, not each, of these codes.)

Use of modifier -59 to indicate different procedures/surgeries does not require a different diagnosis for each HCPCS/CPT coded procedure/surgery. Additionally, different diagnoses are not adequate criteria for use of modifier -59. The HCPCS/CPT codes remain bundled unless the procedures/surgeries are performed at different anatomic sites or separate patient encounters.

From an NCCI perspective, the definition of different anatomic sites includes different organs, different anatomic regions, or different lesions in the same organ. It does not include treatment of contiguous structures of the same organ. For example, treatment of the nail, nail bed, and adjacent soft tissue constitutes treatment of a single anatomic site. Treatment of posterior segment structures in the ipsilateral eye constitutes treatment of a single anatomic site. Arthroscopic treatment of a shoulder injury in adjoining areas of the ipsilateral shoulder constitutes treatment of a single anatomic site.

If the same procedure is performed at different anatomic sites, it does not necessarily imply that a HCPCS/CPT code may be reported with more than one unit of service (UOS) for the procedure. Determining whether additional UOS may be reported depends in part upon the HCPCS/CPT code descriptor including the definition of the code's unit of service, when present.

Example #1: The column one/column two code edit with column one CPT code 38221 (*Diagnostic* bone marrow biopsy) and column two CPT code 38220 (*Diagnostic* bone marrow, aspiration) includes two distinct procedures when performed at separate anatomic sites *(e.g., contralateral iliac bones)* or separate patient encounters. In these circumstances, it would be acceptable to use modifier -59. However, if both 38221 and 38220 are performed *on* the same *iliac bone* at the same patient encounter which is the usual practice, modifier -59 *shall* NOT be used. Although CMS does not allow separate payment for CPT code 38220 with CPT code 38221 when bone marrow aspiration and biopsy are performed *on* the same *iliac bone* at a single patient encounter, *a physician may report CPT code 38222 Diagnostic* bone marrow; biopsy*(ies) and aspiration(s).*

Example #2: The procedure to procedure edit with column one CPT code 11055 (paring or cutting of benign hyperkeratotic lesion ...) and column two CPT code 11720 (debridement of nail(s) by any method; 1 to 5) may be bypassed with modifier 59 only if the paring/cutting of a benign hyperkeratotic lesion is performed on a different digit (e.g., toe) than one that has nail debridement. Modifier 59 *shall* not be used to bypass the edit if the two procedures are performed on the same digit.

e) Modifiers XE, XS, XP, XU: These modifiers were effective January 1, 2015. These modifiers were developed to provide greater reporting specificity in situations where modifier 59 was previously reported and may be utilized in lieu of modifier 59 whenever possible. (Modifier 59 should only be utilized if no other more specific modifier is appropriate.) Although NCCI will eventually require use of these modifiers rather than modifier 59 with certain edits, physicians may begin using them for claims with dates of service on or after January 1, 2015. The modifiers are defined as follows:

XE – "Separate encounter, A service that is distinct because it occurred during a separate encounter" This modifier *shall* only be used to describe separate encounters on the same date of service.

XS – "Separate Structure, A service that is distinct because it was performed on a separate organ/structure"

XP – "Separate Practitioner, A service that is distinct because it was performed by a different practitioner"

XU – "Unusual Non-Overlapping Service, The use of a service that is distinct because it does not overlap usual components of the main service"

F. Standard Preparation/Monitoring Services for Anesthesia

With few exceptions anesthesia HCPCS/CPT codes do not specify the mode of anesthesia for a particular procedure. Regardless of the mode of anesthesia, preparation and monitoring services are not separately reportable with anesthesia service HCPCS/CPT codes when performed in association with the anesthesia service. However, if the provider of the anesthesia service performs one or more of these services prior to and unrelated to the anticipated anesthesia service or after the patient is released from the anesthesia practitioner's postoperative care, the service may be separately reportable with modifier -59.

G. Anesthesia Service Included in the Surgical Procedure

Under the CMS Anesthesia Rules, with limited exceptions, Medicare does not allow separate payment for anesthesia services performed by the physician who also furnishes the medical or surgical service. In this case, payment for the anesthesia service is included in the payment for the medical or surgical procedure. For example, separate payment is not allowed for the physician's performance of local, regional, or most other anesthesia including nerve blocks if the physician also performs the medical or surgical procedure. However, Medicare allows separate reporting for moderate conscious sedation services (CPT codes 99151-99153) when provided by same physician performing a medical or surgical procedure except for those procedures listed in Appendix G of the *CPT Manual.*

CPT codes describing anesthesia services (00100-01999) or services that are bundled into anesthesia *shall* not be reported in addition to the surgical or medical procedure requiring the anesthesia services if performed by the same physician. Examples of improperly reported services that are bundled into the anesthesia service when anesthesia is provided by the physician performing the medical or surgical procedure include introduction of needle or intracatheter into a vein (CPT code 36000), venipuncture (CPT code 36410), intravenous infusion/injection (CPT codes 96360-96368, 96374-96377) or cardiac assessment (e.g., CPT codes 93000-93010, 93040-93042). However, if these services are not related to the delivery of an anesthetic agent, or are not an inherent component of the procedure or global service, they may be reported separately.

The physician performing a surgical or medical procedure *shall* not report an epidural/subarachnoid injection (CPT codes 62320-62327) or nerve block (CPT codes 64400-64530) for anesthesia for that procedure.

H. HCPCS/CPT Procedure Code Definition

The HCPCS/CPT code descriptors of two codes are often the basis of an NCCI PTP edit. If two HCPCS/CPT codes describe redundant services, they *shall* not be reported separately. Several general principles follow:

1. A family of CPT codes may include a CPT code followed by one or more indented CPT codes. The first CPT code descriptor includes a semicolon. The portion of the descriptor of the first code in the family preceding the semicolon is a common part of the descriptor for each subsequent code of the family. For example,

   CPT code 70120 Radiologic examination, mastoids; less than 3 views per side
   CPT code 70130 Complete, minimum of 3 views per side

The portion of the descriptor preceding the semicolon ("Radiologic examination, mastoids") is common to both CPT codes 70120 and 70130. The difference between the two codes is the portion of the descriptors following the semicolon. Often as in this case, two codes from a family may not be reported separately. A physician cannot report CPT codes 70120 and 70130 for a procedure performed on ipsilateral mastoids at the same patient encounter. It is important to recognize, however, that there are numerous circumstances when it may be appropriate to report more than one code from a family of codes. For example, CPT codes 70120 and 70130 may be reported separately if the two procedures are performed on contralateral mastoids or at two separate patient encounters on the same date of service.

2. If a HCPCS/CPT code is reported, it includes all components of the procedure defined by the descriptor. For example, CPT code 58291 includes a vaginal hysterectomy with "removal of tube(s) and/or ovary(s)." A physician cannot report a salpingo-oophorectomy (CPT code 58720) separately with CPT code 58291.
3. CPT code descriptors often define correct coding relationships where two codes may not be reported separately with one another at the same anatomic site and/or same patient encounter. A few examples follow:
   a) A "partial" procedure is not separately reportable with a "complete" procedure.
   b) A "partial" procedure is not separately reportable with a "total" procedure.
   c) A "unilateral" procedure is not separately reportable with a "bilateral" procedure.
   d) A "single" procedure is not separately reportable with a "multiple" procedure.
   e) A "with" procedure is not separately reportable with a "without" procedure.
   f) An "initial" procedure is not separately reportable with a "subsequent" procedure.

I. *CPT Manual* and CMS Coding Manual Instructions

CMS often publishes coding instructions in its rules, manuals, and notices. Physicians must utilize these instructions when reporting services rendered to Medicare patients.

The *CPT Manual* also includes coding instructions which may be found in the "Introduction", individual chapters, and appendices. In individual chapters the instructions may appear at the beginning of a chapter, at the beginning of a subsection of the chapter, or after specific CPT codes. Physicians should follow *CPT Manual* instructions unless CMS has provided different coding or reporting instructions.

The American Medical Association publishes *CPT Assistant* which contains coding guidelines. CMS does not review nor approve the information in this publication. In the development of NCCI PTP edits, CMS occasionally disagrees with the information in this publication. If a physician utilizes information from *CPT Assistant* to report services rendered to Medicare patients, it is possible that Medicare Carriers (A/B MACs processing practitioner service claims) and Fiscal Intermediaries may utilize different criteria to process claims.

J. CPT "Separate Procedure" Definition

If a CPT code descriptor includes the term "separate procedure", the CPT code may not be reported separately with a related procedure. CMS interprets this designation to prohibit the separate reporting of a "separate procedure" when performed with another procedure in an anatomically related region often through the same skin incision, orifice, or surgical approach.

A CPT code with the "separate procedure" designation may be reported with another procedure if it is performed at a separate patient encounter on the same date of service or at the same patient encounter in an anatomically unrelated area often through a separate skin incision, orifice, or surgical approach. Modifier -59 or a more specific modifier (e.g., anatomic modifier) may be appended to the "separate procedure" CPT code to indicate that it qualifies as a separately reportable service.

K. Family of Codes

The *CPT Manual* often contains a group of codes that describe related procedures that may be performed in various combinations. Some codes describe limited component services, and other codes describe various combinations of component services. Physicians must utilize several principles in selecting the correct code to report:

1. A HCPCS/CPT code may be reported if and only if all services described by the code are performed.

2. The HCPCS/CPT code describing the services performed *shall* be reported. A physician *shall* not report multiple codes corresponding to component services if a single comprehensive code describes the services performed. There are limited exceptions to this rule which are specifically identified in this Manual.
3. HCPCS/CPT code(s) corresponding to component service(s) of other more comprehensive HCPCS/CPT code(s) *shall* not be reported separately with the more comprehensive HCPCS/CPT code(s) that include the component service(s).
4. If the HCPCS/CPT codes do not correctly describe the procedure(s) performed, the physician *shall* report a "not otherwise specified" CPT code rather than a HCPCS/CPT code that most closely describes the procedure(s) performed.

L. More Extensive Procedure

The *CPT Manual* often describes groups of similar codes differing in the complexity of the service. Unless services are performed at separate patient encounters or at separate anatomic sites, the less complex service is included in the more complex service and is not separately reportable. Several examples of this principle follow:

1. If two procedures only differ in that one is described as a "simple" procedure and the other as a "complex" procedure, the "simple" procedure is included in the "complex" procedure and is not separately reportable unless the two procedures are performed at separate patient encounters or at separate anatomic sites.
2. If two procedures only differ in that one is described as a "simple" procedure and the other as a "complicated" procedure, the "simple" procedure is included in the "complicated" procedure and is not separately reportable unless the two procedures are performed at separate patient encounters or at separate anatomic sites.
3. If two procedures only differ in that one is described as a "limited" procedure and the other as a "complete" procedure, the "limited" procedure is included in the "complete" procedure and is not separately reportable unless the two procedures are performed at separate patient encounters or at separate anatomic sites.
4. If two procedures only differ in that one is described as an "intermediate" procedure and the other as a "comprehensive" procedure, the "intermediate" procedure is included in the "comprehensive" procedure and is not separately reportable unless the two procedures are performed at separate patient encounters or at separate anatomic sites.
5. If two procedures only differ in that one is described as a "superficial" procedure and the other as a "deep" procedure, the "superficial" procedure is included in the "deep" procedure and is not separately reportable unless the two procedures are performed at separate patient encounters or at separate anatomic sites.
6. If two procedures only differ in that one is described as an "incomplete" procedure and the other as a "complete" procedure, the "incomplete" procedure is included in the "complete" procedure and is not separately reportable unless the two procedures are performed at separate patient encounters or at separate anatomic sites.
7. If two procedures only differ in that one is described as an "external" procedure and the other as an "internal" procedure, the "external" procedure is included in the "internal" procedure and is not separately reportable unless the two procedures are performed at separate patient encounters or at separate anatomic sites.

M. Sequential Procedure

Some surgical procedures may be performed by different surgical approaches. If an initial surgical approach to a procedure fails and a second surgical approach is utilized at the same patient encounter, only the HCPCS/CPT code corresponding to the second surgical approach may be reported. If there are different HCPCS/CPT codes for the two different surgical approaches, the two procedures are considered "sequential", and only the HCPCS/CPT code corresponding to the second surgical approach may be reported. For example, a physician may begin a cholecystectomy procedure utilizing a laparoscopic approach and have to convert the procedure to an open abdominal approach. Only the CPT code for the open cholecystectomy may be reported. The CPT code for the failed laparoscopic cholecystectomy is not separately reportable.

N. Laboratory Panel

The *CPT Manual* defines organ and disease specific panels of laboratory tests. If a laboratory performs all tests included in one of these panels, the laboratory may report the CPT code for the panel or the CPT codes for the individual tests. If the laboratory repeats one of these component tests as a medically reasonable and necessary service on the same date of service, the CPT code corresponding to the repeat laboratory test may be reported with modifier -91 appended.

O. Misuse of Column Two Code with Column One Code (Misuse of Code Edit Rationale)

CMS manuals and instructions often describe groups of HCPCS/CPT codes that should not be reported together for the Medicare program. Edits based on these instructions are often included as misuse of column two code with column one code.

A HCPCS/CPT code descriptor does not include exhaustive information about the code. Physicians who are not familiar with a HCPCS/CPT code may incorrectly report the code in a context different than intended. The NCCI has identified HCPCS/CPT codes that are incorrectly reported with other HCPCS/CPT codes as a result of the misuse of the column two code with the column one code. If these edits allow use of NCCI-associated modifiers (modifier indicator of "1"), there are limited circumstances when the column two code may be reported on the same date of service as the column one code. Two examples follow:

1. Three or more HCPCS/CPT codes may be reported on the same date of service. Although the column two code is misused if reported as a service associated with the column one code, the column two code may be appropriately reported with a third HCPCS/CPT code reported on the same date of service. For example, CMS limits separate payment for use of the operating microscope for microsurgical techniques (CPT code 69990) to a group of procedures listed in the online *Claims Processing Manual* (Chapter 12, Section

20.4.5 (Allowable Adjustments)). The NCCI has edits with column one codes of surgical procedures not listed in this section of the manual and column two CPT code of 69990. Some of these edits allow use of NCCI-associated modifiers because the two services listed in the edit may be performed at the same patient encounter as a third procedure for which CPT code 69990 is separately reportable.

2. There may be limited circumstances when the column two code is separately reportable with the column one code. For example, the NCCI has an edit with column one CPT code of 80061 (lipid profile) and column two CPT code of 83721 (LDL cholesterol by direct measurement). If the triglyceride level is less than 400 mg/dl, the LDL is a calculated value utilizing the results from the lipid profile for the calculation, and CPT code 83721 is not separately reportable. However, if the triglyceride level is greater than 400 mg/dl, the LDL may be measured directly and may be separately reportable with CPT code 83721 utilizing an NCCI-associated modifier to bypass the edit.

Misuse of code as an edit rationale may be applied to procedure to procedure edits where the column two code is not separately reportable with the column one code based on the nature of the column one coded procedure. This edit rationale may also be applied to code pairs where use of the column two code with the column one code is deemed to be a coding error.

P. Mutually Exclusive Procedures

Many procedure codes cannot be reported together because they are mutually exclusive of each other. Mutually exclusive procedures cannot reasonably be performed at the same anatomic site or same patient encounter. An example of a mutually exclusive situation is the repair of an organ that can be performed by two different methods. Only one method can be chosen to repair the organ. A second example is a service that can be reported as an "initial" service or a "subsequent" service. With the exception of drug administration services, the initial service and subsequent service cannot be reported at the same patient encounter.

Q. Gender-Specific Procedures (formerly Designation of Sex)

The descriptor of some HCPCS/CPT codes includes a gender-specific restriction on the use of the code. HCPCS/CPT codes specific for one gender should not be reported with HCPCS/CPT codes for the opposite gender. For example, CPT code 53210 describes a total urethrectomy including cystostomy in a female, and CPT code 53215 describes the same procedure in a male. Since the patient cannot have both the male and female procedures performed, the two CPT codes cannot be reported together.

R. Add-on Codes

Some codes in the *CPT Manual* are identified as "add-on" codes which describe a service that can only be reported in addition to a primary procedure. *CPT Manual* instructions specify the primary procedure code(s) for most add-on codes. For other add-on codes, the primary procedure code(s) is(are) not specified. When the *CPT Manual* identifies specific primary codes, the add-on code *shall* not be reported as a supplemental service for other HCPCS/CPT codes not listed as a primary code.

Add-on codes permit the reporting of significant supplemental services commonly performed in addition to the primary procedure. By contrast, incidental services that are necessary to accomplish the primary procedure (e.g., lysis of adhesions in the course of an open cholecystectomy) are not separately reportable with an add-on code. Similarly, complications inherent in an invasive procedure occurring during the procedure are not separately reportable. For example, control of bleeding during an invasive procedure is considered part of the procedure and is not separately reportable.

In general, NCCI procedure to procedure edits do not include edits with most add-on codes because edits related to the primary procedure(s) are adequate to prevent inappropriate payment for an add-on coded procedure. (I.e., if an edit prevents payment of the primary procedure code, the add-on code *shall* not be paid.) However, NCCI does include edits for some add-on codes when coding edits related to the primary procedures must be supplemented. Examples include edits with add-on HCPCS/CPT codes 69990 (microsurgical techniques requiring use of operating microscope) and 95940/95941/G0453 (intraoperative neurophysiology testing).

HCPCS/CPT codes that are not designated as add-on codes *shall* not be misused as an add-on code to report a supplemental service. A HCPCS/CPT code may be reported if and only if all services described by the CPT code are performed. A HCPCS/CPT code *shall* not be reported with another service because a portion of the service described by the HCPCS/CPT code was performed with the other procedure. For example: If an ejection fraction is estimated from an echocardiogram study, it would be inappropriate to additionally report CPT code 78472 (cardiac blood pool imaging with ejection fraction) with the echocardiography (CPT code 93307). Although the procedure described by CPT code 78472 includes an ejection fraction, it is measured by gated equilibrium with a radionuclide which is not utilized in echocardiography.

S. Excluded Service

The NCCI does not address issues related to HCPCS/CPT codes describing services that are excluded from Medicare coverage or are not otherwise recognized for payment under the Medicare program.

T. Unlisted Procedure Codes

The *CPT Manual* includes codes to identify services or procedures not described by other HCPCS/CPT codes. These unlisted procedure codes are generally identified as XXX99 or XXXX9 codes and are located at the end of each section or subsection of the manual. If a physician provides a service that is not accurately described by other HCPCS/CPT codes, the service *shall* be reported utilizing an unlisted procedure code. A physician *shall* not report a CPT code for a specific procedure if it does not accurately describe the service performed. It is inappropriate to report the best fit HCPCS/CPT code unless it accurately describes the service performed, and all components of the HCPCS/CPT code were performed. Since unlisted procedure codes may be reported for a very diverse group of services, the NCCI generally does not include edits with these codes.

U. Modified, Deleted, and Added Code Pairs/Edits

Information moved to Introduction chapter, Section (Purpose), Page Intro-5 of this Manual.

V. Medically Unlikely Edits (MUEs)

To lower the Medicare Fee-For-Service Paid Claims Error Rate, CMS has established units of service edits referred to as Medically Unlikely Edit(s) (MUEs).

An MUE for a HCPCS/CPT code is the maximum number of units of service (UOS) under most circumstances allowable by the same provider for the same beneficiary on the same date of service. The ideal MUE value for a HCPCS/CPT code is the unit of service that allows the vast majority of appropriately coded claims to pass the MUE.

All practitioner claims submitted to Carriers (A/B MACs processing practitioner service claims), outpatient facility services claims (Type of Bill 13X, 14X, 85X) submitted to Fiscal Intermediaries (A/B MACs processing facility claims), and supplier claims submitted to Durable Medical Equipment (DME) MACs are tested against MUEs.

Prior to April 1, 2013, each line of a claim was adjudicated separately against the MUE value for the HCPCS/CPT code reported on that claim line. If the units of service on that claim line exceeded the MUE value, the entire claim line was denied.

In the April 1, 2013 version of MUE*s*, CMS began introducing date of service (DOS) MUEs. Over time CMS will convert many, but not all, MUEs to DOS MUEs. Since April 1, 2013, MUEs are adjudicated either as claim line edits or DOS edits. If the MUE is adjudicated as a claim line edit, the units of service (UOS) on each claim line are compared to the MUE value for the HCPCS/CPT code on that claim line. If the UOS exceed the MUE value, all UOS on that claim line are denied. If the MUE is adjudicated as a DOS MUE, all UOS on each claim line for the same date of service for the same HCPCS/CPT code are summed, and the sum is compared to the MUE value. If the summed UOS exceed the MUE value, all UOS for the HCPCS/CPT code for that date of service are denied. Denials due to claim line MUEs or DOS MUEs may be appealed to the local claims processing contractor. DOS MUEs are utilized for HCPCS/CPT codes where it would be extremely unlikely that more UOS than the MUE value would ever be performed on the same date of service for the same patient.

The MUE files on the CMS NCCI website display an "MUE Adjudication Indicator" (MAI) for each HCPCS/CPT code. An MAI of "1" indicates that the edit is a claim line MUE. An MAI of "2" or "3" indicates that the edit is a DOS MUE.

If a HCPCS/CPT code has an MUE that is adjudicated as a claim line edit, appropriate use of CPT modifiers (e.g., -59, -76, -77, -91, anatomic) may be used to the same HCPCS/CPT code on separate lines of a claim. Each line of the claim with that HCPCS/CPT code will be separately adjudicated against the MUE value for that HCPCS/CPT code. Claims processing contractors have rules limiting use of these modifiers with some HCPCS/CPT codes.

MUEs for HCPCS codes with an MAI of "2" are absolute date of service edits. These are "per day edits based on policy". HCPCS codes with an MAI of "2" have been rigorously reviewed and vetted within CMS and obtain this MAI designation because UOS on the same date of service (DOS) in excess of the MUE value would be considered impossible because it was contrary to statute, regulation or subregulatory guidance. This subregulatory guidance includes clear correct coding policy that is binding on both providers and CMS claims processing contractors. Limitations created by anatomical or coding limitations are incorporated in correct coding policy, both in the HIPAA mandated coding descriptors and CMS approved coding guidance as well as specific guidance in CMS and NCCI manuals. For example, it would be contrary to correct coding policy to report more than one unit of service for CPT 94002 "ventilation assist and management . . . initial day" because such usage could not accurately describe two initial days of management occurring on the same date of service as would be required by the code descriptor. As a result, claims processing contractors are instructed that an MAI of "2" denotes a claims processing restriction for which override during processing, reopening, or redetermination would be contrary to CMS policy.

MUEs for HCPCS codes with an MAI of "3" are "per day edits based on clinical benchmarks". MUEs assigned an MAI of "3" are based on criteria (e.g., nature of service, prescribing information) combined with data such that it would be possible but medically highly unlikely that higher values would represent correctly reported medically necessary services. If contractors have evidence (e.g., medical review) that UOS in excess of the MUE value were actually provided, were correctly coded and were medically necessary, the contractor may bypass the MUE for a HCPCS code with an MAI of "3" during claim processing, reopening or redetermination, or in response to effectuation instructions from a reconsideration or higher level appeal.

Both the MAI and MUE value for each HCPCS/CPT code are based on one or more of the following criteria:

(1) Anatomic considerations may limit units of service based on anatomic structures. For example,
   a) The MUE value for an appendectomy is "1" since there is only one appendix.
   b) The MUE for a knee brace is "2" because there are two knees and Medicare policy does not cover back-up equipment.
   c) The MUE value for a lumbar spine procedure reported per lumbar vertebra or per lumbar interspace cannot exceed "5" since there are only five lumbar vertebrae or interspaces.
   d) The MUE value for a procedure reported per lung lobe cannot exceed "5" since there are only five lung lobes (three in right lung and two in left Lung).

(2) CPT code descriptors/CPT coding instructions in the *CPT Manual* may limit units of service. For example,
   a) A procedure described as the "initial 30 minutes" would have an MUE value of 1 because of the use of the term "initial". *A different code may be reported for additional time.*
   b) If a code descriptor uses the plural form of the procedure, it must not be reported with multiple units of service. For example, if the code descriptor states "biopsies", the code is reported with "1" unit of service regardless of the number of biopsies performed.
   c) The MUE value for a procedure with "per day", "per week", or "per month" in its code descriptor is "1" because MUEs are based on number of services per day of service.

d) *The MUE value of a code for a procedure described as "unilateral" is "1" if there is a different code for the procedure described as "bilateral".*

e) *The code descriptors of a family of codes may define different levels of service, each having an MUE of "1".*

For example, CPT codes 78102-78104 describe bone marrow imaging. CPT code 78102 is reported for imaging a "limited area". CPT code 78103 is reported for imaging "multiple areas". CPT code 78104 is reported for imaging the "whole body".

f) *The MUE value for CPT code 86021 (Antibody identification; leukocyte antibodies) is "1" because the code descriptor is plural including testing for any and all leukocyte antibodies. On a single date of service only one specimen from a patient would be tested for leukocyte antibodies.*

(3) Edits based on established CMS policies may limit units of service *(UOS)*. For example,

a) *The MUE value for a surgical or diagnostic procedure may be based on* the bilateral surgery indicator on the Medicare Physician Fee Schedule Database(MPFSDB)

i. *If the bilateral surgery indicator is "0", a bilateral procedure must be reported with "1" UOS. There is no additional payment for the code if reported as a unilateral or bilateral procedure because of anatomy or physiology. Alternatively, the code descriptor may specifically state that the procedure is a unilateral procedure, and there is a separate code for a bilateral procedure.*

ii. *If the bilateral surgery indicator is "1", a bilateral surgical procedure must be reported with "1" UOS and modifier 50 (bilateral modifier). A bilateral diagnostic procedure may be reported with "2" UOS on one claim line, "1" UOS and modifier 50 on one claim line, or "1" UOS with modifier RT on one claim line plus "1" UOS and modifier LT on a second claim line.*

iii. *If the bilateral surgery indicator is "2", a bilateral procedure must be reported with "1" UOS. The procedure is priced as a bilateral procedure because (1) the code descriptor defines the procedure as bilateral; (2) the code descriptor states that the procedure is performed unilaterally or bilaterally; or (3) the procedure is usually performed as a bilateral procedure.*

iv. *If the bilateral surgery indicator is "3", a bilateral surgical procedure must be reported with "1" UOS and modifier 50 (bilateral modifier). A bilateral diagnostic procedure may be reported with "2" UOS on one claim line, "1" UOS and modifier 50 on one claim line, or 1 UOS with modifier RT on one claim line plus "1" UOS and modifier LT on a second claim line.*

b) *The MUE value for a code may be "1" where the code descriptor does not specify a UOS and CMS considers the default UOS to be "per day".*

c) *The MUE value for a code may be "0" because the code is listed as invalid, not covered, bundled, not separately payable, statutorily excluded, not reasonable and necessary, etc. based on*

i. *The Medicare Physician Fee Schedule Database*
ii. *Outpatient Prospective Payment System Addendum B*
iii. *Alpha-Numeric HCPCS Code File*
iv. *DMEPOS Jurisdiction List*
v. *Medicare Internet-Only Manual*

(4) The nature of an analyte may limit units of service and is in general determined by one of three considerations:

a) The nature of the specimen may limit the units of service. *For example, CPT code 81575 describes a creatinine clearance test and has an MUE of "1" because the test requires a 24 hour urine collection.*

b) The physiology, pathophysiology, or clinical application of the analyte is such that a maximum unit of service for a single date of service can be determined. For example, the MUE for *CPT code 82747 (*RBC folic acid*)* is *"1" because the test result would not be expected to change during a single day, and thus it is not necessary to perform the test more than once on a single date of service.*

(5) The nature of a procedure/service may limit units of service and is in general determined by the amount of time required to perform a procedure/service (e.g., overnight sleep studies) or clinical application of a procedure/service (e.g., motion analysis tests).

a) *The MUE for many surgical or medical procedures is "1" because the procedure is rarely, if ever, performed more than one time per day (e.g., colonoscopy, motion analysis tests).*

b) *The MUE value for a procedure is "1" because of the amount of time required to perform the procedure (e.g., overnight sleep study).*

(6) The nature of equipment may limit units of service and is in general determined by the number of items of equipment that would be utilized (e.g., cochlear implant or wheelchair). *For example, the MUE value for a wheelchair code is "1" because only one wheelchair is used at one time and Medicare policy does not cover back-up equipment.*

*(7) Although c*linical judgment considerations and determinations are based on input from numerous physicians and certified coders *are sometimes initially utilized to establish some MUE values, these values are subsequently validated or changed based on submitted and/or paid claims data.*

(8) Prescribing information is based on FDA labeling as well as off-label information published in CMS approved drug compendia. *See below for additional information about how prescribing information is utilized in determining MUE values.*

(9) Submitted *and paid* claims data (100%) from a six month period is utilized to ascertain the distribution pattern of UOS typically *reported* for a given HCPCS/CPT code.

(10) Published policies of the Durable Medical Equipment (DME) Medicare Administrative Contractors (MACs) may limit units of service for some durable medical equipment, prosthetics, orthotics, and supplies (DMEPOS). For example,

a) *The MUE values for many ostomy and urological supply codes, nebulizer codes, and CPAP accessory codes are typically based on a three month supply of items.*

b) *The MUE values for surgical dressings, parenteral and enteral nutrition, immunosuppressive drugs, and oral anti-cancer drugs are typically based on a one month supply.*

c) *The MUE values take into account the requirement for reporting certain codes with date spans.*

d) *The MUE value of a code may be 0 if the item is noncovered, not medically necessary, or not separately payable.*

e) *The MUE value of a code may be 0 if the code is invalid for claim submission to the DME MAC.*

UOS denied based on an MUE may be appealed. Because a denial of services due to an MUE is a coding denial, not a medical necessity denial, the presence of an Advanced Beneficiary Notice of Noncoverage (ABN) shall not shift liability to the beneficiary for UOS denied based on an MUE. If during reopening or redetermination medical records are provided with respect to an MUE denial for an edit with an MAI of "3", contractors *will* review the records to determine if the provider actually furnished units in excess of the MUE, if the codes were used correctly, and whether the services were medically reasonable and necessary. If the units were actually provided but one of the other conditions is not met, a change in denial reason may be warranted (for example, a change from the MUE denial based on incorrect coding to a determination that the item/service is not reasonable and necessary under section 1862(a)(1)). This may also be true for certain edits with an MAI of "1". CMS interprets the notice delivery requirements under §1879 of the Social Security Act (the Act) as applying to situations in which a provider expects the initial claim determination to be a reasonable and necessary denial. Consistent with NCCI guidance, denials resulting from MUEs are not based on any of the statutory provisions that give liability protection to beneficiaries under section 1879 of the Social Security Act. Thus, ABN issuance based on an MUE is NOT appropriate. A provider/ supplier may not issue an ABN in connection with services denied due to an MUE and cannot bill the beneficiary for units of service denied based on an MUE.

HCPCS J code and drug related C and Q code MUEs are based on prescribing information and 100% claims data for a six month period of time. Utilizing the prescribing information the highest total daily dose for each drug was determined. This dose and its corresponding units of service were evaluated against paid and submitted claims data. Some of the guiding principles utilized in developing these edits are as follows:

(1) If the prescribing information defined a maximum daily dose, this value was used to determine the MUE value. For some drugs there is an absolute maximum daily dose. For others there is a maximum "recommended" or "usual" dose. In the latter of the two cases, the daily dose calculation was evaluated against claims data.
(2) If the maximum daily dose calculation is based on actual body weight, a dose based on a weight range of 110-150 kg was evaluated against the claims data. If the maximum daily dose calculation is based on ideal body weight, a dose based on a weight range of 90-110 kg was evaluated against claims data. If the maximum daily dose calculation is based on body surface area (BSA), a dose based on a BSA range of 2.4-3.0 square meters was evaluated against claims data.
(3) For "as needed" (PRN) drugs and drugs where maximum daily dose is based on patient response, prescribing information and claims data were utilized to establish MUE values.
(4) Published off label usage of a drug was considered for the maximum daily dose calculation.
(5) The MUE values for some drug codes are set to 0. The rationale for such values include but are not limited to: discontinued manufacture of drug, non-FDA approved compounded drug, practitioner MUE values for oral anti-neoplastic, oral anti-emetic, and oral immune suppressive drugs which should be billed to the DME MACs, and outpatient hospital MUE values for inhalation drugs which should be billed to the DME MACs, and Practitioner/ASC MUE values for HCPCS C codes describing medications that would not be related to a procedure performed in an ASC.

Non-drug related HCPCS/CPT codes may be assigned an MUE of 0 for a variety of reasons including, but not limited to: outpatient hospital MUE value for surgical procedure only performed as an inpatient procedure, noncovered service, bundled service, or packaged service.

The MUE files on the CMS NCCI website display an "Edit Rationale" for each HCPCS/CPT code. Although an MUE may be based on several rationales, only one is displayed on the website. One of the listed rationales is "Data." This rationale indicates that 100% claims data from a six month period of time was the major factor in determining the MUE value. If a physician appeals an MUE denial for a HCPCS/CPT code where the MUE is based on "Data," the reviewer will usually confirm that (1) the correct code is reported; (2) the correct UOS is utilized; (3) the number of reported UOS were performed; and (4) all UOS were medically reasonable and necessary.

The first MUEs were implemented January 1, 2007. Additional MUEs are added on a quarterly basis on the same schedule as NCCI updates. Prior to implementation proposed MUEs are sent to numerous national healthcare organizations for a sixty day review and comment period.

Many surgical procedures may be performed bilaterally. Instructions in the CMS *Internet-only Manual* (Publication 100-04 *Medicare Claims Processing Manual,* Chapter 12 (Physicians/Nonphysician Practitioners), Section 40.7.B. and Chapter 4 (Part B Hospital (Including Inpatient Hospital Part B and OPPS)), Section 20.6.2 require that bilateral surgical procedures be reported using modifier 50 with one unit of service. If a bilateral surgical procedure is performed at different sites bilaterally, one unit of service may be reported for each site. That is, the HCPCS/CPT code may be reported with modifier 50 and one unit of service for each site at which it was performed bilaterally.

Some A/B MACs allow providers to report repetitive services performed over a range of dates on a single line of a claim with multiple units of service. If a provider reports services in this fashion, the provider should report the "from date" and "to date" on the claim line. Contractors are instructed to divide the units of service reported on the claim line by the number of days in the date span and round to the nearest whole number. This number is compared to the MUE value for the code on the claim line.

Suppliers billing services to the DME MACs typically report some HCPCS codes for supply items for a period exceeding a single day. The DME MACs have billing rules for these codes. For some codes the DME MACs require that the "from date" and "to date" be reported. The MUEs for these codes are based on the maximum number of units of service that may be reported for a single date of service. For other codes the DME MACs permit multiple days' supply items to be reported on a single claim line where the "from date" and "to date" are the same. The DME MACs have rules allowing supply items for a maximum number of days to be reported at one time for each of these types of codes. The MUE values for these codes are based on the maximum number of days that may be reported at one time. As with all MUEs, the MUE value does not represent a utilization guideline. Suppliers *shall* not assume that they may report units of service up to the MUE value on each date of service. Suppliers may only report supply items that are medically reasonable and necessary.

Most MUE values are set so that a provider or supplier would only very occasionally have a claim line denied. If a provider encounters a code with frequent denials due to the MUE, or frequent use of a CPT modifier to bypass the MUE, the provider or supplier should consider the following: (1) Is the HCPCS/CPT code being used correctly? (2) Is the unit of service being counted correctly? (3) Are all reported services medically reasonable and necessary? and (4) Why does the provider's or supplier's practice differ from national patterns? A provider or supplier may choose to discuss these questions with the local Medicare contractor or a national healthcare organization whose members frequently perform the procedure.

Most MUE values are published on the CMS MUE webpage *https://www.cms.gov/Medicare/Coding/NationalCorrectCodInitEd/MUE.html.* However, some MUE values are not published and are confidential. These values *shall* not be published in oral or written form by any party that acquires one or more of them.

MUEs are not utilization edits. Although the MUE value for some codes may represent the commonly reported units of service (e.g., MUE of "1" for appendectomy), the usual units of service for many HCPCS/CPT codes is less than the MUE value. Claims reporting units of service less than the MUE value may be subject to review by claims processing contractors, Program Safeguard Contractors (PSCs), Zoned Program Integrity Contractors (ZPICs), Recovery Audit Contractors (RACs), and Department of Justice (DOJ).

Since MUEs are coding edits rather than medical necessity edits, claims processing contractors may have units of service edits that are more restrictive than MUEs. In such cases, the more restrictive claims processing contractor edit would be applied to the claim. Similarly, if the MUE is more restrictive than a claims processing contractor edit, the more restrictive MUE would apply.

A provider, supplier, healthcare organization, or other interested party may request reconsideration of an MUE value for a HCPCS/CPT code. A written request proposing an alternative MUE with rationale may be sent to:

National Correct Coding Initiative
Correct Coding Solutions, LLC
P.O. Box 907
Carmel, IN 46082-0907
Fax: 317-571-1745

W. Add-on Code Edit Tables

Add-on codes are discussed in Chapter I, Section R (Add-on Codes). CMS publishes a list of add-on codes and their primary codes annually prior to January 1. The list is updated quarterly based on the AMA's "CPT Errata" documents or implementation of new HCPCS/CPT add-on codes. CMS identifies add-on codes and their primary codes based on CPT Manual instructions, CMS interpretation of HCPCS/CPT codes, and CMS coding instructions.

The NCCI program includes three Add-on Code Edit Tables, one table for each of three "Types" of add-on codes. Each table lists the add-on code with its primary codes. An add-on code, with one exception, is eligible for payment if and only if one of its primary codes is also eligible for payment.

The "Type I Add-on Code Edit Table" lists add-on codes for which the CPT Manual or HCPCS tables define all acceptable primary codes. Claims processing contractors should not allow other primary codes with Type I add-on codes. CPT code 99292 (Critical care, evaluation and management of the critically ill or critically injured patient; each additional 30 minutes (List separately in addition to code for primary service)) is included as a Type I add-on code since its only primary code is CPT code 99291 (Critical care, evaluation and management of the critically ill or critically injured patient; first 30-74 minutes). For Medicare purposes, CPT code 99292 may be eligible for payment to a physician without CPT code 99291 if another physician of the same specialty and physician group reports and is paid for CPT code 99291.

The "Type II Add-on Code Edit Table" lists add-on codes for which the CPT Manual and HCPCS tables do not define any primary codes. Claims processing contractors should develop their own lists of acceptable primary codes.

The "Type III Add-on Code Edit Table" lists add-on codes for which the CPT Manual or HCPCS tables define some, but not all, acceptable primary codes. Claims processing contractors should allow the listed primary codes for these add-on codes but may develop their own lists of additional acceptable primary codes.

Although the add-on code and primary code are normally reported for the same date of service, there are unusual circumstances where the two services may be reported for different dates of service (e.g., CPT codes 99291 and 99292).

The first Add-On Code edit tables were implemented April 1, 2013. For subsequent years, new Add-On Code edit tables will be published to be effective for January 1 of the new year based on changes in the new year's CPT Manual. CMS also issues quarterly updates to the Add-On Code edit tables if required due to publication of new HCPCS/CPT codes or changes in add-on codes or their primary codes. The changes in the quarterly update files (April 1, July 1, or October 1) are retroactive to the implementation date of that year's annual Add-On Code edit files unless the files specify a different effective date for a change. Since the first Add-On Code edit files were implemented on April 1, 2013, changes in the July 1 and October 1 quarterly updates for 2013 were retroactive to April 1, 2013 unless the files specified a different effective date for a change.

FIGURE CREDITS

1. From Little J et al: *Dental management of the medically compromised patient,* ed 9, St. Louis, 2017, Mosby. *(Courtesy Medtronic, Minneapolis)*
2. From Franklin I, Dawson P, Rodway A: *Essentials of Clinical Surgery*, ed 2, 2012, Saunders.
3. Modified from Grosfeld J et al: *Pediatric surgery,* ed 7, Philadelphia, 2012, Mosby.
4. Modified from Hsu J, Michael J, Fisk J: *AAOS atlas of orthoses and assistive devices,* ed 4, Philadelphia, 2008, Mosby.
5. From Wold G: *Basic Geriatric Nursing*, ed 5, St. Louis, 2011, Mosby.
6. Modified from Roberts J, Hedges J: *Clinical procedures in emergency medicine,* ed 6, St. Louis, 2013, Saunders.
7. From Auerbach P: *Wilderness medicine,* ed 7, Philadelphia, 2016, Mosby. (Courtesy Black Diamond Equipment, Ltd.)
8. *(Original to book).*
9. Modified from Abeloff M et al: *Clinical oncology,* ed 5, Philadelphia, 2013, Churchill Livingstone.
10. *(Original to book).*
11. Modified from Duthie E, Katz P, Malone M: *Practice of geriatrics,* ed 4, Philadelphia, 2007, Saunders.
12. Modified from Roberts J, Hedges J: *Clinical procedures in emergency medicine,* ed 6, St. Louis, 2013, Saunders.
13. From Young A, Proctor D: *Kinn's the medical assistant,* ed 13, St. Louis, 2016, Saunders.
14. From Bonewit-West K: *Clinical procedures for medical assistants,* ed 9, Philadelphia, 2015, WB Saunders.
15. From Roberts J, Hedges J: *Clinical procedures in emergency medicine,* ed 6, St. Louis, 2013, Saunders.
16. From Yeo: *Shackelford's surgery of the alimentary tract,* ed 7, Philadelphia, 2012, Saunders.
17. Redrawn from Bragg D, Rubin P, Hricak H: *Oncologic imaging,* ed 2, 2002, Saunders.
18. From Roberts J, Hedges J: *Clinical procedures in emergency medicine,* ed 6, St. Louis, 2013, Saunders. *(Courtesy Atrium Medical Corp., Hudson, NH 03051)*
19. **A** From Auerbach P: *Wilderness medicine,* ed 7, Philadelphia, 2016, Mosby. **B** Modified from Hsu J, Michael J, Fisk J: *AAOS atlas of orthoses and assistive devices,* ed 4, Philadelphia, 2008, Mosby.
20. Modified from Lusardi M, Nielsen C: *Orthotics and prosthetics in rehabilitation,* ed 3, St. Louis, 2013, Butterworth-Heinemann.
21. Modified from Lusardi M, Nielsen C: *Orthotics and prosthetics in rehabilitation,* ed 3, St. Louis, 2013, Butterworth-Heinemann.
22. Modified from Lusardi M, Nielsen C: *Orthotics and prosthetics in rehabilitation,* ed 3, St. Louis, 2013, Butterworth-Heinemann.
23. From Buck C: *The Next Step, Advanced Medical Coding 2019/2020 edition,* St. Louis, 2017, Saunders.
24. From Jardins T: *Clinical Manifestations and Assessment of Respiratory Disease,* ed 7, St. Louis, 2015, Elsevier.
25. From Hsu J, Michael J, Fisk J: *AAOS atlas of orthoses and assistive devices,* ed 4, Philadelphia, 2008, Mosby.
26. Modified from Hsu J, Michael J, Fisk J: *AAOS atlas of orthoses and assistive devices,* ed 4, Philadelphia, 2008, Mosby.
27. Modified from Hsu J, Michael J, Fisk J: *AAOS atlas of orthoses and assistive devices,* ed 4, Philadelphia, 2008, Mosby.
28. From Didomenico, Lawrence A., and Nik Gatalyak. "End-Stage Ankle Arthritis." *Clinics in Podiatric Medicine and Surgery* 29.3 (2012): 391-412.
29. Cameron, Michelle H., and Linda G. Monroe. *Physical Rehabilitation for the Physical Therapist Assistant,* ed 1, St. Louis, 2011, Saunders.
30. From Rowe, Dale E., and Avinash L. Jadhav. "Care of the Adolescent with Spina Bifida." *Pediatric Clinics of North America* 55.6 (2008): 1359-374.
31. Modified from Lusardi M, Nielsen C: *Orthotics and prosthetics in rehabilitation,* ed 3, St. Louis, 2013, Butterworth-Heinemann.
32. From Hsu J, Michael J, Fisk J: *AAOS atlas of orthoses and assistive devices,* ed 4, Philadelphia, 2008, Mosby.
33. *(Original to book.)*
34. From Hochberg, Marc C. *Rheumatology,* ed 5, Philadelphia, 2011, Mosby.
35. Modified from Hsu J, Michael J, Fisk J: *AAOS atlas of orthoses and assistive devices,* ed 4, Philadelphia, 2008, Mosby.
36. From Coughlin, Michael J., Roger A. Mann, and Charles L. Saltzman. *Surgery of the Foot and Ankle,* ed 9, Philadelphia, 2013, Mosby.
37. From Canale S: *Campbell's operative orthopaedics,* ed 12, St. Louis, 2012, Mosby.
38. From Sorrentino, Sheila A., and Bernie Gorek. *Mosby's Textbook for Long-term Care Nursing Assistants,* ed 7, St. Louis, 2014, Mosby.
39. From Pedretti, Lorraine Williams, Heidi McHugh. Pendleton, and Winifred Schultz-Krohn. *Pedretti's Occupational Therapy: Practice Skills for Physical Dysfunction,* ed 7, St. Louis, 2013, Elsevier.
40. From Skirven, Terri M. *Rehabilitation of the Hand and Upper Extremity,* ed 6, Philadelphia, 2010, Mosby.
41. From Lusardi M, Nielsen C: *Orthotics and prosthetics in rehabilitation,* ed 3, St. Louis, 2013, Butterworth-Heinemann. *(Courtesy Michael Curtain)*
42. Schickendantz, Mark S. "Diagnosis and Treatment of Elbow Disorders in the Overhead Athlete." *Hand Clinics* 18.1 (2002): 65-75.
43. Modified from Bland K, Copeland E: *The breast: comprehensive management of benign and malignant disorders,* ed 4, St. Louis, 2009, Saunders.
44. From Shah, Jatin P., Snehal G. Patel, Bhuvanesh Singh, and Jatin P. Shah. *Jatin Shah's Head and Neck Surgery and Oncology,* ed 4, Philadelphia, 2012, Mosby, 2012. From Subburaj, K., C. Nair, S. Rajesh, S.m. Meshram, and B. Ravi. "Rapid Development of Auricular Prosthesis Using CAD and Rapid Prototyping Technologies." *International Journal of Oral and Maxillofacial Surgery* 36.10 (2007): 938-43.
45. From Weinzweig J: *Plastic surgery secrets,* ed 2, Philadelphia, 2010, Hanley & Belfus, p 543.
46. Modified from Mann D: *Heart failure: a companion to Braunwald's heart disease,* ed 3, Philadelphia, 2015, Saunders.
47. Modified from Roberts J, Hedges J: *Clinical procedures in emergency medicine,* ed 6, Philadelphia, 2013, Saunders.
48. From Yanoff M, Duker J: *Ophthalmology,* ed 4, St. Louis, 2014, Mosby.
49. From Feldman M, Friedman L, Brandt L: *Sleisenger and Fordtran's gastrointestinal and liver disease,* ed 10, Philadelphia, 2015, Saunders.
50. From Katz V et al: *Comprehensive gynecology,* ed 7, Philadelphia, 2016, Mosby.
51. From Young A, Proctor D: *Kinn's the medical assistant,* ed 13, St. Louis, 2016, Saunders.
52. From Yanoff M, Duker J: *Ophthalmology,* ed 4, St. Louis, 2014, Mosby.

Teacher's Book

A RESOURCE FOR PLANNING AND TEACHING

Level 3.1 Enjoy

Introductory Selection: **Miss Nelson Is Missing!**

Theme 1 **Oink, Oink, Oink**

Theme 2 **Community Ties**

Theme 3 **Disaster!**

Theme 4 **What's Cooking?**

Theme 5 **Weather Watch**

Theme 6 **What a Day!**

Senior Authors
J. David Cooper
John J. Pikulski

Authors
Kathryn H. Au
Margarita Calderón
Jacqueline C. Comas
Marjorie Y. Lipson
J. Sabrina Mims
Susan E. Page
Sheila W. Valencia
MaryEllen Vogt

Consultants
Dolores Malcolm
Tina Saldivar
Shane Templeton

INVITATIONS TO LITERACY

Houghton Mifflin Company • Boston
Atlanta • Dallas • Geneva, Illinois • Palo Alto • Princeton

Literature Reviewers

Librarians: **Consuelo Harris,** Public Library of Cincinnati, Cincinnati, Ohio; **Sarah Jones,** Elko County Library, Elko, Nevada; **Maeve Visser Knoth,** Cambridge Public Library, Cambridge, Massachusetts; **Valerie Lennox,** Highlands Branch Library, Jacksonville, Florida; **Margaret Miles,** Central Library, Sacramento, California; **Danilta Nichols,** Fordham Library, New York, New York; **Patricia O'Malley,** Hartford Public Library, Hartford, Connecticut; **Rob Reid,** L.E. Phillips Memorial Public Library, Eau Claire, Wisconsin; **Mary Calletto Rife,** Kalamazoo Public Library, Kalamazoo, Michigan

Teachers: **Debora Adam,** South Dover Elementary School, Dover, Delaware; **Linda Chick,** Paloma School, San Marcos, California; **Bea Garcia,** Kolfax Elementary School, Denver, Colorado; **Flavia Gordon-Gunther,** Morningside Elementary School, Atlanta, Georgia; **Linda Macy,** Washington Elementary School, Wichita, Kansas; **Paul Warnke,** Onate Elementary School, Albuquerque, New Mexico; **Margaret White,** Hilton Head Elementary School, Hilton Head, South Carolina

Program Reviewers

Debora Adam, South Dover Elementary School, Dover, Delaware; **Sue Bradley,** Ardmore Elementary School, Bellevue, Washington; **Marsha Kiefer,** Truman Elementary School, Rolla, Missouri; **Paul Warnke,** Onate Elementary School, Albuquerque, New Mexico

Be a Writer Feature

Special thanks to the following teachers whose students' compositions are included in the Be a Writer features in this level:

David Burton, Blake Lower School, Hopkins, Minnesota; **Linda Chick,** Paloma Elementary School, San Marcos, California; **Debora Adam,** South Dover Elementary School, Dover, Delaware

Printed in the U.S.A.

ISBN 0-395-74748-1

23456789-WC-99 98 97 96 95

Credits

Photography: Tracy Wheeler Studio, pp. 6A, 34D, 34G, 34H, 60A, 60K, 60L, 60O, 88A, 88N, 114A, 114C, 114H, 114K, 114M, 114N, 117B, 117E, 119A, 119C

Banta Digital Group, pp. 34C, 35B, 60K, 60N, 88C, 88O, 114N, 114O, 117E, 119C

Harry Allard, p. 8A; F. Damm (ZEFA/The Stock Market), p.67D; Francois Gohier (Photo Researchers Inc.), p.88N; Ross Humphreys, p.67A; Don King (The Image Bank), p.114M; Stephen J. Krasemann (DRK Photo), p.67D; Charles Krebs (Tony Stone Images), p.67D; Glenn Kremer, p.34H; Donivee Martin Laird, p.91A; Renee Lynn (Tony Stone Images), p.35F; Roy Morsch (The Stock Market), p.67D; Marc Romanelli (The Image Bank) p.99M; Eugene Trivizas, p.35C; Art Wolfe (Tony Stone Images), p. 60M, 88N

Illustration: James Marshall, Title Page

Acknowledgments

Special thanks to David E. Freeman and Yvonne S. Freeman for their contribution to the development of the instructional support for students acquiring English.

Grateful acknowledgment is made for permission to reprint copyrighted material as follows:

"August," by Sandra Liatsos. Copyright © 1990 by Sandra Liatsos. Reprinted by permission of Marian Reiner for the author.

Launching the Program
with
Miss Nelson Is Missing!

INTRODUCTORY SELECTION

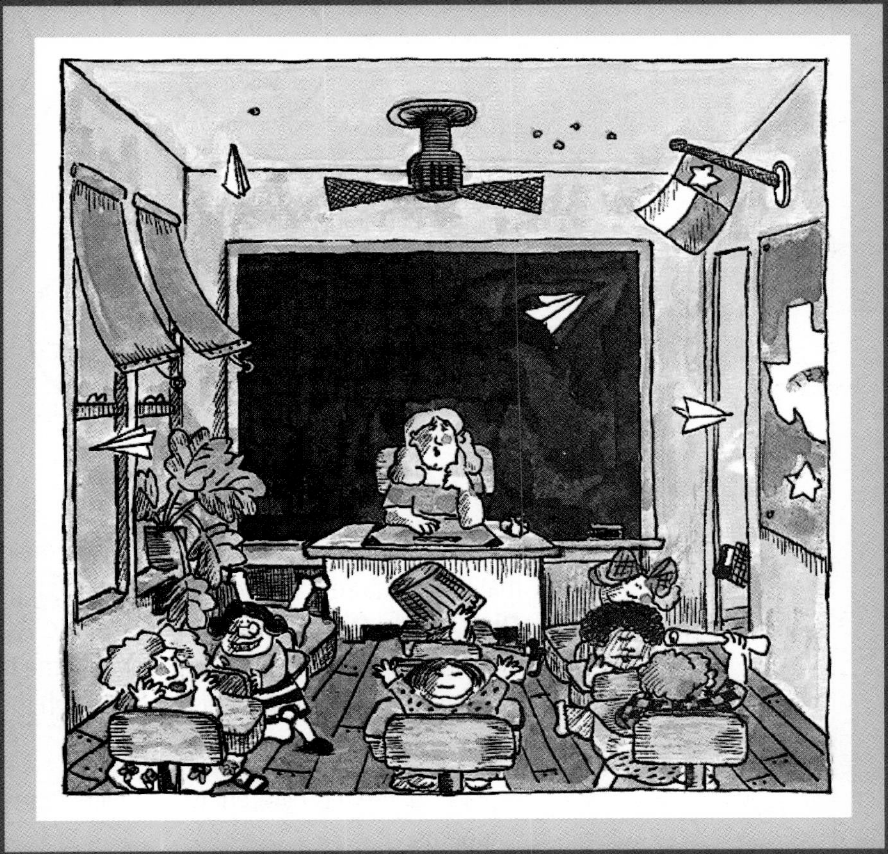

INVITATIONS TO LITERACY

Launching the Program

Managing Instruction

Grouping

Use a variety of group sizes to meet individual needs.

- **Whole class** for concepts all students need to learn.
- **Small groups** of three or more for meeting special needs.
- **Cooperative groups** with partners for completing a common task.
- **Individual activities** for focusing on a special need or individual choice.

INTERACTIVE LEARNING

Previewing the Literature

Cooperative Learning

Ask students to look through their anthologies and to work with partners to complete the graphic organizer. Discuss students' responses.

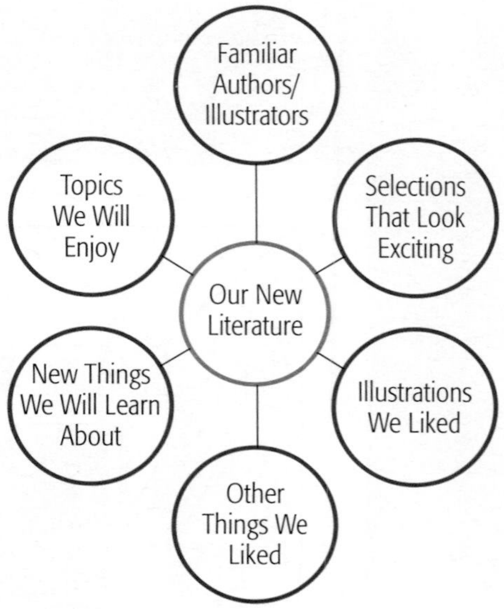
Familiar Authors/ Illustrators
Topics We Will Enjoy
Selections That Look Exciting
Our New Literature
New Things We Will Learn About
Illustrations We Liked
Other Things We Liked

Discussing Themes

Direct students to the table of contents of their anthologies and point out that the literature is organized in groups that go together called themes–**Oink, Oink, Oink, Community Ties,** etc. Ask volunteers to read the theme titles. Have the class select one theme to preview. Divide the class into small groups. As students look through the theme, bring out the following points in discussion:

- Each theme has different types of literature–stories, information, poems.
- There are activities for responding to the literature.
- Author/illustrator information is given.
- **Be a Writer** is a place where student writers share their work.

Making a Collage About Me

Invite students to make a collage that tells about themselves by gluing pictures on a piece of paper. Suggest that they cut out pictures that show:

- what they like to do for fun
- their favorite foods
- how they feel
- things they would like to learn
- their interests

Put names on the backs of collages and display them for others to see. You may want to make and display your own collage. As everyone gets to know each other, have students guess which collage belongs to which student.

Materials
- magazines
- safety scissors
- construction paper
- markers or crayons
- glue

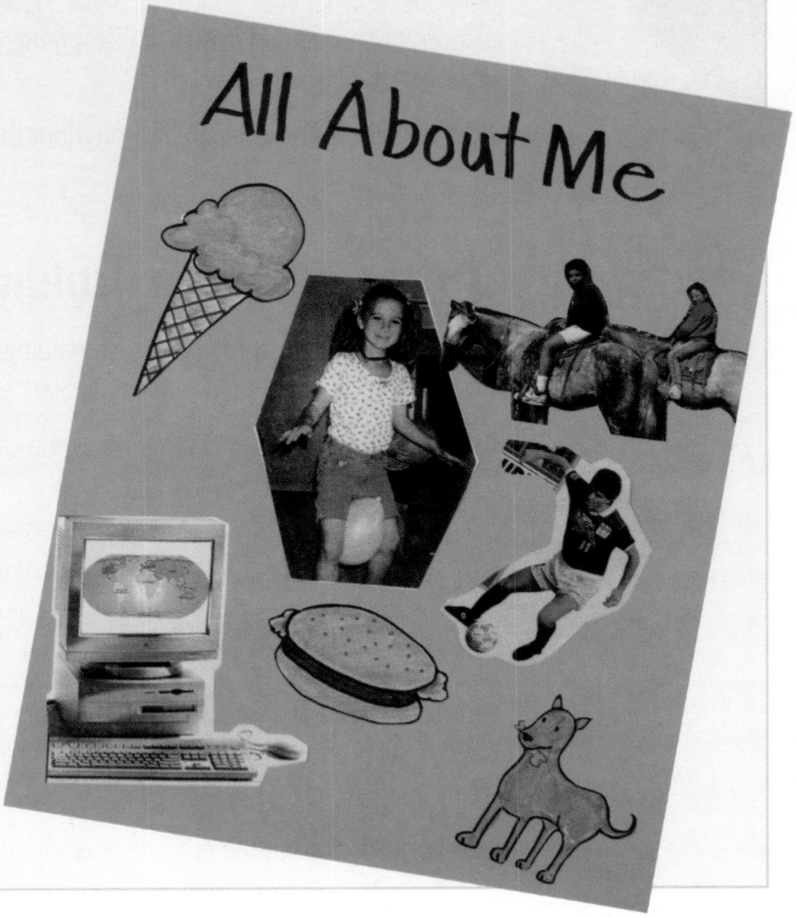
All About Me

Managing Assessment

Getting to Know Your Students

Question: How can I use this introductory time to get to know my students?

Answer: Try these ideas:

- Note how students work with each other to complete activities.
- Note how students express themselves during small group and whole class discussions.
- Note whether students are excited about the literature and seem familiar with particular authors and illustrators.
- Look at each student's collage to identify interests and attitudes.
- Observe students' writing, looking for strengths and things to improve (see Responding, pages 29–29A and Reading-Writing Workshop, pages 29B–30A).
- Observe students' reading, looking for strengths and things to improve in fluency (oral reading) and comprehension (responding and discussing).

Give the Baseline Group Test or the Informal Reading Inventory, if needed. See the *Teacher's Assessment Handbook.*

Portfolio Opportunity

Save students' collages for a record of their interests and favorite activities.

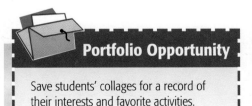

A Literacy-Centered Classroom

INTERACTIVE LEARNING

A Reading-Writing Area

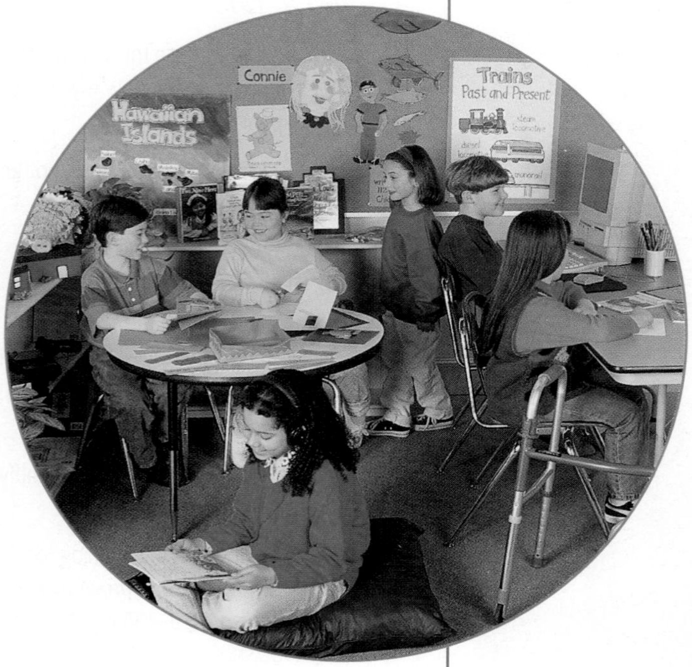
Connie
Hawaiian Islands
Trains
Past and Present

Discuss with students the importance of having a place in the classroom where reading and writing get special attention.

Brainstorm with students a list of things the Reading-Writing area might have:

- books to check out
- comfortable chairs and pillows
- a rug or carpet
- a bulletin board to display things written about books students have read and student-written books
- tables
- writing materials—paper, pencils, pens, markers
- magazines and newspapers
- a checkout system for books
- a plant or other things to make the area attractive
- posters

Create the Reading-Writing area in your classroom by having students help decide what your space will allow. Have students sign up to be responsible for certain tasks such as arranging book displays, organizing writing materials, etc.

Add to and change the area throughout the year.

Literacy Areas Across the Curriculum

Discuss with students how they use reading, writing, listening, speaking, viewing, and thinking skills in every subject and in everyday life.

Brainstorm with students other areas the classroom might include to help them become more literate:

- a listening area
- a display area for science and social studies activities
- a math manipulatives table
- an area for painting and other art projects
- a computer area

Create other areas by having students help decide what the class needs. Have small groups of students be responsible for helping to arrange the area.

Add to and change the areas throughout the year.

Independent Work

Making an Independent Reading-Writing Chart

Explain to students that there will be time each day for independent reading as well as independent writing. Ask students to share their ideas about what everyone should do during these times. Record responses on a chart to display in the classroom.

Reading	Writing
• Everyone reads during reading time. • Select reading materials before the special time. • The teacher may talk and read with the students. • Keep a record of books read. • Share with a friend what has been read.	• Everyone writes during writing time. • Write stories, letters, cartoons, and other things. • There may be teacher/student conferences. • Have a folder to keep writing. • Share your writing with a friend.

Making a Journal

Discuss with students that a journal is a place for them to keep their thoughts, questions, and feelings about what they have read. Journals may also include a list of new words, things they have written, and a list of stories they would like to read independently.

Materials
- writing paper
- construction paper or notebooks
- stapler
- yarn
- markers or crayons

Invite students to create their own journals and decorate the covers. Have them divide their journals into sections:

- Reading
- Vocabulary
- Writing
- Independent Reading

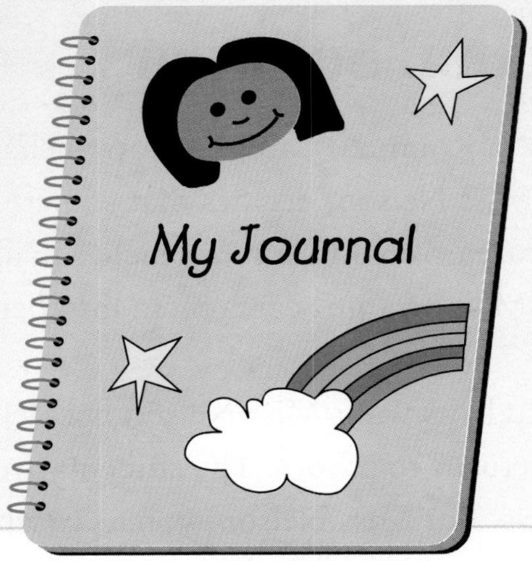
My Journal

Managing Instruction

Independent Reading and Writing

Schedule daily time for independent reading and independent writing. Build time up to 15–20 minutes per day for each.

Give these times special names:

- DIRT, Daily Independent Reading Time
- WART, Writing and Reading Time
- DEAR, Drop Everything and Read

Managing Instruction

Journals

There are many different ways to use journals.

Encourage students to:

- record thoughts and feelings about what they read
- write or draw responses
- keep a list of new/interesting words
- write predictions or questions about their reading

Read students' journals and write responses to their entries.

Have students read a partner's journal and write a response.

INTRODUCTORY SELECTION:

Miss Nelson Is Missing!

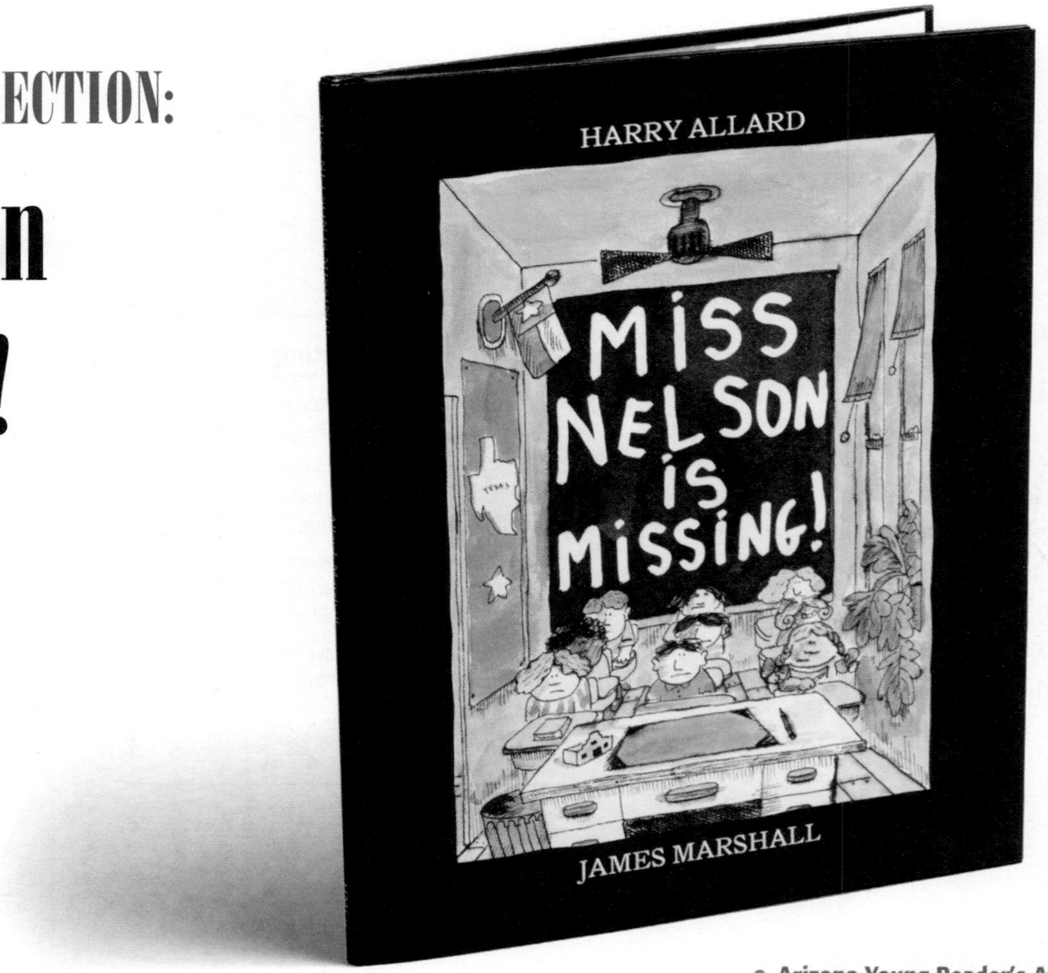
HARRY ALLARD
MISS NELSON IS MISSING!
JAMES MARSHALL

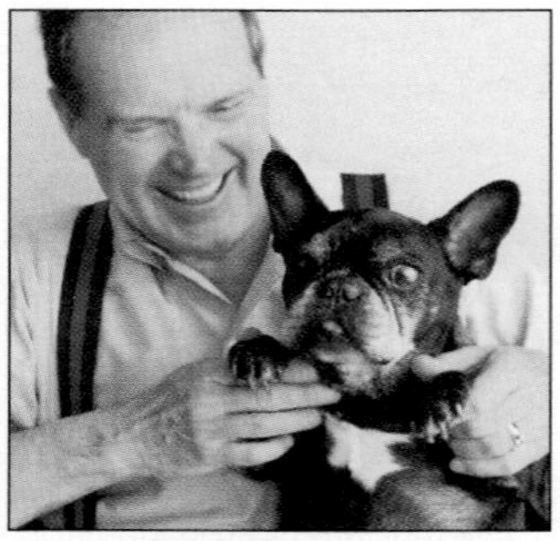

by Harry Allard

Other Books by the Author

Miss Nelson Is Back
The Stupids Step Out
The Stupids Take Off

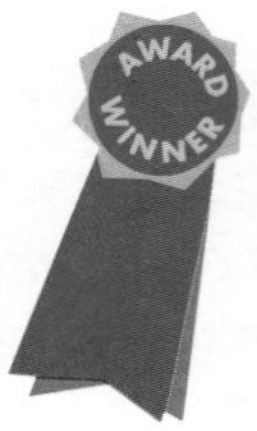
AWARD WINNER

- Arizona Young Reader's Award
- California Young Reader Medal
- Georgia Children's Picture Storybook Award

Selection Summary

The kids in Room 207 are the worst-behaved class in the school. Their teacher, Miss Nelson, decides that something must be done. One day the students are greeted by a new teacher in an ugly black dress—Miss Viola Swamp. Miss Swamp scares them into behaving and loads them down with work.

The students want Miss Nelson back! Just as they are losing hope, Miss Nelson returns to school. The students are overjoyed and, of course, behave like angels. But Miss Nelson won't say where she has been. And when she returns home that night, she hangs up her coat beside an ugly black dress.

Lesson Planning Guide

	Skill/Strategy Instruction	Meeting Individual Needs	Lesson Resources
1 Introduce *the* Literature *Pacing: 1 day*	**Preparing to Read and Write** Introducing a Reading Strategy, 10A Prior Knowledge/Building Background, 10A **Selection Vocabulary,** 11A • misbehaving • detective • worst-behaved • change • act up • rapped • secret	**Other Choices for Building Background,** 11A	***Literacy Activity Book,*** Reading Strategies, p. 1; Vocabulary, p. 2 **Transparency,** Vocabulary, IS–1
2 Interact *with* Literature *Pacing: 1–3 days*	**Reading Strategies** Predict/Infer, 13 Think About Words, 17 Self-Question, 19 Monitor, 21 Evaluate, 23 Summarize, 27	**Choices for Reading,** 12 **Students Acquiring English,** 13, 14, 17, 25, 29 **Extra Support,** 15 **Minilessons** Predict/Infer, 13 Think About Words, 17 Self-Question, 19 Monitor, 21 Evaluate, 23 Summarize, 27	**Reading-Writing Workshop,** 29B-30A ***Literacy Activity Book*** Comprehension, p. 3; Prewriting, pp. 4–5; Revising, p. 6 The Learning Company's new elementary writing center software
Reading-Writing Workshop *Pacing: 3 days*	**About the Workshop,** 29B Prewriting, 29C–29D Drafting, 29E Revising, 29E–29F Proofreading, 29G Publishing and Sharing, 30A	**Students Acquiring English,** 29E Minilessons Prewriting, 29D Drafting, 29E Revising, 29E–29F Proofreading, 29G Publishing and Sharing, 30A	***Literacy Activity Book*** Prewriting, pp. 4–5; Revising, p. 6 The Learning Company's new elementary writing center software

Introduce *the* Literature

Preparing to Read and Write

INTERACTIVE LEARNING

Introducing a Reading Strategy

Have students work with a partner to brainstorm what they think good readers do as they read. Share and discuss students' ideas.

Direct partners to compare their ideas to the checklist on *Literacy Activity Book* page 1. As students review the checklist, bring out the following points.

- Good readers use these strategies whenever they read.
- Different strategies are used before, during, and after reading.
- As readers are learning to use strategies, they must think about how each strategy will help them.

Ask students to read the points under each strategy and discuss what they mean. Suggest that students use this checklist as they read.

Literacy Activity Book, p. 1

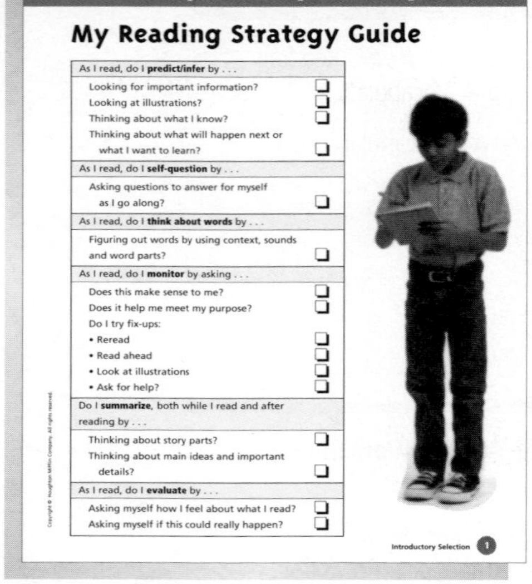

My Reading Strategy Guide

As I read, do I **predict/infer** by . . .
Looking for important information? ❑
Looking at illustrations? ❑
Thinking about what I know? ❑
Thinking about what will happen next or what I want to learn? ❑

As I read, do I **self-question** by . . .
Asking questions to answer for myself as I go along? ❑

As I read, do I **think about words** by . . .
Figuring out words by using context, sounds and word parts? ❑

As I read, do I **monitor** by asking . . .
Does this make sense to me? ❑
Does it help me meet my purpose? ❑
Do I try fix-ups:
• Reread ❑
• Read ahead ❑
• Look at illustrations ❑
• Ask for help? ❑

Do I **summarize**, both while I read and after reading by . . .
Thinking about story parts? ❑
Thinking about main ideas and important details? ❑

As I read, do I **evaluate** by . . .
Asking myself how I feel about what I read? ❑
Asking myself if this could really happen? ❑

Copyright © Houghton Mifflin Company. All rights reserved.

Introductory Selection 1

Prior Knowledge/Building Background

Key Concept

Understanding how students behave in class

Reproduce the chart below. Ask students to work with a partner to suggest ways they should behave in school. Then construct a class chart by having students share ideas. Invite students to predict what might happen if students did not behave properly in school.

How We Should Act in School

During Lessons	During Storytime	In the Halls

Managing Instruction

Reading Strategies

- At the beginning of and throughout each selection, students will be directed in thinking about each of the reading strategies.
- In this selection, minilessons are provided to give practice with each strategy. Use these as needed to help students learn the strategies.

Other Choices for Building Background

Quick-Write: The World's Best Teacher

Ask students to think about what the "best teacher in the world" might be like. Invite them to write a short description of this teacher in their journal. Have volunteers share their answers.

Teacher Read Aloud

Students Acquiring English Read aloud page 13 of *Miss Nelson Is Missing!* Have students use the illustration to describe the things that the "worst-behaved class in the whole school" might do.

Transparency IS–1

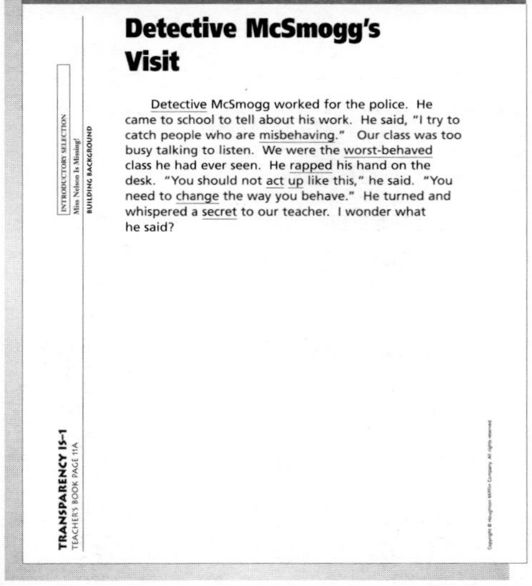
Detective McSmogg's Visit

Detective McSmogg worked for the police. He came to school to tell about his work. He said, "I try to catch people who are misbehaving." Our class was too busy talking to listen. We were the worst-behaved class he had ever seen. He rapped his hand on the desk. "You should not act up like this," he said. "You need to change the way you behave." He turned and whispered a secret to our teacher. I wonder what he said?

TRANSPARENCY IS–1
TEACHER'S BOOK PAGE 11A

INTERACTIVE LEARNING

Selection Vocabulary

Key Words

- **misbehaving**
- **worst-behaved**
- **detective**
- **change**
- **act up**
- **rapped**
- **secret**

Display Transparency IS–1. Read it aloud and then have students take turns reading it aloud with partners. Encourage students to use the context and their own knowledge to discuss the meanings of the underlined words.

You may wish to check students' understanding of the Key Words by asking these questions:

What word means information you don't want someone else to know?	secret
Who has a job of finding out other people's secrets?	detective
What words have to do with people acting bad or improperly?	misbehaving, worst-behaved, act up
What word means hit or struck sharply?	rapped
What would a bad person have to do to turn into a good person?	change

Vocabulary Practice Have students complete *Literacy Activity Book* page 2.

Literacy Activity Book, p. 2

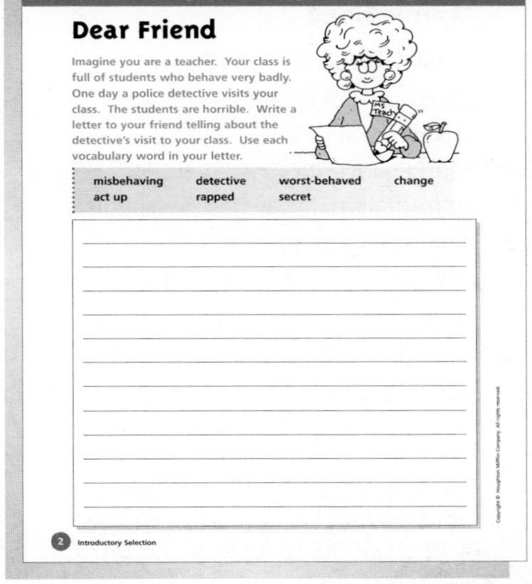
Dear Friend

Imagine you are a teacher. Your class is full of students who behave very badly. One day a police detective visits your class. The students are horrible. Write a letter to your friend telling about the detective's visit to your class. Use each vocabulary word in your letter.

misbehaving, detective, worst-behaved, change, act up, rapped, secret

2 Introductory Selection

Interact *with* Literature

Reading Strategies

- **Predict/Infer**
- **Monitor**
- **Think About Words**
- **Self-Question**
- **Evaluate**
- **Summarize**

Teacher/Modeling Have students look back at their Reading Strategy Guide on *Literacy Activity Book* page 1. Discuss how these strategies can be used together as students read. Model the process with a Think Aloud.

Think Aloud

First, I'll look at the pictures and predict what I think will happen. As I read I will monitor my predictions and change them as I get new information. I may have questions that I want to answer as I read. I'll think about words I don't know. Can I sound them out? As I read and after I read I'll summarize the story and evaluate how I feel about it.

Predicting/Purpose Setting Invite students to look at the pictures on the cover and on page 13. Ask them to predict what they think will happen in the story.

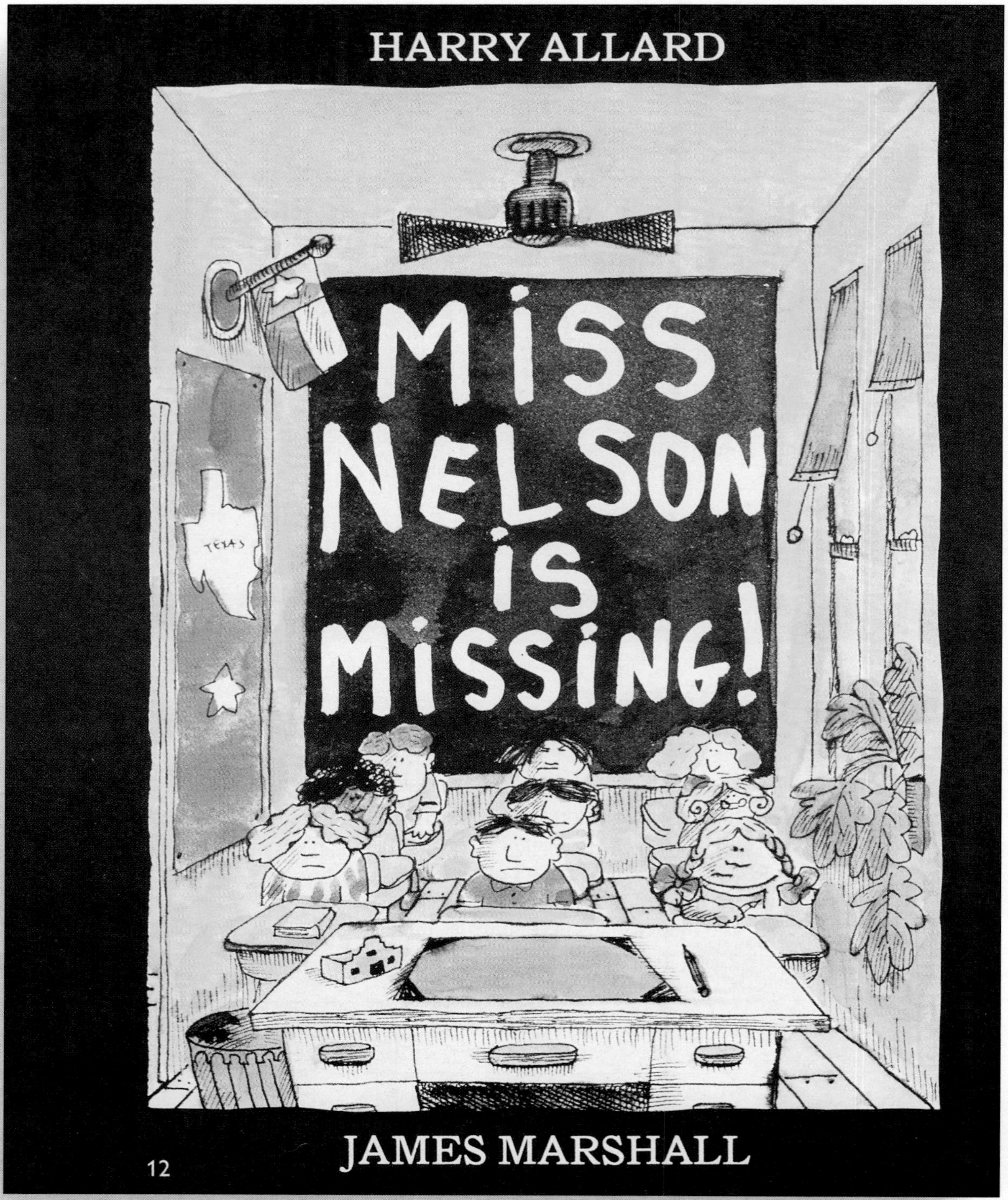
HARRY ALLARD
MISS NELSON IS MISSING!
TEXAS
12
JAMES MARSHALL

Choices for Reading

Independent Reading	Cooperative Reading
Guided Reading	Teacher Read Aloud

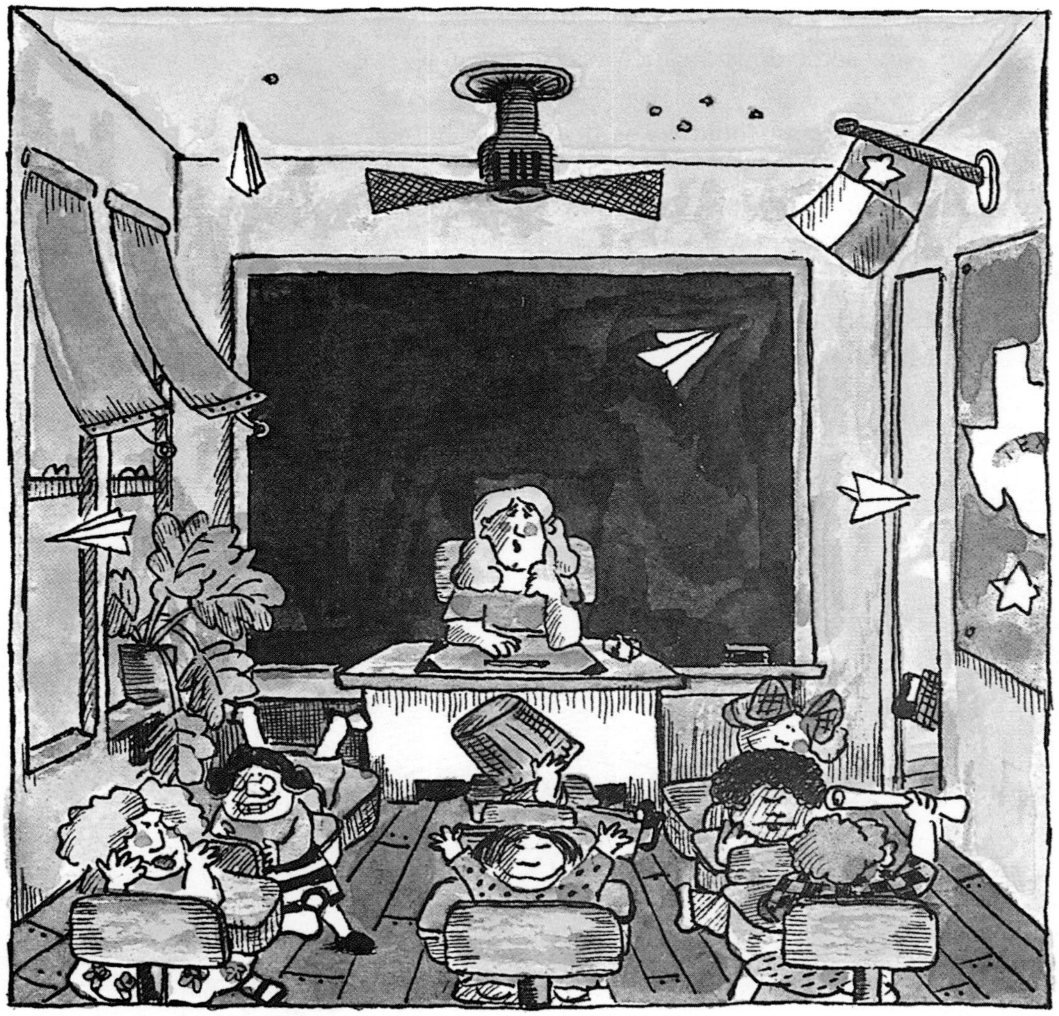

The kids in Room 207 were misbehaving again. Spitballs stuck to the ceiling. Paper planes whizzed through the air. They were the worst-behaved class in the whole school.

13

MINILESSON

Predict/Infer

Teach/Model

Discuss with students whether they try to figure out what might happen next in a story. Point out that good readers use pictures and other details to predict what might happen and to infer, or figure out, things that the author doesn't say directly. Model this with a Think Aloud.

Think Aloud

As I read the title of the book, look at the pictures, and read the first page, I can tell the teacher is having a tough time. The kids are awful. I can infer that this is Miss Nelson. I predict that she is going to leave.

Practice/Apply

Ask students to read pages 14–15, look at the pictures, and predict what will happen next. Have volunteers tell what clues they used to make their predictions.

QuickREFERENCE

Journal

Have students write predictions in their journals. Encourage them to check and revise their predictions as they continue reading.

MEETING INDIVIDUAL NEEDS

Students Acquiring English

Encourage students to use the illustrations to tell the story in small groups. Students might also write speech balloons for the characters in the illustrations.

"Now settle down," said Miss Nelson in a sweet voice.

But the class would *not* settle down. They whispered and giggled. They squirmed and made faces. They were even rude during story hour. And they always refused to do their lessons.

"Something will have to be done," said Miss Nelson.

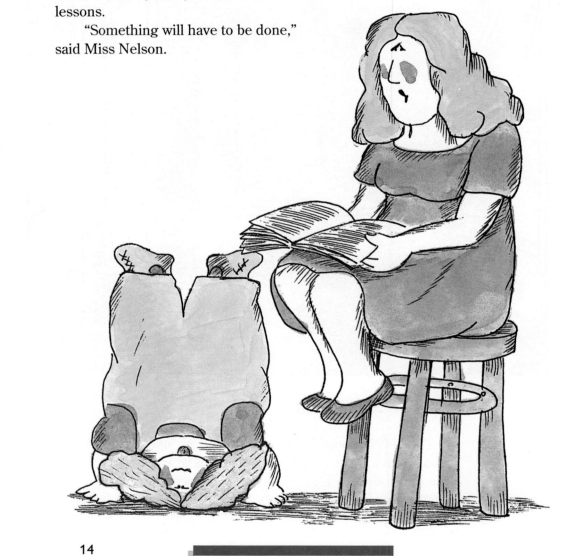

14

QuickREFERENCE

Students Acquiring English

To further comprehension, invite students to role-play both the kids and Miss Nelson in the scene.

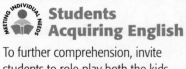

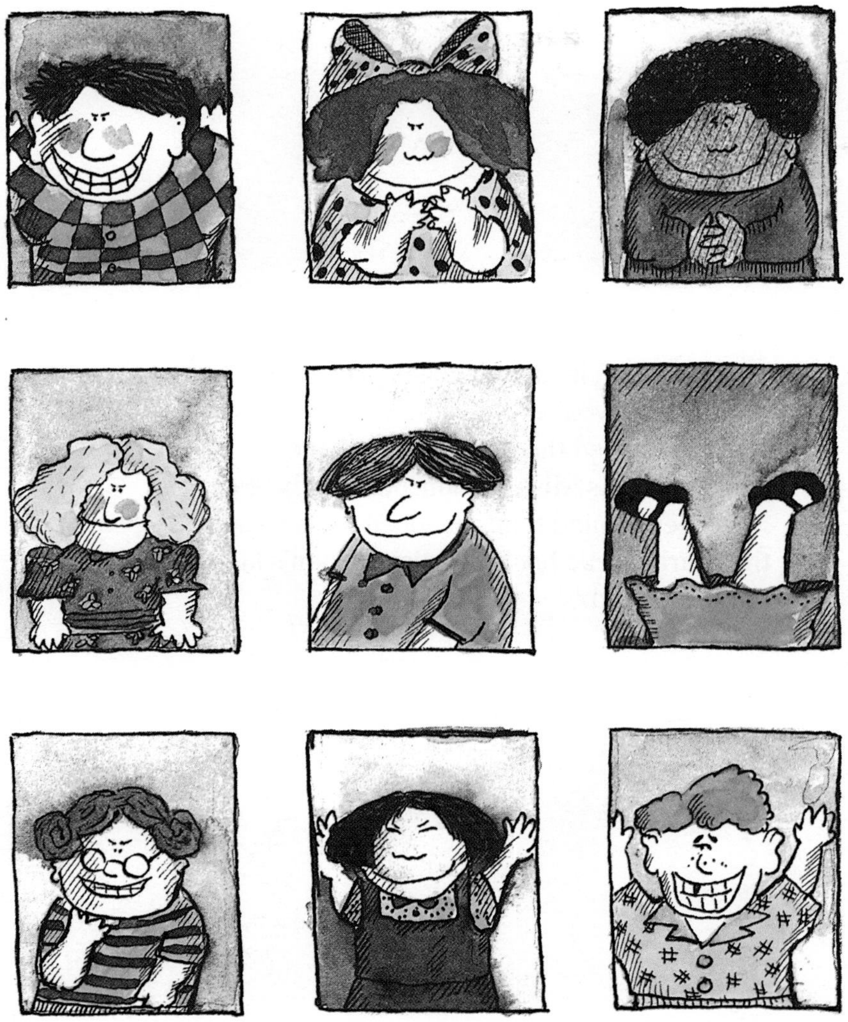

The next morning Miss Nelson did not come to school. "Wow!" yelled the kids. "Now we can *really* act up!" They began to make more spitballs and paper planes. "Today let's be just terrible!" they said.

"Not so fast!" hissed an unpleasant voice.

15

Multicultural Link

Schools Have students who have attended schools in other countries share their experiences with the class.

Extra Support

Vocabulary Some students may need help with the words *squirmed* and *hissed*. Have volunteers demonstrate how the kids *squirmed*. Read aloud the line that is *hissed* by an unpleasant voice.

Interact *with* Literature

A woman in an ugly black dress stood before them. "I am your new teacher, Miss Viola Swamp." And she rapped the desk with her ruler.

"Where is Miss Nelson?" asked the kids.

"Never mind that!" snapped Miss Swamp. "Open those arithmetic books!" Miss Nelson's kids did as they were told.

16

Informal Assessment

As students read, make notes about how well they stick to the task and whether they seem to be enjoying the story. If any students are reading aloud, note how well they decode difficult words.

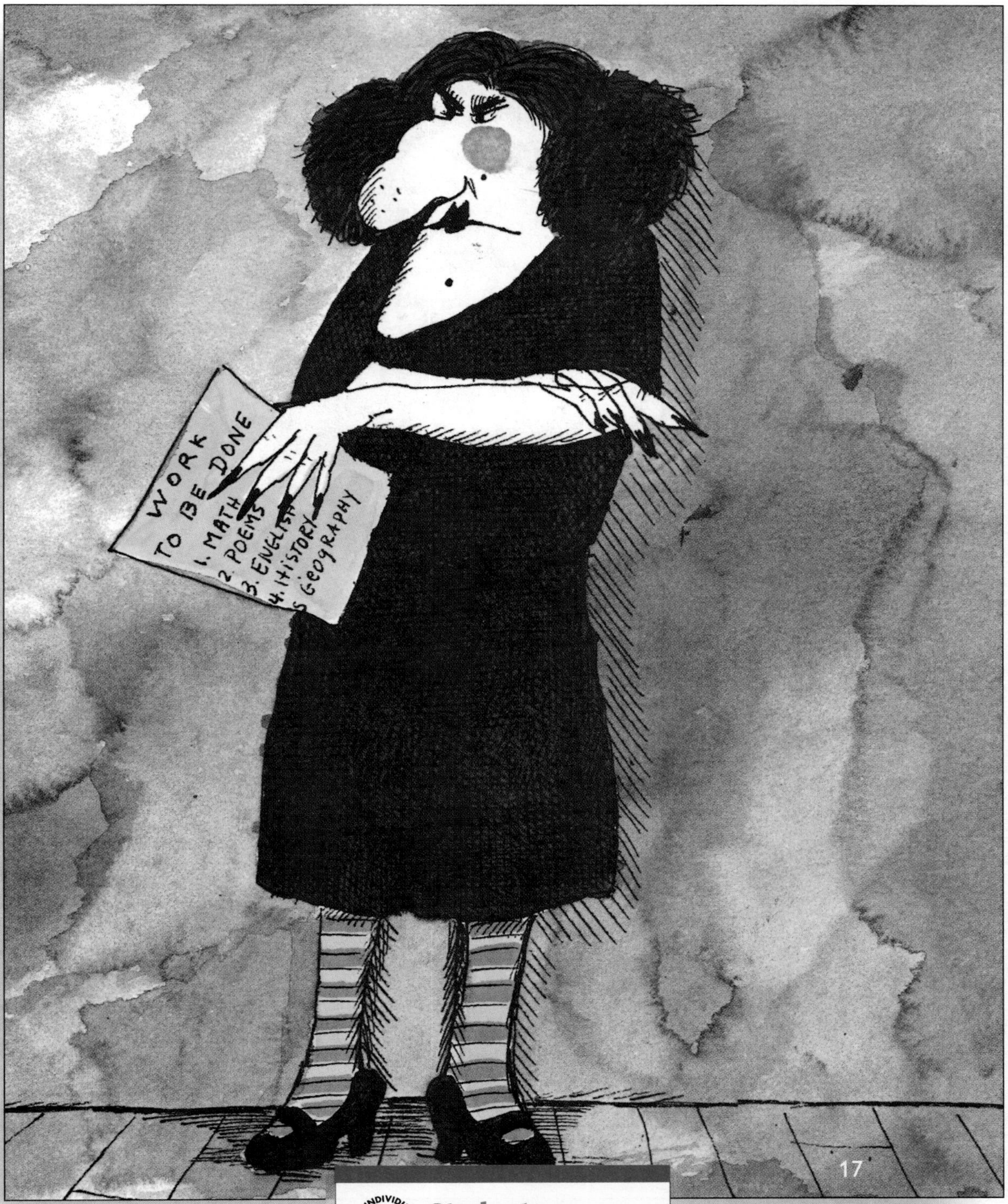
WORK
TO BE DONE
1. MATH
2. POEMS
3. ENGLISH
4. HISTORY
5. GEOGRAPHY
17

Students Acquiring English

Have students begin a profile of Miss Viola Swamp by creating a word web of words related to her. Students can start by describing details in the illustration on page 17. Encourage them to add to their webs as they read.

QuickREFERENCE

MINILESSON

Think About Words

Teach/Model

Point out that readers always come across new words. Good readers use clues to figure out how to say the word and what it means. Discuss these hints:

Find out what makes sense. Read to the end of the sentence or paragraph to see if this helps. Sometimes the words around a new word can help you.

Sound out letters or word parts. How does the word begin? How does the word end? What word parts do you know?

Look for other clues. Look at pictures or think of other words that look like the new word.

Think Aloud

As I read page 16, I come to the word *rapped,* a word that I don't know. I read to the end of the sentence. I know what a ruler is. What could Miss Swamp do to the desk with a ruler? She could hit it to make a noise. *Rapped* must be another word for *hit*. And it makes sense when I reread the sentence.

Practice/Apply

Have students work with partners to select another word in the story and tell how they could figure out what it means and how to pronounce it.

Interact *with* Literature

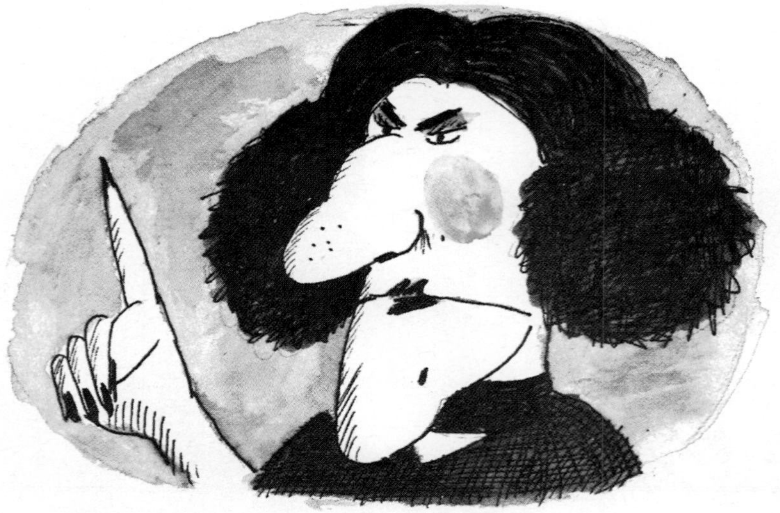

They could see that Miss Swamp was a real witch. She meant business.

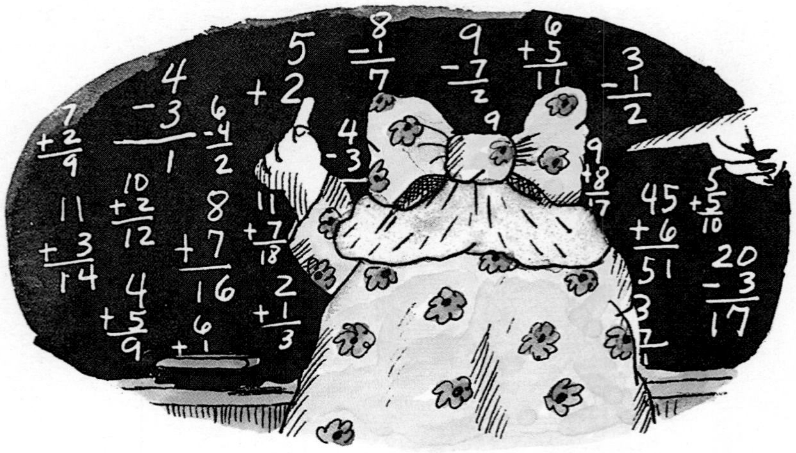
11 + 3 14
8 + 7 16
45 + 6 51
20 − 3 17

Right away she put them to work. And she loaded them down with homework.

18

Self-Assessment

Ask students how they are helping themselves with their reading. Encourage them to ask themselves:

- Am I understanding the story?
- Am I thinking about words and making predictions?
- How do I feel about the story so far?

QuickREFERENCE

Math Link

Sums Encourage students to work out the sums pictured on the chalkboard to see if Miss Nelson's kids arrived at the correct answers.

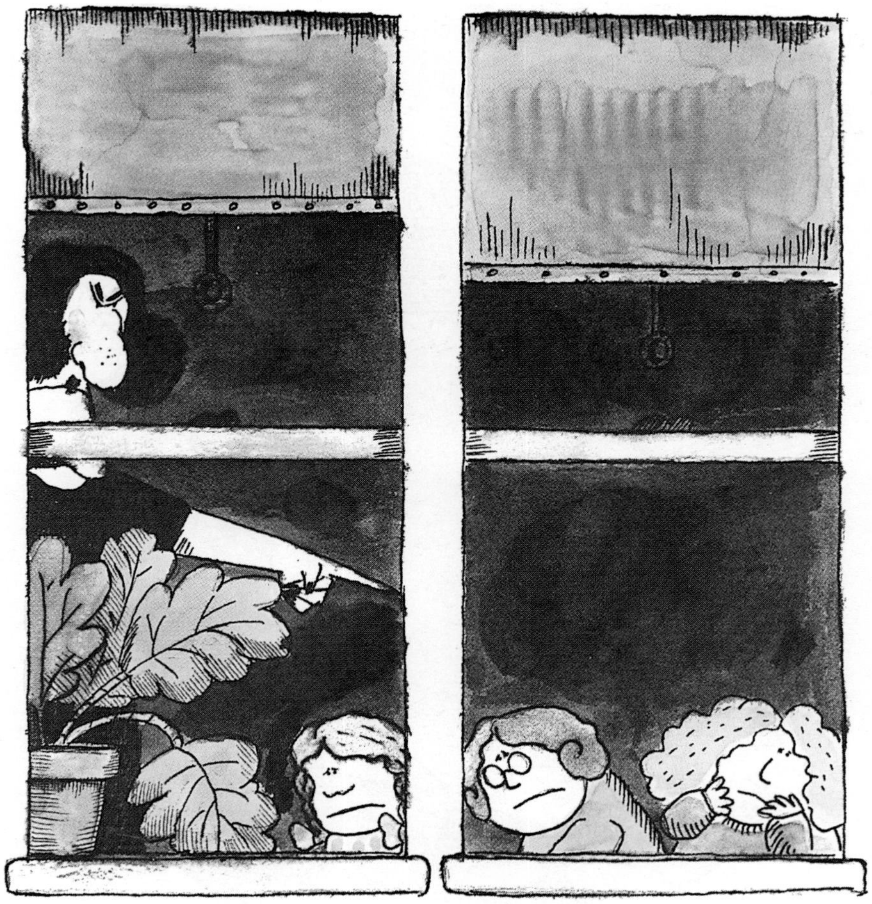

"We'll have no story hour today," said Miss Swamp.

"Keep your mouths shut," said Miss Swamp.

"Sit perfectly still," said Miss Swamp.

"And if you misbehave, you'll be sorry," said Miss Swamp.

The kids in Room 207 had *never* worked so hard.

Days went by and there was no sign of Miss Nelson. The kids *missed* Miss Nelson!

19

MINILESSON

Self-Question

Teach/Model

Ask students what questions they have about the story so far. Record responses on the board. Explain that good readers ask questions as they read, and they keep reading to find the answers.

Practice/Apply

Ask volunteers to tell what questions they want to have answered as they read more of the story. Examples might include

- Where is Miss Nelson?
- Who is Miss Swamp?

Interact *with* Literature

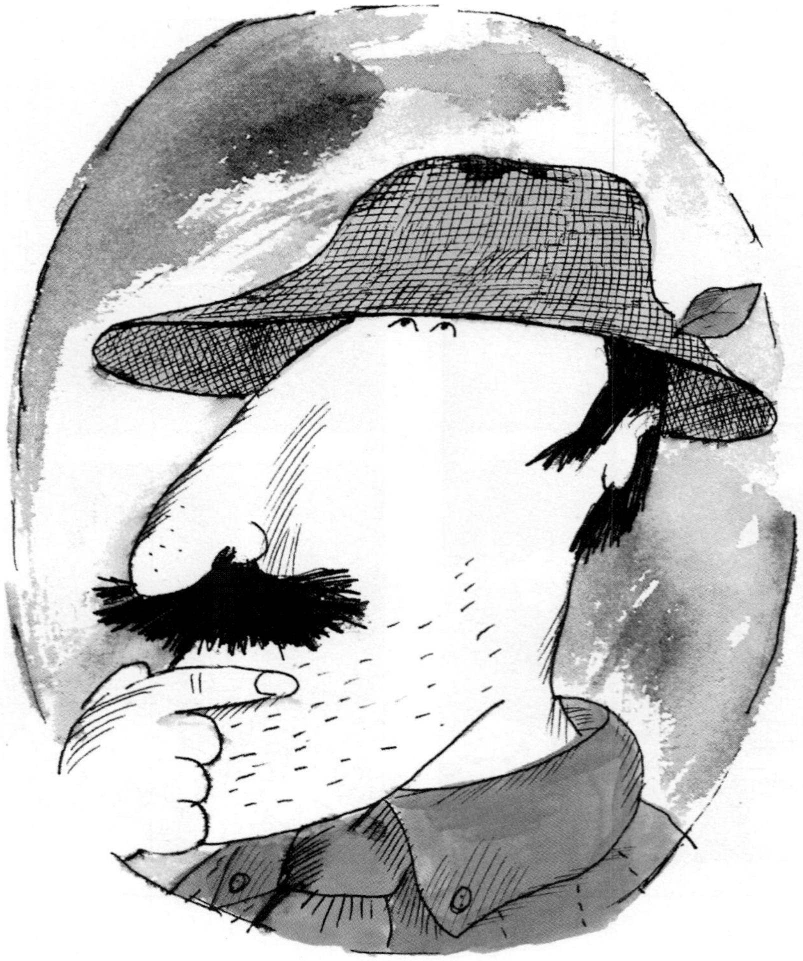

"Maybe we should try to find her," they said. Some of them went to the police.

Detective McSmogg was assigned to the case. He listened to their story. He scratched his chin. "Hmmmm," he said. "Hmmm. I think Miss Nelson is missing."

Detective McSmogg would not be much help.

20

Informal Assessment

If you notice that students reading independently are having difficulty, suggest that they complete their reading cooperatively. Have partners take turns reading pages aloud.

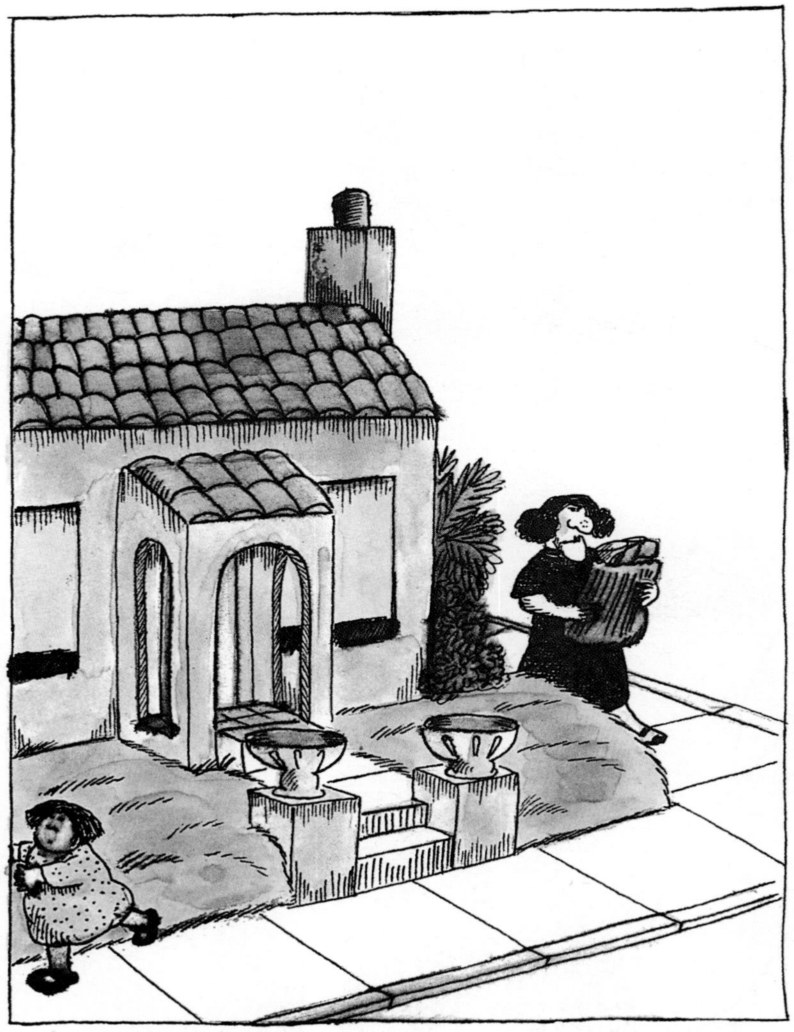

Other kids went to Miss Nelson's house. The shades were tightly drawn, and no one answered the door. In fact, the only person they *did* see was the wicked Miss Viola Swamp, coming up the street.

"If she sees us, she'll give us more homework." They got away just in time.

21

MINILESSON

Monitor

Teach/Model

Explain that when you monitor something, you keep watch over it. Readers monitor their reading to make sure they understand what they read. Discuss with students how rereading, finding answers to questions, checking predictions, and reading further can help readers understand a selection.

Think Aloud

As I first read page 20, I don't understand why Detective McSmogg won't be much help. After I reread the page and think about what I already know, I realize that he only tells the kids what they already know.

Practice/Apply

Ask students to work with partners to read page 21 and discuss things that might not make sense to them. Have them tell how they could monitor their reading to clear up what they don't understand.

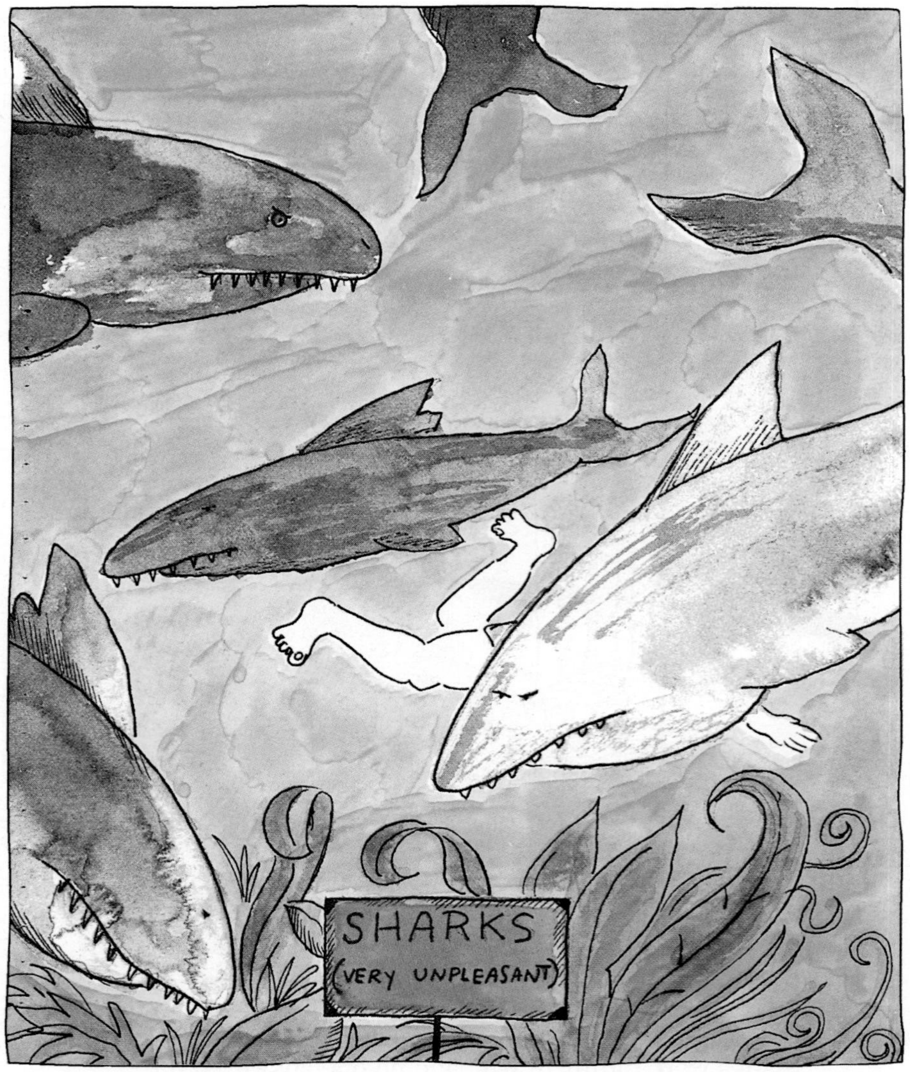
SHARKS
(VERY UNPLEASANT)

Maybe something *terrible* happened to Miss Nelson! "Maybe she was gobbled up by a shark!" said one of the kids. But that didn't seem likely.

22

Informal Assessment

Ask students to read aloud pages 22–23 to check decoding. Students should be allowed to first read the pages silently. See the Oral Reading Checklist in the *Teacher's Assessment Handbook*.

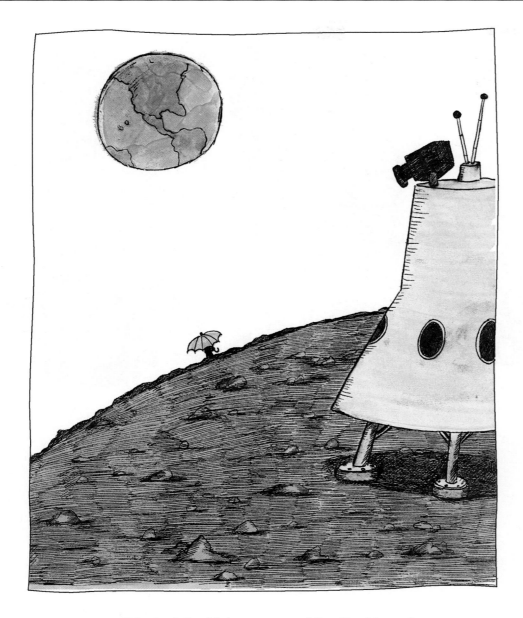

"Maybe Miss Nelson went to Mars!" said another kid. But that didn't seem likely either.

23

MINILESSON

Evaluate

Teach/Model

Ask a volunteer how he or she feels about the story so far. Then explain that the student has just evaluated the story. Good readers evaluate what they read by asking questions such as:

- How do I feel about this story? Why?
- Do I believe this could really happen?

Practice/Apply

Ask students to read pages 22–23. Then ask volunteers what they think of the kids' ideas. Could these things really happen? Would the story be as interesting if the kids had come up with more everyday ideas?

QuickREFERENCE

Science Link

Mars Invite students to tell what they know about Mars. Share these facts:

- It is the fourth planet from the sun.
- It was named after the Roman god of war, *Mars*, because of its reddish color.
- A Martian year is equal to 687 Earth days.
- The mean temperature on Mars is -23 degrees C (-9.4 degrees F).
- It has the largest known volcano in the solar system, Olympus Mons, which is 375 miles (600 kilometers) in diameter and over 65,600 feet (20,000 meters) high.

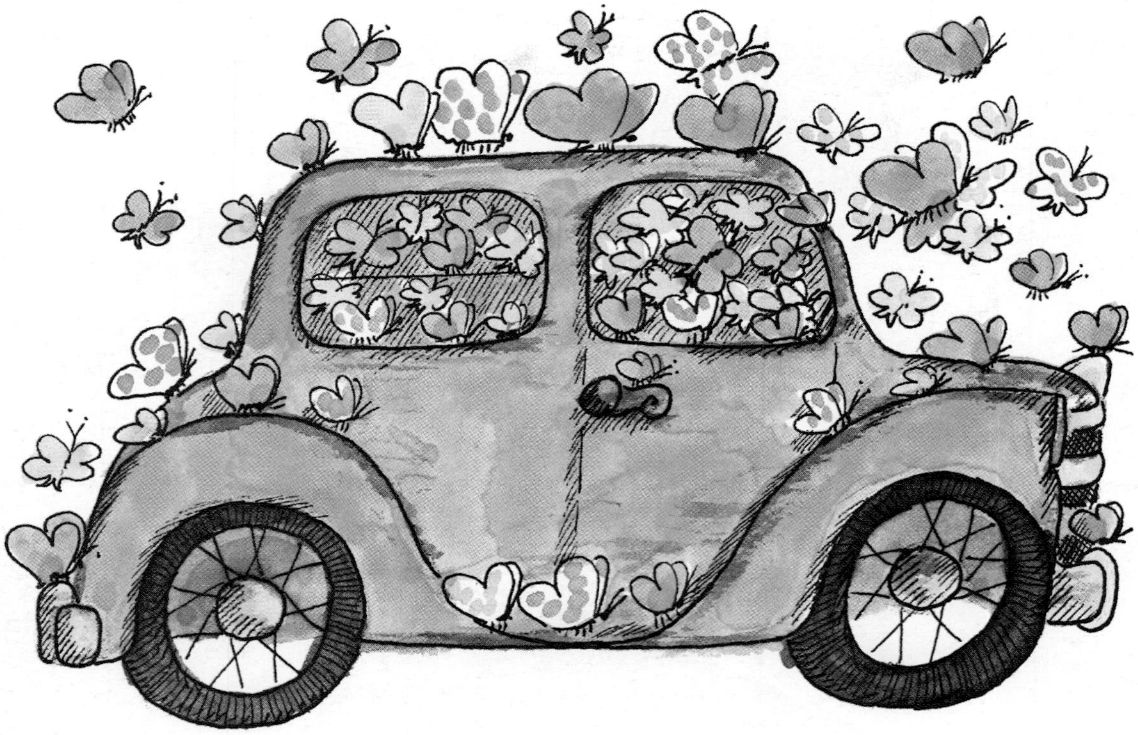

"I know!" exclaimed one know-it-all. "Maybe Miss Nelson's car was carried off by a swarm of angry butterflies!" But that was the least likely of all.

24

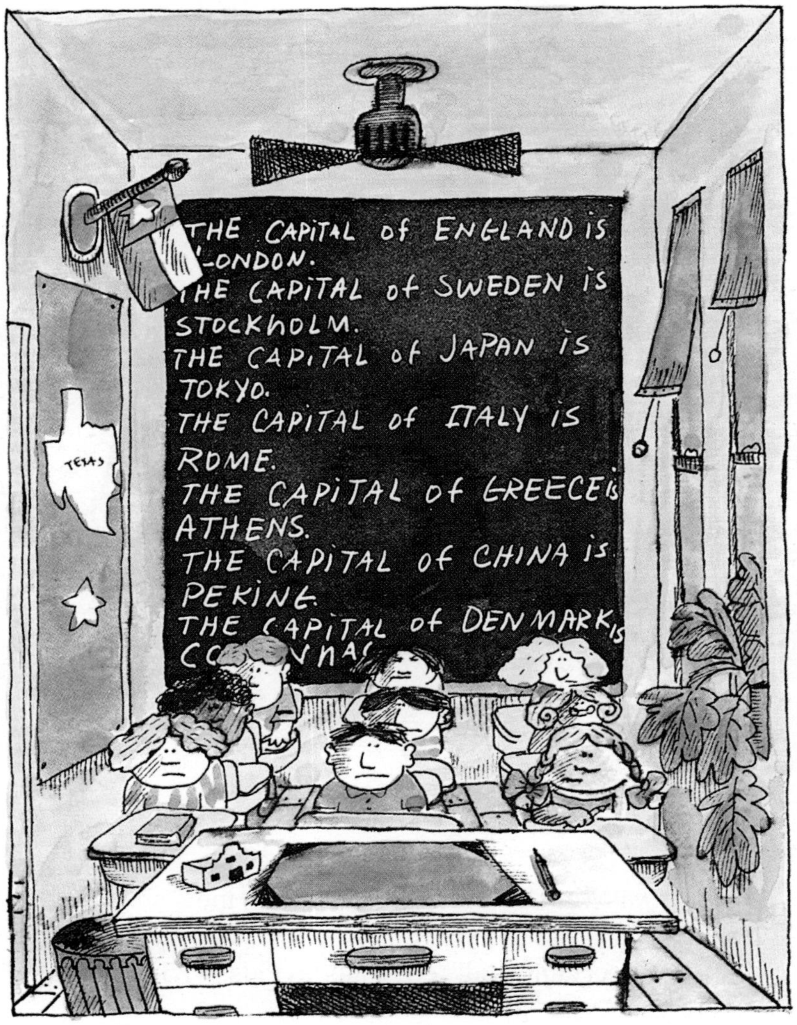
THE CAPITAL of ENGLAND IS LONDON.
THE CAPITAL of SWEDEN IS STOCKHOLM.
THE CAPITAL of JAPAN IS TOKYO.
THE CAPITAL of ITALY IS ROME.
THE CAPITAL of GREECE IS ATHENS.
THE CAPITAL of CHINA IS PEKING.
THE CAPITAL of DENMARK IS

The kids in Room 207 became very discouraged. It seemed that Miss Nelson was never coming back. And they would be stuck with Miss Viola Swamp forever.

They heard footsteps in the hall. "Here comes the witch," they whispered.

"Hello, children," someone said in a sweet voice.

25

QuickREFERENCE

Social Studies Link

China In the illustration the capital of China is given as Peking. *Peking* is the old spelling of what is known today in English as *Beijing*. (This story was written in 1977, when the old spelling was still in use.)

Students Acquiring English

Invite students to role-play this scene of the discouraged kids in Room 207. Have them make up dialogue that the kids might say. For a contrast, suggest that they role-play the scene on page 26, when Miss Nelson returns.

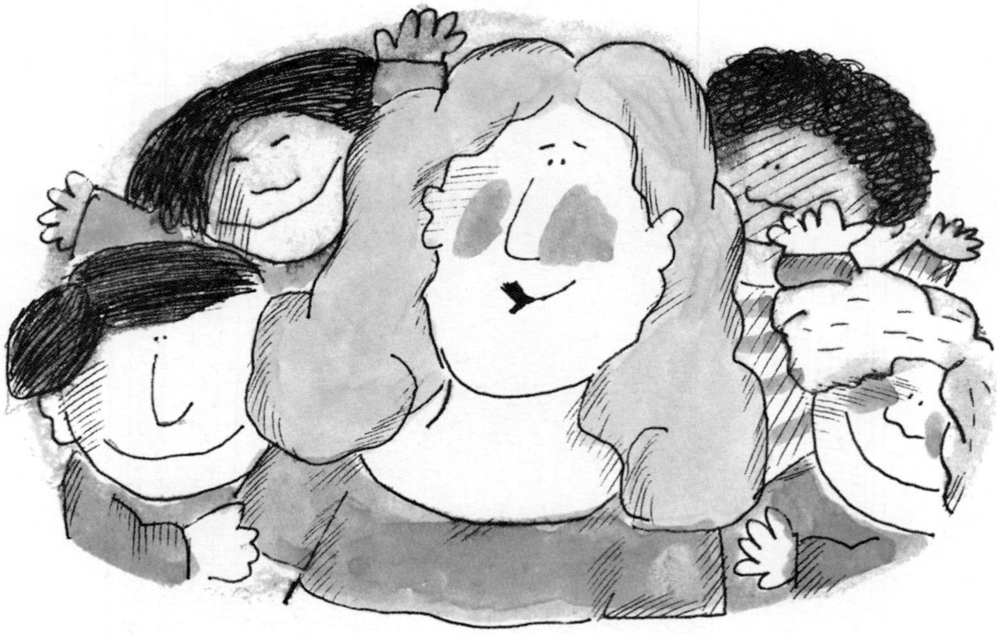

It was Miss Nelson! "Did you miss me?" she asked.

"We certainly did!" cried all the kids. "Where were you?"

"That's my little secret," said Miss Nelson. "How about a story hour?"

"Oh, yes!" cried the kids.

Miss Nelson noticed that during story hour no one was rude or silly. "What brought about this lovely change?" she asked.

"That's *our* little secret," said the kids.

26

Self-Assessment

Reflecting Ask students to talk about reading the story. Have them answer questions about the experience:

- Did I think the story was easy or difficult? What made it easy/difficult?
- What parts did I like best? Why?

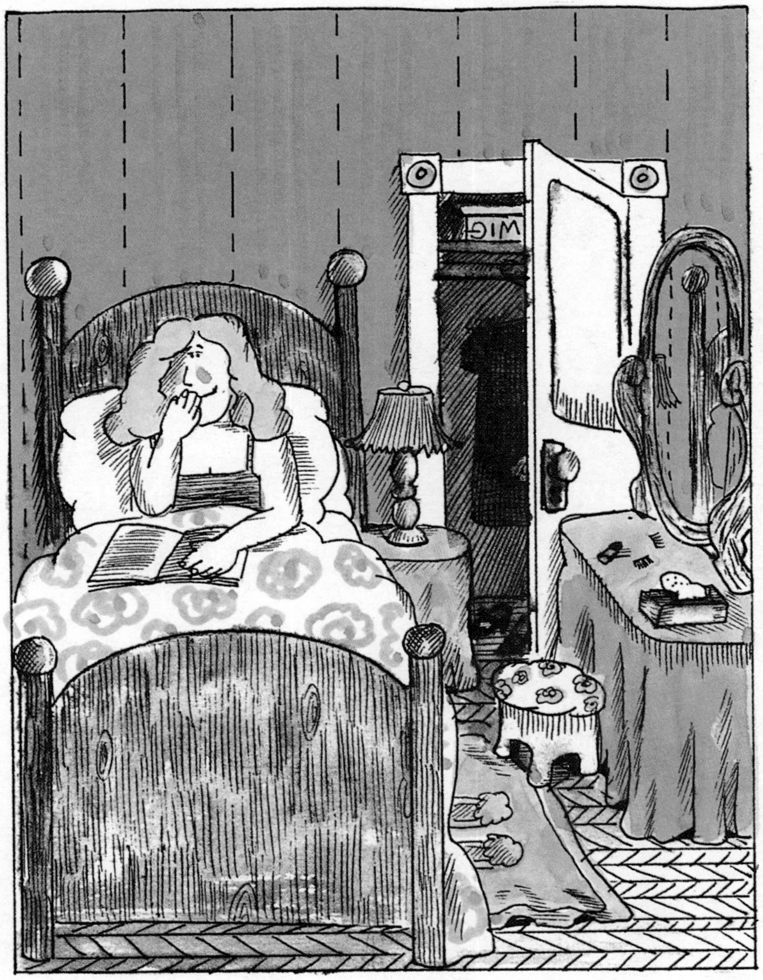

Back home Miss Nelson took off her coat and hung it in the closet (right next to an ugly black dress).

When it was time for bed she sang a little song. "I'll never tell," she said to herself with a smile.

P. S. Detective McSmogg is working on a new case. He is *now* looking for Miss Viola Swamp.

27

MINILESSON

Summarizing

Teach/Model

Explain that a summary tells the main points of a selection. To summarize a story like *Miss Nelson Is Missing!*, a reader thinks about story parts. Draw the chart below and use a Think Aloud to help students begin to fill it in. Have students complete the chart on their own. Then ask volunteers to summarize the story.

Characters
Setting
Problem
Events
Ending

Think Aloud

I know that Miss Nelson, Miss Viola Swamp, and the students are main characters. The story takes place at school. The problem is that the students behave badly in class, and Miss Nelson doesn't know what to do.

Practice/Apply

Have students work with partners to complete a chart on a well-known story. Have pairs share their summaries with the class.

Interact *with* Literature

More About the Author

Harry Allard

When you read a book by Harry Allard, don't look for the message. "I hate anything with a message," says Allard. His children's books are strictly for fun.

Allard's first book, *The Stupids Step Out*, was inspired by the drawings of James Marshall. *The Stupids* and the *Miss Nelson* series are among the many popular books Allard and Marshall created together.

More About the Illustrator

James Marshall

James Marshall had a gift for seeing the ridiculous—especially in his own life. The evil Miss Viola Swamp was inspired by his second grade teacher, who squelched his budding interest in art. It was only by accident—literally—that Marshall rediscovered his talent. He was studying the viola (from which Miss Swamp got her name) when a hand injury ended his plans for a career in music. He became a teacher instead and began drawing for fun in his free time. At a friend's urging, Marshall showed his drawings to a publisher. Some of them were only sketches on paper napkins—but they sparked a career that soon had millions of readers giggling over characters like George and Martha, the Stupids, Miss Nelson, Fox, and the Cut-Ups.

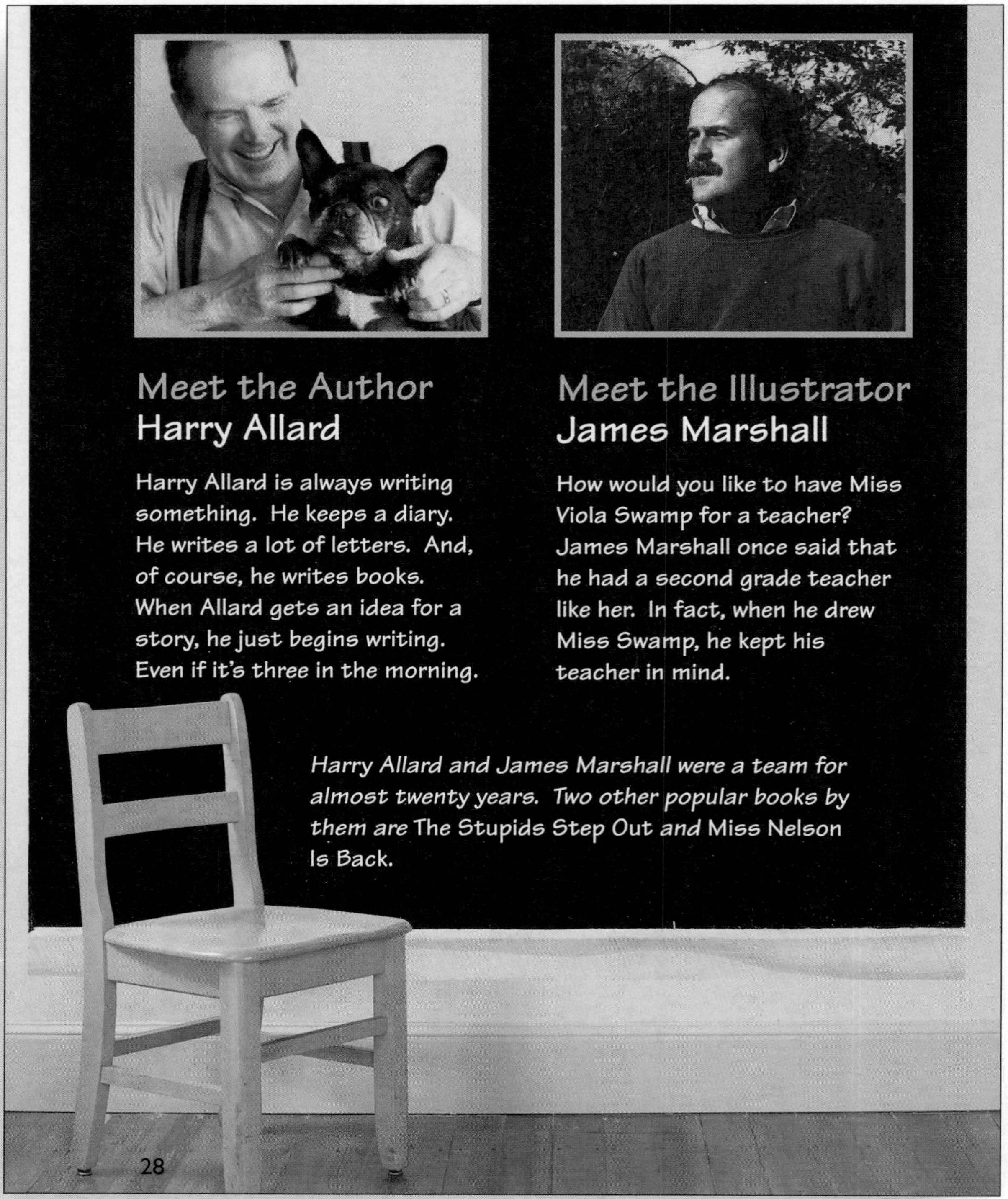

Meet the Author
Harry Allard

Harry Allard is always writing something. He keeps a diary. He writes a lot of letters. And, of course, he writes books. When Allard gets an idea for a story, he just begins writing. Even if it's three in the morning.

Meet the Illustrator
James Marshall

How would you like to have Miss Viola Swamp for a teacher? James Marshall once said that he had a second grade teacher like her. In fact, when he drew Miss Swamp, he kept his teacher in mind.

Harry Allard and James Marshall were a team for almost twenty years. Two other popular books by them are The Stupids Step Out *and* Miss Nelson Is Back.

28

RESPONDING

Investigating the Story

Put On a Puppet Show

Settle Down, Class!

What might Miss Nelson and Miss Swamp say to *your* class? Make puppets of them. Then, with a partner, make up things for them to say.

Make a Poster

Wanted: Miss Viola Swamp

Help Detective McSmogg find Miss Viola Swamp. Create a "Wanted" poster. Be sure to include a picture of her and a description of the way she acts.

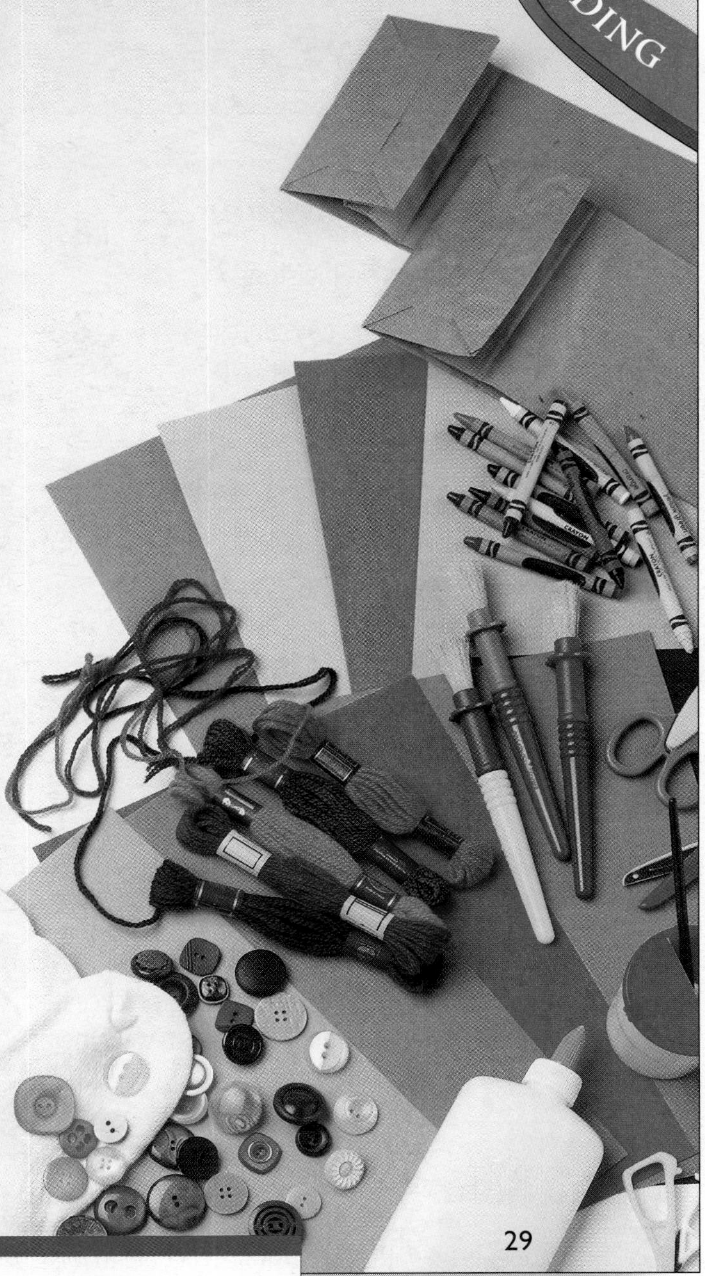

29

Responding Activities

Personal Response

Have students write about and/or draw their favorite part of the story.

Anthology Activities

Students can choose one of the activities on page 29 to do alone or with a partner.

QuickREFERENCE

Home Connection

Have students interview someone older at home to find out who their best teacher was and what he or she was like. Encourage students to share and discuss their findings.

MEETING INDIVIDUAL NEEDS

Student Acquiring English

Invite students to use the puppets made in "Settle Down, Class!" to retell the story.

Informal Assessment

Use students' responses to assess general understanding of the story. If you need more information about each student's comprehension, have them individually retell the story. See the *Teacher's Assessment Handbook*.

Interact *with* Literature

Responding

Comprehension Check

Use *Literacy Activity Book* page 3 and/or the following questions to check comprehension:

1. Who comes to take Miss Nelson's place? (Miss Viola Swamp)
2. Why did someone come to take Miss Nelson's place? (The class was misbehaving and they didn't appreciate Miss Nelson.)
3. Who do you think Miss Swamp was? Why? (Sample: Miss Nelson. She had an ugly black dress and a wig in her closet.)

Literacy Activity Book, p. 3

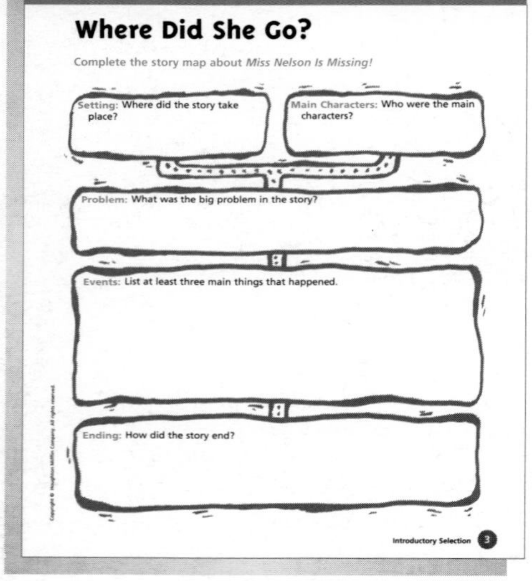

Where Did She Go?

Complete the story map about *Miss Nelson Is Missing!*

Setting: Where did the story take place?

Main Characters: Who were the main characters?

Problem: What was the big problem in the story?

Events: List at least three main things that happened.

Ending: How did the story end?

Introductory Selection 3

Portfolio Opportunity

- For a record of selection comprehension, save *Literacy Activity Book* page 3.
- For a writing sample, save students' personal response.

More Choices for Responding

Literature Discussion

- What surprised you in the story?
- What do you think the boys and girls learned from their encounter with Miss Viola Swamp?
- Have you ever had a teacher like Miss Nelson? Have you had one like Miss Viola Swamp? Describe them.
- What other things could Miss Nelson have tried to get her class to behave better? If you were a student in her class, what could you have done to get your classmates to behave better?

Making a Mural

Invite interested students to make "before and after" murals depicting scenes from the story. You might suggest murals showing

- the kids in Room 207 before and after Miss Viola Swamp's visit
- Miss Nelson before and after transforming herself into Miss Viola Swamp

Students Acquiring English Students can refer to the murals to help them retell the story orally.

Putting On a Skit

Have students work in small groups to develop and perform a skit for *Miss Nelson Is Missing!* Encourage students to practice their skits several times. They might want to invite another class to view their performances.

The Return of Miss Viola Swamp

Invite students to write and illustrate a sequel to *Miss Nelson Is Missing!* If students have difficulty getting started, you might propose the following scenarios:

- Detective McSmogg is missing and Miss Viola Swamp takes over his job.
- Miss Viola Swamp becomes principal at the school.

Afterward, students may enjoy reading the two sequels produced by the team of Harry Allard and James Marshall, *Miss Nelson Is Back* and *Miss Nelson Has a Field Day.*

Reading-Writing Workshop

A CLASS BOOK

About the Workshop

The Reading-Writing Workshops throughout *Invitations to Literacy* are designed to help you guide students through a writing project, using the writing process. Within the guidelines of each workshop, students can develop writing on topics of their own choosing. Minilessons offer brief, point-of-use instruction on specific writing techniques or elements. In this introductory workshop, students write and publish a class book about themselves. The minilessons focus on the stages of the writing process to build background on the process approach.

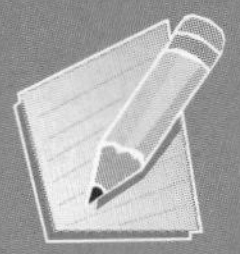

In this and other workshops, keep these points in mind:

- **Writing Process**
Encourage students to use the writing process as a guide, not as a rigid sequence of steps.
- **Selecting Topics**
Give students freedom to select their own topics. Each workshop suggests ways for them to think of topics they want to write about.
- **Switching Topics**
Allow students to abandon an unsatisfying or frustrating piece and begin again, switching topics or using a different technique.
- **Work Environment**
Provide a comfortable atmosphere for students to work at their own pace.
- **Minilessons**
Use minilessons as needed for whole-class or small-group instruction.
- **Peer Support**
Encourage students to help each other throughout the process, especially in peer conferences.
- **Publishing**
Celebrate students' writing by providing many different opportunities for publishing and sharing.
- **Independent Writing**
Provide time each day for students to write independently, as well as time to continue their workshop activities.

Connecting to *Miss Nelson Is Missing!*

Ask students what new children in school might have thought of Miss Nelson's class at the beginning of the story. Have them list ways that students new to a school can get to know their classmates. What suggestions do they have for ways that all students in a class can get to know each other and their teacher at the start of a new school year?

Reading-Writing Workshop
A Class Book

Warm-Up
Shared Writing

Brainstorm with students a list of things they would like to know about each other and about you. Suggestions may include such things as names, birthdays, interests, favorite things, and after-school activities. Record responses on the chalkboard. Guide students to see that writing a class book would be a good way to put all the information together.

Prewriting

LAB, pp. 4, 5

Choose a Topic

Students narrow their topic choices and select their own topics.

- **Narrow the Choices** Using the brainstorm list, discuss parts students will include on their page. Then invite students to choose one additional topic. Encourage them to choose a topic that they think is important for others to know about them.
- **Talk and Think About It** Have partners explore their topic choices, answering these questions about each one: Why do I want to write about this topic? Is this important for others to know about me?
- **Settle on a Topic** Bring the class back together to finalize their choices.

Help with Topics

Class Clown?

Encourage students to think about whether they will tell something funny or something serious about themselves. Discuss how this might affect what they write.

Topics for Two

MEETING INDIVIDUAL NEEDS

Students Acquiring English
Some students may benefit from working with a partner to gain needed vocabulary to write about particular topics.

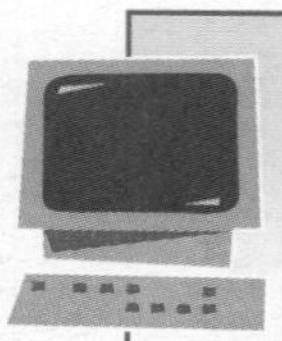

Students can use The Learning Company's new elementary writing center to brainstorm and organize their ideas.

Prewriting *(continued)*

Plan Your Writing

Students plan their page of the book, listing and organizing their ideas.

- **Main Ideas and Details** Encourage students to jot down their main ideas, leaving plenty of space between them. Under each idea, have them note smaller ideas that go with it – reasons, examples, and details.

Help with Planning

Cut and Paste

Students can cut their lists apart and tape them in a new order.

TECH TIPS Students using a word processor can use the Cut and Paste features to reorganize ideas.

What Order Works?

Help students think of how to put their ideas in the best order. For example, talk about how they might organize a description of themselves or a family member.

Literacy Activity Book, p. 4

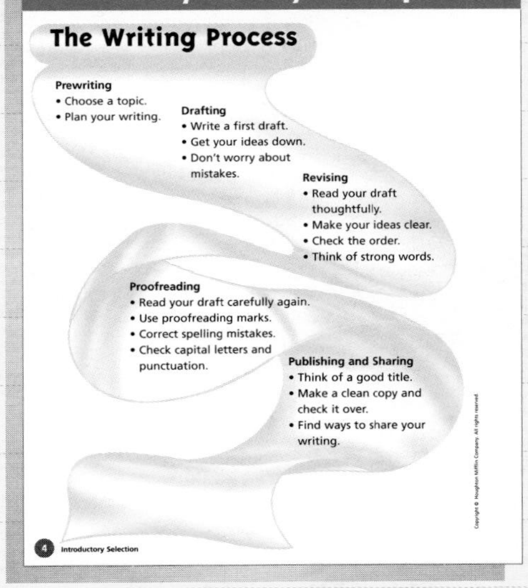

The Writing Process

Prewriting
- Choose a topic.
- Plan your writing.

Drafting
- Write a first draft.
- Get your ideas down.
- Don't worry about mistakes.

Revising
- Read your draft thoughtfully.
- Make your ideas clear.
- Check the order.
- Think of strong words.

Proofreading
- Read your draft carefully again.
- Use proofreading marks.
- Correct spelling mistakes.
- Check capital letters and punctuation.

Publishing and Sharing
- Think of a good title.
- Make a clean copy and check it over.
- Find ways to share your writing.

4 Introductory Selection

Literacy Activity Book, p. 5

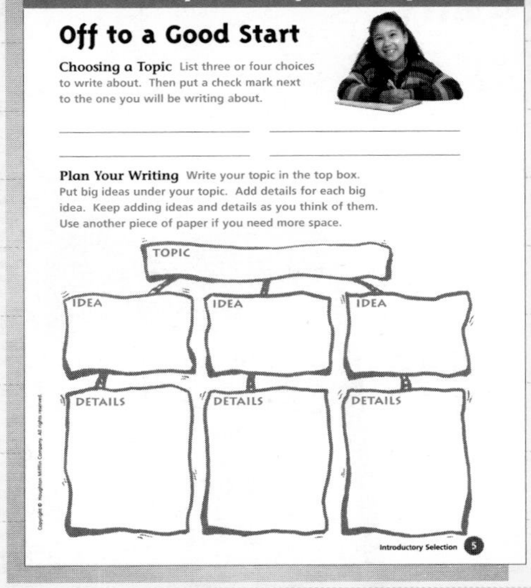

Off to a Good Start

Choosing a Topic List three or four choices to write about. Then put a check mark next to the one you will be writing about.

Plan Your Writing Write your topic in the top box. Put big ideas under your topic. Add details for each big idea. Keep adding ideas and details as you think of them. Use another piece of paper if you need more space.

TOPIC

IDEA / IDEA / IDEA

DETAILS / DETAILS / DETAILS

Introductory Selection 5

MINILESSON

Prewriting

LAB, p. 4

Use *Literacy Activity Book* page 4 to review the writing process with students. Encourage them to use this page as a reminder not to try to do everything at once.

Now have students discuss how to get started writing. Elicit that a good topic is one you're interested in, know something about, or want to learn about. Ask how to get topic ideas:

- brainstorm
- make lists
- look at journal or photo album
- answer a partner's questions
- make a cluster or web of experiences and interests

You may want to model one of the prewriting strategies for your page of the class book.

Next, discuss what to do with a topic once it's chosen.

- list ideas and details
- make a cluster or web
- think about a good order
- draw a picture

Continue modeling your own prewriting. Emphasize to students that there isn't a right or wrong method. Encourage them to try different ways to see what works best for them and their topic.

Reading-Writing Workshop *(continued)*

A Class Book

MINILESSON

Drafting

Ask students to compare two ways of taking a trip: (1) using a map and knowing where you're headed; and (2) just starting off, with no map or plan. Compare prewriting with planning a trip. With a plan, writing a first draft should go smoothly.

Be sure students understand the term *first draft.* Emphasize the word *first* and that drafting is simply getting ideas into words and onto paper. Assure them they'll have plenty of time to make changes and corrections later.

Give students these guidelines for writing a first draft:

- Think about your purpose and who your readers will be.
- Write down your ideas as quickly as you can.
- Don't worry if your paper is messy.
- Don't worry about spelling or punctuation. You can fix them later.

Discuss with students what to do if they get stuck during drafting. Remind them to do more prewriting for additional ideas or details.

Self-Assessment

Have students evaluate their book page, using the Revising Checklist on *Literacy Activity Book* page 6.

Drafting

Students use their prewriting notes to write a first draft.

- **Getting Ideas Down** Remind students that the purpose of a first draft is to get ideas on paper. They shouldn't worry about mistakes now.

Help with Drafting

Tips for Drafting

Urge students to write on every other line. Writing on only one side of their paper will allow them to cut and paste during revising, if they wish.

Keep On Writing!

MEETING INDIVIDUAL NEEDS

Students Acquiring English Encourage students to keep writing, even if they're unsure about how to say something. Invite them to ask questions when they need to.

Revising

LAB, p. 6

Students revise their drafts and discuss them in writing conferences.

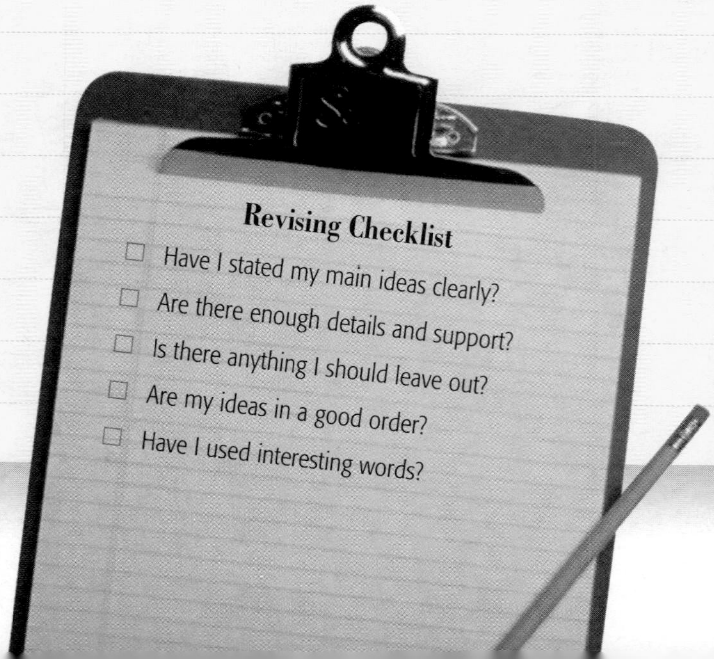
Revising Checklist
☐ Have I stated my main ideas clearly?
☐ Are there enough details and support?
☐ Is there anything I should leave out?
☐ Are my ideas in a good order?
☐ Have I used interesting words?

Revising *(continued)*

Writing Conference

Cooperative Learning Have students read aloud their revised draft and discuss it with you or a classmate. When they've listened to a partner's writing, they can use questions such as these, which appear on *Literacy Activity Book* page 6. You may need to modify the questions so that they are specific to the writing your students are doing.

Questions for a Writing Conference

- What is the best thing about this piece?
- Does it stay on the topic?
- Does it seem well organized?
- Does it help me get to know this person?
- What additional information would a new friend like to have?
- Does it end in a strong way?

Help with Revising

Mark It Up!

Ask students to cross out and write new words in the space above instead of erasing.

Conference Cues

Remind students to be positive and helpful in their writing conferences. Encourage them to ask one another questions and make suggestions.

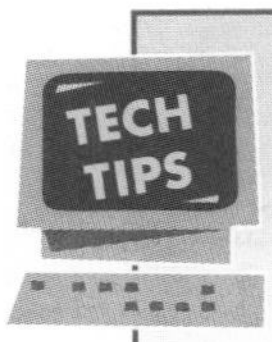
TECH TIPS

Students writing at a computer may find it helpful to read their draft on a printout. They can cut and paste either on paper or on the computer.

MINILESSON

Revising

Provide a sample of writing from your own draft page for the class book. Be sure that your sample is in first draft form, with obvious need for revision.

Ask volunteers to suggest ways you could revise your writing. Model how to use questions from the revising checklist as you work through the sample. Encourage students to think of interesting words and to point out where additional details would help.

Using students' suggestions, model how to revise by using arrows and crossing out words. Have a volunteer read the revision aloud. Elicit that the writing is clearer. Discuss that revising is a way to help readers know what the writer really means.

Literacy Activity Book, p. 6

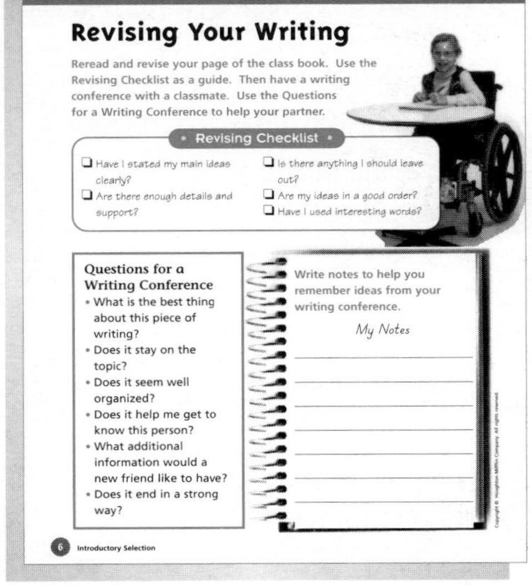

Revising Your Writing

Reread and revise your page of the class book. Use the Revising Checklist as a guide. Then have a writing conference with a classmate. Use the Questions for a Writing Conference to help your partner.

Revising Checklist

- ❑ Have I stated my main ideas clearly?
- ❑ Are there enough details and support?
- ❑ Is there anything I should leave out?
- ❑ Are my ideas in a good order?
- ❑ Have I used interesting words?

Questions for a Writing Conference
- What is the best thing about this piece of writing?
- Does it stay on the topic?
- Does it seem well organized?
- Does it help me get to know this person?
- What additional information would a new friend like to have?
- Does it end in a strong way?

Write notes to help you remember ideas from your writing conference.

My Notes

6 Introductory Selection

Reading-Writing Workshop *(continued)*
A Class Book

MINILESSON

Proofreading

Congratulate students on their revised drafts. Tell them that now is the time to check for mistakes in spelling, capital letters, and punctuation marks. Elicit that correcting mistakes will make their reader's job easier and more pleasant.

Review proofreading marks with students. They can refer to the list in the Handbook at the back of the *Literacy Activity Book*. Write these marks on the chalkboard:

- ¶ Indent new paragraph
- ∧ Add something
- ℘ Take out something
- ≡ Capitalize
- / Make lowercase letter

Next, write these sentences on the chalkboard without the corrections.

i enjoy teaching because. I make so many knew Friends.

Then ask volunteers to use proofreading marks and make corrections at the board.

Proofreading

Students proofread their revised drafts, correcting errors in spelling, capitalization, and punctuation.

Grammar and Spelling Connections

- **Checking Sentences** Remind students to be sure each sentence begins with a capital letter and ends with the right punctuation.
- **Special Nouns** Have students check that special names of people and places begin with capital letters.
- **Spelling** Have them check each word for spelling, especially words with *-ed* and *-ing* endings.

Help with Proofreading

Proofreading Marks

Refer students to the proofreading marks in the Handbook at the back of the *Literacy Activity Book*. They may need to practice making paragraph symbols and delete marks.

Using a Checklist

A proofreading checklist is in the Handbook at the back of the *Literacy Activity Book.* Encourage students to add to the checklist as they find mistakes in their own writing.

Checking It Twice

Urge students to proofread their writing more than once to be sure of catching everything that needs correction.

Publishing and Sharing

Students make a clean copy of their writing and combine pieces to form a class book.

- Have the class decide on a title and discuss how they want their finished book to appear.
- ***Cooperative Learning*** Invite volunteers to form teams to create a cover design, write a table of contents, and make illustrations for the book.
- Discuss ways of making the book available to new students, classroom visitors, and parents.

Ideas for Publishing and Sharing

Making Copies

Elicit suggestions and volunteers for making multiple copies of the book. Volunteers might photocopy the inside pages and have each student make a cover for one of the copies.

Showing It Off

Have students suggest ways to share their book with readers beyond their own classroom.

Open House

If your school holds a parents night or an open house, copies of the class book might be distributed.

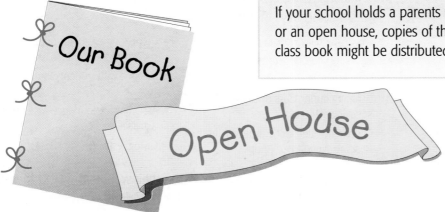
Our Book
Open House

MINILESSON

Publishing and Sharing

- Ask a volunteer what the word *publish* means. Invite students to list things that are published. Use the classroom as a starting point, but also include real-world publications, such as newspapers, magazines, newsletters, posters, brochures, and calendars, along with many kinds of books.
- Review with students the list of people who might use their class book. Remind them that all their hard work has a purpose when they share it.
- Invite students to suggest other kinds of writing they may do this year and the ways they can share their writing with readers beyond the classroom.

Portfolio Opportunity

You may wish to save students' writing as an example of their written work early in the year. You might attach their notes and drafts to indicate their use of the writing process.

Selection Wrap-Up

Managing Assessment

Portfolios

Question: How can I get students interested in portfolios?

Answer: Try these suggestions:

- If possible, share an example of a portfolio from another class or a previous year. Model for students how you might evaluate the contents:
  1. Compare two pieces of writing from different times during the year. Point out ways in which the student's work improved over time.
  2. Discuss a piece of work the student selected for inclusion in the portfolio. Point out what it shows about the student's interests and strengths.
- Explain that a portfolio includes many different samples of a student's work. Discuss how a variety of work samples provides a better picture of student's growth than, for example, a single test score.
- Note that during the first theme students will make collection folders to hold all their work, and that later they will take part in selecting samples of their work to be put in their portfolios.

ASSESSMENT

Reflecting/Self-Assessment

Ask students how well they did during the reading of *Miss Nelson Is Missing!* Use prompts such as these to help them think about their work:

- How well did you understand the story?
- How did you use strategies to help your reading?
- What worked well in your writing? What worked less well?
- How much did you take part in class discussions?

Have students copy and fill in the graphic organizer below. Help individuals identify strengths and areas for improvement.

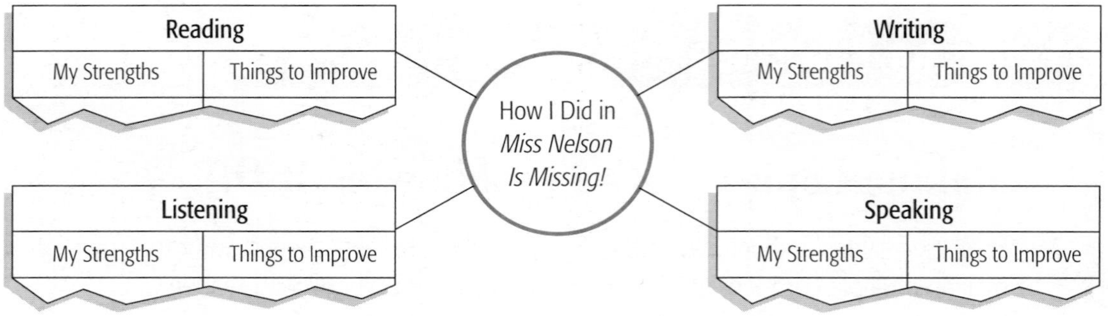
Reading
My Strengths
Things to Improve
Writing
My Strengths
Things to Improve
How I Did in Miss Nelson Is Missing!
Listening
My Strengths
Things to Improve
Speaking
My Strengths
Things to Improve

Discussing Literacy Assessment

Explain to students that during the year you and they will use many ways to evaluate their growth as readers, writers, speakers, and listeners. List some of these ways on the board:

- Observing daily work in class
- Checking *Literacy Activity Book* pages
- Listening as students read aloud
- Listening during class discussions and speaking activities
- Checking written work, especially from Reading-Writing Workshops
- Comparing examples of past and present work
- Meeting with students to discuss their work
- Assigning Performance Assessment activities
- Giving tests

Note that they will be saving samples of their work throughout the year. Invite them to save one piece of work they did during *Miss Nelson Is Missing!* Talk with students about creating collection folders and portfolios to hold their work. (See Managing Assessment note on left.)

Oink, Oink, Oink

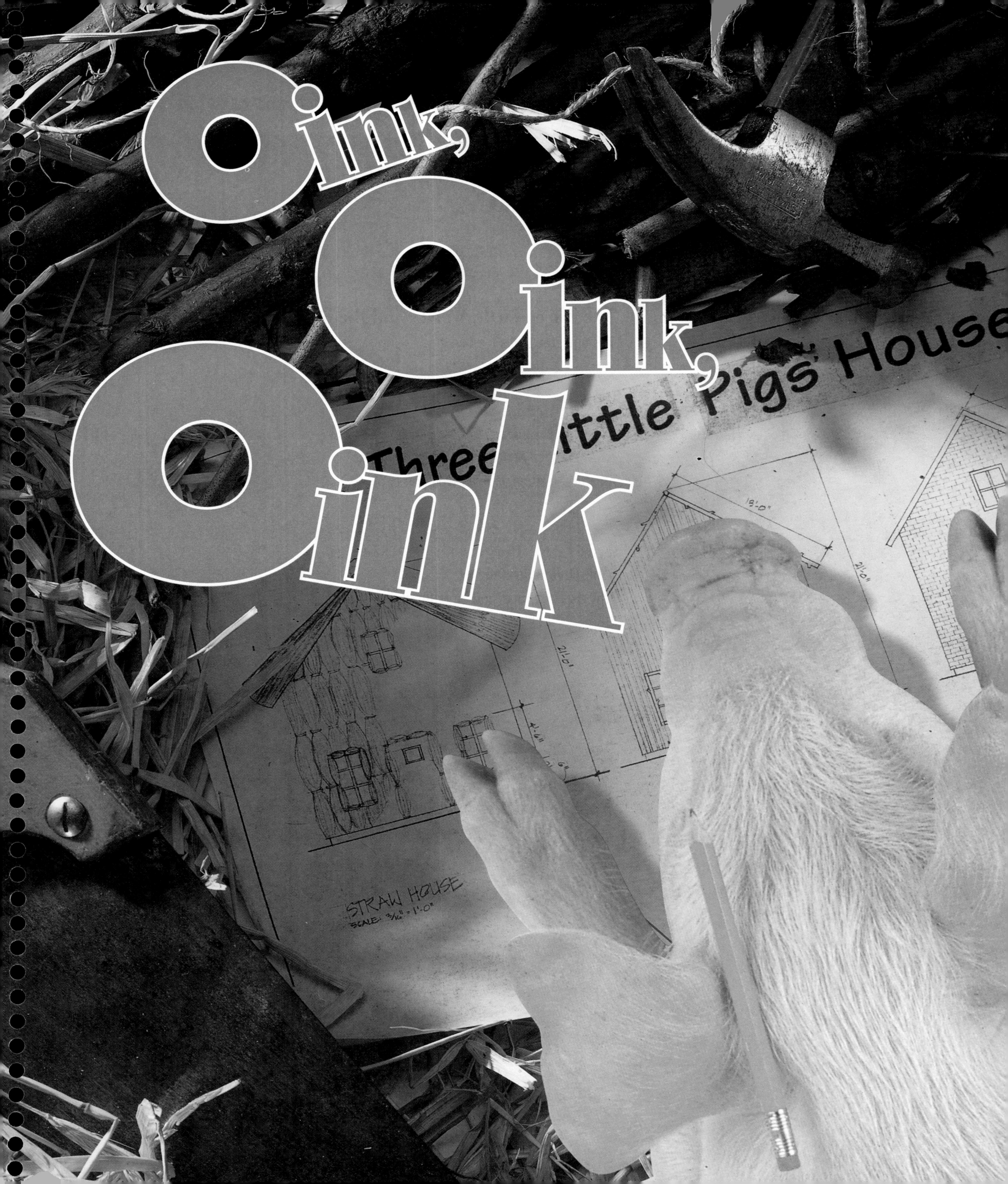

Three Little Pigs' House
STRAW HOUSE
SCALE: 3/16" = 1'-0"

Table of Contents

THEME: Oink, Oink, Oink

Anthology

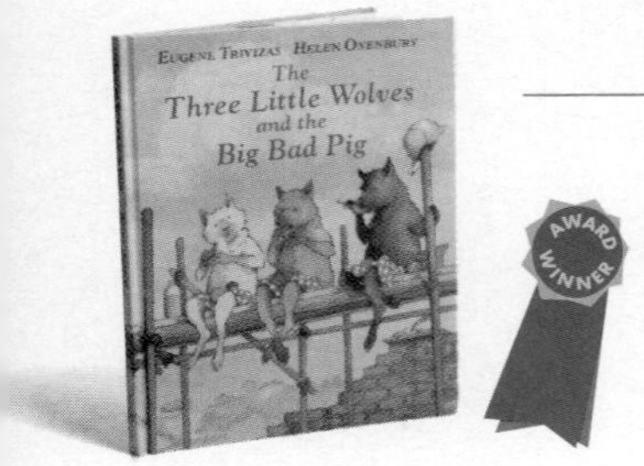

The Three Little Wolves and the Big Bad Pig
AWARD WINNER

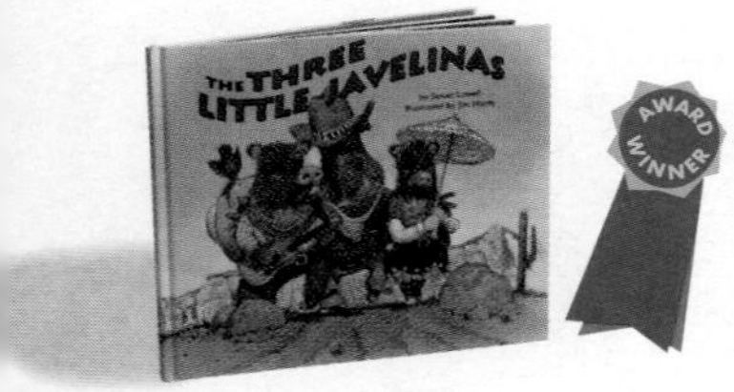

THE THREE LITTLE JAVELINAS
AWARD WINNER

PAPERBACK **PLUS**

EASY

Sidney Rella and the Glass Sneaker

When Sidney wants to be a football star, his fairy godfather helps out.

In the same book . . .
The original "Cinderella," plus a photo guessing game to keep you on your toes.

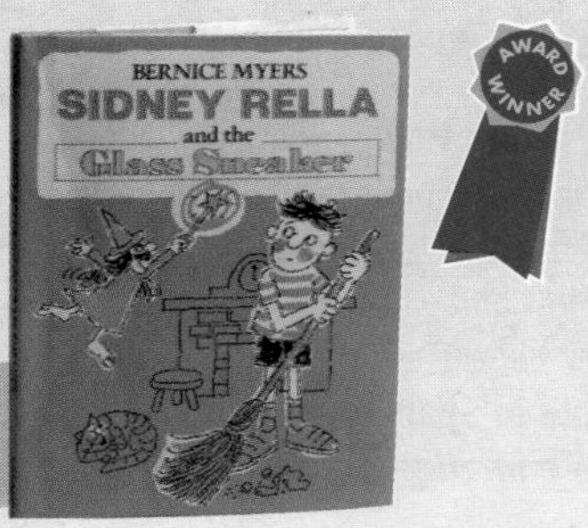
BERNICE MYERS
SIDNEY RELLA
and the
Glass Sneaker
AWARD WINNER

Best Books for Children

written and illustrated by Bernice Myers

AVERAGE/CHALLENGING

Sleeping Ugly

Plain Jane's no beauty. Will the prince awaken her?

In the same book . . .
The unfractured version, plus some tired old jokes.

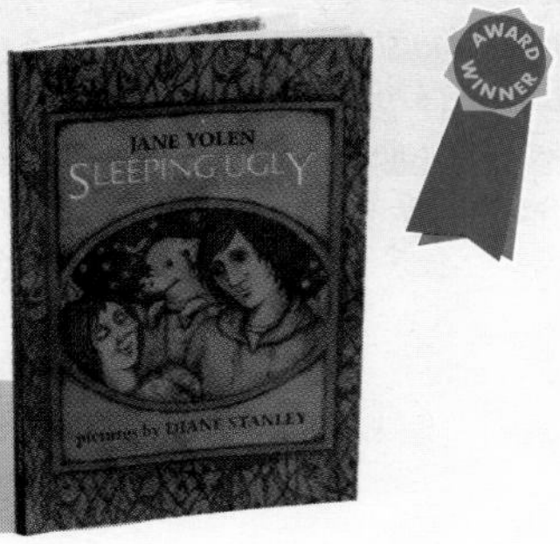
JANE YOLEN
SLEEPING UGLY
pictures by DIANE STANLEY
AWARD WINNER

Best Books for Children

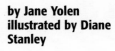

by Jane Yolen
illustrated by Diane Stanley

Bibliography

Books for Independent Reading

- *Multicultural*
- *Science/Health*
- *Math*
- *Social Studies*
- *Music*
- *Art*

VERY EASY

Pig
by Mary Ling
Dorling 1993 (24p)
The growth of a pig from birth to adulthood.

Rockabye, Crocodile
by Jose Aruego and Ariane Dewey Greenwillow 1988 (32p) 1993 paper
A Philippine fable about two boars who learn how attitude determines success.

Pigs From 1 to 10
by Arthur Geisert
Houghton 1992 (32p)
Readers search for hidden numerals in this story about 10 piglet brothers.

Pigs From A to Z
by Arthur Geisert
Houghton 1986 (32p)
Readers must find the letters hidden in Geisert's illustrations.

Smart, Clean Pigs
by Allan Fowler
Childrens 1993 (32p) paper
How and where pigs live and why they behave as they do. **Available in Spanish as *Los limpios e inteligentes cerdos.***

Somebody and the Three Blairs
by Marilyn Tolhurst
Orchard 1991 (32p) 1994 paper
In a reversal of roles, a bear visits the home of three humans.

EASY

All Pigs Are Beautiful
by Dick King-Smith
Candlewick 1993 (32p)
A famous author tells why he loves pigs.

Pigs Will Be Pigs
by Amy Axelrod
Four Winds 1994 (32p)
The Pigs search their house for money to eat out. Menu and prices included.

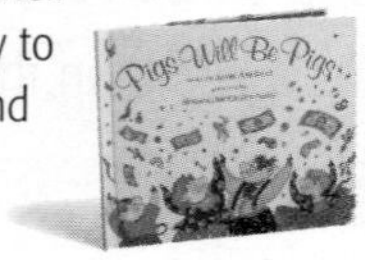
Pigs Will Be Pigs

The Fourth Little Pig
by Teresa Celsi
Raintree 1990 (24p) paper
A visit from their sister changes the three little pigs' attitude.

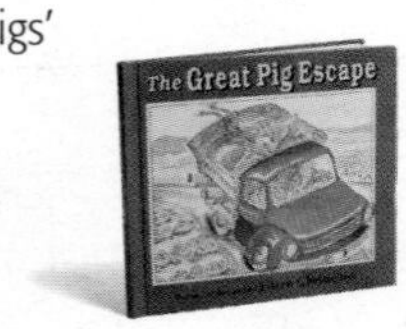
The Great Pig Escape

The Great Pig Escape
by Eileen Christelow
Clarion 1994 (32p)
Pigs on their way to the market escape to Florida.

Pigs Aplenty, Pigs Galore!
by David McPhail
Dutton 1993 (32p)
As the narrator tries to read, several pigs wreak havoc in his home.

Mrs. Goat and Her Seven Little Kids
by Tony Ross
Atheneum 1990 (32p)
A cheerful, satirical updating of the well-known Grimm classic.

Cinder Edna
by Ellen Jackson
Lothrop 1994 (32p)
Cinderella could learn something from her feisty neighbor, Cinder Edna.

Piggybook
by Anthony Browne
Knopf 1986 (32p)
Mrs. Piggot's husband and sons are such "pigs."

Pigsty
by Mark Teague
Scholastic 1994 (32p)
Wendell Fultz's room looks like a pigsty, so several pigs move in.

The Gruff Brothers
by William Hooks
Bantam 1990 (32p) paper
A new twist to the Three Billy Goats Gruff.

The Pigs' Wedding
by Helme Heine
McElderry 1988 (32p) 1991 paper
Curlytail and Porker get married and have a wild wedding reception.

Los tres lobitos y el cochino feroz (The Three Little Wolves and the Big Bad Pig)
by Eugene Trivizas
Text in Spanish.

AVERAGE

The True Story of the Three Little Pigs
by Jon Scieszka
Viking
1991 (32p)

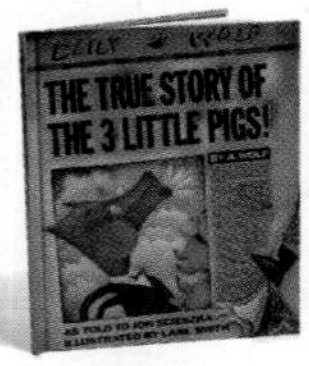
THE TRUE STORY OF THE 3 LITTLE PIGS!

A. Wolf gives his version of what really happened in the famous tale. **Available in Spanish as *La verdadera historia de los tres cerditos.***

The Tortoise and the Jackrabbit
by Susan Lowell
Chronicle 1994 (32p)
A humorous retelling set in the Southwest.

Princess Furball
by Charlotte Huck
Greenwillow 1989 (40p) also paper
A strong-willed princess overcomes many obstacles in this Cinderella variant.

Tales of Amanda Pig
by Jean Van Leeuwen
Dial 1982 (56p) Puffin 1994 paper
Five stories about Amanda Pig and her brother Oliver. **Available in Spanish as *Cuentos de la cerdita Amanda.*** See others in series.

Piggins
by Jane Yolen
Harcourt 1987 (32p) 1992 paper
Piggins, the very proper butler, keeps things running smoothly. See others in series.

The Frog Prince, Continued
by Jon Scieszka
Viking 1991 (32p) Puffin 1994 paper
The honeymoon is over for the princess and the frog.

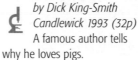

The Amazing Bone
by William Steig
Farrar 1983 (32p) 1993 paper
Pearl the pig needs help outwitting robbers *and* a hungry fox.
Available in Spanish as *El hueso prodigioso.*

Wild Boars
by Daniel Nicholson
Carolrhoda 1987 (48p)
A photo essay about the pig's wild relative.

The Three Little Pigs and the Fox
by William Hooks
Macmillan 1989 (32p)
Appalachian variant

Garth Pig Steals the Show
by Mary Rayner
Dutton 1993 (32p)
More hilarious adventures of Garth Pig and the Pig family band. See others in series.

Cinder-Elly
by Frances Minters
Viking 1994 (32p)
Cinder-Elly stays home while her sisters attend a basketball game in this urban retelling.

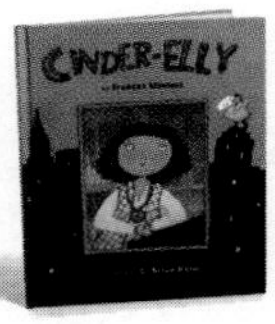
CINDER-ELLY

Parents in the Pigpen, Pigs in the Tub
by Amy Ehrlich
Dial 1993 (40p)
When the pasture gate is left open, farm animals move into the house.

Piggies, Piggies, Piggies: A Treasury of Stories, Songs, and Poems
by Walter Retan
Simon 1993 (96p)
An assortment of selections, some illustrated, about pigs.

Peeping Beauty
by Mary Jane Auch
Holiday 1993 (32p)
Poulette Pig wants to become a ballerina, but the fox has other ideas.

Ruthann and Her Pig
by Barbara Ann Porte
Orchard 1989 (84p)
Ruthann's cousin Frank wants to borrow her pet pig for protection from bullies.

Hooray for the Golly Sisters
by Betsy Byars
Harper 1990 (64p)
Sisters May-May and Rose share adventures that include disappearing pigs.

Dear Peter Rabbit
by Alma Flor Ada
Atheneum 1994 (32p)
Peter Rabbit, Goldilocks, Red Riding Hood, and friends exchange letters.
Available in Spanish as *Querido Pedrín.*

Chester the Worldly Pig
by Bill Peet
Houghton 1978 paper
When Chester joins the circus, he quickly learns that farm life isn't so bad.

CHALLENGING

Quentin Corn
by Mary Stolz
Godine 1985 (128p)
Learning he will soon become a meal, Quentin disguises himself and runs away.

King Emmett the Second
by Mary Stolz
Greenwillow 1991 (56p)
Emmett Murphy moves from New York to Ohio and misses his friends, especially his pet pig.

Pigs Might Fly
by Dick King-Smith
Viking 1982 (158p)
Daggie Dogfoot, a runt piglet with a deformity, becomes the hero of the farm.

Farmer Palmer's Wagon Ride
by William Steig
Farrar 1974 (32p) 1992 paper
Farmer Palmer's return trip from the market is full of obstacles.

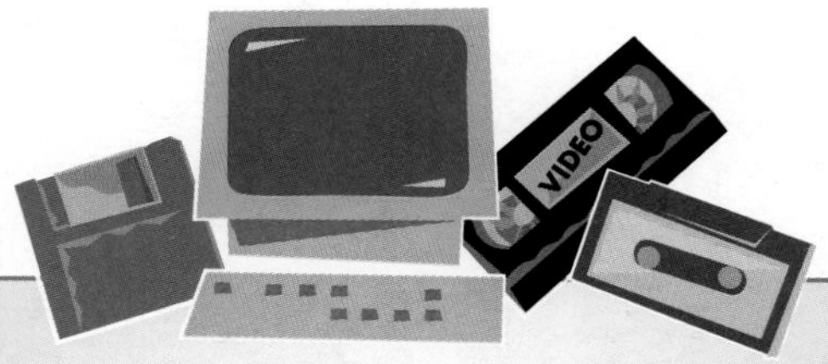
VIDEO

Technology Resources

Software

Great Start™ Macintosh or Windows CD-ROM software. Includes story summaries, background building, and vocabulary support for each selection in the theme. Houghton Mifflin Company.

Channel R.E.A.D. Videodiscs "License to Drive" and "The Ordinary Princess." Houghton Mifflin Company.

Writing Software The Learning Company's new elementary writing center. Macintosh or Windows software. The Learning Company®.

Internet See the Houghton Mifflin Internet resources for additional bibliographic entries and theme-related activities.

Teacher's Resource Disk Macintosh or Windows software. Houghton Mifflin Company.

Video Cassettes

Princess Furball, *by Charlotte Huck. Weston Woods*

The Three Little Pigs, *by James Marshall. Weston Woods*

The Pigs' Wedding, *by Helme Heine. Weston Woods*

The Pigs' Picnic, by Keiko Kasza. Amer. Sch. Pub.

The Amazing Bone, by William Steig. Weston Woods

Audio Cassettes

Princess Furball, *by Charlotte Huck. Weston Woods*

The Three Little Pigs, *by James Marshall. Weston Woods*

The Pigs' Wedding, by Helme Heine. Weston Woods

The True Story of the Three Little Pigs, *by Jon Scieszka. Viking*

Audio Tapes for Oink, Oink, Oink. Houghton Mifflin Company.

AV addresses are on pages H7–H8.

Books for Teacher Read Aloud

Zeke Pippin
by William Steig
Harper 1994 (32p)
When Zeke the pig plays his harmonica, everyone falls asleep.

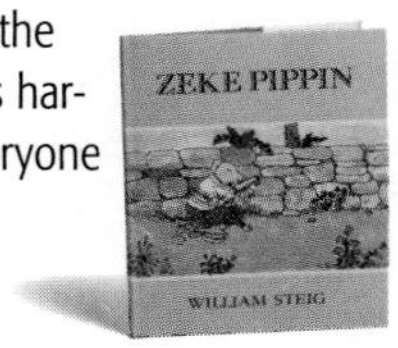
ZEKE PIPPIN
WILLIAM STEIG

That Extraordinary Pig of Paris
by Roni Schotter
Philomel 1994 (32p)
Monsieur Cochôn, a pig in Paris, has quite a day when he gets too close to a pastry shop.

Mrs. Pig Gets Cross
by Mary Rayner
Dutton 1986 (64p)
Seven short stories about Mr. and Mrs. Pig and their ten children.

Theme at a Glance

	Reading		Writing and Language Arts	
Selections	**Comprehension Skills and Strategies**	**Word Skills**	**Responding**	**Writing**
The Three Little Wolves and the Big Bad Pig	Genre: Fantasy, 41 ✓ Summarizing: Story Structure, 45, 60B–60C Making Judgments, 47 Fantasy/Realism, 57 Reading Strategies, 38, 44, 48, 50	✓ Base Words, 60F–60G Short Vowels, 60G	Personal Response, 60 Anthology Activities, 60 Home Connection, 60 Literature Discussion, 60A Selection Connection, 60A	Character Role Reversal, 59 ✓ Writing a Sentence, 60D
What's Up, Pup?	Making Comparisons, 60P			Narrative Nonfiction, 61
This Little Piggy!	Predict/Infer, 64		Home Connection, 66	
The Three Little Javelinas	✓ Compare and Contrast, 75, 88B–88C Predicting Outcomes, 79 Summarizing: Story Structure, 83 Reading Strategies, 70, 72, 76, 78, 80, 84	✓ Inflected Endings *-ed* and *-ing,* 88F–88G Long Vowel Pairs and Vowel-Consonant *-e,* 88G	Personal Response, 88 Anthology Activities, 88 Home Connection, 88 Literature Discussion, 88A Selection Connection, 88A	✓ Setting, 85 Writing a Book Report, 88D
My Hairy Neighbors	K-W-L Chart, 88P Photo Essay, 89		Home Connection, 89, 91 Literature Discussion, 90	Author's Voice, 89
The Three Little Hawaiian Pigs and the Magic Shark	✓ Fantasy/Realism, 95, 114B–114C Compare and Contrast, 103 Sequence, 107 Reading Strategies, 94, 98, 100, 108	✓ Using Context, 114F–114G Alphabetical Order, 114G	Personal Response, 114 Anthology Activities, 114 Home Connection, 114 Literature Discussion, 114A Selection Connection, 114A	Anthropomorphism, 97 ✓ Combining Sentences: Compound Sentences, 114D
Pigs	Reading a Poem, 114P		Home Connection, 115	
Reading-Writing Workshop **Be a Writer: Surprise, Surprise**				**Reading-Writing Workshop** A Story, 116–117F; Workshop Minilessons: Characters and Setting, 117A; Beginning, Middle, and End, 117B; Dialogue, 117C
The Wild Boar & the Fox	Genre: Plays, 119			

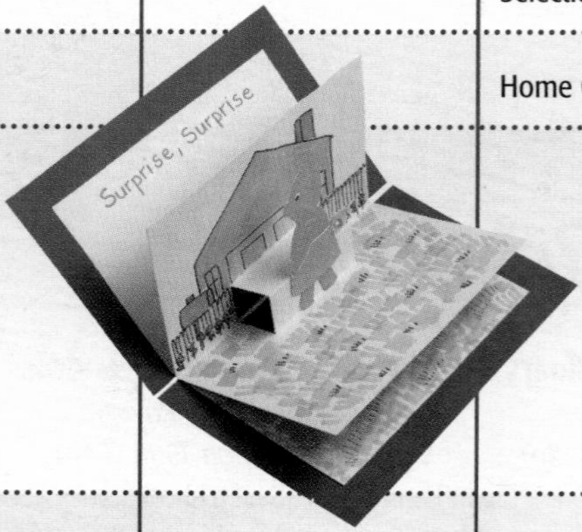
Surprise, Surprise

✓ ***Indicates Tested Skills.*** *See page 34F for assessment options.*

Theme Concept

Traditional stories can be retold in a variety of humorous, altered versions.

Pacing

This theme is designed to take 4 to 6 weeks, depending on your students' needs.

Multi-Age Classroom

Related theme from:
Grade 2 – Tell Me a Tale
Grade 4 – Super Sleuths

Cross-Curricular

Spelling	Grammar, Usage and Mechanics	Listening and Speaking	Viewing	Study Skills	Content Area
✓ Short Vowels, 60I	✓ Subjects and Predicates, 60J–60K	Storytelling, 60L Interviewing the Big Bad Pig, 60L	Watching a Video, 60M Using Facial Expressions and Body Language, 60M Examining Real Wolves and Pigs, 60M		**Science:** Careers in Construction, Tools of the Trade, Building Your School, Looking at Blueprints, 60N **Math:** Playing a Huff and Puff Game, 60O **Dance:** Dancing the Tarantella, 60O
				✓ Taking Notes, 63	
				K-W-L, 65	**Science:** Animal Myths, 67 **Health:** Staying Cool, 67 **Social Studies:** Finding Habitats, 67
✓ Vowel-Consonant -*e*, 88I	✓ Correcting Run-on Sentences, 88J–88K	Listening to a Poetic Picture, 88L Building a Language Tree, 88L Hearing a Range of Sounds, 88M	Watching a Video of Desert Life, 88M Taking a Walking Tour, 88M		**Science:** Making a Desert Terrarium, Exploring the Saguaro Cactus, 88N **Art:** Designing Outfits, 88O **Math:** Graphing Desert Weather, 88O
					Math: A Javelina's Height, 91 **Science:** Omnivorous Animals, 91
✓ Long *a* and Long *e*, 114I	✓ Kinds of Sentences, 114J–114K	Literature Discussion Guidelines, 114L Hawaiian Music, 114L	A Game of Disguise, 114M Let's Visit Hawaii, 114M Hula Hands, 114M		**Social Studies:** Discovering Tropical Fruits, Making a Relief Map of Hawaii, 114N **Science:** Collecting Shark Facts, Making a Food Chain Mobile, 114O
		Reading a Poem, 114P			
					Social Studies: Symbols, 115; **Music:** Song, 115 **Art:** Class Book, 115
		Reading a Play, 118			

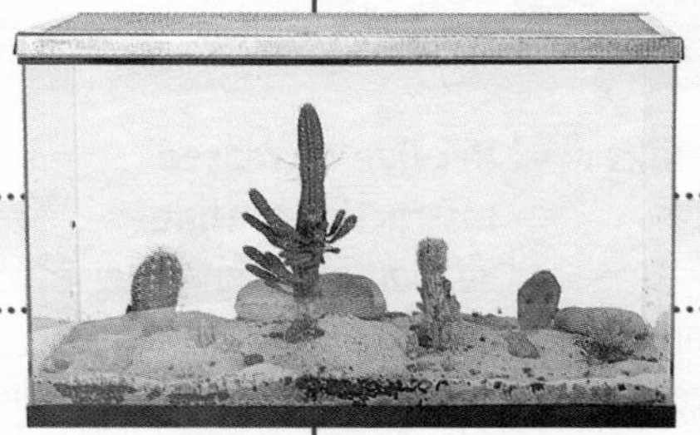

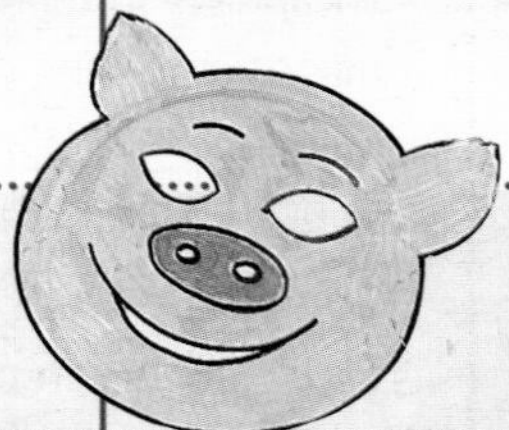

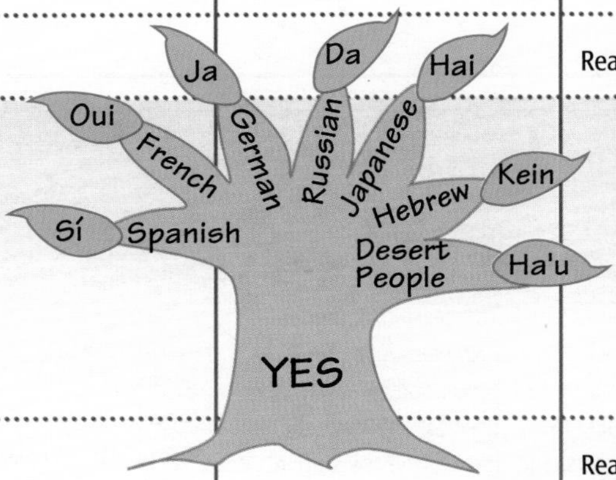
Ja
Da
Hai
Oui
French
German
Russian
Japanese
Kein
Hebrew
Sí
Spanish
Desert People
Ha'u
YES

Meeting Individual Needs

Key to Meeting Individual Needs

Students Acquiring English

Activities/notes throughout the lesson plans offer strategies to help students understand the selections and lessons.

Challenge

Challenge activities and notes throughout the lesson plans suggest additional activities to stimulate critical and creative thinking.

Extra Support

Activities and notes throughout the book lesson plans offer additional strategies to help students experience success.

During this theme, all students will learn to

- *Recognize when and how a story can be altered for humorous effect*
- *Write a story*
- *Summarize fiction stories*
- *Compare fiction selections by completing a chart*
- *Edit writing with an emphasis on sentence variety*

Students Acquiring English	Challenge	Extra Support
• **Discuss Key Concepts** Support in Advance suggestions help students focus on key concepts through making word wall charts, drawing pictures, and taking an advance look at illustrations.	• **Apply Critical Thinking Skills** Opportunities to apply critical thinking include discussing Spanish influences in the southwestern United States and reading a poem aloud with and without punctuation.	• **Receive Increased Instructional Time** Support in Advance suggestions help students develop background. Skills minilessons allow students to receive small group instruction.
• **Expand Vocabulary** Opportunities for expanding vocabulary include charting definitions and using context clues. Students use graphic organizers to build word knowledge.	• **Analyze the Author's Craft** Students learn how a writer can make a traditional tale fresh by reversing roles or changing settings.	• **Increase Independent Reading** The use of interactive bulletin boards motivates students to read independently after school and at home.
• **Contribute to Group Project** Each student can make creative contributions when they work with others on building a house.	• **Engage in Creative Thinking** Opportunities for creative expression include making blueprints for a house and retelling a traditional folktale.	• **Learn Challenging Material** Completing the Selection Connection chart will help students think critically as they compare selections across a theme.
• **Act as a Resource** Students can draw on their backgrounds to share attitudes and beliefs.	• **Create Environments** Students make relief maps; create desert terrariums; draw blueprints.	

Managing Instruction

Small Group Instruction

For some instructional work, whole class instruction is appropriate; for other lessons, small flexible groups will work better. Use whole class instruction if the content of the lesson will benefit everyone and if the format involves all students. To increase involvement, use cooperative teams and engage students in writing, drawing, or working with graphic organizers.

Additional Resources

Extra Support Handbook
Includes additional theme, skill, and language support for program literature plus strategies for increasing reading fluency and self-selected reading and writing.

Students Acquiring English Handbook
Provides general guidelines, as well as specific strategies and additional instruction for students acquiring English.

Great Start CD-ROM Software
Provides extra support in English and Spanish. Includes story summaries, background building to develop key concepts, and vocabulary support for each selection in the theme.

Writing Software
The Learning Company's new elementary writing center software. Can be used for independent writing activities by students of all ability levels.

Channel R.E.A.D. Videodiscs
- "License to Drive"
- "The Ordinary Princess"

Provides additional instruction in English and Spanish for students needing extra support.

Planning for Assessment

Teaching CHOICES

Informal Assessment

Informal Assessment Checklist

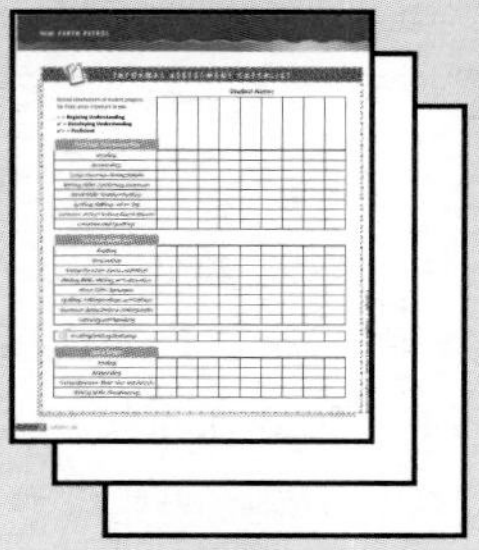

- Reading and Responding
- Summarizing: Story Structure, Compare and Contrast, Fantasy/Realism
- Writing Sentences, Comparison/ Contrast Paragraphs
- Word Skills and Strategies
- Grammar
- Attitudes and Habits

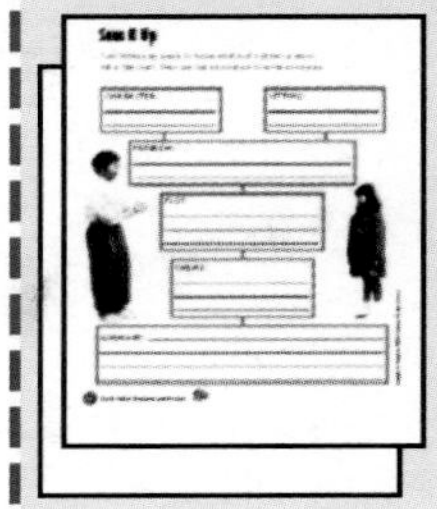

Literacy Activity Book

- Selection Connections, p. 34G
- Comprehension Check, pp. 60A, 88A, 114A
- Comprehension Skills, pp. 60C, 88C, 114C
- Writing Skills, pp. 60E, 88E, 114E
- Word Skills, pp. 60F, 88F, 114F

Reading–Writing Workshop

- Writing a Story, p. 116
- Scoring Rubric, p. 117F

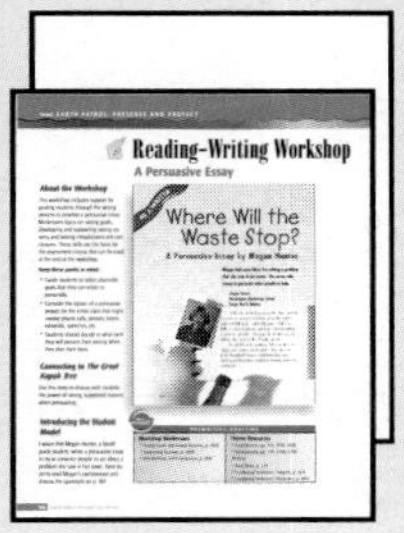
Reading-Writing Workshop
A Persuasive Essay
Where Will the Waste Stop?

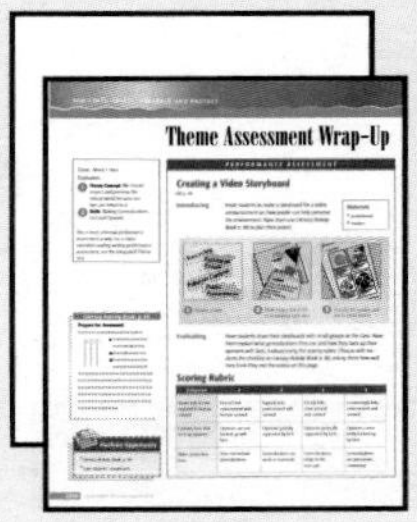
Theme Assessment Wrap-Up

Performance Assessment

- Creating a Story Strip, p. 119A
- Scoring Rubric, p. 119A

Retellings–Oral/Written

- *Teacher's Assessment Handbook*

Formal Assessment

Integrated Theme Test

Test applies the following theme skills to a new reading selection:

- Reading Strategies
- Summarizing: Story Structure, Compare and Contrast, Fantasy/Realism
- Word Skills and Strategies
- Writing Fluency
- Grammar and Spelling (optional)
- Self-Assessment

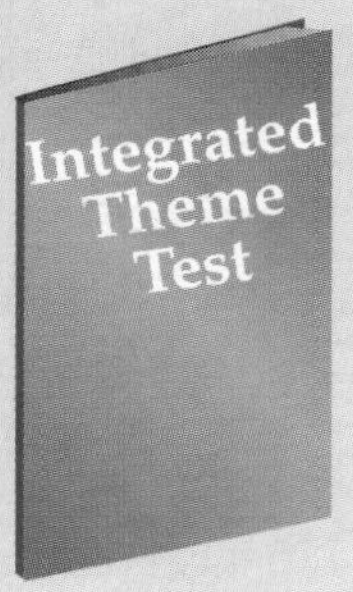
Integrated Theme Test

Theme Skills Test

- Summarizing: Story Structure, Compare and Contrast, Fantasy/Realism
- Base Words, Inflected Endings *-ed* and *-ing*, Context
- Writing Skills
- Study Skills
- Spelling
- Grammar

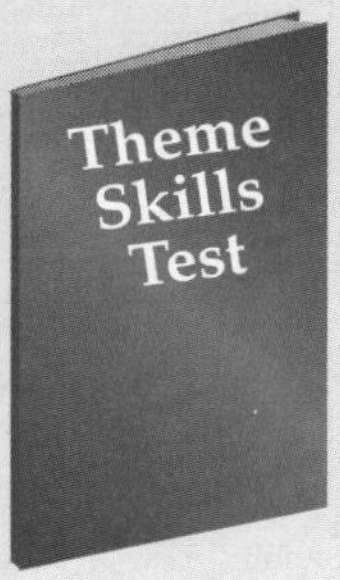
Theme Skills Test

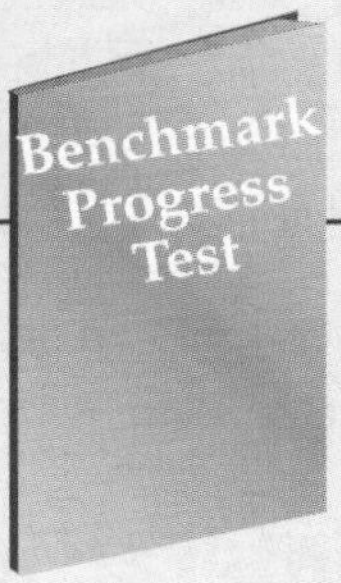
Benchmark Progress Test

Benchmark Progress Test

- Give a *Benchmark Progress Test* two or three times a year to measure student growth in reading and writing.

Managing Assessment

Theme Checklists

Question: How can I best use the Informal Assessment Checklist?

Answer: The Informal Assessment Checklist can help you keep track of informal observations you make throughout the theme. These tips can keep it simple to use:

- The Checklist has individual and group forms. Use the group form to monitor most students. Use the individual form for students who are a focus of concern.
- Don't try to check all categories for all students. For many students, occasional checks during a theme will be sufficient to document their progress or to note any difficulties in particular areas. For students needing more support, plan more observations, focused on the categories of concern.
- Some teachers keep the Checklist on a clipboard and make notes as they teach. Others take a moment at the end of the day or week to reflect and record their observations. Experiment to find the way that works for you.

For more information on this and other topics, see the *Teacher's Assessment Handbook*.

Portfolio Assessment

The portfolio icon signals portfolio opportunities throughout the theme.

Additional Portfolio tips:

- Introducing Portfolios to the Class, p. 119B
- Selecting Materials for the Portfolio, p. 119B
- Grading Work in Portfolios, p. 119B

Launching the Theme

INTERACTIVE LEARNING

Theme Concept Traditional stories can be retold in a variety of humorous, altered versions.

Setting the Scene

Teacher Read Aloud

Ask students if they are familiar with "The Three Little Pigs." Read aloud one of the popular versions of the story (such as James Marshall's), or use the version that appears on page 35A. Note: The story is also available in Spanish (*Tres cerditos,* Addison Wesley 1989; *Tres cochinitos,* Western 1993).

Fractured Tales

Note that the stories in "Oink, Oink, Oink" are versions of "The Three Little Pigs" that have been fractured to make them funny. Explain that *fractured* is another word for *broken.* Speculate how a story might be fractured. Have students complete *Literacy Activity Book* page 7.

Students Acquiring English Make sure students know that *oink* is the English word for the sound that pigs make.

Dramatizing a Tale

Let students bring the original version of "The Three Little Pigs" to life by creating and performing their own play version. Then encourage them to fracture the title of that story and improvise the play that results. Suggest such titles as "The Three Enormous Pigs" or "The Three Little Pigs and the Hyena."

Students Acquiring English Give parts with repetitive lines to students acquiring English and allow them to rehearse.

Interactive Bulletin Board

Help students to recall folktales they know or to make up new ones. Invite them to write or draw these stories and post them. During the theme, encourage students to create fractured versions of these stories and add them to the bulletin board.

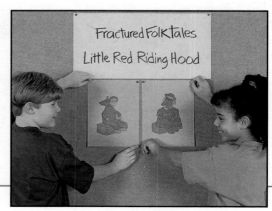
Fractured Folktales
Little Red Riding Hood

Literacy Activity Book, p. 8

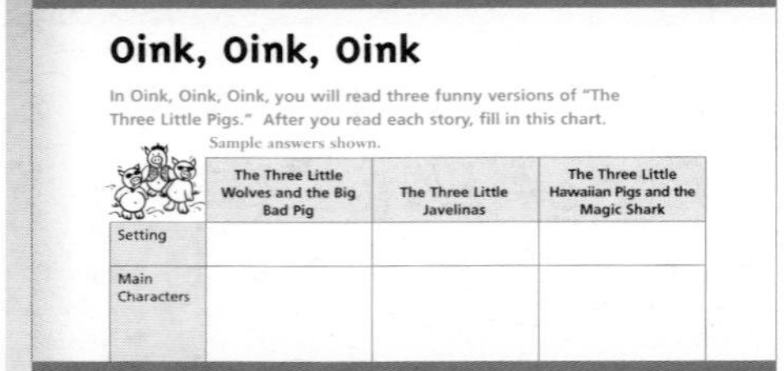

Oink, Oink, Oink

In Oink, Oink, Oink, you will read three funny versions of "The Three Little Pigs." After you read each story, fill in this chart.

Sample answers shown.

	The Three Little Wolves and the Big Bad Pig	The Three Little Javelinas	The Three Little Hawaiian Pigs and the Magic Shark
Setting			
Main Characters			

Literacy Activity Book, p. 7

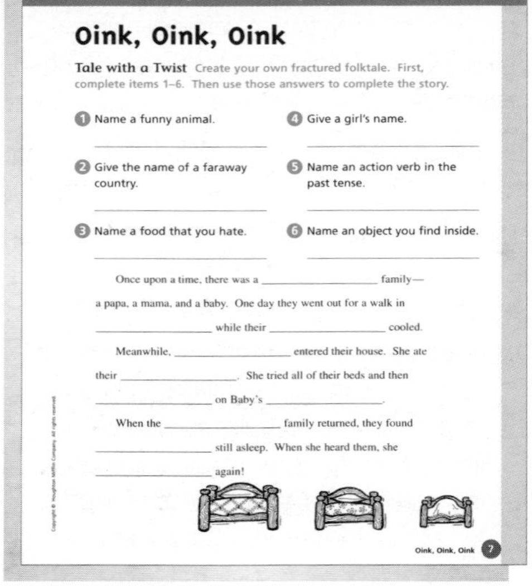

Oink, Oink, Oink

Tale with a Twist Create your own fractured folktale. First, complete items 1–6. Then use those answers to complete the story.

1. Name a funny animal. ______
2. Give the name of a faraway country. ______
3. Name a food that you hate. ______
4. Give a girl's name. ______
5. Name an action verb in the past tense. ______
6. Name an object you find inside. ______

Once upon a time, there was a ______ family—a papa, a mama, and a baby. One day they went out for a walk in ______ while their ______ cooled.

Meanwhile, ______ entered their house. She ate their ______. She tried all of their beds and then ______ on Baby's ______.

When the ______ family returned, they found ______ still asleep. When she heard them, she ______ again!

Copyright © Houghton Mifflin Company. All rights reserved.

Oink, Oink, Oink 7

Selection Connections

Discuss with students the Selection Connections on *Literacy Activity Book* page 8. Students should note that they will return to the chart after each selection and at the end of the theme.

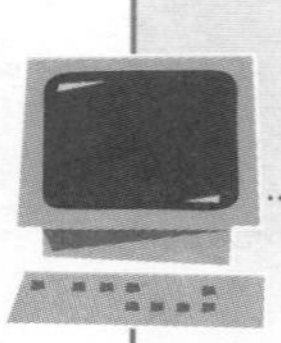

See the Houghton Mifflin **Internet** resources for additional activities.

See the **Teacher's Resource Disk** for theme-related support material.

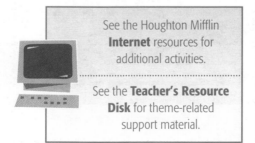

Choices for Projects

Building Your Own House

Cooperative Learning

Each of the three little pigs used a different material to build his house. Students may enjoy making their own houses out of readily available materials, such as packing peanuts, buttons, or popsicle sticks. Have groups of three choose one material and use it to build a house. Later, students can compare their projects and explain their choice of material.

Materials

- packing peanuts, buttons, or popsicle sticks
- cardboard
- glue or two-sided sticky paper
- scissors

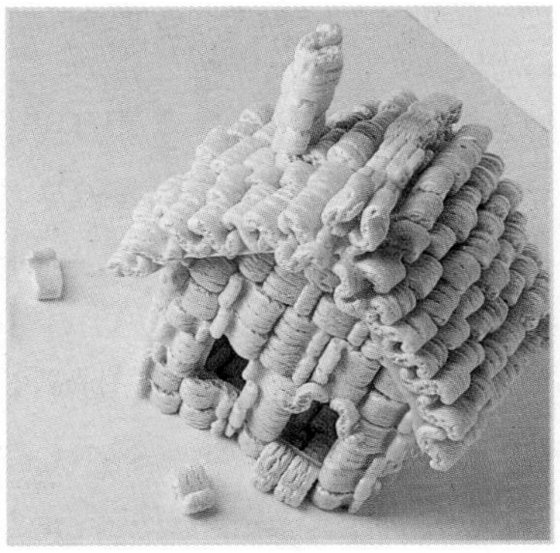

- Glue together a cardboard frame of a house, with the windows and door already cut.
- Cover the house with glue, or apply two-sided sticky paper.
- Attach materials to the house.

Making a Fractured Flip Book

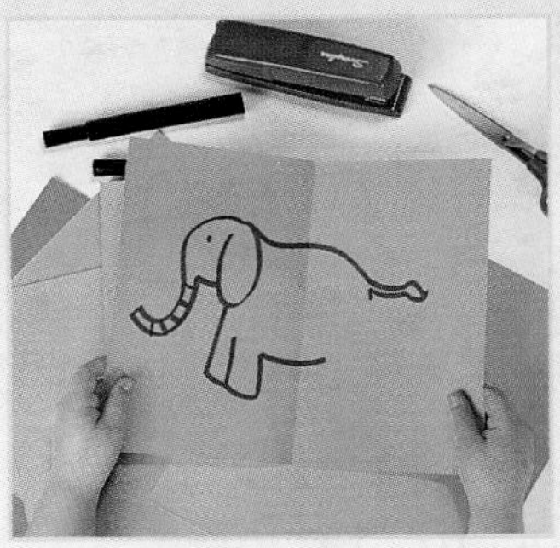

1 Hold sheets of paper horizontally and fold them in half, side to side. Unfold them. Then on each sheet draw a picture of a favorite animal, making sure the fold runs down the center of the drawing.

2 Collect the pictures into a book. Add a cover and secure with staples across the top.

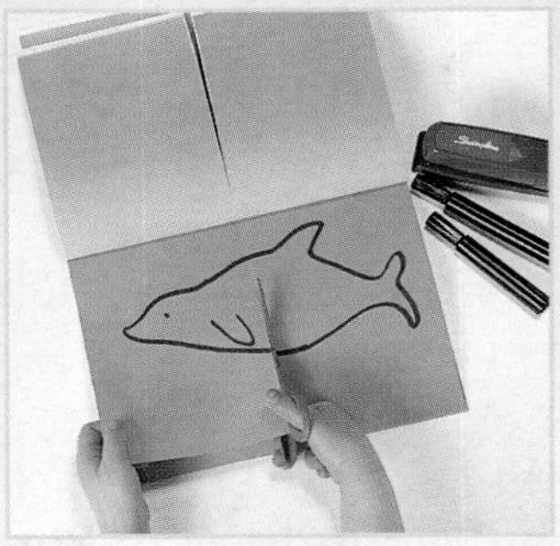

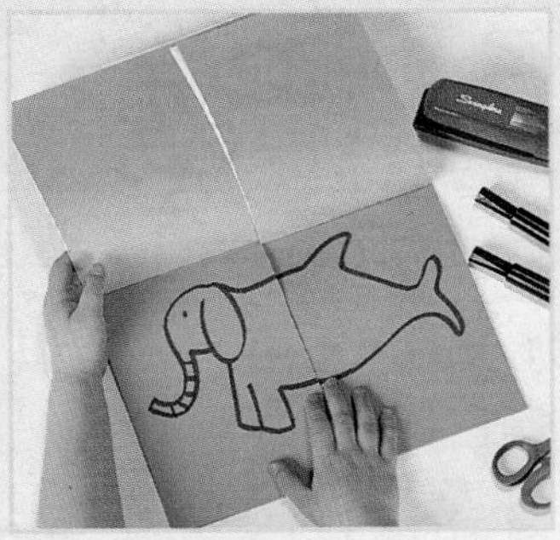

3 Cut the pages in half along the folds. Flip through the pages to create funny new combination animals.

Encourage discussion about why these unusual pairings are silly. Challenge volunteers to make up stories about some of the fractured animals.

Materials

- markers or crayons
- paper
- stapler
- scissors

Independent Reading and Writing

One fun way to foster independent reading and writing each day is to have a Drop-Everything break. All other work stops for a specified time so that individuals can read and/or write on their own. For independent reading, invite students to go to the library and select their own books, provide books from the Bibliography on pages 34A–34B, or encourage students to read one of the Paperback Plus books for this theme.

Easy reading: *Sidney Rella and the Glass Sneaker* by Bernice Myers

Average/challenging reading: *Sleeping Ugly* by Jane Yolen.

For independent writing, encourage students to choose their own activities. For those who need help getting started, suggest one or more of the activities on pages 60E, 88E, and 114E.

See the *Home/Community Connections Booklet* for materials related to this theme.

Portfolio Opportunity

- Save *Literacy Activity Book* page 8 to show students' ability to compare selections.
- The Portfolio Assessment icon highlights other portfolio opportunities throughout the theme.

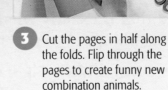

THE CLASSIC TALE

The Three Little Pigs

Teacher Read Aloud

Once upon a time, there were three little pigs, who lived with their mother in a cottage in the woods. Although she struggled to make ends meet, the pigs' mother grew poorer and poorer. And so one morning she sent the three little pigs out into the world to make their own way. As she kissed them good-bye, she said, "Watch out for the Big Bad Wolf. He eats little piggies like you!"

Now the First Little Pig hadn't gone very far when he met a man carrying a bundle of straw. He asked the man for some straw so that he could build a house. The man agreed. The First Little Pig built his house quickly, and then he went out to play. He played all morning, and so by lunchtime he was very hungry. As he was fixing himself something to eat, he heard a knock at the door. The First Little Pig peeked out the window, and lo and behold there stood the Big Bad Wolf.

"Little Pig, Little Pig, let me come in," said the wolf.

Remembering his mother's warning, the pig said, "Not by the hair of my chinny-chin-chin."

"Then I'll huff and I'll puff and I'll BLOW your house in," said the wolf.

And that is exactly what he did. After which, he ate the First Little Pig all up.

The Second Little Pig hadn't gone very far when he met a man with a cartload of sticks. The Second Little Pig asked for some sticks so he could build himself a house. The man agreed, and before long the Second Little Pig had a fine stick house. Then he went out to play. He played all day, and so he was very hungry by suppertime. As he was fixing his dinner, he heard a knock at the door. When he peeked out the window, who do you think he saw? The Big Bad Wolf!

"Little Pig, Little Pig, let me come in," said the wolf.

"Not by the hair of my chinny-chin-chin," said the pig.

"Then I'll huff and I'll puff and I'll BLOW your house in," said the wolf.

The wolf blew down the house and ate up the Second Little Pig.

The Third Little Pig met a man with a wagonload of bricks. He asked the man for some bricks so that he could build himself a house. The man agreed, and so the Third Little Pig got to work building himself the best house he could. He worked long and hard, and by the end of the day he was very tired. He was just crawling into bed, when he heard a knock at the door. And he heard a voice that said, "Little Pig, Little Pig, let me come in."

The Third Little Pig looked out his bedroom window and saw the Big Bad Wolf at his doorstep.

"Oh, no," said the pig. "Not by the hair of my chinny-chin-chin."

"Then I'll huff and I'll puff and I'll BLOW your house in," said the wolf.

The Big Bad Wolf huffed and puffed, but he couldn't blow the brick house down. So he crawled up onto the roof, intending to go down the chimney to get that third little piggy. But the pig heard the wolf pawing around on his roof, and he guessed what the wolf had in mind. He put a big kettle of water in the fireplace, and he lit a fire under it. When the wolf came down the chimney, he landed with a HOWL in the boiling water.

That was the end of the Big Bad Wolf. The Third Little Pig lived happily ever after.

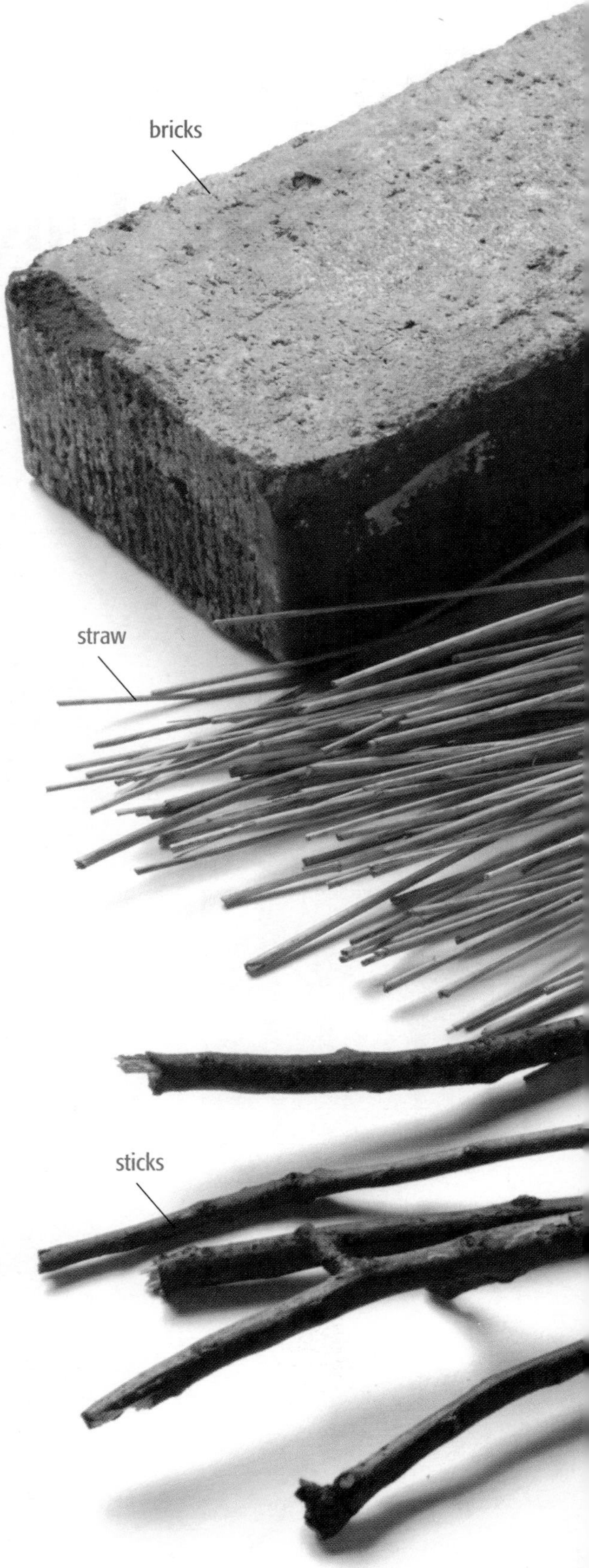
bricks
straw
sticks

SELECTION:

The Three Little Wolves and the Big Bad Pig

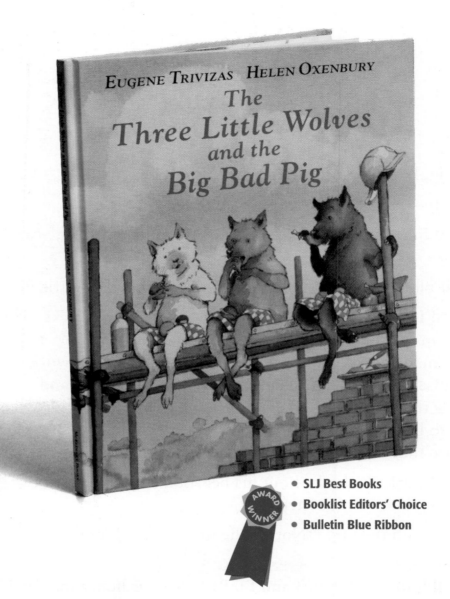
EUGENE TRIVIZAS HELEN OXENBURY
The Three Little Wolves and the Big Bad Pig

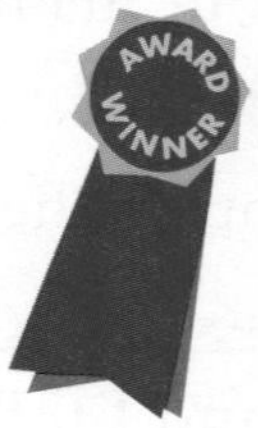
AWARD WINNER

- **SLJ Best Books**
- **Booklist Editors' Choice**
- **Bulletin Blue Ribbon**

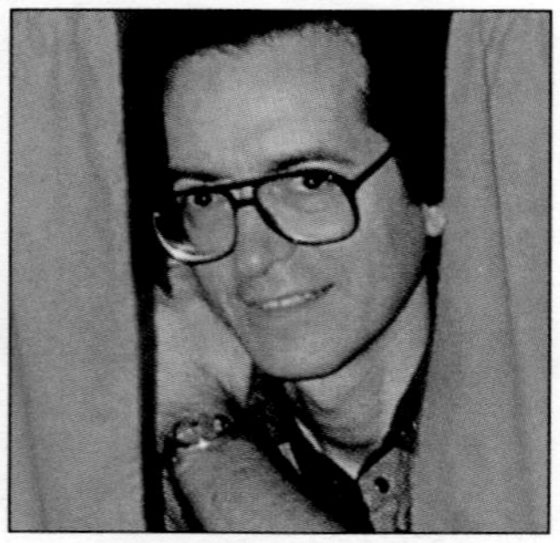

by Eugene Trivizas

Selection Summary

A mother wolf sends her three little wolves out into the world with this warning: Beware of the big bad pig!

The wolves build a house of brick that is demolished by the sledge-hammer-wielding big bad pig. The little wolves build again and again, each time with stronger materials, but the pig always finds a way to destroy their work.

Finally, they build a house of flowers. When the pig inhales its beautiful scent, he has a change of heart and mends his ways. Seeing that the pig has changed, the wolves invite him in for tea, and he becomes a member of the family.

Lesson Planning Guide

	Skill/Strategy Instruction	Meeting Individual Needs	Lesson Resources
1 Introduce *the* Literature *Pacing: 1 day*	**Preparing to Read and Write** Prior Knowledge/Building Background, 35E **Selection Vocabulary,** 35F • prowling • grunted • crumbled • trembling • scorched **Spelling Pretest,** 60I • ask • next • mix • smell • black • shut • lock • truck	**Support in Advance,** 35E **Students Acquiring English,** 35E **Other Choices for Building Background,** 35E **Spelling Challenge Words:** • knock • scent • plenty • fetch	***Literacy Activity Book*** Vocabulary, p. 9 **Transparency:** Vocabulary, 1–1 **Great Start** CD-ROM software, "Oink, Oink, Oink" CD
2 Interact *with* Literature *Pacing: 1-3 days*	**Reading Strategies:** Monitor, 38, 44 Predict/Infer, 38, 48 Think about Words, 48 **Minilessons:** Fantasy, 41 ✓ Summarizing: Story Structure, 45 Making Judgments, 47 Fantasy/Realism, 57 Writer's Craft: Role Reversal, 59	**Choices for Reading,** 38 **Guided Reading,** 38 Comprehension/Critical Thinking, 42, 46, 52, 58 **Students Acquiring English,** 39, 41, 43, 46, 49, 55, 56, 60 **Extra Support,** 38, 40, 49, 55, 59 **Challenge,** 48, 54, 57	**Reading-Writing Workshop** A Story, 116–117F ***Literacy Activity Book,*** pp. 40–42 The Learning Company's new elementary writing center software
3 Instruct *and* Integrate *Pacing: 1-3 days*	✓ **Comprehension:** Summarizing: Story Structure, 60B ✓ **Writing:** Writing a Sentence, 60D **Word Skills and Strategies:** ✓ Structural Analysis: Base Words, 60F Phonics Review: Short Vowels, 60G **Building Vocabulary:** Vocabulary Activities, 60H ✓ **Spelling:** Short Vowels, 60I ✓ **Grammar:** Subjects and Predicates, 60J–60K **Communication Activities:** Listening and Speaking, 60L; Viewing, 60M **Cross-Curricular Activities:** Science, 60N; Math, 60O; Dance, 60O	**Reteaching:** Summarizing: Story Structure, 60C **Activity Choices:** Shared Writing: A Reversed Tale, 60E; Write a Song, 60E; Give Directions, 60E **Reteaching:** Base Words, 60G **Activity Choices:** Synonyms for *big* and *bad*, Classifying/Categorizing, 60H **Challenge Words Practice,** 60I **Reteaching:** Subjects and Predicates, 60K **Activity Choices:** Listening and Speaking, 60L; Viewing, 60M **Activity Choices:** Science, 60N; Math, 60O; Dance, 60O	**Reading-Writing Workshop** A Story, 116–117F **Transparencies:** Comprehension, 1–2; Writing, 1–3; Grammar, 1–4 ***Literacy Activity Book*** Comprehension, p.11; Writing, p.12; Word Skills, p.13; Building Vocabulary, p.14; Spelling, p. 15–16; Grammar, p.17, 19 **Channel R.E.A.D.** videodisc: "License to Drive" **Audio Tape** for Oink, Oink, Oink: *The Three Little Wolves and the Big Bad Pig* The Learning Company's new elementary writing center software

✓ *Indicates Tested Skills*

Introduce *the* Literature

Preparing to Read and Write

Support in Advance

MEETING INDIVIDUAL NEEDS

Use this activity for students who need extra support before participating in the whole-class activity.

Animal Characterizations Discuss how different animals are depicted as good and evil in stories. Ask students to give examples from their own reading and TV viewing.

Management Tip
Students not participating in Support in Advance can engage in self-selected writing or silent reading.

Students Acquiring English
Begin a wall chart of words about building and construction. Invite students to contribute words they know. As students read, add words such as these from the story: *bricks, concrete, sledgehammer, barbed wire, padlocks,* and *Plexiglas.*

Note: Some terms, such as *padlocks* and *barbed wire,* may be distressing for children from war-torn areas.

INTERACTIVE LEARNING

Prior Knowledge/Building Background

Key Concept
Wolves vs. Pigs

Semantic Chart Discuss how the wolf and the pig are depicted in "The Three Little Pigs."

Wolf	• big and bad	• sneaky	• hunts alone
Three Pigs	• cute and fun-loving	• clever	• work together

Tell students that the next selection turns the original folktale upside down: in this story, it's a pig who's the villain and three little wolves who are being chased. Explain that folktales that have been turned around like this are called *fractured tales.*

Key Concept
Being Bad

Semantic Map Discuss with students the meaning of the word *bad* as it is used in the phrase *big bad pig.* You may wish to use a semantic map like the following for this purpose.

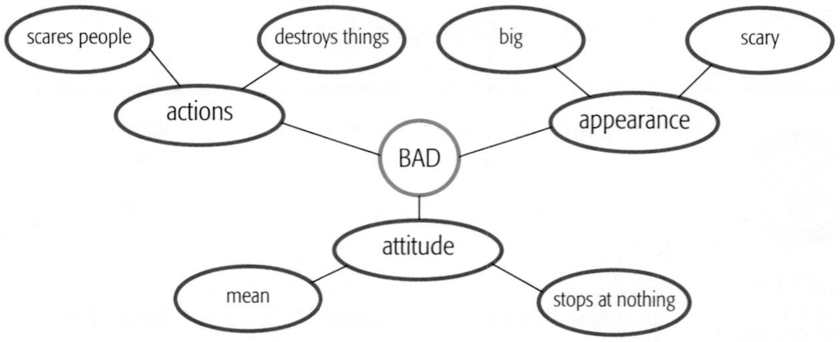
scares people
destroys things
big
scary
actions
appearance
BAD
attitude
mean
stops at nothing

Other Choices for Building Background

Quick Writing

MEETING INDIVIDUAL NEEDS

Challenge Ask students to write about how "The Three Little Pigs" might have turned out if the big bad wolf had been a big *good* wolf.

Describing Words

Cooperative Learning

Ask students to make lists of words that describe both friendly animals (soft, fluffy) and fierce animals (mean, angry).

Great Start
For students needing extra support with key concepts and vocabulary, use the "Oink, Oink, Oink" CD.

Spelling

You may want to give the Spelling Pretest on page 60-I before students read the selection.

Daily Language Practice

Use the sentences on page 60K as daily practice of the spelling and grammar skills taught with this selection.

INTERACTIVE LEARNING

Selection Vocabulary

Key Words

- prowling
- grunted
- crumbled
- trembling

Display Transparency 1–1. Note that students will encounter the underlined words in the story. Have students read each sentence aloud and substitute their own words and phrases for the underlined words. If necessary, discuss the meaning of the underlined words. For example:

The three little pigs felt safe in their new house. But then the big bad wolf came prowling down the road.	**But then the big bad wolf came creeping down the road.**

Students can continue the story in their journals. Or, as they read the selection, they can jot down other words they would like to study. Later, these can be added to their journals, together with definitions.

Students Acquiring English You might wish to introduce these additional words: *escape, secure, strong,* and *fragile.*

Vocabulary Practice Have students work independently or in pairs to complete the activity on page 9 of the *Literacy Activity Book.*

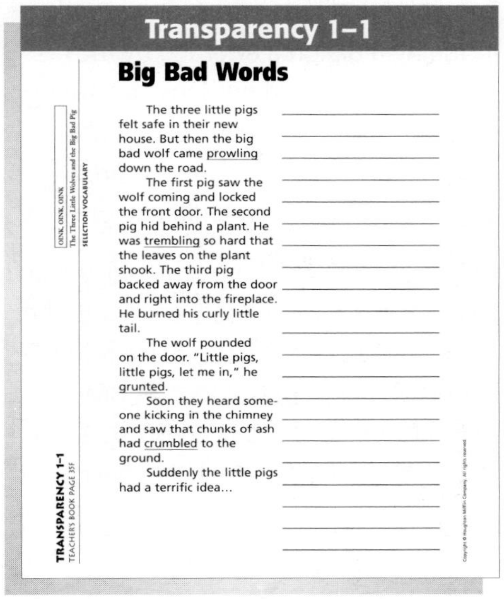
Transparency 1–1

Big Bad Words

The three little pigs felt safe in their new house. But then the big bad wolf came prowling down the road.

The first pig saw the wolf coming and locked the front door. The second pig hid behind a plant. He was trembling so hard that the leaves on the plant shook. The third pig backed away from the door and right into the fireplace. He burned his curly little tail.

The wolf pounded on the door. "Little pigs, little pigs, let me in," he grunted.

Soon they heard someone kicking in the chimney and saw that chunks of ash had crumbled to the ground.

Suddenly the little pigs had a terrific idea...

OINK, OINK, OINK
The Three Little Wolves and the Big Bad Pig
SELECTION VOCABULARY

TRANSPARENCY 1–1
TEACHER'S BOOK PAGE 35F

Copyright © Houghton Mifflin Company. All rights reserved.

Science

Teacher FactFile

Wolves: did you know. . .

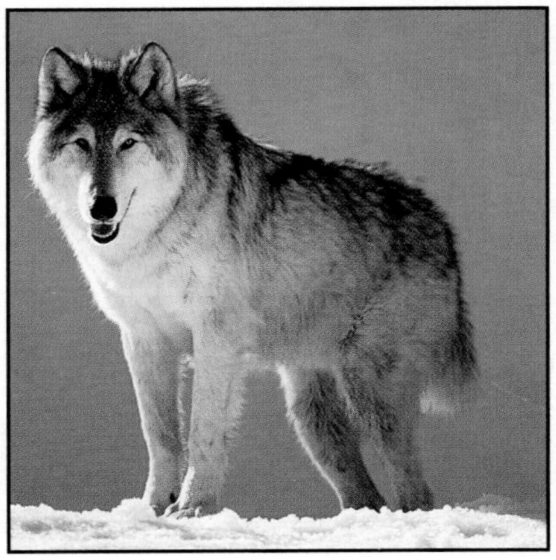

The expression "to eat like a wolf" derives from the fact that an adult wolf can eat 20 pounds of meat at one feeding.

Wolves helped primitive people track down fleet-footed animals. For their reward they received leftover bones and meat scraps.

Wolves hunt everything from moose to mice. They sometimes travel 40 to 50 miles a day looking for food.

Wolves share responsibility for raising their pups. Adult wolves will take turns bringing food to the pups.

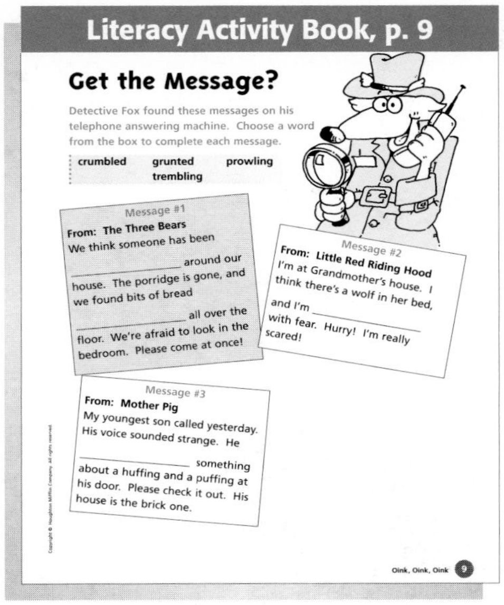
Literacy Activity Book, p. 9

Get the Message?

Detective Fox found these messages on his telephone answering machine. Choose a word from the box to complete each message.

crumbled grunted prowling trembling

Message #1
From: The Three Bears
We think someone has been ______ around our house. The porridge is gone, and we found bits of bread ______ all over the floor. We're afraid to look in the bedroom. Please come at once!

Message #2
From: Little Red Riding Hood
I'm at Grandmother's house. I think there's a wolf in her bed, and I'm ______ with fear. Hurry! I'm really scared!

Message #3
From: Mother Pig
My youngest son called yesterday. His voice sounded strange. He ______ something about a huffing and a puffing at his door. Please check it out. His house is the brick one.

Copyright © Houghton Mifflin Company. All rights reserved.

Oink, Oink, Oink 9

More About the Author

Eugene Trivizas

Eugene Trivizas is a leading writer for children in Greece. In that country his books have been the inspiration for comics, television series, and plays. He has won numerous prizes for his work, including a diploma awarded by IBBY (International Board on Books for Young People) for excellence in writing. *The Three Little Wolves and the Big Bad Pig* is the first story he has written in English.

Dr. Trivizas also teaches criminology and has served as an honorary advisor to the Minister of Justice in Greece. He is the author of papers on subjects as diverse as football, hooliganism, censorship, and the effect of diet on criminal behavior.

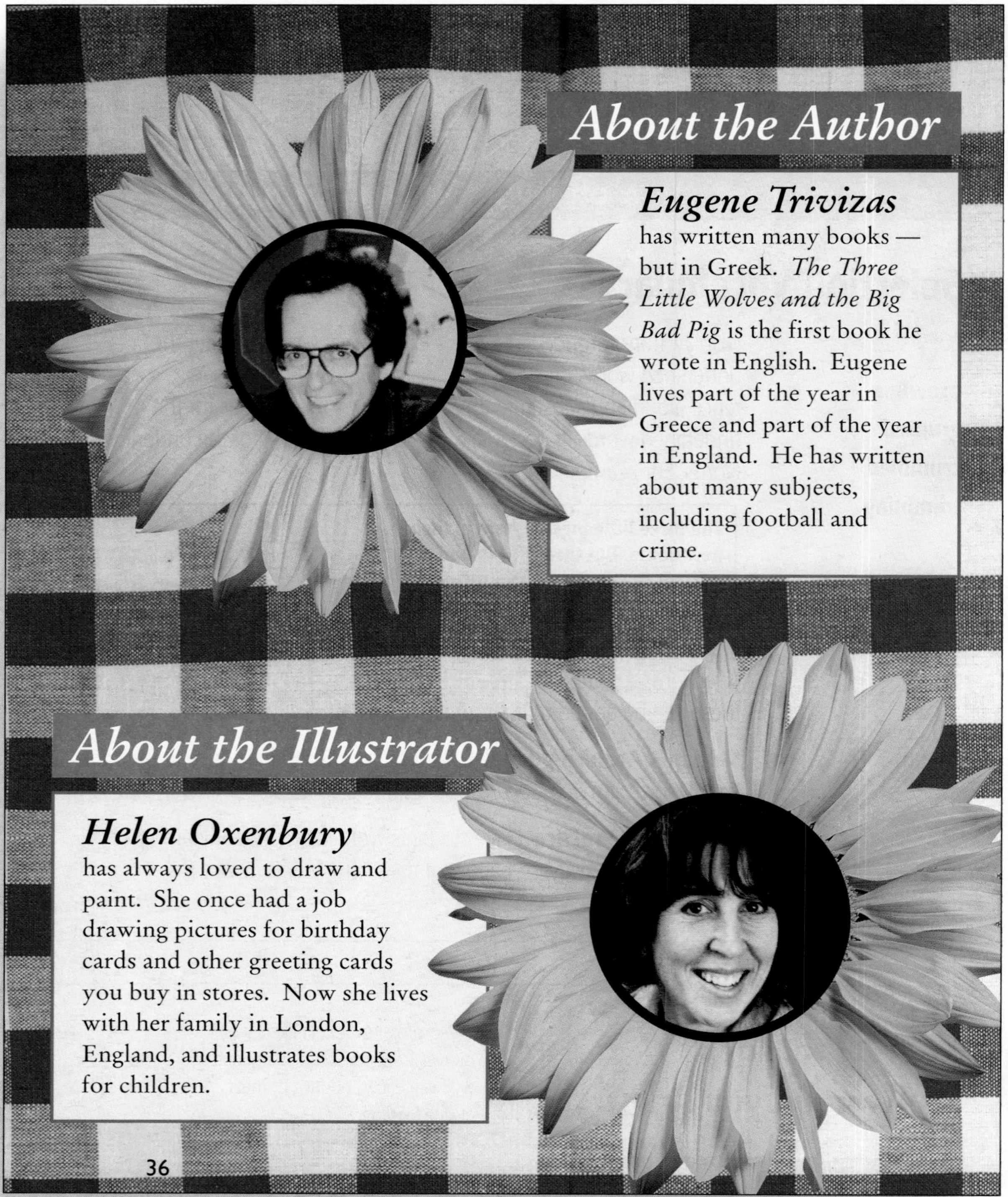

About the Author

Eugene Trivizas has written many books — but in Greek. *The Three Little Wolves and the Big Bad Pig* is the first book he wrote in English. Eugene lives part of the year in Greece and part of the year in England. He has written about many subjects, including football and crime.

About the Illustrator

Helen Oxenbury has always loved to draw and paint. She once had a job drawing pictures for birthday cards and other greeting cards you buy in stores. Now she lives with her family in London, England, and illustrates books for children.

36

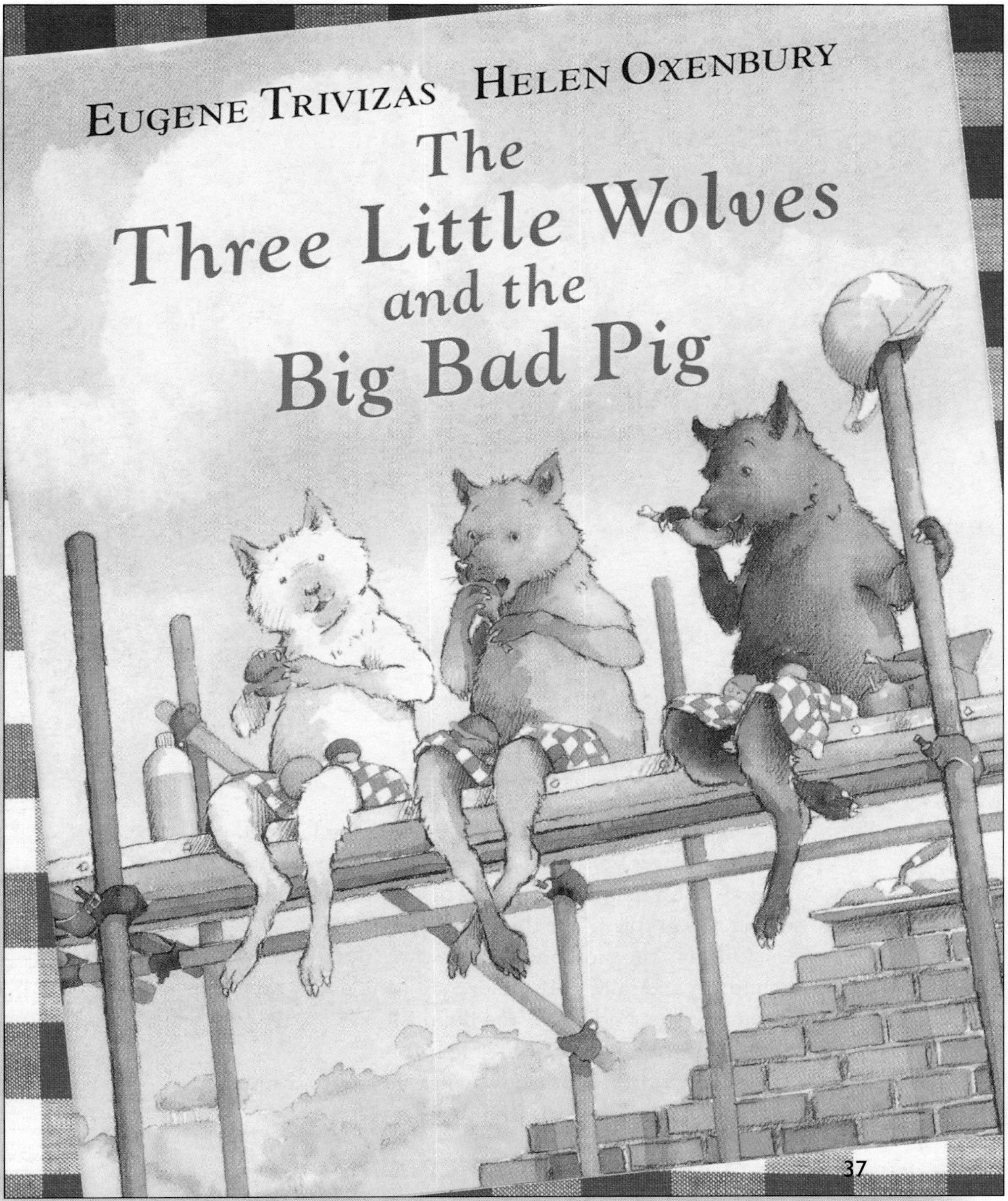
EUGENE TRIVIZAS HELEN OXENBURY
The Three Little Wolves and the Big Bad Pig
37

More About the Illustrator

Helen Oxenbury

British illustrator Helen Oxenbury had a background in theater design before she began illustrating children's books. Her main inspiration for entering the field was "the fact that I [as a young mother] couldn't find any books to show my baby."

She quickly became known for picture books but, as her children grew, she became interested in doing books for older children who "can appreciate things like atmosphere and detail."

No matter what age group Oxenbury aims to reach, she respects her audience. "I believe children to be very canny people who immediately sense if adults talk, write, or illustrate down to them," she says.

Interact *with* Literature

Reading Strategies

Predict/Infer Monitor

Teacher Modeling Discuss how good readers pay attention while reading and make adjustments if they need to. Model the use of strategies using a Think Aloud.

Think Aloud

The title says the pig is big and bad, and in the picture the three little wolves look friendly. That's the opposite of the story I know. I can predict that a lot of things in this story will be backwards. I'll have to monitor, or pay attention, as I read, so I won't get confused.

Predicting/Purpose Setting

Have students predict what will happen to the three wolves. Then suggest that they read and check if their predictions are correct.

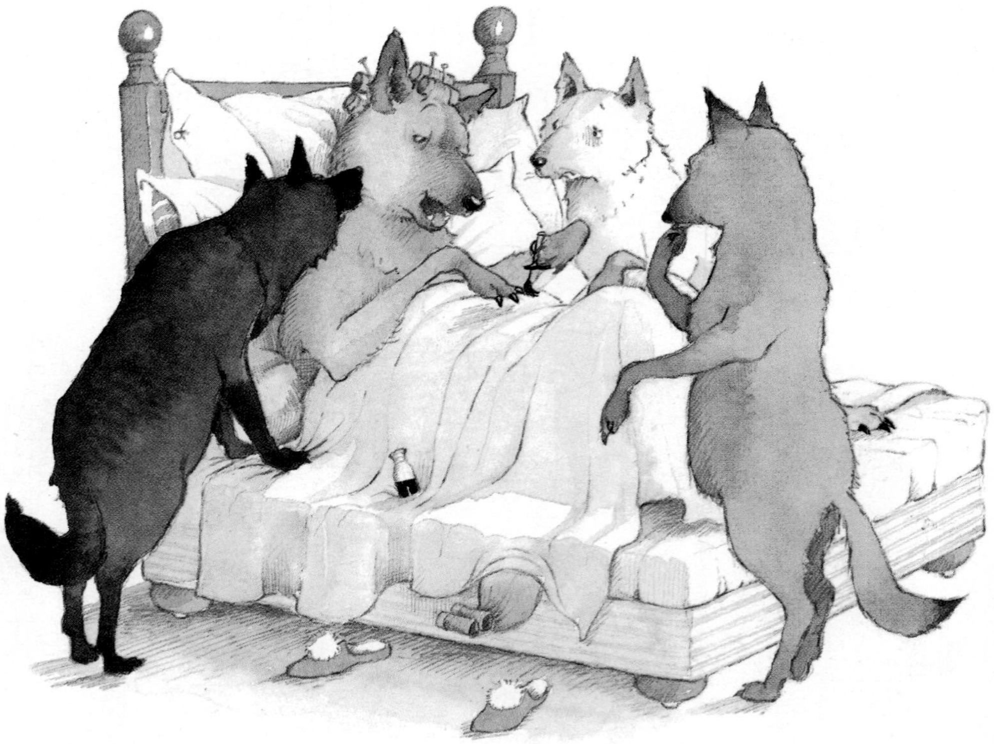

Once upon a time, there were three cuddly little wolves with soft fur and fluffy tails who lived with their mother. The first was black, the second was gray, and the third was white.

One day the mother called the three little wolves around her and said, "My children, it is time for you to go out into the world. Go and build a house for yourselves. But beware of the big bad pig."

"Don't worry, Mother, we will watch out for him," said the three little wolves, and they set off.

38

Choices for Reading

Independent Reading	Cooperative Reading
Guided Reading	Teacher Read Aloud

Meeting Individual Needs: Guided Reading

Have students using the Guided Reading option read to the end of page 43. Use the questions on page 42 to check comprehension.

QuickREFERENCE

Math Link

Calculating Ages Young wolves are usually cared for by their mothers until they're two months old. Ask students to estimate the ages of these little wolves in weeks (eight) and days (sixty).

Meeting Individual Needs: Extra Support

Story Review If students do not know "The Three Little Pigs," you may wish to
- read the story aloud on pages 35A–35B
- play a videotape of the story
- have other students tell the story

Soon they met a kangaroo who was pushing a wheelbarrow full of red and yellow bricks.

"Please, will you give us some of your bricks?" asked the three little wolves.

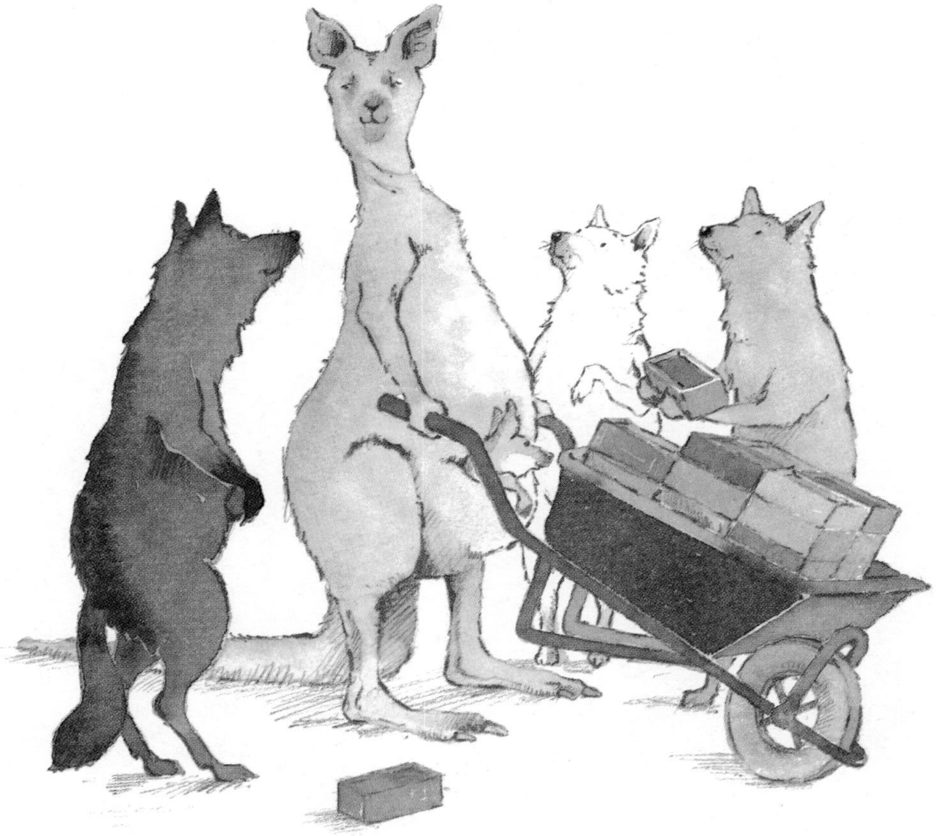

"Certainly," said the kangaroo, and she gave them lots of red and yellow bricks.

So the three little wolves built themselves a house of bricks.

39

Students Acquiring English

Idioms Explain that the wolves *go out into the world* because their mother thinks they are old enough to leave home and live on their own. Note that in some cultures this moment only comes when the children are ready to marry.

Social Studies Link

Gray wolves, once plentiful in North America, now mostly survive in Canada and Alaska. Many hunters regard wolves as competition for game. But wolves only hunt the weak members of a herd, leaving ample game for humans.

Interact *with* Literature

The very next day the big bad pig came prowling down the road and saw the house of bricks that the little wolves had built.

The three little wolves were playing croquet in the garden. When they saw the big bad pig coming, they ran inside the house and locked the door.

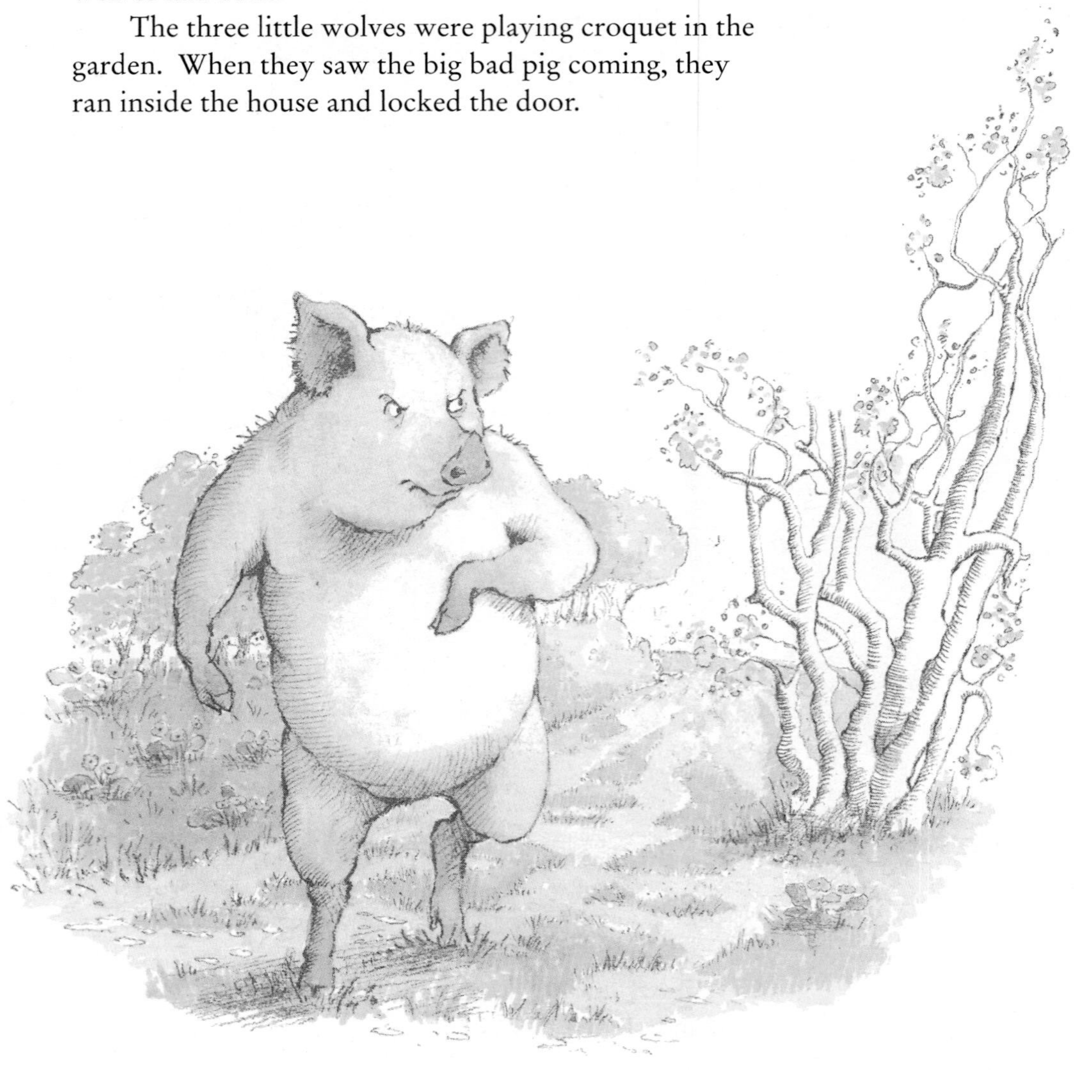

40

QuickREFERENCE

Multicultural Link

Games Often games vary from culture to culture. For example, the English "London Bridge" is known as "The Hen Runs" in Chile or "The Fountain" in Cuba. Ask students to share information about games they know.

Extra Support

Croquet Explain that croquet players use a mallet—originally a *crochet*, or "crooked stick" in French—to hit a ball through wire rungs, or wickets. Have students who have played croquet demonstrate how it is played.

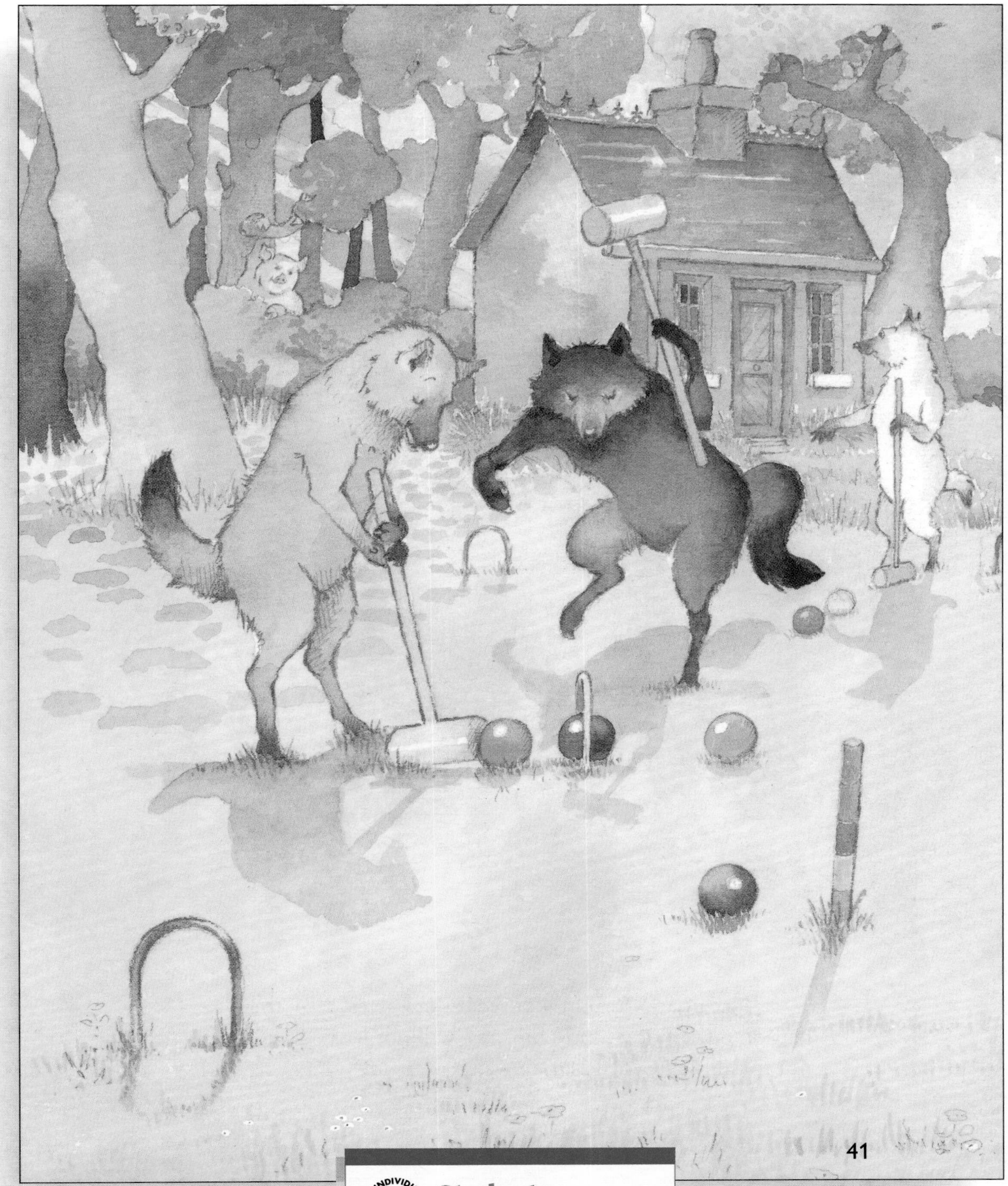

MINILESSON

Genre

Fantasy

Teach/Model

Remind students that *The Three Little Wolves and the Big Bad Pig* is a fantasy. Discuss what parts of the story are make-believe.

Explain that there are many different kinds of fantasies. Model by putting this chart on the board.

Three Kinds of Fantasies
With Animal Characters: *Goldilocks and the Three Bears* *Charlotte's Web*
With Toys or Dolls: *Pinocchio* *Winnie the Pooh*
With Characters That Have Special Powers: *Mary Poppins* *Pippi Longstocking*

Other types of fantasies that you might want to add to the list include ones with tiny characters (such as *The Borrowers*) and ones involving time travel.

Practice/Apply

Invite students to copy the chart and add additional categories and stories from their own reading.

Visual Literacy

Dimension Have students name figures in the foreground of the illustration (the gray and black wolves) and the background (the white wolf, the pig). Discuss how the figures get smaller from the foreground to the background.

MEETING INDIVIDUAL NEEDS

Students Acquiring English

To help students keep track of the narrative, suggest that they make a chart with these two headings: *Type of House* and *What Happens?* Each time the wolves build a new house, have students paraphrase what happens and then fill in the chart.

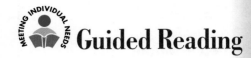

Interact *with* Literature

Guided Reading

Comprehension/Critical Thinking

1. How is the story different from the original tale of "The Three Little Pigs"? (Roles are reversed; three little wolves must watch out for a big bad pig; also, the three wolves stick together instead of going their separate ways.)
2. Why do you think the big bad pig is so dangerous? (He is much bigger and stronger than the wolves. He will stop at nothing to try to catch them.)
3. What else could the wolves do to try to stop the pig? (Sample answer: Perhaps build a fence around the house, or get a watchdog.)

Predicting/Purpose Setting

Discuss with students whether their earlier predictions were accurate. Then ask them to predict what the big bad pig will do next. Have students read pages 44–47 to find out if their predictions are correct.

The pig knocked on the door and grunted, "Little wolves, little wolves, let me come in!"

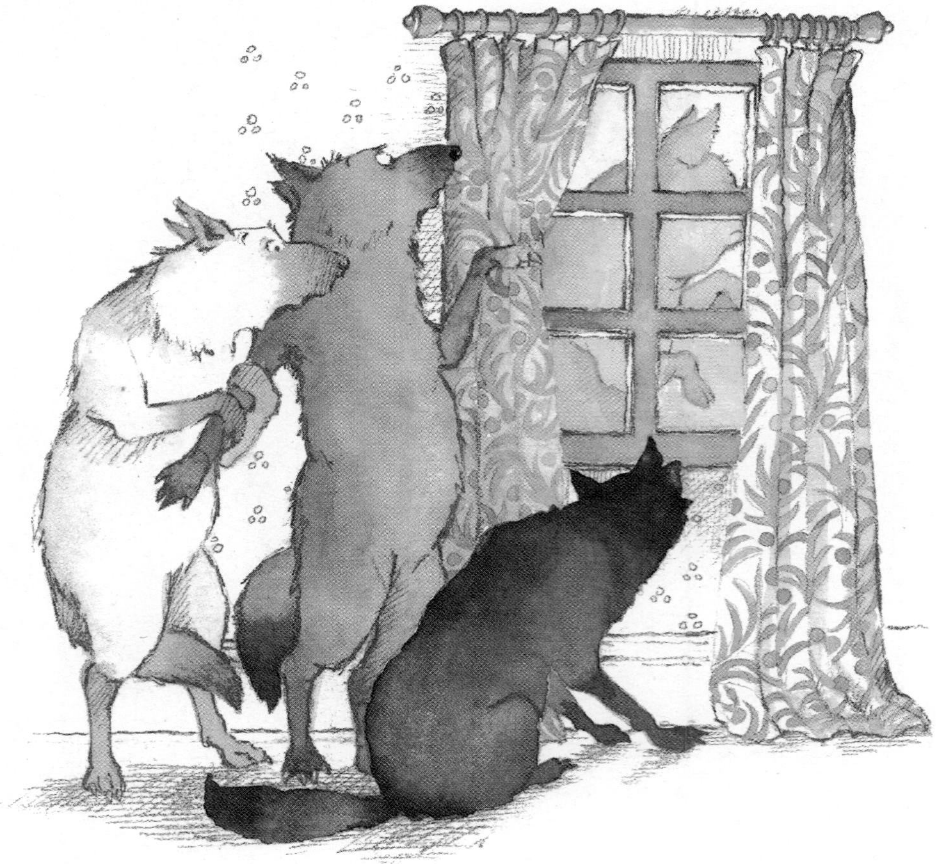

"No, no, no," said the three little wolves. "By the hair on our chinny-chin-chins, we will not let you in, not for all the tea leaves in our china teapot!"

42

Informal Assessment

If students' responses indicate that they understand that the pig is the villain in this story, have them finish reading the story independently or cooperatively.

QuickREFERENCE

Multicultural Link

Wolves Although the wolf is seen as evil in many folktales, there are exceptions, such as the Sarcee legend "How the Indians Obtained Dogs," in which a wolf helps feed a family. Ask students to explain how their cultures view wolves.

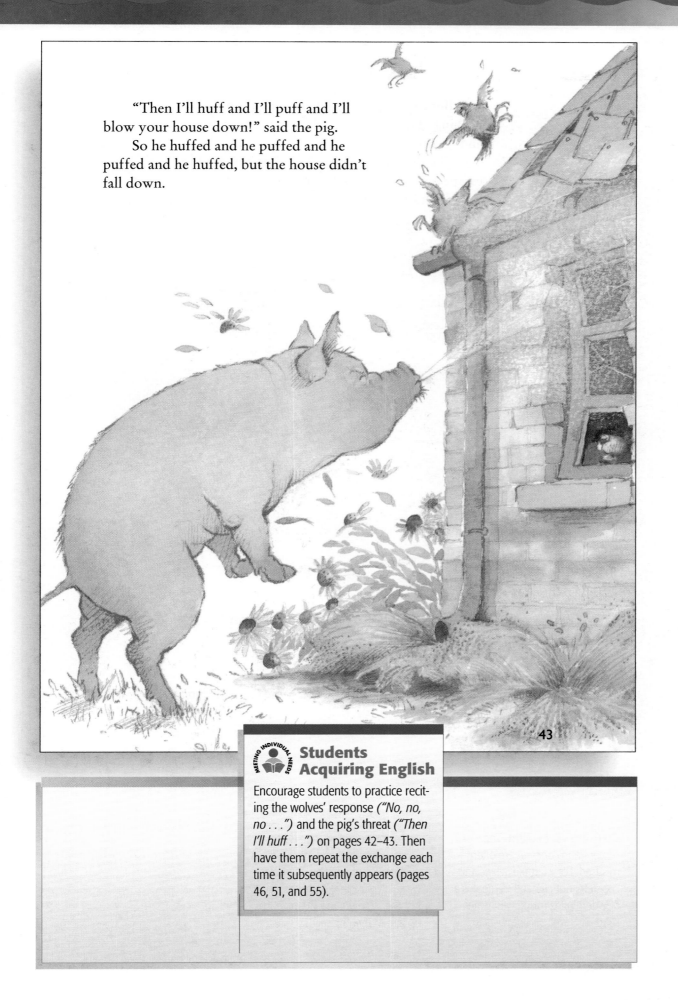

"Then I'll huff and I'll puff and I'll blow your house down!" said the pig.

So he huffed and he puffed and he puffed and he huffed, but the house didn't fall down.

43

Students Acquiring English

Encourage students to practice reciting the wolves' response *("No, no, no . . .")* and the pig's threat *("Then I'll huff . . .")* on pages 42–43. Then have them repeat the exchange each time it subsequently appears (pages 46, 51, and 55).

Interact *with* Literature

Reading Strategies

Monitor

Use a Think Aloud such as the following to model how readers monitor their reading.

Think Aloud

In this part of the story I was confused because I thought brick and concrete were equally hard. I couldn't understand how the wolves were improving their situation. But then I thought about concrete slabs. They are much larger and heavier than bricks. You can hold bricks in your hand, and they can crack if they're thrown on concrete. So concrete is a more solid material.

But the pig wasn't called big and bad for nothing. He went and fetched his sledgehammer, and he knocked the house down.

The three little wolves only just managed to escape before the bricks crumbled, and they were very frightened indeed.

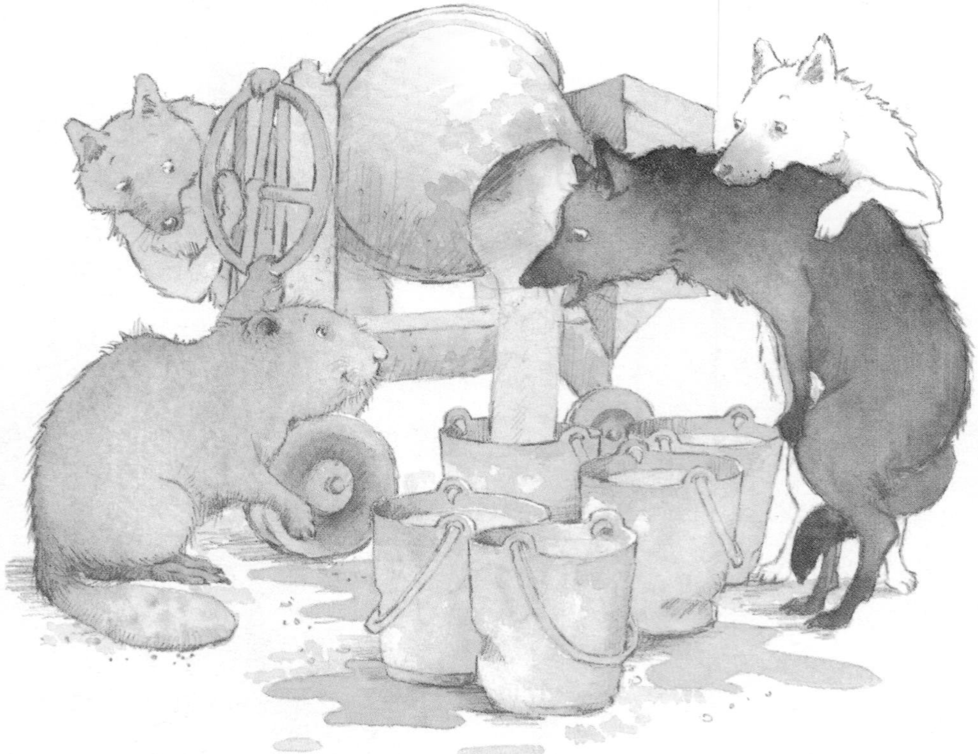

"We shall have to build a stronger house," they said.

Just then they saw a beaver who was mixing concrete in a concrete mixer.

"Please, will you give us some of your concrete?" asked the three little wolves.

44

Informal Assessment

Oral Reading To check oral reading fluency, have individual students read pages 44–45 aloud.

Students should be allowed to first read the pages silently. Use the Oral Reading Checklist in the *Teacher's Assessment Handbook* as a guide for assessment.

QuickREFERENCE

Background: FYI

Concrete vs. Cement The words *cement* and *concrete* are often misused. For example, a sidewalk is concrete, not cement. Cement is a powder that is mixed with water, sand or gravel, and pebbles to make concrete. Concrete is fireproof, watertight, and relatively inexpensive. If you have concrete walls in your class, invite students to test the strength and examine the texture of them.

"Certainly," said the beaver, and he gave them buckets and buckets full of messy, slurry concrete.

So the three little wolves built themselves a house of concrete.

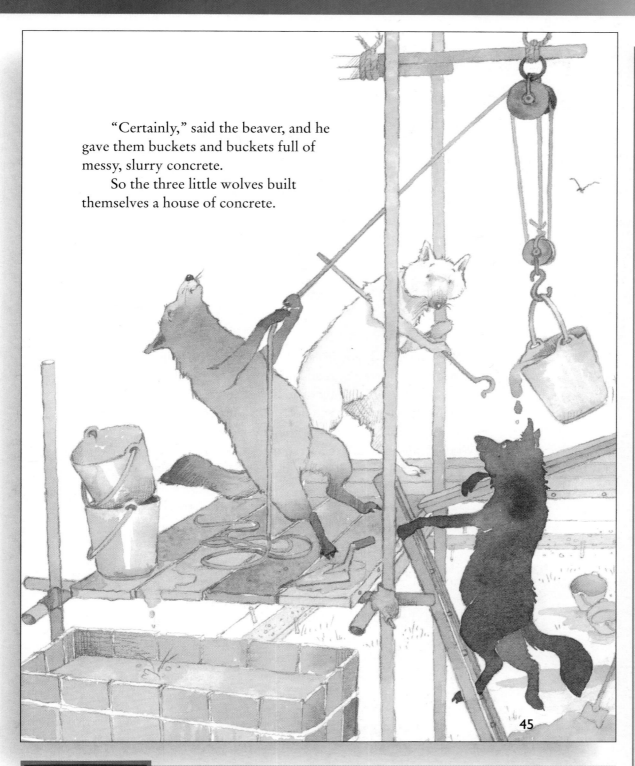

45

QuickREFERENCE

Home Connection

Public Works Is road work being done in your area? Suggest that students go with family members on a field trip to these sights. Students acquiring English may want to make a list of the tools and equipment being used.

MINILESSON

Summarizing: Story Structure

TESTED SKILL

Teach/Model

Explain that a story's structure can be used to summarize, or retell, it.

Begin reviewing story elements using this chart.

Characters	*who* is in the story
Setting	*where* or *when* the story happens
Problem	*what* needs to be solved
Events	*what* happens
Ending	*how* the problem is solved

Practice/Apply

Have students use the chart as a guide for summarizing a story they have read recently. You may wish to model with this example.

"The Three Little Pigs" is about three little pigs and a big bad wolf. The wolf wants to eat the pigs, so the pigs try to build strong houses to avoid him. He easily destroys their houses of straw and sticks but, when he can't get into their brick house, he slips down the chimney. The pigs are ready for him, though. The wolf falls into boiling water and is no longer a danger to the pigs.

Afterward, discuss the details that were excluded from the summary and why you left them out.

SKILL FINDER

Full lesson/Reteaching, pp. 60B–60C

Minilessons, p. 83; Theme 2, p. 207

Interact *with* Literature

Guided Reading

Comprehension/Critical Thinking

1. How did the big bad pig destroy the house of bricks? (with a sledgehammer)
2. Why did the wolves build a concrete house? (Concrete is stronger than brick; the wolves knew they needed a safer house.)
3. Do you think the wolves would have been better off if they had split up and built separate houses? (Have students support their answers by listing reasons.)

Predicting/Purpose Setting

Allow students to discuss whether any of their predictions were correct. Then ask what they think the pig will do next and how the wolves will counteract. Have them read pages 48–51.

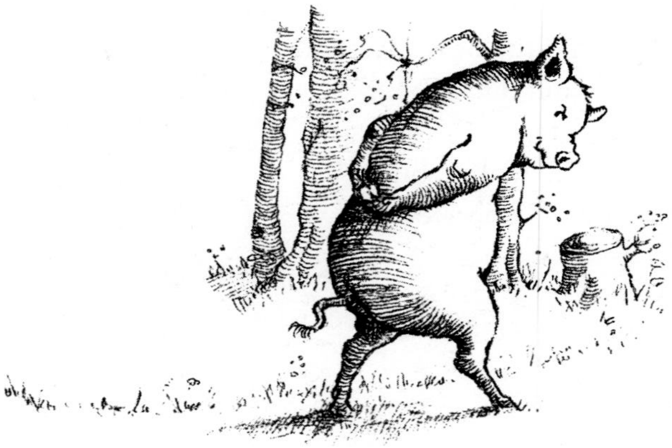

No sooner had they finished than the big bad pig came prowling down the road and saw the house of concrete that the little wolves had built.

They were playing battledore and shuttlecock in the garden, and when they saw the big bad pig coming, they ran inside their house and shut the door.

The pig rang the bell and said, "Little frightened wolves, let me come in!"

"No, no, no," said the three little wolves. "By the hair on our chinny-chin-chins, we will not let you in, not for all the tea leaves in our china teapot."

"Then I'll huff and I'll puff and I'll blow your house down!" said the pig.

So he huffed and he puffed and he puffed and he huffed, but the house didn't fall down.

46

Students Acquiring English

Students may enjoy role-playing the scene on pages 46–48 between the wolves and the pig. Encourage them to make up additional dialogue to show what the characters are thinking and feeling.

QuickREFERENCE

Multicultural Link

Badminton Battledore and shuttlecock, a British game, is an early form of badminton. A *battledore* is the paddle, and *shuttlecock* is the birdie. Ask students who have played badminton to describe the game briefly.

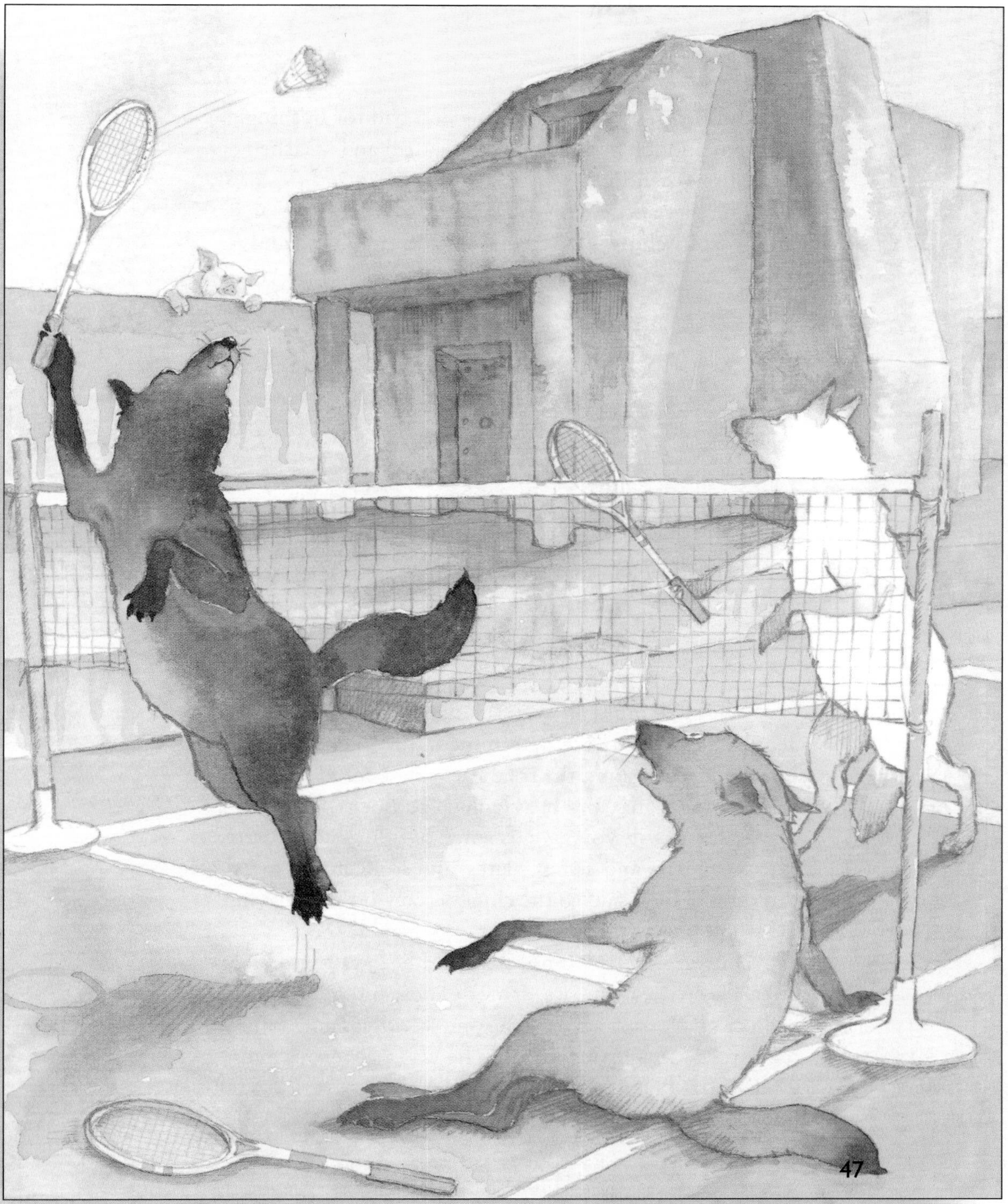
47

MINILESSON

Making Judgments

REVIEW & MAINTAIN

Teach/Model

Explain that readers make judgments based upon the evidence—what the characters do and say. Model with this Think Aloud.

Think Aloud

It's easy to make the judgment that the pig is big and bad. But I'm interested in collecting evidence to learn just how big and bad he is. I'll review what he's said and done.

Big Bad Pig	
Words	• threatened wolves
Actions	• prowled
	• destroyed houses

Discuss how this evidence leads to the judgment that the pig is "bad" in the sense of being menacing.

Practice/Apply

Cooperative Learning In small groups, have students use a chart to judge how well the little wolves defended themselves.

Little Wolves	
Words	• refused to come out
Actions	• received help • built several solid houses • escaped from pig • built flower house

SKILL FINDER

Full lesson/Reteaching, Theme 6, pp. 255C–255D

Minilessons, Theme 4, p. 27; Theme 6, pp. 239, 285

Visual Literacy

Discuss the illustration on page 47. Ask students to point out features of the concrete house that would seemingly protect the wolves without fail. Discuss how each wolf's posture indicates whether he is aware of the pig's presence.

Interact *with* Literature

Reading Strategies

Think About Words

Use these questions to prompt students to think about what *Plexiglas* is (a transparent, weather-resistant plastic).

- What common word is "hidden" in the word *Plexiglas*? *(glass)*
- How do you know Plexiglas must be strong? (It is being used with iron bars, padlocks, and other strong material.)
- Why is the first letter in *Plexiglas* capitalized? (It is a proper noun, like the brand name *Kleenex*.)

Reading Strategies

Predict/Infer

Use these questions to prompt students to make inferences and predictions.

- Will it be easier or more difficult for the pig to destroy the wolves' new house? Why? (more difficult; wolves are using barbed wire and armor plates)
- If the pig had to use a pneumatic drill the last time, what do you think he will use now? (Answers will vary, but should show an understanding that a more powerful tool is required.)

But the pig wasn't called big and bad for nothing. He went and fetched his pneumatic drill and smashed the house down.

The three little wolves managed to escape, but their chinny-chin-chins were trembling and trembling and trembling.

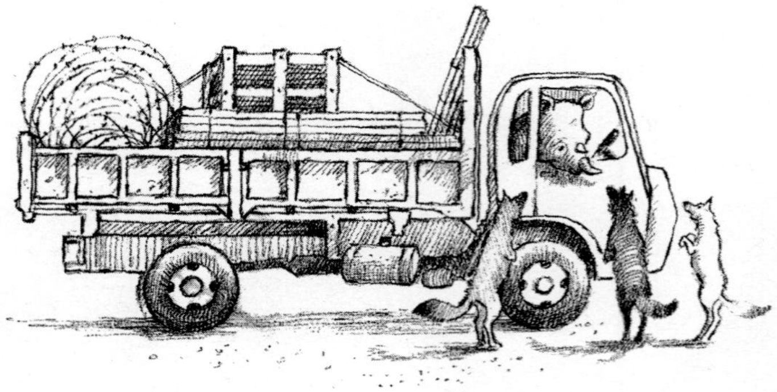

"We shall build an even stronger house," they said, because they were very determined. Just then they saw a truck coming along the road carrying barbed wire, iron bars, armor plates, and heavy metal padlocks.

"Please, will you give us some of your barbed wire, a few iron bars and armor plates, and some heavy metal padlocks?" they said to the rhinoceros who was driving the truck.

"Sure," said the rhinoceros, and he gave them plenty of barbed wire, iron bars, armor plates, and heavy metal padlocks. He also gave them some Plexiglas and some reinforced steel chains, because he was a generous and kind-hearted rhinoceros.

48

QuickREFERENCE

Vocabulary

Silent Letters Explain that the letter *p* in the word *pneumatic* is silent. Ask different students to pronounce the word (noo–MA–tik).

MEETING INDIVIDUAL NEEDS

Challenge

Analogies A pneumatic drill is run by compressed air. Challenge students to draw analogies among *pneumatic* and *pneumonia* (a lung disease) and *automatic* (self-operating). How are these words related to *pneumatic*?

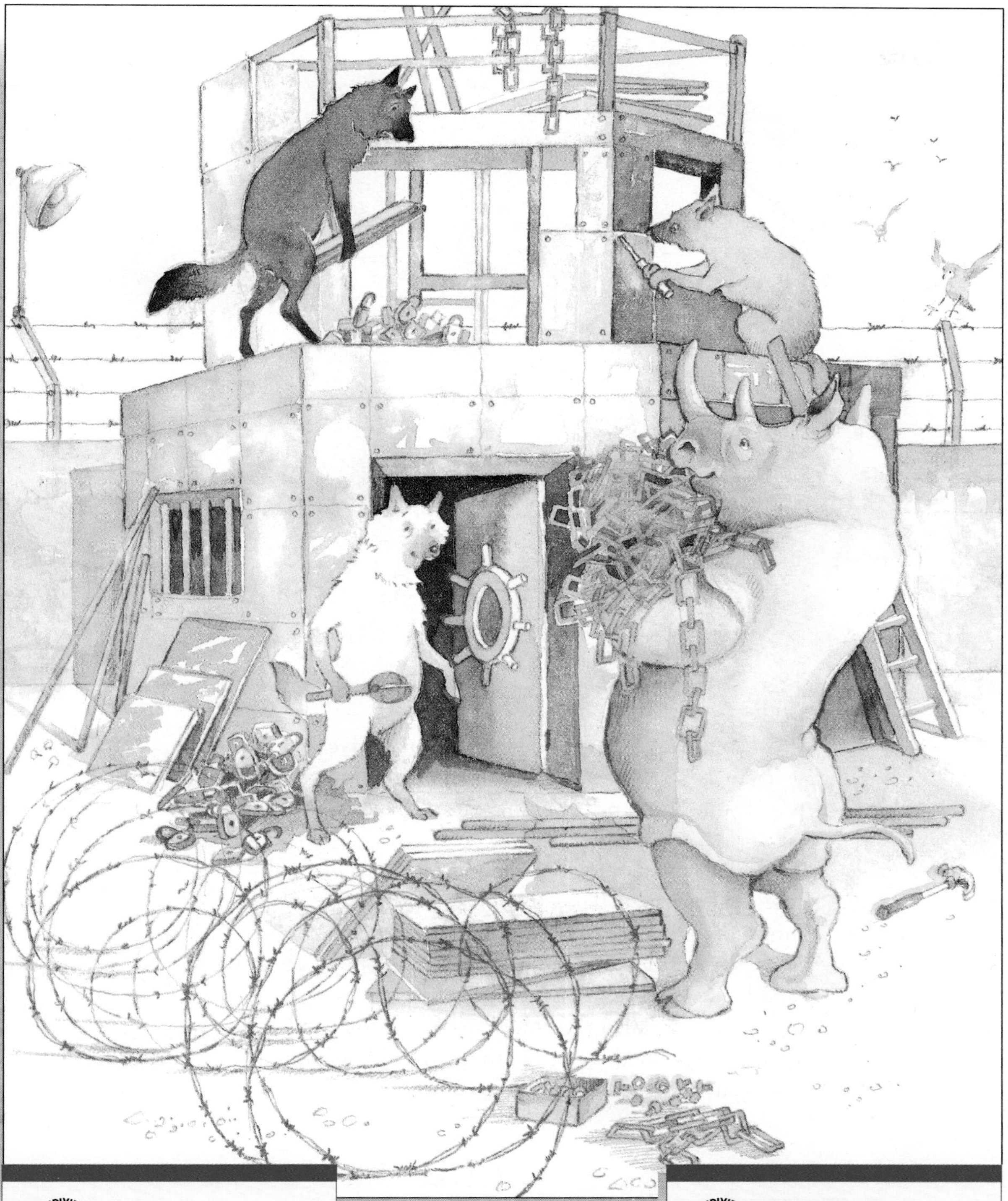

Extra Support

Oral Reading To check fluency, ask students to read aloud the last three paragraphs on page 48. Allow students to first reread these paragraphs silently. Students acquiring English may benefit from reading with a strong reader in English.

Journal

Categorizing Suggest that students list words they come across in the story that can be categorized under the following headings: animals, games, flowers.

Students Acquiring English

Word Meaning Students can use the illustration on page 49 to identify the following words and add them to the vocabulary wall chart: *barbed wire, iron bars, armor plates, metal padlocks,* and *reinforced steel chains*.

Interact with Literature

Guided Reading

MEETING INDIVIDUAL NEEDS

Comprehension/Critical Thinking

1. How did the pig destroy the concrete house? (with a pneumatic drill)
2. What kind of house did the wolves build next? (a house with iron bars, armor plates, metal padlocks, and barbed wire)
3. What did the pig do this time to prove he wasn't called *big and bad for nothing?* (He used a crane with a wrecking ball.)
4. If the iron bars and armor plates fail, what material do you think the wolves should try next? Why? (Accept responses that show an understanding of the wolves' predicament.)

Predicting/Purpose Setting

Have students review and modify their predictions if necessary. Ask what they think will happen next. Then have students read to the end of the story (page 59).

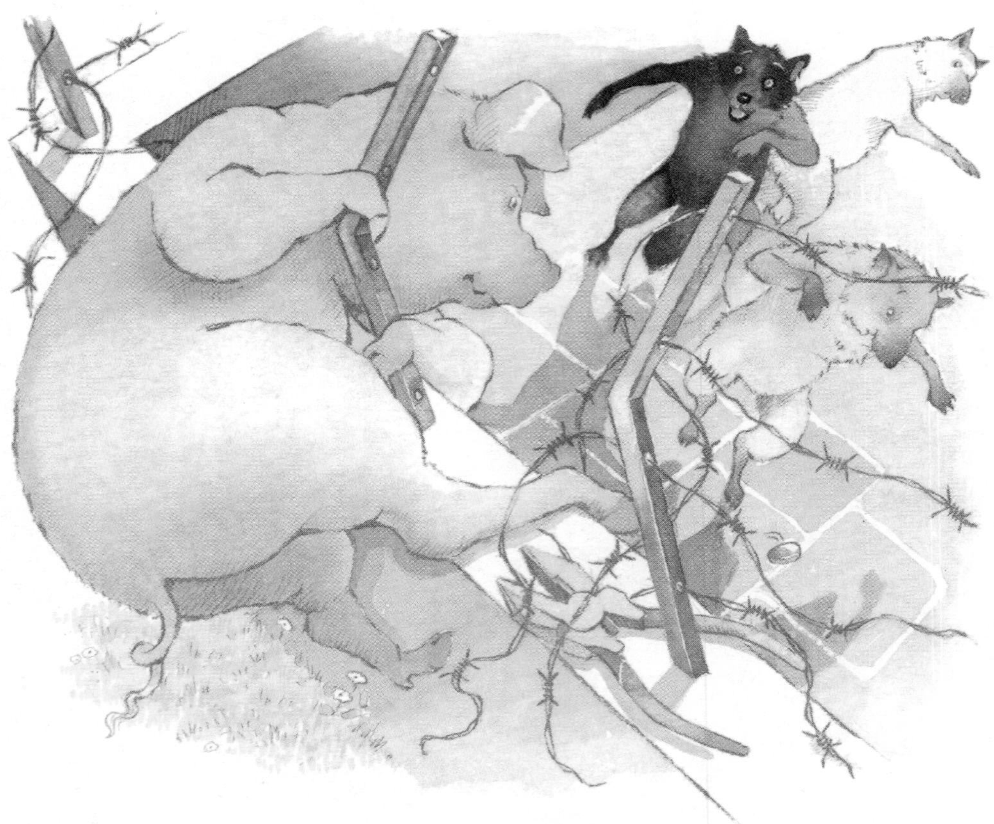

So the three little wolves built themselves an extremely strong house. It was the strongest, securest house one could possibly imagine. They felt absolutely safe.

The next day the big bad pig came prowling along the road as usual. The three little wolves were playing hopscotch in the garden. When they saw the big bad pig coming, they ran inside their house, bolted the door, and locked all the thirty-seven padlocks.

The pig dialed the video entrance phone and said, "Little frightened wolves with the trembling chins, let me come in!"

50

Self-Assessment

Reflecting Invite students to reflect on their reading with questions such as

- How has making predictions helped me understand the story?
- Have I been thinking about the story's structure?
- Have I thought of ways to figure out the meanings of words I don't know?
- What makes this story funny?

QuickREFERENCE

Vocabulary

Have students reread aloud the sentences describing the wolves' new house. Ask them to point to words containing the *-est* ending. Discuss how one can use the ending to figure out the words' meanings. (the *most* strong, the *most* secure)

Multicultural Link

Hopscotch is played all over the world. An ancient hopscotch diagram can be found in the Forum in Rome. Students might describe how they play this game or a similar game. (Variations: the shape of the board; the way players hop.)

"No, no, no!" said the little wolves. "By the hair on our chinny-chin-chins, we will not let you in, not for all the tea leaves in our china teapot."

"Then I'll huff and I'll puff and I'll blow your house down!" said the pig.

So he huffed and he puffed and he puffed and he huffed, but the house didn't fall down.

But the pig wasn't called big and bad for nothing. He rented a crane, drove it to the house, swung the wrecking ball as high as it could go, and . . .

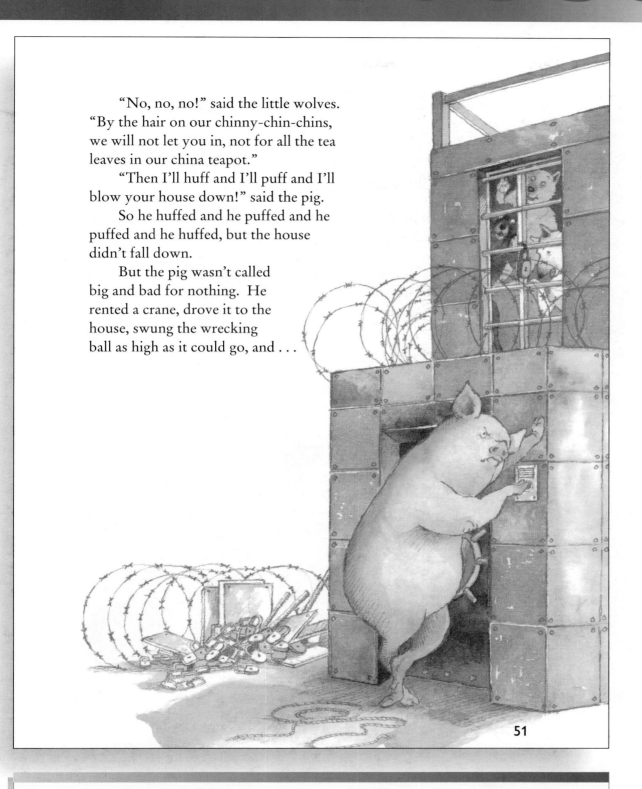

51

Technology Link

Video Entrance Phones By use of a hidden camera, a video entrance phone enables people to observe who is at their door. Ask students to name places where they have seen these phones in use.

he demolished the house. The three little wolves just managed to escape with their fluffy tails flattened.

"Something must be wrong with our building materials," they said. "We have to try something different. But *what?*"

At that moment they saw a flamingo coming along pushing a wheelbarrow full of flowers.

"Please, will you give us some flowers?" asked the little wolves.

"With pleasure," said the flamingo, and he gave them lots of flowers. So the three little wolves built themselves a house of flowers.

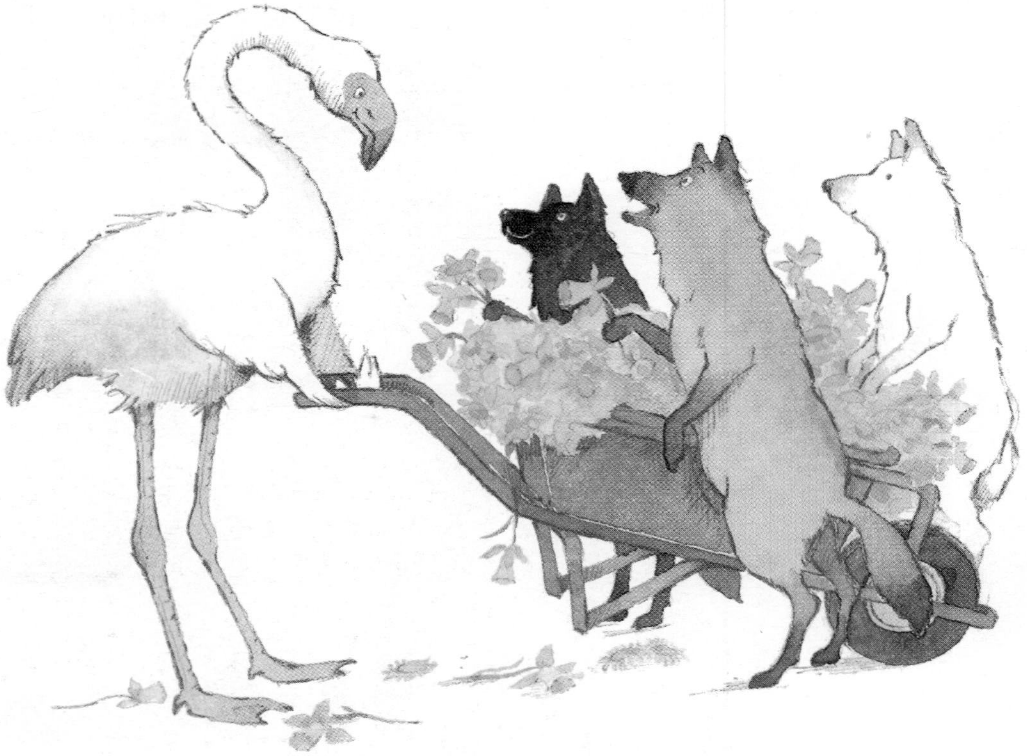

52

QuickREFERENCE

Home Connection

Students may enjoy sharing both the original story of "The Three Little Pigs" and this new version with their families. Students might also ask family members if they know any other versions of the story.

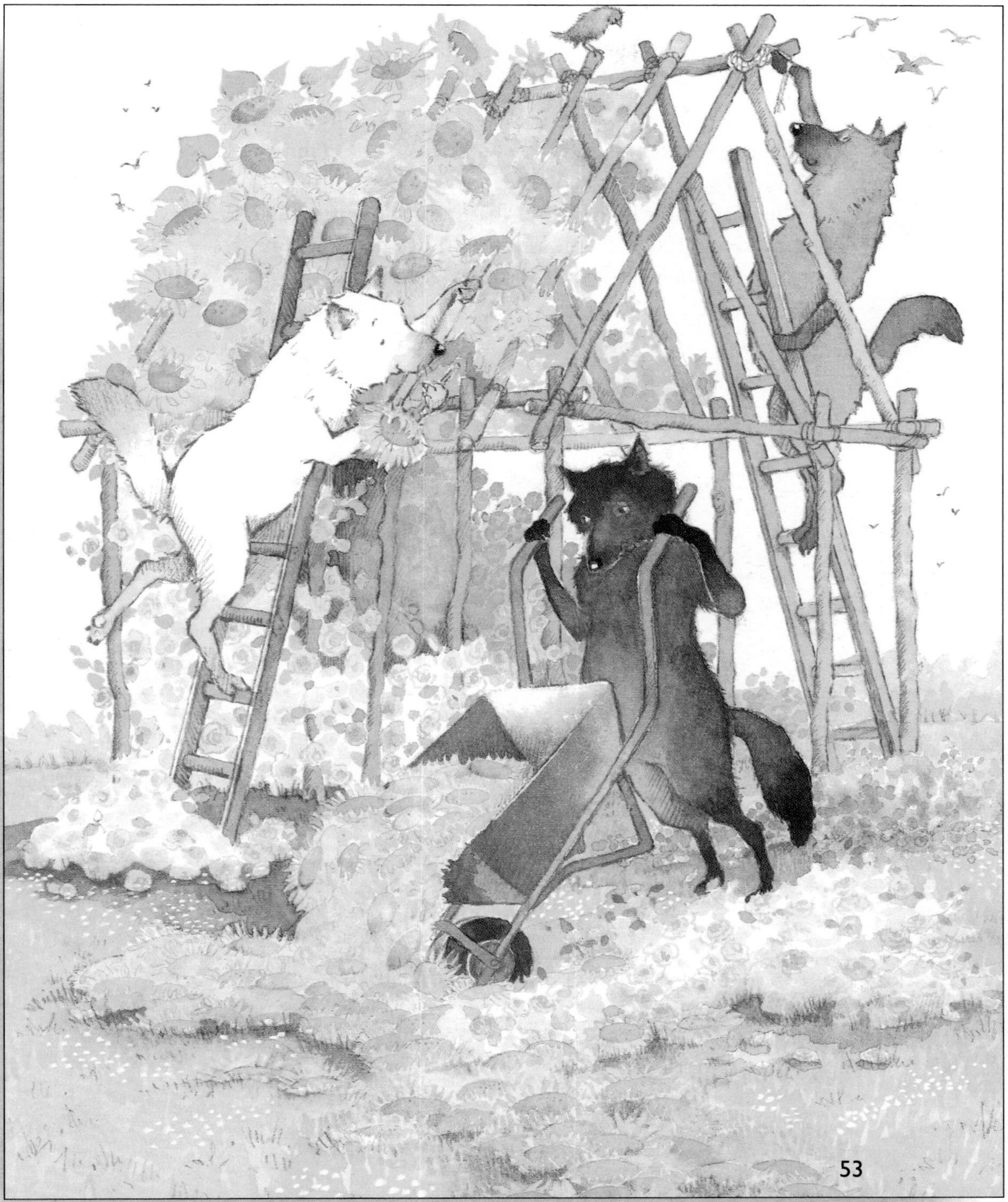

Art Link

Flower Houses Making a flower house is a fun project for students. They can

- use pictures of flowers cut from magazines or nursery catalogs
- make three-dimensional models, using colored tissue paper

Visual Literacy

Ask a volunteer to reread the first paragraph on page 54 aloud while the rest of the class studies the illustration on page 53. Have students point out each of the flowers mentioned, and discuss how the frame of the house was constructed.

Interact *with* Literature

One wall was of marigolds, one of daffodils, one of pink roses, and one of cherry blossoms. The ceiling was made of sunflowers, and the floor was a carpet of daisies. They had water lilies in their bathtub, and buttercups in their refrigerator. It was a rather fragile house and it swayed in the wind, but it was very beautiful.

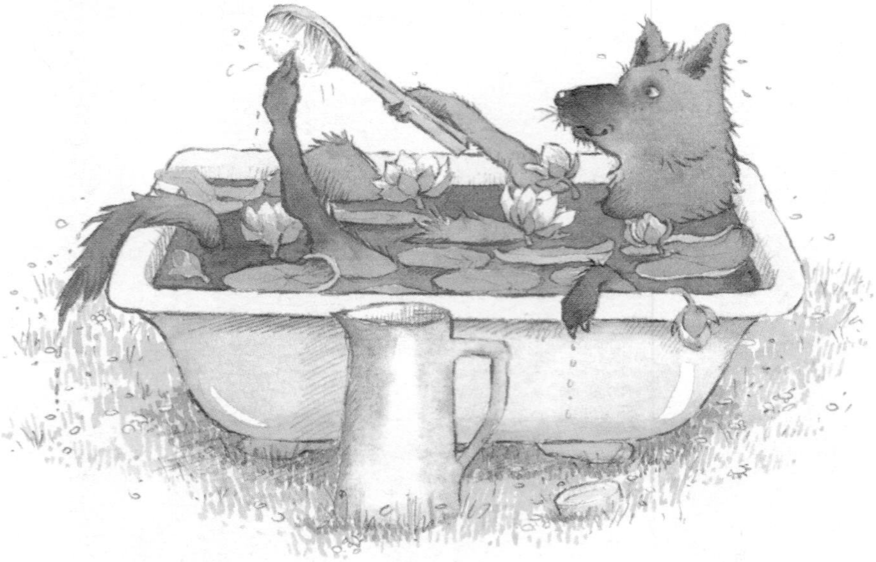

Next day the big bad pig came prowling down the road and saw the house of flowers that the three little wolves had built.

54

QuickREFERENCE

MEETING INDIVIDUAL NEEDS **Challenge**

Researching Flowers Invite students to research other varieties of flowers and recommend additional flowers for the wolves' new house. Students might want to draw pictures of their flowers to share with their classmates.

He rang the bluebell at the door and said, "Little frightened wolves with the trembling chins and the flattened tails, let me come in!"

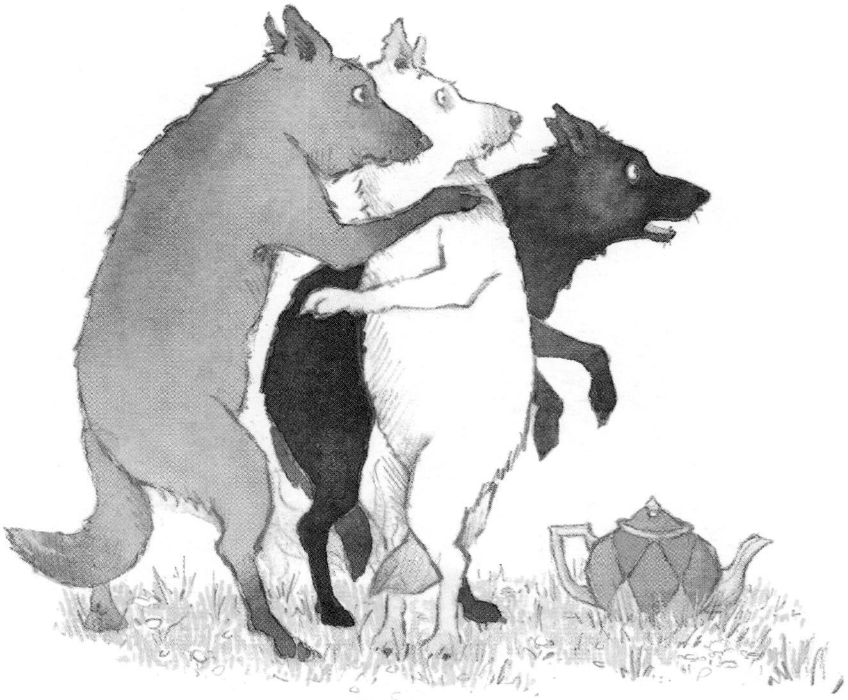

"No, no, no," said the three little wolves. "By the hair on our chinny-chin-chins, we will not let you in, not for all the tea leaves in our china teapot!"

"Then I'll huff and I'll puff and I'll blow your house down!" said the pig.

Students Acquiring English

To build on comprehension, ask students to imagine what the three little wolves might be thinking at this point in the story. Students can express their ideas by writing thought balloons for the characters in the illustration.

Extra Support

Cooperative Learning Ask volunteers to prepare an oral presentation of the text on pages 55–56. As students read, another volunteer might pantomime the pig's actions.

Interact *with* Literature

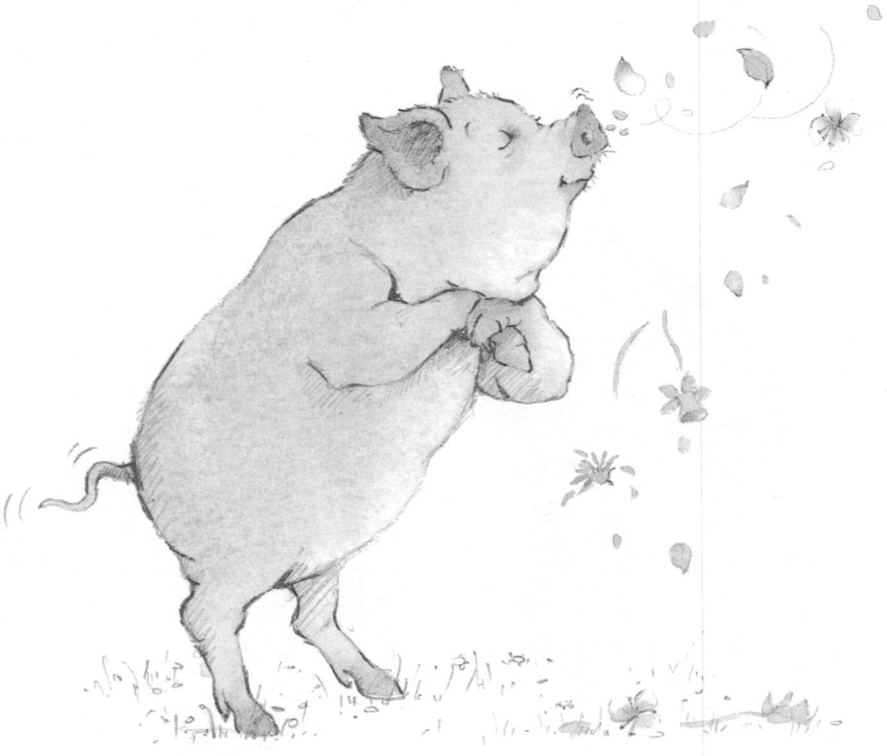

But as he took a deep breath, ready to huff and puff, he smelled the soft scent of the flowers. It was fantastic. And because the scent was so lovely, the pig took another breath and then another. Instead of huffing and puffing, he began to sniff.

He sniffed deeper and deeper until he was quite filled with the fragrant scent. His heart grew tender, and he realized how horrible he had been. Right then he decided to become a big *good* pig.

He started to sing and to dance the tarantella.

56

QuickREFERENCE

Music Link

Mood Have students imagine music for this story. What would the music sound like as the pig is threatening the wolves on pages 42, 46, and 50? How would it change after he sniffs the flowers on page 56?

Students Acquiring English

MEETING INDIVIDUAL NEEDS

Invite students to pantomime the scene of the pig's transformation on pages 56–59. Encourage discussion about the actions and emotions of both the pig and the wolves. Have students contrast this scene with the one on pages 46–48.

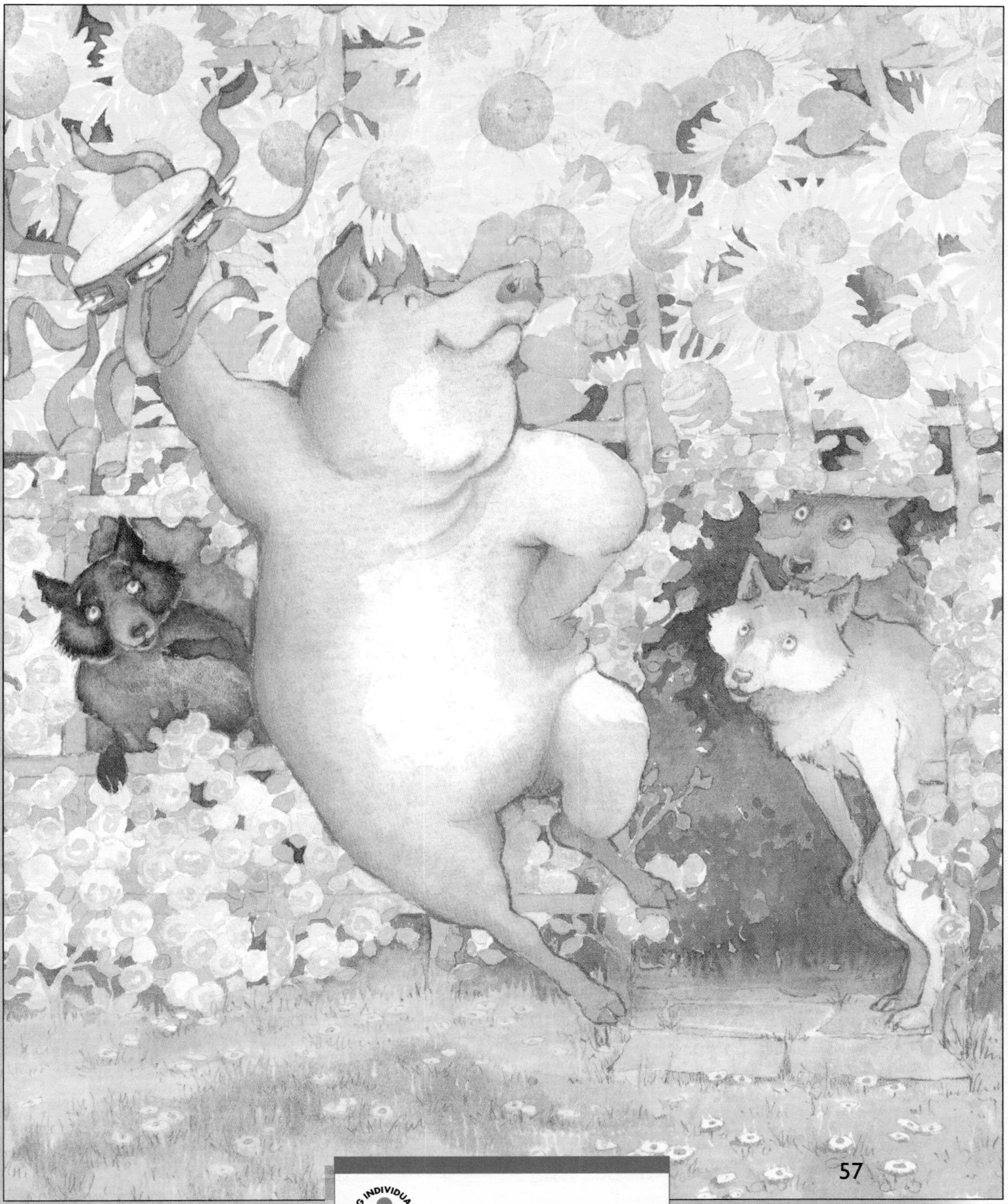

MINILESSON

Fantasy/ Realism

REVIEW & MAINTAIN

Teach/Model

Discuss how fantasy has both real and make-believe elements in it. For example, in this selection the fact that there are wolves building a house is fantasy, but the materials they use are real.

Practice/Apply

Invite students to pick out other story elements and events that are real and fantasy. You might list their responses in a chart.

Real	Fantasy
wheelbarrow	kangaroo talking
croquet	wolves playing it
sledgehammer	pig demolishing house
wire, iron bars	wolves building house
crane	wolves escape

End by discussing how mixing fantasy with realistic elements adds to the humor of the story.

SKILL FINDER

Full lesson/Reteaching, pp. 114B–114C

Minilessons, p. 95; Theme 5, p. 211

MEETING INDIVIDUAL NEEDS

Challenge

The Tarantella Explain that the tarantella is from southern Italy. A person dancing it would be whirling and spinning. Challenge students to learn the origin of this word, especially as it relates to *tarantism* (an uncontrollable urge to dance).

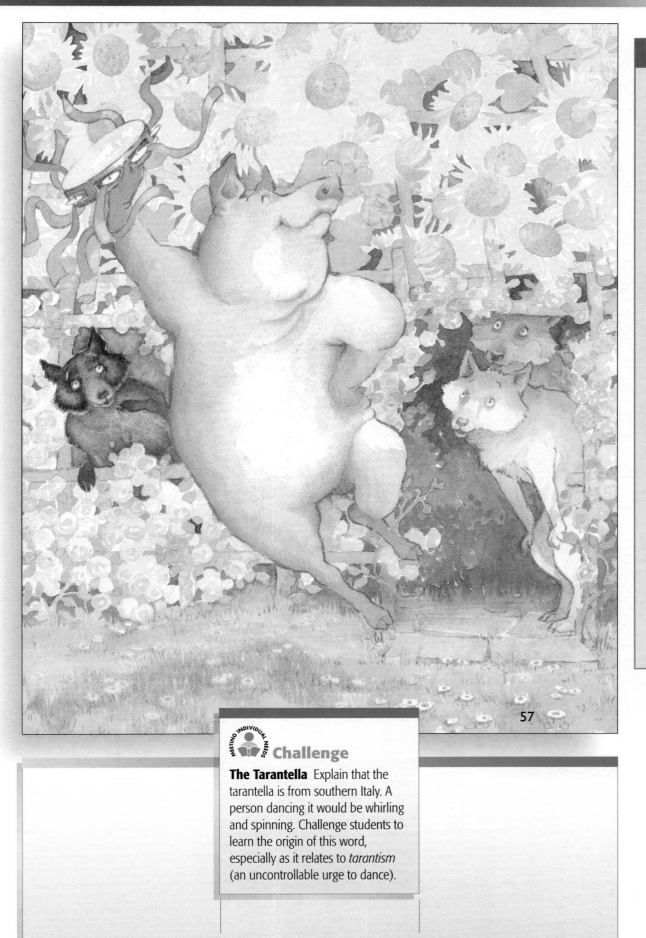

Interact with Literature

Guided Reading

Comprehension/Critical Thinking

1. What kind of house did the wolves build next? Why? (They built a house of flowers; they needed a different solution to their problem with the pig.)
2. Was the house of flowers strong? Describe this house. (Students might paraphrase page 54: *It was a rather fragile house and it swayed in the wind, but it was very beautiful.*)
3. What happened when the pig tried to blow down the house? (The scent of the flowers made his heart grow tender. He began to dance.)
4. What if the house of flowers *hadn't* worked? What do you think the wolves could have done next? (Answers should show an awareness of the difficulties of the wolves' predicament.)

At first the three little wolves were a bit worried. It might be a trick. But soon they realized that the pig had truly changed, so they came running out of the house.

They started playing games with him.

First they played pig-pog and then piggy-in-the-middle, and when they were all tired, they invited him into the house.

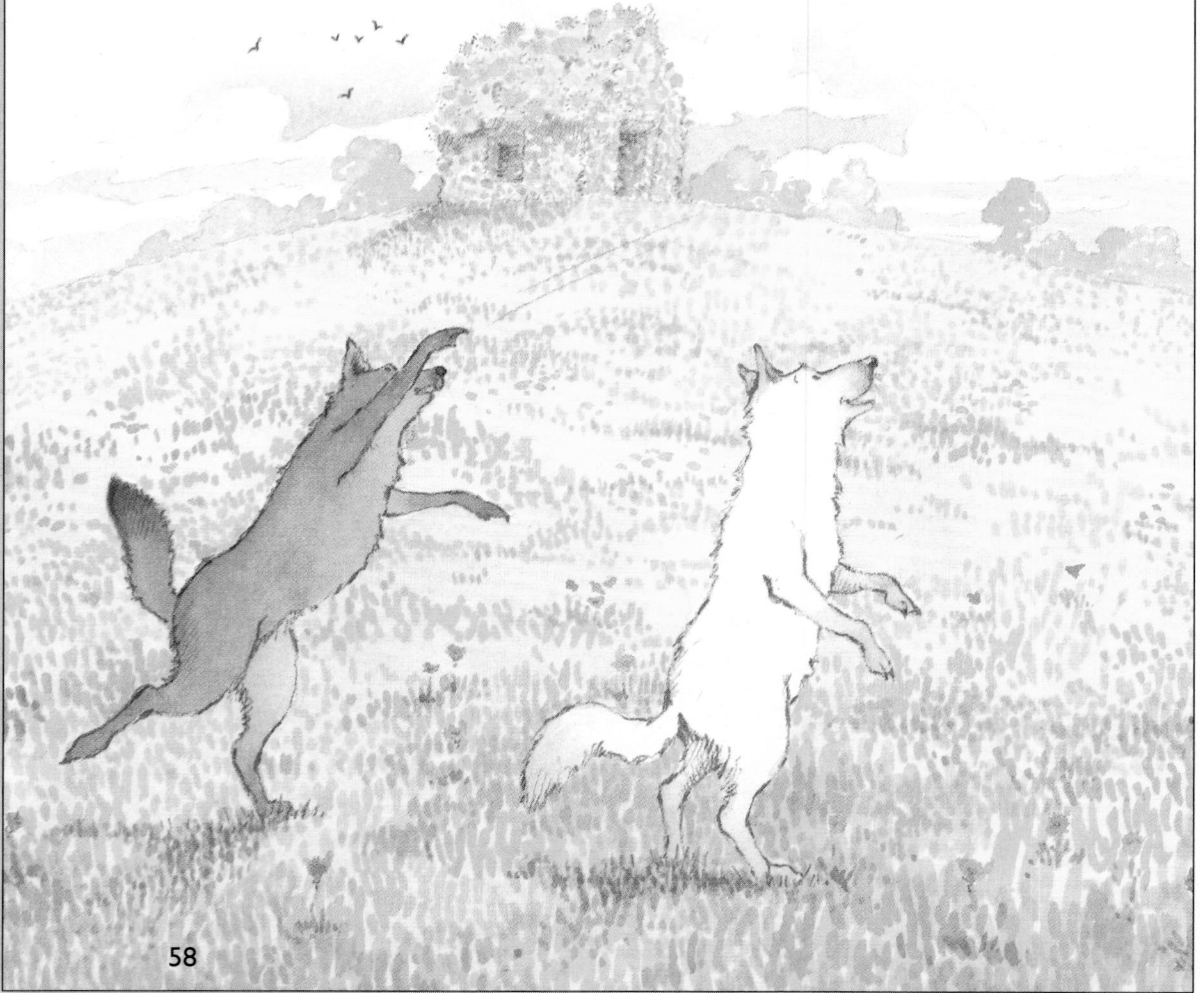

58

Self-Assessment

Ask students to assess their reading using these questions:

- How did monitoring my thinking while reading help me better understand this story?
- How well did I predict and infer actions and events in the story?
- How did knowing the original version of "The Three Little Pigs" help me predict events in this story?
- Would the story still be funny without the role reversals?

QuickREFERENCE

Health Link

Sports Croquet, battledore and shuttlecock (badminton), hopscotch, and piggy-(monkey)-in-the-middle are games that the three little wolves enjoy playing. Ask students what game they think the characters are playing on pages 58 and 59.

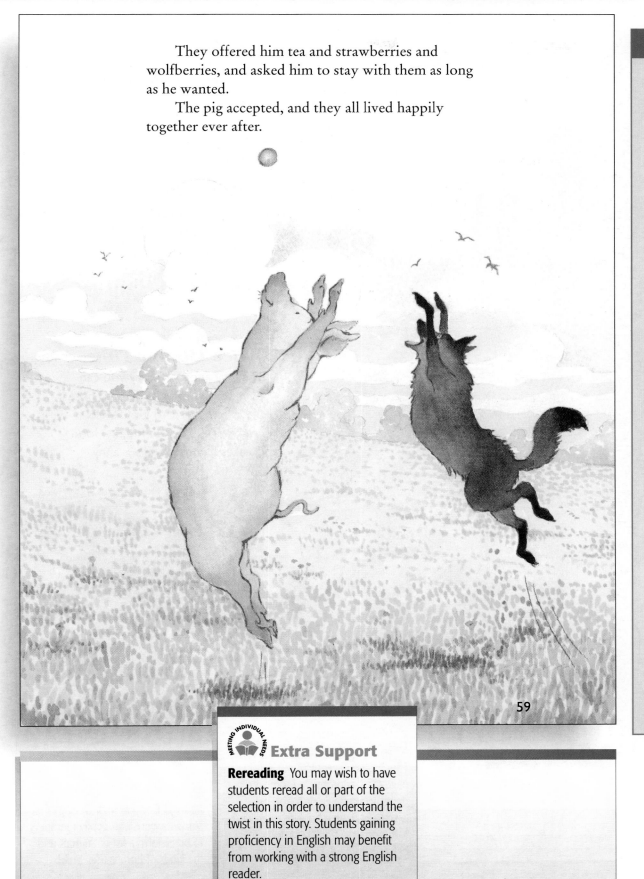

They offered him tea and strawberries and wolfberries, and asked him to stay with them as long as he wanted.

The pig accepted, and they all lived happily together ever after.

59

MINILESSON

Writer's Craft

Character Role Reversal

Teach/Model

Discuss how author Eugene Trivizas has enlivened a familiar tale by reversing the roles of the main characters and giving it a contemporary setting.

Practice/Apply

Recall with students details from the traditional tale that have been altered in the modern version. You may wish to place responses in a chart like the following.

Little Pigs	Big Bad Pig
small →	large
sweet →	mean
leave mother →	no mother

Big Bad Wolf	Little Wolves
menacing →	fun-loving
eats pigs →	drink tea
will stop at nothing →	want peace

Discuss how other familiar folk or fairy tales could be altered in a similar way.

SKILL FINDER

Writing Activities: A Reversed Tale, p. 60E

Reading-Writing Workshop, pp. 116–117F

MEETING INDIVIDUAL NEEDS

Extra Support

Rereading You may wish to have students reread all or part of the selection in order to understand the twist in this story. Students gaining proficiency in English may benefit from working with a strong English reader.

Responding Activities

Personal Response

Invite students to write or tell their feelings about the story's ending. Were they glad that the big bad pig, unlike the big bad wolf, was not hurt?

Anthology Activities

Choose, or have students choose, a response activity from page 60. For students acquiring English, discuss why the second activity is called "Twice Upon a Time." Also explain the idea of turning something *inside out.* Relate it to the concept of role reversal.

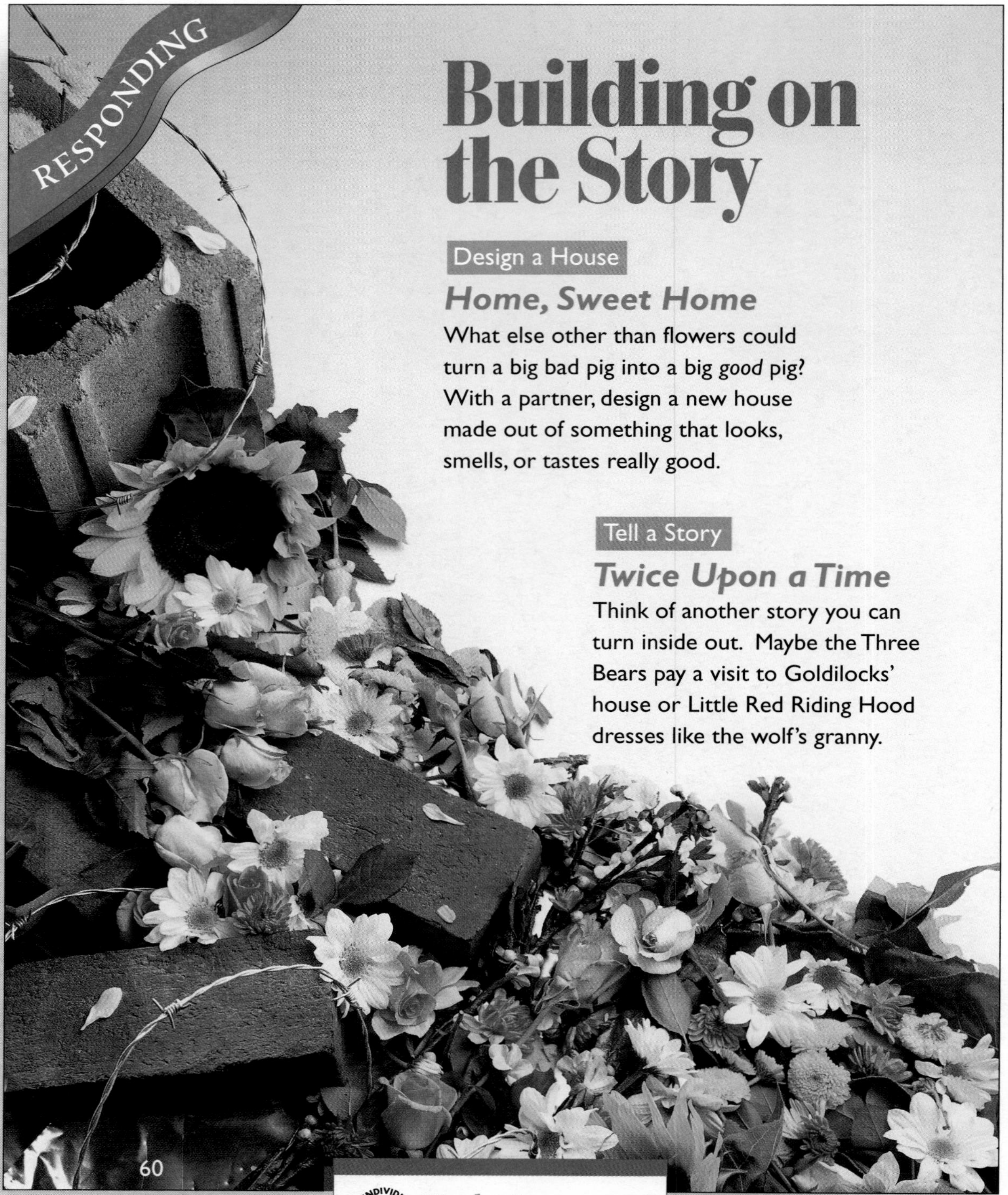
RESPONDING

Building on the Story

Design a House

Home, Sweet Home

What else other than flowers could turn a big bad pig into a big *good* pig? With a partner, design a new house made out of something that looks, smells, or tastes really good.

Tell a Story

Twice Upon a Time

Think of another story you can turn inside out. Maybe the Three Bears pay a visit to Goldilocks' house or Little Red Riding Hood dresses like the wolf's granny.

60

Informal Assessment

Check students' responses for a general understanding of the selection and how it relates to the original story of "The Three Little Pigs."

Additional Support:

- Use Guided Reading questions or the Summarizing: Story Structure minilesson to review.
- Have students work cooperatively to complete a Venn diagram comparing this story with the traditional tale.

QuickREFERENCE

Students Acquiring English

MEETING INDIVIDUAL NEEDS

The "Home, Sweet Home" activity on page 60 is appropriate for most students acquiring English. You may wish to bring in a book or magazine with pictures of different houses to help get students thinking.

Home Connection

Animal Contractors Suggest that students work with family members to brainstorm a list of animals and the kinds of homes they build. (beavers/dams, spiders/webs, birds/nests, and so on)

More Choices for Responding

Thank-You Notes

Materials
- construction paper
- scissors
- stapler
- markers or crayons

As the three little wolves, students can write notes to the other story characters to thank them for the building supplies and to tell what happened to the homes the wolves built.

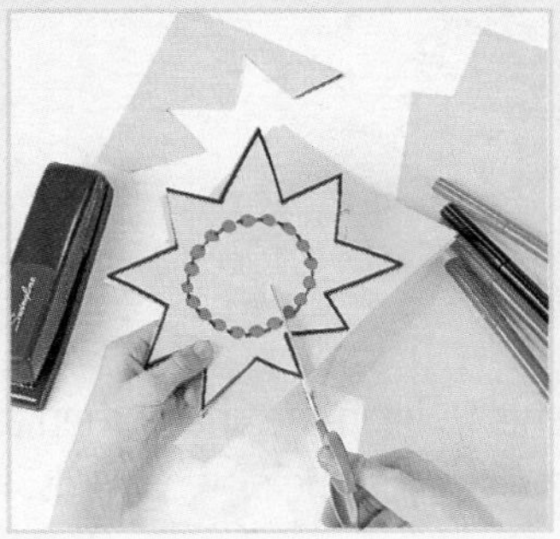

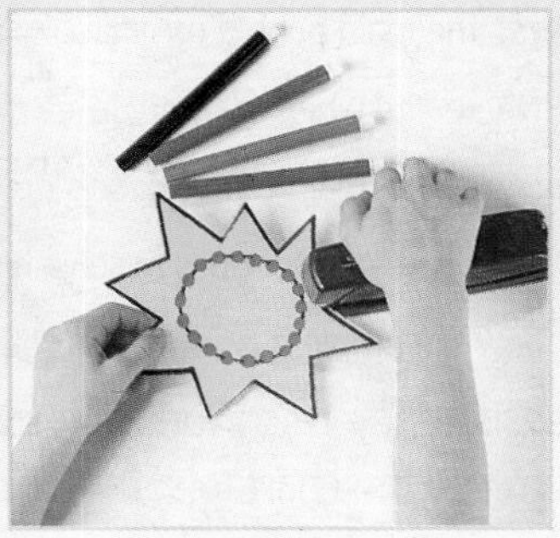

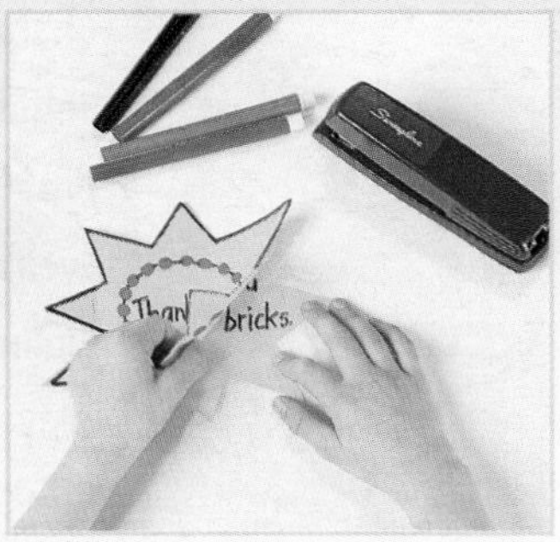

1. Have students use 2 pieces of paper together to cut out flower shapes.
2. Have students staple the flower shapes together.
3. Then have students write their messages inside.

Share Favorite Things

In their response to the pig, the wolves always say *"not for all the tea leaves in our china teapot."* Ask students to think of a favorite thing they own that they would never want to give up. Students could bring their valued objects in and share why these objects are so important to them.

Selection Connections

LAB, p. 8

Have students complete the portion of the chart relating to *The Three Little Wolves and the Big Bad Pig.*

Literature Discussion

- Tell about a time that you met someone who, like the big bad pig, was unfriendly at first but later became your friend. What happened that turned you into friends?
- What do you think the wolves' mother would say if she visited the flower house and saw her children living with the pig?
- How long do you think the big bad pig will stay and live with the three little wolves? What could he do for the wolves to show them that he has changed for good?

Comprehension Check

To check selection comprehension, use the following questions and/or have students complete *Literacy Activity Book* page 10.

1. What does the pig do in this story to prove that he is big and bad? (He demolishes three houses in his tireless pursuit of the little wolves.)
2. Why do you think the wolves didn't try to hurt the big bad pig? Was this a good idea or not? (It only would have made the pig madder and provided him with a reason to continue to attack them.)

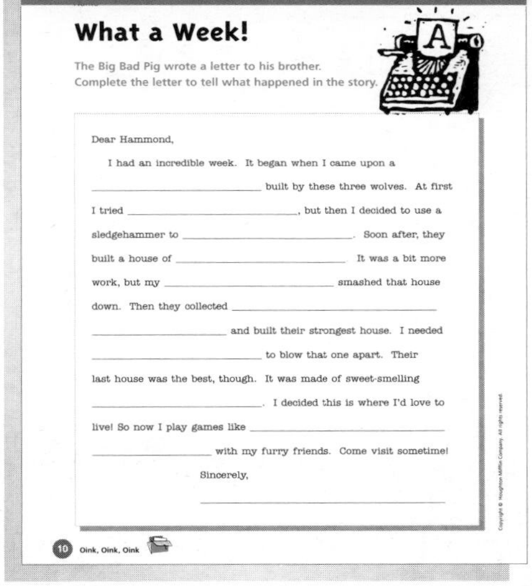

Literacy Activity Book, p. 10

What a Week!

The Big Bad Pig wrote a letter to his brother.
Complete the letter to tell what happened in the story.

Dear Hammond,

I had an incredible week. It began when I came upon a ________ built by these three wolves. At first I tried ________, but then I decided to use a sledgehammer to ________. Soon after, they built a house of ________ It was a bit more work, but my ________ smashed that house down. Then they collected ________ ________ and built their strongest house. I needed ________ to blow that one apart. Their last house was the best, though. It was made of sweet-smelling ________. I decided this is where I'd love to live! So now I play games like ________ ________ with my furry friends. Come visit sometime!

Sincerely,

____

Copyright © Houghton Mifflin Company. All rights reserved.

10 Oink, Oink, Oink

Portfolio Opportunity

- Selection comprehension: Save *Literacy Activity Book* page 10.
- Writing samples: Save thank-you notes or responses to other writing activities.

Instruct *and* Integrate

Comprehension

Transparency 1–2

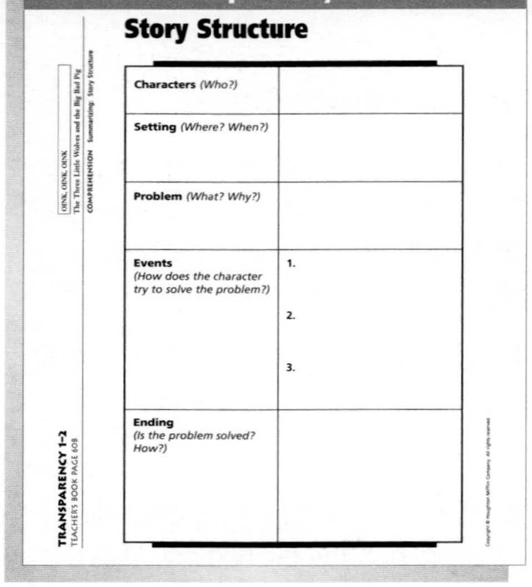
Story Structure

Characters *(Who?)*	
Setting *(Where? When?)*	
Problem *(What? Why?)*	
Events *(How does the character try to solve the problem?)*	1. 2. 3.
Ending *(Is the problem solved? How?)*	

TRANSPARENCY 1–2
TEACHER'S BOOK PAGE 60B

Literacy Activity Book, p. 11

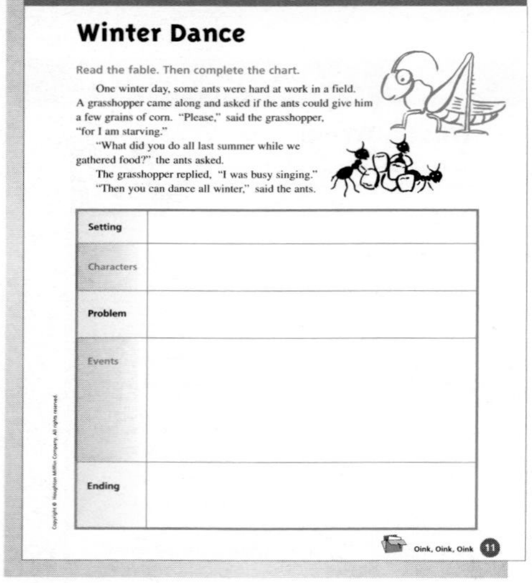
Winter Dance

Read the fable. Then complete the chart.

One winter day, some ants were hard at work in a field. A grasshopper came along and asked if the ants could give him a few grains of corn. "Please," said the grasshopper, "for I am starving."

"What did you do all last summer while we gathered food?" the ants asked.

The grasshopper replied, "I was busy singing."

"Then you can dance all winter," said the ants.

Setting	
Characters	
Problem	
Events	
Ending	

Oink, Oink, Oink 11

INTERACTIVE LEARNING

Summarizing: Story Structure

TESTED SKILL

LAB, p. 11

Teach/Model

Discuss how focusing on the following elements of a story can help readers organize their thoughts when they want to summarize.

- **Characters:** the main people (or animals) in the story
- **Setting:** where and when the story takes place
- **Problem:** what the main character sets out to do
- **Events:** what the character does to solve his/her problem
- **Ending:** how the problem is (or is not) solved

Display Transparency 1–2. Work with students to fill in the chart. Then ask volunteers to use the chart to summarize the story in their own words. If necessary, model with this summary.

Think Aloud

This version of "The Three Little Pigs" is about three little wolves and a big bad pig. The pig in this story does more than huff and puff. He uses different tools to smash the wolves' houses. The wolves finally decide to build a house of flowers, and it works: the pig loves flowers, and he becomes their friend.

Characters	3 wolves, a pig
Setting	a wooded area, Once Upon a Time
Problem	Wolves must avoid Big Bad Pig.
Events	1. Wolves build brick house, but pig hammers it down.
	2. Wolves try cement house, but pig uses pneumatic drill.
	3. Wolves build secure house, but pig uses a crane.
Ending	Wolves build a house of flowers, and pig, who loves flowers, becomes their friend.

Practice/Apply

- Have students complete *Literacy Activity Book* page 11.
- Have students summarize another story they know well.

SKILL FINDER
Minilessons, pp. 45, 83; Theme 2, p. 207

Informal Assessment

Check the discussion portion of the lesson and/or *Literacy Activity Book* page 11 for an assessment of students' ability to summarize.

Additional Support:

Reteaching, p. 60C
Minilessons, pp. 45, 83; Theme 2, p. 207

Reteaching

Summarizing: Story Structure

MEETING INDIVIDUAL NEEDS

Cooperative Learning

Read the classic version of "The Three Little Pigs" on pages 35A–35B. Divide students into four small groups and assign a story element to each group. Have students listen carefully and draw every element except the problem (which can be stated in a sentence or two). You may wish to reuse Transparency 1–2 for this activity or make a chart on the bulletin board. Tape students' pictures in the appropriate rows and discuss how each artist chose to capture a story element.

Students can use the **Channel R.E.A.D.** videodisc "License to Drive" for additional support with Summarizing: Story Structure.

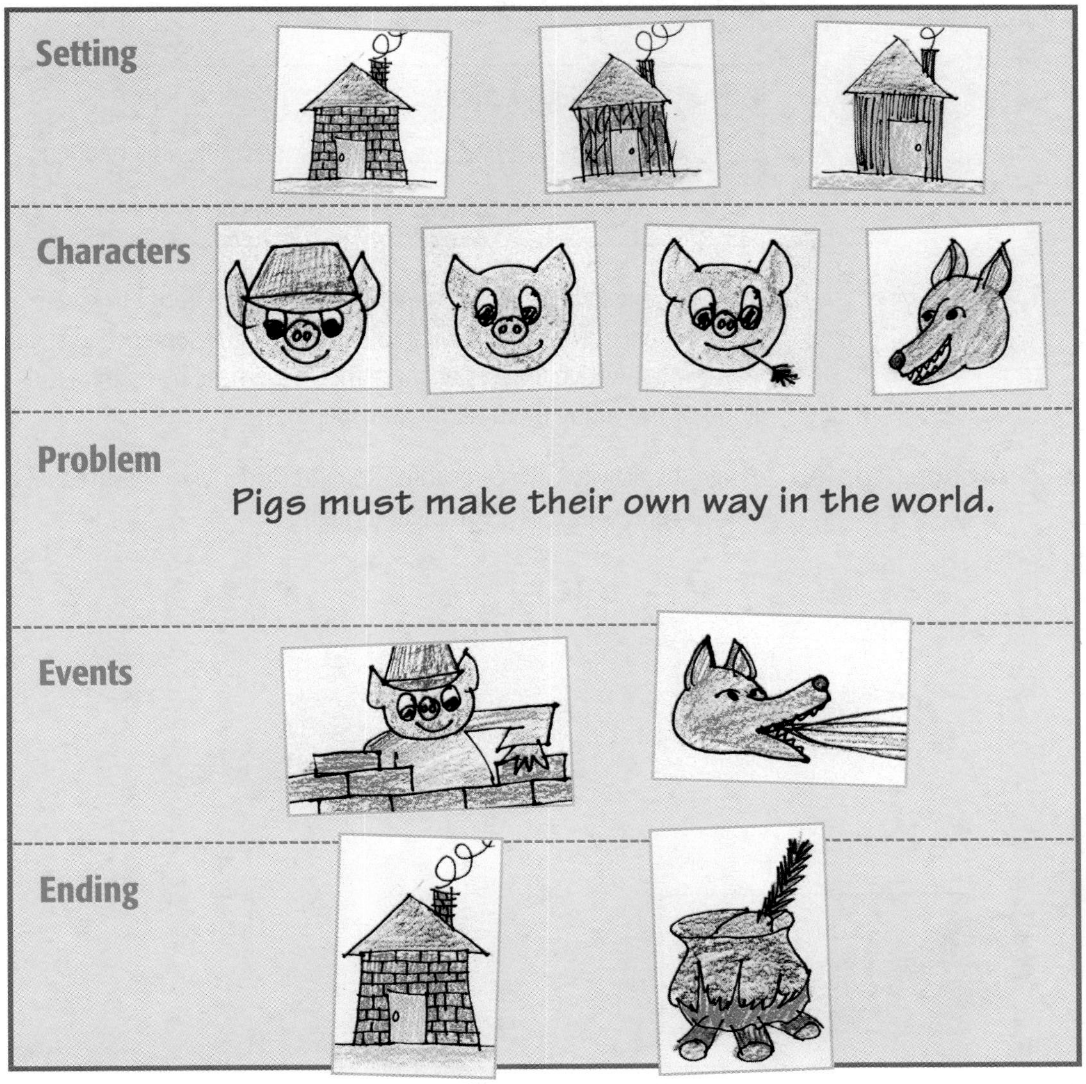
Setting
Characters
Problem
Pigs must make their own way in the world.
Events
Ending

Portfolio Opportunity

- Save *Literacy Activity Book* page 11 to record students' understanding of story structure and summarizing.

Instruct *and* Integrate

Writing Skills and Activities

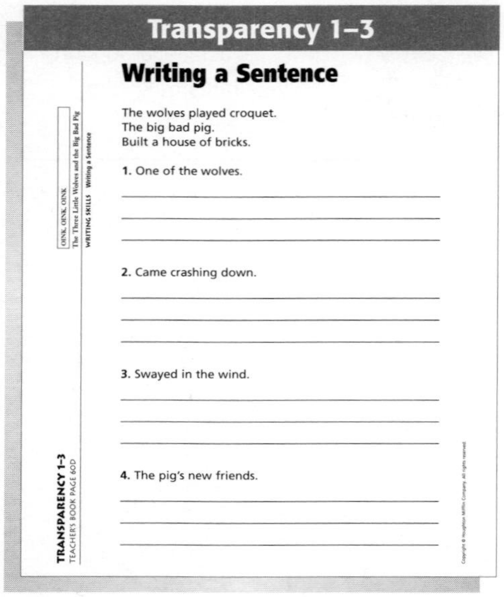
Transparency 1–3

Writing a Sentence

The wolves played croquet.
The big bad pig.
Built a house of bricks.

1. One of the wolves.
2. Came crashing down.
3. Swayed in the wind.
4. The pig's new friends.

TRANSPARENCY 1–3

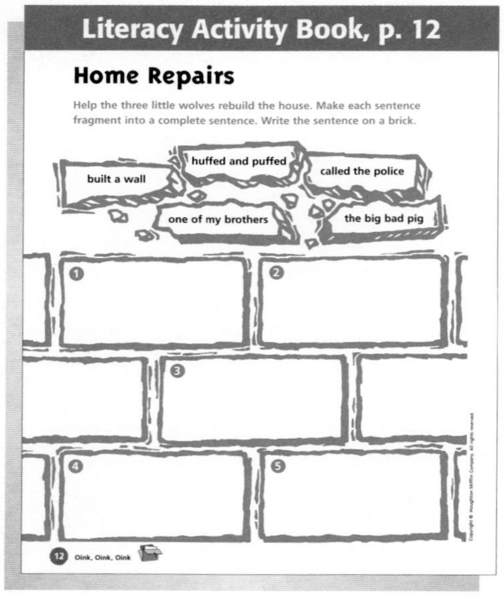
Literacy Activity Book, p. 12

Home Repairs

Help the three little wolves rebuild the house. Make each sentence fragment into a complete sentence. Write the sentence on a brick.

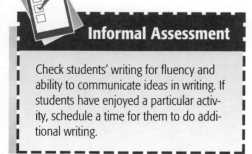

built a wall
huffed and puffed
called the police
one of my brothers
the big bad pig

Informal Assessment

Check students' writing for fluency and ability to communicate ideas in writing. If students have enjoyed a particular activity, schedule a time for them to do additional writing.

INTERACTIVE LEARNING

Writing a Sentence

TESTED SKILL

LAB, p.12

Teach/Model

Display Transparency 1–3. Have students read the three groups of words at the top of the transparency. Ask which group of words is a sentence. (the first) Remind students that a sentence is a group of words that tells a complete thought—it tells who or what the sentence is about and what happens. Ask students to explain why the second group of words is not a sentence. (It doesn't tell what happens—what the pig did.) Ask the same question about the third group. (It doesn't tell who or what built the house.)

Explain that it is important for writers to use complete sentences so their readers are not confused.

The wolves played croquet.	complete sentence
The big bad pig.	doesn't tell what happens
Built a house of bricks.	doesn't tell who built the house

Have students add to each fragment on the transparency to create a complete sentence. They might want to complete each sentence in several different ways. Ask volunteers to share their sentences by reading them aloud or by writing them on the transparency.

Practice/Apply

Assign the activity Give Directions. Remind students to be sure that each of their sentences tells a complete thought.

SKILL FINDER

Grammar, pp. 60J–60K
Reading-Writing Workshop, p. 116–117F

Writing Activities

Shared Writing: A Reversed Tale

Work with students to write a story, reversing the roles in another traditional tale. Use one of the following ideas or brainstorm ideas together.

- The Three Trolls and the Billy Goat Gruff
- Baby Bear and the Goldilocks Family
- Rotten Red Riding Hood and the Little Wolf

(See the Writer's Craft Minilesson on page 59.)

Write a Song

Cooperative Learning

Remind students that when the big bad pig smelled the flowers, he started to sing and dance the tarantella. Have students work in small groups to write a song that the pig might have sung. Have volunteers perform their songs for the class.

Give Directions

Remind students that the three little wolves enjoyed playing games, including croquet, battledore and shuttlecock, hopscotch, pig-pog, and piggy-in-the-middle. Have each student select a favorite game and write a set of directions for playing it.

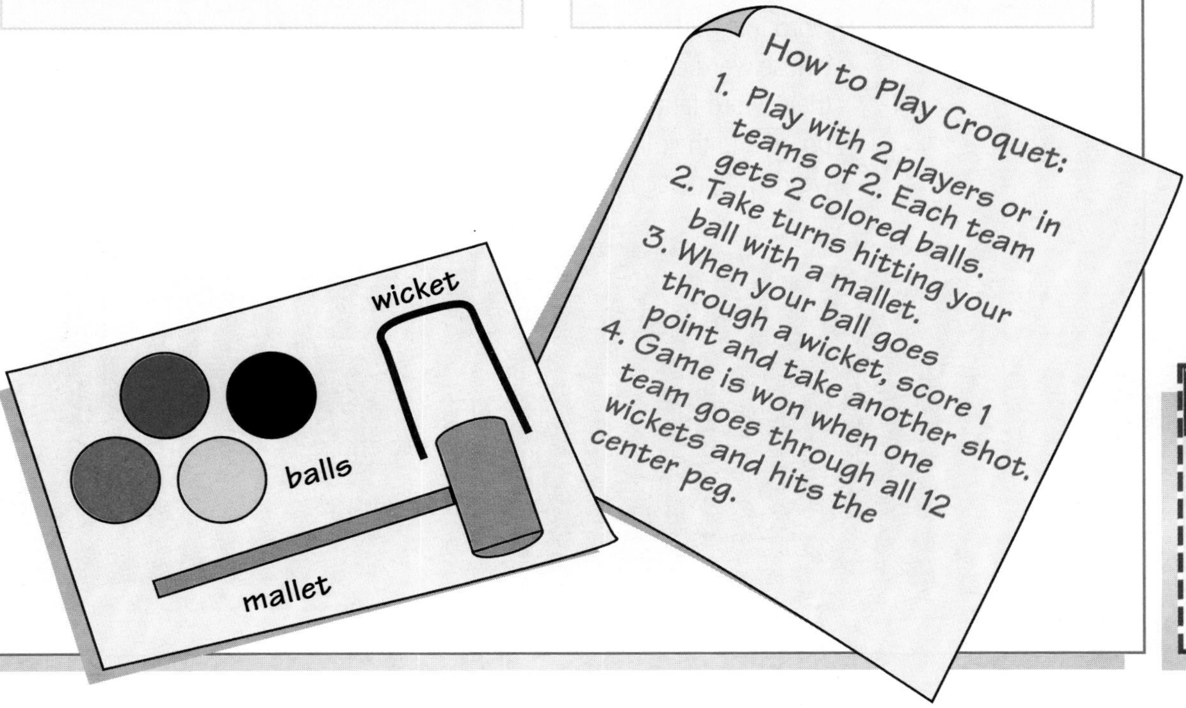
wicket
balls
mallet
How to Play Croquet:
1. Play with 2 players or in teams of 2. Each team gets 2 colored balls.
2. Take turns hitting your ball with a mallet.
3. When your ball goes through a wicket, score 1 point and take another shot.
4. Game is won when one team goes through all 12 wickets and hits the center peg.

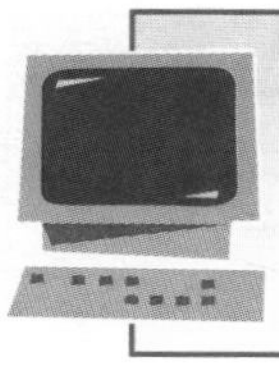

Students can use The Learning Company's new elementary writing center for all their writing activities.

Portfolio Opportunity

- Save *Literacy Activity Book* page 12 to record students' understanding of writing complete sentences.
- Save responses to activities on this page for writing samples.

Word Skills and Strategies

Literacy Activity Book, p. 13

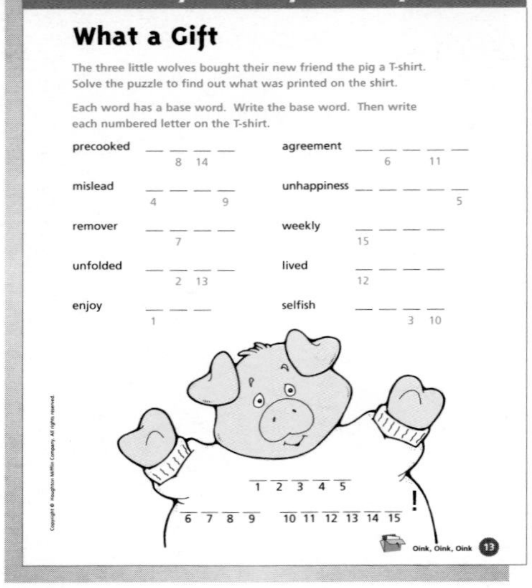
What a Gift

The three little wolves bought their new friend the pig a T-shirt. Solve the puzzle to find out what was printed on the shirt.

Each word has a base word. Write the base word. Then write each numbered letter on the T-shirt.

precooked ___ ___ ___ ___ (8, 14)
agreement ___ ___ ___ ___ ___ (6, 11)
mislead ___ ___ ___ ___ (4, 9)
unhappiness ___ ___ ___ ___ ___ (5)
remover ___ ___ ___ ___ (7)
weekly ___ ___ ___ ___ (15)
unfolded ___ ___ ___ ___ (2, 13)
lived ___ ___ ___ ___ (12)
enjoy ___ ___ ___ (1)
selfish ___ ___ ___ ___ (3, 10)

1 2 3 4 5
6 7 8 9 10 11 12 13 14 15 !

INTERACTIVE LEARNING

TESTED SKILL

Structural Analysis
Base Words

LAB, p. 13

Teach/Model

Write this sentence on the board.

The little wolves were getting tired of rebuilding their house.

Ask students if they can find a word in the sentence that is made from the smaller word *build.* Repeat with *get, wolf,* and *tire.* As they find each word, write the base word above it. Tell students that many words are created by adding beginnings and endings to smaller words. Explain that the smaller words are called base words. Point out that the spelling of the base word sometimes changes when an ending is added, as in *wolf* and *wolves.*

Tell students that many words can be made from the same base word. Under *rebuilding* on the board, add *builds* and *builder.* Explain that *rebuilding, builds,* and *builder* are all part of the word family for *build.* Tell students that all of the words in a word family are related in meaning, for example, a builder is a person who builds. Point out that when students come across an unfamiliar word in their reading, finding the base word can be a clue to figuring out the meaning of the word.

Practice/Apply

Write each word below on an index card (not including the base words) and give one card to each student. Have students determine the base word that their word comes from and then find the other four students whose word comes from the same base word. Once students have found their "word-family members," have them write their base word on the board and their individual words beneath it. As a class, discuss how the words within each family are related in meaning.

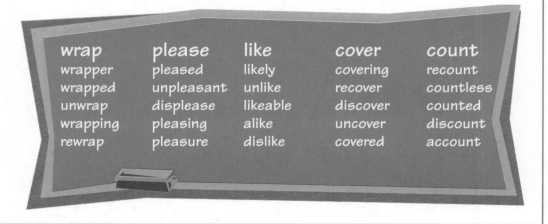

wrap	please	like	cover	count
wrapper	pleased	likely	covering	recount
wrapped	unpleasant	unlike	recover	countless
unwrap	displease	likeable	discover	counted
wrapping	pleasing	alike	uncover	discount
rewrap	pleasure	dislike	covered	account

MEETING INDIVIDUAL NEEDS

Extra Support

Point out to students that the meaning of a base word is closely related to the meaning of the longer word. Make sure they understand that not every group of letters that happens to form a word within a longer word is a base word. For instance, *neigh* is not a base word in *neighbor.*

Informal Assessment

Use Practice/Apply to check students' understanding of base words.

Additional support:

Reteaching, p. 60G

Reteaching

Base Words

Draw three houses and mailboxes on the board. Label the mailboxes *lock, trust,* and *fair.* Remind students that many words come from a smaller base word, and that words that come from the same base words are all part of the same word family. Write each word below on the board in random order and ask students which word family it belongs to. Have a volunteer write the word in the appropriate house.

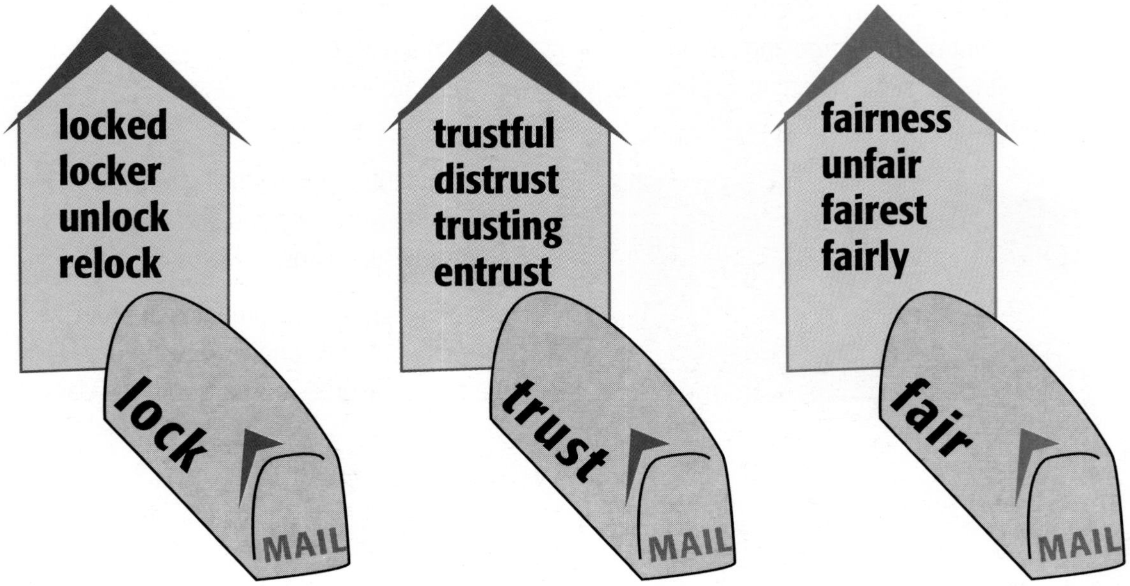
locked
locker
unlock
relock
lock
MAIL
trustful
distrust
trusting
entrust
trust
MAIL
fairness
unfair
fairest
fairly
fair
MAIL

MINILESSON

Reviewing Short Vowels

Teach/Model Write this sentence on the board.

Nice pigs do not huff and puff to be let in!

Ask students which word or words in the sentence have the short *a* sound. *(and)* The short *e* sound? *(let)* The short *i* sound? *(pigs, in)* The short *o* sound? *(not)* The short *u* sound? *(huff, puff)*

Practice/Apply ***Cooperative Learning*** Divide the class into five groups and assign each group a short vowel sound. Have each group hunt for words in the story that contain their vowel sound. Write the headings *and, let, pigs, not,* and *puff* on the board. As students share their words with the class, write each word under the heading with the appropriate vowel sound.

Portfolio Opportunity

Use *Literacy Activity Book* page 13 to record students' understanding of base words.

Building Vocabulary

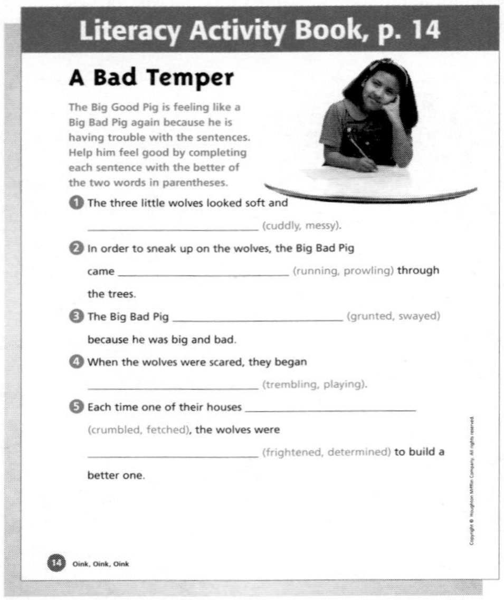
Literacy Activity Book, p. 14

A Bad Temper

The Big Good Pig is feeling like a Big Bad Pig again because he is having trouble with the sentences. Help him feel good by completing each sentence with the better of the two words in parentheses.

1. The three little wolves looked soft and ________ (cuddly, messy).
2. In order to sneak up on the wolves, the Big Bad Pig came ________ (running, prowling) through the trees.
3. The Big Bad Pig ________ (grunted, swayed) because he was big and bad.
4. When the wolves were scared, they began ________ (trembling, playing).
5. Each time one of their houses ________ (crumbled, fetched), the wolves were ________ (frightened, determined) to build a better one.

14 Oink, Oink, Oink

Use this page to review Selection Vocabulary.

Vocabulary Activities

Synonyms for *big* and *bad*

Cooperative Learning

On the board, write the title *The Three Little Wolves and the Big Bad Pig.* Then cross out the words *Big* and *Bad* and above them write *Large Wicked*. Ask students whether or not you've changed the meaning of the title. Point out that *large* and *big* are synonyms–words that have the same or nearly the same meaning. Explain that *wicked* and *bad* are also synonyms.

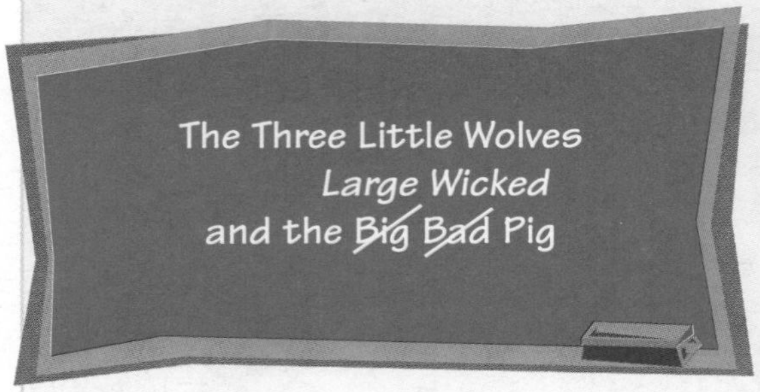
The Three Little Wolves
Large Wicked
and the ~~Big Bad~~ Pig

Have students work in small groups to replace the words *big* and *bad* with more interesting synonyms.

Encourage groups to come up with several versions of the title and then to choose one or two favorites to share with the class.

Classifying/Categorizing

Remind students that the big bad pig couldn't destroy the little wolves' houses with his bare hoofs–he had to rely on tools such as a sledgehammer and a pneumatic drill. Ask students to describe these tools. Point out that a tool is a hand-held object designed to do a certain kind of work.

Tell students that when the pig became good and moved in with the wolves, he needed tools for being helpful rather than harmful. Set up posters around the room with the labels *Workbench, Gardening Shed, Cleaning Closet, Sewing Box,* and *Kitchen Drawer.* Have students move independently from poster to poster, listing tools that the pig should keep in each area of his new home. Encourage students to read what their classmates have written and to think of new words.

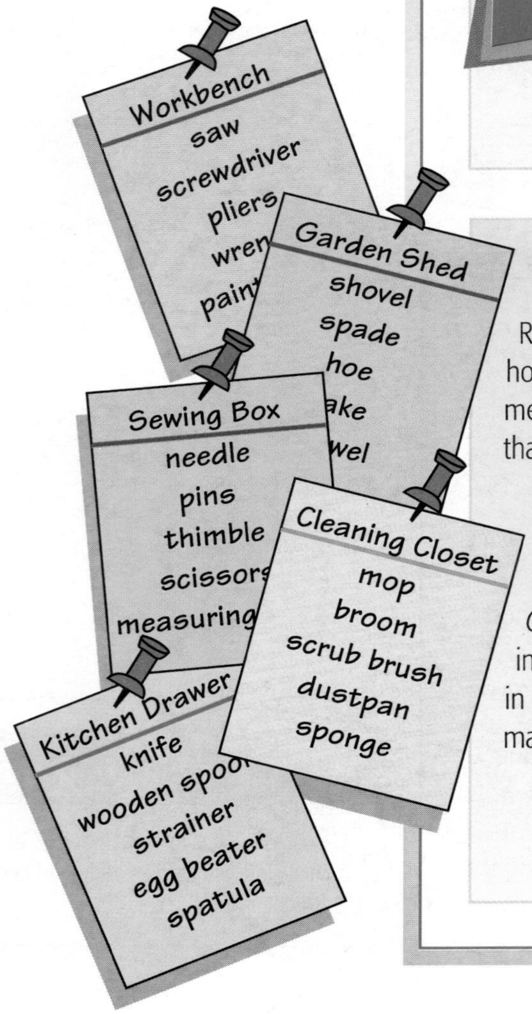
Workbench
saw
screwdriver
pliers
Garden Shed
shovel
spade
hoe
Sewing Box
needle
pins
thimble
Cleaning Closet
mop
broom
scrub brush
dustpan
sponge
Kitchen Drawer
knife
strainer
egg beater
spatula

Spelling

MINILESSON

Spelling Words

*ask
*next
*mix
*smell
*black
*shut
*lock
*truck

Challenge Words

*knock
*scent
*plenty
*fetch

*Starred words or forms of the words appear in *The Three Little Wolves and the Big Bad Pig.*

TESTED SKILL

Short Vowels

LAB, pp. 15–16

- Say the word *ask.* Have students repeat the word. Ask them what vowel sound they hear in *ask.* (ă). Then write *ask* on the board. Have a volunteer tell how the vowel sound is spelled. (*a*) Underline the vowel.
- Introduce the /ĕ/, /ĭ/, /ŏ/, and /ŭ/, sounds, using *next, mix, lock,* and *shut.*
- Write the Spelling Words on the board. Tell students that each Spelling Word has a short vowel sound. Say the Spelling Word and have students repeat them.
- Encourage students to add to their Study List some words that they have misspelled in their own writing.

Spelling Assessment

Pretest

Say each underlined word, read the sentence, and then repeat the word. Have students write only the underlined words.

1. Before you open the door, ask who it is.
2. What happens next in the story?
3. The first step is to mix the flour and the sugar.
4. Do you smell something burning?
5. Wolves can be black, white, or gray.
6. Remember to shut the windows.
7. It's a good idea to lock your door at night.
8. That truck is full of bricks.

Test

Spelling Words Use the Pretest sentences.

Challenge Words

9. Please fetch me some water.
10. Do you hear a knock at the door?
11. The scent of roses is in the air.
12. There is plenty of time to catch the bus.

SKILL FINDER

Daily Language Practice, p. 60K
Reading-Writing Workshop, p. 117E

Literacy Activity Book, p. 15

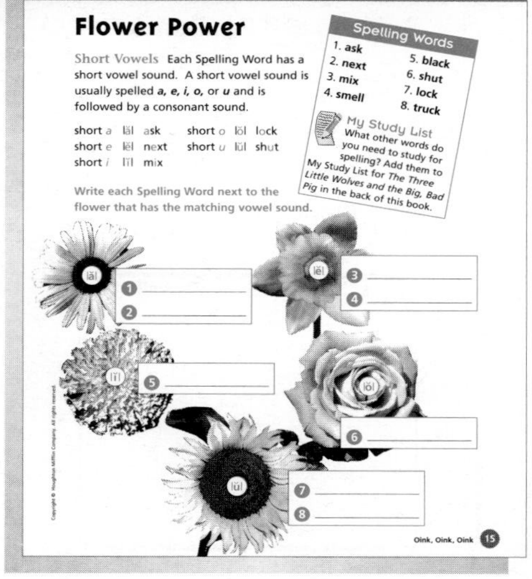
Flower Power

Short Vowels Each Spelling Word has a short vowel sound. A short vowel sound is usually spelled *a, e, i, o,* or *u* and is followed by a consonant sound.

short *a* /ă/ ask
short *e* /ĕ/ next
short *i* /ĭ/ mix
short *o* /ŏ/ lock
short *u* /ŭ/ shut

Spelling Words: 1. ask 2. next 3. mix 4. smell 5. black 6. shut 7. lock 8. truck

My Study List What other words do you need to study for spelling? Add them to My Study List for *The Three Little Wolves and the Big, Bad Pig* in the back of this book.

Write each Spelling Word next to the flower that has the matching vowel sound.

/ă/ 1 2
/ĕ/ 3 4
/ĭ/ 5
/ŏ/ 6
/ŭ/ 7 8

Oink, Oink, Oink 15

Literacy Activity Book, p. 16

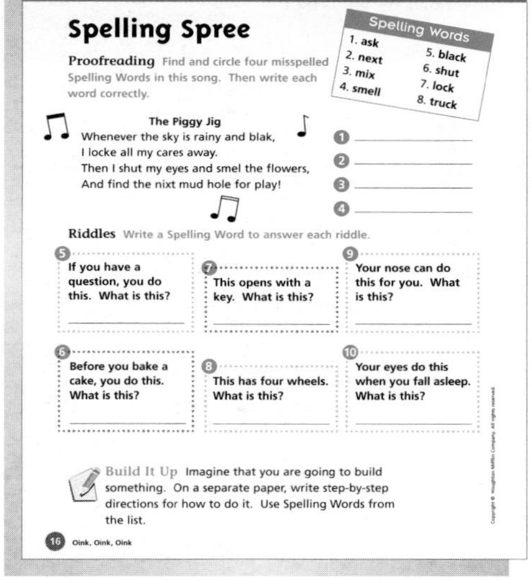
Spelling Spree

Spelling Words: 1. ask 2. next 3. mix 4. smell 5. black 6. shut 7. lock 8. truck

Proofreading Find and circle four misspelled Spelling Words in this song. Then write each word correctly.

The Piggy Jig
Whenever the sky is rainy and blak,
I locke all my cares away.
Then I shut my eyes and smel the flowers,
And find the nixt mud hole for play!

Riddles Write a Spelling Word to answer each riddle.

5. If you have a question, you do this. What is this?
6. Before you bake a cake, you do this. What is this?
7. This opens with a key. What is this?
8. This has four wheels. What is this?
9. Your nose can do this for you. What is this?
10. Your eyes do this when you fall asleep. What is this?

Build It Up Imagine that you are going to build something. On a separate paper, write step-by-step directions for how to do it. Use Spelling Words from the list.

16 Oink, Oink, Oink

MEETING INDIVIDUAL NEEDS

Challenge

Challenge Words Practice Have students use the Challenge Words to write tongue twisters.

Instruct *and* Integrate

Grammar

Transparency 1–4

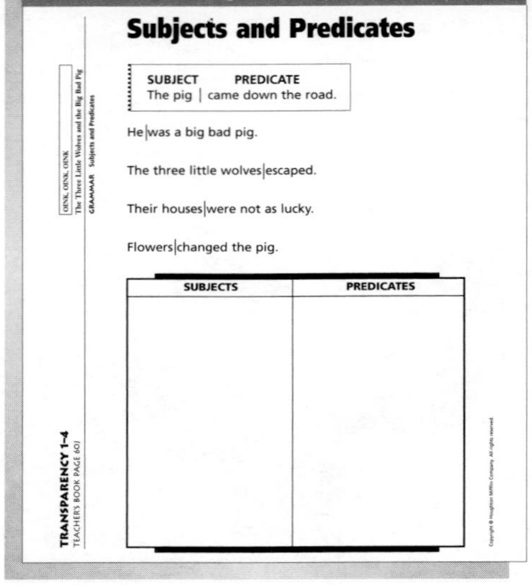

Subjects and Predicates

SUBJECT PREDICATE
The pig | came down the road.

He|was a big bad pig.

The three little wolves|escaped.

Their houses|were not as lucky.

Flowers|changed the pig.

SUBJECTS	PREDICATES

OINK, OINK, OINK
The Three Little Wolves and the Big Bad Pig
GRAMMAR Subjects and Predicates

TRANSPARENCY 1–4
TEACHER'S BOOK PAGE 60J

Copyright © Houghton Mifflin Company. All rights reserved.

Literacy Activity Book, p. 19

Literacy Activity Book, p. 17

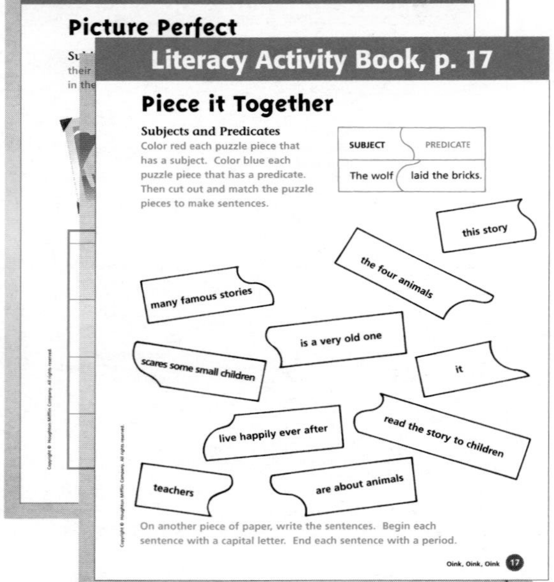

Picture Perfect

Piece it Together

Subjects and Predicates
Color red each puzzle piece that has a subject. Color blue each puzzle piece that has a predicate. Then cut out and match the puzzle pieces to make sentences.

SUBJECT	PREDICATE
The wolf	laid the bricks.

this story
the four animals
many famous stories
is a very old one
scares some small children
it
live happily ever after
read the story to children
teachers
are about animals

On another piece of paper, write the sentences. Begin each sentence with a capital letter. End each sentence with a period.

Oink, Oink, Oink 17

Copyright © Houghton Mifflin Company. All rights reserved.

Informal Assessment

Responses to the activities should indicate a general understanding of subjects and predicates.

Additional Support:

Reteaching, p. 60K.

INTERACTIVE LEARNING

TESTED SKILL

Subjects and Predicates

LAB, pp. 17, 19

Every sentence has two parts.

- The **subject** tells whom or what the sentence is about.
- The **predicate** tells what the subject does or is.

Teach/Model

Write the following sentences on the chalkboard, and ask volunteers to role-play each one.

The pig huffed and puffed.
The wolves are scared.

Ask the class to tell who or what each sentence is about (pig, wolves) and then what the sentences say about the pig or the wolves (huffed and puffed; are scared). Introduce the terms *subject* and *predicate* and underline them in each sentence. Explain that every sentence has a subject and a predicate.

Show Transparency 1–4. Direct students to the example sentence. Have volunteers draw a line between the subject and the predicate in each of the other sentences. Point out that a subject and a predicate can be made up of one word or several words.

Divide the class into Subjects and Predicates. Have the Subjects take turns giving a subject to start a sentence, and have the Predicates take turns finishing it. Write their sentences on the transparency.

Note that a sentence begins with a capital letter and ends with an end mark.

Practice/Apply

Cooperative Learning: **Build the Brick House** Have students work in small groups to build "brick houses" of subjects and predicates. Write the sentences below on the board. Have each group cut out sixteen "bricks" and write subjects and predicates from the eight sentences.

The wolves | lived with their mother.
Tea | was their favorite drink.
She | sent them into the world.
Other animals | gave them supplies.
Their first three houses | fell.
The flowers | were a great idea.
The big bad pig | became a big good pig.
The last house | was a flower house.

SKILL FINDER
Reading-Writing Workshop, p. 117E
Writing a Sentence, p. 60D

INTERACTIVE LEARNING *(continued)*

Practice/Apply

Cooperative Learning: **Build the Brick House** (*continued*) Then ask students to match each subject with the correct predicate. Help students draw the outline of a house large enough to hold eight rows of bricks. Have students glue the bricks onto a sheet of paper, "stacking" them to create a "wall." When all groups are finished, students can check one another's subjects and predicates.

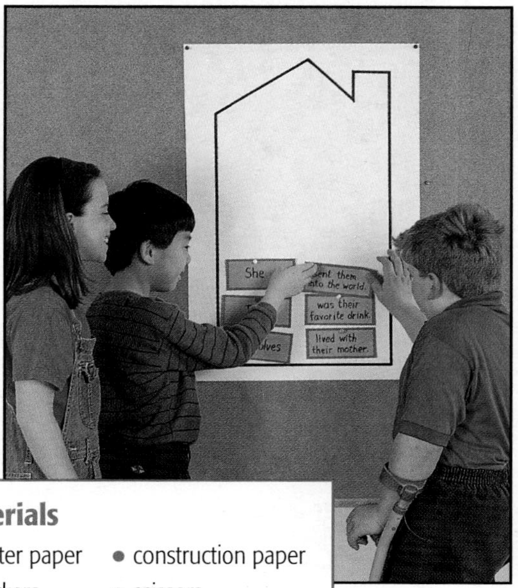
She
was their favorite drink.
lived with their mother.

Writing Application: Paragraph About a Character Invite students to write a paragraph about their favorite story character. Remind them to be sure that each sentence has a subject and a predicate.

Students' Writing Have students look at a piece of writing they have done or are working on to make sure that all sentences have subjects and predicates.

Materials

- poster paper
- markers
- construction paper
- scissors

Reteaching Subjects and Predicates

MEETING INDIVIDUAL NEEDS

Have students work in pairs to draw picture sentences. First, ask them to draw a picture of the subject of a sentence, such as a dog. Next, ask them to draw a picture of the subject doing something, such as chasing a car. Then have them write the sentence shown in the pictures.

Ask each pair to share their pictures and sentences with the group and to identify who or what the sentence is about and what that person/animal/object is or is doing. Reinforce the terms *subject* and *predicate,* and have each pair identify them in their written sentences.

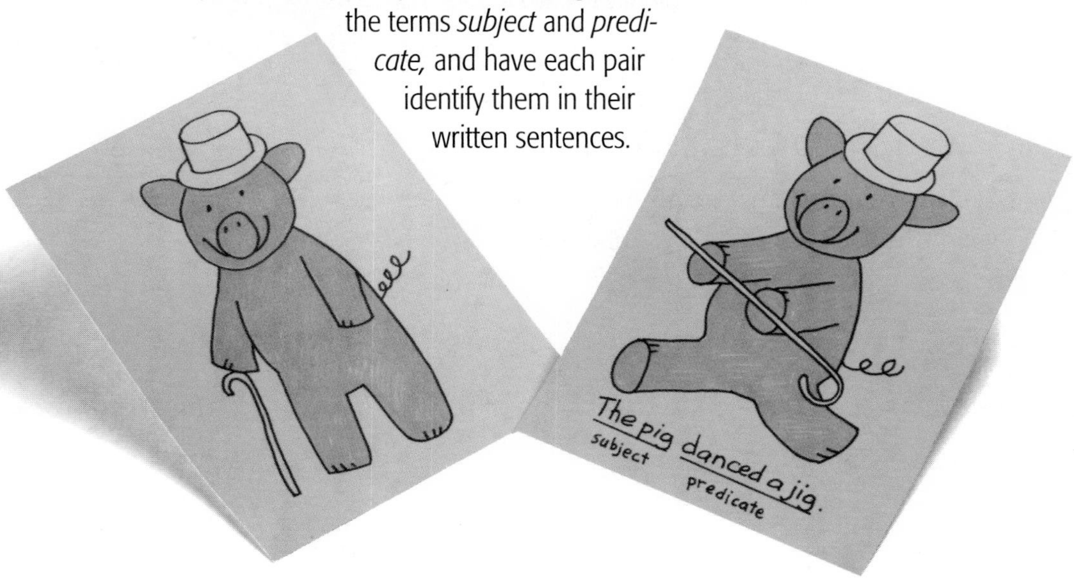
The pig danced a jig.
subject
predicate

Daily Language Practice

Focus Skills

Grammar: Subjects and Predicates

Spelling: Short Vowel Sounds

Every day write one sentence fragment on the chalkboard. Tell students that each sentence is missing a subject or a predicate. Ask them to add the missing part. Remind them to begin each sentence with a capital letter and to end it with a period. Tell students also to check for misspelled words. Have each student write the sentence correctly on a sheet of paper. Have students correct their own papers as a volunteer corrects the sentence on the chalkboard.

Students Acquiring English: Have these students work with fluent English-speaking partners.

Sample responses:

1. Were gray and white and blak.
   The little wolves were gray and white and **black.**
2. Had only one loc and key.
   Their brick house had only one **lock** and key.
3. Their nixt house.
   Their **next** house **was stronger.**
4. A shutt door.
   A **shut** door **did not keep out the big bad pig.**
5. Loved the smel of flowers.
   The pig loved the **smell** of flowers.

Communication Activities

Listening and Speaking

Audio Tape
for Oink, Oink, Oink: *The Three Little Wolves and the Big Bad Pig*

Storytelling

Cooperative Learning

Suggest that students work in small groups to retell either *The Three Little Wolves and the Big Bad Pig* or some other once-upon-a-time tale. Provide the titles of several tales on chart paper and have students sign up for their retelling. Share and discuss the guidelines before they begin.

Students Acquiring English Students acquiring English can speak the refrain or other patterned parts of the story.

Tales to Retell:

- Cinderella
- Juan Bobo
- Jack and the Beanstalk
- The Princess and the Pea

Guidelines for Storytelling

Read the story several times. Try telling it aloud without looking at the book. Practice out loud to yourself or a friend.

Divide the story into big sections, such as beginning, middle, and end.

Do not memorize the story. Use your own words. Memorize only key phrases or rhymes, such as "huff and puff."

Speak loudly and clearly. Use your hands and body to show expression.

Consider using a prop, such as a hat or a scarf.

Interviewing the Big Bad Pig

Cooperative Learning

Invite students to plan a TV or radio talk show interview with the Big Bad Pig. They can work together to develop a list of possible questions. For example,

- Why did you behave so violently toward the wolves?
- What made you change?
- What advice do you have for other pigs?

Students can take turns playing either host or guest. The audience can also ask questions.

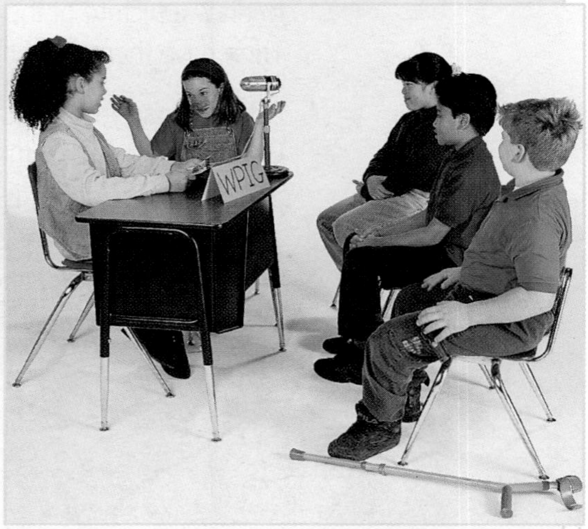
WPIG

Informal Assessment

Use the Guidelines for Storytelling to evaluate students' storytelling presentations.

Additional Support:

- Review the guidelines.
- Have students work in pairs to practice the story before sharing it with the group.

Viewing

Watching a Video

There are several videotape versions of the original story of "The Three Little Pigs." If students have the opportunity to watch one, have them discuss the difference between reading a story and watching one on television.

Resources
The Three Little Pigs by James Marshall. Weston Woods.
The Three Little Pigs by Erik Blegvad. Weston Woods.

Using Facial Expressions and Body Language

MEETING INDIVIDUAL NEEDS

Students Acquiring English You can learn a lot about how a person feels by examining his or her body language and facial expressions. Encourage students to look at the following illustrations from *The Three Little Wolves and the Big Bad Pig:* pages 40, 42, and 51. What emotions are being expressed? Invite volunteers to pantomime emotions, such as the ones listed in the box, as other students guess what feeling is being expressed.

anger	hate
fear	joy
surprise	confusion
sadness	love

Note: Body language and expressions vary in meaning from culture to culture.

Examining Real Wolves and Pigs

Cooperative Learning

What do real wolves and pigs look like? Provide several nonfiction books on wolves and pigs. Students can also refer to the articles "What's Up, Pup?" (page 61) and "This Little Piggy" (page 64). They can work in small groups to compare pictures of real wolves and pigs with the story illustrations.

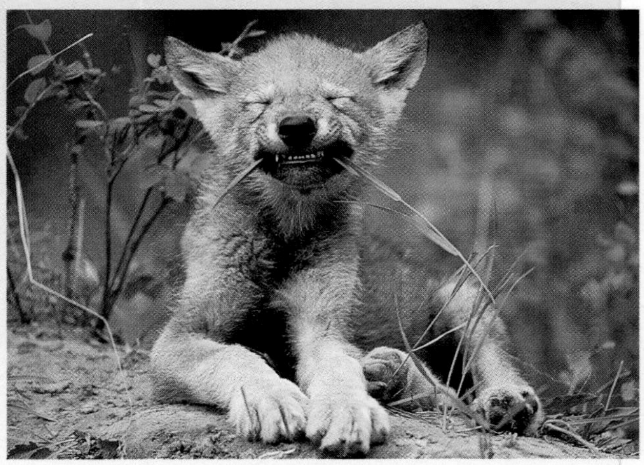

Portfolio Opportunity

Film or tape-record students' storytelling sessions.

Cross-Curricular Activities

Book List

Science

Unbuilding
by David Macaulay

Hammers, Nails, Planks and Paint: How a House Is Built
by Thomas Campbell Jackson

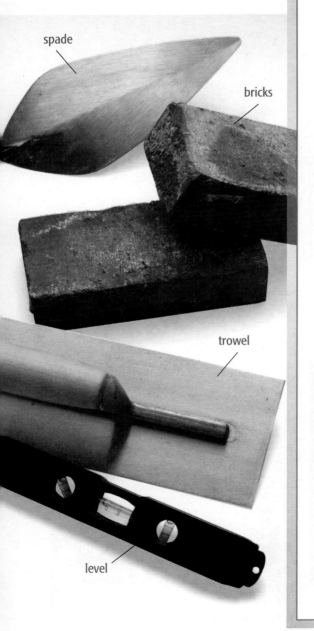
spade
bricks
trowel
level

Choices for Science

Careers in Construction

Brainstorm with students the different professions on a construction site. (carpenters, electricians, insulation workers, plasterers, plumbers, etc.) What kind of expertise is required for each job? Encourage students to interview family or friends in these professions and report back to the class.

Students Acquiring English Encourage students to work with a partner to prepare interview questions beforehand.

Tools of the Trade

Students Acquiring English If possible, visit a hardware store or lumberyard with students. Perhaps an employee can explain the construction tools and materials to students. Alternatively, show students the photos of tools on this page, and discuss each tool's name and function.

Looking at Blueprints

Challenge Give students the opportunity to study the blueprint on pages 30 and 31 and to draw blueprints for a room of their own at home.

Students Acquiring English Students can draw or explain types of houses found in their birthplaces. Discuss how the houses are similar and different.

Building Your School

Lead students on a discovery tour of your school, examining the walls, floors, and ceilings to determine what materials were used. Then invite a knowledgeable person (town engineer, school maintenance employee, architect, or construction worker) to describe the less visible features of the building. Perhaps students can recommend repairs or improvements to the building.

Cross Section of a Foundation

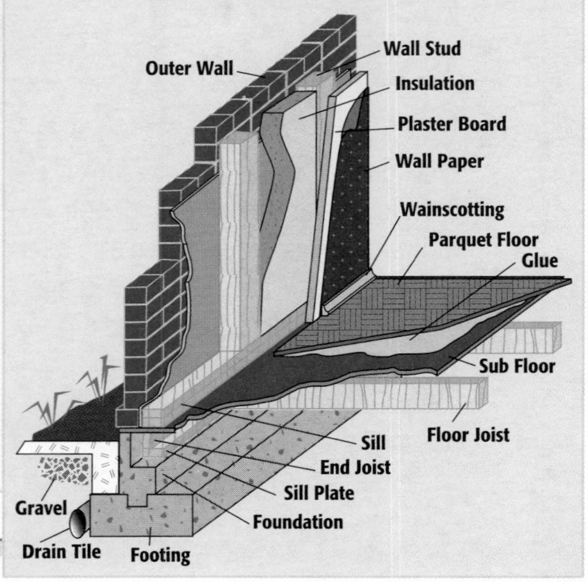
Outer Wall
Wall Stud
Insulation
Plaster Board
Wall Paper
Wainscotting
Parquet Floor
Glue
Sub Floor
Floor Joist
Sill
End Joist
Sill Plate
Foundation
Gravel
Drain Tile
Footing

Math

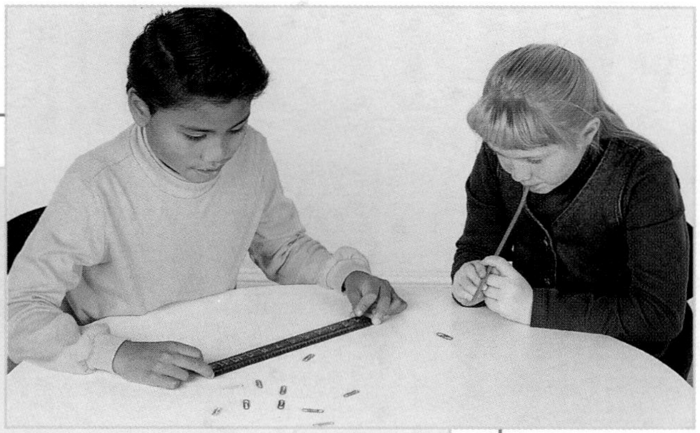

Playing a Huff-and-Puff Game

Cooperative Learning

Ask students to collect objects they think will not be able to withstand a strong gust of air. Students can then use their measurement skills to play Huff-and-Puff in teams.

Rules:

1. Take turns using a straw to blow the objects across a desk top.
2. Measure the distances traveled.
3. After several rounds, add up team totals to determine a winner.

Materials

- drinking straws
- objects such as paper clips and bottle caps
- measuring tape or ruler

Dance

Dancing the Tarantella

Did you know that the tarantella was originally danced as a cure for the bite of a tarantula spider? Teach students this dance using a famous tarantella by Liszt, Chopin, or Weber.

Resources

Jorge Bolet Plays Liszt, London/Decca Chamber Music series

Arthur Rubinstein—The Chopin Collection, RCA Victor Gold Seal

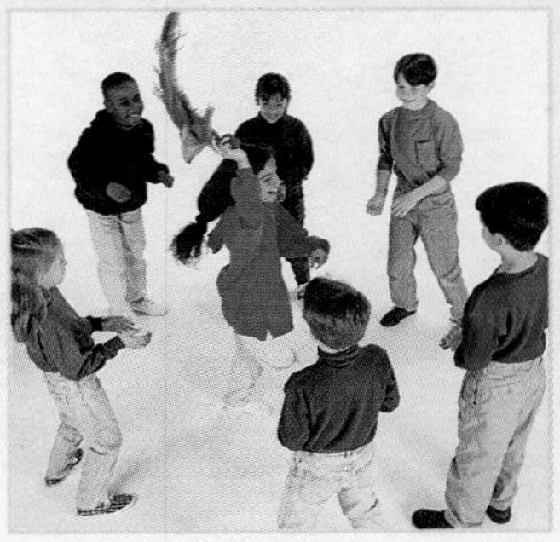

1 Do a simple hop or double hop while waving a scarf. Move in a wide circle.

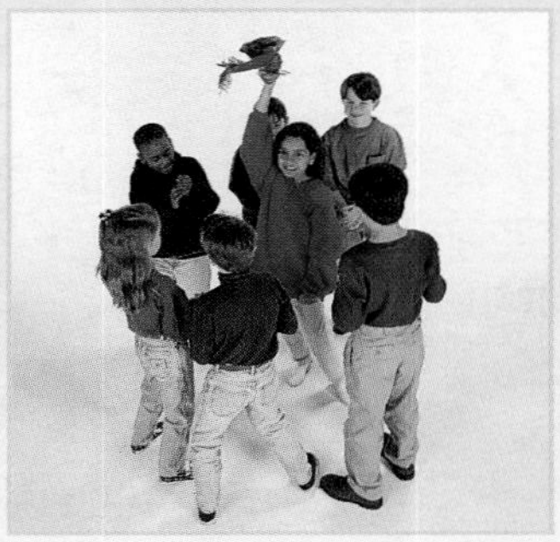

2 Continue to dance in smaller and smaller circles as your audience closes in.

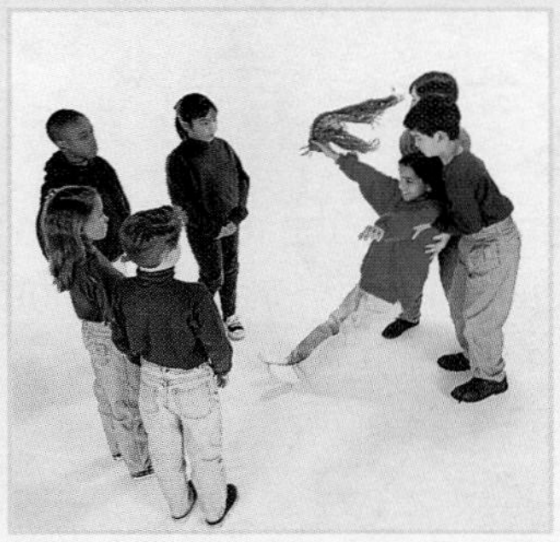

3 As the music slows and the dance ends, fall into the arms of your audience.

Students Acquiring English Students may enjoy teaching a dance from their culture.

Materials

- colorful scarf
- tape or CD player

What's Up, Pup?

Introduce the Literature

Building Background

Previewing/Predicting

Ask students to examine the photographs and use them as the basis for making predictions about how wolves are alike and different from dogs. You might use a Venn diagram like this.

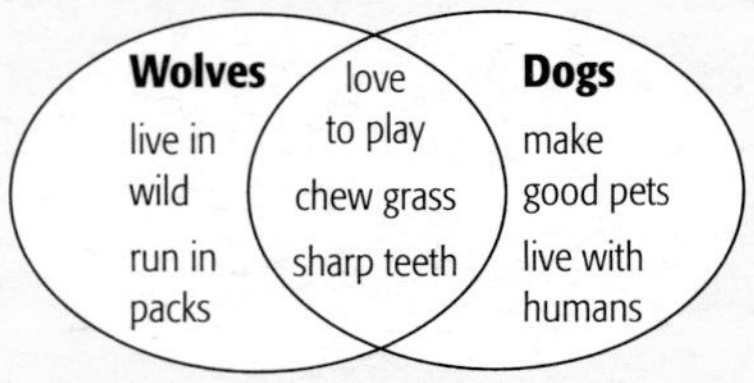
Wolves
live in wild
run in packs
love to play
chew grass
sharp teeth
Dogs
make good pets
live with humans

Selection Vocabulary

You may wish to review the following vocabulary before students begin to read. Invite students to make up sentences using each word.

romp: to play in a lively way

mischief: naughty or bad behavior

autumn: the season that follows summer

Students Acquiring English

Students may not be familiar with the female name *Gretta*. Tell them it is a short form of the name *Margaret*. It is derived from *margaron*, a word meaning "pearl."

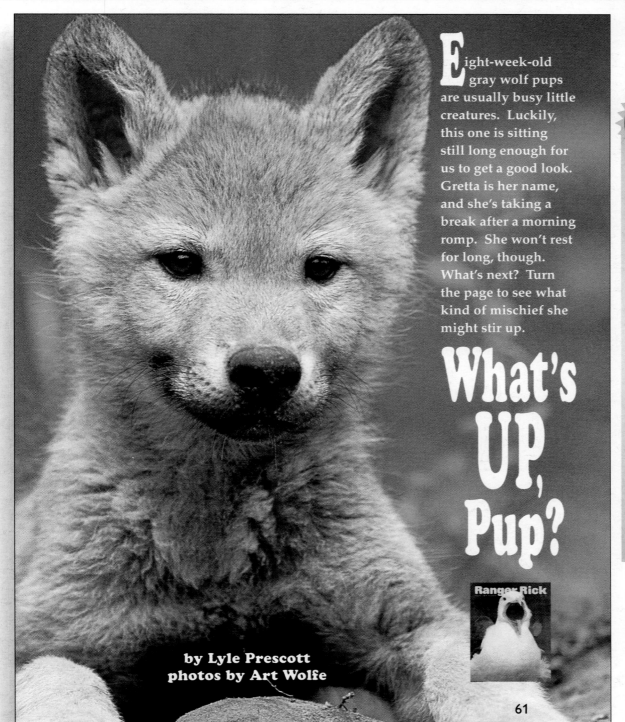

Eight-week-old gray wolf pups are usually busy little creatures. Luckily, this one is sitting still long enough for us to get a good look. Gretta is her name, and she's taking a break after a morning romp. She won't rest for long, though. What's next? Turn the page to see what kind of mischief she might stir up.

What's UP, Pup?

by Lyle Prescott
photos by Art Wolfe

Ranger Rick

61

Interact with Literature

Writer's Craft

Narrative Nonfiction Ask students whether or not they think Gretta is a good name for a wolf pup. Discuss how naming the pup makes the article immediately more appealing. Why is nonfiction that reads like a story often easier to read?

Media Literacy

Magazines Ask students if they have ever read *Ranger Rick* before. If they haven't, ask them to examine the cover and speculate what subjects a magazine like *Ranger Rick* might cover.

Interact with Literature

Extra Support

Parentheses Point out the directional words in parentheses throughout the article. Discuss with students how helpful it is for an author to include this information in an article with many photos.

Challenge

Observations Ask students to make two lists–one of Gretta's behaviors that a scientist could observe, and the other of thoughts and actions the writer assigns to Gretta.

Science Link

Canines Explain that *canine* is the name of an animal family that includes foxes and dogs. Ask students to identify dogs that look like wolves. If possible, bring in pictures of different dog breeds for students to look through.

Chomp! "OK, grass — you haven't got a chance against a tough wolf like me," Gretta might be thinking (**right**). Like other young wolf pups, she likes to play with and explore almost everything around her. (She may even eat the grass after she finishes "attacking" it.)

Gretta is also practicing using her teeth. See those pointy ones at the sides of her mouth? They're called *canines* (KAY-nines), and they'll help her hunt when she gets older.

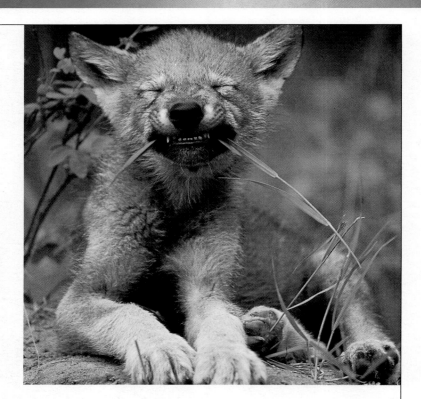

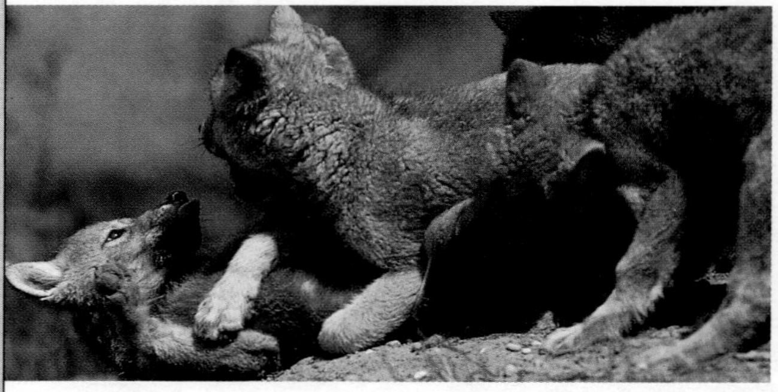

Every day, wolf pups tumble and wrestle together (**left**). Playing like this helps the pups figure out which ones will later be bosses and which ones will get bossed around. Plus, the fast-growing pups need to exercise their muscles. By the time autumn comes, they'll have to be strong enough to join the adults at hunting time.

62

Interact with Literature

Social Studies Link

Wolf Survival Discuss how wolves were once plentiful in the United States, but now many of them live in protected areas. If possible, bring in maps and information about the range of wolves. Have volunteers point to areas where wolves remain in significant numbers.

The other frisky wolf pups have dashed off without Gretta. They couldn't have gone far — but where are they? She throws back her head and lets out a long, sad howl (**right**). "Hey, guys, you left me here all alone — *please* come back," the little pup seems to be calling.

A wolf may howl alone, or a pack may howl together in a chorus. Either way, the sounds can carry for a long distance. Sometimes wolves may howl messages to each other from a mile or two apart.

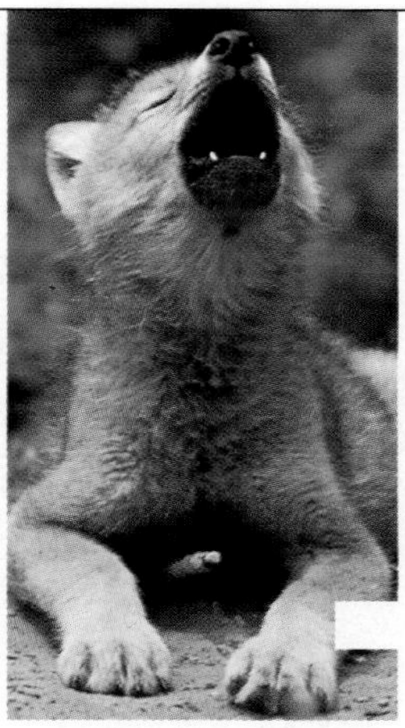

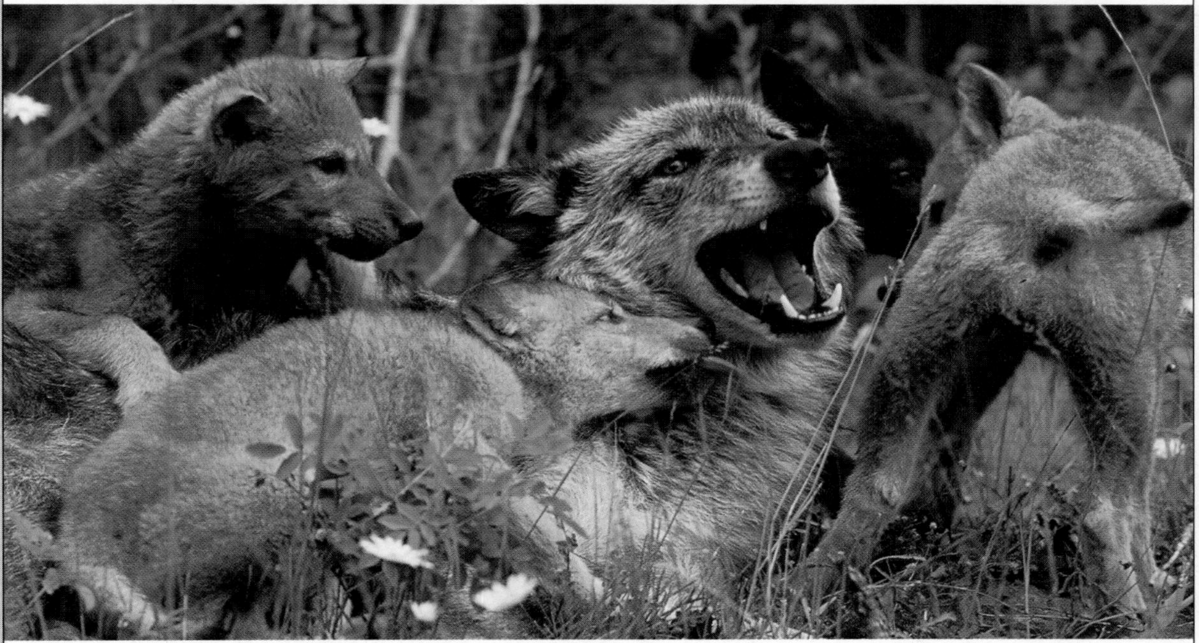

The wolf pups like to hang out all over Mom (**above**). That's Gretta in front, giving Mom a lick. Luckily for the little pups, the adult wolves are never too old to play.

63

Instruct and Integrate

MINILESSON

Study Skill

Taking Notes

TESTED SKILL

Teach/Model

Explain that the article describes not only what wolf pups do, but why they do it. Discuss how taking notes is a good strategy when you have a lot of information. Then model with this Think Aloud.

Think Aloud

If I don't write down the reasons why Gretta does different things, I know I'll forget them. I don't need to write everything down, just the most important facts. I think making a chart will be easier than writing sentences.

What She Does	Why She Does It
eats grass	to strengthen teeth
wrestles	to exercise muscles; to determine who is boss

Begin filling in a chart like this.

Practice/Apply

Have students continue taking notes on why Gretta howls (to tell where she is) and why she plays with her mom (to show affection).

SKILL FINDER Full lesson, p. H2

Interact with Literature

MEETING INDIVIDUAL NEEDS

Students Acquiring English

Punctuation/Expressions Be sure students understand that the dialogue is set off by quotation marks. Also point out the punctuation. Explain that to *hang out* is slang meaning "to keep company."

Introduce the Literature

Building Background

Have students recite the rhyme "This Little Piggy." Discuss how this rhyme is usually recited. (by pinching a person's toes) Have students preview the article. Ask if, given the title and format of the article, they think this selection will be fun facts or serious information.

Discuss the questions listed at the beginning of the article. Ask students to suggest possible answers. List the questions and students' responses on chart paper, and save for future use.

Reading Strategies

Predict/Infer

Ask students what they expect to find out as they read the selection. Then have them preview the selection, paying special attention to the key words (in larger type) in the headlines. Students should be able to predict that the selection will give answers to the questions at the beginning. Have them read to find out the answers.

It oinks! It wallows! It hangs out with the litter! Here's all the dirt on . . .

This Little Piggy!

by Linda Granfield

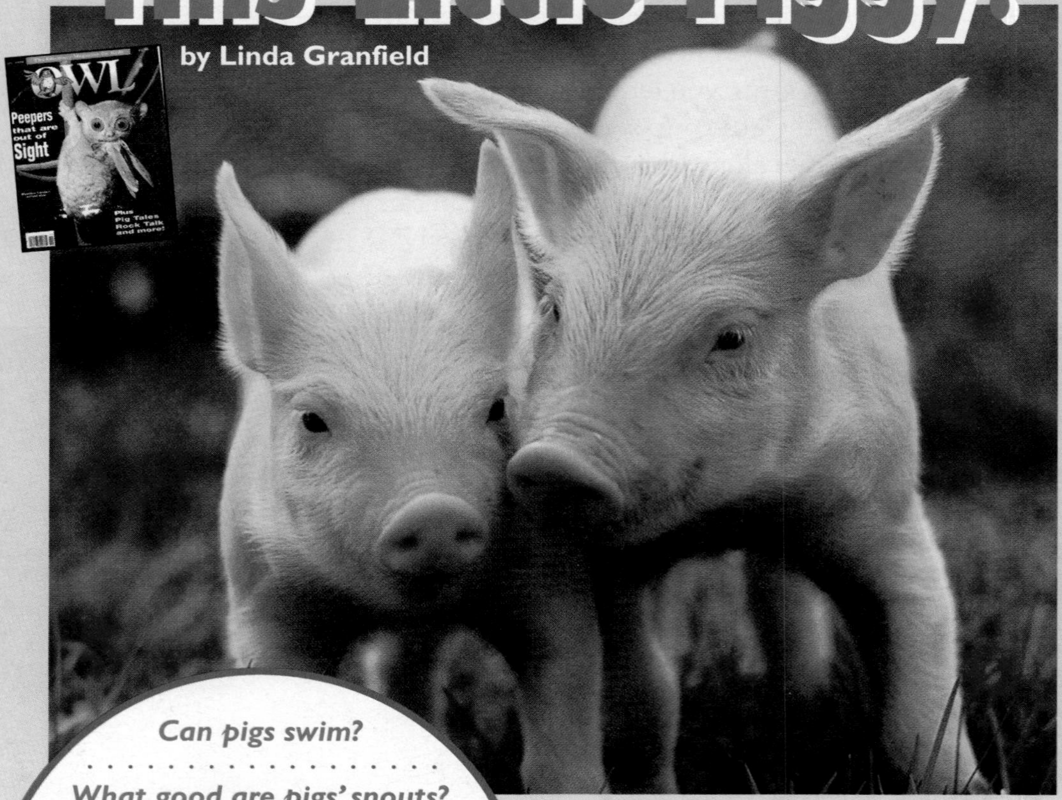
OWL
Peepers that are out of Sight

Can pigs swim?

What good are pigs' snouts?

Are pigs smart?

Are all pigs born with curly tails?

Do pigs prefer to be dirty?

Do pigs really make pigs of themselves?

Go hog wild. Take a look at these questions and see how many you can answer. If you think pigs are hard to peg down, you're right!

64

Interact with Literature

Students Acquiring English

MEETING INDIVIDUAL NEEDS

Expressions Ask students what it means to *go hog wild*. Explain that *to make a pig of yourself* is to eat too much and *hard to peg down* means "difficult to understand." Point out that these expressions are like the ones listed in the box on page 65.

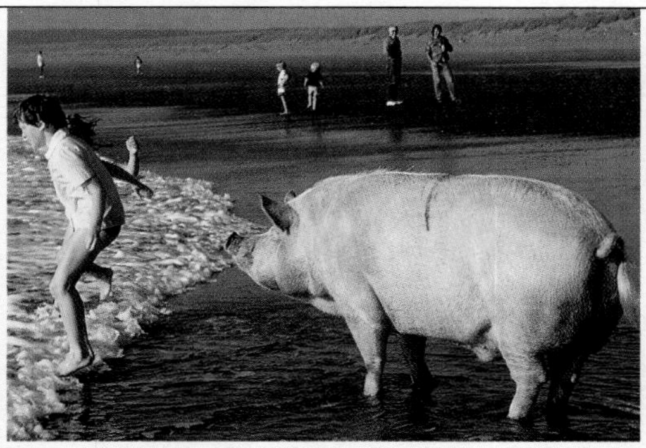

Pigs swim on hot, sunny days.

You might be surprised to know that pigs are great dog paddlers! Sometimes, they'll escape the burning sun by taking a swim at a water hole. The large amount of fat in their bodies helps keep even heavy pigs floating in the water. Pigs are such good swimmers they can cross rivers many kilometers (miles) wide.

A pig's snout is a pig's best friend.

Sure, a pig's snout is used for breathing — but it's also great for sweating, digging, and reaching out to other pigs! Like a dog, a pig sweats through its nose instead of its skin. A pig counts on its snout's flat front and bony upper rim as it digs in the dirt and unearths tasty roots. But all that digging doesn't harden a pig's nose. It remains moist and tender — perfect for greeting another pig snout-to-snout when they meet!

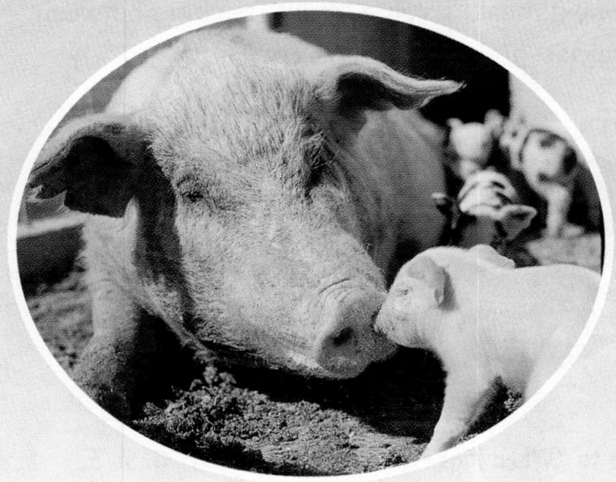

When Pigs Fly

Pigs have trotted their way into many of our expressions. See if you can match each of these with its meaning. Then check your answers on page 66.

1. pigpen	a. stubborn
2. pig-headed	b. braid
3. go whole hog	c. living well
4. pigtail	d. never
5. high off the hog	e. messy place
6. when pigs fly	f. take to the limit

65

Interact with Literature

Meeting Individual Needs

Extra Support

Expressions You may want to have students work with partners to match the expressions with their meanings. Afterward ask students which expressions they've heard before. In each case, what or who was being described?

Instruct and Integrate

MINILESSON

Study Skill
K-W-L

Teach/Model

Explain to students that K-W-L is a strategy that will enable them to understand, organize, and remember information in nonfiction selections. The *K* stands for what students already know, the *W* stands for what they want to know, and the *L* stands for what they learn. Model with this Think Aloud.

Think Aloud

I know some obvious things about pigs–that they're big and they like mud–but I still have a lot of questions. I'll put these questions in a chart like this and when I find the answers, I'll write them in the column titled "What I Learned About Pigs."

What I Know About Pigs	What I Want to Know About Pigs	What I Learned About Pigs
Pigs are big.	Do they eat a lot?	
Pigs like mud.	Why do they like it?	

Practice/Apply

Have students work in small groups to list other things they know about pigs and questions they have about pigs. Afterward have them list what they have learned and share their findings.

SKILL FINDER Full lesson, p. H3

Interact with Literature

Visual Literacy

Advertisements Ask students to compare the way the advertisement on page 66 presents information with the way the article "This Little Piggy!" does. Discuss how large type and exclamation marks are an effective way of attracting a reader's attention.

Students Acquiring English

Word Meaning Discuss the meaning of *stuff themselves silly*. (eat much too much) Point out these other meanings of *stuff*:

- to pack something (a bag) tightly
- to fill with a soft material, or stuffing
- to stop up, as in a nose being stuffed

Ask students to recall an occasion on which they ate too much. How did it make them feel? Did they also feel like napping afterward?

Point out that *curly* and *kinky* are synonyms. Ask a volunteer to demonstrate the meaning of *clockwise*. (You might also use the face of a clock for this purpose.)

Also, explain that a *maze* is a complicated network of passages and paths.

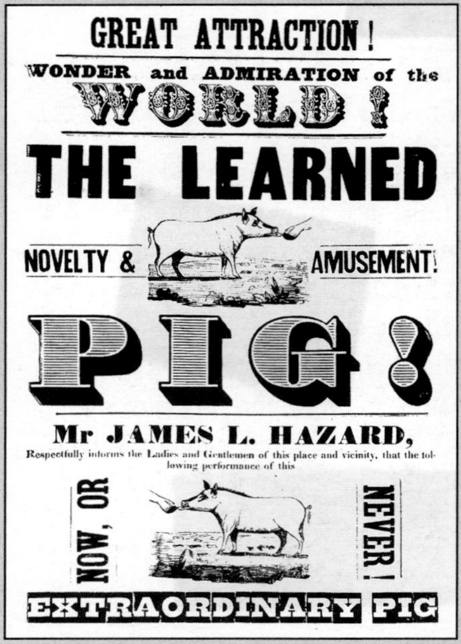
GREAT ATTRACTION!
WONDER and ADMIRATION of the
WORLD!
THE LEARNED
NOVELTY & AMUSEMENT!
PIG!
Mr JAMES L. HAZARD,
Respectfully informs the Ladies and Gentlemen of this place and vicinity, that the following performance of this
NOW, OR
NEVER!
EXTRAORDINARY PIG

Pigs are smarter than you think!

Pigs were one of the first animals to be trained by people. In 1785, a famous hog, called the Learned Pig, was taught to spell words, tell time, and solve math problems with the help of rewards. Today, some scientists believe that pigs are very intelligent and easier to train than dogs. They report that pigs can easily find their way through mazes that prove too difficult for many other animals.

Straight or curly pig tails tell tales.

Many, but not all breeds of pigs are born with curly tails. But when a kinky-tailed pig is scared or not feeling well, its tail may straighten out. Do all curly pig tails curl in the same direction? One old American saying claims that pigs' tails in the south twist clockwise, while pigs' tails in the north twist the opposite way.

Pigs won't stuff themselves silly.

Pigs will eat almost anything — even snow! But that doesn't mean pigs go hog wild over food. Unlike cows and horses, which will eat until they are ill, pigs stop when they feel full. After they have eaten, they usually nap until the next meal. Even without snacking between breakfast and dinner, pigs grow very quickly!

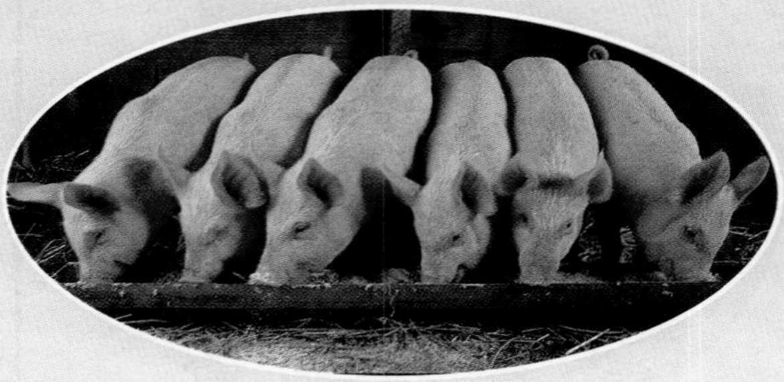

Answers to "When Pigs Fly": 1. e 2. a 3. f 4. b 5. c 6. d

66

Interact with Literature

Home Connection

Animal Stories What are students' experiences with animals? Have they ever owned one, or visited a zoo? Invite them to share their experiences, and to compare their animals with pigs.

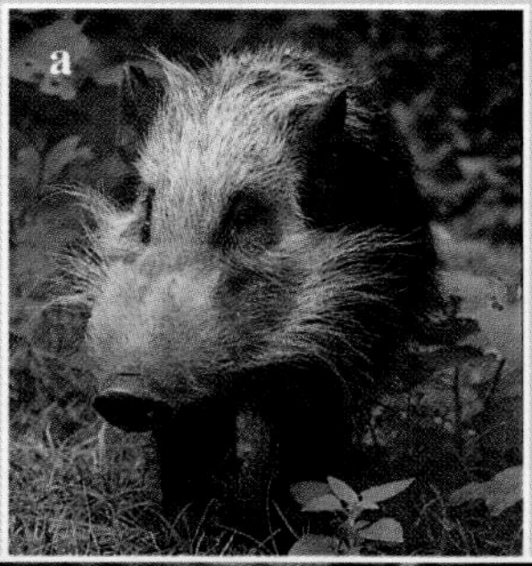
a

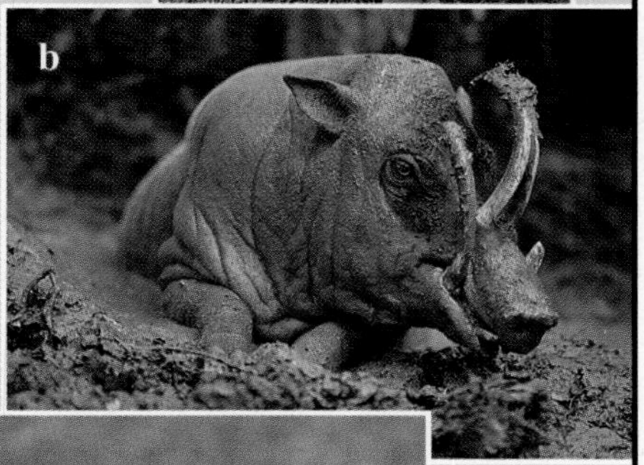
b

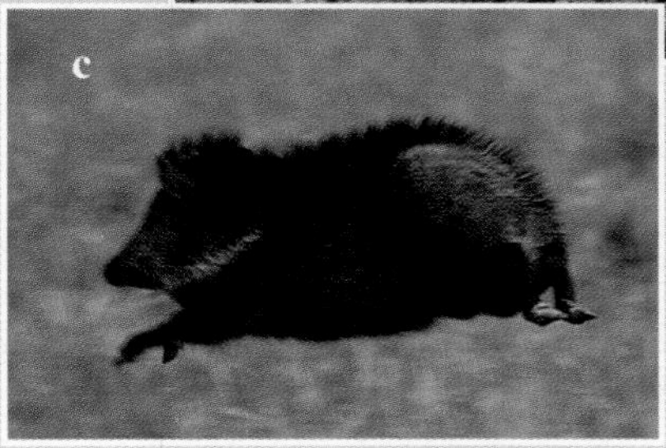
c

Picks of the Litter

Whether you're in Africa or Asia or somewhere in South America, you'll find a wild pig cousin or two! The **bush pig (a)** lives in the grasslands of Africa and Madagascar. Like a wart hog (another African wild pig), male bush pigs have warts on their faces. These warts help protect their faces from the tusks of other bush pigs when they fight. The **babirusa (b)** makes its home in southeast Asia. Its teeth, which can be longer than your foot, grow through the roof of its mouth and out the top of its snout. The **collared peccary (c)**, from South and Central America, is a more distant pig relation. A peccary will "woof" like a dog when its enemy the jaguar is nearby.

Pigs look dirty but really they're cool.

If you visit a farm, you'll probably find pigs covered with dried, caked mud. But it's not because pigs want to be dirty. They need the moisture found in mud. Pigs are very sensitive to heat but have no sweat glands to help them cool off. A coating of mud lowers their body temperature and stops sunburn. If there's clean water nearby, pigs will use that, too.

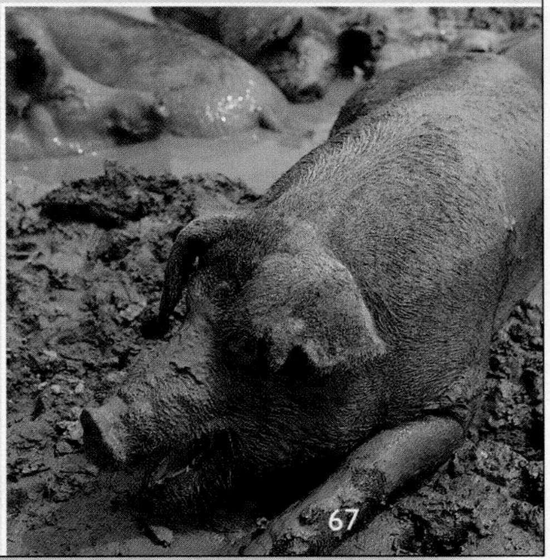

67

Interact with Literature

Students Acquiring English

Word Meaning Discuss the meaning of the phrase *sensitive to heat*. Ask students how they feel when playing outside on very hot days. What do they do to cool off? Also, explain that wart hogs have many warts—hard, rough lumps that grow on the skin.

Instruct and Integrate

Science Link

Animal Myths Have students create bulletin board displays that highlight myths about animals and present the true facts. Students might write the myth on the face of file cards and put factual information on the back.

Health Link

Staying Cool Discuss the ways human beings can stay cool in hot weather. (Encourage students acquiring English to share ways to stay cool associated with their cultural groups.) How can someone avoid sunburn? What foods are good to eat on a hot day?

Social Studies Link

Habitats Using a map or globe, help students locate the habitats of the bush pig (Africa and Madagascar) and the collared peccary (South and Central America). Invite students acquiring English to share stories and descriptions of wild pigs or pig-like animals from their native countries.

Journal

Have students list more animal expressions in their journals. Allow students time to share these expressions and to explain when they might be used.

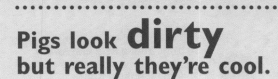

SELECTION: The Three Little Javelinas

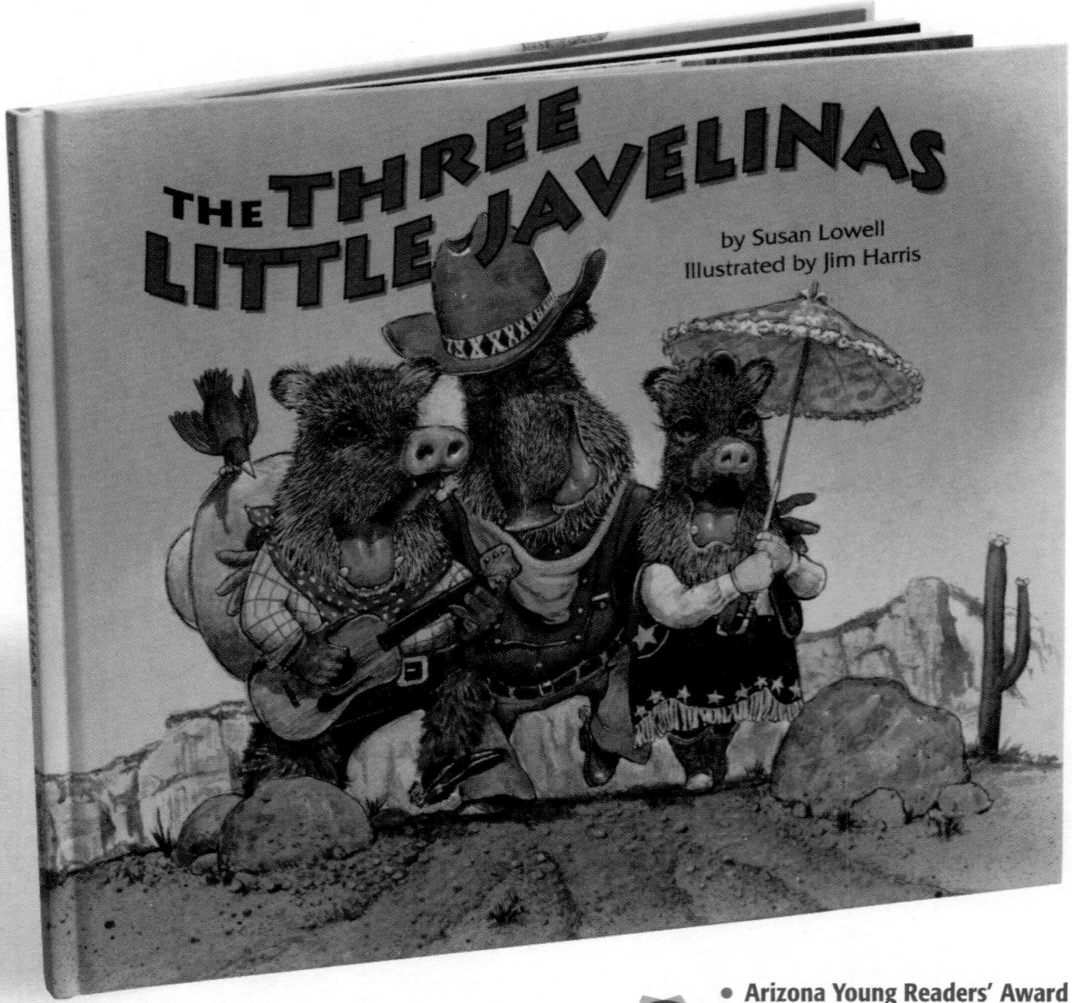
THE THREE LITTLE JAVELINAS
by Susan Lowell
Illustrated by Jim Harris

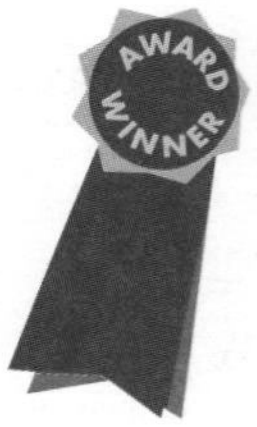
AWARD WINNER

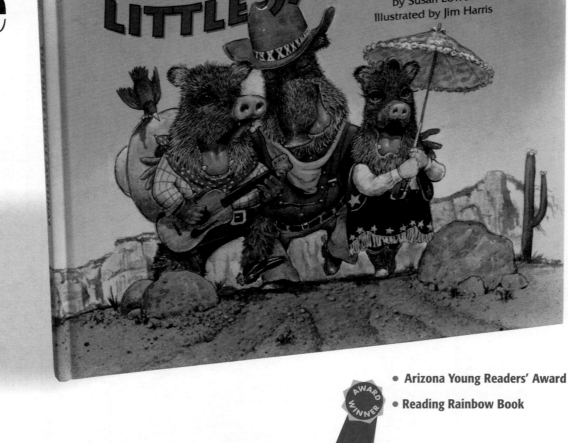

- Arizona Young Readers' Award
- Reading Rainbow Book

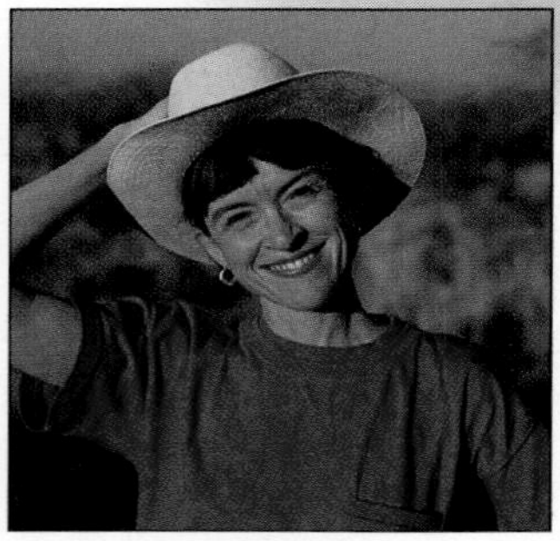

by Susan Lowell

Other Books by the Author

The Tortoise and the Jackrabbit

Selection Summary

Three little javelinas (pronounced ha-ve-LEE-nas)—"wild, hairy, southwestern cousins of pigs"—set out to seek their fortunes in the desert. As in the traditional tale, each little javelina builds a house. But the materials they use are true to the desert. The first house is of tumbleweed, the second, saguaro (sa–WA–ro) ribs (sticks from the inside of a dried-up cactus), and the third, adobe (a–DOE–be) bricks.

Of course, only the adobe house can withstand the huffing and puffing of their tireless foe, Coyote. As he tries to enter the house through the stove pipe, the third little javelina lights a fire in the stove, and Coyote takes off in a puff of smoke.

Lesson Planning Guide

	Skill/Strategy Instruction	Meeting Individual Needs	Lesson Resources
1 Introduce *the* Literature *Pacing: 1 day*	**Preparing to Read and Write** Prior Knowledge/Building Background, 67C **Selection Vocabulary,** 67D • desert • dust storm • whirlwind • tumbleweeds • cactus • adobe **Spelling Pretest,** 88I • nose • these • shade • use • mice • smoke • snake • ripe	**Support in Advance,** 67C **Students Acquiring English,** 67C **Other Choices for Building Background,** 67C **Spelling Challenge Words:** • escape • amaze • arrive • fortune	***Literacy Activity Book:*** Vocabulary, p. 20 **Transparency:** Vocabulary, 1–5 **Great Start** CD-ROM software, "Oink, Oink, Oink" CD
2 Interact *with* Literature *Pacing: 1–3 days*	**Reading Strategies:** Predict/Infer, 70, 72 Monitor, 70, 78 Think About Words, 76 Summarize, 80 Evaluate, 84 **Minilessons:** ✓ Compare and Contrast, 75 Predicting Outcomes, 79 Summarizing: Story Structure, 83 Writer's Craft: Setting, 85	**Choices for Reading,** 70 **Guided Reading,** 70 Comprehension/Critical Thinking, 74, 78, 86 **Students Acquiring English,** 69, 70, 72, 75, 77, 80, 82, 83, 85, 86, 88 **Extra Support,** 73, 74, 78, 87 **Challenge,** 76, 81	**Reading-Writing Workshop** A Story, 116–117F ***Literacy Activity Book,*** p. 40–42 The Learning Company's new elementary writing center software
3 Instruct *and* Integrate *Pacing: 1–3 days*	✓ **Comprehension:** Compare and Contrast, 88B ✓ **Writing:** Writing a Book Report, 88D **Word Skills and Strategies:** ✓ Structural Analysis: Inflected Endings *-ed* and *-ing*, 88F Phonics Review: Long Vowel Pairs and Vowel-Consonant-*e*, 88G **Building Vocabulary:** Vocabulary Activities, 88H ✓ **Spelling:** Vowel-Consonant-*e*, 88I ✓ **Grammar:** Correcting Run-on Sentences, 88J–88K **Communication Activities:** Listening and Speaking, 88L–88M; Viewing, 88M **Cross-Curricular Activities:** Science, 88N; Art, 88O; Math, 88O	**Reteaching:** Compare and Contrast, 88C **Activity Choices:** Write a Book Report, Shared Writing: Same Plot, Different Setting, Create a Cartoon, 88E **Reteaching:** Inflected Endings *-ed* and *-ing*, 88G **Activity Choices:** Selection Vocabulary Extension, Words from Spanish, Rhyming Words, 88H **Challenge Words Practice,** 88I **Reteaching:** Correcting Run-on Sentences, 88K **Activity Choices:** Listening and Speaking, 88L–88M; Viewing, 88M **Activity Choices:** Science, 88N; Art, 88O; Math, 88O	**Reading-Writing Workshop** A Story, 116–117F **Transparencies:** Comprehension, 1–6, Writing, 1–7, Grammar, 1–8 ***Literacy Activity Book:*** Comprehension, p. 22; Writing, p. 23; Word Skills, p.24; Building Vocabulary, p. 25; Spelling p.26–27; Grammar, p. 28–29 The Learning Company's new elementary writing center software **Video:** *Along Sandy Trails* **Audio Tape** for Oink, Oink, Oink: *The Three Little Javelinas*

✓ ***Indicates Tested Skills.*** *See page 34F for assessment options.*

Preparing to Read and Write

Support in Advance

MEETING INDIVIDUAL NEEDS

Use this activity with students who need extra support before participating in the whole-class activity.

Desert Talk Ask students what they know about the desert. Use the story illustrations, especially on pages 73 and 78, as a guide. You might have students draw pictures of a desert environment and share them with the class.

Management Tip
During this time, have other students describe in their journals one story or TV show that was set in the desert.

Students Acquiring English

This story contains words describing motion, such as *trotted away* and *wandered lazily,* that students may not know. Start a word wall with these words. Have students pantomime them. Students can then add other motion words as they read the story.

INTERACTIVE LEARNING

Prior Knowledge/Building Background

Key Concept
Life in the Desert

Cooperative Learning Have groups of students work together to make lists of the sights, sounds, and feelings a person walking through the desert might experience.

Key Concept
Coyote and Javelinas

Have students preview the illustrations. Note that in this story the pigs have been replaced by javelinas (ha-ve-LEE-nas) and the wolf by a coyote. Have students compare these animals and discuss how they are often depicted in stories.

Why Pigs/Javelinas Are Seen As Good	Why Wolf/Coyote Is Seen As Bad
They have round bodies and are cute-looking.	He is lean and his teeth are sharp and scary.
They help each other out.	He is alone.
They want to live in peace.	He wants to eat them.

Students Acquiring English If possible, show pictures of a desert or a video such as *Let's Explore the Desert* (National Geographic) to build background.

Other Choices for Building Background

Drawing Settings

MEETING INDIVIDUAL NEEDS

Students Acquiring English Have students draw two houses: one in a city setting and one in a desert setting. Ask them to compare and contrast the settings. What special needs would someone who lives in a desert environment have?

Being Prepared

Cooperative Learning

Have students work in small groups to make lists of clothing and other supplies that would help a person survive in the desert. Afterward students can share their lists and combine them into a master list.

Great Start
For students needing extra support with key concepts and vocabulary, use the Oink, Oink, Oink CD.

INTERACTIVE LEARNING

Selection Vocabulary

Key Words

desert

dust storm

whirlwind

tumbleweeds

cactus

adobe

Display Transparency 1–5. After volunteers have read aloud the Key Words, use these questions to discuss the captions.

- What would you need to protect yourself in a dust storm?
- What would it feel like to brush against some tumbleweeds?
- How can a cactus survive in a dry place like the desert? (It absorbs huge amounts of water during occasional desert rains.)
- How is an adobe brick different from a regular brick? (It is baked in the sun, not an oven; adobe is a light color, not red.)

Two Key Words are compounds. Challenge students to define them using the parts of the compound. (Example: *Tumbleweeds* are *weeds* that *tumble*.)

Students Acquiring English You might wish to introduce these additional words: *hooves, hairy, sneaky, shade, heat, magic,* and *suspicious.*

Vocabulary Practice Have students work independently or together to complete the activity on *Literacy Activity Book* page 20.

Spelling

You may want to give the Spelling Pretest on p. 88I before students read the selection.

Daily Language Practice

Use the sentences on page 88K as daily practice of the spelling and grammar skills taught with this selection.

Transparency 1–5

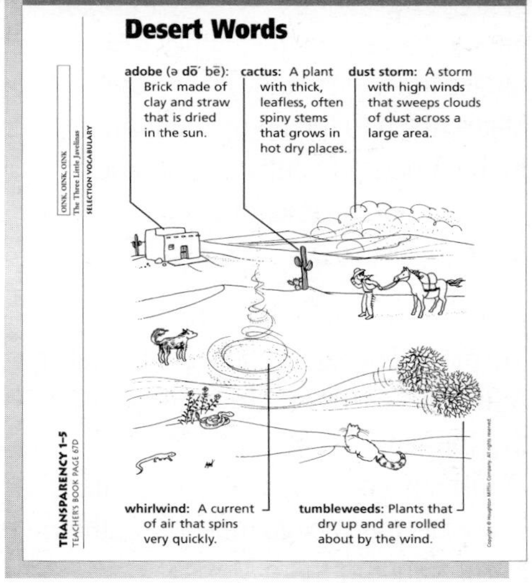
OINK, OINK, OINK
The Three Little Javelinas
SELECTION VOCABULARY

Desert Words

adobe (ə dō′ bē): Brick made of clay and straw that is dried in the sun.

cactus: A plant with thick, leafless, often spiny stems that grows in hot dry places.

dust storm: A storm with high winds that sweeps clouds of dust across a large area.

whirlwind: A current of air that spins very quickly.

tumbleweeds: Plants that dry up and are rolled about by the wind.

TRANSPARENCY 1–5
TEACHER'S BOOK PAGE 67D

Copyright © Houghton Mifflin Company. All rights reserved.

Literacy Activity Book, p. 20

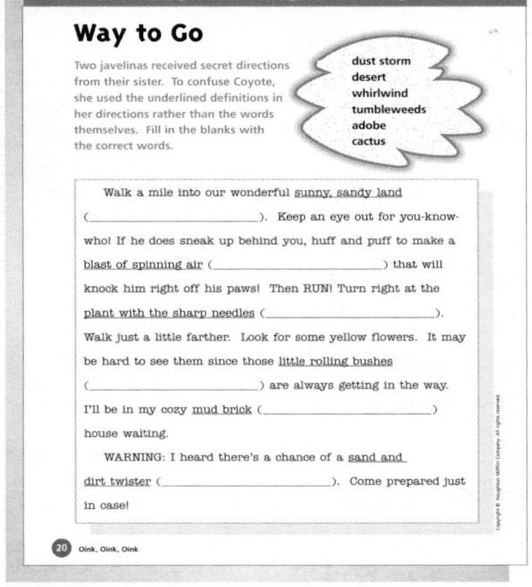
Way to Go

Two javelinas received secret directions from their sister. To confuse Coyote, she used the underlined definitions in her directions rather than the words themselves. Fill in the blanks with the correct words.

dust storm
desert
whirlwind
tumbleweeds
adobe
cactus

Walk a mile into our wonderful sunny, sandy land (__________). Keep an eye out for you-know-who! If he does sneak up behind you, huff and puff to make a blast of spinning air (__________) that will knock him right off his paws! Then RUN! Turn right at the plant with the sharp needles (__________). Walk just a little farther. Look for some yellow flowers. It may be hard to see them since those little rolling bushes (__________) are always getting in the way. I'll be in my cozy mud brick (__________) house waiting.

WARNING: I heard there's a chance of a sand and dirt twister (__________). Come prepared just in case!

20 Oink, Oink, Oink

Copyright © Houghton Mifflin Company. All rights reserved.

Science

Teacher FactFile

Desert Food Chain

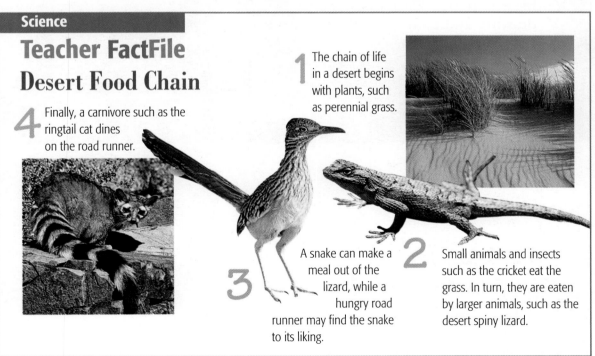

1 The chain of life in a desert begins with plants, such as perennial grass.

2 Small animals and insects such as the cricket eat the grass. In turn, they are eaten by larger animals, such as the desert spiny lizard.

3 A snake can make a meal out of the lizard, while a hungry road runner may find the snake to its liking.

4 Finally, a carnivore such as the ringtail cat dines on the road runner.

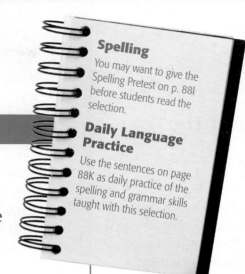

Interact *with* Literature

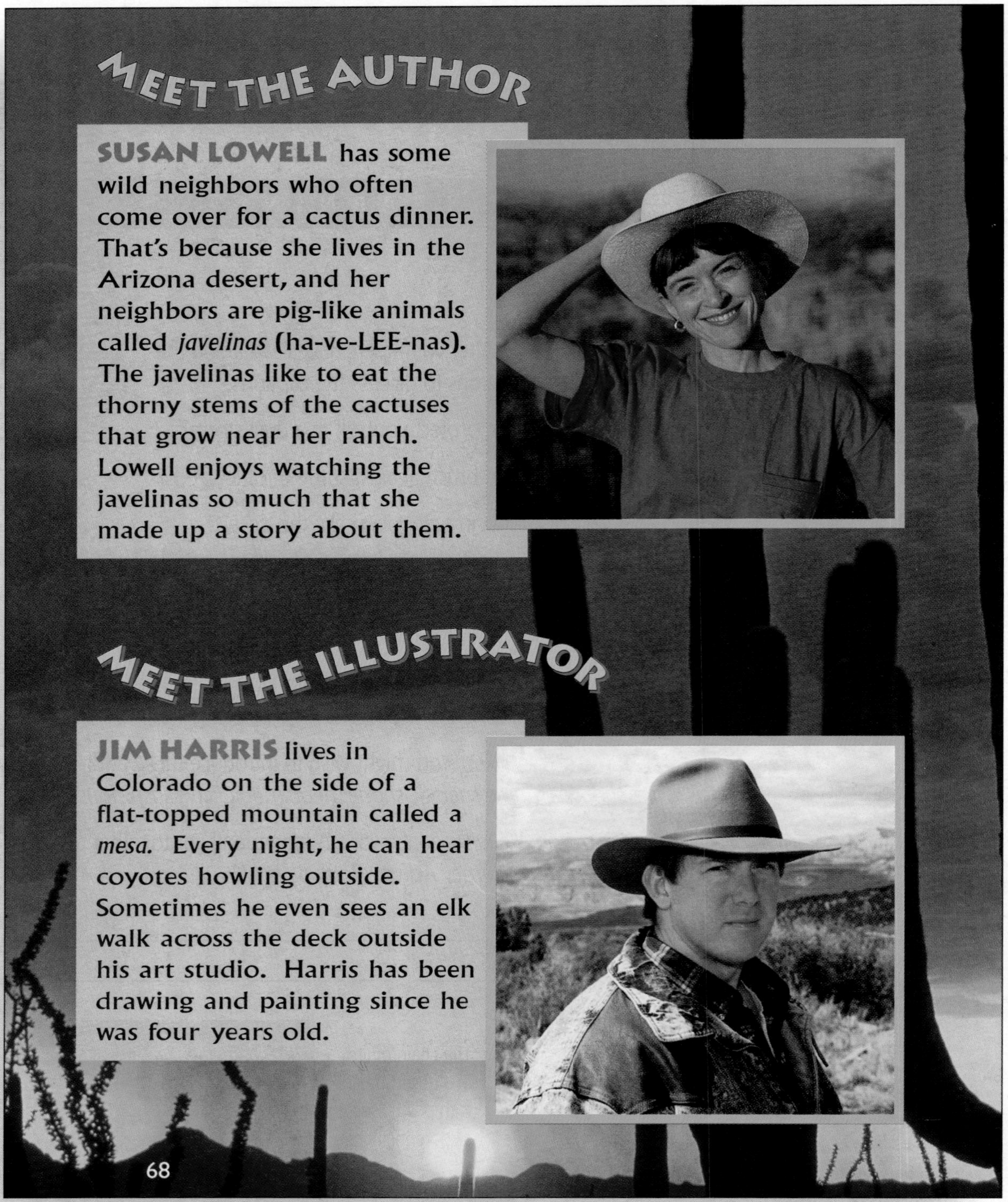

MEET THE AUTHOR

SUSAN LOWELL has some wild neighbors who often come over for a cactus dinner. That's because she lives in the Arizona desert, and her neighbors are pig-like animals called *javelinas* (ha-ve-LEE-nas). The javelinas like to eat the thorny stems of the cactuses that grow near her ranch. Lowell enjoys watching the javelinas so much that she made up a story about them.

MEET THE ILLUSTRATOR

JIM HARRIS lives in Colorado on the side of a flat-topped mountain called a *mesa.* Every night, he can hear coyotes howling outside. Sometimes he even sees an elk walk across the deck outside his art studio. Harris has been drawing and painting since he was four years old.

68

More About the Author

Susan Lowell

Susan Lowell describes javelinas as being "extremely bristly—very hairy on the chinny-chin-chin. Oddly enough, they are also related to the hippopotamus." The name comes from the Spanish word for the collared peccary, a member of the swine family that ranges from the southwestern United States down to the tip of South America. In the American Southwest, another common local name for peccaries, besides javelinas, is "wild pigs."

Lowell's sources for this story include the many Coyote legends told by Native Americans of the Southwest, especially the Tohono O'Odham (toe-HO-no O-OH-tam) or Desert People, formerly known as the Papago tribe, of southern Arizona and northern Mexico.

More About the Illustrator

Jim Harris

The coyote in *The Three Little Javelinas* is no stranger to Jim Harris. The illustrator lives at the end of a dirt road on the slope of a mesa in Colorado. Every night he hears the coyotes howl. Sometimes an elk walks across the deck of his art studio. Harris has been drawing and painting since he was four years old.

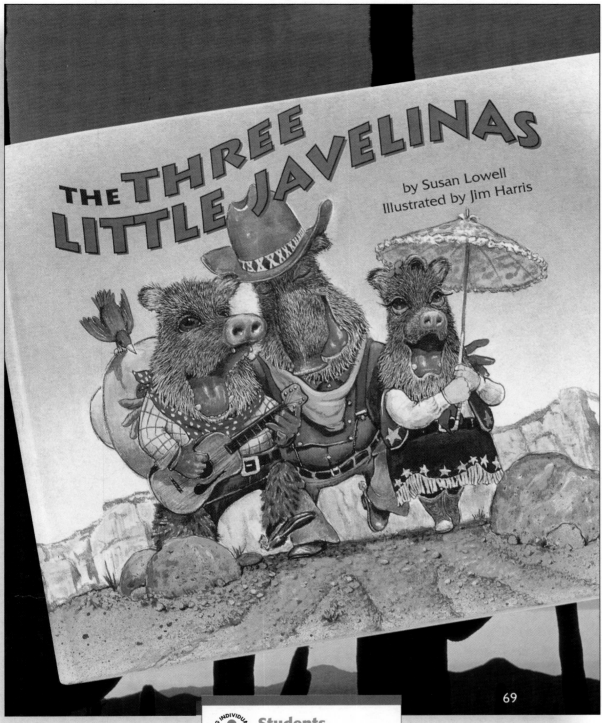
THE THREE LITTLE JAVELINAS
by Susan Lowell
Illustrated by Jim Harris
69

QuickREFERENCE

Science Link

Javelinas Although javelinas look like pigs, they are not. They are classified as peccaries, which are members of the swine family. Have students turn to "My Hairy Neighbors" on page 89 to study photos of real javelinas.

Students Acquiring English

MEETING INDIVIDUAL NEEDS

This story makes use of descriptive words, dialogue, and action that can be acted out or pantomimed by students as they read it.

Visual Literacy

Discuss the javelinas' clothing. Ask why chaps and bandannas are worn. (Chaps protect your legs and bandannas cover your mouth in dust and sand storms.) If you have students from arid countries, ask them to share how people dress.

Interact *with* Literature

Reading Strategies

Monitor
Predict/Infer

Discussion Discuss with students how good readers adjust the way they read depending on the kind of material they are reading.

Ask students what reading strategies might help them with this story. Discuss how the story might be surprising, so they may need to make predictions and monitor their reading.

Predicting/Purpose Setting

Have students summarize the simple structure of the traditional tale "The Three Little Pigs" and predict how *The Three Little Javelinas* will be similar to it.

Choices for Reading

Independent Reading	**Cooperative Reading**
Guided Reading	**Teacher Read Aloud**

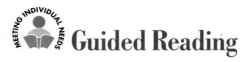

Guided Reading

Students using the Guided Reading option should read to page 75, keeping their predictions in mind as they read. Use the questions on page 74 to check comprehension.

ONCE UPON A TIME, way out in the desert, there were three little javelinas. Javelinas (ha-ve-LEE-nas) are wild, hairy, southwestern cousins of pigs.

Their heads were hairy, their backs were hairy, and their bony legs — all the way down to their hard little hooves — were very hairy. But their snouts were soft and pink.

One day, the three little javelinas trotted away to seek their fortunes. In this hot, dry land, the sky was almost always blue. Steep purple mountains looked down on the desert, where the cactus forests grew.

Soon the little javelinas came to a spot where the path divided, and each one went a different way.

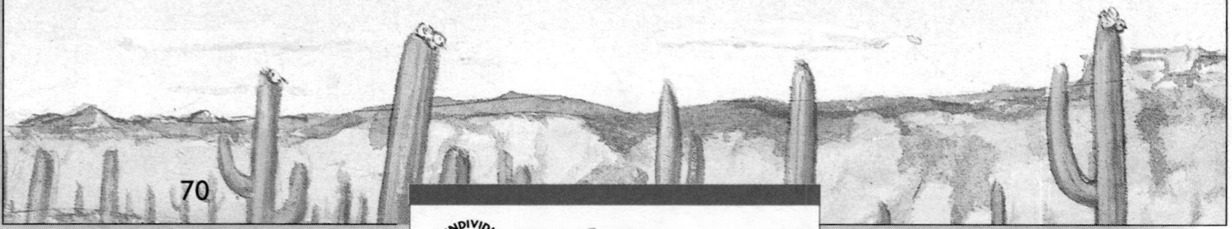

70

QuickREFERENCE

Journal

Encourage students to record their predictions and inferences in their journals. You might also point out the phrase *Once upon a time* and ask students to add it to their journals as a story starter.

Students Acquiring English

Idiom/Multiple-Meaning Word
The phrase *to seek their fortunes* means the javelinas left home to work and look for success. You may want to ask students what success means to them. Also, explain that a *spot* is a place or location.

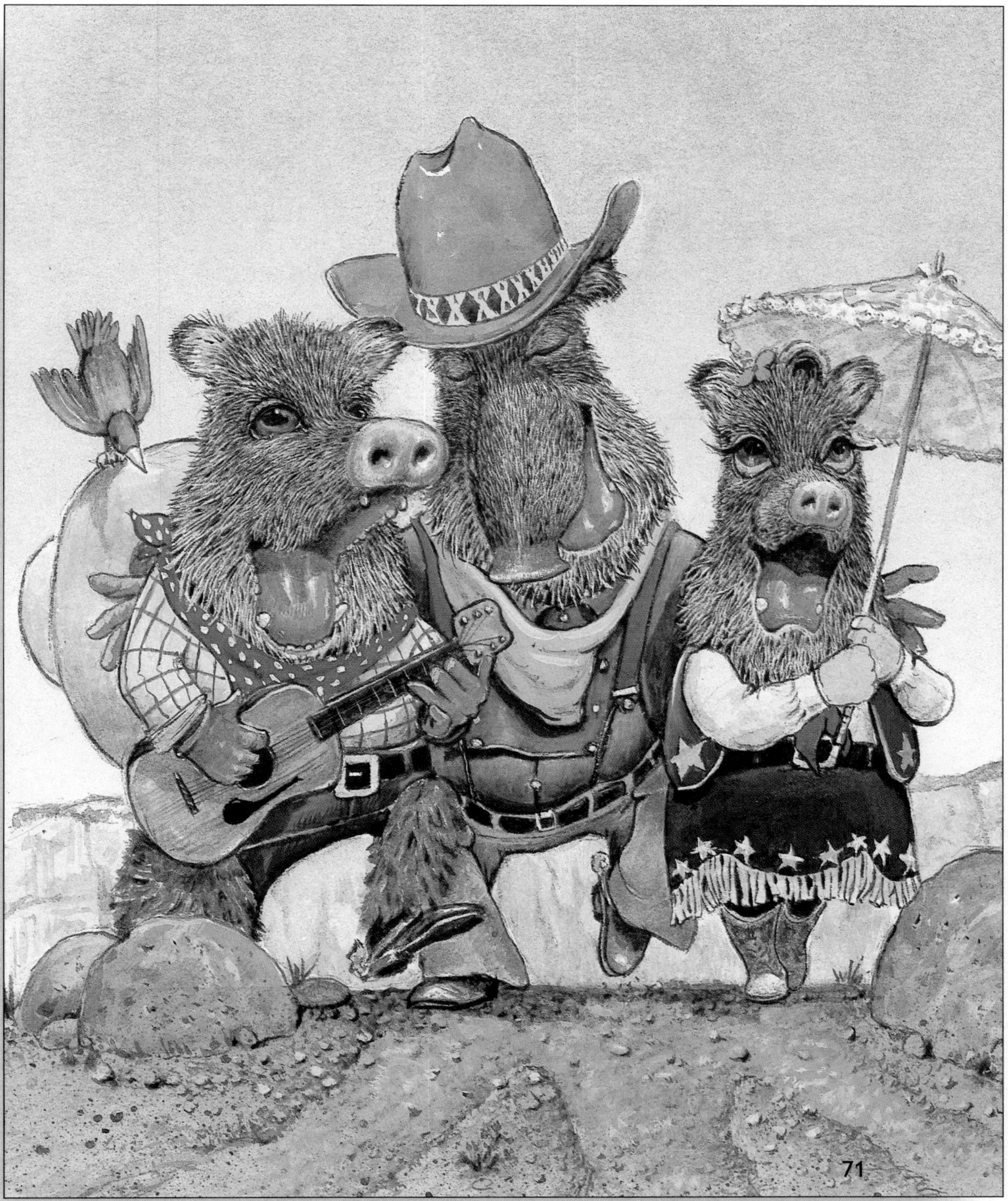
71

Math Link

Numbers vs. Numerals Discuss the difference between a number and a numeral. A number is something said out loud. A numeral is a symbol. When we write a number, we can write the numeral (*3*) or the word for that number (*three*).

Music Link

Cowboy Songs Do students know any cowboy songs, such as "Home on the Range" or "Red River Valley"? During long cattle drives, these songs helped alleviate a cowboy's loneliness. They were also an effective way to quiet the cattle!

Interact *with* Literature

Reading Strategies

Predict/Infer

Remind students that in the original tale the wolf blew the pigs' houses down. Tell them they can use this knowledge to make a prediction about how Coyote will approach the first javelina. Do they think the javelina will escape? Why or why not?

The first little javelina wandered lazily along. He didn't see a dust storm whirling across the desert — until it caught him.

The whirlwind blew away and left the first little javelina sitting in a heap of tumbleweeds. Brushing himself off, he said, "I'll build a house with them!" And in no time at all, he did.

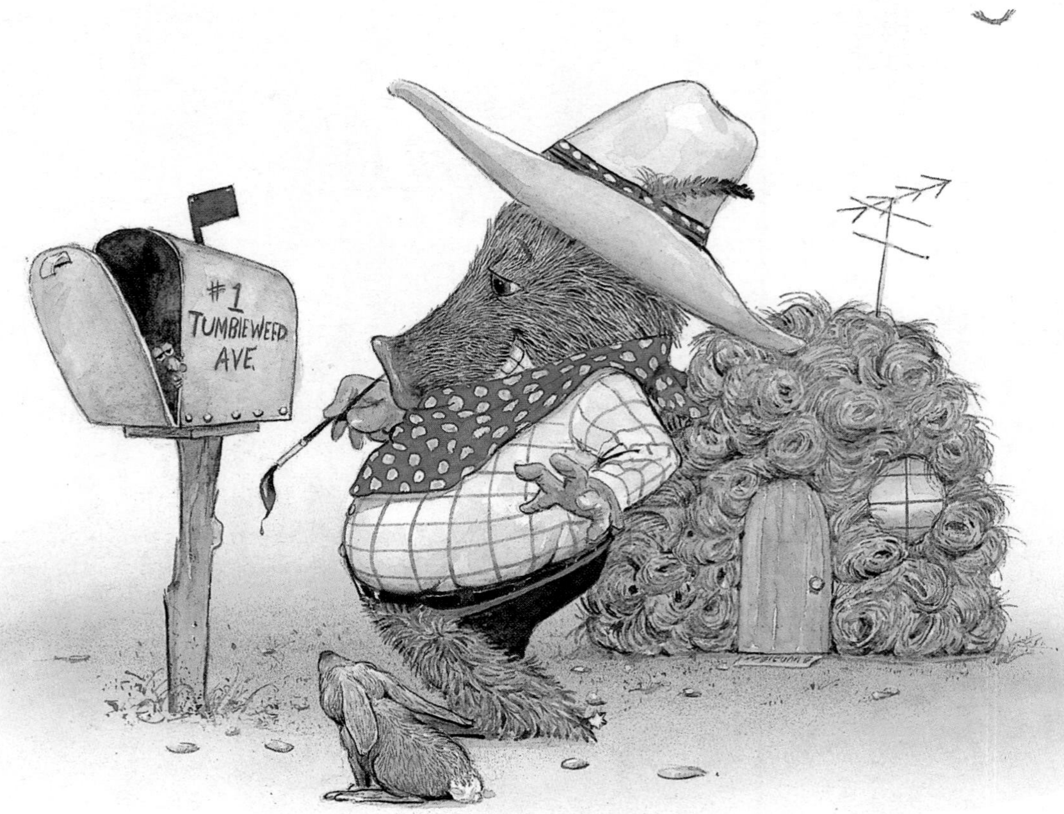
#1
TUMBLEWEED
AVE

72

QuickREFERENCE

Students Acquiring English

Motion Words Have a student pantomime the action of *wandered lazily,* and discuss how its meaning differs from the word *walked.* Explain what it means to be *caught* by something and the meaning of the word *heap.*

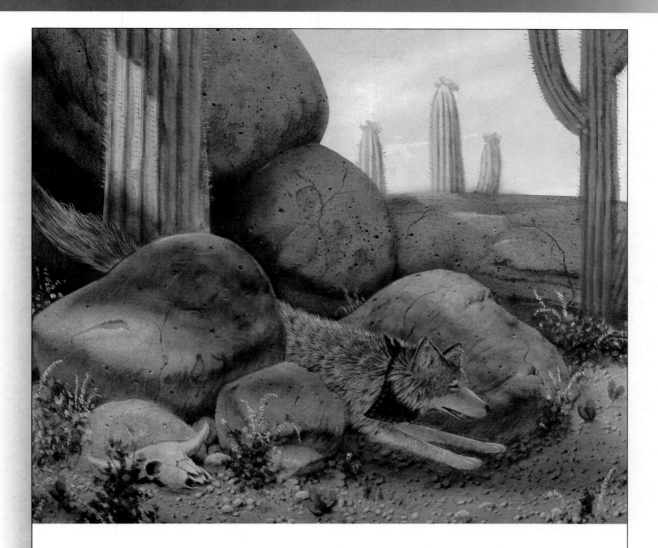

Then along came a coyote. He ran through the desert so quickly and so quietly that he was almost invisible. In fact, this was only one of Coyote's many magical tricks. He laughed when he saw the tumbleweed house and smelled the javelina inside.

"Mmm! A tender juicy piggy!" he thought. Coyote was tired of eating mice and rabbits.

73

Science Link

Prairie Wolves Coyotes are also called *prairie wolves*. Unlike wolves, though, coyotes usually live alone or in pairs. Their main food is rabbits and rodents. But they will also prey upon large animals such as sheep and antelope.

Extra Support

MEETING INDIVIDUAL NEEDS

Pronunciation Explain to students that the word *coyote* can be pronounced two ways: either kie-OH-tee or KIE-ote. Ask students to share how they pronounce it.

Visual Literacy

The story text says the coyote was almost invisible due to his speed and stealth. Ask students to look at the illustration to find another reason. (His coloration blends in with the earth tones of rocks and sand.)

Interact *with* Literature

Guided Reading

Comprehension/Critical Thinking

1. Why is Coyote called sneaky? (He used magic to make himself almost invisible. He tried to fool the first javelina by calling out sweetly. He tiptoed when he moved.)
2. Why did Coyote laugh when he saw the tumbleweed house and smelled the javelina inside? (He knew that the house would not be strong enough to protect the javelina.)
3. Why didn't the first javelina choose something better than tumbleweeds to build with? (He was lazy and chose the first material that he stumbled onto.)

Predicting/Purpose Setting

Ask students to compare the first part of the story with other versions they know. Discuss whether their purpose-setting predictions were correct.
Tell students to revise their predictions, if necessary, and to read to the end of page 79 to find out what happens to the second javelina.

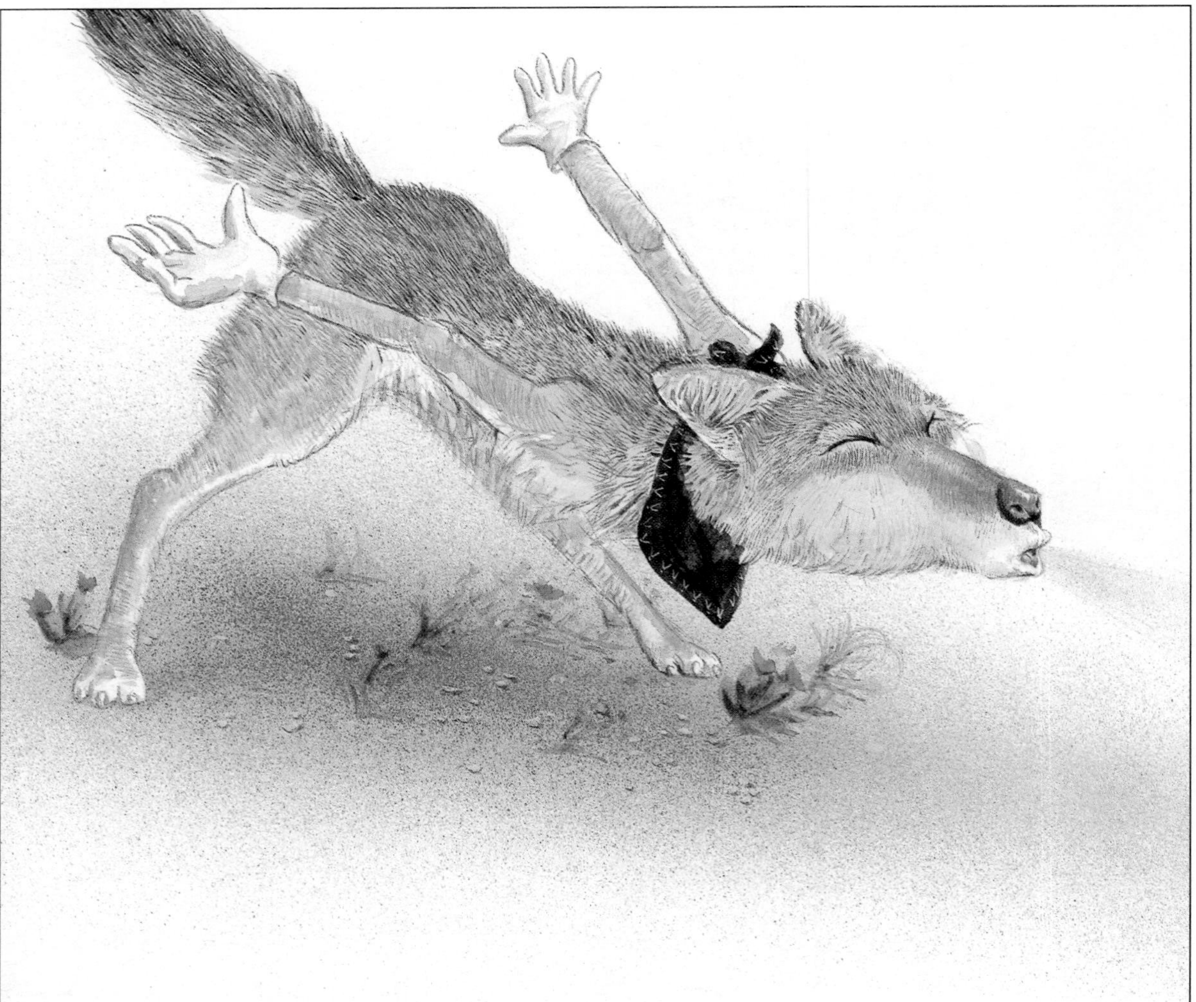

He called out sweetly, "Little pig, little pig, let me come in."

"Not by the hair of my chinny-chin-chin!" shouted the first javelina (who had a lot of hair on his chinny-chin-chin!).

"Then I'll huff, and I'll puff, and I'll blow your house in!" said Coyote.

74

Informal Assessment

If students' responses indicate that they are understanding the story, have them finish reading independently or in a cooperative group.

QuickREFERENCE

Multicultural Link

Tricksters The word *coyote* comes from the Aztec *coyotl.* In many Native American tales Coyote is a trickster who is often outsmarted. Students might enjoy reading *Coyote Steals a Blanket: A Ute Tale* by Janet Stevens.

Extra Support

Rereading Aloud Students may better appreciate the end rhyme and rhythm in the exchange between Coyote and the javelina if they reread the dialogue aloud. Also, discuss the humor in the parenthetical remark.

And he huffed, and he puffed, and he blew the little tumbleweed house away.

But in all the hullabaloo, the first little javelina escaped — and went looking for his brother and sister.

Coyote, who was very sneaky, tiptoed along behind.

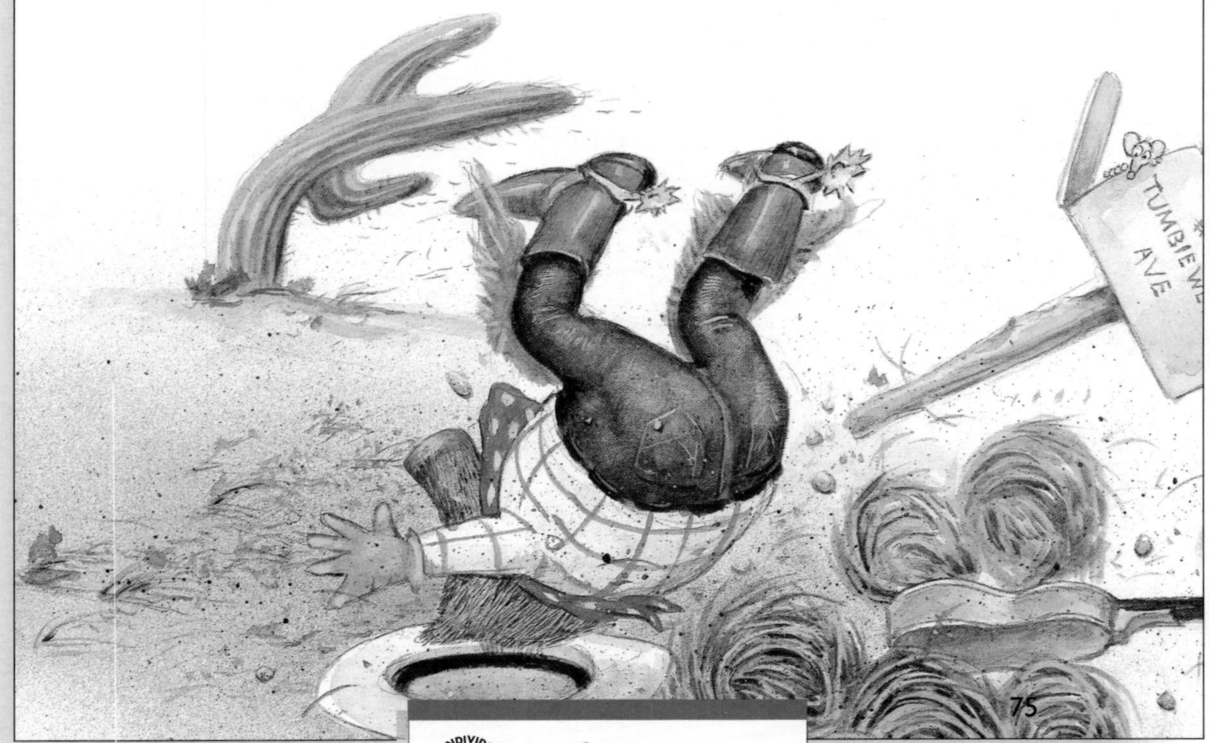

MEETING INDIVIDUAL NEEDS

Students Acquiring English

Word Meaning Explain that *hullabaloo* is a nonsense word that describes a state of confusion.

Motion Words Demonstrate *tiptoed* by tiptoeing in a sneaky way. Then have students add the word to their journals or to the wall chart.

MINILESSON

Compare and Contrast

TESTED SKILL

Teach/Model

Discuss with students how reading different versions of the same tale can be fun. Point out that part of the fun is comparing the new story with the original.

Think Aloud

One big way this story is different from "The Three Little Pigs" is the desert setting. The characters have changed too—there are javelinas instead of pigs, and a coyote has replaced the wolf. The first part is like "The Three Little Pigs" because the coyote asks to be let in and the javelina refuses him in the same way as in the original story.

Practice/Apply

Ask students to point out other ways the traditional tale and *The Three Little Javelinas* are alike and different. Map responses in a Venn diagram.

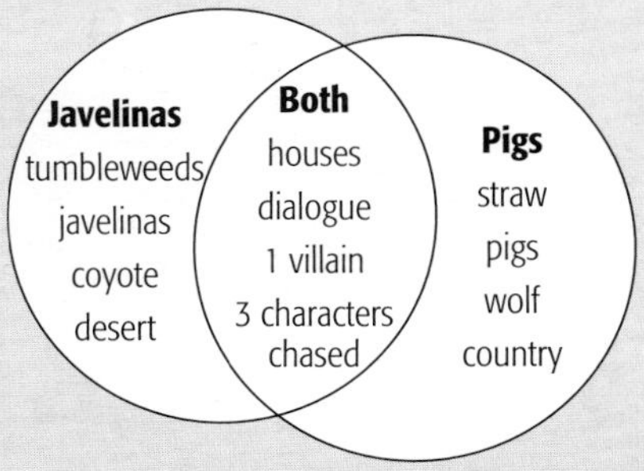
Javelinas
tumbleweeds
javelinas
coyote
desert
Both
houses
dialogue
1 villain
3 characters chased
Pigs
straw
pigs
wolf
country

SKILL FINDER

Full lesson/Reteaching, pp. 88B–88C

Minilessons, p. 103; Theme 4, p. 47

Interact *with* Literature

Reading Strategies

Think About Words

Discuss with students how they can use context clues to figure out the following about saguaros:

- They're tall. (clue: *Giant cactus plants called saguaros*)
- They grow fruit. (clue: *They held their ripe red fruit high in the sky.*)
- Not much grows outward from them. (clue: *But they made almost no shade.*)

The second little javelina walked for miles among giant cactus plants called saguaros (sa-WA-ros). They held their ripe red fruit high in the sky. But they made almost no shade, and the little javelina grew hot.

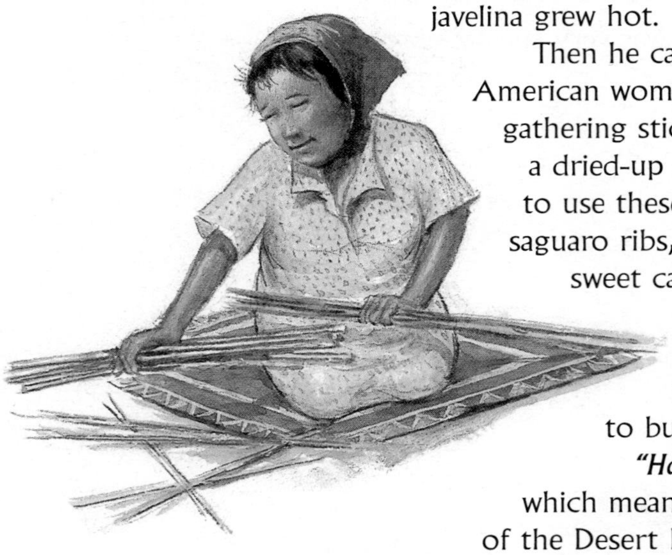

Then he came upon a Native American woman who was gathering sticks from inside a dried-up cactus. She planned to use these long sticks, called saguaro ribs, to knock down the sweet cactus fruit.

The second little javelina said, "Please, may I have some sticks to build a house?"

"Ha'u," (how) she said, which means "yes" in the language of the Desert People.

76

QuickREFERENCE

Multicultural Link

The Tohono O'Odham (toe-HO-no O-OH-tam), or Desert People, conduct a harvest in the early summer, when cactus flowers begin to bear fruit. This harvest was so important that it marked the beginning of the new year.

Challenge

MEETING INDIVIDUAL NEEDS

Saguaros Have students research

- how long saguaros live
- what animals live in them
- the kinds of food they provide

Explain that cactus fruit looks like watermelon when it is broken open.

Multicultural Link

Word Origins Note that the word *saguaros* came from Mexican Spanish. Invite students to research other English words that have been borrowed from other languages and to report back to the class.

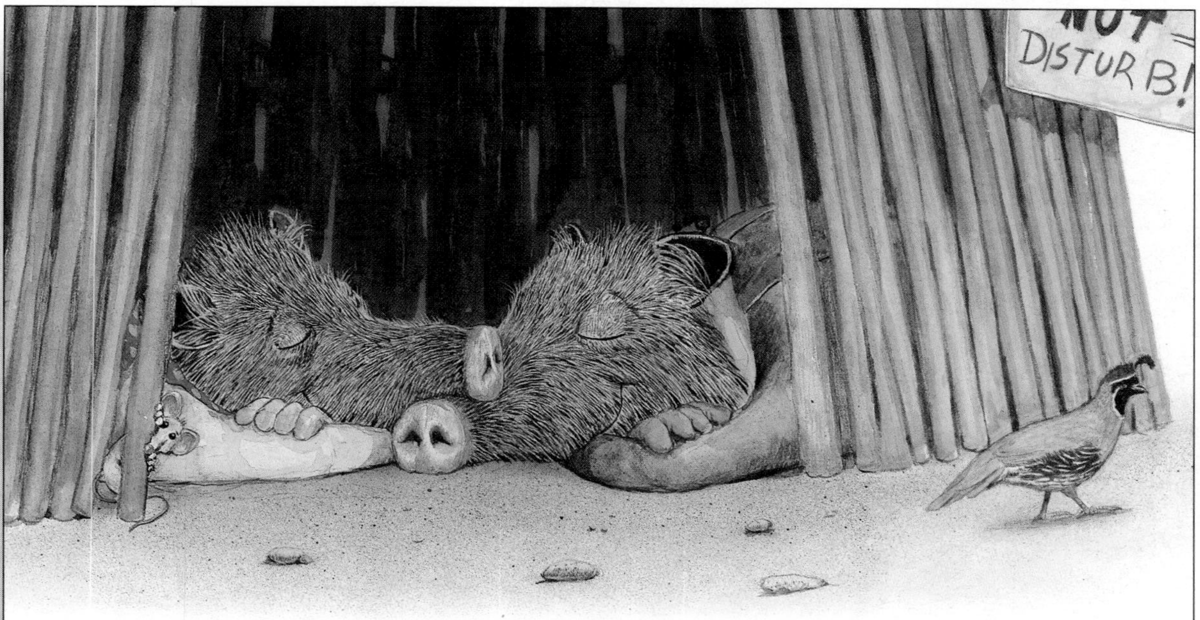
DISTURB!

When he was finished building his house, he lay down in the shade. Then his brother arrived, panting from the heat, and the second little javelina moved over and made a place for him.

77

Students Acquiring English

Word Meaning Have a volunteer demonstrate *panting.* Ask students why animals pant. (to cool off or to catch their breath after running) Also, discuss the phrase *made a place for him*. ("provided a space or area for him to rest")

Visual Literacy

Have students find the mouse on page 77 and then on pages 72 and 75. Discuss how the mouse's facial expressions are a commentary on the story action. Students will enjoy looking for the mouse as they continue to read.

Interact *with* Literature

Reading Strategies

Monitor

Discuss the humor in Coyote's response about not wanting to eat the javelinas' hair. Recall that the author poked fun at the "chinny-chin-chin" response in a parenthetical remark on page 74.

MEETING INDIVIDUAL NEEDS Guided Reading

Comprehension/Critical Thinking

1. Why are saguaro ribs stronger to build with than tumbleweeds? (They are long sticks that are hard enough to knock fruit off a cactus.)
2. Do you think that Coyote is big and bad like the big bad pig? Why or why not? (He is not as big physically, but he's threatening because he is so clever.)

Predicting/Purpose Setting

Have students summarize the story so far. Then ask them to make predictions about the ending. Comprehension questions can be found on page 86.

Self-Assessment

Reflecting Invite students to ask:

- How am I enjoying the story?
- Do I understand everything that has happened so far?
- What was the hardest part so far?

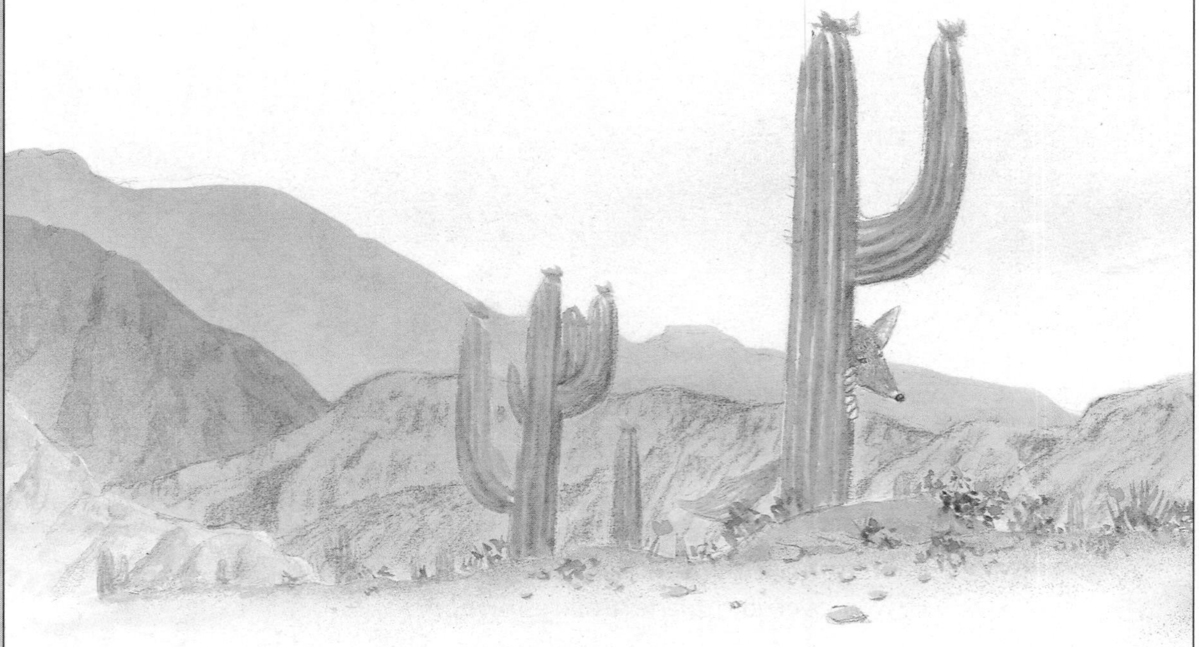

Pretty soon, Coyote found the saguaro rib house. He used his magic to make his voice sound just like another javelina's.

"Little pig, little pig, let me come in!" he called.

But the little javelinas were suspicious. The second one cried, "No! Not by the hair of my chinny-chin-chin!"

"Bah!" thought Coyote. "I am not going to eat your ***hair.***"

78

QuickREFERENCE

Vocabulary

Word Meaning If students have difficulty with *suspicious,* point out context clues: Coyote calls out in a javelina-like voice, but the ones inside don't open the door; they don't completely trust what they're hearing.

MEETING INDIVIDUAL NEEDS Extra Support

Reading Dialogue Point out that Coyote changes his voice to mimic a javelina. Ask students to try reading the dialogue the way either a coyote and a javelina might talk or the way some other animal they know might.

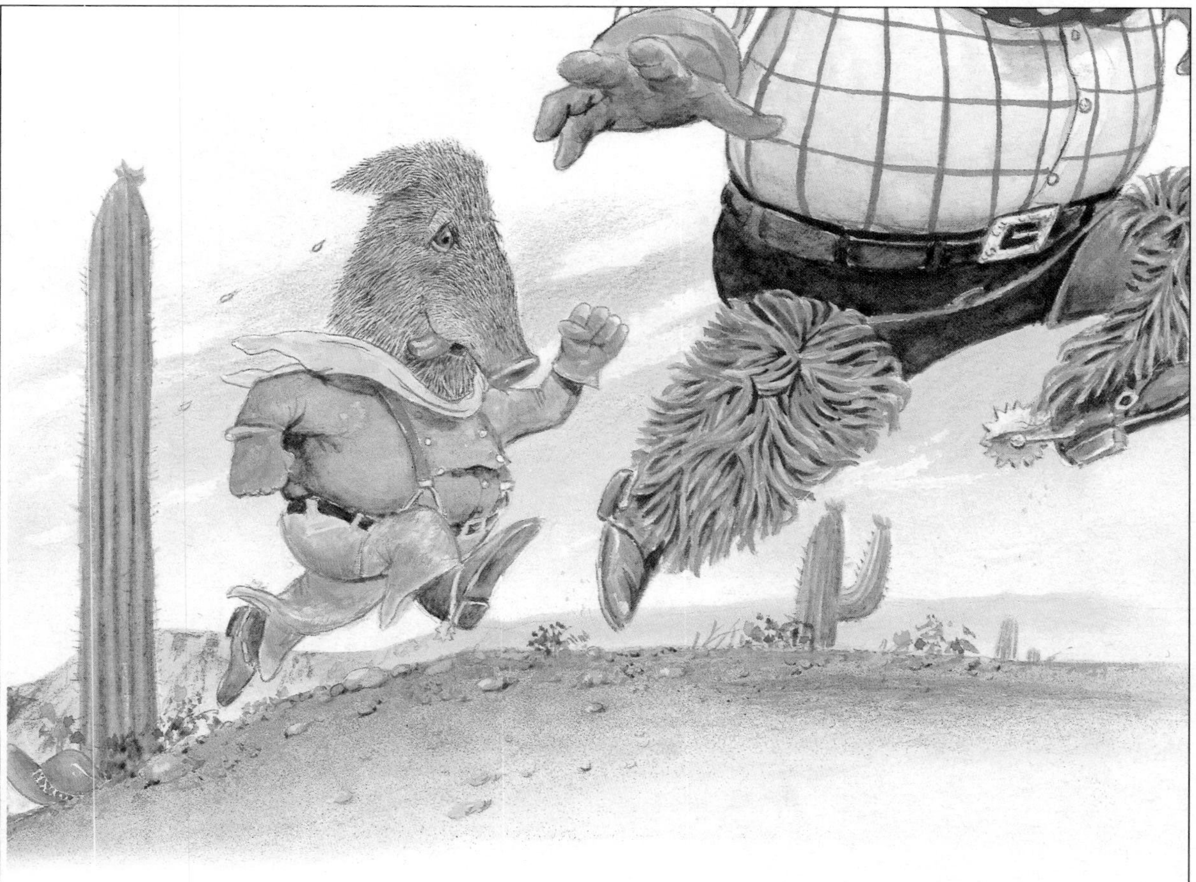

Then Coyote smiled, showing all his sharp teeth: "I'll huff, and I'll puff, and I'll blow your house in!"

So he huffed, and he puffed, and all the saguaro ribs came tumbling down.

But the two little javelinas escaped into the desert.

Still not discouraged, Coyote followed. Sometimes his magic did fail, but then he usually came up with another trick.

79

Journal

Advice If students can think of a better way to trick the javelinas, have them write their words of advice to Coyote in their journals.

MINILESSON

Predicting Outcomes

REVIEW & MAINTAIN

Teach/Model

Discuss how most stories have a sequence of events that result in an outcome. Explain that one way readers can anticipate this outcome is by making predictions. Use this chart to illustrate the process.

What I Learn from the Story	+	What I Know	=	Prediction: What Might Happen

Practice/Apply

Help students predict the outcome of *The Three Little Javelinas* by expanding the chart like this.

What I Learn from the Story	+	What I Know	=	Predicted Outcome
This story is like "The Three Little Pigs."		In the original, the wolf tried to come down the chimney.		Coyote will try the chimney, but, like the wolf, he will fall into boiling water.

Encourage students to develop a similar chart for other stories they read in the future. (You may wish to have them copy the format of the chart above in their journals for reference.)

SKILL FINDER

Full lesson/Reteaching, Theme 4, pp. 58B–58C

Minilessons, Theme 4, pp. 53, 67

Interact *with* Literature

Reading Strategies

Summarize

Ask students to summarize how the javelinas have tried to protect themselves against Coyote thus far. Remind them that in the original story, the houses are built of progressively stronger materials. Have them consider whether Coyote will be able to blow down an adobe house or whether this is the house he will have to enter some other way.

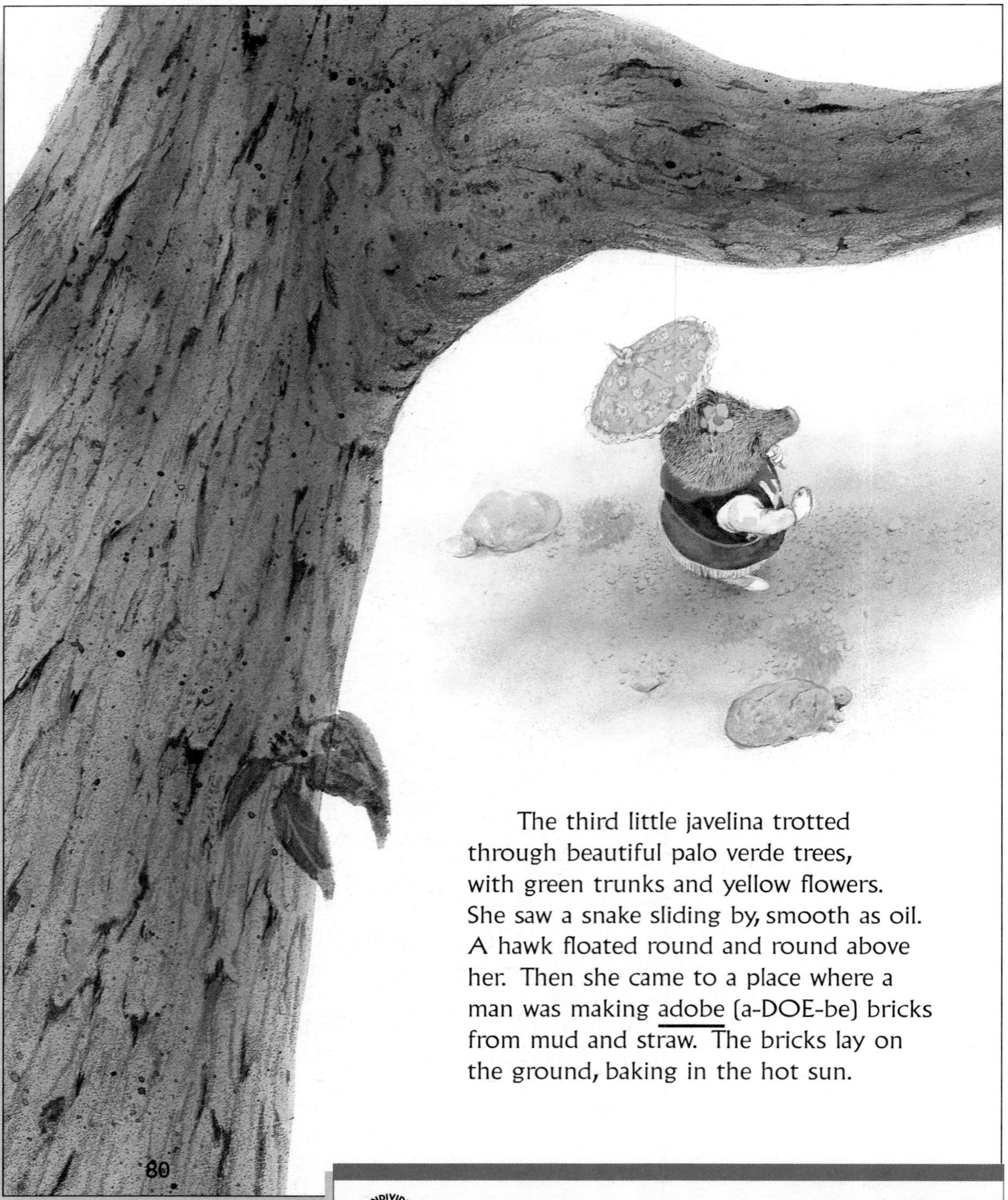

The third little javelina trotted through beautiful palo verde trees, with green trunks and yellow flowers. She saw a snake sliding by, smooth as oil. A hawk floated round and round above her. Then she came to a place where a man was making adobe (a-DOE-be) bricks from mud and straw. The bricks lay on the ground, baking in the hot sun.

80

QuickREFERENCE

Science Link

Palo Verde Trees There are ten species of palo verdes, but all of them bear fruit shaped like a pea-pod. This tree also has spines that jut out like thorns. *Palo verde* is a Spanish phrase that perfectly describes the trees: "green sticks."

Students Acquiring English

Motion Words Discuss with students the mental pictures these images create: *snake sliding by, smooth as oil* and a *hawk floated round and round.* Discuss substitutions for *smooth as oil* and *floated.* What pictures do they make in your mind?

You might wish to bring in pictures and illustrations to reinforce the images, or have a student pantomime the actions.

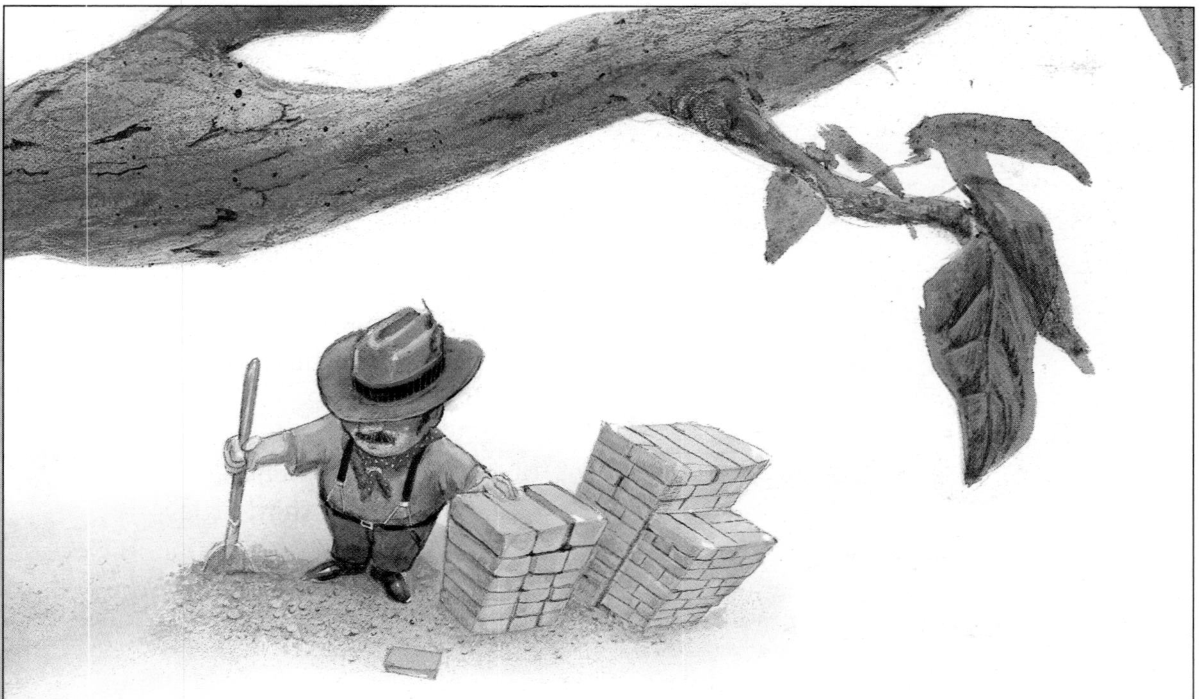

The third little javelina thought for a moment, and said, "May I please have a few adobes to build a house?"

"*Sí,*" answered the man, which means "yes" in Spanish, the brick-maker's language.

So the third javelina built herself a solid little adobe house, cool in summer and warm in winter. When her brothers found her, she welcomed them in and locked the door behind them.

Coyote followed their trail.

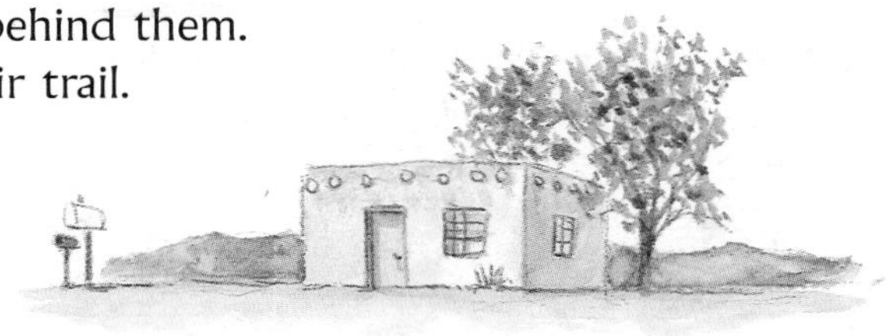

81

Challenge

MEETING INDIVIDUAL NEEDS

The Spanish were the first Europeans to colonize the Southwest. Ask students to research

- Spanish-named cities in the Southwest
- southwestern architecture
- the people of the Southwest

Social Studies Link

Adaptation Adobe houses are one way humans have adapted to life in the desert. Adobe is a better insulator than wood or stone. It's only fit for dry climates because it can crumble in the cold and rain.

Interact *with* Literature

"Little pig, little pig, let me come in!" he called.

The three little javelinas looked out the window. This time Coyote pretended to be very old and weak, with no teeth and a sore paw. But they were not fooled.

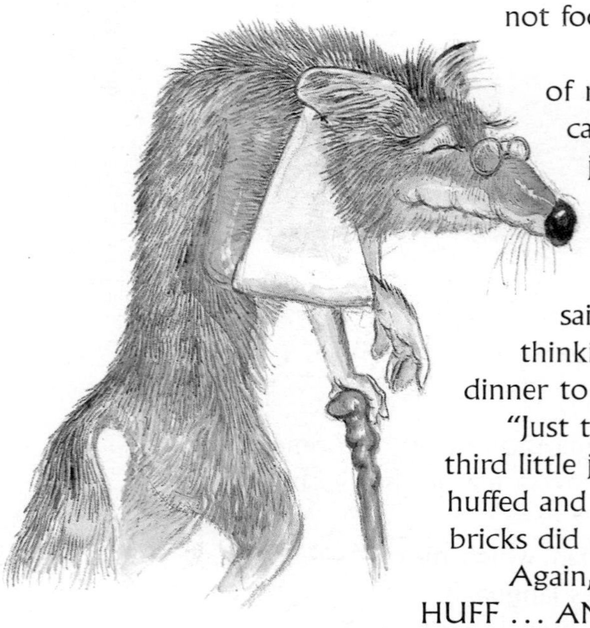

"No! Not by the hair of my chinny-chin-chin," called back the third little javelina.

"Then I'll huff, and I'll puff, and I'll blow your house in!" said Coyote. He grinned, thinking of the wild pig dinner to come.

"Just try it!" shouted the third little javelina. So Coyote huffed and puffed, but the adobe bricks did not budge.

Again, Coyote tried. "I'll HUFF . . . AND I'LL PUFF . . . AND I'LL BLOW YOUR HOUSE IN!"

82

Informal Assessment

Oral Reading Have individual students read aloud pages 82–83 as a check of oral reading fluency. Use the Oral Reading Checklist in the *Teacher's Assessment Handbook* as a guide for assessment.

QuickREFERENCE

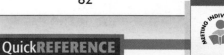

Meeting Individual Needs: Students Acquiring English

Word Meaning Explain that *did not budge* means "did not move slightly." Discuss how this is a humorous word choice by the author because it emphasizes how solid the adobe house is.

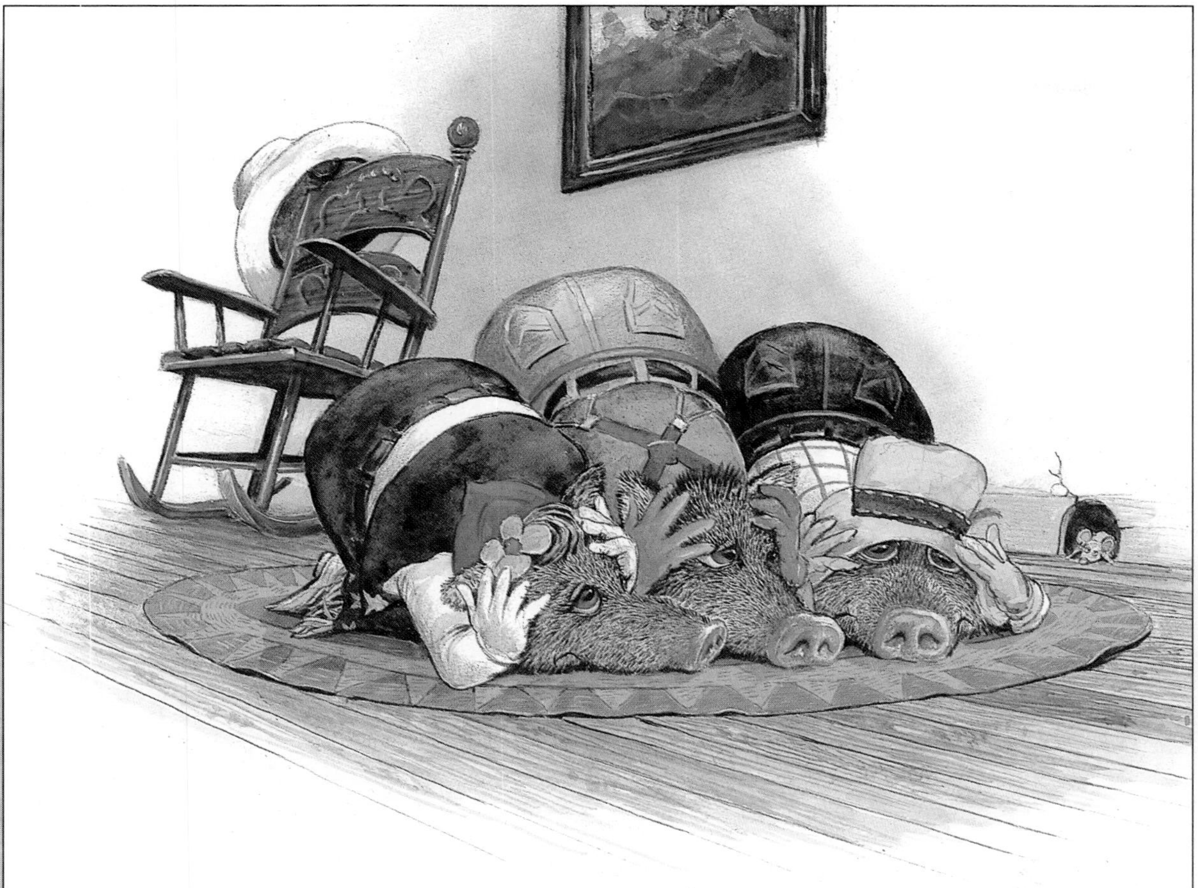

The three little javelinas covered their hairy ears. But nothing happened. The javelinas peeked out the window.

MINILESSON

Summarizing: Story Structure

Teach/Model

REVIEW & MAINTAIN

Review the elements of a story: setting, characters, problem, events, and solution. Discuss how a good story summary includes most of these elements. Then map out *The Three Little Javelinas* like this.

Setting: southwestern U.S.
Characters: Coyote, 3 javelinas
Problem: Three javelinas must escape a clever coyote.
Events: 1. Javelinas leave to seek fortunes. 2. Coyote blows down tumbleweed house. 3. Coyote blows down rib house. 4. Coyote slips through stove pipe in the adobe house.
Solution: Javelinas light fire in stove that chases Coyote away.

Practice/Apply

Have students use the chart to summarize. Here is an example.

This version of "The Three Little Pigs" takes place in the Southwest. This time it's a coyote chasing three javelinas. Their houses made of tumbleweed and saguaro ribs are no match for Coyote. But the third house, made of adobe, does the trick. When Coyote tries to enter this house, his tail is scorched and he runs away in pain.

SKILL FINDER

Full lesson/Reteaching, pp. 60B–60C

Minilessons, p. 45; Theme 2, p. 207

MEETING INDIVIDUAL NEEDS

Extra Support

Dialogue Coyote's second warning to the javelinas (page 82) is in all capital letters. Ask students why the words were printed this way. Then have groups of students form a chorus to read the line the way Coyote would say it.

MEETING INDIVIDUAL NEEDS

Students Acquiring English

Word Meaning Explain that to *peek* means "to look quickly or secretly." Ask volunteers to pantomime peeking out a window or door.

Interact *with* Literature

Reading Strategies

Evaluate

Encourage students to evaluate what makes the climactic scene in the story work well. Discuss how the author uses sound words such as *whoosh* and *sizzle.* Point out how she put extra letters in front of the word *sizzle* to emphasize the initial sound. Ask students to reread the line with this word slowly to emphasize the sound.

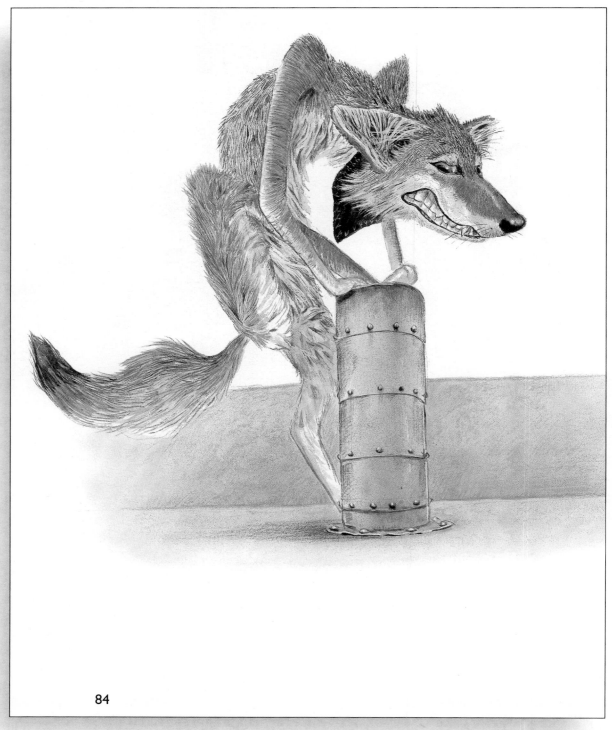

84

The tip of Coyote's raggedy tail whisked right past their noses. He was climbing upon the tin roof. Next, Coyote used his magic to make himself very skinny.

"The stove pipe!" gasped the third little javelina. Quickly she lighted a fire inside her wood stove.

"What a feast it will be!" Coyote said to himself. He squeezed into the stove pipe. "I think I'll eat them with red hot chile sauce!"

Whoosh. S-s-sizzle!

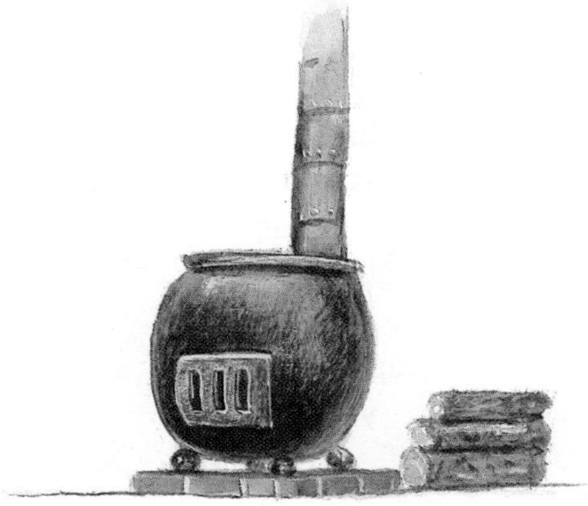

85

MINILESSON

Writer's Craft

Setting

Teach/Model

Ask students to describe where *The Three Little Javelinas* takes place. Spark discussion by asking:

- Where do the javelinas live?
- What is the weather like there?
- What grows there?
- What sounds are there?
- What does the place look like?

Remind students that the setting is where a story takes place. Explain that a rich setting can make a story vivid and interesting.

Practice/Apply

Work together with students to make a chart that compares the setting of *The Three Little Javelinas* with another story. Here is an example.

The Three Little Javelinas	*The Three Little Wolves and the Big Bad Pig*
Sights: javelinas; purple mountains; blue sky; cactus and palo verde trees; flowers; adobe	**Sights:** forest; houses of brick and concrete; gar-dens; trucks; various animals
Sounds: wind blowing dust; panting; howls; differ-ent languages	**Sounds:** animals talking and playing; construction work
Weather: hot; dry	**Weather:** pleasant

SKILL FINDER
Writing Activities: Same Plot, Different Setting, p. 88E
Reading–Writing Workshop, p. 117A

QuickREFERENCE

MEETING INDIVIDUAL NEEDS

Students Acquiring English

Word Meaning Demonstrate or ask a student to demonstrate a *gasp*. Then have students read aloud the sentence *"The stove pipe!" gasped the third little javelina* with appropriate expression.

Interact *with* Literature

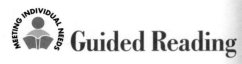

Guided Reading

Meeting Individual Needs

Comprehension/Critical Thinking

1. Why was the noise Coyote made so amazing? (The javelinas had never heard it before. It was a combination of different sounds.)
2. How did the author write down the noise Coyote made? (She broke it into little sounds, and then one long howl.)
3. Coyote was clever but in the end his tricks weren't good enough. How would you describe the third little javelina? (Accept reasonable responses.)
4. Do you think the desert made a good setting? Why or why not? (Students should cite details of the setting in their answers.)

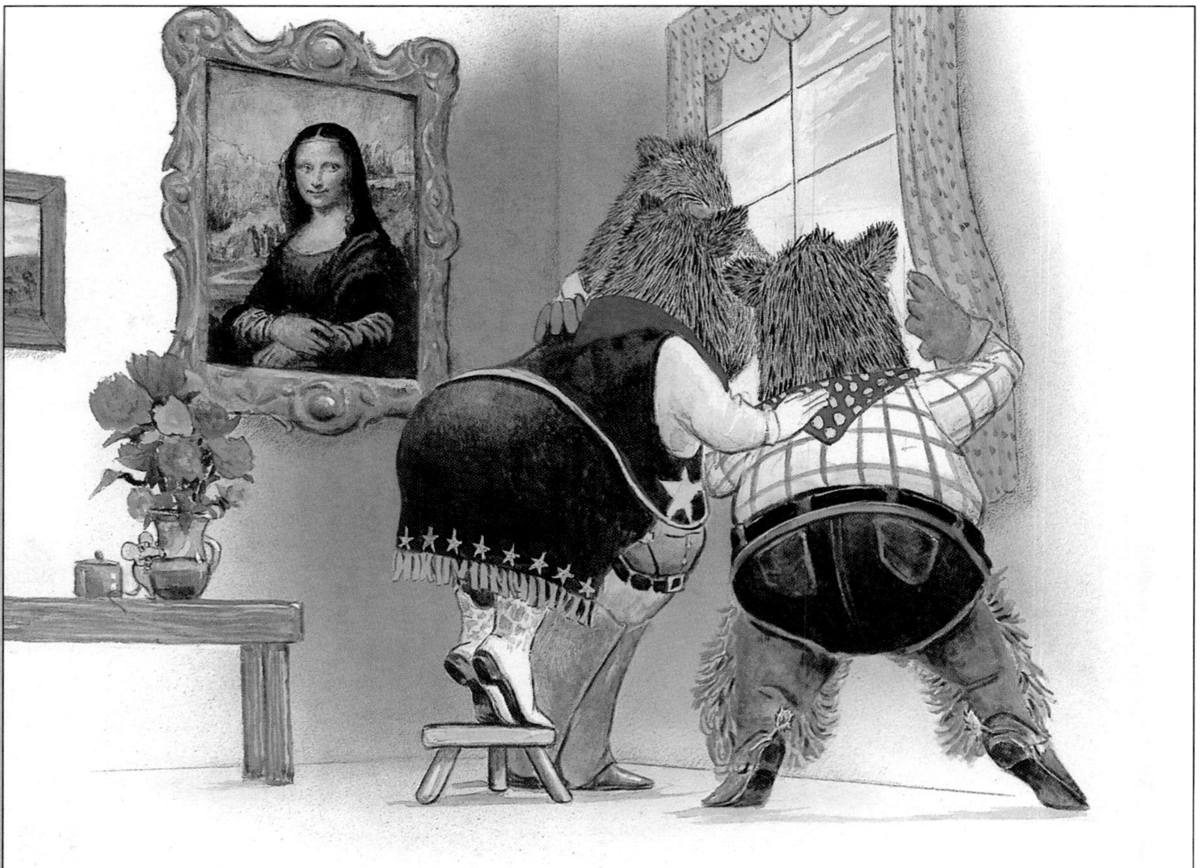

Then the three little javelinas heard an amazing noise. It was not a bark. It was not a cackle. It was not a howl. It was not a scream. It was all of those sounds together.

"Yip
yap
yeep
YEE-OWW-OOOOOOOOOOOOO!"

Away ran a puff of smoke shaped like a coyote.

86

Self-Assessment

Encourage students to assess their own reading by asking

- Did my predictions help me understand the story?
- Were any parts of the story confusing? What did I do to understand them?
- How did knowing the original story help me understand this one?

QuickREFERENCE

Visual Literacy

The *Mona Lisa* Point out that the painting on the wall is called the *Mona Lisa,* by Leonardo da Vinci. Ask students how it adds to the story's humor. (It's a serious work in the middle of a comical and often silly story.)

Students Acquiring English

Meeting Individual Needs

Vocabulary Discuss the words *bark, howl, cackle,* and *scream,* and have volunteers demonstrate how each sound differs. You may wish to make a list of these and other related sound words for students to add to their journals.

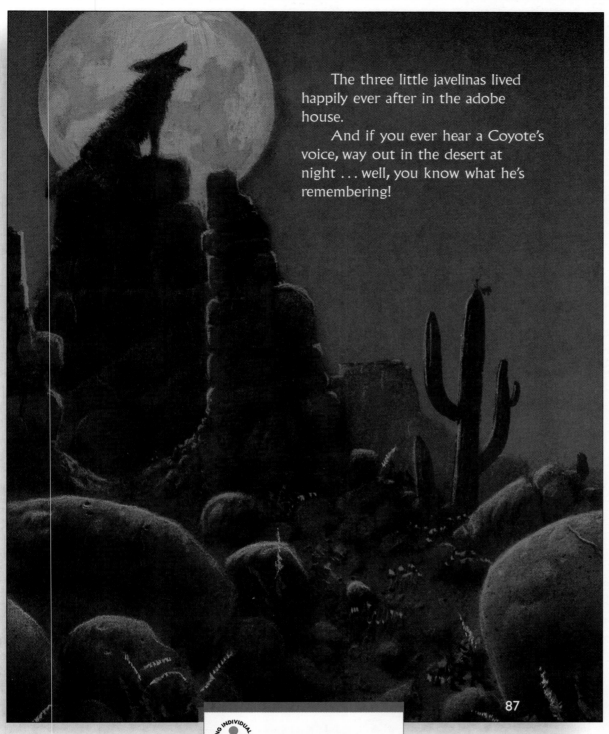

The three little javelinas lived happily ever after in the adobe house.

And if you ever hear a Coyote's voice, way out in the desert at night . . . well, you know what he's remembering!

87

Extra Support

Oral Rereading To improve comprehension and build fluency you may wish to have students reread parts or all of the story aloud. Pair students acquiring English with proficient English readers.

Science Link

Coyotes The coyote is famous for its evening serenade of howls and yelps. In fact, its scientific name, *Canis latrans*, means "barking dog."

Interact *with* Literature

Responding Activities

Personal Response

- What did students like or dislike about this story? Would they recommend it to a friend? Encourage them to write their thoughts in their journals.
- Allow students to choose their own ways of responding to the selection.

Anthology Activities

Choose, or have students choose, a response activity from page 88.

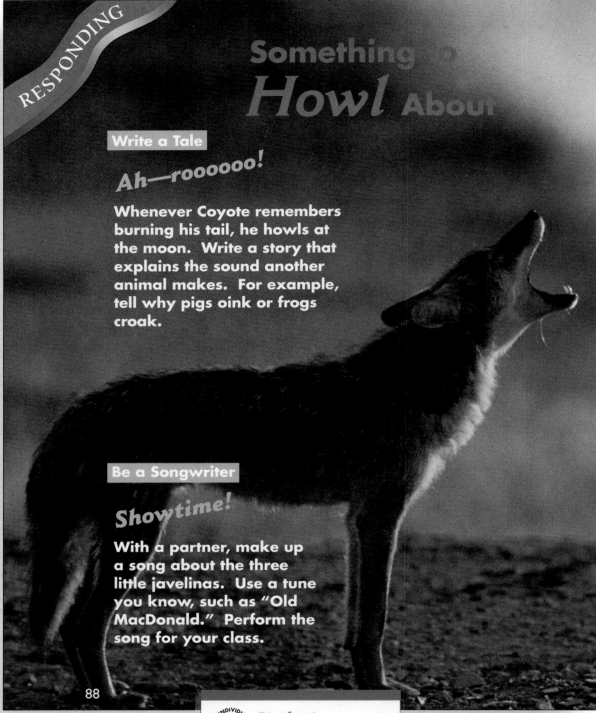

RESPONDING

Something to Howl About

Write a Tale

Ah—roooooo!

Whenever Coyote remembers burning his tail, he howls at the moon. Write a story that explains the sound another animal makes. For example, tell why pigs oink or frogs croak.

Be a Songwriter

Showtime!

With a partner, make up a song about the three little javelinas. Use a tune you know, such as "Old MacDonald." Perform the song for your class.

88

Informal Assessment

Check responses for a general understanding of the selection.

Additional Support:

- Use the Guided Reading questions to review and, if necessary, reread.
- Have students summarize the story or parts of it.
- Reread aloud the original tale on pages 35A–35B and have students compare the selection to it.

QuickREFERENCE

Students Acquiring English

MEETING INDIVIDUAL NEEDS

For the "Create a Refrain" activity on page 88A, encourage students who are acquiring English to create rhymes in their primary language. They can then teach the refrain to the class in their primary language and explain its meaning.

Home Connection

Encourage students to retell the story to their families. Suggest that they think of other stories that involve threes (*Goldilocks and the Three Bears, Three Little Kittens,* and so on).

More Choices for Responding

Conduct an Interview

Cooperative Learning

Have students take the roles of the javelinas, Coyote, and interviewers. Students should probe into the characters' backgrounds, finding out as much as they can about each and taking notes.

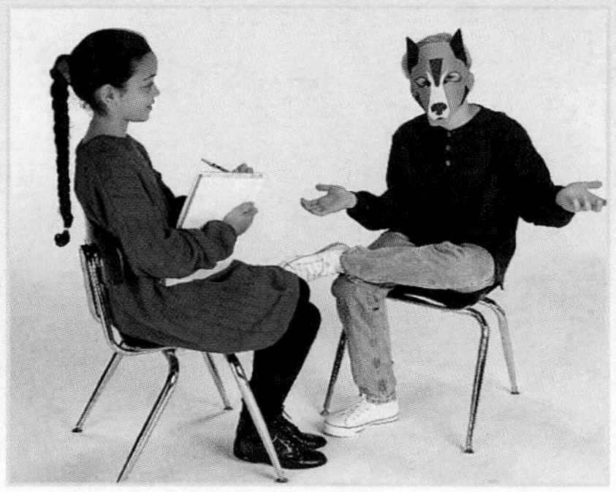

Draw the Coyote in Action

What other kinds of tricks might Coyote have played? Have students draw new possibilities for catching the javelinas.

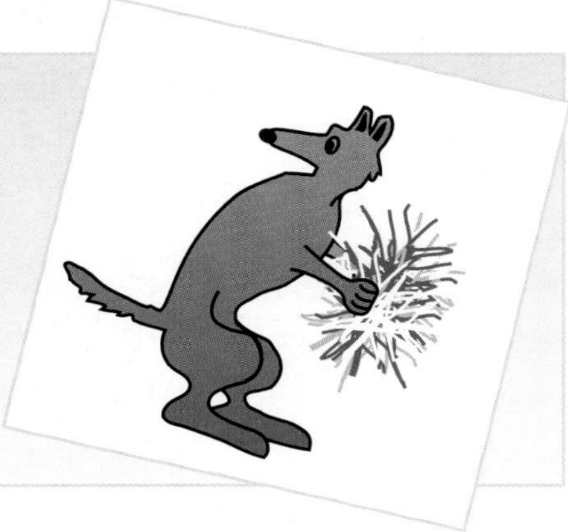

The Tumbleweed Surprise Trick

Create a Refrain

Students may like to think of a new response to Coyote's "*Little pig, little pig, let me come in?*" refrain.

Encourage them to create a refrain that rhymes, as in the original.

Selection Connections

LAB, p. 8

Have students complete the portion of the chart relating to *The Three Little Javelinas.*

Literature Discussion

- Which retelling of "The Three Little Pigs" did you prefer, this one or *The Three Little Wolves and the Big Bad Pig?* Why?
- Would trying to get Coyote to change his mind have worked, or were the javelinas wise to just keep running?
- How was Coyote like the big bad pig? How was he different?

Comprehension Check

Use the following questions and/or *Literacy Activity Book* page 21 to check understanding of the story.

1. What are two ways in which Coyote tried to use his magical powers to catch the javelinas? (He made his voice sound like a javelina's to try to get in the rib house and he made himself skinny enough to fit down the stove pipe.)
2. According to this story, what is a coyote remembering when you hear him howling at night? (He's remembering how he was scorched by the javelinas.)

Literacy Activity Book, p. 21

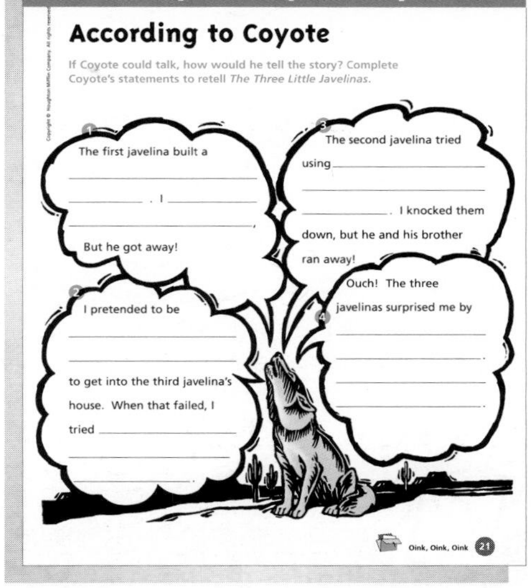

According to Coyote

If Coyote could talk, how would he tell the story? Complete Coyote's statements to retell *The Three Little Javelinas.*

The first javelina built a ______ . I ______ But he got away!

The second javelina tried using ______ . I knocked them down, but he and his brother ran away!

I pretended to be ______ to get into the third javelina's house. When that failed, I tried ______

Ouch! The three javelinas surprised me by ______

Oink, Oink, Oink 21

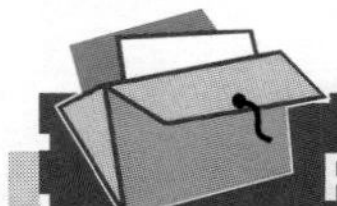

Portfolio Opportunity

- Selection comprehension: Save *Literacy Activity Book* page 21.
- Writing samples: Save responses to other responding activities.

Comprehension

Literacy Activity Book, p. 22

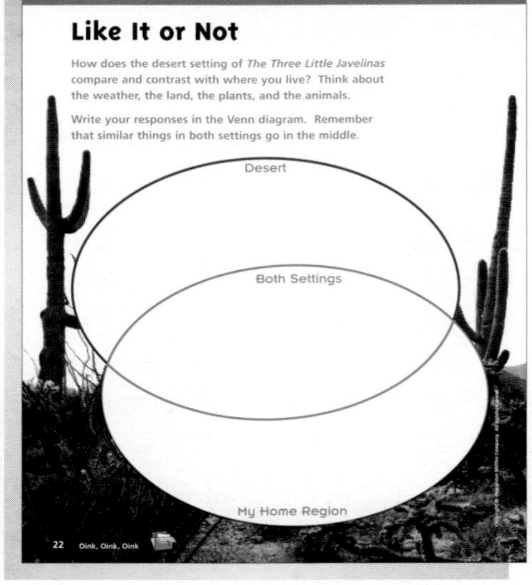

Like It or Not

How does the desert setting of *The Three Little Javelinas* compare and contrast with where you live? Think about the weather, the land, the plants, and the animals.

Write your responses in the Venn diagram. Remember that similar things in both settings go in the middle.

Desert

Both Settings

My Home Region

22 Oink, Oink, Oink

Informal Assessment

During Practice/Apply, circulate to check whether students are making accurate comparisons.

Additional Support:

Reteaching, p. 88C

Minilessons, pp. 75; 103; Theme 4, p. 47

INTERACTIVE LEARNING

TESTED SKILL

Compare and Contrast

LAB, p. 22

Teach/Model

Discuss with students how appreciating a good story often involves comparing it to other stories. Tell students that good readers often compare and contrast story details. They stop and ask themselves questions like:

- Does this character remind me of a character from another story I've read? Are the story events similar?
- How is this story different from other stories I've read? What do I think of these differences?

Read aloud the original version of "The Three Little Pigs" on pages 35A–35B. Then have students compare and contrast it with *The Three Little Javelinas.* Use these prompts. Chart students' responses.

- Which stories have animal characters? human characters?
- What building materials are used in each story?
- What happens to the villain in each story?
- In which stories does the wolf huff and puff and the pigs say *"not by the hair of my chinny-chin-chin"*?

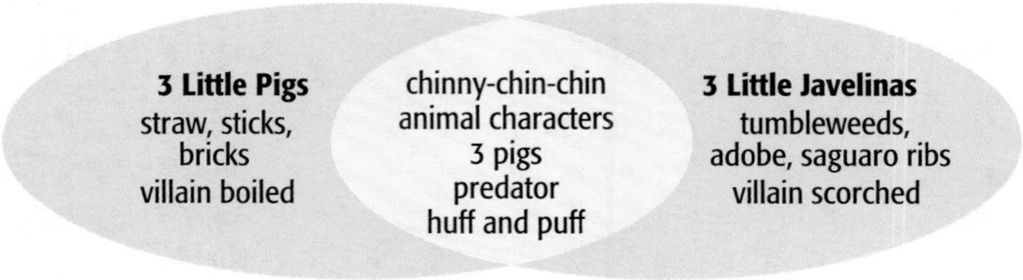
3 Little Pigs
straw, sticks, bricks
villain boiled
chinny-chin-chin
animal characters
3 pigs
predator
huff and puff
3 Little Javelinas
tumbleweeds, adobe, saguaro ribs
villain scorched

Practice/Apply

- Have students use *Literacy Activity Book* page 22 to compare and contrast the desert setting of *The Three Little Javelinas* with the setting (region) in which they live.
- Have small groups use a Venn diagram to compare and contrast the illustrations in *The Three Little Wolves and the Big Bad Pig* and *The Three Little Javelinas.* Students might analyze the colors used and what makes each style of illustration funny.

SKILL FINDER

Minilessons, pp. 75; 103; Theme 4, p. 47

Reteaching

Compare and Contrast

Cooperative Learning Divide students into small groups. Assign one of the following animals to each group: pigs, javelinas, coyotes, and wolves. Have students work together to describe different features of the animals. Students should use illustrations and photos from the stories and articles such as "This Little Piggy!" as guidance.

Encourage them to ask themselves questions like the following:

- hair: is it furry? rough? short? long?
- eyes: are they large? narrow?
- body size: is the animal large or small? fast or slow?
- ears: are they pointy or flat? how big are they?

Afterward display Transparency 1–6. Have the groups make comparisons and then fill in the chart. For example:

	Javelinas	Pigs	Wolves	Coyotes
pointy ears			+	+
curly tails	+	+		
big snouts	+	+		

Additionally, you might invite students to make animal riddle cards. Tell them to take one feature of the animal they chose, and think of another animal that has the same feature. They should then write the riddle on the face of the card and answer it inside.

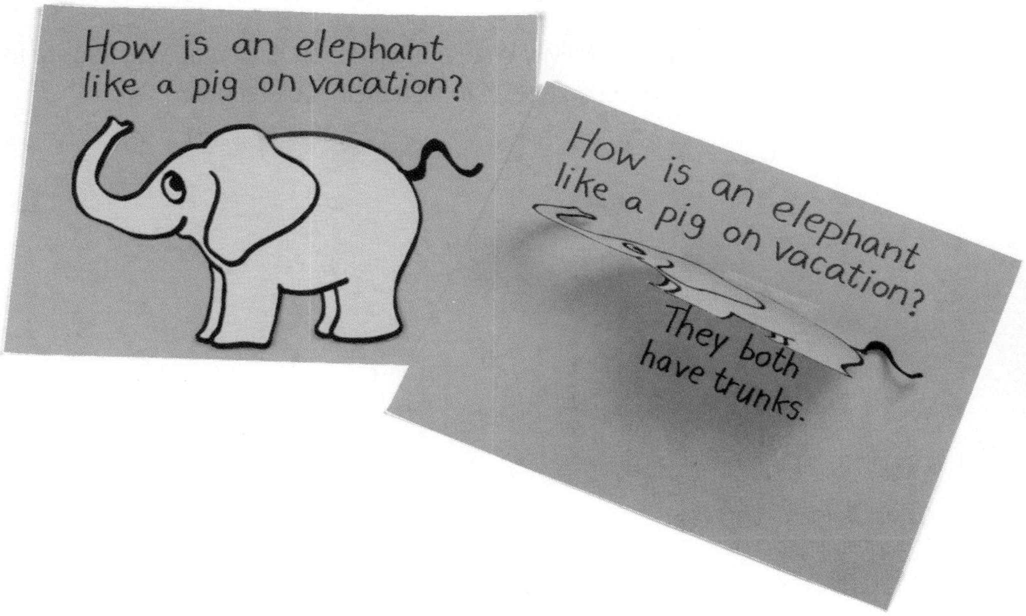
How is an elephant like a pig on vacation?
How is an elephant like a pig on vacation?
They both have trunks.

Transparency 1–6

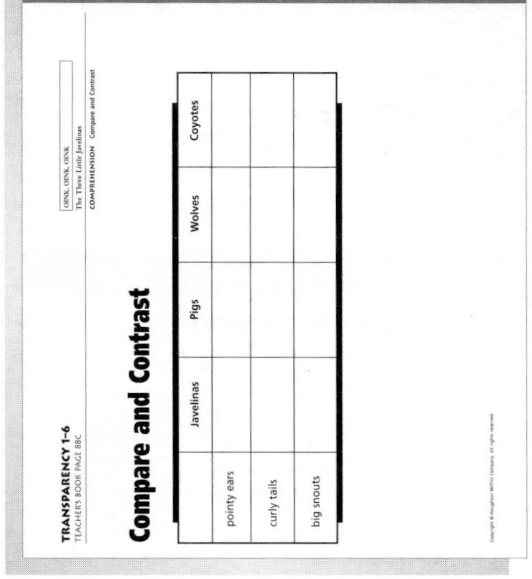

TRANSPARENCY 1-6

Compare and Contrast

	Javelinas	Pigs	Wolves	Coyotes
pointy ears				
curly tails				
big snouts				

Portfolio Opportunity

Save *Literacy Activity Book* page 22 to record students' understanding of comparison and contrast.

Instruct *and* Integrate

Writing Skills and Activities

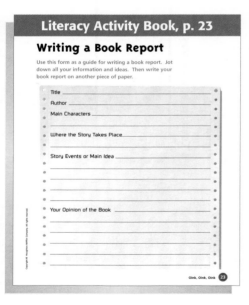

INTERACTIVE LEARNING

Writing a Book Report

LAB, p. 23

Teach/Model Hold up a storybook that is a favorite of yours and identify it as such. Tell students that one way to share your thoughts about a book is to write a book report. Explain that a book report tells what the book is about and also gives your opinion of the book.

Display Transparency 1–7 and read the model book report aloud as students follow along. Then ask the following questions:

- What does this student tell about the story?
- What is this student's opinion of *The Three Little Javelinas?*

Discuss with students these guidelines for writing a good book report.

Guidelines for Writing a Book Report

- Tell the title of the book and the author's name.
- Tell a little about the main characters and where the story takes place.
- Tell about important events or the story's main idea. Don't give away the ending.
- Give your opinion of the book.

Practice/Apply Assign the activity Write a Book Report. Encourage students to use *Literacy Activity Book* page 23 to plan their book reports.

Transparency 1–7

Book Report

OINK, OINK, OINK
The Three Little Javelinas
WRITING SKILLS Writing a Book Report

The Three Little Javelinas

The Three Little Javelinas was written by Susan Lowell. This book is a lot like the story of the three little pigs, only it takes place in the desert. Javelinas are animals that are like pigs. These three little javelinas are chased by a coyote. The coyote wants to eat them, so he keeps blowing down their houses. Does he get them? You'll have to read the book to find out.

There are some funny parts in this book, and they will make you laugh. The art is funny, too. I really like this book.

TRANSPARENCY 1–7
TEACHER'S BOOK PAGE 88D

Literacy Activity Book, p. 23

Writing a Book Report

Use this form as a guide for writing a book report. Jot down all your information and ideas. Then write your book report on another piece of paper.

Title ____________________

Author ____________________

Main Characters ____________________

Where the Story Takes Place ____________________

Story Events or Main Idea ____________________

Your Opinion of the Book ____________________

Oink, Oink, Oink 23

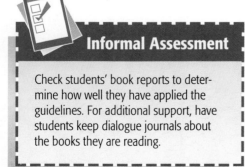

Informal Assessment

Check students' book reports to determine how well they have applied the guidelines. For additional support, have students keep dialogue journals about the books they are reading.

Writing Activities

Create a Cartoon

Suggest that students write and draw cartoons telling the story of *The Three Little Javelinas.* Students might tell the whole story individually or work in small groups to divide up scenes and cartoon frames.

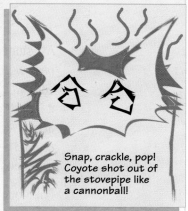

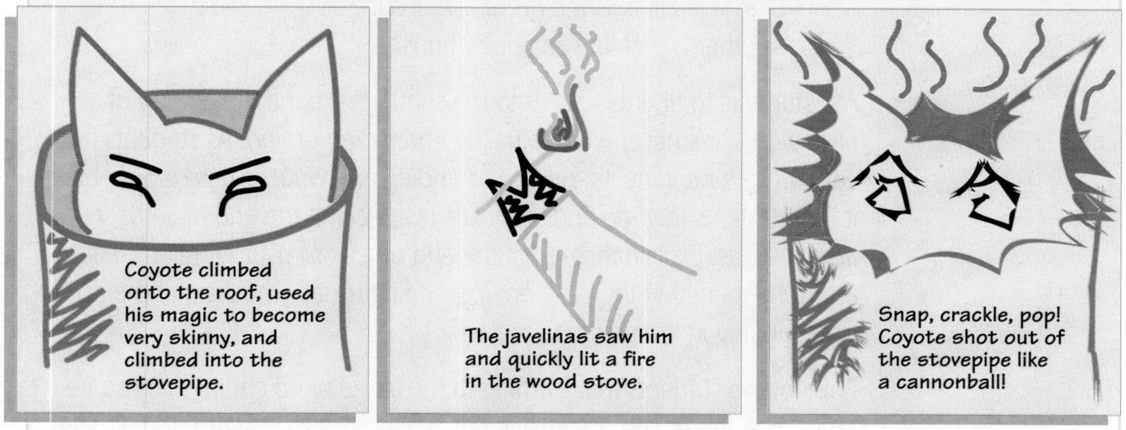
Coyote climbed onto the roof, used his magic to become very skinny, and climbed into the stovepipe.
The javelinas saw him and quickly lit a fire in the wood stove.
Snap, crackle, pop! Coyote shot out of the stovepipe like a cannonball!

Write a Book Report

Have students write a book report about a book they have read recently. Collect their book reports in a loose-leaf notebook and keep it in an accessible place in the classroom. Encourage students to look in the notebook for ideas for books to read and to add book reports whenever they want to share their opinions about books they have read.

Shared Writing: Same Plot, Different Setting

Work with students to write the three little pigs story in another story setting. Remind them that the story characters, building materials, and other story elements might have to change to fit the new setting. A polar cap setting might involve three little penguins and a big bad bear, for example. You might want to try several ideas and brainstorm for each before choosing one and beginning to write. (*See the Writer's Craft Minilesson on page 85.*)

Students can use The Learning Company's new elementary writing center for all their writing activities.

Portfolio Opportunity

Save responses to activities on this page for writing samples.

Instruct *and* Integrate

Word Skills and Strategies

Literacy Activity Book, p. 24

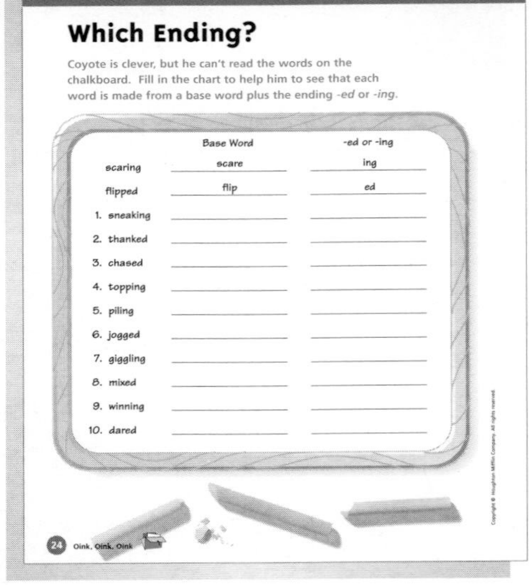
Which Ending?

Coyote is clever, but he can't read the words on the chalkboard. Fill in the chart to help him to see that each word is made from a base word plus the ending *-ed* or *-ing*.

	Base Word	*-ed* or *-ing*
scaring	scare	ing
flipped	flip	ed
1. sneaking		
2. thanked		
3. chased		
4. topping		
5. piling		
6. jogged		
7. giggling		
8. mixed		
9. winning		
10. dared		

24 Oink, Oink, Oink

MEETING INDIVIDUAL NEEDS

Extra Support

Be sure students understand that not every word that ends with the letters *ed* or *ing* is made up of a base word and ending. Use the words *red, tumbleweed,* and *nothing* as examples.

Informal Assessment

Use Practice/Apply to check students' understanding of the endings *-ed* and *-ing*.

Additional Support:

Reteaching, p. 88G

INTERACTIVE LEARNING

TESTED SKILL

Structural Analysis
Inflected Endings *-ed* and *-ing*

LAB, p. 24

Teach/Model Write these sentences on the board.

> One javelina finished his house of sticks.
> Another is building an adobe house.

Ask students to find the words in the sentences that are made up of a base word, or smaller word, plus the ending *-ed* or *-ing*. As students find each word, underline its *-ed* or *-ing* ending and write its base word above it. Tell students that *-ed* and *-ing* usually appear at the end of verbs, or action words. Explain that *-ed* at the end of a word usually means that the action happened in the past. An *-ing* ending usually means that the action is happening in the present.

Point out to students that learning to recognize word endings can sometimes help them read unfamiliar words. Once they recognize the ending, they may discover that they know the base word as well.

Practice/Apply ***Cooperative Learning*** Divide the class into small groups. For each group, divide a sheet of paper into two columns. Label one column *-ed* and the other *-ing*. Have the students in each group search through the story to find words with *-ed* or *-ing* endings and list them in the columns. When they have listed all the words they can, have them identify each base word.

-ed	-ing
trotted	whirling
looked	brushing
divided	eating
wandered	looking
laughed	gathering
smelled	building
tired	panting
called	showing
shouted	tumbling

SKILL FINDER Spelling, Theme 5

Reteaching

Inflected Endings *-ed* and *-ing*

MEETING INDIVIDUAL NEEDS

Write the words *walked, dropped, running,* and *taking* on the board. Remind students that many words are made up of a smaller word and the ending *-ed* or *-ing*. Have volunteers break apart the words on the board by writing each base word and ending.

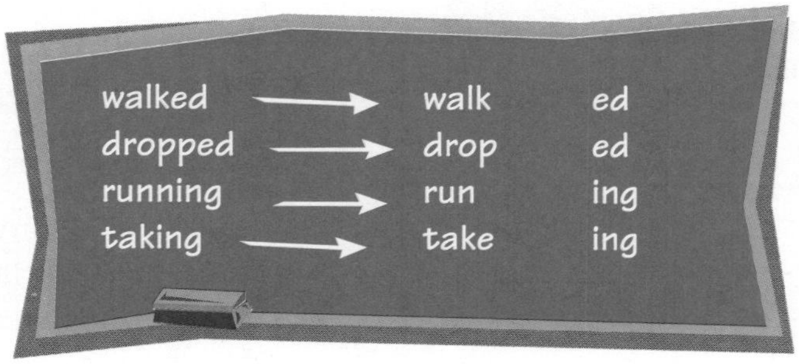
walked → walk ed
dropped → drop ed
running → run ing
taking → take ing

Then have students look in a favorite storybook for more examples.

MINILESSON

Phonics Review
Long Vowel Pairs and Vowel-Consonant-*e*

Teach/Model Write these nonsense words on the board. Tell students that the words don't mean anything but to try pronouncing them anyway.

tweel   jeam   chay   blail   prew   bife

Remind students that they can often make good guesses about the pronunciation of a new word by looking for familiar groups of letters. Discuss the letters students based their guesses on. *(ee* and *ea* often have the long *e* sound; *ay* and *ai* often have the long *a* sound; *ew* often has the long *u* sound; any vowel followed by a single consonant and *e* usually has the long vowel sound.) Circle each pair of vowels and *ife* in *bife.* Point out that by knowing vowel patterns, they can pronounce unfamiliar words or even nonsense words!

Practice/Apply ***Cooperative Learning*** Divide the class into small groups. Have each group try to be the first to find three words in *The Three Little Javelinas* that follow each vowel pattern on the board.

Possible responses:

ee	*ea*	*ay*	*ai*	vowel-consonant-*e*		
three	each	way	fail	came	divided	fire
seek	heap	day	trail	escaped	inside	like
steep	eating	lay	tail	shade	tired	coyote
tumbleweeds	sneaky			make/made	mice	adobe
sweetly	heat			snake	miles	stove
teeth	please			place	ripe	noses
trees	weak			bake	arrived	smoke
green	feast			shaped	smiled	used
peeked	scream			these	sometimes	
squeezed				time	pipe	

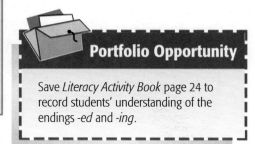

Portfolio Opportunity

Save *Literacy Activity Book* page 24 to record students' understanding of the endings *-ed* and *-ing*.

Building Vocabulary

Literacy Activity Book, p. 25

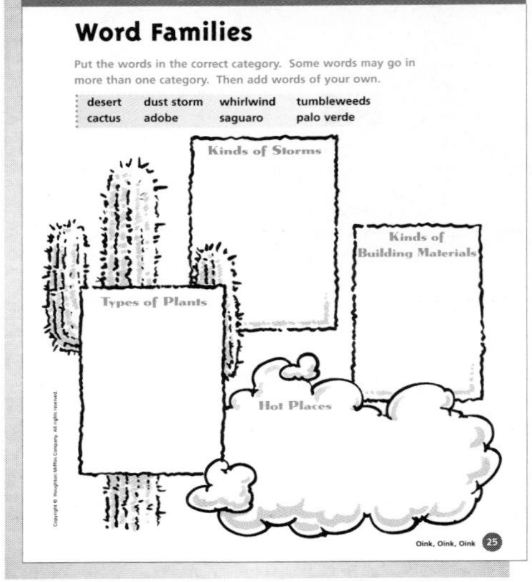
Word Families

Put the words in the correct category. Some words may go in more than one category. Then add words of your own.

desert	dust storm	whirlwind	tumbleweeds
cactus	adobe	saguaro	palo verde

Kinds of Storms
Kinds of Building Materials
Types of Plants
Hot Places
Oink, Oink, Oink 25

Use this page to review Selection Vocabulary.

tornado
plaza
siesta
fiesta
burro
hammock
chocolate
alligator
tomato
patio
cargo
poncho
cocoa
vanilla
pueblo

iguana
saguaro
mesa
stampede
chile
lariat
bronco
barbecue
jaguar
mosquito
avocado
coyote
cafeteria
pimento
adobe

Vocabulary Activities

Rhyming Words

Cooperative Learning

Ask students what rhyming words the coyote used each time he came to the house of a little javelina. (*huff and puff*) Point out to students that words rhyme when they begin with different sounds but end with the same sound. Have the class brainstorm for other words that rhyme with huff and puff, and write the words on the board. (*stuff, muff, cuff, fluff, gruff, bluff, scuff, rough, enough, tough*)

Divide students into small teams. Tell them that when you say "Go," they will have one minute to list words that rhyme with *trick*. When the time is up, have the team with the most words read their list. Write the words on the board, and ask the other teams to mention words on their own list that the winning team did not include. Repeat the game two more times, having students rhyme with *snake* and then *heat*.

Words from Spanish

Tell students that many Spanish words have become part of the English language. Then tell them that they will each create one page of a Words from Spanish pictionary.

Write each word on the list to the left on a slip of paper and put the slips in a bag. Have students pick a word, write it on a sheet of paper, and draw a picture to show what it means. Help students use a dictionary or encyclopedia if they are not sure what the word means or how to illustrate it. Have them show and explain their drawings to the class. Then bind the drawings into a book to display in the classroom.

Selection Vocabulary Extension

Display again Transparency 1–5 and review the Selection Vocabulary Words, *desert, dust storm, whirlwind, tumbleweeds, cactus,* and *adobe.*

Encourage students to add other desert-related words to the list. To think of words have them look at the transparency, revisit *The Three Little Javelinas,* and use their own knowledge of deserts.

partial word list:

saguaro, coyote, javelina, hawk, lizard, scorpion, sand, oasis, mesa, butte, dunes, mirage

Spelling

MINILESSON

Spelling Words

*nose
*these
*shade
*use
*mice
*smoke
*snake
*ripe

Challenge Words

*escape
*amaze
*arrive
*fortune

*Starred words or forms of the words appear in *The Three Little Javelinas*.

TESTED SKILL

Vowel-Consonant-*e*

LAB, pp. 26–27

- Write the words *rip* and *ripe* on the board. Say the words, and have students repeat them. Have a volunteer name the vowel sound in *rip*. (/ĭ/)
- Ask students if the vowel sounds in *rip* and *ripe* are the same or different. (different) Explain that the word *ripe* has the /ī/ sound because it ends in the vowel-consonant-*e* pattern. Underline the letters *ipe*.
- Introduce the /ā/, /ē/, /ō/, and /yōō/ sounds, using the words *shade, these, nose,* and *use*. Point out that the vowel sound in the *u*-consonant-*e* pattern can be pronounced /ōō/, or /yōō/, as in *use*.
- Write the Spelling Words on the board. Tell students that each Spelling Word has the vowel-consonant-*e* pattern. Say the Spelling Words and have students repeat them.

Spelling Assessment

Pretest

Say each underlined word, read the sentence, and then repeat the word. Have students write only the underlined words.

1. A pig's nose is called a snout.
2. Where do these animals live?
3. It's hard to find shade in the desert.
4. They will use bricks to build a house.
5. The wolf was tired of eating mice.
6. The fire sent smoke up the chimney.
7. The snake slid along the sand.
8. Those berries look ripe to me.

Test

Spelling Words Use the Pretest sentences.

Challenge Words

9. This story will really amaze you!
10. We must find a way to escape from the wolf.
11. The sailor went to seek his fortune.
12. Plan to arrive at my house by six.

SKILL FINDER

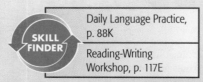

Daily Language Practice, p. 88K
Reading-Writing Workshop, p. 117E

Literacy Activity Book, p. 26

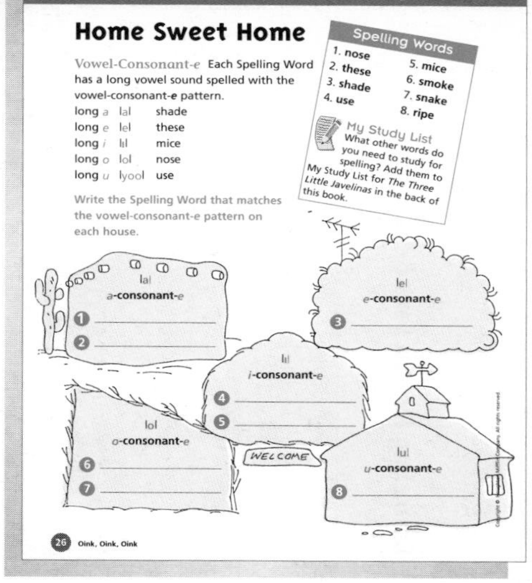
Home Sweet Home

Spelling Words: 1. nose 2. these 3. shade 4. use 5. mice 6. smoke 7. snake 8. ripe

Vowel-Consonant-*e* Each Spelling Word has a long vowel sound spelled with the vowel-consonant-*e* pattern.

long *a* /ā/ shade
long *e* /ē/ these
long *i* /ī/ mice
long *o* /ō/ nose
long *u* /yōō/ use

My Study List What other words do you need to study for spelling? Add them to My Study List for The Three Little Javelinas in the back of this book.

Write the Spelling Word that matches the vowel-consonant-e pattern on each house.

/ā/ *a*-consonant-*e* 1 2
/ē/ *e*-consonant-*e* 3
/ī/ *i*-consonant-*e* 4 5
/ō/ *o*-consonant-*e* 6 7
/ū/ *u*-consonant-*e* 8

26 Oink, Oink, Oink

Literacy Activity Book, p. 27

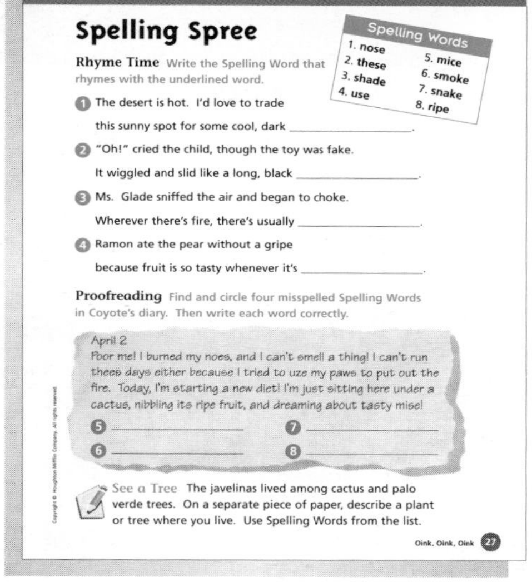
Spelling Spree

Spelling Words: 1. nose 2. these 3. shade 4. use 5. mice 6. smoke 7. snake 8. ripe

Rhyme Time Write the Spelling Word that rhymes with the underlined word.

1. The desert is hot. I'd love to trade this sunny spot for some cool, dark ______.
2. "Oh!" cried the child, though the toy was fake. It wiggled and slid like a long, black ______.
3. Ms. Glade sniffed the air and began to choke. Wherever there's fire, there's usually ______.
4. Ramon ate the pear without a gripe because fruit is so tasty whenever it's ______.

Proofreading Find and circle four misspelled Spelling Words in Coyote's diary. Then write each word correctly.

April 2
Poor me! I burned my noes, and I can't smell a thing! I can't run thees days either because I tried to uze my paws to put out the fire. Today, I'm starting a new diet! I'm just sitting here under a cactus, nibbling its ripe fruit, and dreaming about tasty mise!

5 ______ 6 ______ 7 ______ 8 ______

See a Tree The javelinas lived among cactus and palo verde trees. On a separate piece of paper, describe a plant or tree where you live. Use Spelling Words from the list.

Oink, Oink, Oink 27

MEETING INDIVIDUAL NEEDS

Challenge

Challenge Words Practice Have students use the Challenge Words to write newspaper headlines.

Grammar

Transparency 1–8

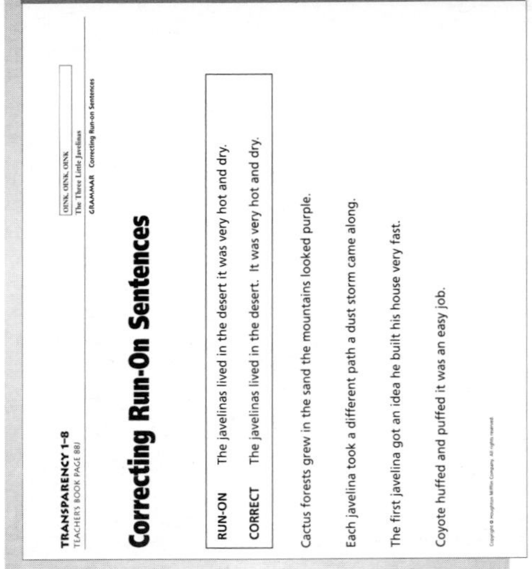
TRANSPARENCY 1–8
TEACHER'S BOOK PAGE 88J
Correcting Run-On Sentences
RUN-ON The javelinas lived in the desert it was very hot and dry.
CORRECT The javelinas lived in the desert. It was very hot and dry.
Cactus forests grew in the sand the mountains looked purple.
Each javelina took a different path a dust storm came along.
The first javelina got an idea he built his house very fast.
Coyote huffed and puffed it was an easy job.

Literacy Activity Book, p. 29

Literacy Activity Book, p. 28

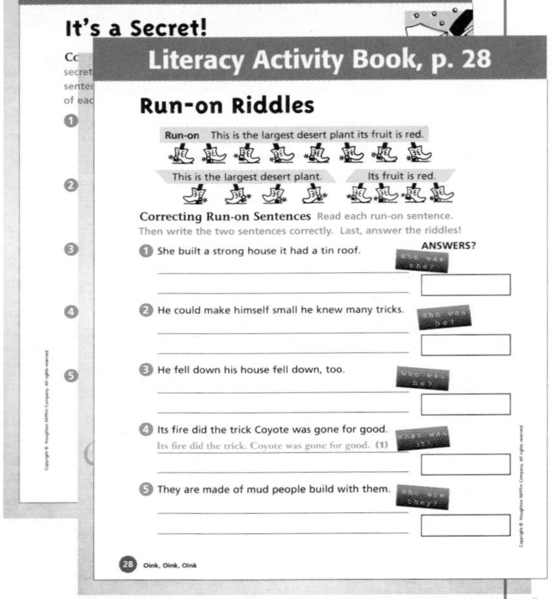
It's a Secret!
Run-on Riddles
Run-on This is the largest desert plant its fruit is red.
This is the largest desert plant.
Its fruit is red.
Correcting Run-on Sentences Read each run-on sentence. Then write the two sentences correctly. Last, answer the riddles!
ANSWERS?
1 She built a strong house it had a tin roof.
2 He could make himself small he knew many tricks.
3 He fell down his house fell down, too.
4 Its fire did the trick Coyote was gone for good.
Its fire did the trick. Coyote was gone for good. (1)
5 They are made of mud people build with them.
28 Oink, Oink, Oink

Informal Assessment

Responses to the activities should indicate students' ability to recognize and correct run-on sentences.

Additional Support:

Use Reteaching, p. 88K.

INTERACTIVE LEARNING

TESTED SKILL

Correcting Run-on Sentences

LAB, pp. 28–29

Two or more sentences that run together form a **run-on sentence.** Correct run-on sentences by adding end marks and capital letters.

Teach/Model

Invite volunteers to make up two or three sentences about the story. Write students' sentences on the chalkboard as a run-on sentence. Read the run-on sentence rapidly without any pauses or vocal inflections to indicate the end of any sentence other than the run-on one.

Elicit from students that run-on sentences are confusing because they lack the signals that tell where one sentence ends and another begins—end marks and capital letters.

Ask volunteers to draw lines separating the run-on sentence into individual sentences. Ask other volunteers to add periods and capital letters.

Display Transparency 1–8. Point out that two or more sentences that run together make a *run-on sentence.* Ask the class to help you rewrite these run-on sentences. Have students read each run-on sentence aloud with you. Then call on volunteers to draw a line between the complete thoughts. If the class agrees, invite other volunteers to add capital letters and end marks. Point out that this is what they should do when they proofread their work.

Practice/Apply

Cooperative Learning: **Correcting a Letter** Duplicate the following letter, and distribute copies to small groups of students. Explain that the javelina did not understand about run-on sentences. Have each group work together to correct the letter. Then have each student create a decorated sheet of stationery and write the corrected letter on it.

Dear Friend,

I now live with my brother and sister in an adobe brick house the coyote tried to trick us and eat us he was burned by the fire in the stove we played in the desert every day I hope you come to visit me soon you will be safe because the coyote is gone.

Sincerely,
A. Javelina

SKILL FINDER

Reading-Writing Workshop, p. 117E

INTERACTIVE LEARNING *(continued)*

Practice/Apply

Writing Application: A Place Ask students to imagine that the javelinas could change their voices or appearance the way Coyote did. What trick would they play to scare him away? Suggest that students write a plan describing what the javelinas could do. Remind them to avoid run-on sentences.

Students' Writing Encourage students to check their works in progress for run-on sentences. Point out that one way to proofread for this kind of error is to read their sentences aloud, listening for the beginning and the end of each complete thought.

Reteaching

Correcting Run-on Sentences

MEETING INDIVIDUAL NEEDS

Write the run-on sentences below on sentence strips. Display the first sentence strip, and have students read it aloud with you. Discuss with students what is wrong with it, and review the term *run-on sentence*. Then have students tell where the sentence should be cut apart and where the end mark and capital letter are needed. Invite different volunteers to cut apart the sentence strip and to write the correct end mark and capital letter. Repeat for the other run-on sentences. Post the cut-apart sentences.

cut apart here — capital letter here

People helped the javelinas | they gave sticks and bricks.

end mark needed here

The sticks came from a cactus the bricks baked in the sun.

The stick house fell quickly it was not strong enough.

Coyote found the brick house he huffed and puffed as usual.

Adobe bricks are strong the little javelinas were safe.

Daily Language Practice

Focus skills

Grammar: Correcting Run-on Sentences

Spelling: Vowel-Consonant-*e*

Every day write one run-on sentence on the chalkboard. Have each student write the sentence correctly on a sheet of paper. Tell students to separate the sentences in the run-on sentence by adding an end mark and a capital letter. Tell students also to correct any misspelled words. Have students correct their own papers as a volunteer corrects the sentence on the chalkboard.

1. The sand is hot there is almost no shaade.
   The sand is hot**. T**here is almost no **shade.**
2. A snake crossed our path mise also live here.
   A snake crossed our path**. Mice** also live here.
3. People build cool houses they uze mud bricks.
   People build cool houses**. T**hey **use** mud bricks.
4. The cactus has rype fruit people get it down with sticks.
   The cactus has **ripe** fruit**. P**eople get it down with sticks.
5. The dust storm looks like smok you must cover your nose.
   The dust storm looks like **smoke. Y**ou must cover your nose.

Communication Activities

Audio Tape
for Oink, Oink, Oink: *The Three Little Javelinas*

August

The desert sun of August
Is shimmering my street
And turning houses into dunes
That glitter in the heat.
One tree is my oasis.
I need the ice cream man!
His truck comes just as slowly
As a camel caravan.

by Sandra Liatsos

Listening and Speaking

Listening to a Poetic Picture

Read aloud "August" for students' listening pleasure. Invite them to share their reactions. Then tell students the first listening guideline, and read the poem again. Ask students to focus on that point. Encourage them to discuss the word picture drawn by the poet. Use this same method with the other guidelines.

Invite each student to bring a poem to class to share. They can then pair up with a listening partner or in small groups, read the poem aloud, practice their listening skills, and discuss how the guidelines apply to their poem.

Guidelines for Listening to Poetry

Listen for feelings that the poet expresses. What words does he or she use to describe them?

Think about how the poet's experiences are like yours. Have you ever felt the same way?

Listen for something ordinary that the poet describes in a new and fresh way.

Listen for when the poet uses the word *like* or *as* to make a comparison. What is being compared?

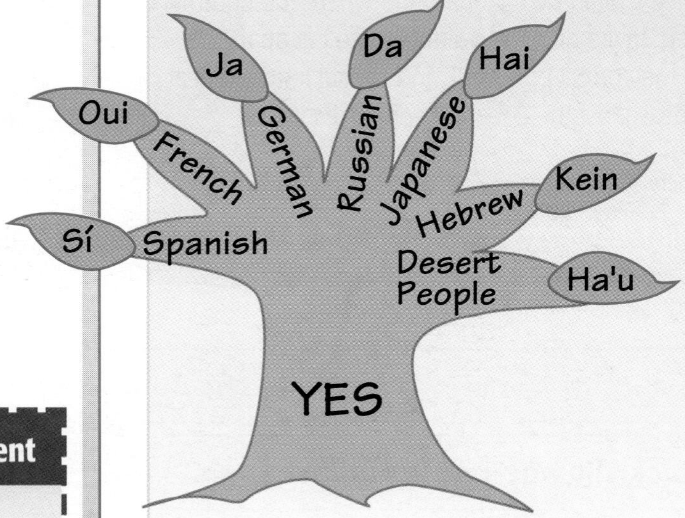
Ja
Da
Hai
Oui
French
German
Russian
Japanese
Kein
Hebrew
Sí
Spanish
Desert People
Ha'u
YES

Building a Language Tree

Multicultural Link Students tap into their own diverse backgrounds by creating a language tree. First, have them recall the people in the desert who said *yes* to the javelinas. Then volunteers draw a tree on poster board and label two branches "Spanish" and "Desert People." They write *sí* and *ha'u* on leaves off these branches. Invite them to share how to say *yes* in other languages and to add these words and languages to the tree.

Informal Assessment

Circulate among the listening groups, and encourage students to use the "Guidelines for Listening to Poetry" as the basis of their discussions.

Listening and Speaking continued

Hearing a Range of Sounds

Resources
Listen to the Desert
by Pat Mora

Challenge students to focus on desert sounds. First, they can rehearse and present a choral reading of Pat Mora's book *Listen to the Desert.* Then they can work in small groups to recreate a desert sound, such as an animal sound, desert rain, thunder, or wind. Each group presents its sound alone and then together with other groups as you orchestrate.

Viewing

Watching a Video of Desert Life

VIDEO *Along Sandy Trails*
by Ann Nolan Clark

There are many fine videos about the desert. Ask your school librarian or media specialist for a suggestion, or consider showing *Along Sandy Trails,* by Ann Nolan Clark, which depicts desert life as it is experienced by a young Tohono O'Odham (Papago) girl on a walk with her grandmother. Before watching the video, use a K-W-L chart to brainstorm questions.

DESERTS		
What do you KNOW?	What do you WANT to find out?	What did you LEARN?

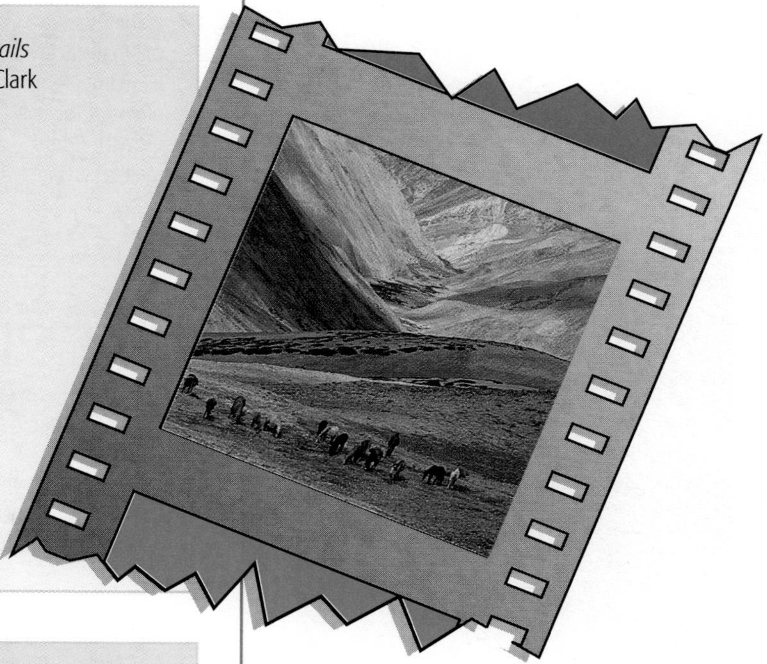

Taking a Walking Tour

Lead students on a walking tour of the buildings in your community. Have students use a chart to group the buildings into general types, such as wood houses, brick apartment buildings, etc.

Portfolio Opportunity

Save the language tree from Building a Language Tree in a class portfolio.

Cross-Curricular Activities

Book List

Science

Cactus Hotel
by Brenda Z. Guiberson

Choices for Science

Making a Desert Terrarium

Students may enjoy building their own desert terrarium.

Materials

- glass or plastic container
- pebbles
- watering can
- water
- sponge or paper towels
- cactus soil—available in garden centers or hardware stores
- sand
- cacti
- rocks or other props
- mesh cover—available at pet shops

1 Line a tank with small pebbles for drainage. Carefully add a layer of commercial cactus soil—a handful at a time.

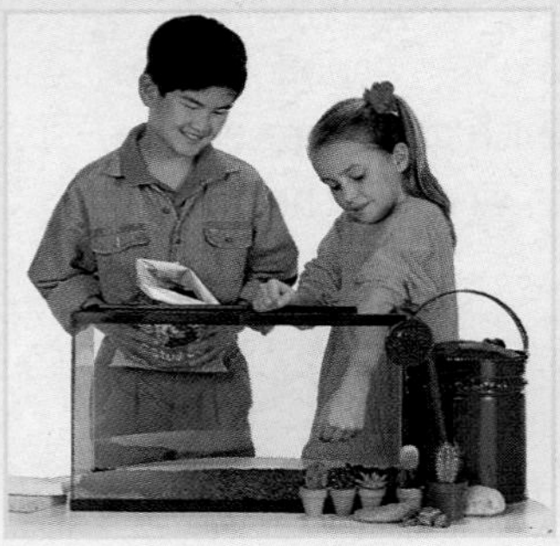

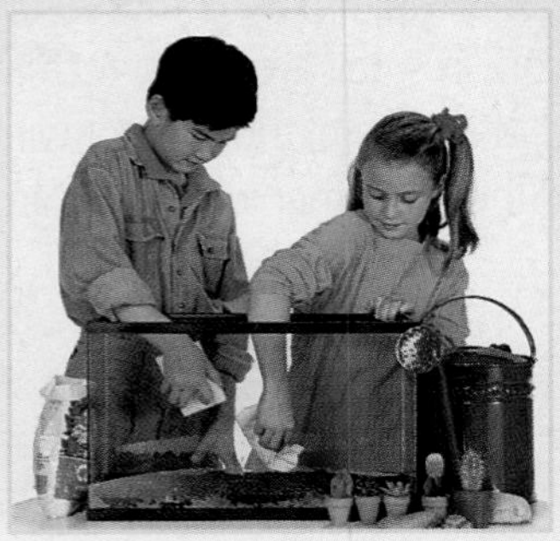

2 Moisten the soil. Clean the sides of the tank.

3 Plant a variety of small cacti, allowing plenty of space for growth. Add $^{1}/_{4}$ inch layer of sand.

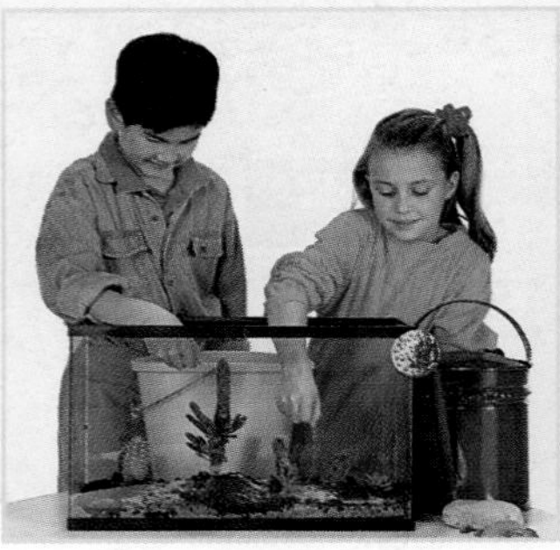

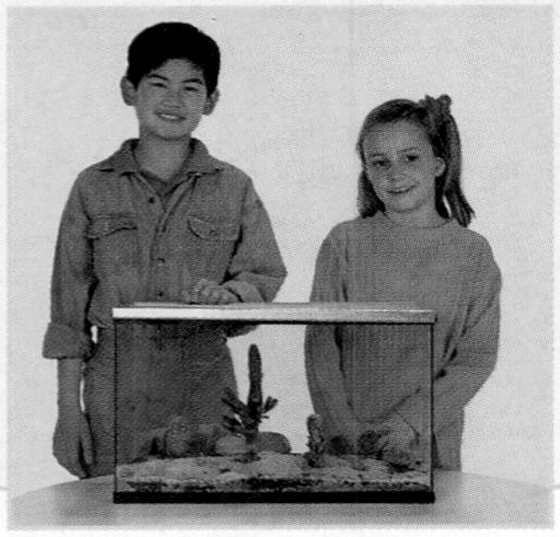

4 Add props or rocks. Protect the plants with a mesh cover that allows air in. Set in a sunny spot.

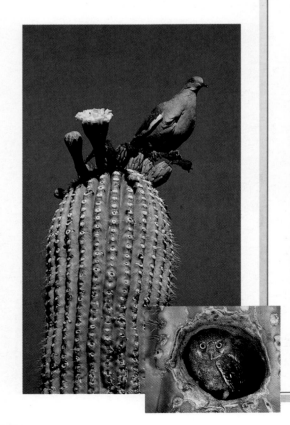

Exploring the Saguaro Cactus

MEETING INDIVIDUAL NEEDS

Challenge The saguaro is a commanding presence in the Sonoran Desert because of its size and longevity. Invite students to research the saguaro cactus and report on questions such as

- Where do saguaros grow?
- What are the average height and weight of mature saguaros? How old do they get?
- What animals live in or near saguaros?

Students can then collaborate on a saguaro poster for classroom display. They can draw one life-size saguaro or several at different stages of growth. Some students can draw birds in nest holes and Sonoran Desert animals.

Resource
Saguaro National Monument
3693 South Old Spanish Trail
Tucson, AZ 85730-5699

Materials

- encyclopedias or other reference books
- poster board or butcher paper
- markers

Art

Designing Outfits

Cooperative Learning

Students can work in small groups. Each group draws a pig and creates outfits for desert, Arctic, country, and city settings. (The illustrations in *The Three Little Javelinas* can serve as a starting point.)

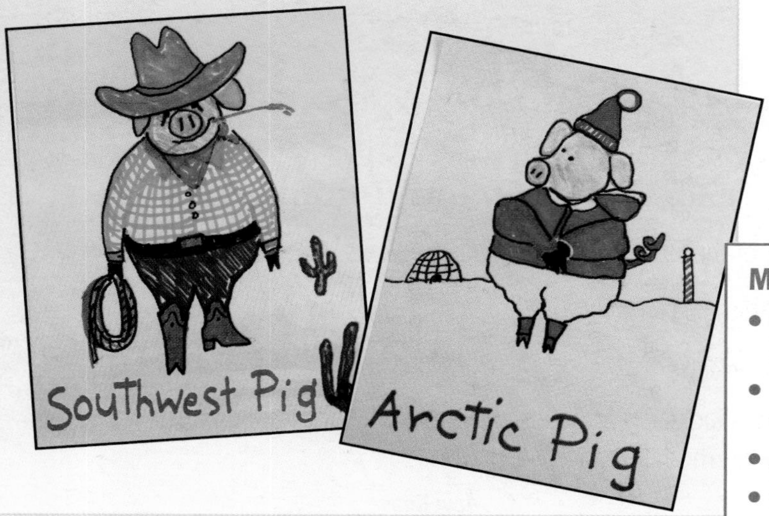

Southwest Pig
Arctic Pig

Materials

- construction paper
- markers or crayons
- glue
- yarn
- clothing scraps
- cotton balls

Math

Graphing Desert Weather

Cooperative Learning

The Sonoran Desert is spread across southern Arizona and the Mexican state of Sonora. Have students work in teams to collect temperature and rainfall data for Tucson and four other major U.S. cities of their choice. Have students develop graphs and post them on a bulletin board.

Resource

The Arizona-Sonora Desert Museum
2021 North Kinney Road
Tucson, AZ 85743

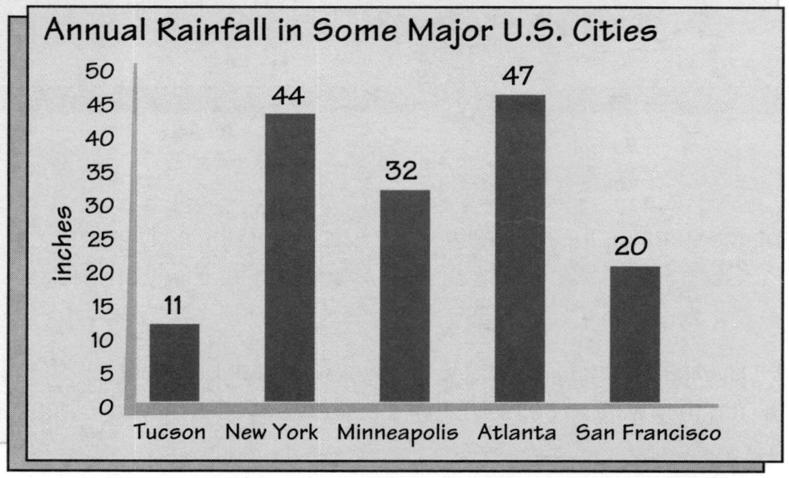

Annual Rainfall in Some Major U.S. Cities
50
45
40
35
30
25
20
15
10
5
0
inches
11
44
32
47
20
Tucson
New York
Minneapolis
Atlanta
San Francisco

My Hairy Neighbors

Introduce the Literature

Building Background/Prior Knowledge

Remind students of the story *The Three Little Javelinas*. Ask:

- What kind of animal is a javelina? (a wild, hairy, piglike animal)
- Where do javelinas live? (southwestern United States)

Point out that this is factual information they learned while reading a story. Use this information to begin modeling a K-W-L chart.

Javelinas

What I Know	What I Want to Find Out	What I Learned
wild and hairy piglike live in Southwest		

Cooperative Learning Tell students the article they are about to read will contain many more facts about javelinas. Have small groups of students work together to fill out their own K-W-L charts. Tell them to list in the second column other things they would like to know about javelinas. Then have students read the selection, and meet again to fill out the third column of their charts.

Interact with Literature

Background: FYI

Feeding Time During the summer, the collared peccary eats only in the early morning or evening, when it's cool. During the day the collared peccary rests under shady bushes for over ten hours.

Bristles Explain that a javelina's long hair is bristly, or coarse and stiff. Compare it with the bristles on a hairbrush. You may want to point out that a peccary's bristles may be as long as seven inches!

Expanding Literacy
Science Feature

My Hairy Neighbors

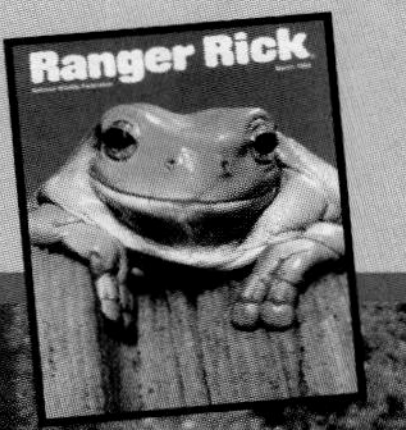
Ranger Rick

by Susan Lowell

photos by
Thomas A. Wiewandt

Meet some pig-like animals that "talk" with stinky smells!

Welcome to my ranch. I live deep in a rocky canyon way out in the Arizona desert. I have many wild neighbors. At the end of a summer day, three of my favorites often come for dinner. Just watch!

There — a hairy animal is peeking through the bushes. And another. And another. It's Juan, José, and Josefina!

The animals are each about 20 inches (50 cm) high, with rounded backs. And they look and act a bit like pigs. But they're *peccaries* (PECK-a-rees). Some people around here also call them *javelinas* (ha-ve-LEE-nas).

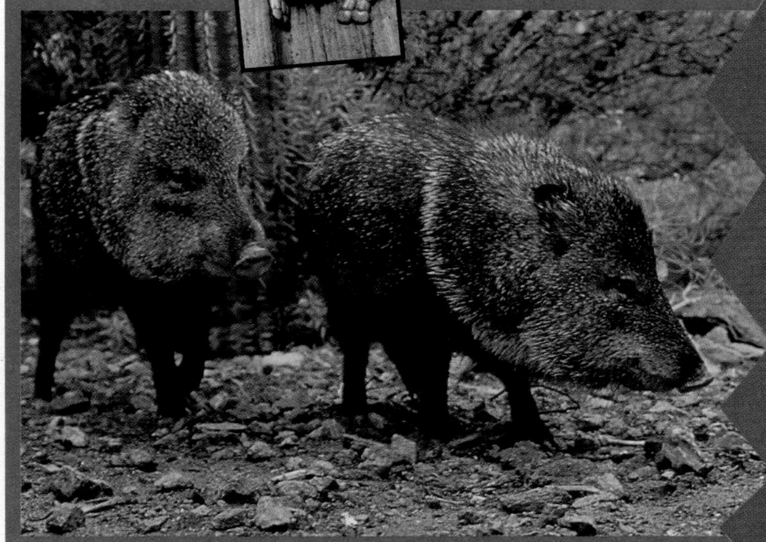

Check out the rings of light hair around the necks of these peccaries. They look like collars, don't they? That's why the animals are called *collared peccaries*.

89

Interact with Literature

Media Literacy

Photo Essays Explain that in a photo essay, words and pictures work hand-in-hand to give information. Words alone do not tell the whole story, nor do the photographs alone. Both are equally important.

Extra Support

Meeting Individual Needs

Quotations What is different about the use of quotations around the word *talk* in the introduction? Discuss how quotations can sometimes mean "not exactly" or "in a different way." Why might this motivate someone to continue reading the article?

Students Acquiring English

Meeting Individual Needs

Author's Voice Explain that *check it out* is a casual way of saying "Look here!" Ask students why Susan Lowell adopts this voice. What if she had written *The Three Little Javelinas* using the same voice? Would the story be the same?

Interact with Literature

Home Connection

Ask students what animals they might see outside their windows at home. What is interesting about observing animals?

Visual Literacy

Ask students to compare the photos here with Jim Harris' illustrations.

A peccary can use its long, sharp teeth to bite a prickly pear cactus. Those teeth may look nasty, but this animal is probably just yawning.

Peccaries live in groups called *herds*, which helps them protect each other from their enemies. And when it's snooze time, the herd snuggles close together.

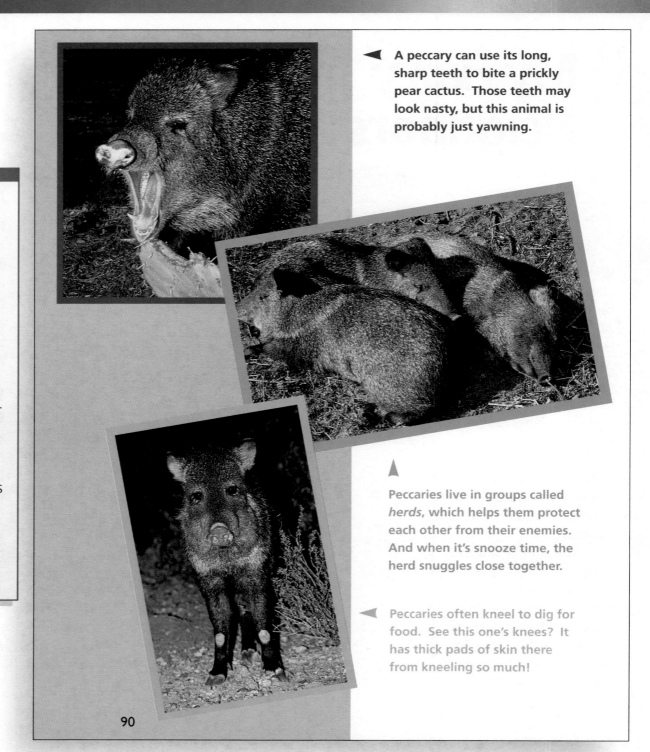

Peccaries often kneel to dig for food. See this one's knees? It has thick pads of skin there from kneeling so much!

90

Interact with Literature

Discussion

- Why are javelinas called collared peccaries? (because of the ring of light hair around their necks)
- Why does a javelina need sharp teeth? (because it has to gnaw through hard surfaces, such as prickly pear cactuses)
- Why do you think javelinas snuggle together when they sleep? (to keep each other warm and also to make sure they're all safe)
- Can you name any other animals that travel in herds? (elephants, horses, cattle, etc.)
- How do javelinas communicate? (by rubbing musk on one another)

Interact with Literature

MEETING INDIVIDUAL NEEDS

Students Acquiring English

Word Meaning Students may enjoy saying the word *snooze* several times, drawing it out so that the relationship of the sound of the word to its meaning is clearer. Explain that *snooze time* is merely a more colorful way of saying "time to sleep."

Expanding Literacy
Science Feature

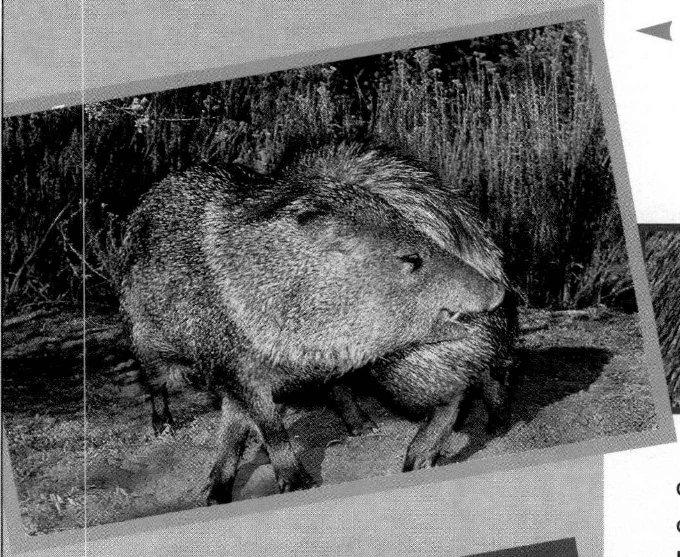

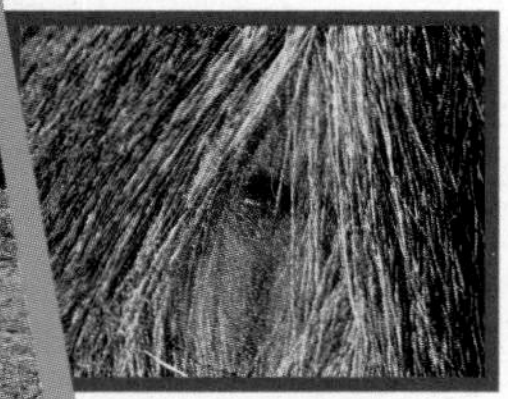

A drippy hole on the javelina's back oozes a smelly liquid called *musk*. Family members rub the musk on each other. That helps them keep track of each other.

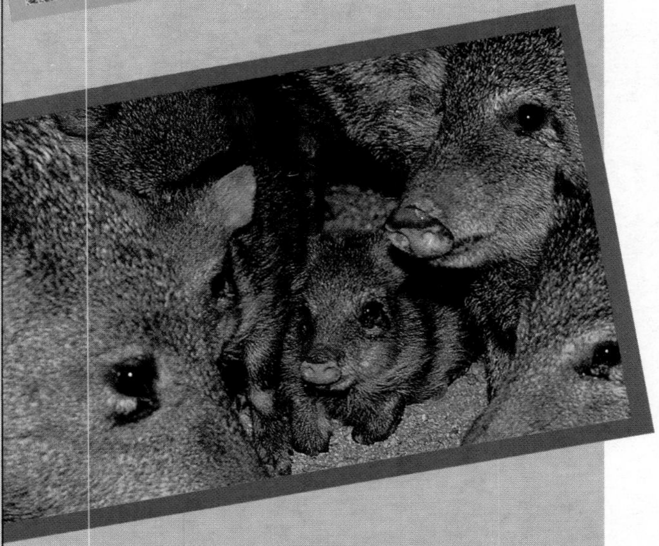

Peccary herds stick close together. This young one found a safe place in its herd — right in the thick of things.

Peccaries don't live just in deserts. In Mexico and much of South America, they also can be found in mountains and rain forests. They live only in wild areas. But some of those wild areas are very close to the homes of people.

As I go into my house, I suddenly hear some loud noise. *Clang! Bang! Clatter!*

What's that? Uh-oh! Outside my ranch house, Josefina just knocked over one of the trash cans. Her babies poke their snouts inside it and sniff for something good to eat.

"Shoo!" I say. "No junk food! Go find some nice cactus fruit." Josefina grunts. Together the herd starts moving. "Good night!" I call to them. Then I watch the herd gallop off into the desert darkness.

91

Instruct and Integrate

Math Link

A Javelina's Height Ask students to read aloud the sentence that tells how high a peccary is. Ask them to identify objects in the classroom that are about 20 inches (50 cm) high. Have students compare their own heights with the height of a typical peccary. Is the peccary as tall? Almost as tall? Half as tall?

Science Link

Omnivorous Animals A javelina's snout enables it to uproot logs and dig in the ground for roots and underground stems. Javelinas are omnivorous—they eat anything that is available. Ask students to brainstorm what plants and animals a javelina might find in a desert or forest. (snakes, eggs, fruit, cactus, acorns)

Home Connection

Wild Areas What is the "wild area" nearest your school? The front section of your phone book is a good place to find a listing of parks and preserves in your area. Ask students if they have ever visited these places. What wild animals are there?

Interact with Literature

Meeting Individual Needs

Students Acquiring English

Expressions Explain the meaning of the phrase *keep track of*. Ask students what things they try to keep track of. Point out that this caption explains the comment made at the top of page 89 about how javelinas "talk."

Explain that *in the thick of things* means "right in the middle of what is going on." Point out that *thick* also refers to the peccaries' thick, hairy coats.

SELECTION:
The Three Little Hawaiian Pigs and the Magic Shark

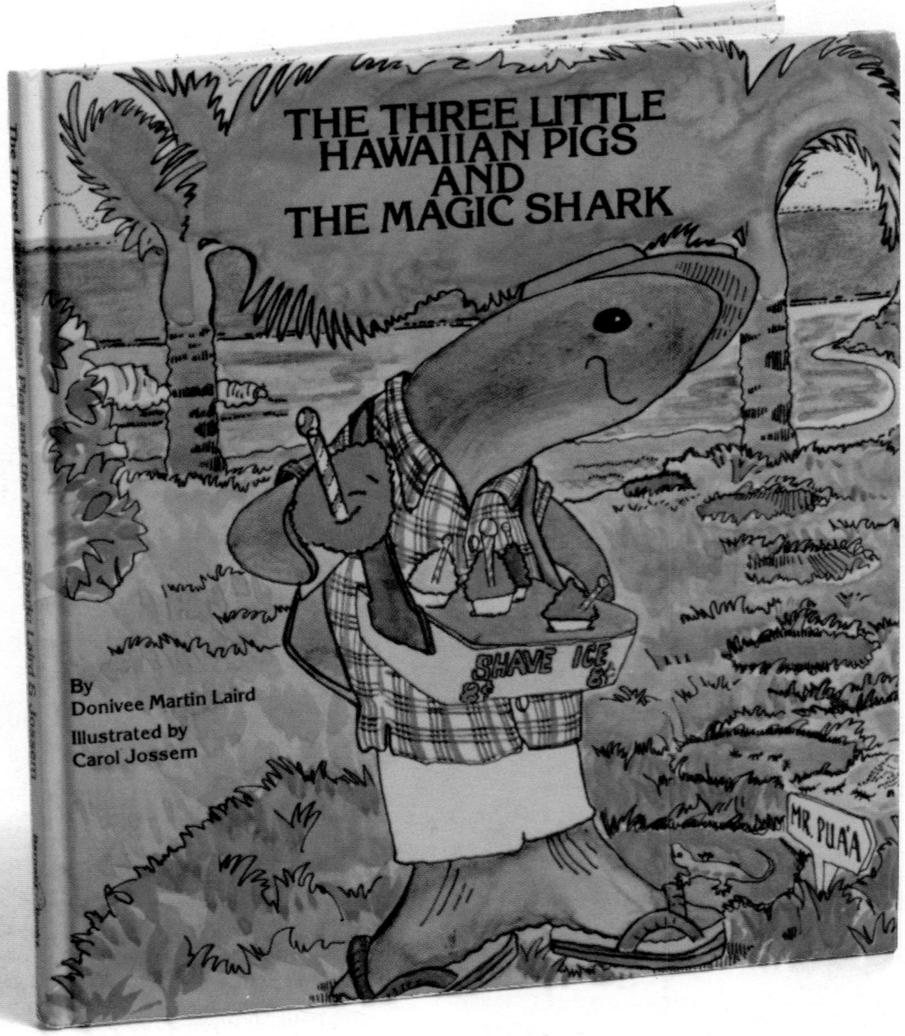
THE THREE LITTLE HAWAIIAN PIGS AND THE MAGIC SHARK
By
Donivee Martin Laird
Illustrated by
Carol Jossem
SHAVE ICE
MR. PUA'A

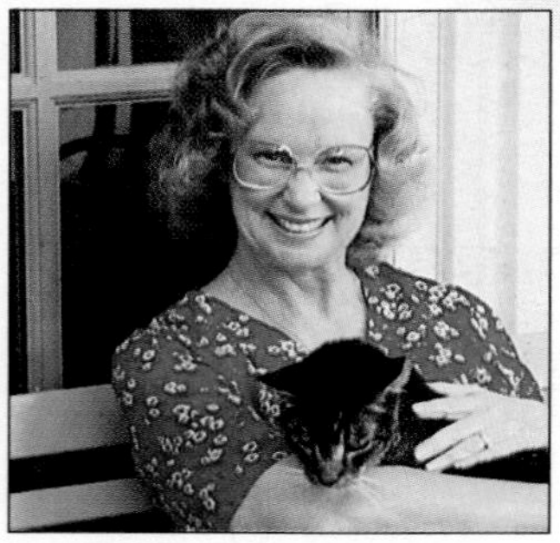

by Donivee Martin Laird

Other Books by the Author

Keaka and the Liliko'i Vine

Wili Wai Kula and the Three Mongooses

Selection Summary

The story of "The Three Little Pigs" moves to Hawaii, where the first two little pigs quickly build their houses out of pili grass and driftwood, respectively. The third pig takes the time to build a sturdy house of lava rock before joining his brothers on the beach.

A magic shark sees them surfing and craves a pig dinner. Disguised first as a shave ice man and then as a beachboy, he cannot con his way into the first and second little pigs' houses; so he blows their houses down as the pigs escape. Frustrated and hungry, the shark goes as a lei seller to the third pig's house but still cannot fool the pigs. This time, the magic shark futilely huffs and puffs until he is out of air and the pigs can dispose of him like a rug.

Lesson Planning Guide

	Skill/Strategy Instruction	Meeting Individual Needs	Lesson Resources
1 Introduce the Literature *Pacing: 1 day*	**Preparing to Read and Write** Prior Knowledge/Building Background, 91C **Selection Vocabulary,** 91D • craving • anxiously • plot • scheme • pangs • furious **Spelling Pretest,** 114I • three • tail • beach • play • deep • away • please • chain	**Support in Advance,** 91C **Students Acquiring English,** 91C **Other Choices for Building Background,** 91C **Spelling Challenge Words:** • easy • really • reef • creature	***Literacy Activity Book:*** Vocabulary, p. 30 **Transparencies:** Building Background, 1–9, Vocabulary, 1–10 **Great Start** CD-ROM software, "Oink, Oink, Oink" CD
2 Interact with Literature *Pacing: 1-3 days*	**Reading Strategies:** Monitor, 94, 98, 100 Think About Words, 94, 108 **Minilessons:** ✓ Fantasy/Realism, 95 Writer's Craft: Anthropomorphism, 97 Compare and Contrast, 103 Sequence, 107	**Choices for Reading,** 94 **Guided Reading,** 94 Comprehension/Critical Thinking, 96, 102, 106, 112 **Students Acquiring English,** 94, 95, 96, 97, 98, 99, 102, 105, 106, 109, 110, 112, 114 **Extra Support,** 100, 111, 113 **Challenge,** 103	**Reading-Writing Workshop** A Story, 116–117F ***Literacy Activity Book,*** p. 40–42 The Learning Company's new elementary writing center software
3 Instruct and Integrate *Pacing: 1-3 days*	✓ **Comprehension:** Fantasy/Realism, 114B ✓ **Writing:** Combining Sentences: Compound Sentences, 114D **Word Skills and Strategies:** ✓ Using Context, 114F Dictionary: Alphabetical Order, 114G **Building Vocabulary:** Vocabulary Activities, 114H ✓ **Spelling:** Long *a* and Long *e*, 114I ✓ **Grammar:** Kinds of Sentences, 114J–114K **Communication Activities:** Listening and Speaking, 114L; Viewing, 114M **Cross-Curricular Activities:** Social Studies, 114N; Science, 114O	**Reteaching:** Fantasy/Realism, 114C **Activity Choices:** Creative Writing: Animal Characters, 114E; Plan a House, 114E; Write a Poem, 114E **Reteaching:** Using Context, 114G **Activity Choices:** Selection Vocabulary Extension, Synonym Search, Vocabulary Notebook, 114H **Challenge Words Practice,** 114I **Reteaching:** Kinds of Sentences, 114K **Activity Choices:** Listening and Speaking, 114L; Viewing, 114M **Activity Choices:** Social Studies, 114N; Science, 114O	**Reading-Writing Workshop** A Story, 116–117F **Transparencies:** Comprehension, 1–11; Writing, 1–12; Grammar, 1–13 ***Literacy Activity Book:*** Comprehension, p. 32; Writing, p. 33; Word Skills, p. 34; Building Vocabulary, p. 35; Spelling, p. 36–37; Grammar, p. 38–39 **Audio Tape** for "Oink, Oink, Oink": *The Three Hawaiian Pigs and the Magic Shark* **Channel R.E.A.D.** videodisc: "The Ordinary Princess" The Learning Company's new elementary writing center software

✓ ***Indicates Tested Skills.*** *See page 34F for assessment options.*

Introduce *the* Literature

Preparing to Read and Write

Support in Advance

Use this activity for students who need extra support before participating in the whole-class activity.

Picture Walk Preview the illustrations with students and make a web using words such as *ocean, reef, ukulele, surfboard,* and *lei.*

Management Tip
Suggest that other students spend a few minutes writing a description of a tropical place in their journals.

Students Acquiring English
This story has boxes that help define many Hawaiian words. Preview them with students to build background.

Transparency 1–9

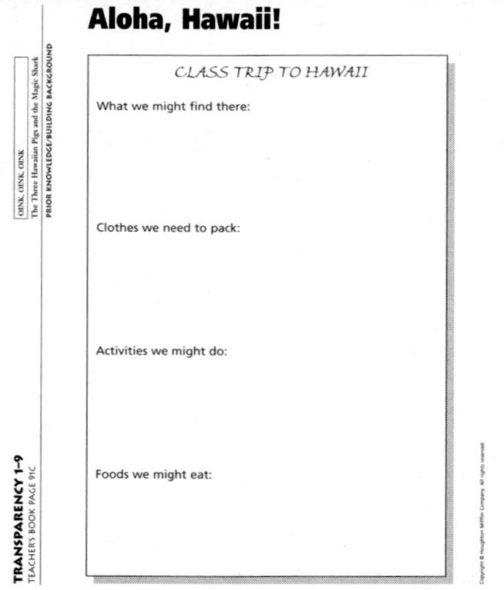
Aloha, Hawaii!

CLASS TRIP TO HAWAII

What we might find there:

Clothes we need to pack:

Activities we might do:

Foods we might eat:

OINK, OINK, OINK
The Three Hawaiian Pigs and the Magic Shark
PRIOR KNOWLEDGE/BUILDING BACKGROUND

TRANSPARENCY 1–9
TEACHER'S BOOK PAGE 91C

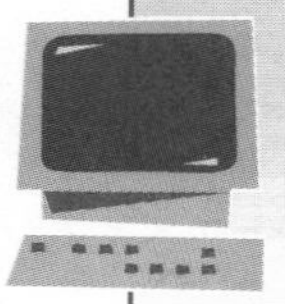

Great Start
For students needing extra support with key concepts and vocabulary, use the "Oink, Oink, Oink" CD.

INTERACTIVE LEARNING

Prior Knowledge/Building Background

Key Concept
Hawaii

Ask students to share what they know about Hawaii. Tell them that the next version of "The Three Little Pigs" takes place in Hawaii. Ask:

- If you were building a house out of things you could find in Hawaii, what would you use?
- What kind of animal in Hawaii would make a good villain for this story?

Then work with the class to plan a "trip" to Hawaii. Organize the trip by completing the planner on Transparency 1–9 with students.

Class Trip to Hawaii

What we might find there:	Clothes we need to pack:
ocean, palm trees, mountains	T-shirts, shorts, sandals

Other Choices for Building Background

Rehearsing the Lines

Students Acquiring English Reread the traditional tale (pages 35A–35B). Invite students to chime in on (or recite from memory) the dialogue between the wolf and the pigs.

Map Study

Challenge Have students find Hawaii on a map. Then ask: Where is Hawaii? What is it near? What other places are about the same size as Hawaii? Which states are closest to Hawaii?

Quick Writing

Cooperative Learning

Have students work in small groups to brainstorm a list of ways the story of "The Three Little Pigs" might change when it is set in Hawaii.

Spelling
You may want to give the Spelling Pretest on page 114I before students read the selection.

Daily Language Practice
Use the sentences on page 114K as a daily practice of the spelling and grammar skills taught with this selection.

INTERACTIVE LEARNING

Selection Vocabulary

Key Words

- craving
- anxiously
- plot
- scheme
- pangs
- furious

Display Transparency 1–10. Point out that all the words are used in the story to tell about the villain, or evil character. Read each of these sentences aloud and ask students to place the underlined words on the map based on how they are used in the sentence.

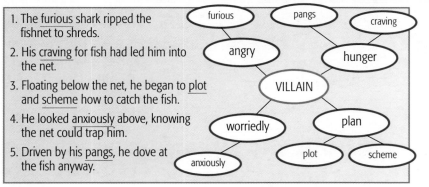

1. The furious shark ripped the fishnet to shreds.
2. His craving for fish had led him into the net.
3. Floating below the net, he began to plot and scheme how to catch the fish.
4. He looked anxiously above, knowing the net could trap him.
5. Driven by his pangs, he dove at the fish anyway.

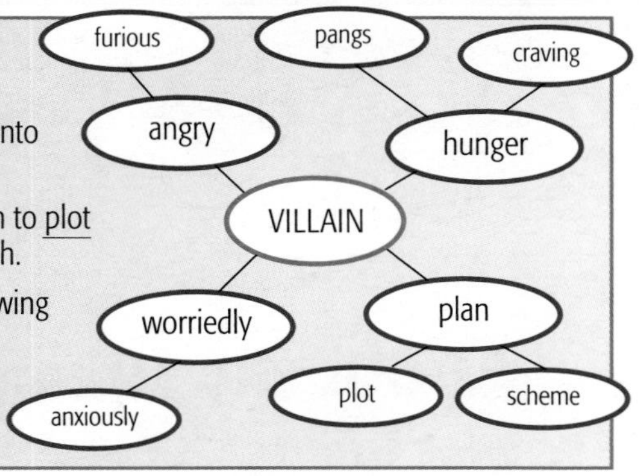

furious
pangs
craving
angry
hunger
VILLAIN
worriedly
plan
anxiously
plot
scheme

Vocabulary Practice Students can work independently or in pairs to complete the activity on *Literacy Activity Book* page 30.

Transparency 1–10

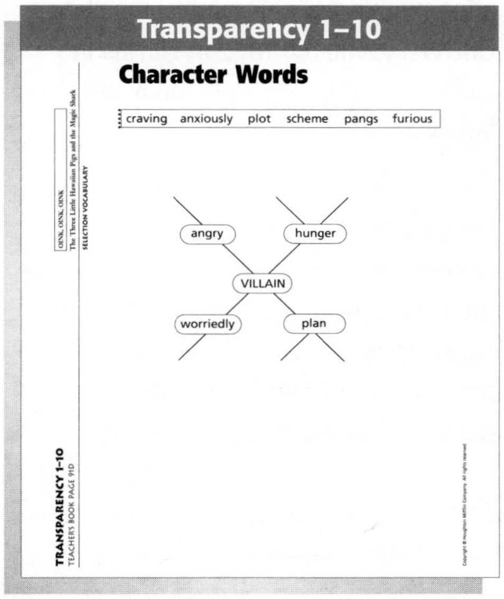

Character Words
craving anxiously plot scheme pangs furious
angry
hunger
VILLAIN
worriedly
plan
TRANSPARENCY 1-10

Multicultural

Teacher FactFile

Hawaiian Islands

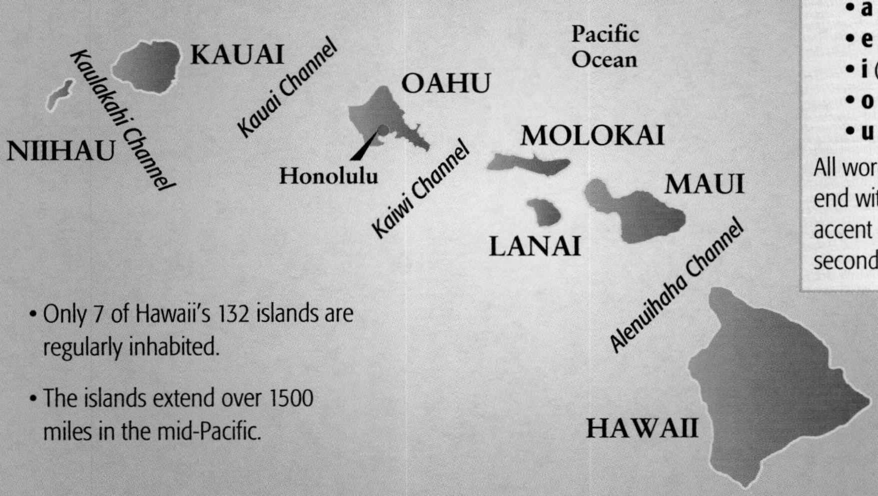

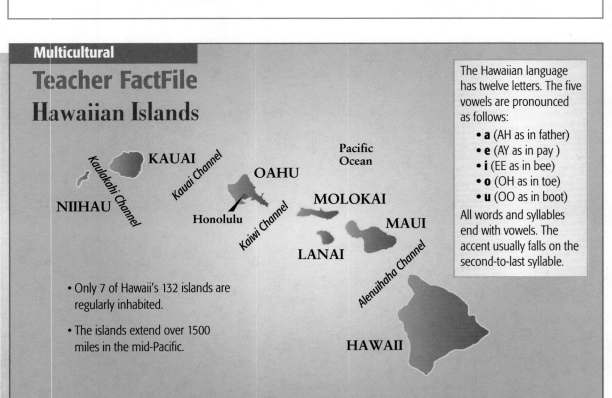

KAUAI
Kaulakahi Channel
NIIHAU
Kauai Channel
OAHU
Honolulu
Kaiwi Channel
Pacific Ocean
MOLOKAI
MAUI
LANAI
Alenuihaha Channel
HAWAII

- Only 7 of Hawaii's 132 islands are regularly inhabited.
- The islands extend over 1500 miles in the mid-Pacific.

The Hawaiian language has twelve letters. The five vowels are pronounced as follows:

- **a** (AH as in father)
- **e** (AY as in pay)
- **i** (EE as in bee)
- **o** (OH as in toe)
- **u** (OO as in boot)

All words and syllables end with vowels. The accent usually falls on the second-to-last syllable.

Literacy Activity Book, p. 30

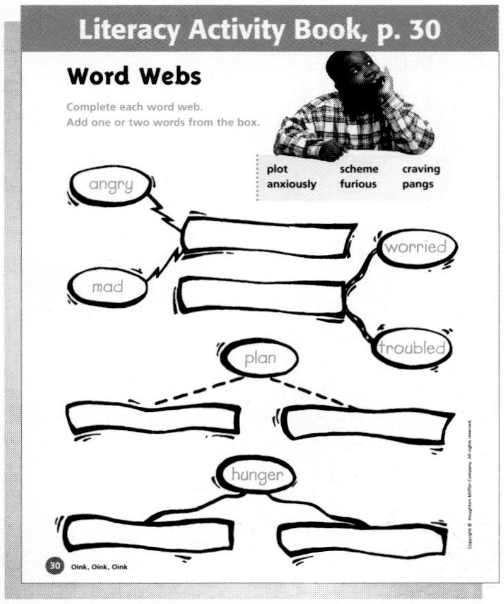

Word Webs
Complete each word web.
Add one or two words from the box.
plot
anxiously
scheme
furious
craving
pangs
angry
worried
mad
troubled
plan
hunger
30 Oink, Oink, Oink

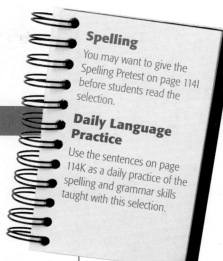

Interact *with* Literature

More About the Author

Donivee Martin Laird

Donivee Martin Laird grew up in Hawaii, which she describes as "one of the most beautiful places in the world." After living in Puerto Rico for several years, and then attending school at Pennsylvania State University, she returned to Hawaii in 1973, where she still lives today with her family.

A teacher in Honolulu since 1977, Laird began writing children's stories to fill a void in contemporary Hawaiian literature for the early grades. She began experimenting with Hawaiian adaptations of well-known folktales, using her own classroom as her "laboratory." Her books, including *Wili Wai Kula and the Three Mongooses* (Hawaii's own "Goldilocks and the Three Bears") and *'Ula Li'i and the Magic Shark* (a Hawaiian "Little Red Riding Hood"), have been well-received by teachers and schoolchildren.

About the Author

Donivee Martin Laird

The beautiful state of Hawaii is home to Donivee Martin Laird. She was born there and lives there today with her family and a mongoose named Custard. Laird has written several Hawaiian versions of popular tales, such as *Wili Wai Kula and the Three Mongooses*, a Hawaiian "Goldilocks and the Three Bears."

About the Illustrator

Don Stuart

Don Stuart didn't have any brothers or sisters growing up, so he used to entertain himself by drawing. Making his own comic books was a favorite thing to do. Among the illustrators Stuart admires today is Lane Smith, the illustrator of *The True Story of the 3 Little Pigs*.

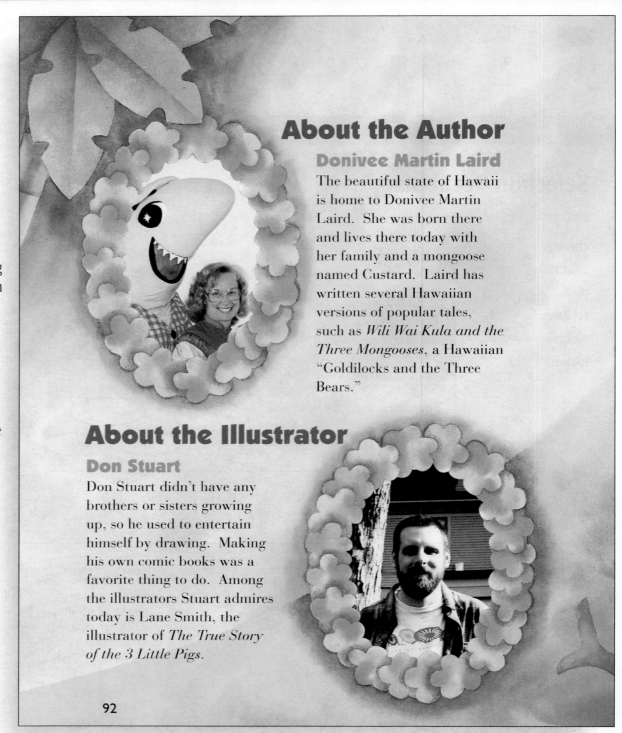

92

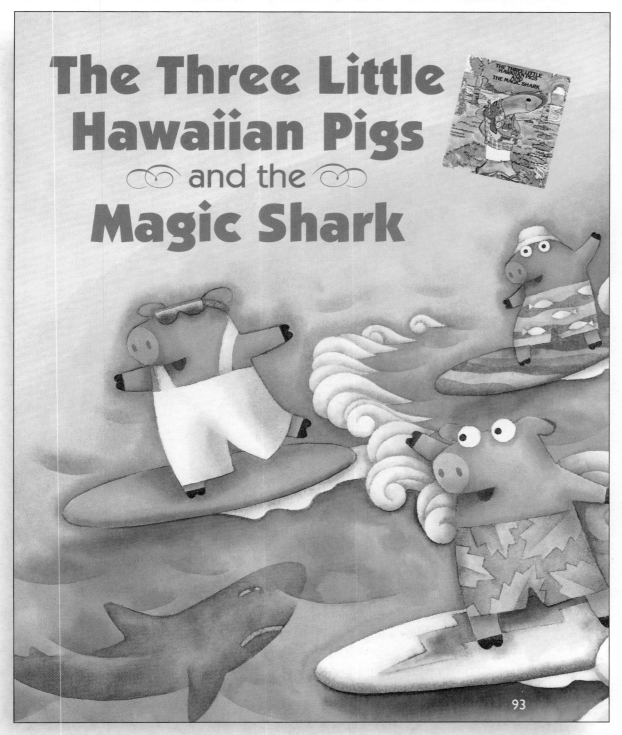
The Three Little
Hawaiian Pigs
and the
Magic Shark
93

More About the Illustrator

Don Stuart

Growing up as an only child, Don Stuart entertained himself by writing and drawing his own comic books. Although he says he frequently got into trouble for drawing during class, he credits a high school art teacher with putting the idea into his head that he could one day make a living at something he enjoyed so much.

Today, Stuart lives in Ohio with his wife and three sons, all of whom spend a lot of time drawing. "I think there's at least one artist among them," he says. For the illustrations for *The Three Little Hawaiian Pigs and the Magic Shark*, Stuart used bright liquid watercolors called luma dyes.

Interact *with* Literature

Reading Strategies

Think About Words
Monitor

Student Application

Ask students to preview the selection and talk about what strategies they think will be useful in understanding it. If necessary, lead students to note that since the story is set on an island, there may be details that will confuse them at first, so they should monitor their reading. Also, discuss how thinking about the Hawaiian words that are in boxes may be necessary.

Predicting/Purpose Setting

Have students make predictions on how the shark will try to catch the pigs. Have them read to find out.

Choices for Reading

Independent Reading	**Cooperative Reading**
Guided Reading	**Teacher Read Aloud**

Guided Reading

Because of the Hawaiian words in this story, you may wish to read aloud parts of the story. Pronunciations are found in boxes. Have students read to the end of page 97, keeping their purpose in mind. Then use the questions on page 96 to check comprehension.

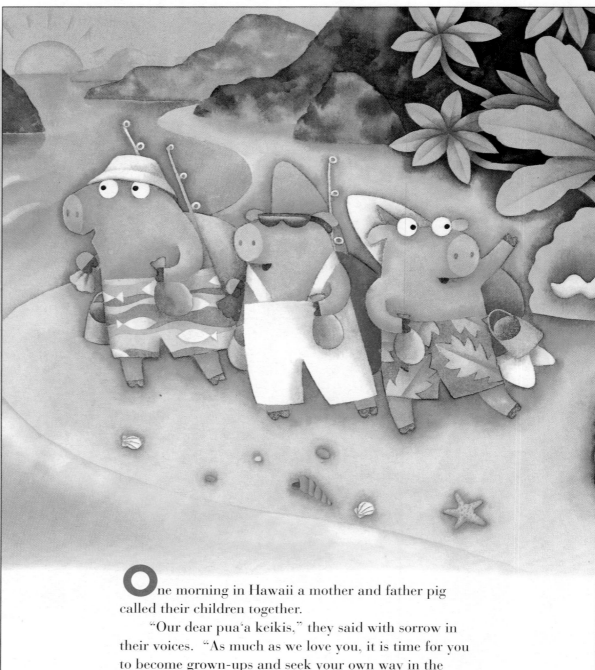

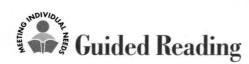

One morning in Hawaii a mother and father pig called their children together.

"Our dear pua'a keikis," they said with sorrow in their voices. "As much as we love you, it is time for you to become grown-ups and seek your own way in the

94

QuickREFERENCE

Multicultural Link

Most Hawaiians speak English but some incorporate words from the Hawaiian language into their everyday speech. The language sounds very melodic to English speakers, perhaps because words are made up mostly of vowels.

Students Acquiring English

Expressions Note that the phrase *seek your own way in the world* has the same meaning as *seek your fortune*: to leave home and earn money on one's own.

Journal

Encourage students to explore their thinking by writing in their journals. In their entries they could discuss
- questions they had while reading
- evaluations they made
- how they figured out word meanings

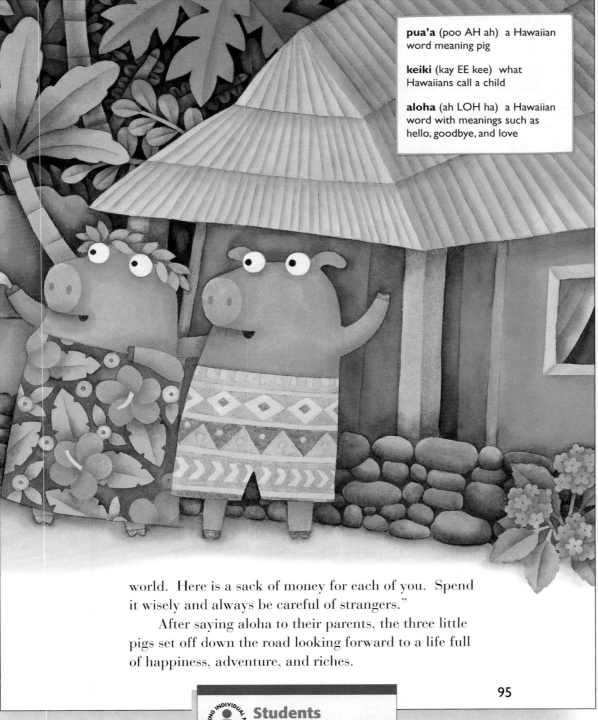

pua'a (poo AH ah) a Hawaiian word meaning pig

keiki (kay EE kee) what Hawaiians call a child

aloha (ah LOH ha) a Hawaiian word with meanings such as hello, goodbye, and love

world. Here is a sack of money for each of you. Spend it wisely and always be careful of strangers."

After saying aloha to their parents, the three little pigs set off down the road looking forward to a life full of happiness, adventure, and riches.

95

MINILESSON

Fantasy/ Realism

TESTED SKILL

Teach/Model

Remind students that fantasies contain both real and make-believe elements. Begin mapping them out for this story using the illustration on pages 94–95.

Real	Fantasy
palm trees	pigs dressed like people

Then reread the text on these two pages with students. Ask:

- Can pigs really talk?
- Can pigs collect riches?

Add these details to the Fantasy column. To add to the Real column, students can pull out elements such as the buckets and fishing rods from the illustration.

Practice/Apply

Have students review the story and add other real and make-believe details to the chart.

SKILL FINDER

Full lesson/Reteaching, p. 114B–114C

Minilessons, p. 57; Theme 5, p. 211

MEETING INDIVIDUAL NEEDS

Students Acquiring English

Pronunciations Since Hawaiian vowels approximate those in most European languages, you may want to have students who speak these languages give their classmates help with the pronunciations of the Hawaiian words in this story.

Interact *with* Literature

Guided Reading

Comprehension/Critical Thinking

1. What has happened in the story so far? (The little pigs left their parents and built their own homes. The first pig built a house out of pili grass, while the second built his out of driftwood.)
2. Why were the first two pigs able to build their houses so quickly? (The materials they used were light.)
3. Do you think they spent their money wisely? What other material could they have chosen? (Have students cite alternate materials that could be found on an island.)
4. What kind of house do you think the third Hawaiian pig will build? (one that is stronger than a pili grass house or a driftwood house)

Predicting/Purpose Setting

Ask students to predict whether the first two pigs' houses will be strong enough to stop the villain. Then have them read to the end of page 102 to find out what the third pig does.

pili (PEE lee) **grass** a grass used to thatch grass houses in old Hawaii

opihi (oh PEE hee) a shallow, cone-shaped limpet shell whose animal is prized eating

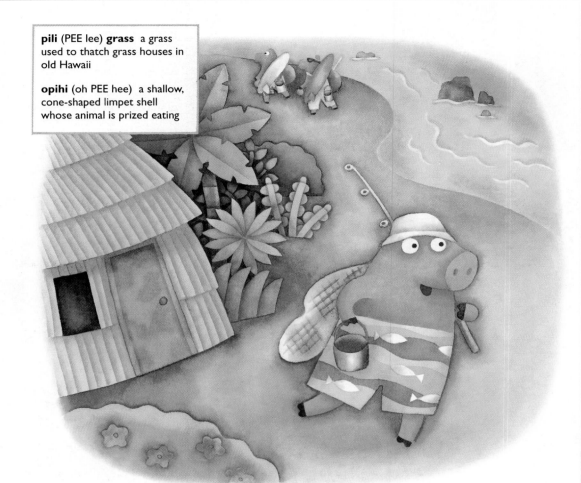

They had gone only a short distance when they met a man with a load of pili grass. "Ah ha," said the first little pig. "This is for me. I will build myself a grass house and live beside the sea."

So, he bought the pili grass and happily headed towards the beach where he built his house. It was finished quickly and he took his pole, his net, his small bucket for opihi, and he went fishing.

96

Informal Assessment

If students' responses indicate that they are understanding the effect the setting has on the story, have them finish reading the story independently or with partners.

QuickREFERENCE

Vocabulary

Pronunciations Model for students the pronunciations on page 96 and then have them try. Ask them what a reader could infer about the sound of the vowel *i* in Hawaiian from the pronunciations of *pili* and *opihi.*

Students Acquiring English

Word Meaning Point out that to *live beside the sea* means "to live near the water." Have students demonstrate standing *beside* their desks. Ask students why the pigs want to live by the sea.

Social Studies Link

Physical Features Ask students if they know these words, used to describe mountainous areas:

- *plateau:* an area of flat land that is higher than the land around it
- *valley:* a long, narrow area of low land between mountains

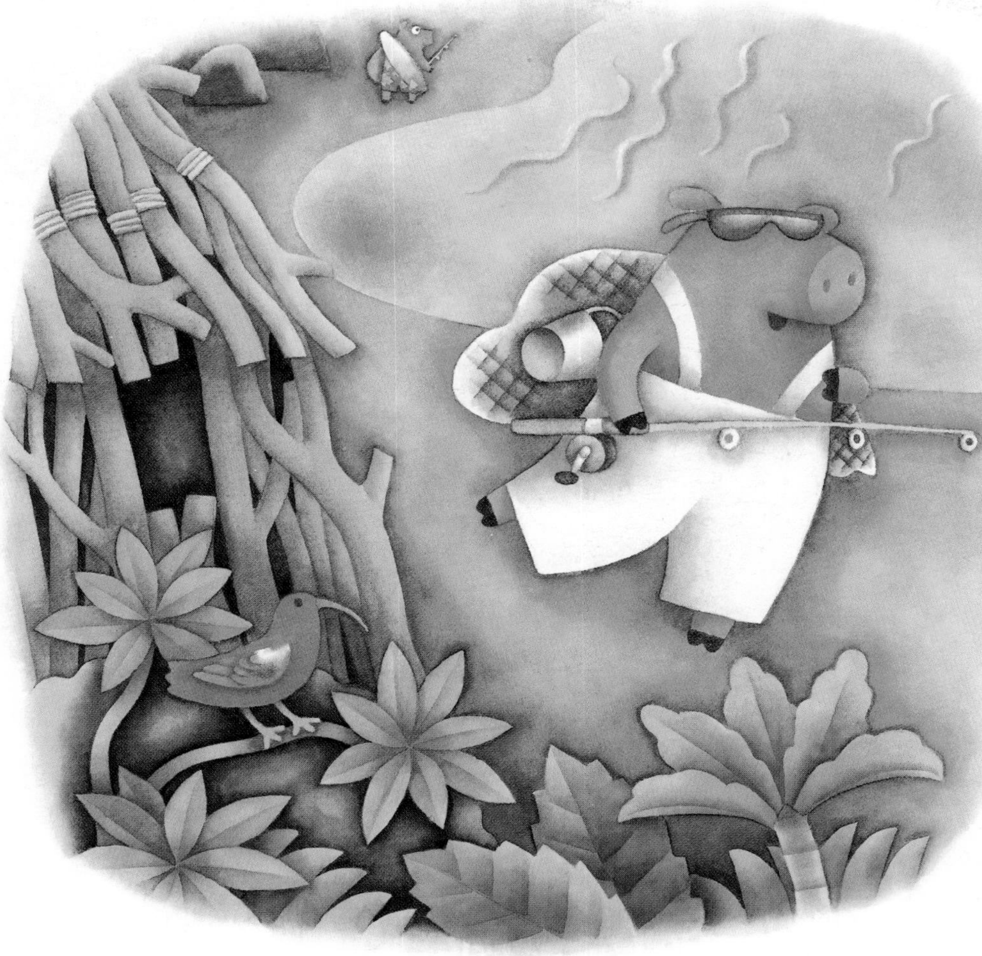

The other two little pigs went on until they met a man selling driftwood. "Ah ha," said the second little pig. "This is for me. I will build myself a house of driftwood and live beside the sea."

Feeling pleased with himself, he quickly built his house and went to join the first little pig fishing and scraping opihi off the slippery rocks.

97

MINILESSON

Writer's Craft

Anthropomorphism

Teach/Model

Tell students that the pigs in this story do many things that real-life pigs could never do. Spark discussion by asking:

- What is funny about the idea of a pig fishing?
- What would the story be like if the pigs acted like real pigs do?
- What is your favorite story with talking animals? Why do you like it?

Point out that in fantasies, animals often do things that only people can do in real life, and this is called *anthropomorphism.* This adds to the humor of the story.

Practice/Apply

Have students make a list of all the things the pigs do in this story that are make-believe. Suggest that they draw a smiling face next to those actions (such as pigs surfing) that they think help make the story a funny one.

SKILL FINDER
Writing Activities: Animal Characters, p. 114E
Reading–Writing Workshop, pp. 116–117F

Science Link

Opihi Opihi are mollusks—animals that usually live in water and have a hard outer shell. Ask students if they know the names of any other sea animals that live inside shells, such as clams, oysters, or limpets.

MEETING INDIVIDUAL NEEDS

Students Acquiring English

Word Meaning Explain that opihi cling to rocks. Have a student demonstrate *scraping*. Discuss objects that serve as good scrapers. Ask students what it would sound like if they were scraping a rock with a knife.

Interact *with* Literature

Reading Strategies

Monitor

Ask students why, even though they may know little about pili grass, driftwood, and lava rock, they can still conclude that the third pig's house is probably the strongest. Volunteers might cite these clues:

- the original story of "The Three Little Pigs" (The first two houses were built out of weaker materials than the third.)
- the materials the first two Hawaiian pigs used (Pili grass and driftwood can fall apart easily.)
- how quickly the pigs finished building their houses (The first two pigs finished quickly, while the third pig worked longer on his house.)

Discuss how these clues come to the surface when a reader stops and rereads. Ask students what other steps a reader can take when a story becomes confusing. (read further to see if the story becomes clearer; study the illustrations)

lava rock formed by a volcano

pau (POW) finished, all done

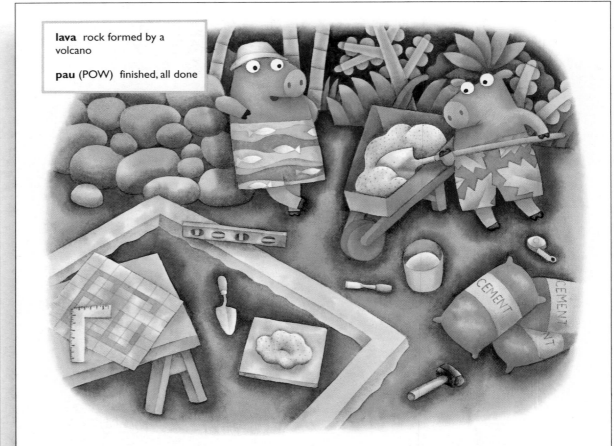
CEMENT
CEMENT

The third little pig went on until he met a man selling lava rock. "Ah ha," said the third little pig. "This is for me. I will build myself a house of lava rock and live beside the sea and go fishing with my brothers."

It took many days to build the house and before it was done, one brother came to visit the third little pig.

"Why are you wasting your time on such a hard house to build?" he asked. "We are pau with our houses and have time to fish and take it easy surfing and playing. Forget this house, come with us."

The third little pig just shook his head and said he would rather take his time and build a strong house.

98

Students Acquiring English

Word Meaning Use the illustration on page 98 to discuss why the house is *hard* (difficult) to build. Point out that since it is *hard* (solid), it will also be difficult to destroy. Use the illustration on page 102 to explain what *surfing* is.

QuickREFERENCE

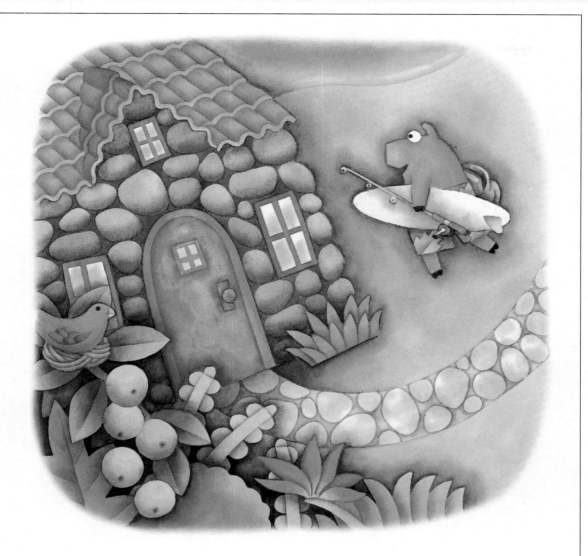

After many days of hard work, the lava rock house was finished. It was sturdy and strong and the third little pig was pleased with his work. He checked his doors and windows carefully to be sure his house was snug and safe.

Then off he went to join his brothers beside the sea.

99

Science Link

Volcanoes The Hawaiian islands were formed from volcanoes. At least two volcanoes, Mauna Loa and Kilauea, are still active.

Students Acquiring English

Pantomime Have a student pantomime the action of checking doors and windows. Discuss the meaning of *snug and safe*.

Multicultural Link

Ancestry The first Hawaiians were Polynesian, but now many people of European and Japanese descent live there. Have students study a map and name different Pacific islands where the first Hawaiians came from.

Interact *with* Literature

Reading Strategies

Monitor

Ask students if they have had difficulty understanding any part of the story thus far. For example, has the setting made the story harder to understand? If so, encourage students to discuss how they have dealt with these difficulties. Have they tried rereading certain parts? Have they used the illustrations? Have they asked a reading partner for help?

yellow tang a small bright yellow reef fish

humuhumu (hoo moo HOO moo) a member of the trigger fish family; one of whom is the humuhumu-nukunuku-a-pua'a or fish with a snout like a pig, made famous in a popular Hawaiian song

he'e (HAY ay) the Hawaiian word for octopus

puhi paka (POOK hee PAH kah) a ferocious eel with sharp teeth

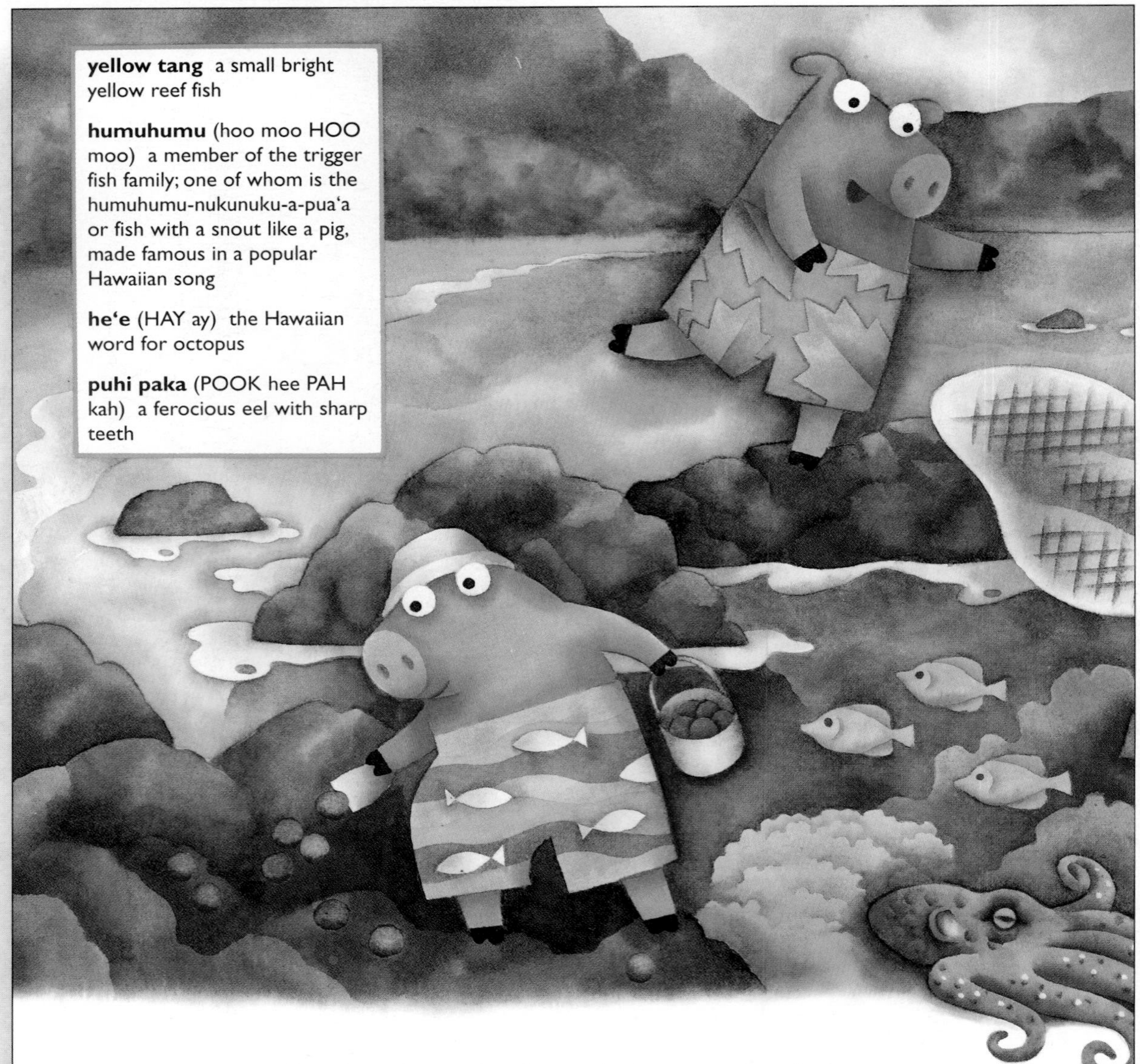

The three little pigs threw their nets and pulled in reef creatures like the brilliant yellow tang, the horned humuhumu, or the slimy octopus, he'e. They climbed over the wet rocks scraping off the delicious opihi and once in a while they caught puhi paka, the fierce fanged eel.

100

QuickREFERENCE

Visual Literacy

Ask students to identify fish in the illustration using
- the definitions in the box
- context clues such as *brilliant, horned, slimy, delicious,* and *fierce fanged*
- their prior knowledge of fish

MEETING INDIVIDUAL NEEDS

Extra Support

Word Meaning If necessary, explain that a *reef* is a strip of rock, sand, or coral that rises close to the surface of the sea. *Tide pools* are puddles of water that the sea leaves behind when the tide goes out.

Science Link

Tropical Fish The yellow tang and the opihi live in reefs because reefs provide a food source (they eat growths on the coral reef) and offer them protection. Can students name other animals that hide in caves or holes to avoid enemies?

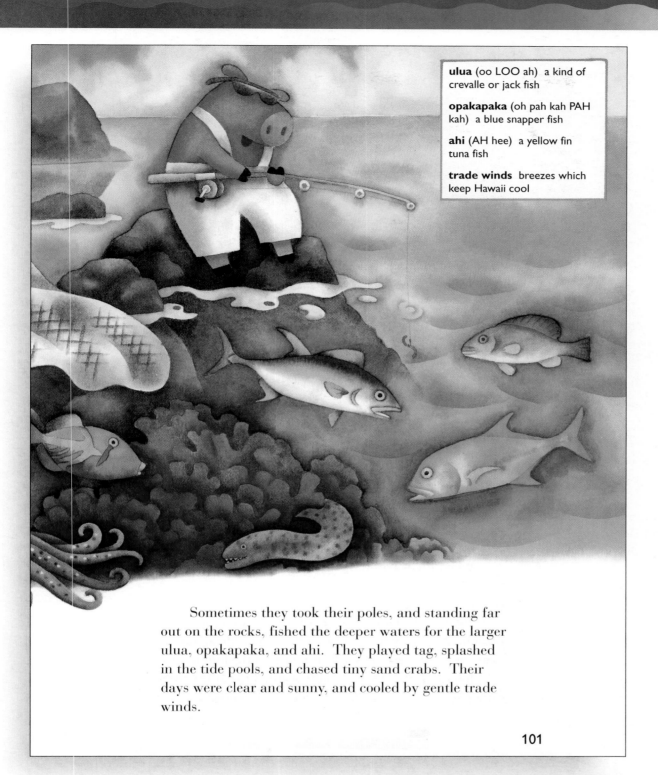

ulua (oo LOO ah) a kind of crevalle or jack fish

opakapaka (oh pah kah PAH kah) a blue snapper fish

ahi (AH hee) a yellow fin tuna fish

trade winds breezes which keep Hawaii cool

Sometimes they took their poles, and standing far out on the rocks, fished the deeper waters for the larger ulua, opakapaka, and ahi. They played tag, splashed in the tide pools, and chased tiny sand crabs. Their days were clear and sunny, and cooled by gentle trade winds.

101

Vocabulary

Ask students what sound the vowel *u* makes in Hawaiian, based on the pronunciations of *humuhumu, puhi paka,* and *ulua*. (It makes the sound *oo*.) Some students acquiring English will enjoy helping others pronounce these words.

Interact *with* Literature

Guided Reading

Comprehension/Critical Thinking

1. How would you summarize this part of the story? (The third pig built a strong house of lava rock; then he went to fish and surf with his brothers. An evil shark saw the pigs and wanted to eat them.)
2. Why couldn't the shark catch the pigs on the lava rocks? (They were too quick; the lava was sharp.)
3. How does the author describe the shark? Do you think he is scary? (Students should cite details such as the shark's teeth and his drooling.)

Predicting/Purpose Setting

Ask students to make predictions about what the shark may do. Then have them read to the end of page 107 to find out what scheme the shark chooses.

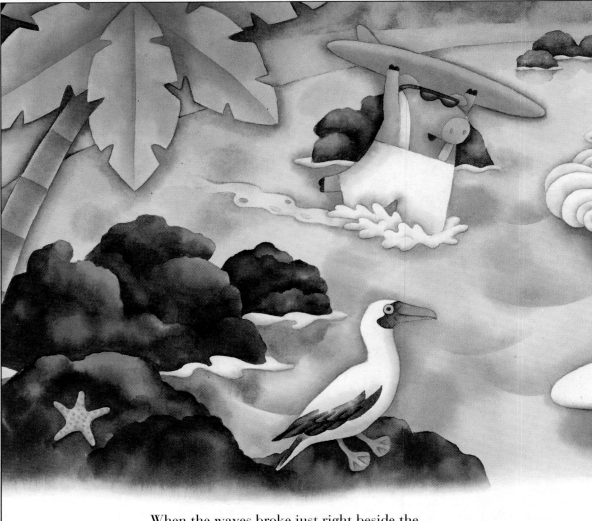

When the waves broke just right beside the reef, they took their surfboards and caught long breathtaking rides to the beach.

Meanwhile, an evil magic shark watched them from deep down where the water is green. Back and forth swam the magic shark, his long teeth shining in the gloomy water. He especially wanted to eat the three little pigs since they looked so sweet and tender.

102

Self-Assessment

Reflecting Ask students if they are thinking about how late the villain appears in this version of "The Three Little Pigs." How might this make his first appearance more suspenseful?

QuickREFERENCE

Students Acquiring English

Word Meaning Discuss the meaning of *the waves broke just right*. Point out that surfers look for waves they can ride for long distances. Ask why such a ride might be exciting. If necessary, demonstrate *breath-taking*.

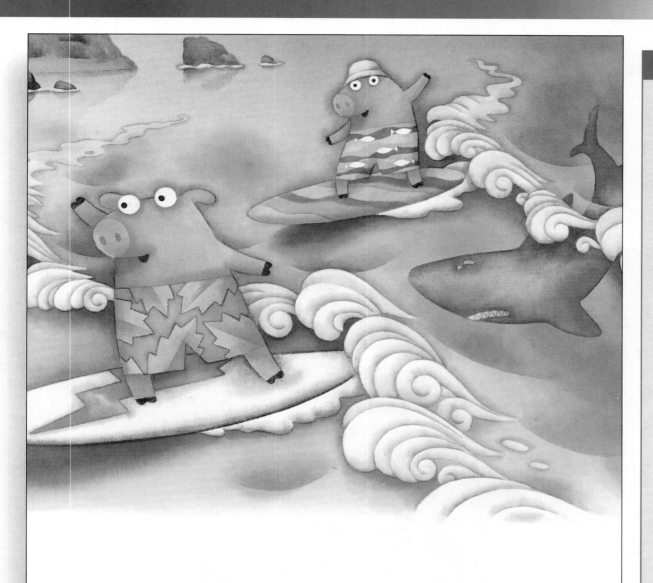

He knew he couldn't catch them on the rocks, for the lava was sharp and the pigs too quick. He wished they would fall off their surfboards, but the pigs were too good and went too fast through the rough water.

So, watching and planning, the magic shark drooled and thought of the yummy little pigs.

103

MEETING INDIVIDUAL NEEDS

Challenge

Waves Invite students to research how ocean waves are created (by wind) and what *tsunamis* are (tidal waves caused by earthquakes). If possible, let students tie a jump rope to a stationary object and demonstrate how waves move.

MINILESSON

Compare and Contrast

REVIEW & MAINTAIN

Teach/Model

Work with students to complete a chart that compares and contrasts the building materials used by the pigs in the following stories.

House

Tale	#1	#2	#3
3 Hawaiian Pigs	pili grass	driftwood	lava rock
3 little javelinas	tumble-weeds	saguaro ribs	adobe
traditional 3 little pigs	straw	sticks	brick

Discuss how comparing and contrasting these details helps readers better understand the relative strength of these materials. Point out that it also helps a reader remember what he or she has read.

Practice/Apply

Have students prepare a chart like the following that compares the villains' strategies in the different versions of "The Three Little Pigs."

Villain	Prey	Strategy
wolf	pigs	huff and puff
coyote	javelinas	magic
shark	pigs	disguise

SKILL FINDER

Full lesson/Reteaching, pp. 88B–88C

Minilessons, p. 75; Theme 4, p. 47

shave ice powdery ice shavings put in a paper cone and covered with sweet, flavored syrup

One morning, unable to stand his craving any longer, the magic shark disguised himself as a shave ice man and knocked on the door of the first little pig's house. "Little Pig, Little Pig, let me come in," he called. "I have plenty shave ice!"

The little pig peeked out of the window. He was hot and thirsty and the cool, colorful shave ice looked so tasty. He grabbed his money and started to open the door.

But, just in time, he saw a fin on the shave ice man's back and he knew it was really the magic shark. He quickly shut and locked the door.

The shark knocked harder and called, "Little Pig, Little Pig, let me come in."

"Oh no," cried the little pig. "Not by the hair on my chinny, chin, chin."

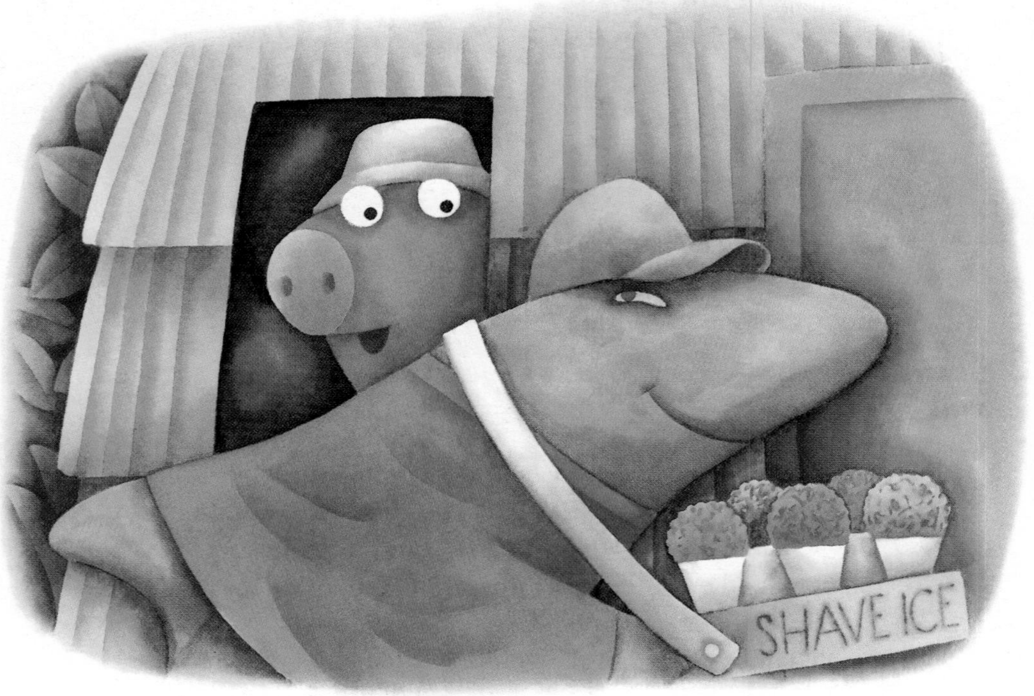
SHAVE ICE

104

Informal Assessment

Oral Reading Have individual students read aloud pages 104–105 as a check of oral reading fluency. Use the Oral Reading Checklist in the *Teacher's Assessment Handbook* as a guide for assessment.

QuickREFERENCE

Vocabulary

Word Meaning Ask students if they have ever eaten *shave ice* or a similar treat such as snowcones. What kinds of tropical fruits might be used as the syrup in shave ice? What are the colors of the fruits?

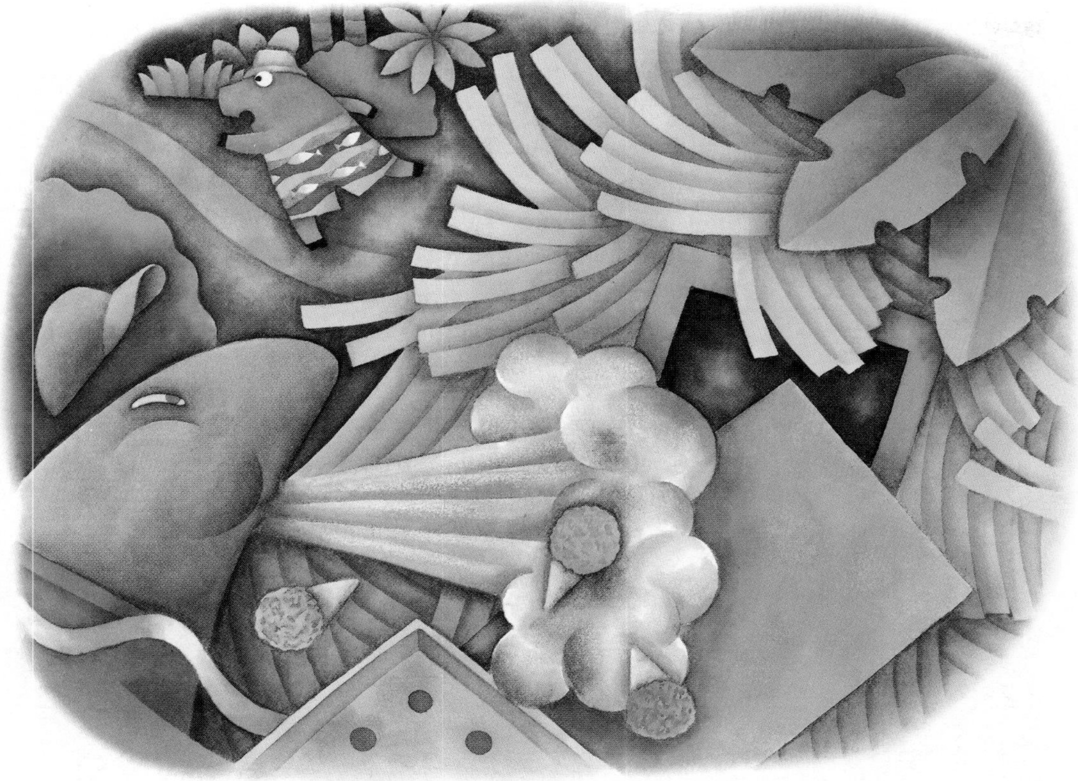

The magic shark was hot and hungry and the little pig's answer made him very mad. He yelled, "Little Pig, Little Pig, let me come in or I will huff and I will puff and I will blow your house down."

The little pig did not open his door. (After all he wasn't crazy, he knew what the magic shark wanted.)

So, the very mad magic shark huffed and the very mad magic shark puffed and the very mad magic shark blew down the first little pig's house.

The first little pig ran out of the back door and down the path to the house of the second little pig. The very mad magic shark went back to the ocean to cool off and make a new plan.

Students Acquiring English

Idioms Explain that *to stand* in this context means "to put up with" or "to endure." The expression *to cool off* can mean to calm down or to do something–such as swimming–that will make one feel less hot.

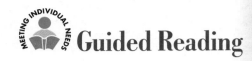

Interact *with* Literature

Guided Reading

Comprehension/Critical Thinking

1. What happened to the first two little pigs? (The shark blew down the first pig's pili grass house and the second pig's driftwood house. The pigs ran to the lava house of the third little pig.)
2. What tricks did the shark try and how well did they work? (He disguised himself as a shave ice man and a beachboy. Neither disguise fooled the pigs.)
3. What do you think of the two pigs so far? (Answers will vary.)
4. Why must the magic shark plan so much more than the big bad pig or Coyote did? (He is not as strong as the big bad pig or as clever as Coyote. Also, he is a sea animal rather than a land animal, and, given his great hunger, his attack must be quick and effective.)

Predicting/Purpose Setting

Ask if students' predictions were accurate. Have them read to the end of the story to find out what the shark does and how the story ends.

lei (LAY) a garland (usually of flowers)

ukulele (oo koo LAY lay) a four stringed instrument played by strumming, 'uke' is short for ukulele

nose flute a flute like instrument played by blowing air with the nose

In a few days, the magic shark was hungry for little pigs again. This time he dressed up as a beachboy, wearing white pants, a coconut leaf hat, and a lei around his neck. He knocked on the door of the second little pig's house and called, "Little Pig, Little Pig, let's talk story and play ukes."

The little pigs grabbed their ukulele and nose flute and opened the door. The beachboy smiled and the little pigs saw rows and rows of long, sharp white teeth and just in time, they slammed the door.

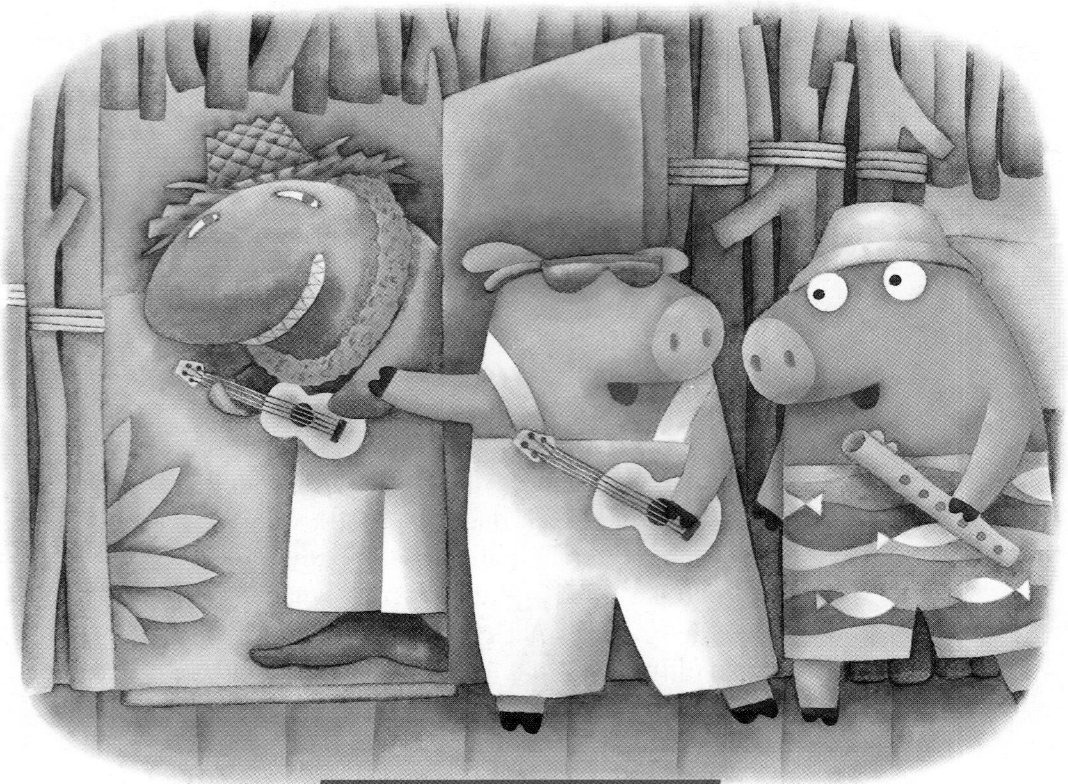

106

Students Acquiring English

Word Meaning As necessary, explain the following:

- A *beachboy* is someone who spends a lot of time at the beach, surfing and swimming and relaxing in the sun.
- *Ukes* is short for *ukuleles*.

QuickREFERENCE

Multicultural Link

Folktales Tell students that to *talk story* means to tell stories. Explain that many folktales were originally passed down from generation to generation by word of mouth. They were often polished and embellished with each retelling.

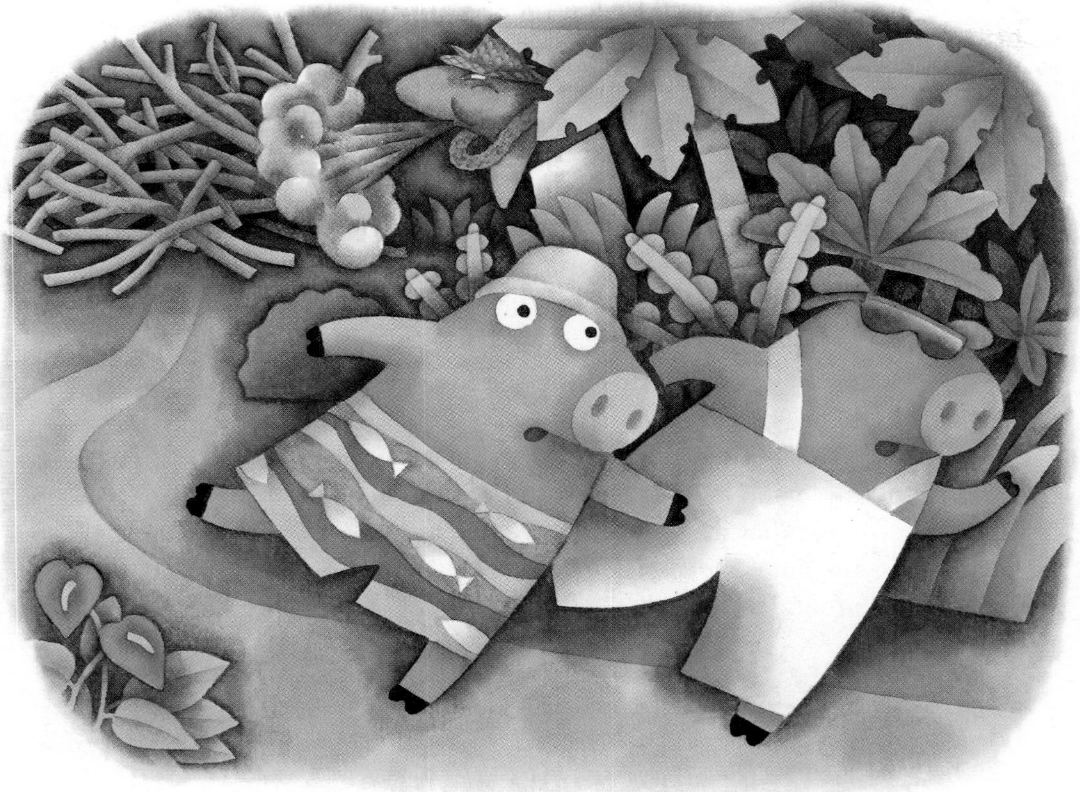

"Little Pig, Little Pig, let me come in," called the hot and hungry magic shark anxiously.

"Oh no," cried the little pigs. (They knew that was no friendly beachboy out on the steps.) "Not by the hairs on our chinny, chin, chins."

This made the magic shark upset so he roared, "Then I will huff and I will puff and I will blow your house down." Just as he said he would, the very upset magic shark huffed and the very upset magic shark puffed and the very upset magic shark blew down the house of the second little pig.

The little pig and his brother jumped out of the window and ran down the path to the house of the third little pig.

107

MINILESSON

Sequence

REVIEW & MAINTAIN

Teach/Model

Tell students that noting the sequence of events in a story makes it easier to understand.

Write these sentences on the board and ask students what's wrong with the sequence of events. Then have students rearrange the events in the proper order.

1. The first two little pigs ran to their brother's lava rock house.
2. The shark blew down the house of the second little pig.
3. Disguised as a beachboy, the shark knocked on the second pig's door.

Discuss how remembering the sequence in a story helps a reader summarize. Ask students what they could do if they failed to remember the sequence of events in a story. (reread; review with someone who's also read it)

Practice/Apply

After students have read pages 108–111, ask them to list the events in the order in which they occur. You may want to leave the list from this lesson on the board for reference.

SKILL FINDER

Full lesson/Reteaching, Theme 4, pp. 84B–84C

Minilessons, Theme 4, pp. 33, 77

Music Link

Ukulele The word *ukulele* means "leaping flea" in Hawaiian because the instrument is played as if a person's fingers are jumping off the strings. If possible, share some ukulele music with the class, such as *Hawaiian Mood* by Ohta-San.

Interact *with* Literature

Reading Strategies

Think About Words

Have a volunteer model the kinds of questions a reader might ask in order to figure out the meaning of the word *pangs*. For example:

- What word or words are around *pangs* that might provide a clue to its meaning? (*Hunger* modifies it. Hunger is a feeling, so perhaps *pangs* has something to do with feeling.)
- What happens when I try to substitute *feeling* for *pangs*? Does it make sense? (Yes. The sentence would read: *After a few days his hunger* feeling *was so bad that the magic shark decided to try again.*)

mu'u mu'u (MOO oo MOO oo) a long, loose fitting woman's dress

lauhala (loo HAH lah) leaf of the hala or Pandanus tree; used in weaving hats, rugs, and baskets

Once more the magic shark, hot and still hungry, swam angrily down to his watery home to plot and scheme. After a few days his hunger pangs were so bad that the magic shark decided to try again.

This time he went pretending to be a lei seller. He knocked on the third little pig's door and called sweetly, "Little Pig, Little Pig, let me come in. I have leis to sell."

The three little pigs loved to wear leis and were happy to hear a sweet voice calling.

They looked out and saw the lei seller in her mu'u mu'u and lauhala hat, with flower leis on her arms. But then, they also saw a shark's tail sticking out from under the mu'u mu'u. They knew who that was so they rushed around locking the doors and windows.

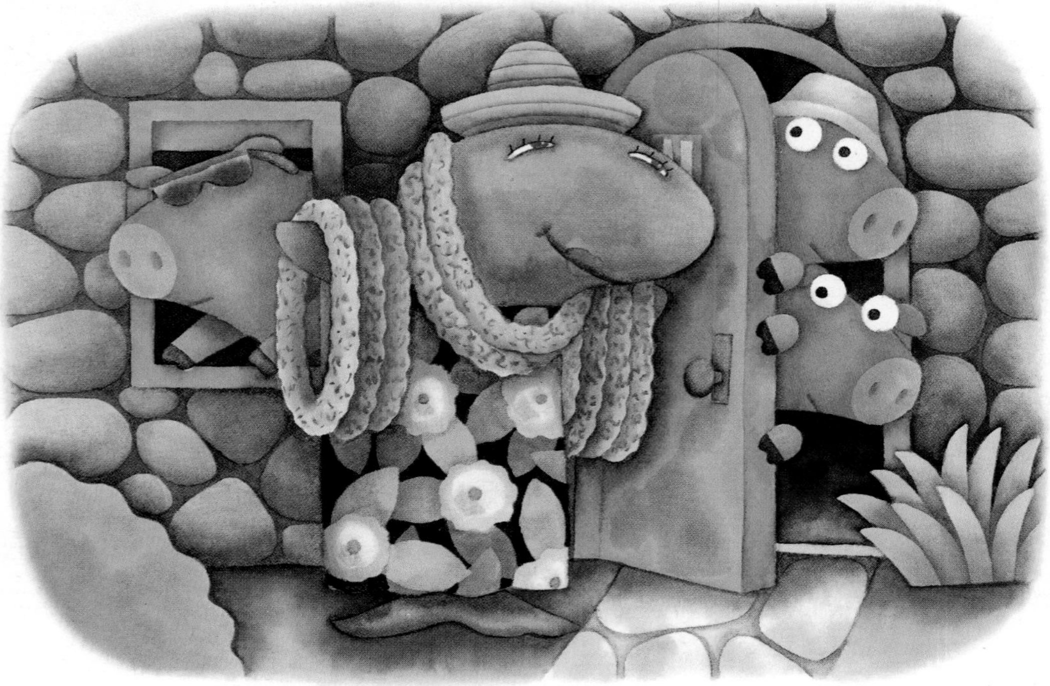

108

QuickREFERENCE

Journal

Saying "Welcome" Visitors to Hawaii are often greeted with leis made from orchids, carnations, and/or jasmines. Have students acquiring English share customs and greetings in their primary languages. Then invite students to write in their journals about other ways of saying "welcome" to someone. Have they ever greeted a person by giving him or her a gift?

"Little Pig, Little Pig, let me come in," called the magic shark, growing upset.

"Oh no," answered the little pigs. "Not by the hairs on our chinny, chin, chins."

"You will be sorry!" screamed the furious magic shark in his loudest voice. "I will huff and I will puff and I will blow your house down." No one answered and no one opened the door, so the furious magic shark huffed and the furious magic shark puffed and he huffed and he puffed and he blew . . . and nothing happened!

Again he huffed and he puffed and he huffed and he puffed and he blew and he blew and still nothing happened.

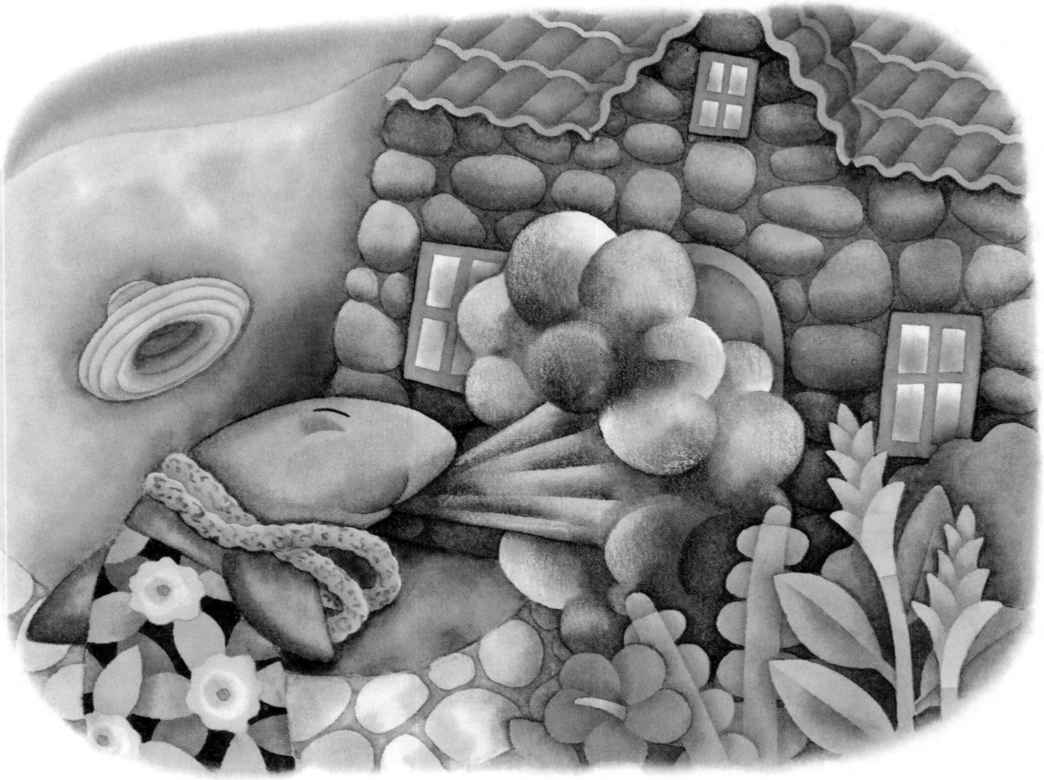

109

Students Acquiring English

Reading Aloud Invite students to practice reading aloud the shark's dialogue. Discuss how his anger increases and how a reader can tell this latest outburst is worse than those on pages 105 and 107.

Interact *with* Literature

Once more the furious magic shark huffed and the furious magic shark puffed and the furious magic shark huffed and the furious magic shark puffed and the furious magic shark blew and blew and still . . . the lava rock house stood firm.

Now this made the magic shark extremely furious. So, gathering up all of his air, the extremely furious magic shark huffed and puffed and huffed and puffed and huffed and puffed

and blew
and blew
and blew
and blew
and blew
and blew
and blew

until . . . whoosh; ker-splat, he fell on the ground all out of air looking like a flat balloon!

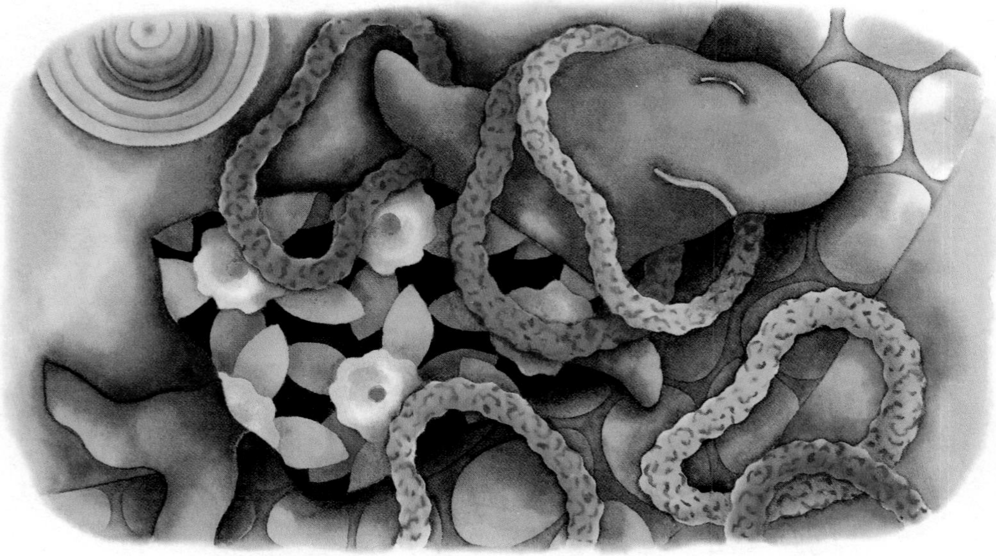

110

Students Acquiring English

Explain that *stood firm* means that the lava house remained standing. Have students demonstrate the sound words *whoosh* and *ker-splat*. Invite them to give examples of other sound words in several languages and in English.

QuickREFERENCE

Journal

Have students describe in their journals how the author builds suspense by

- repeating *huffed* and *puffed*
- unusual line breaks
- sound words such as *ker-splat*

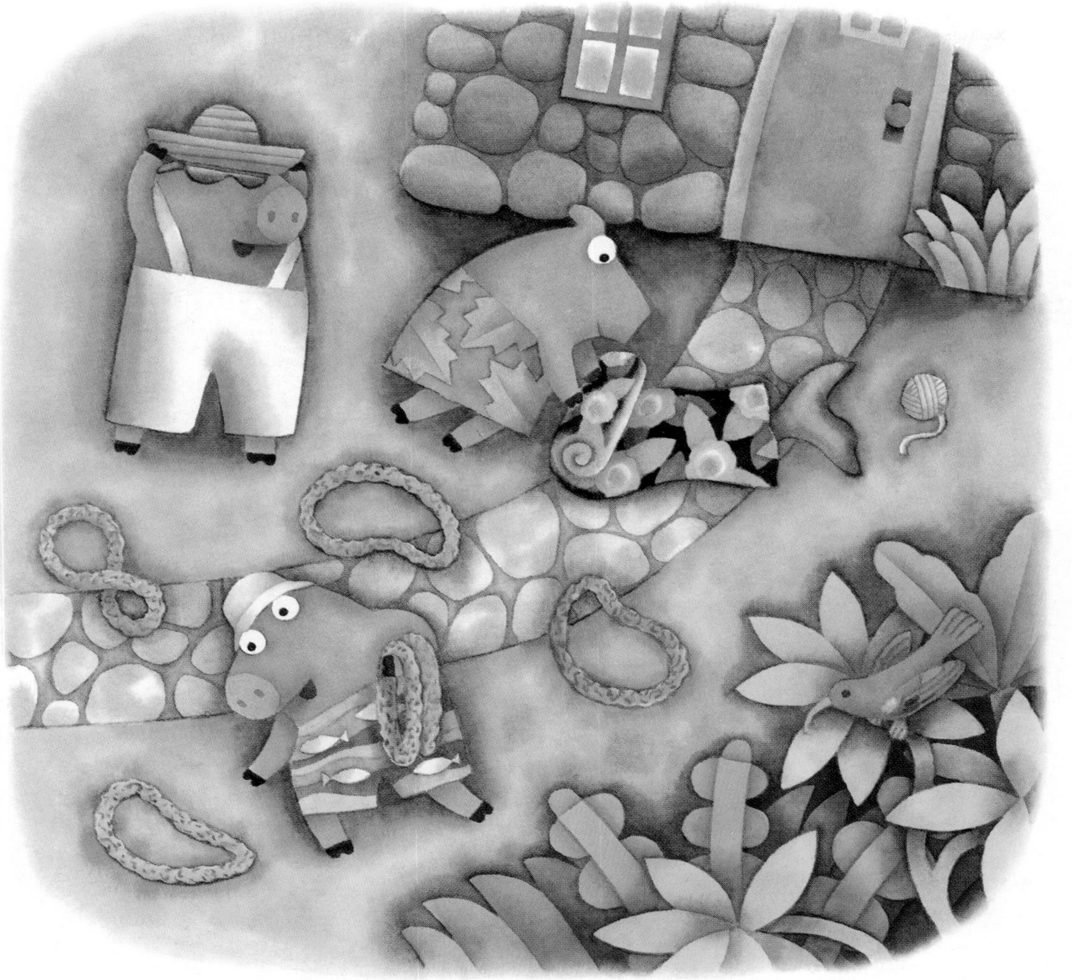

It was quiet and still and the three little pigs cautiously peeked out of the house. Seeing the very flat magic shark, they quickly ran outside, rolled him up like a straw mat, and tied a string around him.

Then . . . taking him off to the dump they threw him away.

111

Extra Support

Prompt discussion about why the shark looked so flat. Could a shark really end up looking like a flat balloon as a result of so much blowing? If students don't understand what a flat balloon looks like, show them one.

Interact with Literature

Guided Reading

Comprehension/Critical Thinking

1. What happened to the magic shark at the end of this story? (He blew so hard trying to knock down the lava house that he blew himself all out of air; he ended up looking like a flat balloon; the pigs rolled him up and took him to the dump.)
2. Why is an island a fun place for a party? (Answers will vary, but students might cite a variety of outdoor activities.)
3. What would the pigs' parents think of where their children are living? (They would be happy because the little pigs are safe and living close to one another.)

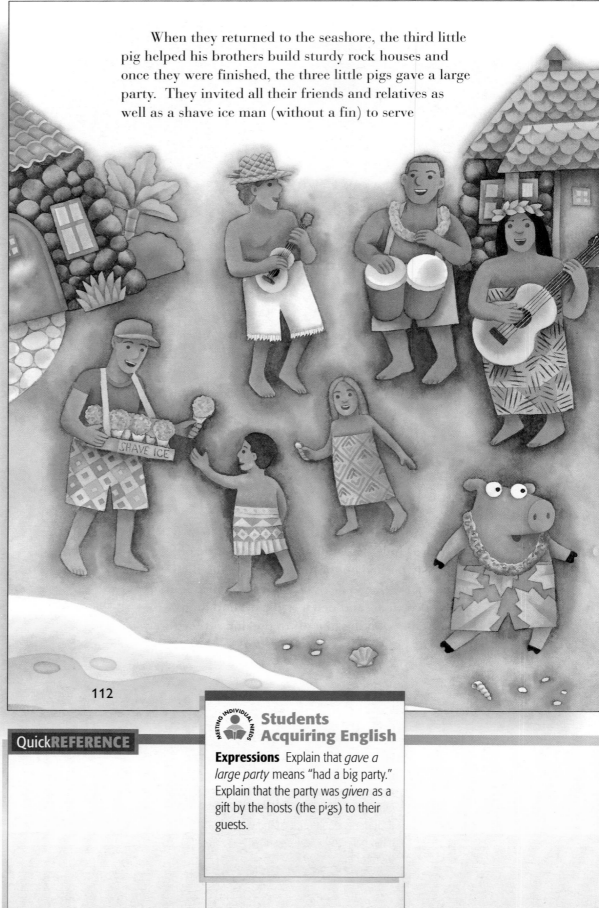

When they returned to the seashore, the third little pig helped his brothers build sturdy rock houses and once they were finished, the three little pigs gave a large party. They invited all their friends and relatives as well as a shave ice man (without a fin) to serve

SHAVE ICE

112

Self-Assessment

Ask students to assess their reading with questions such as the following:

- Were there any places where I had trouble understanding the story? What did I do?
- How did I handle the hard words in the story?
- Do I think this is a good story?

QuickREFERENCE

Students Acquiring English

Expressions Explain that *gave a large party* means "had a big party." Explain that the party was *given* as a gift by the hosts (the pigs) to their guests.

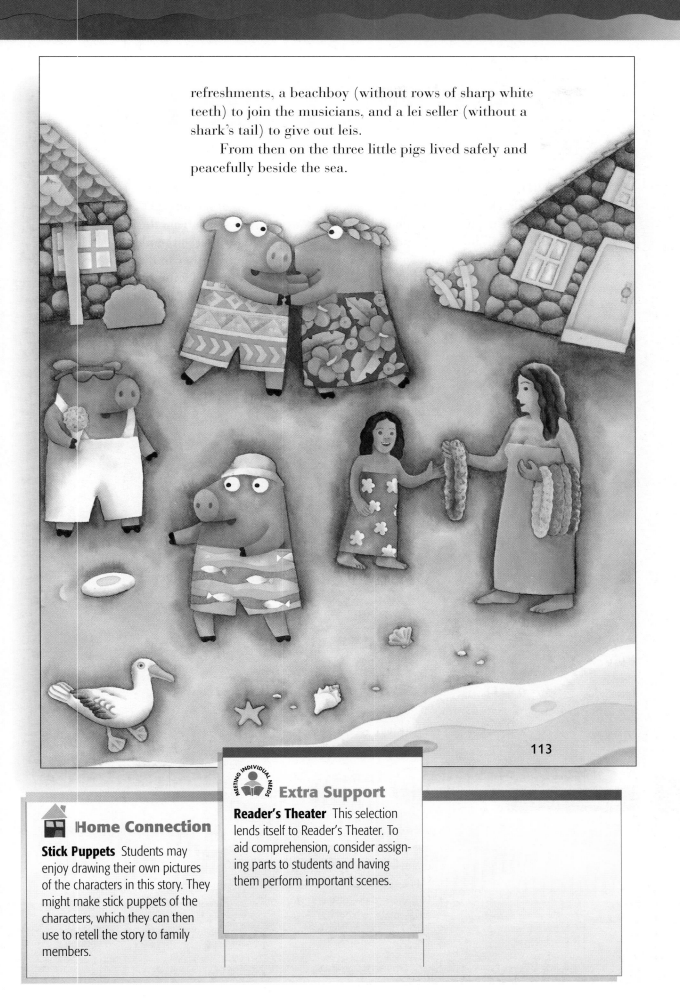

refreshments, a beachboy (without rows of sharp white teeth) to join the musicians, and a lei seller (without a shark's tail) to give out leis.

From then on the three little pigs lived safely and peacefully beside the sea.

113

Home Connection

Stick Puppets Students may enjoy drawing their own pictures of the characters in this story. They might make stick puppets of the characters, which they can then use to retell the story to family members.

Extra Support

Reader's Theater This selection lends itself to Reader's Theater. To aid comprehension, consider assigning parts to students and having them perform important scenes.

Interact *with* Literature

Responding Activities

Personal Response

- Suggest that students choose a favorite part of the story to describe in their journals.
- Allow students to choose their own way of responding to the selection.

Anthology Activities

Choose one of the activities on page 114 for students to do or have them choose one independently.

RESPONDING

Aloha, Little Pigs

Write a Paragraph

Dear Magic Shark

The shark didn't have much luck fooling the pigs. Can you think of a better disguise he could have used? Write a paragraph to give the shark advice on what to wear and how to act.

Act Out a Scene

Let Me Come In!

With a group of friends, act out your favorite scene from the story. You'll need one person to play each part and another to be the narrator. It might be fun to make props to help you tell the story.

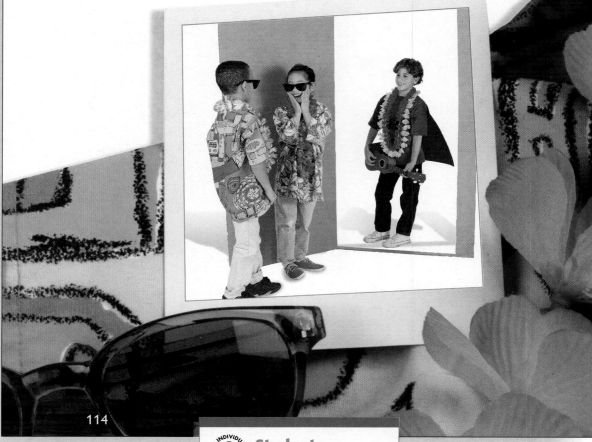

114

Informal Assessment

Responses should indicate a general understanding of the story and its structure.

Additional Support:

- Use the Guided Reading questions to review and if necessary reread.
- Have students summarize the story.
- Reread confusing sections aloud.

Quick**REFERENCE**

MEETING INDIVIDUAL NEEDS

Students Acquiring English

Students who are gaining proficiency with written English may respond by role-playing or by drawing. For example, for the activity "Dear Magic Shark," students can draw a picture of a shark in disguise and work with a classmate to label it.

Home Connection

News from Hawaii Encourage students to work with family members to find magazine and/or newspaper articles about Hawaii.

More Responding Activities

Make Masks

Cooperative Learning

Students may enjoy working together to make masks of the story characters. These can be used to re-enact the story.

Materials
- paper plates
- scissors
- string or yarn
- markers or crayons

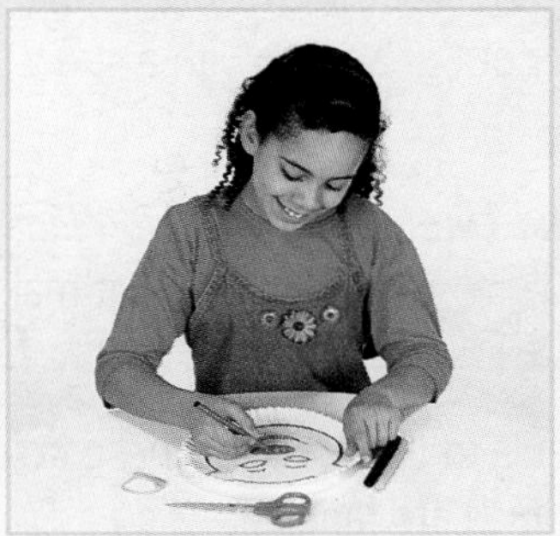

1. Draw a pig or a shark face on a paper plate.

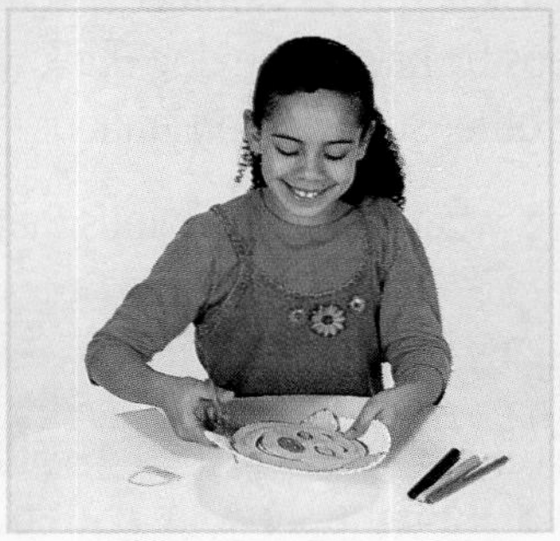

2. Cut out the face and eyes. Make holes on the side for string.

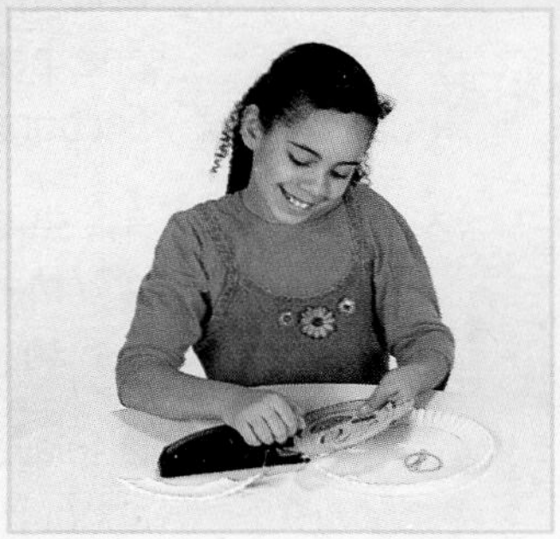

3. Run the string through the side holes and secure with knots or staples.

Literature Discussion

Note: Guidelines for conducting a literature discussion can be found on page 114L.

- Were you satisfied with the ending of this story, or can you think of a different ending?
- Who is the trickiest villain—the big bad pig, Coyote, or the shark? Why?

Selection Connections

LAB, p. 8

Have students complete the portion of the chart relating to the story.

Compose a Song

Invite students to write a song that the three Hawaiian pigs might sing at the party. For example: "Ding, Dong, the Shark Is Dead"; "He'll Be Comin' Round the Coral Reef When He Comes"; "He's Huffing, He's Puffing" (melody: "It's Raining, It's Pouring").

Comprehension Check

To check selection comprehension use these questions and/or *Literacy Activity Book* page 31.

1. What did the Hawaiian pigs do for fun? (They played tag and went fishing and surfing.)
2. Why couldn't the shark catch the pigs when they were on their surfboards? (He knew they were too good at surfing and they traveled very fast.)
3. Why didn't the shark's disguises work? (Parts of the shark showed through, or he smiled and the pigs could tell he was a shark by his teeth.)

Literacy Activity Book, p. 31

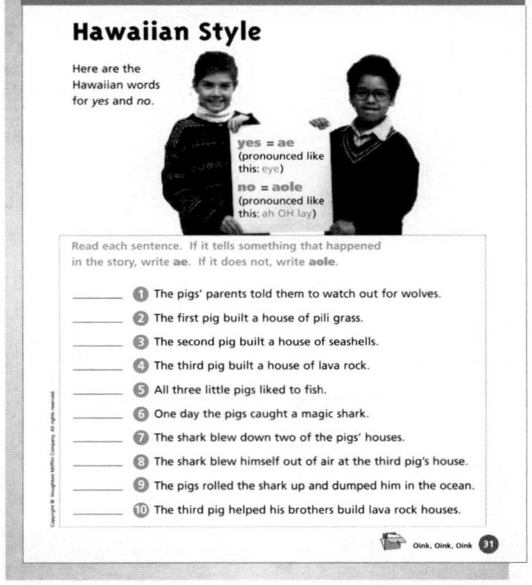

Hawaiian Style

Here are the Hawaiian words for *yes* and *no*.

yes = ae (pronounced like this: eye)

no = aole (pronounced like this: ah OH lay)

Read each sentence. If it tells something that happened in the story, write **ae**. If it does not, write **aole**.

_______ 1. The pigs' parents told them to watch out for wolves.

_______ 2. The first pig built a house of pili grass.

_______ 3. The second pig built a house of seashells.

_______ 4. The third pig built a house of lava rock.

_______ 5. All three little pigs liked to fish.

_______ 6. One day the pigs caught a magic shark.

_______ 7. The shark blew down two of the pigs' houses.

_______ 8. The shark blew himself out of air at the third pig's house.

_______ 9. The pigs rolled the shark up and dumped him in the ocean.

_______ 10. The third pig helped his brothers build lava rock houses.

Oink, Oink, Oink 31

Portfolio Opportunity

- Selection comprehension: Save *Literacy Activity Book* p. 31.
- Writing samples: Save responses to other responding activities.

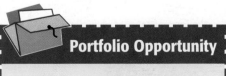

Instruct *and* Integrate

Comprehension

Literacy Activity Book, p. 32

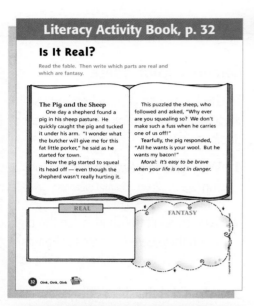
Is It Real?

Read the fable. Then write which parts are real and which are fantasy.

The Pig and the Sheep

One day a shepherd found a pig in his sheep pasture. He quickly caught the pig and tucked it under his arm. "I wonder what the butcher will give me for this fat little porker," he said as he started for town.

Now the pig started to squeal its head off — even though the shepherd wasn't really hurting it.

This puzzled the sheep, who followed and asked, "Why ever are you squealing so? We don't make such a fuss when he carries one of us off!"

Tearfully, the pig responded, "All he wants is your wool. But he wants my bacon!"

Moral: It's easy to be brave when your life is not in danger.

REAL

FANTASY

32 Oink, Oink, Oink

Transparency 1–11

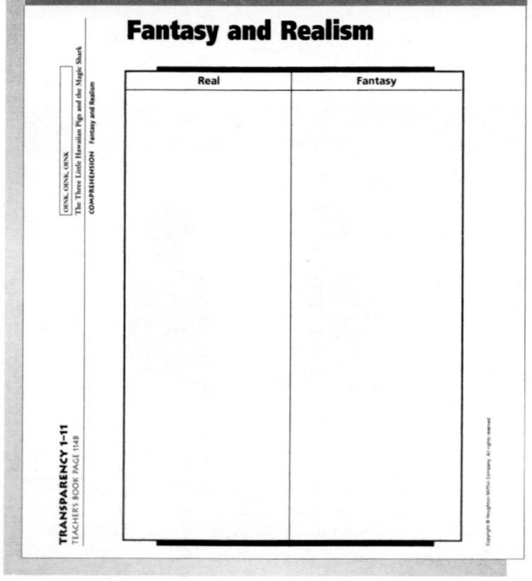
Fantasy and Realism

Real	Fantasy

TRANSPARENCY 1–11
TEACHER'S BOOK PAGE 114B

Informal Assessment

Check students' responses during discussion or on *Literacy Activity Book* page 32 to see if they demonstrate an understanding of fantasy and realism.

Additional Support:

Reteaching, p. 114C

Minilessons, pp. 57; 95;
Theme 5, p. 211

INTERACTIVE LEARNING

TESTED SKILL

Fantasy/Realism

LAB, p. 32

Teach/Model

Invite students to role-play the difference between realism and fantasy. For example, have a volunteer role-play a dog drinking water out of a dog dish. Then ask another volunteer to turn this realistic scene into a fantasy one, perhaps by having the dog drink water out of a glass with a straw. Encourage other such demonstrations.

Ask students what makes it obvious that *The Three Little Hawaiian Pigs and the Magic Shark* is a fantasy. (animals talking) Then discuss what makes the story funny. (the animals do many things humans do)

Display Transparency 1–11. Then ask students to tell which of these details about Hawaii from the story are real and which are fantasy.

- **beaches**
- **pigs having money**
- **ocean**
- **pigs building houses**
- **tropical fish**
- **magic shark**
- **fishing nets**
- **tide pools**
- **pigs surfing**

Real	Fantasy
beaches	pigs having money
ocean	pigs building houses

Explain that the real details were not made up—they actually exist. Add that although the fantasy details use some part of reality—there are pigs—they contain other parts that were made up by the author.

Practice/Apply

- Have students use *Literacy Activity Book* page 32 to identify the fable as a fantasy.
- Have students classify several fiction books from the classroom library as fantasy or realism.

SKILL FINDER Minilessons, pp. 57; 95; Theme 5, p. 211

Reteaching Fantasy/Realism

Fantasy and reality are an integral part of comic strips, and the following activity capitalizes on this fact.

Cut out two kinds of comic strips from your daily newspaper: ones that are set in the "real world" and ones that employ fantasy elements, such as talking animals and robots. Then put the strips in a box.

Invite students to select a strip from the box and identify the strip as an example of realism or fantasy. Ask them to name elements that are real and fantastical in each strip. You might use the questions in the box below to prompt students' responses.

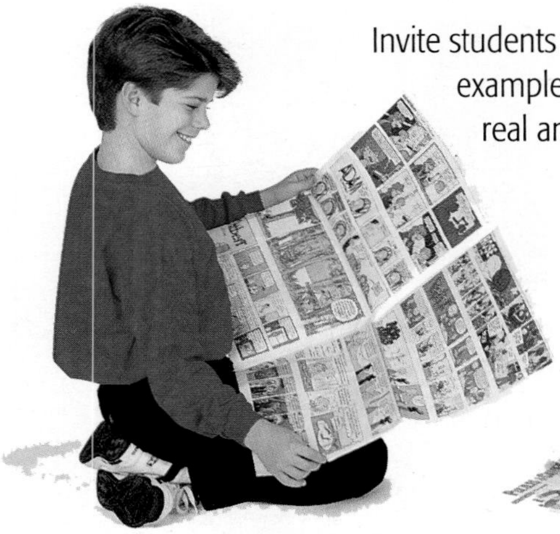

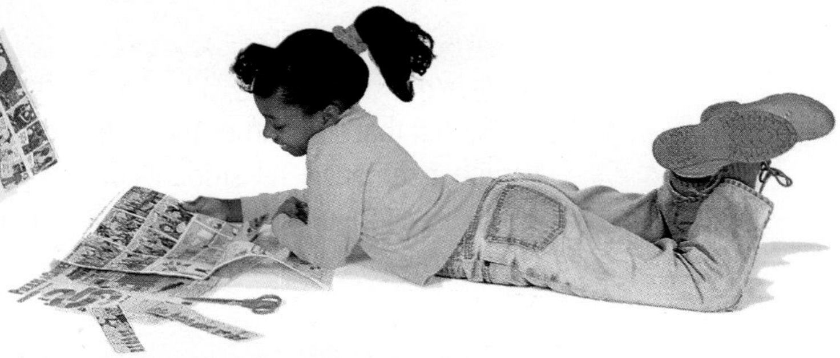

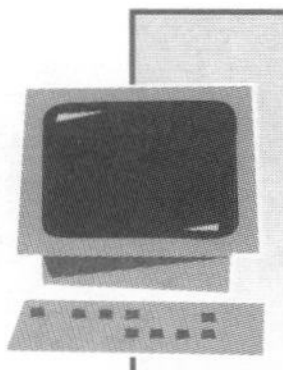

Students can use the **Channel R.E.A.D.** videodisc "The Ordinary Princess" for additional support with Fantasy/Realism.

To extend this activity, students could:

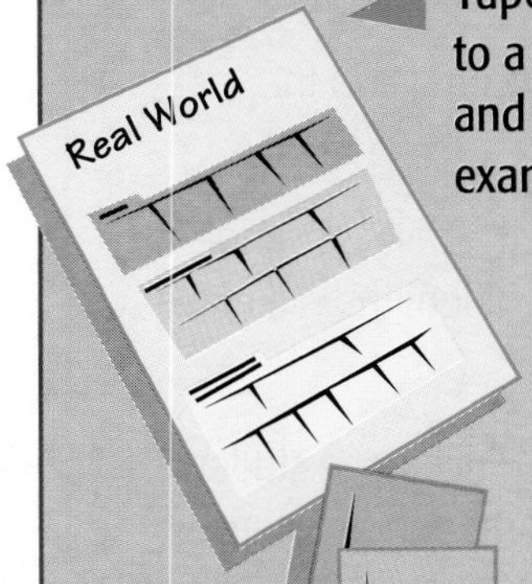
Real World

- Tape each kind of strip to a sheet of chart paper, and then daily add other examples.
- Glue the strip at the top of a sheet of paper and then write a review of it.

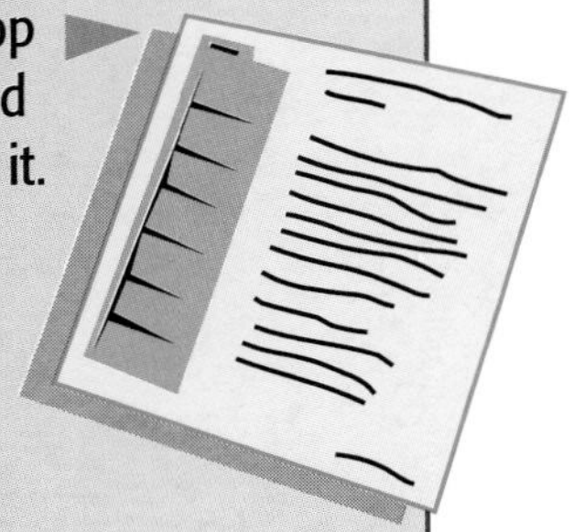

- Find examples of advertising images that employ realistic figures, such as fictional spokespersons, and fantasy creatures, such as talking animals.

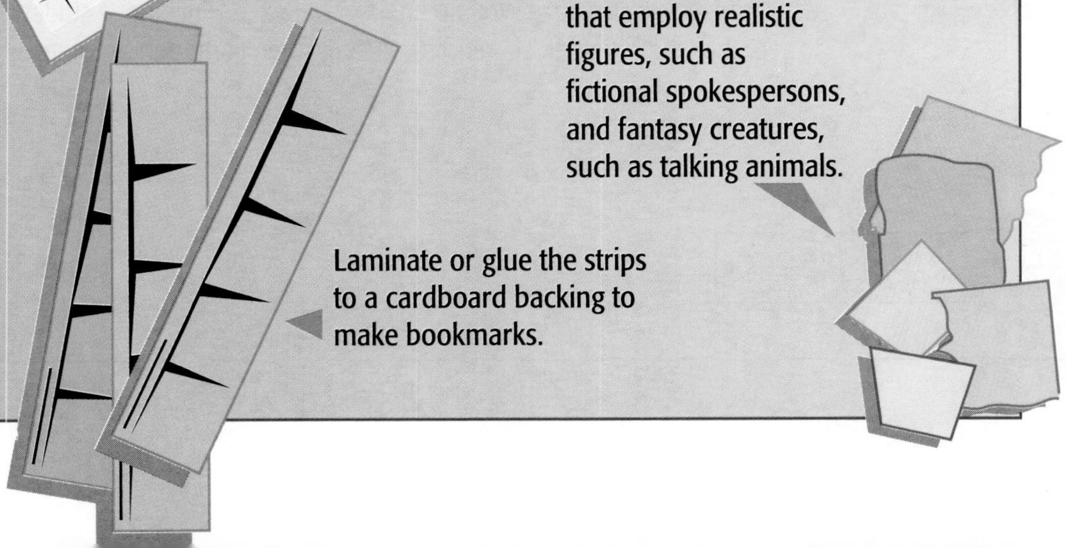

- Laminate or glue the strips to a cardboard backing to make bookmarks.

Questions About Comics

- What is real in the comic strip? What's make-believe?
- Why do you think this comic strip is popular?
- How could you change the comic strip to make it more real (or fantastical)?

Portfolio Opportunity

Save *Literacy Activity Book* p. 32 to record students' understanding of fantasy and realism.

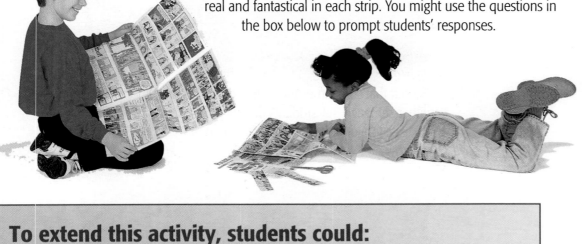

Instruct *and* Integrate

Writing Skills and Activities

INTERACTIVE LEARNING

Combining Sentences: Compound Sentences

TESTED SKILL

LAB, p. 33

Teach/Model Write these sentences on the board.

The pigs surfed.

The shark watched them from below.

Point out that sometimes the idea in one sentence can go with the idea in another sentence. Tell students that they can combine the two sentences to make a longer sentence called a compound sentence. Combine the sentences on the board as shown.

The pigs surfed, and the shark watched them from below.

Explain that the two sentences are joined by using a comma and the word *and.*

Display Transparency 1–12. Have volunteers combine the pairs of simple sentences. Tell students that using sentences of different lengths will make their writing more interesting.

Practice/Apply Assign the activity Creative Writing: Animal Characters. Encourage students to vary the length of their sentences by using some compound sentences.

SKILL FINDER Reading-Writing Workshop, p. 116–117F

Transparency 1–12

OINK, OINK, OINK
The Three Little Hawaiian Pigs and the Magic Shark
WRITING SKILLS Combining Sentences: Compound Sentences

Combining Sentences: Compound Sentences

	Simple Sentences	Compound Sentences
	The pigs surfed. The shark watched them from below.	The pigs surfed, and the shark watched them from below.
1	One little pig built his house. The others went fishing.	
2	The gentle trade winds blew. The sun shined.	
3	The shark knocked on the door. The pig peeked out of the window.	
4	The beachboy played music. The shave ice man served refreshments.	

TRANSPARENCY 1–12
TEACHER'S BOOK PAGE 114D

Two to One

This story is about the three little pigs and the magic shark. Look for five sentences that could be combined. Write them as compound sentences.

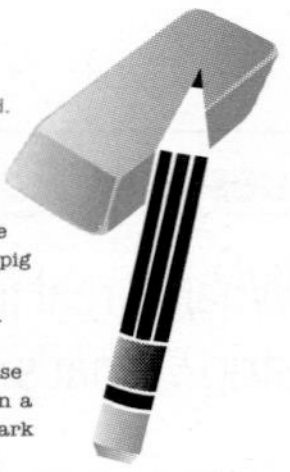

Three Little Heroes

This week, three little pigs have become heroes! They took care of a pesky shark. The shark came into their yard. The pigs ran inside to hide. One pig began closing windows. Another locked the front door. The shark started knocking with his big fin. He was very hungry. The pigs were very scared. The angry shark began to huff and puff. The house shook. Finally, the shark ran out of air. He fell in a heap. The pigs took him off to the dump. The shark won't be bothering them anymore!

1 ______

2 ______

3 ______

4 ______

5 ______

Oink, Oink, Oink 33

Informal Assessment

Check students' writing for creativity and imagination as well as to see if they have included compound sentences. If students have enjoyed a particular activity, suggest they go on with it in their self-selected writing.

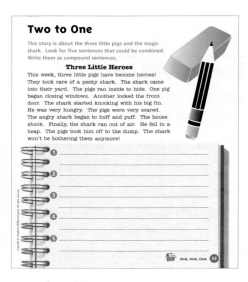

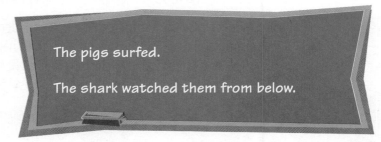

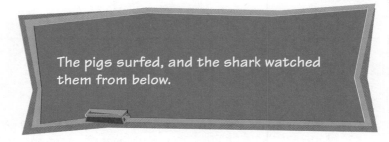

Writing Activities

Plan a House

Remind students that the three Hawaiian pigs built their houses from pili grass, driftwood, and lava rock. Have students write a paragraph of at least five sentences about the kind of house they would want to build.

- What would it be made of?
- What would it look like?
- Where would it be?

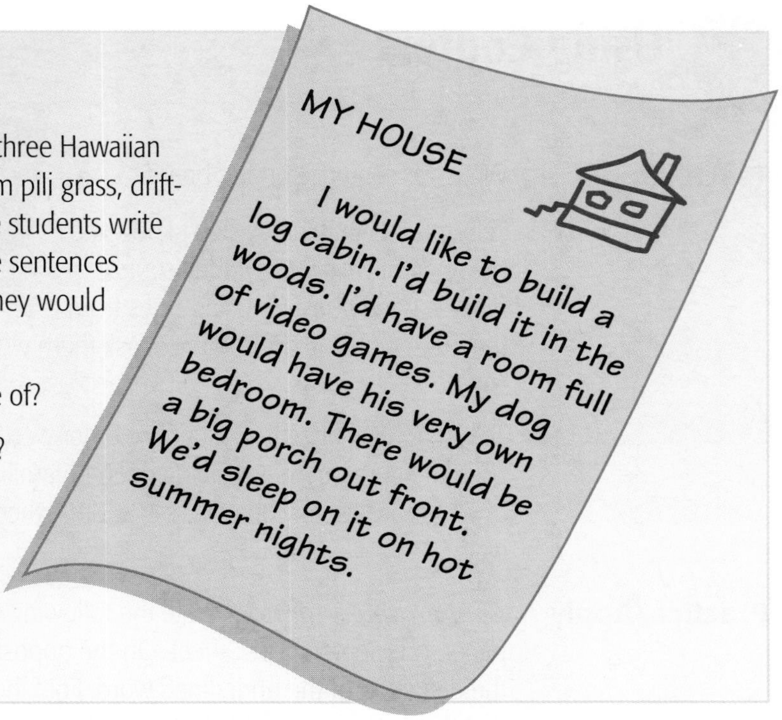
MY HOUSE
I would like to build a log cabin. I'd build it in the woods. I'd have a room full of video games. My dog would have his very own bedroom. There would be a big porch out front. We'd sleep on it on hot summer nights.

Creative Writing: Animal Characters

Suggest that students write their own stories using animal characters. Encourage them to have their characters do some things that only humans could really do. Suggest that in planning their stories, they make a list of human behaviors that might work well with their story idea. (*See the Writer's Craft Minilesson on page 97.*)

Write a Poem

Have students write poems using the Hawaiian words in *The Three Little Hawaiian Pigs and the Magic Shark.* Suggest that they might want to rhyme the Hawaiian words with English ones, but explain that their poems do not have to rhyme at all.

Students can use The Learning Company's new elementary writing center for all their writing activities.

Portfolio Opportunity

- Save *Literacy Activity Book* page 33 to record students' understanding of combining sentences to form compound sentences.
- Save responses to activities on this page for writing samples.

Instruct *and* Integrate

Word Skills and Strategies

INTERACTIVE LEARNING

Literacy Activity Book, p. 34

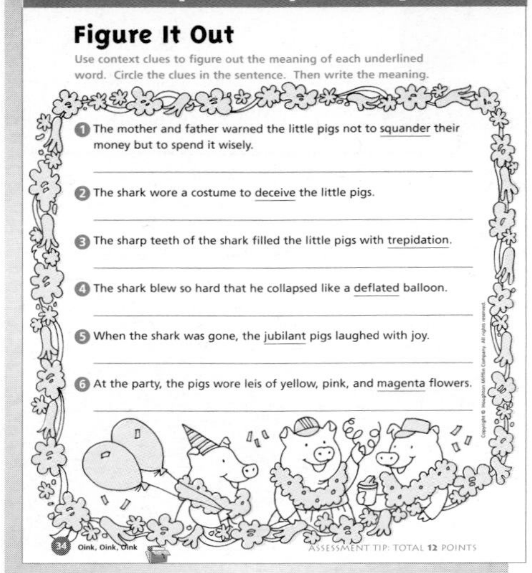
Figure It Out

Use context clues to figure out the meaning of each underlined word. Circle the clues in the sentence. Then write the meaning.

1. The mother and father warned the little pigs not to squander their money but to spend it wisely.
2. The shark wore a costume to deceive the little pigs.
3. The sharp teeth of the shark filled the little pigs with trepidation.
4. The shark blew so hard that he collapsed like a deflated balloon.
5. When the shark was gone, the jubilant pigs laughed with joy.
6. At the party, the pigs wore leis of yellow, pink, and magenta flowers.

34 Oink, Oink, Oink — ASSESSMENT TIP: TOTAL 12 POINTS

Using Context

TESTED SKILL

LAB, p. 34

Teach/Model

Write this sentence on the board.

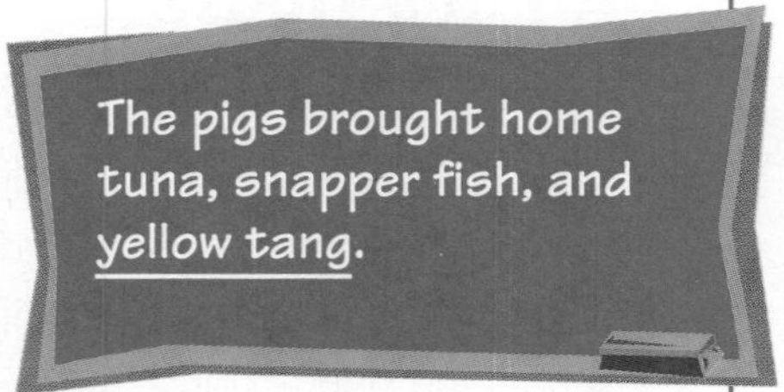
The pigs brought home tuna, snapper fish, and yellow tang.

Tell students that if they don't know the meaning of *yellow tang*, they could make a good guess by using clues from the other words in the sentence. Ask them what clues they would use. (Yellow tang are listed with tuna and snapper fish, so they are probably a kind of fish.)

Tell students that context clues are other words in a sentence that can be used to figure out the meaning of an unfamiliar word. Point out that lists of words are useful context clues but that there are other types of clues as well.

Practice/Apply

Cooperative Learning Write the following sentences on three sheets of paper, one sentence per sheet. On the opposite side of each sheet, write the definition of the underlined word. Fold the sheet and paperclip it so that the sentence is visible but the definition is not. Divide the class into groups and give each group one of the sentences. Have students guess the meaning of the underlined word and identify the clues they used. When the group thinks they have figured out the meaning, have them remove the paperclip to find out if they are right. Then have them reclip the paper and pass the sentence on to another group.

Sentence	Meaning	Clues
The villain was hated by every-one for his nefarious deeds.	evil, wicked	villain, hated
The salad contained leaves of spinach, lettuce, and escarole.	a leafy vegetable	leaves, spinach, lettuce
The winners wore cheerful grins, but the losers looked morose.	gloomy, unhappy	losers opposite of winners suggests morose is opposite of cheerful

Informal Assessment

Use Practice/Apply to check students' understanding of using context clues.

Additional Support:

Reteaching, page 114G

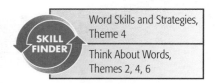

SKILL FINDER

Word Skills and Strategies, Theme 4
Think About Words, Themes 2, 4, 6

Reteaching

Using Context

MEETING INDIVIDUAL NEEDS

Write this sentence on the board and read it aloud.

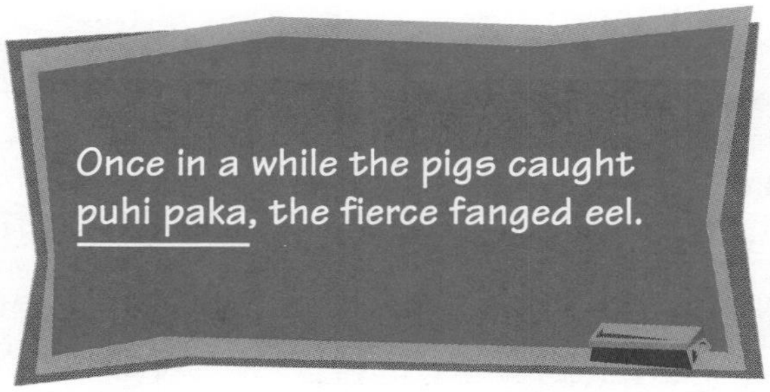
Once in a while the pigs caught
puhi paka, the fierce fanged eel.

Ask students what *puhi paka* means. (a fierce fanged eel)

Point out that the meaning of the word is given in the sentence. Write the sentence below on the board and read it aloud.

The shark was ravenous and
couldn't wait to eat all three pigs.

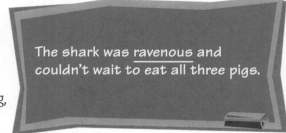

Ask students what they think *ravenous* means. (hungry) Point out that although the sentence doesn't tell the meaning of *ravenous,* some of the words are clues to the meaning. Ask students what clues they used. *(couldn't wait, eat)*

Tell students that when they come to an unfamiliar word in their reading, other words in the sentence will often help them figure it out.

MINILESSON

Dictionary

Alphabetical Order

Teach/Model Write these words in a random cluster on the board.

reason listen butter rent elephant load

Ask students to help you list the words in alphabetical order. Model the process by starting with the first letter of each word, and where the letters are the same, going on to the second letter, and so on.

Practice/Apply Write each of these words on a large index card and group the cards as shown. Divide the class into teams of five, and give each team one set of words. Tell students that when you say "Go," they should each take a word, hold it up for the group to see, and then arrange themselves in alphabetical order. The first group to arrange themselves correctly scores a point. After the first round, have groups exchange words and play again.

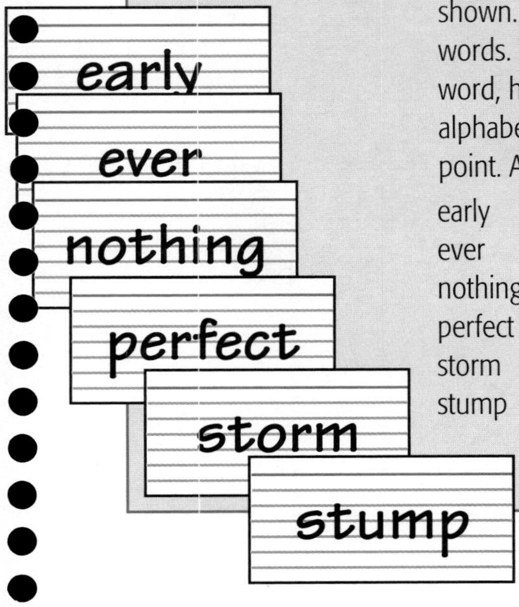
early
ever
nothing
perfect
storm
stump

early	great	nine	clean	order
ever	itch	parent	clover	organ
nothing	quiz	repeat	history	queen
perfect	quote	roam	honey	silly
storm	thank	weather	interest	uncle
stump	toward	went	keep	upset

Portfolio Opportunity

Save *Literacy Activity Book* page 34 to record students' understanding of using context clues.

Building Vocabulary

Literacy Activity Book, p. 35

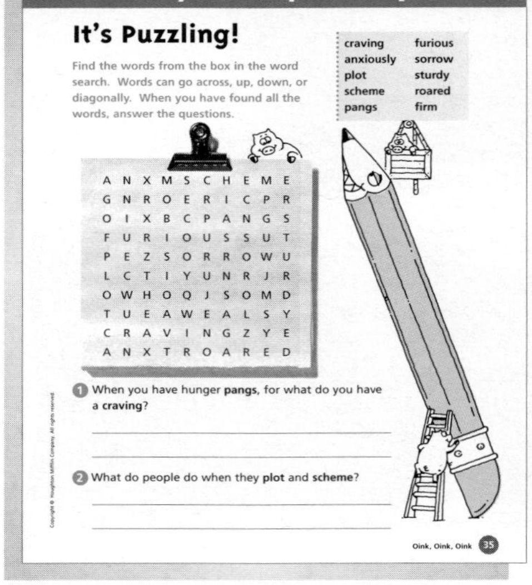

It's Puzzling!

Find the words from the box in the word search. Words can go across, up, down, or diagonally. When you have found all the words, answer the questions.

craving	furious
anxiously	sorrow
plot	sturdy
scheme	roared
pangs	firm

A	N	X	M	S	C	H	E	M	E
G	N	R	O	E	R	I	C	P	R
O	I	X	B	C	P	A	N	G	S
F	U	R	I	O	U	S	S	U	T
P	E	Z	S	O	R	R	O	W	U
L	C	T	I	Y	U	N	R	J	R
O	W	H	O	Q	J	S	O	M	D
T	U	E	A	W	E	A	L	S	Y
C	R	A	V	I	N	G	Z	Y	E
A	N	X	T	R	O	A	R	E	D

1. When you have hunger **pangs**, for what do you have a **craving**?

2. What do people do when they **plot** and **scheme**?

Copyright © Houghton Mifflin Company. All rights reserved.

Oink, Oink, Oink 35

Use this page to review Selection Vocabulary.

Vocabulary Activities

Synonym Search

sorrow 1 **sadness 1**	**plan 2** **plot 2** **scheme 2**	**quickly 2** **speedily 2** **rapidly 2**
sack 1 **bag 1**	**finished 2** **completed 2** **done 2**	**extremely 1** **very 1**
frightened 2 **scared 2** **afraid 2**	**hurt 3** **harmed 3** **damaged 3** **injured 3**	**happily 2** **cheerfully 2** **joyfully 2**
delicious 1 **tasty 1**		**carefully 1** **cautiously 1**
creatures 1 **animals 1**	**strong 1** **sturdy 1**	**certainly 2** **surely 2** **absolutely 2**
shining 2 **gleaming 2** **glowing 2**	**certainly 2** **surely 2** **absolutely 2**	

Remind students that when the little pigs escaped from the shark, the shark was very mad. Write *mad* on the board, and ask students what other words they can think of that have the same or nearly the same meaning. (*annoyed, angry, furious*) Write their responses on the board and draw a circle around all of the words. Tell students that words with the same or nearly the same meaning are called synonyms.

Write each of the words shown (with its corresponding number) on a separate slip of paper, and give one slip to each student. Have students find the other student or students whose words are synonyms for their own word. The number on each slip will tell them how many other students they must find. Once students have formed their synonym pairs or groups, have them write their synonyms on the board and draw a circle around them.

Vocabulary Notebook

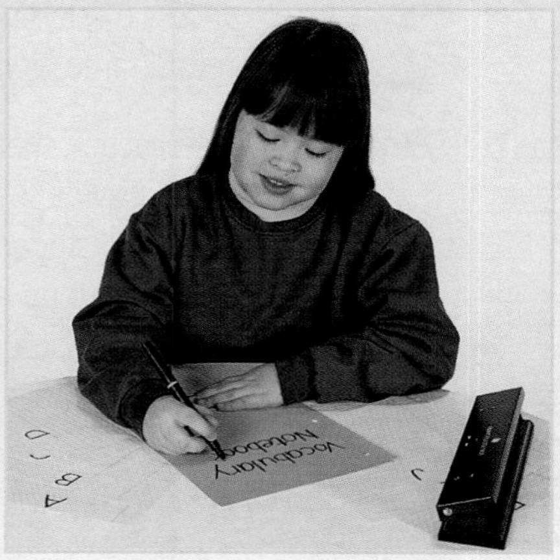
Vocabulary Notebook

Ask students what they would do to remember a friend's telephone number. (write it down) Point out that the same idea can be applied to learning the meaning of a new word.

Tell students that they will be making special notebooks for recording new words that they want to learn or remember. Have each student staple or three-hole punch 26 sheets of lined paper and write a letter of the alphabet at the top of each sheet. Students can use construction paper to make a cover for their notebook.

Suggest that when students record a word, they write it in a sentence and also write down its meaning. They might even want to draw a picture.

Spelling

MINILESSON

Spelling Words
*three
*tail
*beach
*play
*deep
*away
*please
chain

Challenge Words
*easy
*really
*reef
*creature

*Starred words or forms of the words appear in *The Three Little Hawaiian Pigs and the Magic Shark*.

TESTED SKILL

Spelling Long *a* and Long *e*

LAB, pp. 36–37

- Write *chain* and *play* on the board. Say the words and have students repeat them. Ask students to name the vowel sound in each word. (/ā/) Have students tell how the /ā/ sound is spelled in these words. (*ai, ay*) Point out that the *ai* pattern appears in the middle of a word, and the *ay* pattern appears at the end of a word.
- Write *beach* and *deep* on the board. Say the words and have students repeat them. Ask students to name the vowel sound in each word. (/ē/) Elicit the two spelling patterns for the /ē/ sound. (*ea, ee*)
- Write the Spelling Words on the board. Tell students that each Spelling Word has the /ā/ sound or the /ē/ sound. Say the Spelling Words and have students repeat them.

Spelling Assessment

Pretest
Say each underlined word, read the sentence, and then repeat the word. Have students write only the underlined words.

1. The three pigs live by the sea.
2. That pig has a curly tail.
3. Bring your fishing rod to the beach.
4. It's fun to play in the waves!
5. Do sharks stay in deep water?
6. Stay away from the rocks when you surf.
7. Can you please pass me my towel?
8. I lost my gold chain in the sand.

Test
Spelling Words Use the Pretest sentences.

Challenge Words

9. Let's go diving near the coral reef.
10. It's not easy to catch a big fish.
11. What sea creature has eight long arms?
12. Those sand crabs are really fast.

SKILL FINDER
Daily Language Practice, p. 114K
Reading-Writing Workshop, p. 117E

Literacy Activity Book, p. 36

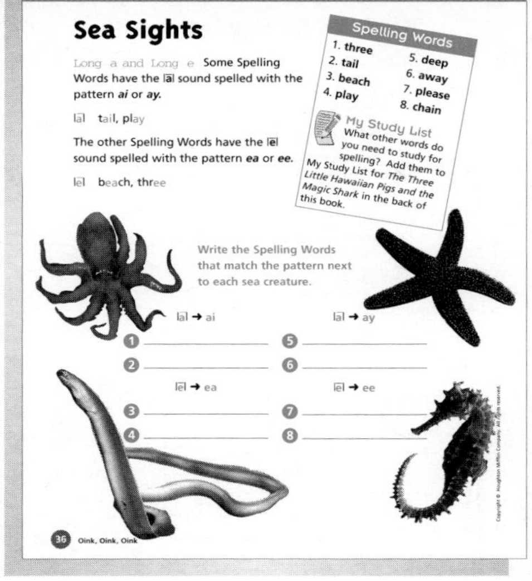
Sea Sights
Spelling Words
1. three
2. tail
3. beach
4. play
5. deep
6. away
7. please
8. chain
Long a and Long e Some Spelling Words have the /ā/ sound spelled with the pattern ai or ay.
tail, play
The other Spelling Words have the /ē/ sound spelled with the pattern ea or ee.
beach, three
My Study List What other words do you need to study for spelling? Add them to My Study List for The Three Little Hawaiian Pigs and the Magic Shark in the back of this book.
Write the Spelling Words that match the pattern next to each sea creature.
/ā/ → ai
/ā/ → ay
/ē/ → ea
/ē/ → ee
36 Oink, Oink, Oink

Literacy Activity Book, p. 37

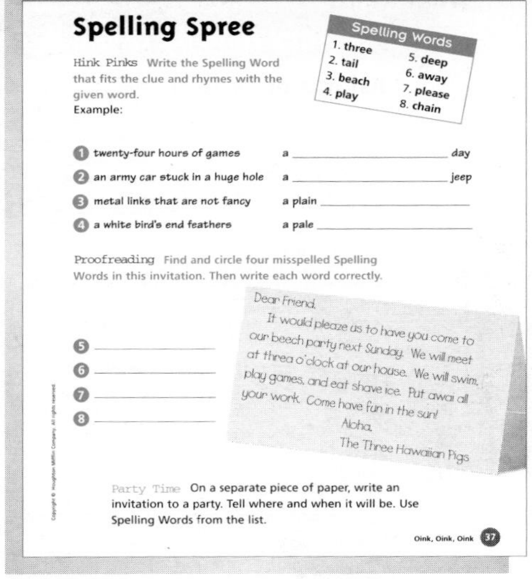
Spelling Spree
Spelling Words
1. three
2. tail
3. beach
4. play
5. deep
6. away
7. please
8. chain
Hink Pinks Write the Spelling Word that fits the clue and rhymes with the given word.
Example:
twenty-four hours of games a day
an army car stuck in a huge hole a jeep
metal links that are not fancy a plain
a white bird's end feathers a pale
Proofreading Find and circle four misspelled Spelling Words in this invitation. Then write each word correctly.
Dear Friend,
It would pleaze us to have you come to our beach party next Sunday. We will meet at threa o'clock at our house. We will swim, play games, and eat shave ice. Put awai all your work. Come have fun in the sun!
Aloha,
The Three Hawaiian Pigs
Party Time On a separate piece of paper, write an invitation to a party. Tell where and when it will be. Use Spelling Words from the list.
Oink, Oink, Oink 37

MEETING INDIVIDUAL NEEDS

Challenge

Challenge Words Practice Have students use the Challenge Words to write safety tips for beachgoers.

Instruct *and* Integrate

Grammar

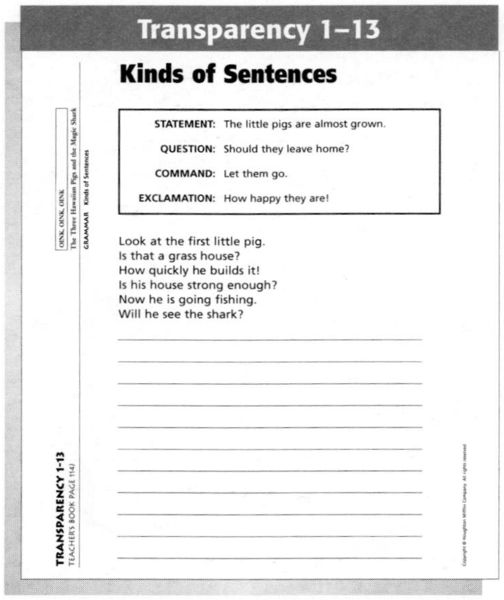
Transparency 1–13

Kinds of Sentences

STATEMENT: The little pigs are almost grown.
QUESTION: Should they leave home?
COMMAND: Let them go.
EXCLAMATION: How happy they are!

Look at the first little pig.
Is that a grass house?
How quickly he builds it!
Is his house strong enough?
Now he is going fishing.
Will he see the shark?

TRANSPARENCY 1–13
TEACHER'S BOOK PAGE 114J

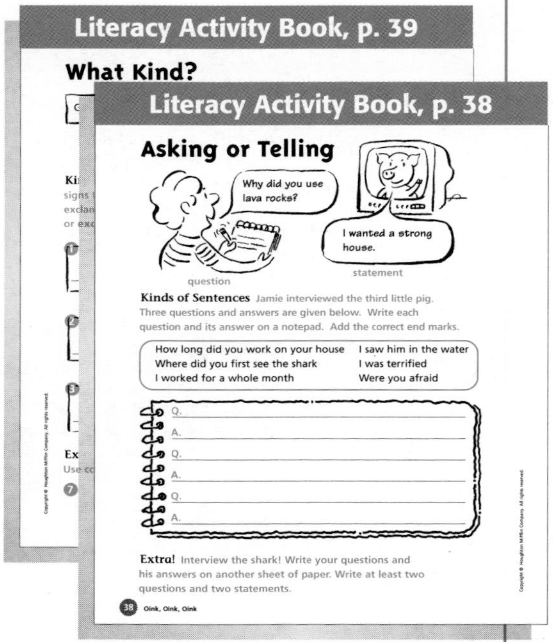
Literacy Activity Book, p. 39

What Kind?

Literacy Activity Book, p. 38

Asking or Telling

Why did you use lava rocks?
I wanted a strong house.
question
statement

Kinds of Sentences Jamie interviewed the third little pig. Three questions and answers are given below. Write each question and its answer on a notepad. Add the correct end marks.

How long did you work on your house
Where did you first see the shark
I worked for a whole month
I saw him in the water
I was terrified
Were you afraid

Q.
A.
Q.
A.
Q.
A.

Extra! Interview the shark! Write your questions and his answers on another sheet of paper. Write at least two questions and two statements.

38 Oink, Oink, Oink

INTERACTIVE LEARNING

TESTED SKILL

Kinds of Sentences

LAB, pp. 38–39

- A **statement** tells something. It ends with a period.
- A **question** asks something. It ends with a question mark.
- A **command** tells someone to do something. It ends with a period.
- An **exclamation** shows strong feeling. It ends with an exclamation point.

Teach/Model Write these quotations from the story on the chalkboard.

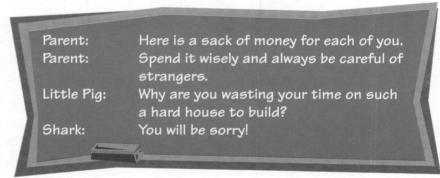

Parent:	Here is a sack of money for each of you.
Parent:	Spend it wisely and always be careful of strangers.
Little Pig:	Why are you wasting your time on such a hard house to build?
Shark:	You will be sorry!

As you ask each pair of questions below, have volunteers go to the chalkboard, point to the appropriate sentence, and name the end mark. Then ask volunteers to read each sentence aloud so as to convey its purpose.

- Which sentence tells someone to do something? What mark does it end with?
- Which sentence asks something? What mark does it end with?
- Which sentence shows strong feeling? What mark does it end with?
- Which sentence tells something? What mark does it end with?

Display Transparency 1–13. Point out the name of each kind of sentence. Review the end mark for each. Read aloud the other sentences. Have volunteers label each sentence and add the end mark. Have students write their own statements, questions, commands, and exclamations.

SKILL FINDER Reading-Writing Workshop, p. 117E

Informal Assessment

Responses to the activities should indicate students' ability to recognize the four kinds of sentences and punctuate them correctly.

Additional Support:

Reteaching, p. 114K

INTERACTIVE LEARNING *(continued)*

Practice/Apply

Literacy Activity Book Page 38 provides practice with statements and questions. Page 39 provides practice with commands and exclamations.

***Cooperative Learning:* A Play** Divide the class into four or more small groups. Assign each group a section of the story to turn into a script. Demonstrate script format, and explain that they will be writing only what the characters say. Students should supplement story dialogue with their own lines and include at least one sentence of each type. When the groups are finished, invite each group to act out its script.

Writing Application: Safety Instructions Suggest that students write a paragraph telling how to play safely at the beach or another place. Ask them to include each of the four types of sentences.

Students' Writing Suggest that students check their work in process to see if they have used correct end marks. Encourage them to use different types of sentences in their writing.

Reteaching

Kinds of Sentences

MEETING INDIVIDUAL NEEDS

Prepare four cards, each with the name of a different kind of sentence and its end mark. Review the purpose of each kind of sentence, and pass out the cards to four students.

Write the sentences below on chart paper. Have students read aloud the first sentence. Ask a volunteer to say what the sentence does (tells something, asks something, etc.) and point to the student holding the card that identifies the kind of sentence. The cardholder reads the card aloud as the volunteer writes the end mark.

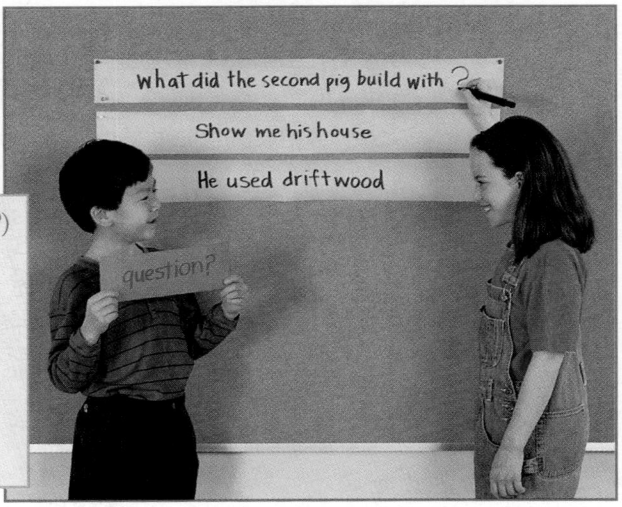
What did the second pig build with ?
Show me his house
He used driftwood
question?

What did the second pig build with (question ?)
Show me his house (command .)
He used driftwood (statement .)
Here comes the shark (exclamation !)
Keep the door closed (command .)
What sharp teeth you have (exclamation !)
What will the pig do now (question ?)
He is running to his brother (statement .)

Daily Language Practice

Focus Skills

Grammar: Kinds of Sentences

Spelling: Long *a* and Long *e*

Every day write one sentence on the chalkboard. Have each student write the sentence correctly on a sheet of paper. Tell students to correct incorrect end marks and misspelled words. Have students correct their own paper as a volunteer corrects the sentence on the chalkboard.

1. Pleeze read us another story?
   Please read us another story**.**
2. Why did the thre little pigs go away!
   Why did the **three** little pigs go away**?**
3. They loved to pley at the beach?
   They loved to **play** at the beach**.**
4. How deap that water looks?
   How **deep** that water looks**!**
5. Could the shark hide his tayl.
   Could the shark hide his **tail?**

Communication Activities

Audio Tape
for Oink, Oink, Oink: *The Three Little Hawaiian Pigs and the Magic Shark*

Listening and Speaking

Literature Discussion Guidelines

1. Listen carefully.
2. Take turns talking.
3. Support your ideas with evidence.
4. Stick to the topic.
5. Be polite!

Invite students to set up guidelines for their Literature Discussion groups.

- Begin by asking them to recall discussions that were especially good—or others that were not so good.
- Brainstorm ideas for good discussions, listing all ideas on the board.
- Encourage students to choose those ideas that are most important and create a chart for display.

Divide the class into small groups to practice guidelines they've set up. Pose this question: Which story in "Oink, Oink, Oink" was the best? Why do you think so?

Hawaiian Music

Multicultural Link Offer students the opportunity to listen to the melodic sounds of the Hawaiian language. Especially recommended is *It's a Small World/Pumehana,* a recording by the youth group Na Mele O Na Opio, which includes a variety of Hawaiian styles.

Resources
It's a Small World/ Pumehana by Na Mele O Na Opio
Na Mele O Paniolo by the Hawaii State Foundation of Culture and the Arts

Informal Assessment

Check students' speaking skills, using the *Literature Discussion Guidelines.* For students who need additional support, plan more speaking activities in small groups.

Viewing

A Game of Disguise

Discuss how the pigs were able to identify the shark each time he visited. Then play a game of disguise.

One student acts as the shark, by changing something about his or her appearance. The volunteer might put on a hat or take off glasses—out of the sight of classmates. Observers must study details carefully both before and after the change. The first student to identify the disguise becomes the next shark.

Let's Visit Hawaii

Hawaii: Stranger in Paradise

Alaska and Hawaii

To further appreciate life in our fiftieth state, students may enjoy comparing and contrasting these two National Geographic videos.

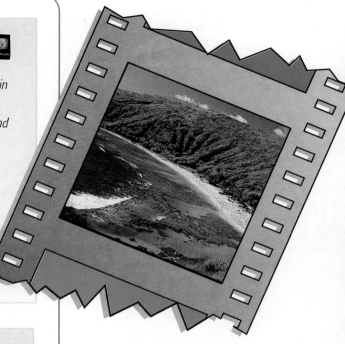

Hula Hands

Most hula dances, especially the ancient ones, tell of historical or legendary events. If possible, invite an expert to demonstrate a few of the hand movements. Students may also enjoy making up their own dance form to tell a story.

1. A rippling motion of the hands and arms is used to show water.

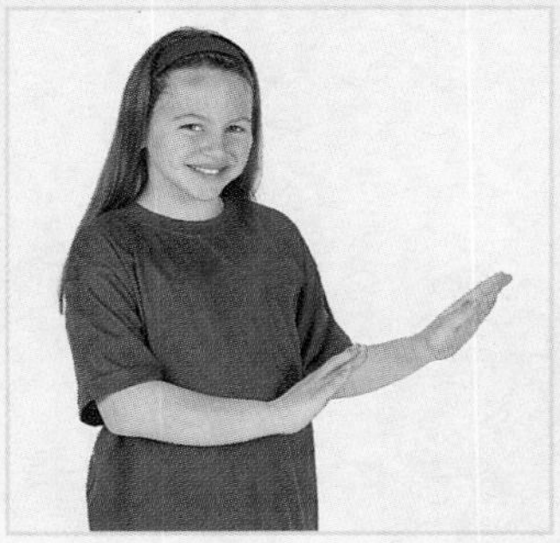

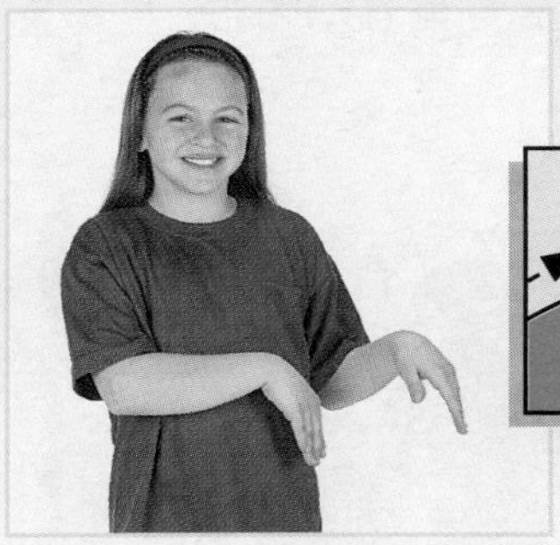

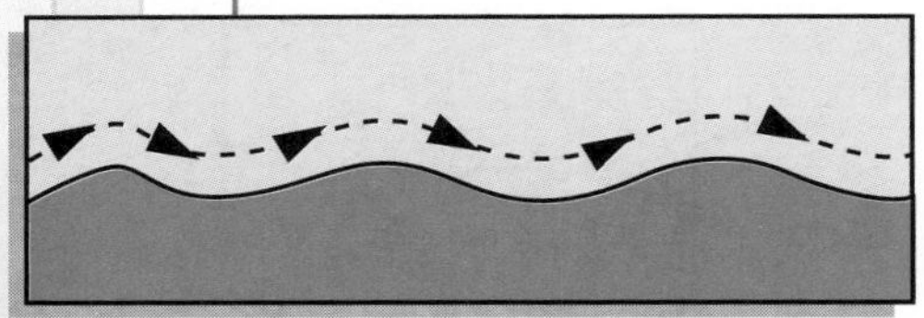

2. Rolling the hands, one over the other, stands for the ocean's roll.

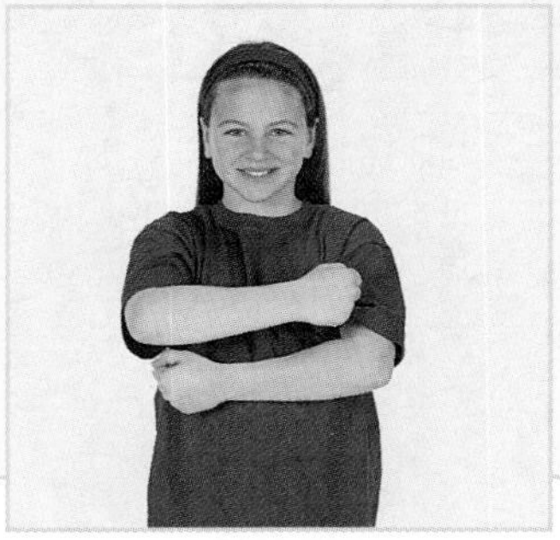

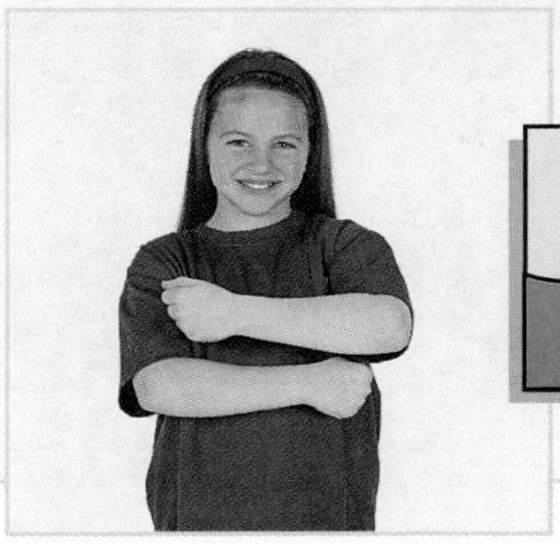

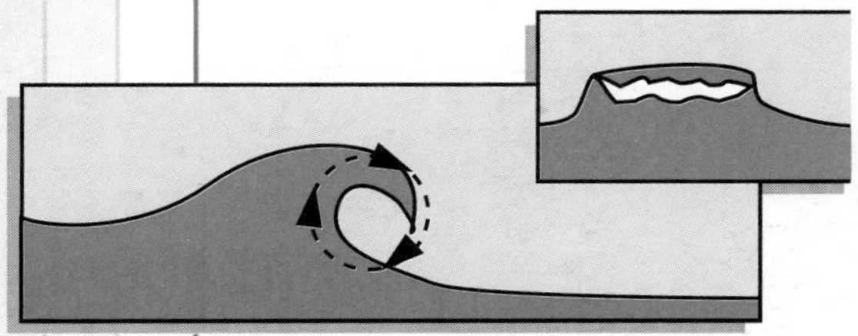

Cross-Curricular Activities

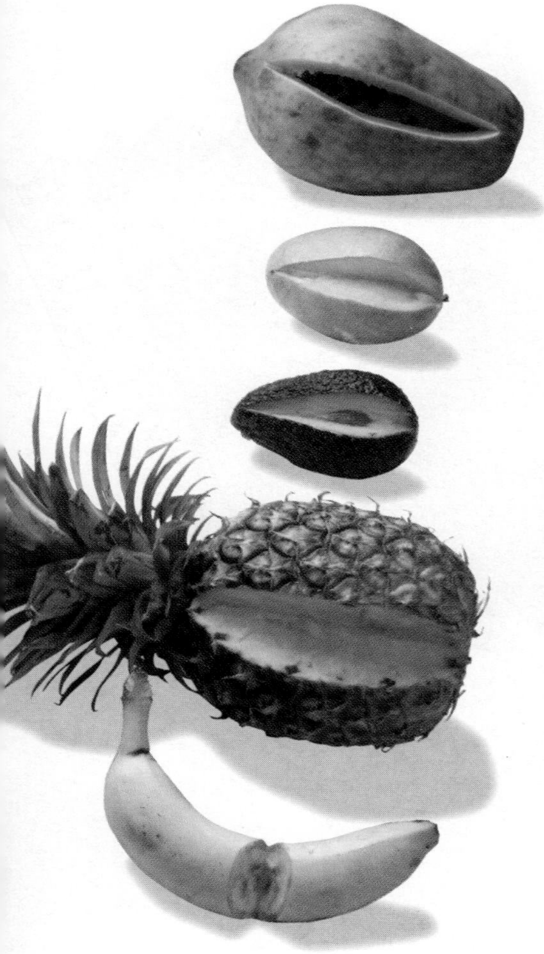

Choices for Social Studies

Discovering Tropical Fruits

MEETING INDIVIDUAL NEEDS

Challenge Invite students to research Hawaiian fruits. Then have them conduct a poll to see how many classmates have tasted these fruits. They can compile their findings on a chart. If possible, provide tropical fruits for the class to taste. Encourage students to compare these fruits to the ones grown in your region.

Have I tasted it?	yes	no
papaya		
guava		
mango		
avocado		
pineapple		
banana		

Making a Relief Map of Hawaii

Cooperative Learning

Students can work together to create a relief map of eight major Hawaiian islands—Hawaii, Maui, Oahu, Kauai, Molokai, Niihau, Lanai, and Kahoolawe. Encourage them to form teams and consult encyclopedias and atlases. Each team collects topographical information about one island and coordinates with the other teams to create one large class map.

To make the dough:

1. Mix the salt and flour in a bowl.
2. Add the water. The dough should look like thick icing.
3. Stir to mix the dough.
4. Use the dough right away.

Materials

- 2 cups salt
- 1 cup flour
- 1 cup water
- heavy cardboard
- pencils and markers
- paint and brushes

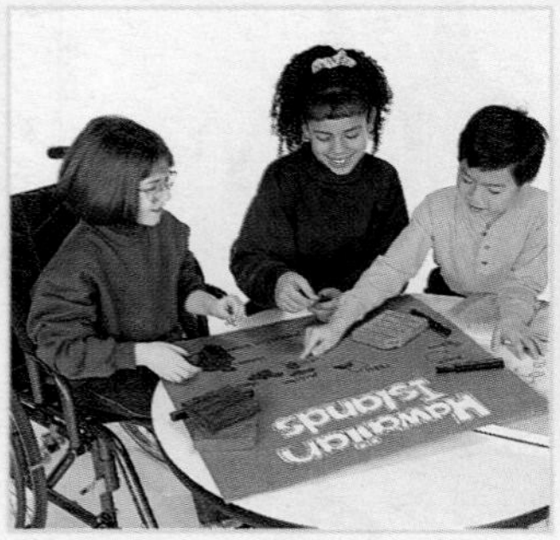

1 Draw an outline of the eight main Hawaiian islands on heavy cardboard. Spread the dough inside the outline.

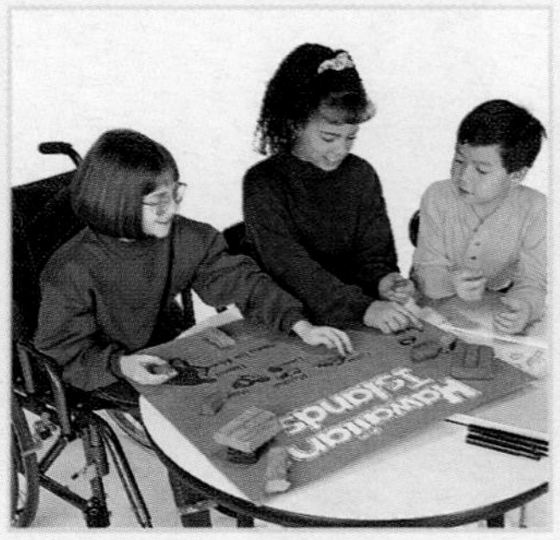

2 Build the mountains a layer at a time. Let each layer dry to prevent cracking.

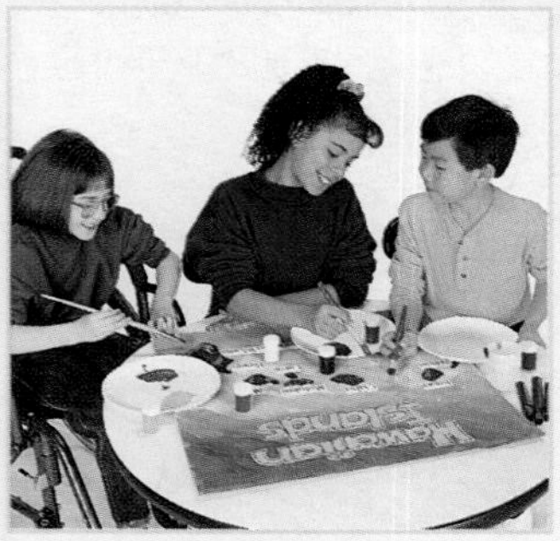

3 Allow 1-3 days for the map to dry. Then paint the cities, the ocean, and other waterways. Label them.

Choices for Science

Collecting Shark Facts

Cooperative Learning

Have the class list ten types of sharks they want to investigate. Then encourage students to work in research teams. Each team selects a type of shark, illustrates it, and then cuts it out. On the flip side of each cutout, the team writes the type of shark and its characteristics, including physical features and behavior. Each team pins up its shark on a blue "ocean" bulletin board and has others guess which kind it is.

Types of Sharks

tiger	great white
thresher	dogfish
nurse	mako
hammerhead	bull
basking	scalloped

Making a Food Chain Mobile

Cooperative Learning

Invite students to construct a mobile illustrating a shark's food chain. Students can work in small groups. Each group selects a type of shark (perhaps the same one chosen for the activity above) and researches the food chain for that specific shark.

Materials
- construction paper
- scissors
- markers or crayons
- stapler
- shredded paper
- yarn
- tape
- coat hanger

1. **Draw** on construction paper the creatures for your food chain. (Omit the plankton.)
2. **Make** each fish a two-sided figure by holding a blank piece of construction paper behind your drawing. Cut through both layers. Use markers to color both sides.
3. **Staple** the two sides together except for a small "fill" hole. Stuff the fish with shredded paper.
4. **For** plankton, use just a single layer of construction paper and no stuffing.
5. **Use** yarn or tape to attach each part of the food chain to a coat hanger for display.

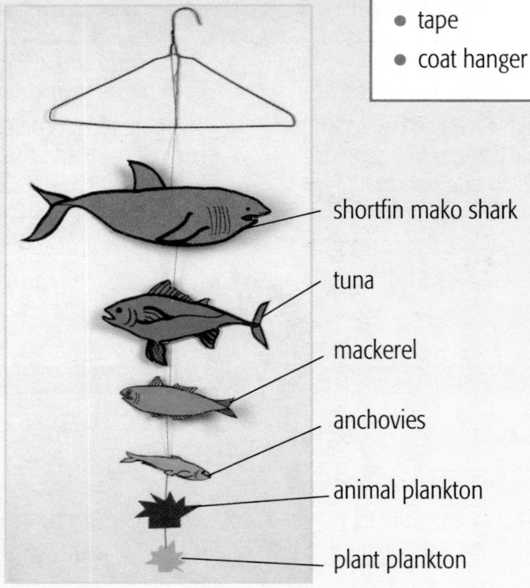
shortfin mako shark
tuna
mackerel
anchovies
animal plankton
plant plankton

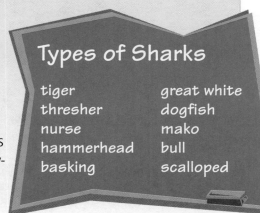

Pigs

Introduce the Literature

Activating Prior Knowledge

Invite students to summarize their knowledge about pigs. Map responses.

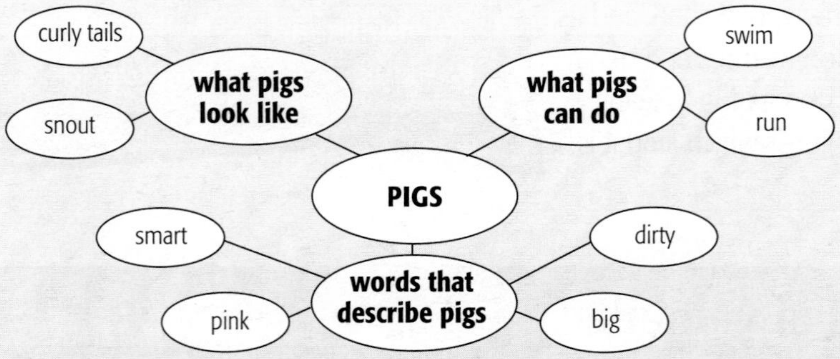
PIGS
what pigs look like
curly tails
snout
what pigs can do
swim
run
words that describe pigs
smart
pink
dirty
big

Keep the map on the board to check which of the traits Charles Ghigna explores in his poem.

Building Background

Discuss with students how a reader can tell immediately that "Pigs" is a poem. Here are elements you may wish to bring out in this discussion.

- It is divided into four groups of lines, or stanzas.
- Although each line begins with a capital letter as in a sentence, there is no end punctuation.
- The second and fourth line of each stanza rhyme.
- The poet repeats different sounds, such as the *p* and the *s* in the word *pigs*.

Interact with Literature

Challenge

Ask students to read the poem aloud twice—once with no punctuation, and once by inserting punctuation where it would ordinarily be. Discuss how the rhythm of the poem is enhanced by leaving out the punctuation.

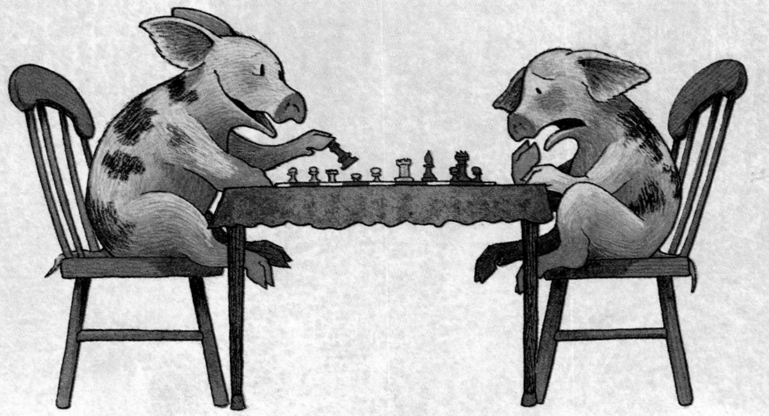

Pigs

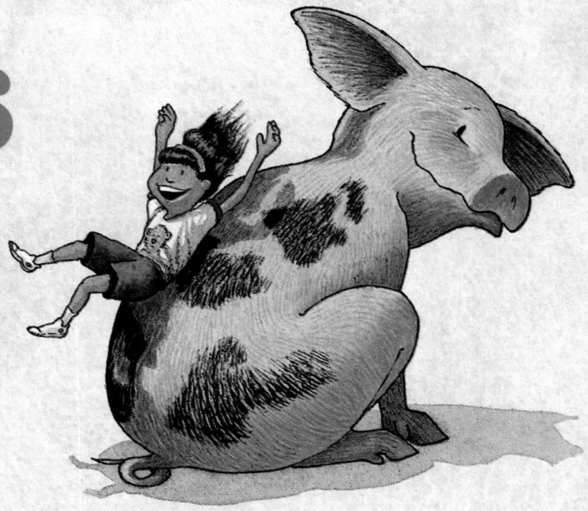

Pigs are playful
Pigs are pink
Pigs are smarter
Than you think

Pigs are slippery
Pigs are stout
Pigs have noses
Called a snout

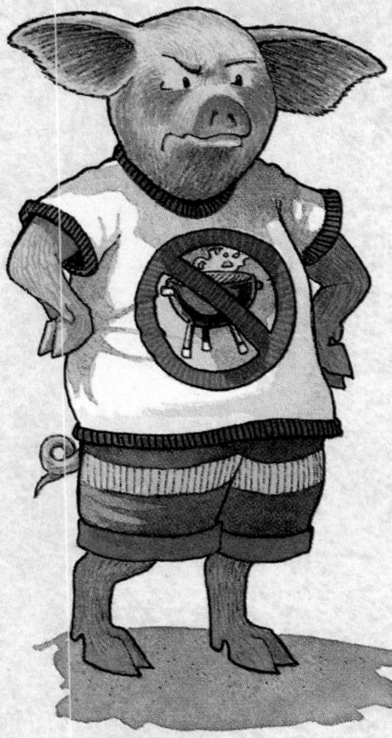

Pigs are pudgy
Pigs are plump
Pigs can run
But never jump

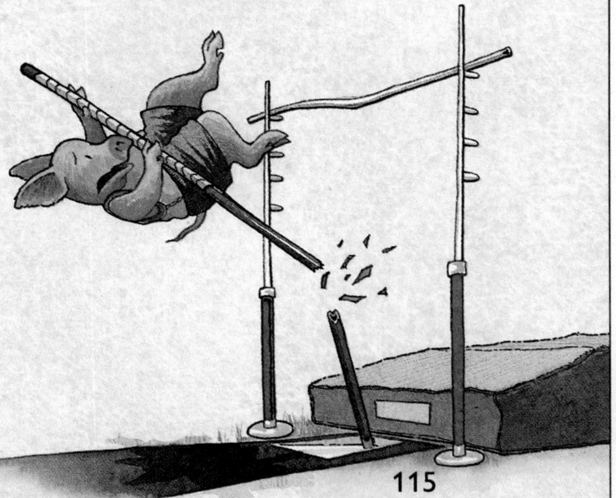

Pigs are loyal
Pigs are true
Pigs don't care for
Barbecue

115

Interact with Literature

Students Acquiring English

Expressions Explain that the phrase *don't care for* means "don't like."

Home Connection

Poetry Students may enjoy reciting the poem to family members. Also encourage students to ask family members to share poems they know.

Instruct and Integrate

Language Arts

Alliteration Have volunteers copy lines of the poem on the board, read them aloud, and then circle any sounds that are repeated.

Visual Literacy

Symbols Pigs are pervasive! Suggest that students keep their eyes out for how pigs are used as icons in advertising and as decoration for stationery and other writing materials. Perhaps students could bring objects to class that show pigs and discuss

- what trait of a pig is emphasized
- elements of the art that makes the pig humorous, sad, etc.

Music Link

Song Students will enjoy using a familiar tune, such as "The Alphabet Song" or "Twinkle, Twinkle, Little Star," to sing the poem.

Art Link

Class Book Have students work in small groups to create their own illustrations for Pigs. They might copy and illustrate each stanza and then compile the pages into a class book.

Reading-Writing Workshop

A Story

About the Workshop

This workshop includes story-specific suggestions and ideas to help you guide students as they use the writing process to write a fictional story.

Minilessons focus on characters and setting, plot, and dialogue. These elements form the assessment criteria at the end of the workshop.

Keep in mind these considerations:

- Friends or stereotypic heroes, heroines, and TV characters may still crop up in students' stories.
- Acknowledge and praise students' progress with the emerging skills of dialogue and description.
- Continue to read aloud quality picture books and guide students to discuss them as both writers and readers.

Connecting to Literature

Have students discuss how different authors used characters, setting, and events to write three different stories based on the traditional story of the three little pigs.

Introducing the Student Model

Explain that Kara Johnson, a third-grade student, wove together characters, setting, and events into an enjoyable story of her own. Have students read Kara's story about Mr. Pig's surprise and discuss the questions on page 117.

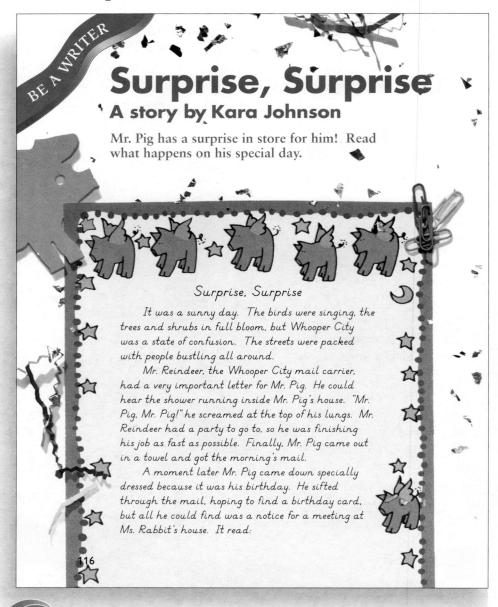

BE A WRITER

Surprise, Surprise

A story by Kara Johnson

Mr. Pig has a surprise in store for him! Read what happens on his special day.

Surprise, Surprise

It was a sunny day. The birds were singing, the trees and shrubs in full bloom, but Whooper City was a state of confusion. The streets were packed with people bustling all around.

Mr. Reindeer, the Whooper City mail carrier, had a very important letter for Mr. Pig. He could hear the shower running inside Mr. Pig's house. "Mr. Pig, Mr. Pig!" he screamed at the top of his lungs. Mr. Reindeer had a party to go to, so he was finishing his job as fast as possible. Finally, Mr. Pig came out in a towel and got the morning's mail.

A moment later Mr. Pig came down specially dressed because it was his birthday. He sifted through the mail, hoping to find a birthday card, but all he could find was a notice for a meeting at Ms. Rabbit's house. It read:

116

SKILL FINDER

PREWRITING/DRAFTING	
Workshop Minilessons • Characters and Settings, p. 117A • Beginning, Middle, End, p. 117B • Dialogue, p. 117C	**Theme Resources** *Writing* • Writing a Sentence, p. 60D • Setting, p. 85

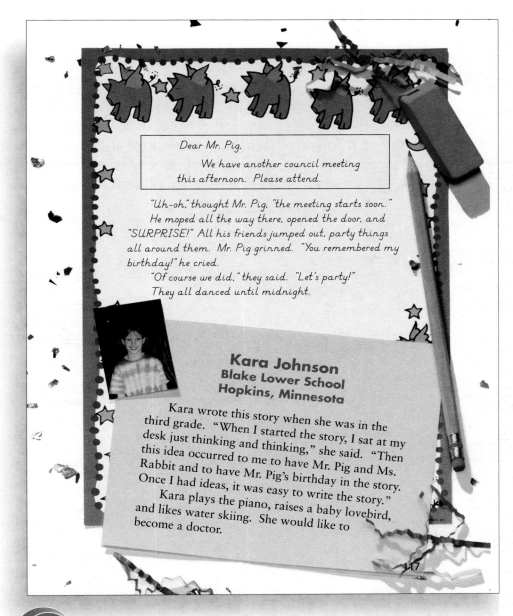

Dear Mr. Pig,

We have another council meeting this afternoon. Please attend.

"Uh-oh," thought Mr. Pig, "the meeting starts soon."

He moped all the way there, opened the door, and "SURPRISE!" All his friends jumped out, party things all around them. Mr. Pig grinned. "You remembered my birthday!" he cried.

"Of course we did," they said. "Let's party!"

They all danced until midnight.

Kara Johnson
Blake Lower School
Hopkins, Minnesota

Kara wrote this story when she was in the third grade. "When I started the story, I sat at my desk just thinking and thinking," she said. "Then this idea occurred to me to have Mr. Pig and Ms. Rabbit and to have Mr. Pig's birthday in the story. Once I had ideas, it was easy to write the story."

Kara plays the piano, raises a baby lovebird, and likes water skiing. She would like to become a doctor.

117

Discussing the Model

Reading and Responding

- What did you like best about Kara's story?
- Were you surprised by the end? Why or why not?
- Have you ever been disappointed in some way but later been happily surprised? Tell about it.

Reading As a Writer

- What is the setting? (Whooper City)
- Who are the characters? (Mr. Pig, Mr. Reindeer)
- How does the beginning catch your interest? (creates a sense of excitement; raises interest in the letter)
- What details help you picture Mr. Pig and Mr. Reindeer? (Mr. Reindeer *screams at the top of his lungs;* Mr. Pig *came out in a towel;* Mr. Pig was *specially dressed;* Mr. Pig *moped.*)
- What problem develops for Mr. Pig? (He thought no one remembered his birthday.) Does the ending solve it in a way that makes sense? How else might the story have ended?

Characteristics of Stories

Help students list these story elements:

- *Purpose*: to tell an original story
- Main characters and a setting
- A beginning, a middle, and an end that focus on a problem and how the characters work it out
- Details that make the characters and events "come alive"

SKILL FINDER

PROOFREADING

Theme Resources	Theme Resources
Grammar	*Spelling*
• Subjects and Predicates, pp. 60J–60K	• Short Vowels, p. 60I
• Run-on Sentences, pp. 88J–88K	• Vowel-consonant-*e*, p. 88I
• Kinds of Sentences, pp. 114J–114K	• Long *a* and Long *e*, p. 114I

Reading-Writing Workshop *(continued)*

A Story

MINILESSON

Characters and Settings

Resource: Anthology pp. 93–113

- Ask students how the author of *The Three Little Hawaiian Pigs and the Magic Shark* let them know what the shark was like. (by the shark's actions, by mean things the shark says)
- Ask students what they know about the pigs based on what they say and do. (like to play at the beach; are smart enough to recognize the magic shark in his disguises; one pig thinks hard-working pig is foolish)
- Help students write questions to use for developing story characters, such as
  1) What do the characters look like?
  2) How do they act?
  3) What do they say?
  4) What kinds of feelings or ideas do they have?
  5) What are their interests?
- Write the setting for each story in this theme on the chalkboard, and have students discuss how the setting does or does not affect the story.

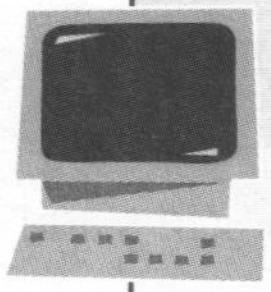

Students can use the prewriting feature in the Learning Company's new elementary writing center to stimulate ideas for their writing.

Warm-up

Shared Writing

As a class, brainstorm an original story. Keep the brainstorming fast-moving and lively. Ask questions about the characters, where the story takes place, and what happens. Write students' ideas on the chalkboard or chart paper. Then become a storyteller, and have students help tell the story as you write it on chart paper. When finished drafting, encourage them to discuss improvements or changes they could make.

Prewriting

LAB, pp. 40–41

Choose a Story Topic

Students brainstorm and narrow possible story topics and then choose one to write about.

- **Make a List** Have each student list three to five story ideas.
- **Talk and Think About It** Have students tell their ideas to a partner, and narrow their choices by answering these questions about each idea: Can I picture the characters and setting clearly? Do I have enough ideas for the beginning, middle, and end? Do I really want to write about this idea?

Help with Topics

Brainstorm

Cooperative Learning

Draw a chart like the one below on the chalkboard. Have students use the questions to interview each other. Record their responses.

Story Ideas

What people, animals, or creatures could be story characters?	Where could stories take place?	What problems could stories be about?

Sources for Ideas

Personal Experiences Invite students to draw pictures of their memorable experiences. Help them see these as story ideas.

Traditional Literature Suggest that students rewrite a traditional story with new plot twists, characters, or settings.

Prewriting *(continued)*

Plan the Story Students plan their stories before they write their first drafts.

- **Think of Details** Have students make a story map or draw detailed pictures of their characters, setting, and beginning, middle, and end.
- **Audience Check** Have students tell their stories to partners.

Help with Planning

Puppet Walk-through

Have students use their fingers or make simple stick puppets to rehearse story ideas with partners. Prompt listeners to ask questions about parts of the plot that may be unclear or distracting.

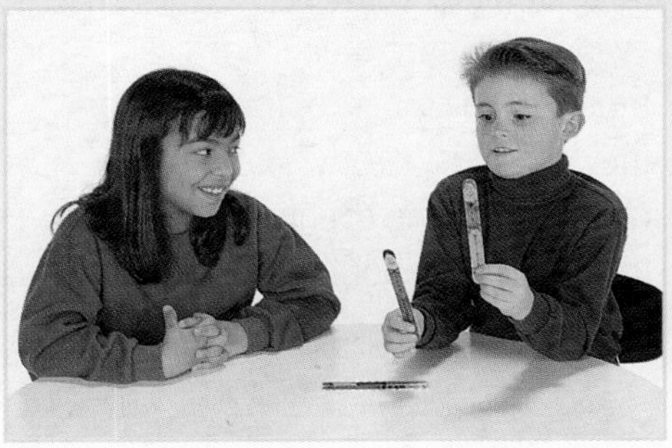

Literacy Activity Book, p. 40

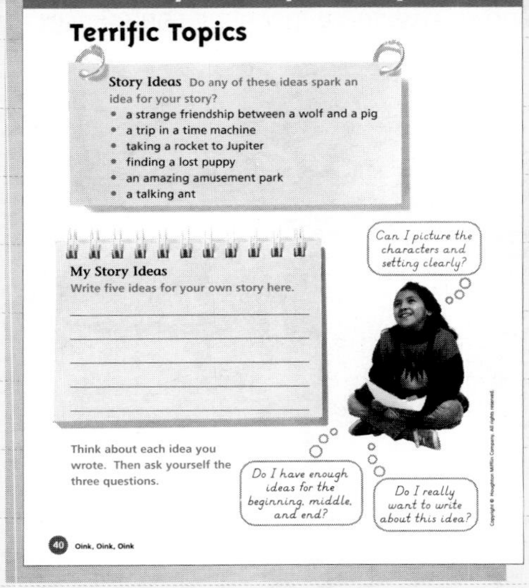

Terrific Topics

Story Ideas Do any of these ideas spark an idea for your story?

- a strange friendship between a wolf and a pig
- a trip in a time machine
- taking a rocket to Jupiter
- finding a lost puppy
- an amazing amusement park
- a talking ant

My Story Ideas
Write five ideas for your own story here.

Think about each idea you wrote. Then ask yourself the three questions.

Can I picture the characters and setting clearly?

Do I have enough ideas for the beginning, middle, and end?

Do I really want to write about this idea?

40 Oink, Oink, Oink

Literacy Activity Book, p. 41

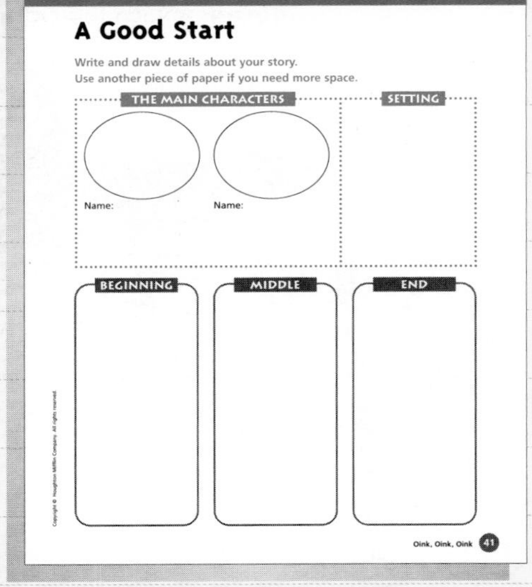

A Good Start

Write and draw details about your story.
Use another piece of paper if you need more space.

THE MAIN CHARACTERS

SETTING

Name:

Name:

BEGINNING

MIDDLE

END

Oink, Oink, Oink 41

M I N I L E S S O N

Beginning, Middle, End

Resource: Anthology pp. 37–59, 69–87, 93–113

- Review the purposes of the main parts of a story.

  Beginning: to introduce the main characters, setting, and a situation or a problem

  Middle: to show how the characters try to work out the situation

  End: to show how the situation works out

  Tell students that these parts form the *plot* of the story.
- Map the beginning, middle, and end of the stories in this theme. Ask students to compare and contrast the main parts.
- Take a class vote to find out which ending students prefer. Ask volunteers to explain their choice. Elicit that each ending works because it makes sense with that story and makes the story feel finished. Contrast the story endings with a weak ending, such as the evil character gives up after only one try, which would end the story too soon and in a disappointing way.

Reading-Writing Workshop *(continued)*

A Story

MINILESSON

Dialogue

Resource: Anthology pp. 93–113

- Invite students to do a Reader's Theater reading of *The Three Little Hawaiian Pigs and the Magic Shark* from the beginning until the shark destroys the first house.
- Help students determine if the examples of dialogue
  1) show what is happening
  2) show what characters think
  3) show what a character is like
- Help students summarize that writers can use dialogue to help tell the story and bring the characters to life.
- Point out that a speaker's exact words are enclosed in *quotation marks* and the writer began a *new paragraph* each time a different character began to speak.

Self-Assessment

Have students evaluate their stories, using the Revising Checklist.

Drafting

Students write the first drafts of their stories, using any pictures, story maps, or other aids they have prepared.

Help with Drafting

Picture It

Suggest that students close their eyes and picture their stories as movies. Which part of the story can they see most clearly? the beginning? one of the events? Encourage them to write about that "scene" first.

Drafting Strategies

Encourage students to write as much as they can and not to worry about grammar and spelling now. Remind them to skip every other line so that they have room to make changes later on.

TECH TIPS Students can set their document for double spacing to allow extra space for revisions.

Revising

LAB, p. 42

Students revise their stories and discuss them in writing conferences.

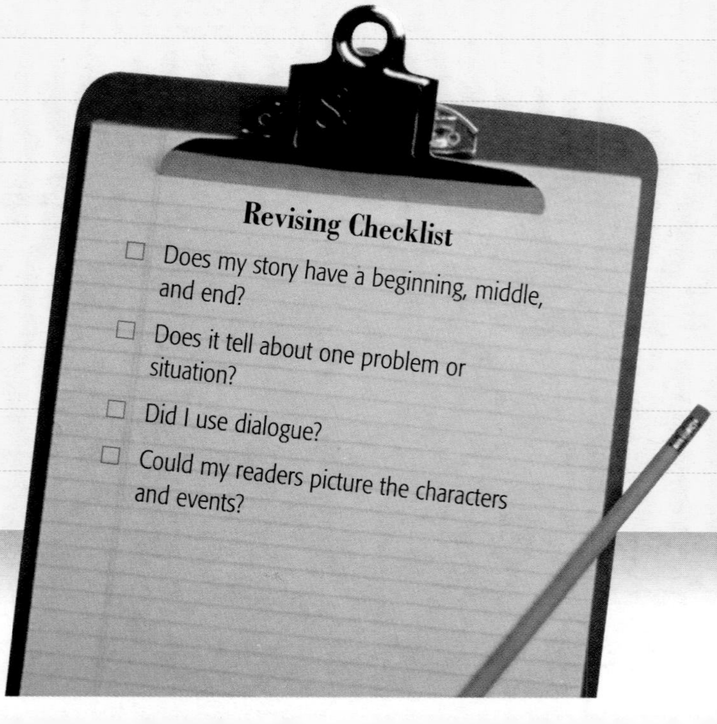
Revising Checklist
☐ Does my story have a beginning, middle, and end?
☐ Does it tell about one problem or situation?
☐ Did I use dialogue?
☐ Could my readers picture the characters and events?

Revising *(continued)*

Writing Conference

Cooperative Learning Encourage students to read their stories aloud to you or to one or more classmates. They can use the Questions for a Writing Conference to guide the discussion.

Questions for a Writing Conference

- Does the story begin in an interesting way?
- Are any parts not clear?
- Do any parts not belong in this story?
- Does the ending make sense? Can it be more interesting?
- What other ways might the story end?

Help with Revising

Author's Chair

Cooperative Learning

Set up a certain time and place each day for students to use an author's chair. Volunteers can use this opportunity to read aloud their drafts and discuss them with the class.

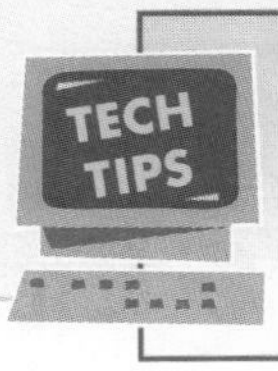
TECH TIPS

Have students record their compliments and suggestions on the computer. They can then print out the notes for the writing conference.

New Ending

Suggest that students write another ending for their stories, present both endings in their writing conference, and choose the one they like better.

Revising Strategies

Demonstrate strategies for revising, such as drawing arrows for moving text, using carets for inserting words or phrases, or taping strips of paper over or beside parts of the story to change or add blocks of text.

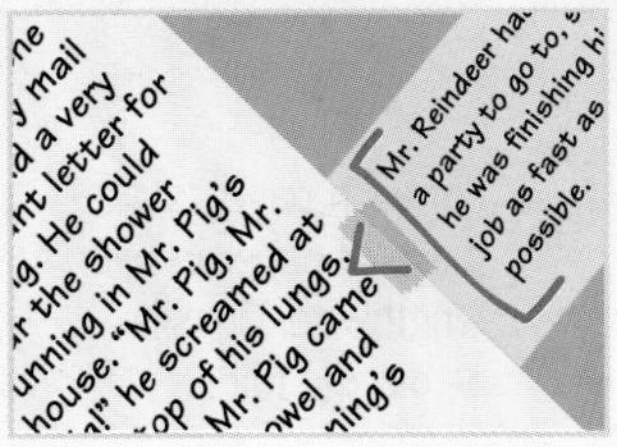

Additional Questions for Writing Conferences

These questions may be useful during teacher-student conferences.

- What happened when . . . ?
- Why did this character [do something, say something]?
- Is [this part] really important to the story?
- What did [this scene, this character] look like? Help me picture it.
- What did this character say when . . . ?
- Can you use dialogue to tell some parts of the story?

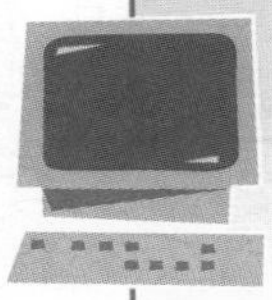

If your class is using the elementary writing center from The Learning Company, you can add comments to your students' work using the sticky notes feature.

Literacy Activity Book, p. 42

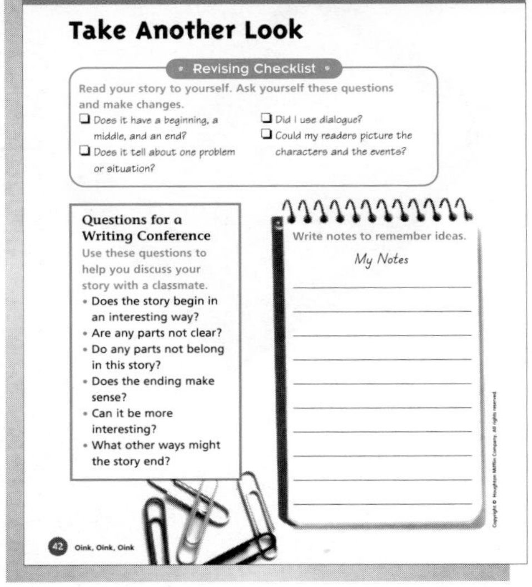

Take Another Look

Revising Checklist

Read your story to yourself. Ask yourself these questions and make changes.

- ❏ Does it have a beginning, a middle, and an end?
- ❏ Does it tell about one problem or situation?
- ❏ Did I use dialogue?
- ❏ Could my readers picture the characters and the events?

Questions for a Writing Conference

Use these questions to help you discuss your story with a classmate.

- Does the story begin in an interesting way?
- Are any parts not clear?
- Do any parts not belong in this story?
- Does the ending make sense?
- Can it be more interesting?
- What other ways might the story end?

Write notes to remember ideas.

My Notes

42 Oink, Oink, Oink

Reading-Writing Workshop *(continued)*
A Story

Proofreading

Students proofread their stories, using the Proofreading Checklist and the proofreading marks in the Handbook of the *Literacy Activity Book*. Encourage students to make as many corrections as they can by themselves or by consulting with classmates.

Grammar/ Spelling Connections

- **Checking Sentences** Remind students to check that every sentence has a subject and a predicate, that they have used correct end marks, and that they have avoided run-on sentences. *pp. 60J–60K, 88J–88K, 114J–114K*
- **Spelling** Remind students to check the spelling of short and long vowel sounds in the words they used. *pp. 60I, 88I, 114I*

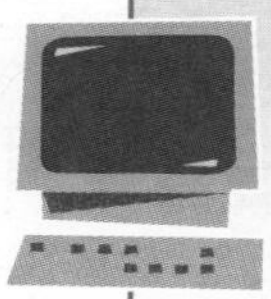

Students using The Learning Company's new elementary writing center can add graphics to their story from the notebook of pictures.

Publishing and Sharing

Students make neat final copies of their stories and choose a way to share them.

Ideas for Publishing and Sharing

Make a Pop-up Book

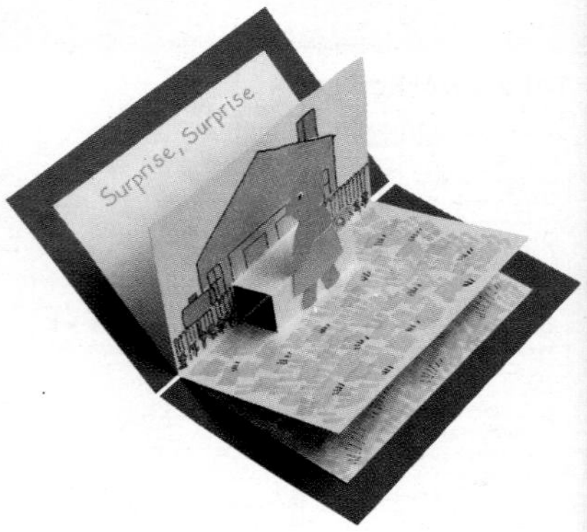
Surprise, Surprise

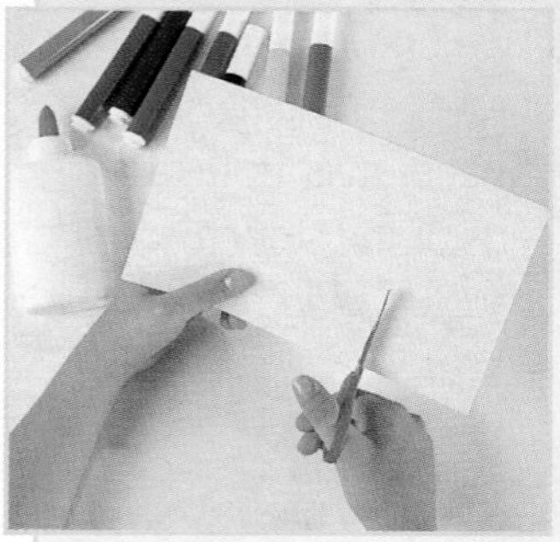

1. For each page, fold a piece of paper in half lengthwise. Cut slits across the fold.

2. Pull out the pop-up tab. Glue a picture to the tab, being careful it does not hang down below the tab.

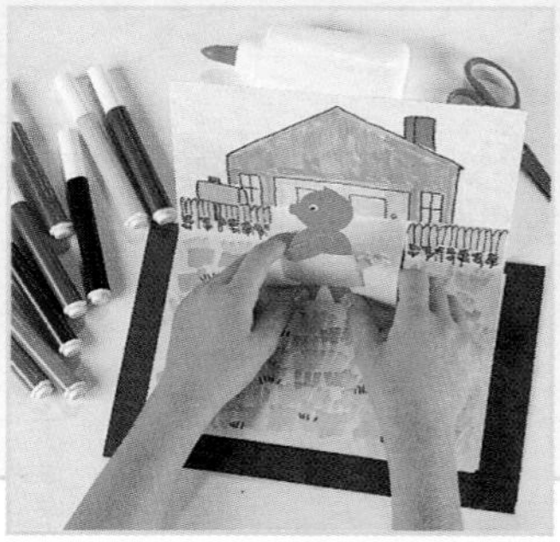

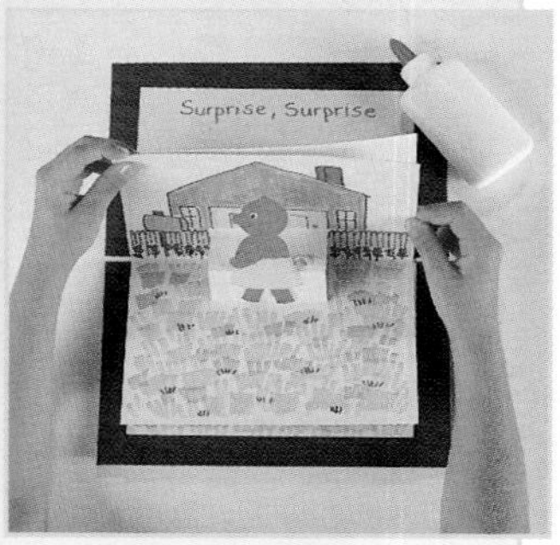
Surprise, Surprise

3. Glue the top half of one page to the bottom half of the next page. Pictures are always inside.

Materials

- construction paper
- scissors
- glue
- magazines for cutting

More Ideas for Publishing and Sharing

Writing Buddies

Form writing partnerships between a student in your class and a younger or older student in the school.

Record a Tape

Record students reading their stories on video- or audiotape. Share the tapes with other classes, or send them home.

Reflecting/Self-Assessment

Use the Self-Assessment questions, or others of your own, to help students reflect on and evaluate their experience writing a story. Students can discuss or write their responses.

Evaluating Writing

Use the criteria below to evaluate students' stories.

Criteria for Evaluating Stories

- The story has a beginning, a middle, and an end that focus on one main problem or situation.
- Details are used to develop the characters, setting, and events.
- Dialogue is used to develop characters and to help tell the story.
- The ending shows how the problem or situation works out and makes the story feel finished.

Sample Scoring Rubric

1	2	3	4
The story meets the criteria only minimally. The characters, setting, and plot are poorly developed, with little or no detail. Events lack a clear sequence and are confusing.	The story is sketchy or inconsistent in some way. There may be minor gaps in the sequence. More details are needed to make the characters, setting, and events come alive.	The story is coherent and detailed, although some parts could be better developed. Nonessential details do not seriously detract. The story might rate a 4 except for significant errors.	The story meets all the evaluation criteria; is unified, clearly sequenced, sufficiently detailed, and has a minimum of spelling or mechanical errors.

Self-Assessment

- What do you like best about your story?
- If you wrote this story again, would you change the beginning, the middle, or the end? Why or why not?
- Which character is developed the best? Why?
- Where did dialogue work the best? Why?
- What might you like to try the next time you write a story?

Portfolio Opportunity

- Save students' final copies to show their understanding of writing a story.
- Save students' planning aids and drafts to show their use of the writing process.

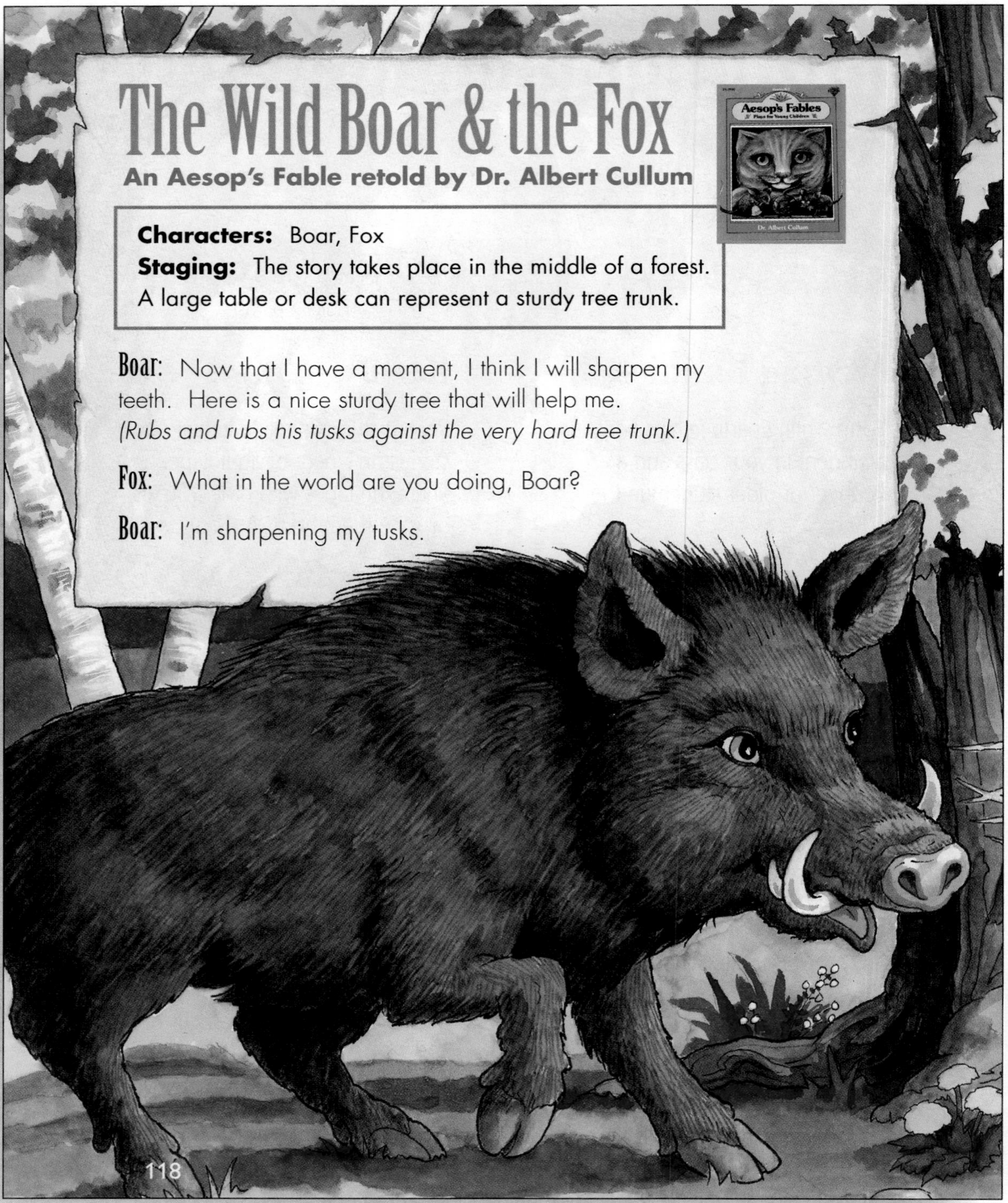

The Wild Boar & the Fox

An Aesop's Fable retold by Dr. Albert Cullum

Characters: Boar, Fox
Staging: The story takes place in the middle of a forest. A large table or desk can represent a sturdy tree trunk.

Boar: Now that I have a moment, I think I will sharpen my teeth. Here is a nice sturdy tree that will help me.
(Rubs and rubs his tusks against the very hard tree trunk.)

Fox: What in the world are you doing, Boar?

Boar: I'm sharpening my tusks.

118

Introduce the Literature

Building Background

Ask students why this play belongs in a theme in which all the stories have pigs or piglike animals as characters. Students might compare the illustration of the boar with the illustrations of the javelinas in *The Three Little Javelinas*.

Explain that a fable often has animal characters that talk and act like humans. It ends with a moral, or lesson.

Meeting Individual Needs **Students Acquiring English** Although this play is short, it will be challenging for students because each line is critical in comprehending the moral. Provide rehearsal time so that students will enjoy acting out the play.

Extra Support Tell students that a play is meant to be read aloud. Ask why it is important to monitor your understanding of the lines before you read them aloud. (It's part of rehearsing for a play.) Then assign each student a partner for oral reading.

Interact with Literature

Background: FYI

Aesop A Greek slave who lived during the sixth century B.C., Aesop is the reputed author of hundreds of fables. Ask students if they know any of Aesop's tales, such as "The Tortoise and the Hare" and "The Ant and the Grasshopper."

Expanding Literacy
Play

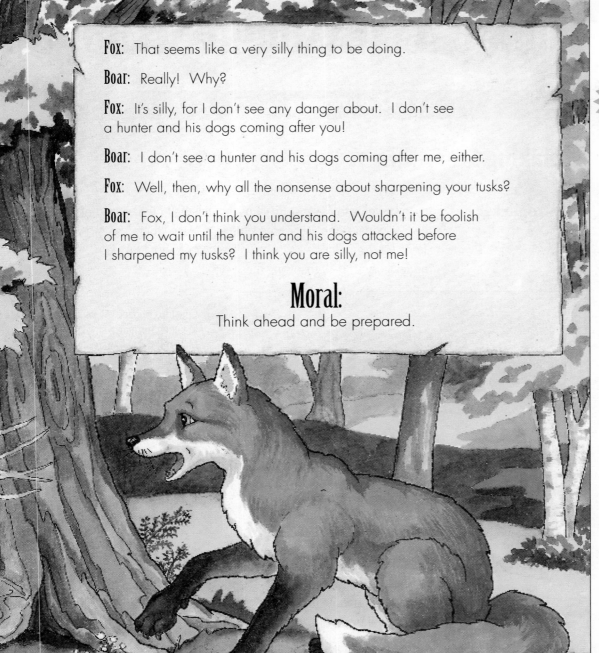

Fox: That seems like a very silly thing to be doing.

Boar: Really! Why?

Fox: It's silly, for I don't see any danger about. I don't see a hunter and his dogs coming after you!

Boar: I don't see a hunter and his dogs coming after me, either.

Fox: Well, then, why all the nonsense about sharpening your tusks?

Boar: Fox, I don't think you understand. Wouldn't it be foolish of me to wait until the hunter and his dogs attacked before I sharpened my tusks? I think you are silly, not me!

Moral:

Think ahead and be prepared.

Interact with Literature

Extra Support

Meeting Individual Needs

Point out the boar's tusks. Ask students to name another animal with tusks and to speculate what the tusks are used for. Discuss how rubbing creates friction, which sharpens the tusks. Have students think of tools or equipment that are sharpened by friction.

Instruct and Integrate

MINILESSON

Genre
Plays

Teach/Model

If any students have acted in a play, ask them to discuss how they prepared for it. Then brainstorm with students how reading a play is different from reading a story.

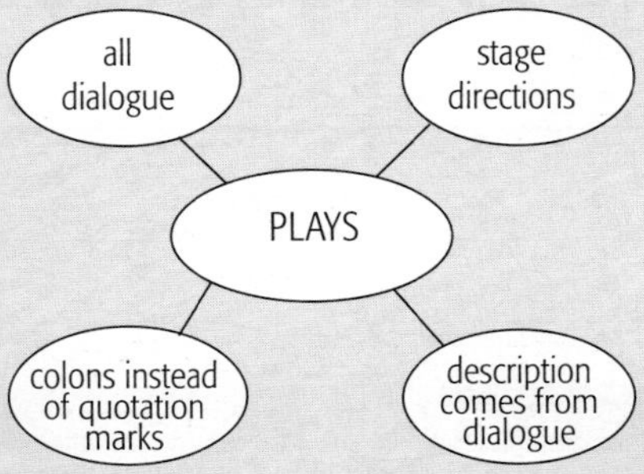
all dialogue
stage directions
PLAYS
colons instead of quotation marks
description comes from dialogue

Discuss how plays are often shorter than stories.

Practice/Apply

Ask volunteers to read the script aloud. Encourage them to read their lines with expression.

Interact with Literature

Discussion

Discuss the moral of the fable with students. Do they agree with it? Do they disagree? Ask students to suggest times when they have thought ahead and were thus prepared for some situation.

Theme Assessment Wrap-Up

Time: About 1 hour

Evaluates:

1. **Theme Concept:** Traditional tales can be retold in a variety of humorous altered versions.
2. **Skills:** Story Structure/ Summarizing, Compare and Contrast

This is a brief, informal performance assessment activity. For a more extended reading-writing performance assessment, see the Integrated Theme Test.

PERFORMANCE ASSESSMENT

Making Story Strips

LAB, p. 43

Materials

- paper
- glue
- tag board
- scissors
- markers

Introducing Invite students to make story strips that tell their own version of the traditional story "The Three Little Pigs." Have them use *Literacy Activity Book* page 43 to plan their project. Make a model story strip by following these steps:

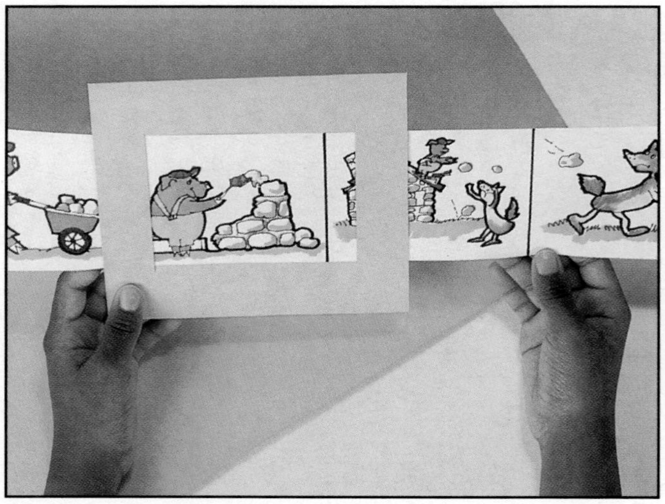

1. Cut strips of paper 3" wide and glue them together, forming a strip about 30" long. Mark off 3"x 4" frames. Illustrate the frames in story order, from left to right.
2. Make a viewing screen from a 6"x 6" sheet of tag board by marking and cutting two 3 1/2" vertical slits, spaced 4" apart.
3. Slide the left end of the strip through the right-hand slit of the screen from back to front. Then pass it through the left-hand slit from front to back.

Evaluating As students slide the strip through the screen, have them summarize their versions of "The Three Little Pigs" for the class. Then have them compare and contrast their version with the traditional story. Evaluate the presentation using the scoring rubric.

Scoring Rubric

Criterion	1	2	3	4
Retells a new version of a traditional tale	Story doesn't resemble traditional tale	Story vaguely resembles traditional tale	Story generally resembles traditional tale	Story is a creative retelling of traditional tale
Shows understanding of story structure	Focuses on single, unconnected elements	Summary is disorganized or incomplete	Summary includes all story elements	Summary is complete and well organized
Compares and contrasts	Does not compare or contrast stories	Gives similarities or differences, but not both	Compares and contrasts tales in a general way	Compares and contrasts several aspects of tales

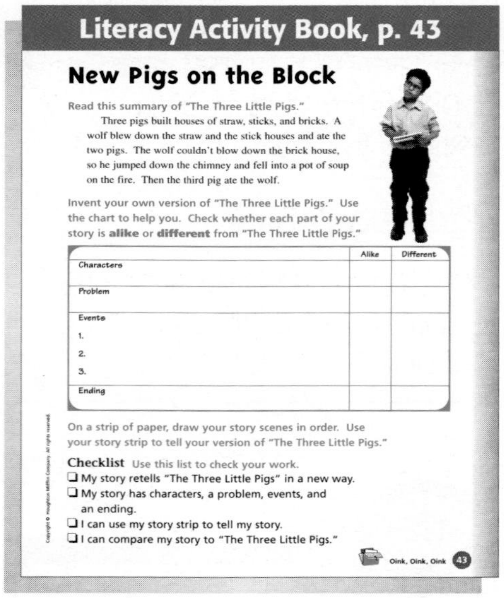
Literacy Activity Book, p. 43

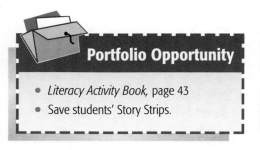

New Pigs on the Block

Read this summary of "The Three Little Pigs."

Three pigs built houses of straw, sticks, and bricks. A wolf blew down the straw and the stick houses and ate the two pigs. The wolf couldn't blow down the brick house, so he jumped down the chimney and fell into a pot of soup on the fire. Then the third pig ate the wolf.

Invent your own version of "The Three Little Pigs." Use the chart to help you. Check whether each part of your story is **alike** or **different** from "The Three Little Pigs."

	Alike	Different
Characters		
Problem		
Events 1. 2. 3.		
Ending		

On a strip of paper, draw your story scenes in order. Use your story strip to tell your version of "The Three Little Pigs."

Checklist Use this list to check your work.

- ❑ My story retells "The Three Little Pigs" in a new way.
- ❑ My story has characters, a problem, events, and an ending.
- ❑ I can use my story strip to tell my story.
- ❑ I can compare my story to "The Three Little Pigs."

Oink, Oink, Oink 43

Portfolio Opportunity

- *Literacy Activity Book,* page 43
- Save students' Story Strips.

Choices for Assessment

Informal Assessment

Review the Informal Assessment Checklist and observation notes to determine the following:

- Did students use the reading strategies at appropriate times during the theme?
- Did students' responses during and after reading indicate comprehension of the selections?
- How well did students follow through with the Writing Process?

Formal Assessment

Select and administer formal tests that meet your classroom needs:

- Integrated Theme Test for Oink, Oink, Oink
- Theme Skills Test for Oink, Oink, Oink
- Benchmark Progress Test

See the *Teacher's Assessment Handbook* for guidelines for administering tests and using answer keys, scoring rubrics, and student sample papers.

Portfolio Assessment

Introducing Portfolios to the Class

Explain to students that their portfolios are like an artist's portfolio: they will show many samples of their work for the year. Portfolios will also show how they improve over time.

- As a first step, have students create temporary collection folders to keep all their work for the theme. Have them decorate their folders using ideas related to the theme.
- Partway through the first theme, have students create their portfolios for special work selected from the collection. Encourage them to decorate their portfolios to express their unique interests.

Selecting Materials for the Portfolio

Meet with students to review the work in their collections, and model the process of selecting work samples for the portfolio. Discuss your criteria as you pick samples that reflect important categories such as writing and comprehension. Also include samples of students' best work and areas of improvement. You may also want to guide students in selecting one sample on their own.

Grading Work in Portfolios

You don't need to grade all the work in portfolios. Both graded and ungraded work can help you understand students' learning. Items you may wish to grade include formal tests, some student writing, and some *Literacy Activity Book* pages. For more information on grading, see Portfolio Assessment notes in Themes 3, 4, and 5, and the *Teacher's Assessment Handbook.*

Managing Assessment

Testing Options

Question How can I assess students' overall progress at the end of a theme?

Answer Invitations to Literacy includes a range of testing options at the end of a theme. Select the options that best meet your needs:

Performance Assessment

The Performance Assessment on page 119A is a hands-on activity that evaluates student understanding of the theme concept and major comprehension skills.

Integrated Theme Test

The Integrated Theme Test provides a new theme-related reading selection. It uses written and multiple-choice formats to evaluate reading strategies, comprehension skills, word skills, writing and language arts.

Theme Skills Test

The Theme Skills Test evaluates discrete literacy skills of the theme, including comprehension, word skills, writing, spelling, grammar, and study skills. Sections of this test can be used to evaluate specific areas of concern.

Benchmark Progress Test

The Benchmark Progress Test can be given two or three times a year to evaluate students' overall progress in reading. It is not theme-related. Many teachers choose to use this test at midyear and at the end of the year.

For more information on this and other topics, see the *Teacher's Assessment Handbook.*

Celebrating the Theme

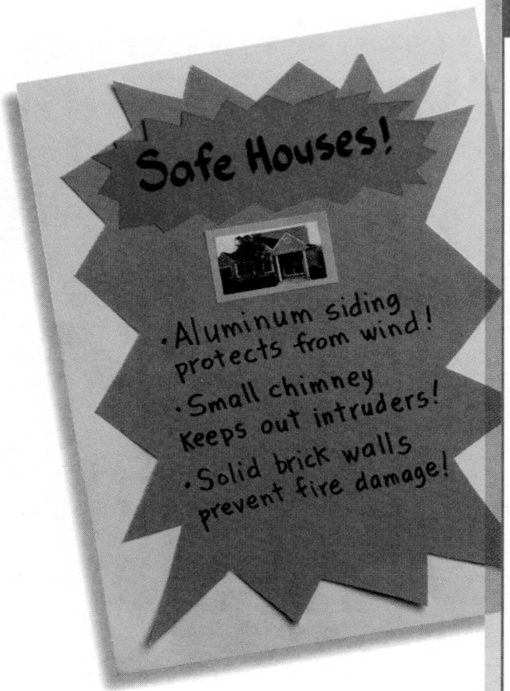
Safe Houses!
·Aluminum siding protects from wind!
·Small chimney keeps out intruders!
·Solid brick walls prevent fire damage!

See the **Teacher's Resource Disk** for theme-related Teacher Support material.

Choices for Celebrating

Design a Real Estate Ad

Ask students to think about houses and buildings in their community that might serve as a safe haven for characters like the three little pigs. Groups of students could make real estate shopping guides featuring photos or drawings of places in their community along with descriptions that emphasize why the pigs would feel safe there.

Home Connection Invite students to work with family members to find photos of homes in their community, perhaps by scanning newspaper real estate ads or taking pictures themselves.

Make a Wanted Poster

Have students celebrate the villains in this theme by making wanted posters of them. You may want to first review the type of information often found on wanted posters, such as

- a photo of the suspect
- information about the crime and previous convictions
- a reward for information
- where the suspect was last seen

A Class Party

Set aside one day to celebrate what students have accomplished during the theme. Invite parents or other classes to attend. Students may enjoy creating a backdrop for the celebration that reflects the theme, such as a fantasy forest. With students, plan a schedule of activities such as

- readings of student writing projects
- displays of artwork or projects
- a dramatization of "The Three Little Pigs"

Students Acquiring English Students can dramatize a story from their culture in their primary language. Perhaps they can teach the class a refrain to repeat.

Fantasy Forest

Hawaiian Islands

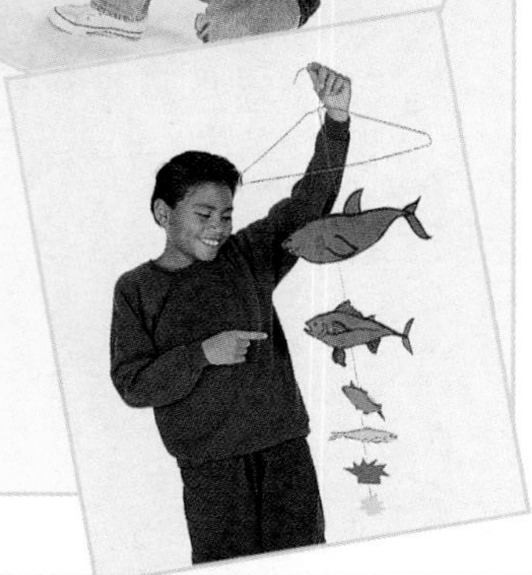

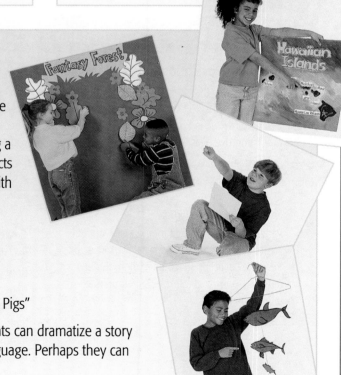

Self-Assessment

Have students meet in small groups to compare and discuss their Selection Connections charts (*Literacy Activity Book*, p. 8). Ask groups to share answers to questions such as the following:

- Which story setting did I learn the most about?
- What things did I learn in this theme that I would like to know more about?
- What other folktales would be fun to reverse the way "The Three Little Pigs" was reversed in this theme? Why?

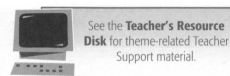

Glossary

Some of the words in this book may have pronunciations or meanings you do not know. This glossary can help you by telling you how to pronounce those words and by telling you the meanings for the words as they are used in this book.

You can find out how to pronounce any glossary word by using the special spelling after the word and the key that runs across the bottom of the glossary pages.

The full pronunciation key on the next page shows how to pronounce each consonant and vowel in a special spelling. The pronunciation key at the bottom of the glossary pages is a shortened form of the full key.

Full Pronunciation Key

Consonant Sounds

b	bib, cabbage	kw	choir, quick	t	tight, stopped
ch	church, stitch	l	lid, needle, tall	th	bath, thin
d	deed, mailed, puddle	m	am, man, dumb	*th*	bathe, this
f	fast, fife, off, phrase, rough	n	no, sudden	v	cave, valve, vine
g	gag, get, finger	ng	thing, ink	w	with, wolf
h	hat, who	p	pop, happy	y	yes, yolk, onion
hw	which, where	r	roar, rhyme	z	rose, size, xylophone, zebra
j	judge, gem	s	miss, sauce, scene, see	zh	garage, pleasure, vision
k	cat, kick, school	sh	dish, ship, sugar, tissue		

Vowel Sounds

ă	rat, laugh	ŏ	horrible, pot	ŭ	cut, flood, rough, some
ā	ape, aid, pay	ō	go, row, toe, though	û	circle, fur, heard, term, turn, urge, word
â	air, care, wear	ô	all, caught, for, paw	yo͝o	cure
ä	father, koala, yard	oi	boy, noise, oil	yo͞o	abuse, use
ĕ	pet, pleasure, any	ou	cow, out	ə	about, silent, pencil, lemon, circus
ē	be, bee, easy, piano	o͝o	full, took, wolf		
ĭ	if, pit, busy	o͞o	boot, fruit, flew		
ī	by, pie, high				
î	dear, deer, fierce, mere				

Stress Marks

Primary Stress ′: bi•ol•o•gy [bī **ŏl′** ə jē]
Secondary Stress ′: bi•o•log•i•cal [bī′ ə **lŏj′** i kəl]

A

ac•cent (**ăk′** sĕnt′) *noun* A small detail that looks different than the things around it, usually added for color or decoration: *The bedroom was blue with pink pillows for **accent**.*

a•do•be (ə **dō′** bē) *noun* Brick that is made from clay and straw and dried in the sun: *Many houses in the southwestern United States are built with **adobe**.*

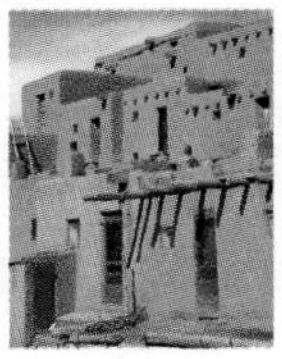

adobe

ADOBE
Adobe is a Spanish word. It goes back to the Arabic word *attoba* meaning "the brick."

an•xious•ly (**ăngk′** shəs lē′) *adverb* In a worried way: *The crowd watched **anxiously** as the firefighter carried the child down the ladder.*

art•ist (**är′** tĭst) *noun* **1.** A person who practices an art, such as painting or music: *The **artist** displayed her paintings in the town hall.* **2.** A person who shows great skill in what he or she does: *Mr. Brown's bake shop has the prettiest wedding cakes in town. He is a true **artist**.*

B

bar•rel (**băr′** əl) *noun* A large, round container with a flat top and bottom: *On the ship, fresh water was stored in large wooden **barrels**.*

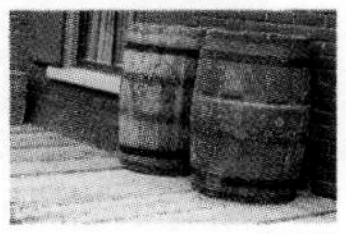

barrels

bel•low (**bĕl′** ō) *verb* To say in a deep, loud voice: *The police officer **bellowed** to the crowd to get away from the burning building.*

brace (brās) *verb* To get ready for something difficult or unpleasant: *As Eric walked toward the lake, he **braced** himself against the shock of the cold water.*

ă rat / ā pay / â care / ä father / ĕ pet / ē be / ĭ pit / ī pie / î fierce / ŏ pot / ō go / ô paw, for / oi oil / o͝o took

bur•y (**bĕr′** ē) *verb* To hide or cover by placing under the ground: *The wind blew sand over the beach and **buried** my sandals.*

C

cac•tus (**kăk′** təs) *noun* A plant with thick, often spiny, leafless stems that grows in hot, dry places.

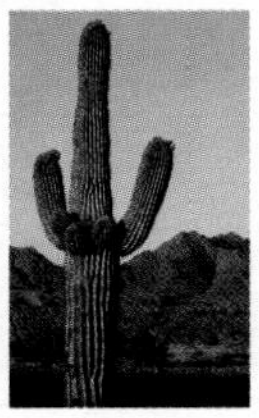

cactus

crav•ing (**krā′** vĭng) *noun* A very strong desire for something: *As I passed the bakery, I suddenly had a **craving** for a piece of apple pie.*

cus•tom (**kŭs′** təm) *noun* Something that members of a group usually do: *One birthday **custom** is to blow out the candles on a birthday cake.*

D

des•ert (**dĕz′** ərt) *noun* A dry area of land that is usually sandy and without trees: *Very few plants grow in the **desert** because it hardly ever rains.*

DESERT
Desert comes from a Latin word meaning "to abandon, or leave behind." When a place was abandoned, it was called a *desert.*

de•sign (dĭ **zīn′**) *noun* A pleasing pattern of lines and shapes: *The wrapping paper was decorated with colorful flower and leaf **designs**.*

di•a•mond (**dī′** ə mənd) *noun* A shape (◊) with four equal sides.

dust storm (dŭst stôrm) *noun* Strong winds that carry clouds of sand and dust across an area: *During the **dust storm**, Dad had to stop the car because he couldn't see to drive.*

E

e•rupt (ĭ **rŭpt′**) *verb* To burst out violently: *The moving van knocked over the fire hydrant, and water **erupted** into the air.*

o͞o boot / ou out / ŭ cut / û fur / hw which / th thin / *th* this / zh vision / ə about, silent, pencil, lemon, circus

F

fu•ri•ous (fyo͝or′ ē əs) *adjective* Full of anger: *Carlos was **furious** when he saw that the puppy had chewed his favorite shoes.*

G

gas (găs) *noun* A poisonous substance that is not liquid or solid and fills the air: *The instructions for the new stove said to call for repairs right away if we smelled **gas**.*

goo•ey (go͞o′ ē) *adjective* Very sticky: *The jar of honey fell off the table and broke into a **gooey** mess on the floor.*

GOOEY
Gooey is the adjective form of the noun *goo* which, in turn, may come from the word *burgoo*. *Burgoo* was a thick kind of oatmeal served to sailors long ago.

grunt (grŭnt) *verb* To say or speak in a short, deep, harsh voice: *Grandpa sleepily **grunted** an answer to my question.*

I

in•spire (ĭn spīr′) *verb* To cause someone to think or act in a particular way: *My grandmother, who made all of her own clothes, **inspired** me to learn to sew.*

M

mar•ket (mär′ kĭt) *noun* A place where people buy and sell goods: *Mr. Choy goes to the **market** each morning to buy fresh fish for his restaurant.*

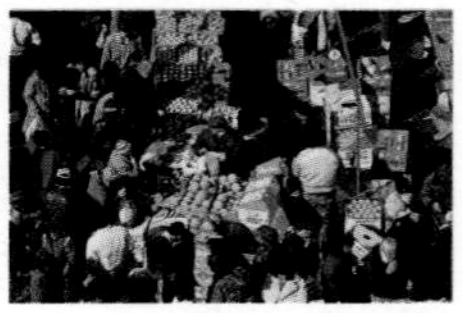
market

ă rat / ā pay / â care / ä father / ĕ pet / ē be / ĭ pit / ī pie / î fierce / ŏ pot / ō go / ô paw, for / oi oil / o͝o took

mo•las•ses (mə lăs′ ĭz) *noun* A thick, sweet syrup: *Marta likes to put **molasses** on her pancakes.*

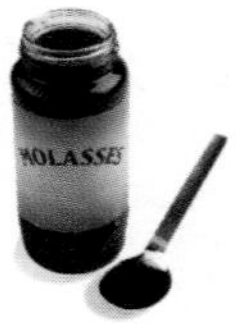
MOLASSES

MOLASSES
Molasses comes from the Portuguese word *melaço*, which means "honey."

O

or•ders (ôr′ dərz) *noun* Certain commands or rules that must be followed: *A soldier must follow the commander's **orders**.*

P

pang (păng) *noun* A short but sharp feeling, as of pain: *Just before dinner, I began having little **pangs** of hunger.*

pas•sen•ger (păs′ ən jər) *noun* A person riding in a vehicle, such as a car, a plane, or a boat: *All the **passengers** in our car must wear their seat belts.*

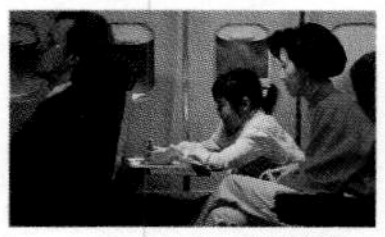
passengers

pitch•er (pĭch′ ər) *noun* A container, usually with a handle, for holding and pouring liquids: *Mom placed a **pitcher** of cold milk on the table.*

plot (plŏt) *verb* To plan secretly: *Dad will **plot** a way to sneak Mom's birthday present into the house without her seeing it.*

poi•son•ous (poi′ zə nəs) *adjective* Causing sickness or death when swallowed or breathed: *The firefighter had to wear a mask to protect him from the **poisonous** air.*

prowl (proul) *verb* To sneak about as if hunting or looking for something: *The stray dog was **prowling** the streets looking for food.*

o͞o boot / ou out / ŭ cut / û fur / hw which / th thin / *th* this / zh vision / ə about, silent, pencil, lemon, circus

pyr•a•mid (pĭr′ ə mĭd) *noun* A figure that has a flat bottom and sides shaped like triangles.

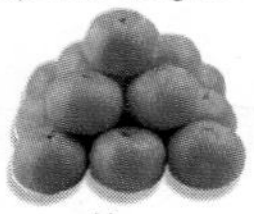
pyramid

R

rec•og•nize (rĕk′ əg nīz′) *verb* To see and know from past experience: *Even from far away, Becky could **recognize** her brother in the crowd by his red cowboy hat.*

res•cue (rĕs′ kyo͞o) *adjective* Being able to save from danger or harm: *The **rescue** team hurried up the mountain to help the hurt hiker.*

S

scene (sēn) *noun* A view of a place: *The photograph showed a **scene** of a cabin by a lake.*

scheme (skēm) *verb* To make up a plan for: *Our team will **scheme** to win the game.*

sur•vi•vor (sər vī′ vər) *noun* Someone who manages to stay alive: *All the **survivors** of the car accident had been wearing seat belts.*

T

tat•tered (tăt′ ərd) *adjective* Torn and ragged looking: *By the time Andy got the stuffed animal away from the puppy, it was torn and **tattered**.*

TATTERED
Tattered comes from the Scandinavian word *tötturr*, which means "rag."

ti•tle (tīt′ l) *noun* A name given to a person to show rank, office, or job: *After finishing medical school, my uncle's new **title** became Doctor.*

ti•tle fight (tīt′ l fīt) *noun* A boxing match to determine the champion: *Joe Louis first won the heavyweight championship in a **title fight** in 1937.*

ă rat / ā pay / â care / ä father / ĕ pet / ē be / ĭ pit / ī pie / î fierce / ŏ pot / ō go / ô paw, for / oi oil / o͝o took

trem•ble (trĕm′ bəl) *verb* **1.** To shake from fear or the cold: *I knew Aunt Shirley was afraid of something when I saw her hands **trembling**.* **2.** To shake: *The earthquake made our house **tremble**.*

tri•an•gle (trī′ ăng′ gəl) A shape (Δ) with three sides.

tum•ble•weed (tŭm′ bəl wēd′) *noun* A plant that breaks off from its roots when it dies and is blown about in the wind.

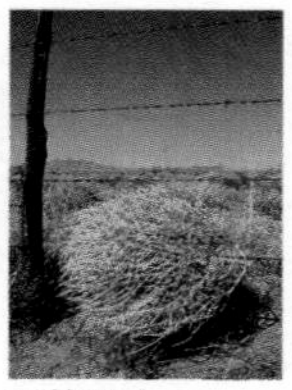
tumbleweed

V

vol•ca•no (vŏl kā′ nō) *noun* An opening in the earth through which lava, ash, and hot gases come out.

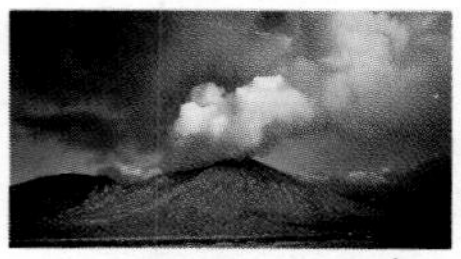
volcano

VOLCANO
Volcano comes from the Latin word *Vulcanus* and the name of a god in Roman mythology. In these myths, *Vulcan*, "the god of fire," was thought to cause volcanoes.

voy•age (voi′ ĭj) A long trip to a far away place: *The Wu family took a long **voyage** across the Pacific Ocean when they moved to the United States.*

W

whirl (wûrl) *verb* To spin around in circles: *The children **whirled** round and round until they felt dizzy.*

whirl•wind (wûrl′ wĭnd′) *noun* A current of air that spins rapidly around: *The **whirlwind** picked up the pile of leaves and spun them around in circles.*

o͞o boot / ou out / ŭ cut / û fur / hw which / th thin / *th* this / zh vision / ə about, silent, pencil, lemon, circus

ACKNOWLEDGMENTS

For each of the selections listed below, grateful acknowledgment is made for permission to excerpt and/or reprint original or copyrighted material, as follows:

Selections

Selection from *Earthwise at school*, by Linda Lowery and Marybeth Lorbiecki. Copyright © 1993 by Linda Lowery and Marybeth Lorbiecki. Reprinted by permission of Carolrhoda Books.

Family Pictures, written and illustrated by Carmen Lomas Garza. Copyright © 1990 by Carmen Lomas Garza. Reprinted by permission of Children's Books Press.

A Fruit & Vegetable Man, by Roni Schotter. Copyright © 1993 by Roni Schotter. Reprinted by permission of Little, Brown and Company.

"History Makers," from June/July 1993 *Kids Discover* magazine. Copyright © 1993 by Kids Discover. Reprinted by permission.

"Make Your Own Erupting Volcano," from *Science Wizardy for Kids*, by Margaret Kenda and Phyllis S. Williams. Copyright © 1992 by Margaret Kenda and Phyllis S. Williams. Reprinted by permission of Barrons Educational Series, Inc., Hauppage, NY.

Miss Nelson Is Missing, by Harry Allard, illustrated by James Marshall. Text copyright © 1977 by Harry Allard. Illustrations copyright © 1977 by James Marshall. Reprinted by permission of Houghton Mifflin Company. All rights reserved.

"Molasses Tank Explosion Injures 50 and Kills 11," from the *Boston Daily Globe*, January 16, 1919. Public domain.

"My Hairy Neighbors," by Susan Lowell, from March 1994 *Ranger Rick* magazine. Copyright © 1994 by the National Wildlife Federation. Reprinted by permission.

Patrick and the Great Molasses Explosion, by Marjorie Stover. Copyright © 1985 by Dillon Press. Reprinted by permission of Silver Burdett Press.

Pompeii . . . Buried Alive! by Edith Kunhardt. Copyright © 1987 by Edith Kunhardt. Reprinted by permission of Random House, Inc.

"Pronunciation Key," from the *American Heritage Children's Dictionary*. Copyright © 1994 by Houghton Mifflin Company. Reprinted by permission. All rights reserved.

"This Little Piggy!" by Linda Granfield, from November 1992 *Owl* magazine. Copyright © 1992 by Linda Granfield. Reprinted by permission of the author.

The Three Little Hawaiian Pigs and the Magic Shark, by Donivee Martin Laird. Copyright © 1981 by Donivee Martin Laird. Reprinted by permission of Barnaby Books, a Hawaii Partnership.

The Three Little Javelinas, by Susan Lowell. Copyright © 1992 by Susan Lowell. Reprinted by permission of Northland Publishing.

The Three Little Wolves and the Big Bad Pig, by Eugene Trivizas. Illustrations by Helen Oxenbury. Text copyright © 1993 by Eugene Trivizas. Illustrations copyright © 1993 by Helen Oxenbury. Reprinted by permission of Margaret K. McElderry Books, Simon & Schuster Children's Publishing Division. First published by Heinemann Young Books in Great Britain.

The Titanic, adapted and arranged by Alan Lomax. Copyright © renewed 1964 by Ludlow Music, Inc., New York, NY. Reprinted by permission.

The Titanic: Lost . . . and Found, by Judy Donnelly. Copyright © 1987 by Judy Donnelly. Reprinted by permission of Random House, Inc.

Titanic Trivia, by A.F.J. Marshello. Copyright © 1987 by A.F.J. Marshello. Reprinted by permission of the Titanic Historical Society, Inc., Indian Orchard, MA 01151.

"What's Up, Pup?" by Lyle Prescott, from July 1994 *Ranger Rick* magazine. Copyright © 1994 by the National Wildlife Federation. Reprinted by permission.

"The Wild Boar & the Fox," from *Aesop's Fables: Plays for Young Children*, by Dr. Albert Cullum. Copyright © 1993 by Fearon Teacher Aids, a Paramount Communications Company. Reprinted by Paramount Communications.

When Jo Louis Won the Title, by Belinda Rochelle, illustrated by Larry Johnson. Text copyright © 1994 by Belinda Rochelle. Illustrations copyright © 1994 by Larry Johnson. Reprinted by permission of Houghton Mifflin Company. All rights reserved.

Poetry

"Away from Town," from *Runny Days, Sunny Days*, by Aileen Fisher. Copyright © 1958 by Aileen Fisher. Reprinted by permission of the author.

"City," by Langston Hughes, from *The Langston Hughes Reader*. Copyright © 1958 by Langston Hughes. Copyright renewed 1986 by George Houston Bass. Reprinted by permission of Harold Ober Associates, Inc.

"Pigs," by Charles Ghigna, from *Ranger Rick* magazine. Copyright © 1993 by Charles Ghigna. Reprinted by permission of the author.

Additional Acknowledgments

Special thanks to the following teachers whose students' compositions are included in the Be a Writer features in this level:

David Burton, Blake Lower School, Hopkins, Minnesota; Linda Chick, Paloma Elementary School, San Marcos, California; Debora Adam, South Dover Elementary School, Dover, Delaware

318

CREDITS

Illustration **12–27** James Marshall; **37–59** Helen Oxenbury; **92–113** Don Stuart; **115** Brian Lies; **118–119** Loretta Lustig; **127–144** Jeanette Winter; **151–179** Carmen Lomas Garza; **181** Pam Rossi; **184** Pam Rossi; **189–210** Larry Johnson; **225–247** John Gamache; **254–274** Robert G. Steele; **284–304** Brad Teare

Photography **28** Courtesy of Harry Allard(tl) **28** Houghton Mifflin Co.(tr) **36** Courtesy of Helen Oxenbury **36** Courtesy of Eugene Trivizas and Reed Childrens Books(t) **36** ©Otto Rogge/The Stock Market(background) **61-63** Art Wolfe **63** Arthur & Elaine Morris (cover) **64** © Andrew Sacks/©Tony Stone Images **65** ©David Falconer/DRK Photo(t) **65** John Colwell/Grant Heilman Photography(b) **66** The Bettmann Archive(t) **66** ©Andrew Sacks/Tony Stone Images(b) **67** ©Stephen J. Krasemann/DRK Photo(t) **67** ©Phil Dotson/Photo Researchers(t) **67** Alain Compost/Bruce Coleman Inc(t) **67** Robert Barclay/Grant Heilman Photography(b) **68** Ross Humphreys/Courtesy of Susan Lowell(t) **68** Courtesy of Jim Harris(b) **68, 69** Mark Muench/©Tony Stone Images **94** Courtesy of Donivee M. Laird(tl) **94** Courtesy of Don Stuart(br) **88** Renee Lynn/Photo Researchers **126** Courtesy of Roni Schotter(tl) **126** Courtesy of Jeanette Winter(br) **146-149** Fred Boyles **182** ©Ken Biggs/©Tony Stone Images **183** ©Ken Biggs/Tony Stone Image **188** Courtesy of Larry Johnson(br) **188** Courtesy of Belinda Rochelle **214** Little, Brown & Co. **215** Francine Seders Gallery LTD **216** National Museum of the American Indian **217** The Cleveland Museum of Art **218-219** Joanna McCarthy/The Image Bank **220-221** G. Brad Lewis/©Tony Stone Images **222-223** G. Brad Lewis/©Tony Stone Images **227** Courtesy of The Mariners Museum, Newport News, Virginia(br) **227** Ken Marschall Collection/The Illustrated London News(br) **228** Courtesy of The Mariners Museum, Newport News, Virginia **228** Brown Brothers(tr) **228** Ken Marschall Collection/Harland & Wolfe(br) **231** Brown Brothers(br) **232** Stock Montage, Inc.(bl) **232** Brown Brothers(bl) **235** Brown Brothers(br) **237** Bruce Dale/National Geographic Society(br) **237** The Bettmann Archive(br) **239** The Illustrated London News Picture Library(br) **240** Brown Brothers(bl) **241** Brown Brothers(m) **241** The Bettmann Archive(m) **241** Hulton Deutsch **242** Stock Montage, Inc. **242** Brown Brothers(m) **243** The Bettmann Archive(ml) **243** The Bettmann Archive(ml) **243** Brown Brothers(mr) **245** R. Sobol/SIPA Press **246** Emory Kristof/(c) National Geographic Society **246-247** (c) Woods Hole Oceanographic Institution **250** Courtesy of The Mariners Museum, Newport News, Virginia(tr) **250** Brown Brothers(mr) **250** The Bettmann Archive(bl)(bm) **251** Ken Marschall Collection/Harland & Wolfe(tr) **254** Courtesy of Edith Kundhardt(t) **254** Courtesy of Robert Steele(b) **271** O. L. Mazzatenta/ (c)National Geographic Society(tl) **271** O. L. Mazzatenta/(c)National Geographic Society(tr) **271** ©David Hiser/Photographers Aspen(b) **272** ©Jonathan Blair/(c)National Geographic Society **273** C M Dixon(ml) **273** David Hiser/Photographers Aspen(b) **274** ©Roy Rainford/Robert Harding Picture Library **276** ©E.R. Degginger/Allstock(bl) **276** Tony Waltham/Robert Harding Picture Library(br) **278** Reuters/Bettmann/The Bettmann Archive(t) **278** ©Sipa Press(tr) **278** The Bettmann Archive(ml) **278** Ralph Perry/Allstock(br) **278** ©Gary Braasch/USDA Forest(bl) **278** The Bettmann Archive(bl) **279** ©Robert Fried/Robert Fried Photography(tr) **279** UPI/Bettmann/The Bettmann Archive(bl) **279** ©Gary Braasch(br) **284** John Stover/ Courtesy of Marjorie Stover(tl) **284** Courtesy of Brad Teare(br) **306** Boston Globe **307-309** Bostonian Society

319

Teacher's Handbook

TABLE OF CONTENTS

Study Skills

Taking Notes

TESTED SKILL

INTERACTIVE LEARNING

Teach/Model

Explain to students that taking notes as they read will help them remember important information. Stress the following points:

- Use a separate page or index card for each topic.
- Write a main heading (a key word or phrase) for each topic.
- Below the heading, write important details about the topic.

Tell the class that they will be doing research and taking notes on particular animals. Use the Think Aloud to model how to use this skill.

Think Aloud

My research topic is pigs. I can probably find this topic in the P book of the encyclopedia. (Some encyclopedias have the information under "Hogs." If so there will be a cross-reference under "Pigs.") I have several sheets of paper for notes. First I think about what I want to learn about pigs, and write these topics as headings on separate pages. For example, I will write the heading "What Pigs Eat" at the top of one page and "Kinds of Pigs" on another page. *(Write these two headings on the chalkboard.)*

Next I will read the article about pigs in the encyclopedia. As I read, I will write down the details I find on the appropriate pages. For example, I read that farmers feed pigs grains such as corn, wheat, rye, and oats. I will write "Corn, wheat, rye, and oats" under "What Pigs Eat." *(Write this on chalkboard.)* I will write other details on that page telling any other foods that pigs eat as well as how much they eat. I will do the same for other topics about pigs.

As I read, I will probably find other interesting topics, such as "Where Pigs Live." Then I will create a separate page of notes–with a heading and details–for each of those topics. When I am done, I will have the information written in a form I can use to study or to write about pigs.

Practice/Apply

Divide the class into small groups and assign each group an animal topic. Monitor students as they research their assigned topics. When they are done, ask questions such as these:

- What is the importance of taking notes?
- When you take notes, how do you group the information?
- What does each detail have to do with the topic?

SKILL FINDER Minilesson, p. 63

Study Skills

K-W-L

INTERACTIVE LEARNING

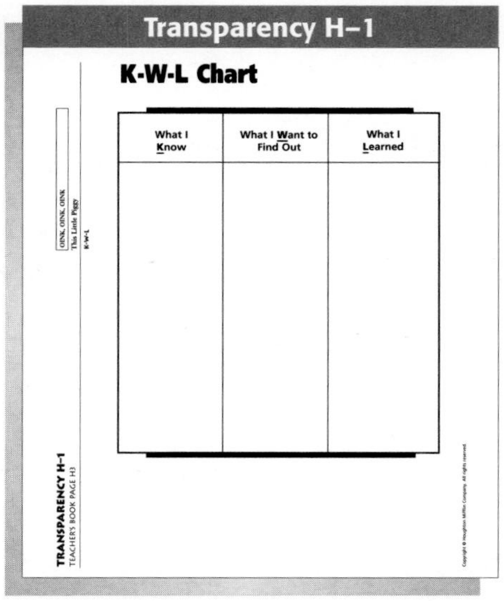
Transparency H–1
K-W-L Chart
What I Know
What I Want to Find Out
What I Learned
TRANSPARENCY H-1

Teach/Model

Write the letters *K W L* on the chalkboard. Tell students that *K* stands for *Know, W* stands for *Want to find out,* and *L* stands for *Learned.* Together these three letters represent a strategy, or plan, that students can use before and after reading to help them understand what they read and remember it better.

Choose a chapter in a classroom text. Display Transparency H-1. Demonstrate how to use the K-W-L strategy by using the Think Aloud. Point to the headings and columns on the K-W-L chart as you explain the strategy.

Think Aloud

I will use the K-W-L chart before and after I read this chapter to help me understand and remember the information. The topic of this chapter is *(name the topic)*. Before I begin reading, I will think about what I already know about this topic. I will write these things in the first column, under the "What I Know" heading. Next, I will thumb through the chapter, thinking about what I want to learn or what I expect to learn about the topic. I will list these things in the second column, under "What I Want to Find Out." Then, as I read the chapter, I will keep on thinking about what I want to learn.

After reading the chapter, I will list what I learned in the third column. Then I will compare this list with my "What I Know" list to see if what I thought I knew turned out to be true. Finally, I will check my "What I Want to Find Out" list to see what questions were not answered yet.

Practice/Apply

Have each student make a K-W-L chart by copying the three column headings on a sheet of paper. Assign another short chapter or section from the same classroom text. Have students fill in their K-W-L charts. Then have them take turns reading one entry from each of the columns on their charts.

Have students summarize what they have learned about the K-W-L strategy by answering these questions.

- What do the letters *K-W-L* stand for?
- What does the K-W-L strategy help a student to do?
- Why is K-W-L a good plan to follow for reading and studying?

SKILL FINDER Minilesson, p. 65

Teaching CHOICES

Study Skills

K-W-L

INTERACTIVE LEARNING

Teach/Model

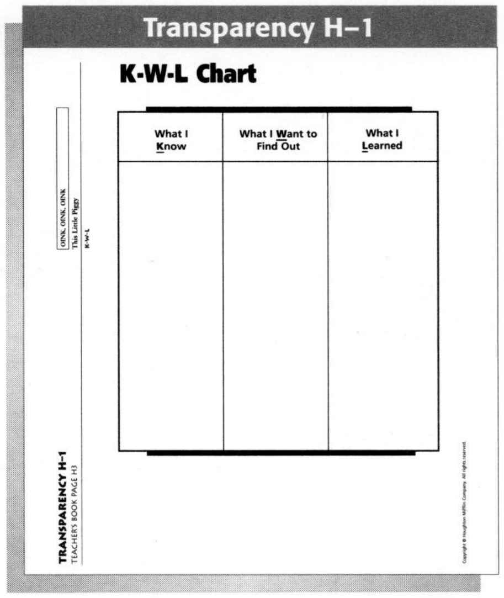
Transparency H–1

K-W-L Chart

What I Know	What I Want to Find Out	What I Learned

INFORMAL ASSESSMENT CHECKLIST

Record observations of student progress for those areas important to you.

– = **Beginning Understanding**
✓ = **Developing Understanding**
✓+ = **Proficient**

Student Names

The Three Little Wolves and the Big Bad Pig									
Reading									
Responding									
Comprehension: Summarizing: Story Structure									
Writing Skills: Writing a Sentence									
Word Skills: Base Words									
Spelling: Short Vowels									
Grammar: Subjects and Predicates									
Listening and Speaking									

The Three Little Javelinas									
Reading									
Responding									
Comprehension: Compare and Contrast									
Writing: Writing a Book Report									
Word Skills: Inflected Endings *-ed, -ing*									
Spelling: Vowel-Consonant-*e*									
Grammar: Correcting Run-on Sentences									
Listening and Speaking									

Reading/Writing Workshop									

INFORMAL ASSESSMENT CHECKLIST

Record observations of student progress for those areas important to you.

– = Beginning Understanding
✔ = Developing Understanding
✔+ = Proficient

The Three Little Hawaiian Pigs and the Magic Shark	Student Names								
Reading									
Responding									
Comprehension: Fantasy/Realism									
Writing Skills: Combining Sentences: Compound Sentences									
Word Skills: Using Context									
Spelling: Long *a* & Long *e*									
Grammar: Kinds of Sentences									
Listening and Speaking									

Performance Assessment									

General Observation									
Independent Reading									
Independent Writing									
Work Habits									
Self Assessment									

Audio-Visual Resources

Adventure Productions
3404 Terry Lake Road
Ft. Collins, CO 80524

AIMS Media
9710 DeSoto Avenue
Chatsworth, CA
91311-4409
800-367-2467

Alfred Higgins Productions
6350 Laurel Canyon Blvd.
N. Hollywood, CA
91606
800-766-5353

American School Publishers/SRA
P.O. Box 543
Blacklick, OH
43004-0543
800-843-8855

Audio Bookshelf
R.R. #1, Box 706
Belfast, ME 04915
800-234-1713

Audio Editions
Box 6930
Auburn, CA 95604-6930
800-231-4261

Audio Partners, Inc.
Box 6930
Auburn, CA 95604-6930
800-231-4261

Bantam Doubleday Dell
1540 Broadway
New York, NY 10036
212-782-9652

Barr Films
12801 Schabarum Ave.
Irwindale, CA 97106
800-234-7878

Bullfrog Films
Box 149
Oley, PA 19547
800-543-3764

Churchill Films
12210 Nebraska Ave.
Los Angeles, CA 90025
800-334-7830

Clearvue/EAV
6465 Avondale Ave.
Chicago, IL 60631
800-253-2788

Coronet/MTI
108 Wilmot Road
Deerfield, IL 60015
800-777-8100

Creative Video Concepts
5758 SW Calusa Loop
Tualatin, OR 97062

Dial Books for Young Readers
375 Hudson St.
New York, NY 10014
800-526-0275

Direct Cinema Ltd.
P.O. Box 10003
Santa Monica, CA 90410
800-525-0000

Disney Educational Production
105 Terry Drive,
Suite 120
Newtown, PA 18940
800-295-5010

Encounter Video
2550 NW Usshur
Portland, OR 97210
800-677-7607

Filmic Archives
The Cinema Center
Botsford, CT 06404
800-366-1920

Films for Humanities and Science
P.O. Box 2053
Princeton, NJ 08543
609-275-1400

Finley-Holiday
12607 E. Philadelphia St.
Whittier, CA 90601

Fulcrum Publishing
350 Indiana St.
Golden, CO 80401

G.K. Hall
Box 500, 100 Front St.
Riverside, NJ 08057

HarperAudio
10 East 53rd Street
New York, NY 10022
212-207-6901

Hi-Tops Video
2730 Wiltshire Blvd.
Suite 500
Santa Monica, CA 90403
213-216-7900

Houghton Mifflin/Clarion
Wayside Road
Burlington, MA 01803
800-225-3362

Idaho Public TV/Echo Films
1455 North Orchard
Boise, ID 83706
800-424-7963

Kidvidz
618 Centre St.
Newton, MA 02158
617-965-3345

L.D.M.I.
P.O. Box 1445,
St. Laurent
Quebec, Canada
H4L 4Z1

Let's Create
50 Cherry Hill Rd.
Parsippany, NJ 07054

Listening Library
One Park Avenue
Old Greenwich, CT
06870
800-243-4504

Live Oak Media
P.O. Box 652
Pine Plains, NY 12567
518-398-1010

Mazon Productions
3821 Medford Circle
Northbrook, IL 60062
708-272-2824

Media Basics
Lighthouse Square
705 Boston Post Road
Guildford, CT 06437
800-542-2505

MGM/UA Home Video
1000 W. Washington Blvd.
Culver City, CA 90232
310-280-6000

Milestone Film and Video
275 W. 96th St.,
Suite 28C
New York, NY 10025

Miramar
200 Second Ave.
Seattle, WA 98119
800-245-6472

Audio-Visual Resources *(continued)*

National Geographic
Educational Services
Washington, DC 20036
800-548-9797

The Nature Company
P.O. Box 188
Florence, KY 41022
800-227-1114

Philomel
1 Grosset Drive
Kirkwood, NY 13795
800-847-5575

Premiere Home Video
755 N. Highland
Hollywood, CA 90038
213-934-8903

Puffin Books
375 Hudson St.
New York, NY 10014

Rabbit Ears
131 Rowayton Avenue
Rowayton, CT 06853
800-800-3277

Rainbow Educational Media
170 Keyland Court
Bohemia, NY 11716
800-331-4047

Random House Media
400 Hahn Road
Westminster, MD 21157
800-733-3000

Reading Adventure
7030 Huntley Road, Unit B
Columbus, OH 43229

Recorded Books
270 Skipjack Road
Prince Frederick, MD 20678
800-638-1304

SelectVideo
7200 E. Dry Creek Rd.
Englewood, CO 80112
800-742-1455

Silo/Alcazar
Box 429, Dept. 318
Waterbury, VT 05676

Spoken Arts
10100 SBF Drive
Pinellas Park, FL 34666
800-126-8090

SRA
P.O. Box 543
Blacklick, OH 43004-0543
800-843-8855

Strand/VCI
3350 Ocean Park Blvd.
Santa Monica, CA 90405
800-922-3827

Taliesin Productions
558 Grove St.
Newton, MA 02162
617-332-7397

Time-Life Education
P.O. Box 85026
Richmond, VA 23285-5026
800-449-2010

Video Project
5332 College Ave.
Oakland, CA 94618
800-475-2638

Warner Home Video
4000 Warner Blvd.
Burbank, CA 91522
818-243-5020

Weston Woods
Weston, CT 06883
800-243-5020

Wilderness Video
P.O. Box 2175
Redondo Beach, CA 90278
310-539-8573

BOOKS AVAILABLE IN SPANISH

Spanish editions of English titles referred to in the Bibliography are available from the following publishers or distributors.

Bilingual Educational Services, Inc.
2514 South Grand Ave.
Los Angeles, CA 90007-9979
800-448-6032

Charlesbridge
85 Main Street
Watertown, MA 02172
617-926-5720

Children's Book Press
6400 Hollis St., Suite 4
Emeryville, CA 94608
510-655-3395

Childrens Press
5440 N. Cumberland Ave.
Chicago, IL 60656-1469
800-621-1115

Econo-Clad Books
P.O. Box 1777
Topeka, KS 66601
800-628-2410

Farrar, Straus, & Giroux
9 Union Square
New York, NY 10003
212-741-6973

Harcourt Brace
6277 Sea Harbor Drive
Orlando, FL 32887
800-225-5425

HarperCollins
10 E. 53rd Street
New York, NY 10022
717-941-1500

Holiday House
425 Madison Ave.
New York, NY 10017
212-688-0085

Kane/Miller
Box 310529
Brooklyn, NY 11231-0529
718-624-5120

Alfred A. Knopf
201 E. 50th St.
New York, NY 10022
800-638-6460

Lectorum
111 Eighth Ave.
New York, NY 10011
800-345-5946

Santillana
901 W. Walnut St.
Compton, CA 90220
800-245-8584

Simon and Schuster
866 Third Avenue
New York, NY 10022
800-223-2336

Viking
357 Hudson Street
New York, NY 10014
212-366-2000

Index

Boldface page references indicate formal strategy and skill instruction.

A

B

C

M

S

T

U

V

W